国际经典影像学译丛

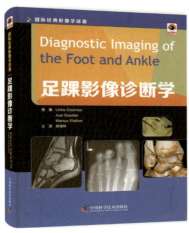

足踝影像诊断学

引进地：德国 Thieme 出版社
定　价：178.00 元（大 16 开精装）
原　著：Ulrike Szeimies 等
主　译：麻增林

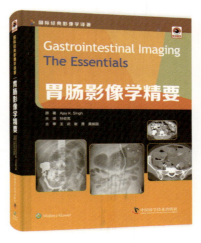

胃肠影像学精要

引进地：荷兰 Wolters Kluwer 出版社
定　价：178.00 元（大 16 开精装）
原　著：Ajay K. Singh
主　译：孙宏亮

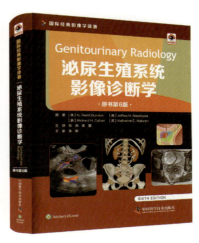

泌尿生殖系统影像诊断学（原书第 6 版）

引进地：荷兰 Wolters Kluwer 出版社
定　价：248.00 元（大 16 开精装）
原　著：N. Reed Dunnick 等
主　译：陈涓　姜蕾

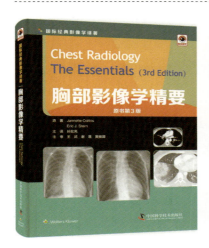

胸部影像学精要（原书第 3 版）

引进地：荷兰 Wolters Kluwer 出版社
定　价：248.00 元（大 16 开精装）
原　著：Jannette Collins 等
主　译：孙宏亮

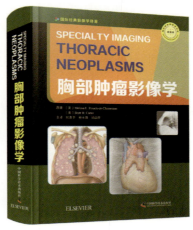

胸部肿瘤影像学

引进地：美国 Elsevier 出版集团
定　价：398.00 元（大 16 开精装）
原　著：Melissa L. Rosado-de-Christenson
　　　　Brett W. Carter
主　译：时惠平　杨本强　刘晶哲

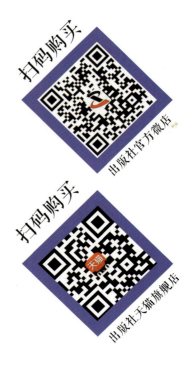

中国科学技术出版社 · 荣誉出品

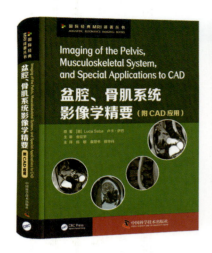
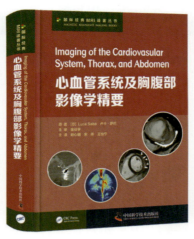
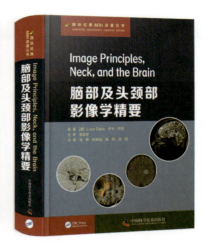

盆腔、骨肌系统影像学精要（附 CAD 应用）
- 引进地：美国 CRC 出版社
- 定　价：298.00 元（大 16 开精装）
- 原　著：Luca Saba
- 主　译：陈敏　袁慧书　薛华丹

心血管系统及胸腹部影像学精要
- 引进地：美国 CRC 出版社
- 定　价：348.00 元（大 16 开精装）
- 原　著：Luca Saba
- 主　译：赵心明　宋伟　王怡宁

脑部及头颈部影像学精要
- 引进地：美国 CRC 出版社
- 定　价：428.00 元（大 16 开精装）
- 原　著：Luca Saba
- 主　译：马林　鲜军舫　娄昕　洪楠

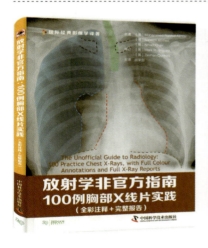

放射学非官方指南：100 例胸部 X 线片实践（全彩注释 + 完整报告）
- 引进地：英国 Zeshan Qureshi 出版社
- 定　价：98.00 元（大 16 开平装）
- 原　著：Mohammed Rashid Akhtar 等
- 主　译：胡荣剑

高分辨率肺部 CT（全新第 5 版）
- 引进地：荷兰 Wolters Kluwer 出版社
- 定　价：295.00 元（大 16 开精装）
- 原　著：W. Richard Webb 等
- 主　译：潘纪成　胡荣剑

致读者

感谢您对我社图书的喜爱和支持。我社是中国科协直属的国家级出版单位，以编辑出版学术专著、科普图书和科学期刊为主业，成立于 1956 年。近年来，我社与多家国际一流出版集团战略合作，在国际医学经典图书出版领域卓有建树。敬请关注我社官方网站（http://www.cspbooks.com.cn）及官方微店。

国际经典 MRI 译著丛书
Magnetic Resonance Imaging bookS

Imaging of the Cardiovascular System, Thorax, and Abdomen

心血管系统及胸腹部影像学精要

原　著　[意] Luca Saba　卢卡·萨巴
主　审　金征宇
主　译　赵心明　宋　伟　王怡宁

中国科学技术出版社
·北　京·

图书在版编目（CIP）数据

心血管系统及胸腹部影像学精要 /（意）卢卡·萨巴（Luca Saba）原著；赵心明，宋伟，王怡宁主译．—北京：中国科学技术出版社，2020.3

（国际经典 MRI 译著丛书）

ISBN 978-7-5046-8571-1

Ⅰ．①心… Ⅱ．①卢… ②赵… ③宋… ④王… Ⅲ．①心脏血管疾病－影像诊断②胸腔疾病－影像诊断③腹腔疾病－影像诊断 Ⅳ．① R540.4 ② R560.4 ③ R572.04

中国版本图书馆 CIP 数据核字 (2020) 第 018939 号

著作权合同登记号：01-2019-6869

策划编辑	焦健姿　王久红
责任编辑	孙　超
装帧设计	华图文轩
责任印制	李晓霖

出　　版	中国科学技术出版社
发　　行	中国科学技术出版社有限公司发行部
地　　址	北京市海淀区中关村南大街 16 号
邮　　编	100081
发行电话	010-62173865
传　　真	010-62179148
网　　址	http://www.cspbooks.com.cn

开　　本	889mm×1194mm　1/16
字　　数	1167 千字
印　　张	41
版　　次	2020 年 3 月第 1 版
印　　次	2020 年 3 月第 1 次印刷
印　　刷	北京威远印刷有限公司
书　　号	ISBN 978-7-5046-8571-1/R・2480
定　　价	348.00 元

（凡购买本社图书，如有缺页、倒页、脱页者，本社发行部负责调换）

版权说明

Imaging of the Cardiovascular System, Thorax, and Abdomen / ISBN: 978-1-4822-1626-4

Copyright © 2017 by Taylor & Francis Group, LLC
CRC Press is an imprint of Taylor & Francis Group, an Informa business
Authorized translation from English language edition published by CRC Press, part of Taylor & Francis Group,LLC; All rights reserved. 本书原版由 Taylor & Francis 出版集团旗下，CRC 出版公司出版，并经其授权翻译出版。版权所有，侵权必究。

Chinese Science and Technology Press(CSTP) is authorized to publish and distribute exclusively the Chinese (Simplified Characters) language edition. This edition is authorized for sale throughout Mainland of China. No part of the publication may be reproduced or distributed by any means, or stored in a database or retrieval system, without the priorwritten permission of the publisher. 本书中文简体翻译版授权由中国科学技术出版社独家出版并仅限在中国大陆地区销售，未经出版者书面许可，不得以任何方式复制或发行本书的任何部分。

Copies of this book sold without a Taylor & Francis sticker on the cover are unauthorized and illegal. 本书封面贴有 Taylor & Francis 公司防伪标签，无标签者不得销售。

内容提要

本书是引进自 CRC 出版社的一部高质量 MRI 影像学著作。全书分 26 章，包括心血管系统和胸腹部两大部分，分别对冠状动脉、心脏、心包、血管、气管及支气管、肺、乳腺、肝脏、胆囊及胆道、脾脏、肾上腺、消化道、腹膜后、腹壁及疝，以及特殊情况下（创伤后及术后）的磁共振影像特点进行了讲解。书中不仅详尽介绍了疾病的 MRI 诊断要点，也对所涉及的 MRI 技术、解剖学、胚胎发育及病理生理过程进行了必要的解释。本书内容翔实，图片精美，语言精练，非常适合该领域的放射科医师及临床医师参考学习。

丛书编译委员会名单

主任委员 金征宇

副主任委员（以姓氏笔画为序）

马 林　王怡宁　宋 伟　陈 敏　赵心明

娄 昕　洪 楠　袁慧书　鲜军舫　薛华丹

委　　员（以姓氏笔画为序）

马霄虹　王 岩　王新艳　李 欣　李世俊

李春媚　郎 宁　姜 虹　隋 昕

分册译者名单

主　审 金征宇

主　译 赵心明　宋 伟　王怡宁

副主译 马霄虹　隋 昕

译　者（以姓氏笔画为序）

王 芬　王 健　王 悦　王 爽　王 磊　代静文　冯 冰

朱 正　朱永健　李 潇　李登峰　杨 阳　杨洁瑾　邱健星

宋 兰　张大明　张红梅　李登峰　林 路　易 妍　郑福玲

赵 蕾　徐 飞　徐晓莉　徐晓娟　曹 剑

学术秘书 冯 冰　曹 剑

原著者寄语

很高兴看到我的这几部磁共振影像学著作翻译为中文版！身为作者，我深知书中内容的复杂程度，在了解到中国影像学界大咖金征宇教授及其团队在翻译工作中所做出的努力后，我坚信本书的中文翻译版一定质量过硬，在学界的影响亦将斐然。我由衷地感谢他们将这些影像学中有趣的新进展介绍给中国的同行们。我还要感谢中国科学技术出版社的引进与出版，感谢他们在医学影像学著作学术传播上做出的努力。

磁共振影像学这几部著作的开始源于数年前，其初衷是希望让国际领域的优秀专家能够以完整广阔的视角、与时俱进的语言、化繁为简的叙述方式来描述磁共振成像在临床中的应用和潜力。这几部著作的撰写历时 3 年左右，众多优秀的同行专家为此投入了大量精力，希望中国读者能够从中得到些许有用的收获。

在这几部磁共振影像学著作中，将展示磁共振成像在临床领域的应用前景，以及备受关注的一些新技术，如灌注技术或高磁场应用（7T）。

衷心希望这几部磁共振影像学著作能给广大读者留下愉快的阅读经历，为大家日常临床实践带来帮助，真切感受磁共振成像在人体疾病诊断中的巨大潜力。

意大利卡利亚里大学诊断成像及放射学系，教授兼主席，医学博士
意大利放射学会（SIRM）撒丁岛分会主席
Neurovascular Imaging 前主编

I write this email to thank you for the wonderful work you have done. It is with great pleasure that I see how the 3 volumes of the "Magnetic Resonance Imaging" have been translated into Chinese to make this great project available also to colleagues who live and work in China.

I would like to thank the China Science and Technology Press Publishing House, for having done this process that will allow a large number of colleagues to approach the latest and most fascinating developments in radiology. I also wish to thank Professor Jin Zhengyu for having carried out, together with his team, the translation of this work of mine; I know how hard and complex it was, but the final result is absolutely spectacular and makes the quality absolutely perfect.

The Magnetic Resonance Imaging project was born a few years ago and immediately was ambitious as the goal was to involve the world's leading experts to be able to describe in a complete, updated but at the same time, simple way, the applications and potential of Magnetic Resonance in the clinical setting. The writing lasted about 3 years, involving numerous colleagues who dedicated great energy to this work. The end result is what you have under your eyes and I hope you enjoy.

In the 3 volumes of this project you will find chapters that include the possible applications of Magnetic Resonance applied in the clinical field, with great attention to newer techniques, such as for example perfusion techniques or applications with very high-field magnetic fields(7 Tesla).

I wish all of you an exciting reading hoping that these books will help you in everyday clinical practice and will guarantee you a moment of reflection for the incredible potential that Magnetic Resonance has in the study of the pathology of the human body.

Luca Saba,MD,Full Professor and Chair
Department of Diagnostic Imaging and Radiology
University of Cagliari
Italy
President of Sardinian Section of the Italian Society of Radiology(SIRM)
Past Editor in Chief of *Neurovascular Imaging*

译者前言

近年来，磁共振成像（MRI）技术发展迅速，随着成像技术不断提高及扫描参数的优化，MRI 在疾病诊断中发挥着重要作用。与 X 线、CT 影像检查相比，MRI 无辐射、软组织分辨率高、对血流信号敏感，故其在心血管系统及胸腹部疾病诊断中具有独特优势。

本书英文原版由 Taylor & Francis 出版集团旗下 CRC 出版社出版，主编为 Luca Saba 教授。本书此次引进国内，由我与宋伟教授共同担任主译。秉承着忠于原著、精益求精的宗旨，在各位译校人员的共同努力下，力求将原著尽可能完美地呈现给国内读者。

本书详细介绍了 MRI 在心血管系统和腹部疾病诊断中的应用，分为 26 章，各章独立而又相互联系。各章开篇均介绍了本章所涉及的 MRI 基本原理、扫描序列及相应参数，正文则简要回顾了各脏器的解剖特点及发育过程，重点介绍了相关疾病的病理及 MRI 表现和特点，并配有相应的典型病例及精美示意图，便于读者理解及记忆。希望本书的中文翻译版能够对该领域放射科同仁及临床医师有所裨益。

赵心明 教授

国家癌症中心 / 中国医学科学院肿瘤医院

原著前言

磁共振成像（MRI）是放射学中可以对体内结构进行准确成像的医学成像技术。与 CT、X 线相比，MRI 这一技术可为不同软组织结构提供极佳的对比度，使其对脑、肌肉、心脏和肿瘤的成像更有价值，因而 MRI 的引入使诊断过程得到根本而深远的改进。

在过去 20 年，随着场强高达 7T 的 MRI 系统的引入，以及各种后处理算法的发展，如扩散张量成像（DTI）、磁共振功能成像（fMRI）和波谱成像，使 MRI 技术得到进一步提升。通过这些发展，实现了绝佳的图像空间分辨率，以及分析各种病理改变的形态和功能的可能性，从而使 MRI 诊断潜能得到显著提升。

本书旨在覆盖使用 MRI 对人体病理进行诊断过程所涉及的工程学及临床获益，包含可获得极高图像分辨率的高场强磁共振扫描仪的序列及潜能。基于磁共振成像领域中这些令人兴奋的发展，我希望这本书可以为该领域日益增多的参考书籍提供及时、完整的补充。

Luca Saba

意大利卡利亚里大学

CONTENTS

目 录

Chapter 1　冠状动脉及心肌灌注磁共振成像概况 ········ 1
　一、冠状动脉 CMR 的技术挑战与一般成像策略 ········ 2
　二、临床应用 ········ 8
　三、心肌灌注成像 ········ 11
　四、总结与未来前景 ········ 13

Chapter 2　心脏影像：心肌磁共振成像 ········ 21
　一、心室功能及容积 ········ 22
　二、区域心肌功能 ········ 23
　三、T_1 及 T_2 加权心肌成像 ········ 24
　四、T_2^* 加权成像 ········ 26
　五、T_1 Mapping 及 T_2 Mapping 心肌组织定量技术 ········ 27
　六、心肌活性 ········ 28

Chapter 3　心包疾病的 CT 和 MR 成像 ········ 33
　一、心包解剖和生理学 ········ 34
　二、CT 和 MR 成像技术 ········ 35
　三、先天性疾病 ········ 37

Chapter 4　头颈部血管成像 ········ 57
　一、血管解剖结构 ········ 58
　二、弓上动脉病变 ········ 62
　三、总结 ········ 87

Chapter 5　主动脉和内脏血管磁共振成像 ········ 93
　一、MR 血管成像技术 ········ 94
　二、主动脉 ········ 99
　三、内脏动脉 ········ 102

四、总结 ··· 106

Chapter 6　周围血管磁共振成像　109

一、磁共振技术 ·· 110
二、无对比剂 MRA：飞行时间序列和稳态自由运动序列 ·· 110
三、对比剂增强 MRA ··· 111
四、时间分辨或四维 MRA ·· 111
五、上肢血管疾病病理学 ·· 112
六、动脉粥样硬化 ·· 112
七、急性动脉闭塞 ·· 112
八、雷诺现象 ··· 112
九、胸廓出口综合征 ··· 113
十、血液透析管 ·· 113
十一、上肢动脉瘤 ·· 113
十二、锁骨下动脉盗血综合征 ·· 114
十三、下肢血管疾病病理学 ··· 114

Chapter 7　磁共振静脉成像　121

一、MRV 技术简介 ·· 122
二、无对比剂增强序列 ·· 123
三、临床应用 ··· 132

Chapter 8　血管畸形　145

一、分类 ··· 146
二、影像 ··· 148
三、治疗 ··· 154
四、总结 ··· 156

Chapter 9　4D 血流成像　159

一、4D 血流磁共振成像 ··· 160
二、4D 血流成像的潜在临床应用 ·· 166
三、先天性心脏病 4D 血流成像 ·· 168
四、4D 血流成像的展望 ··· 176

Chapter 10　气管、支气管及肺部磁共振成像　185

一、肺磁共振成像的影响因素 ·· 186
二、气管 MRI ·· 186

三、气道病变支气管及细支气管磁共振成像 ··· 187
　　四、肺部 MRI ·· 190
　　五、总结 ··· 201

Chapter 11　磁共振成像在肺部的临床应用 ··· 209
　　一、肺部磁共振成像的物理学特点（从磁共振扫描仪角度） ············· 210
　　二、肺部 MR 序列 ··· 217
　　三、现有技术的临床应用 ·· 223

Chapter 12　胸膜和膈 ·· 241
　　一、胸膜 ··· 242
　　二、胸膜肿瘤 ·· 245

Chapter 13　肺及肺血管的功能性磁共振成像 ··· 255
　　一、MR 技术 ·· 256
　　二、临床应用 ·· 260

Chapter 14　乳腺 MRI ··· 275
　　一、乳腺 MRI 的检查适应证 ··· 276
　　二、技术研究 ·· 282
　　三、常见伪影 ·· 286
　　四、正常乳腺的 MRI 解剖 ··· 286
　　五、乳腺 MR 报告及释义 ·· 287
　　六、乳腺 MRI 良性发现 ··· 306
　　七、乳腺 MRI 恶性征象 ··· 312
　　八、乳腺 MRI 上的高危病变 ·· 317
　　九、硅胶乳房植入假体的评价 ·· 317
　　十、MRI 上可疑病变的组织病理学取样 ··· 320
　　十一、总结 ·· 322

Chapter 15　肝脏扫描技术与肝脏弥漫性疾病 ·· 327
　　一、MR 扫描技术 ··· 328
　　二、肝的解剖 ·· 340
　　三、血管解剖与变异 ·· 340
　　四、肝脏弥漫性病变 ·· 341

Chapter 16　肝脏局灶性病变 ·· 361

一、囊性局灶性病变 ··· 362
　　二、肝脏良性局灶性疾病 ·· 365
　　三、其他肝脏良性病变 ·· 376
　　四、肝恶性局灶性病变 ·· 377
　　五、其他肝脏恶性病变 ·· 386
　　六、治疗后评估 ··· 388

Chapter 17　胆囊　401
　　一、正常解剖 ··· 402
　　二、成像技术 ··· 404

Chapter 18　胆道系统磁共振成像　421
　　一、胆道系统 MRI 序列与技术 ··· 422
　　二、胆道的正常解剖表现 ·· 423
　　三、胆道梗阻 ·· 425
　　四、胆道肿瘤 ·· 428
　　五、胆囊的 MRI 表现 ·· 429

Chapter 19　脾脏磁共振成像新进展　437
　　一、解剖 ·· 440
　　二、MRI 技术 ··· 440
　　三、正常 MRI 表现 ·· 442
　　四、正常变异 ·· 442
　　五、多脾综合征 ··· 443
　　六、脾大 ·· 443
　　七、血色沉着病（含铁血黄素沉着症和镰状细胞病） ············· 444
　　八、外伤 ·· 444
　　九、感染性病变（感染） ·· 444
　　十、囊肿 ·· 446
　　十一、血管源性病变 ··· 449
　　十二、非血管源性肿瘤 ··· 459
　　十三、其他脾脏病变 ··· 466
　　十四、总结 ·· 469

Chapter 20　胰腺　473
　　一、正常解剖 ·· 474
　　二、MRI 成像技术 ··· 474

三、发育异常 476
　四、遗传性疾病 476
　五、炎症性疾病 478
　六、胰腺肿瘤 485
　七、实性肿瘤 485
　八、囊性肿瘤 490
　九、外伤 492
　十、胰腺移植 493
　十一、总结 494

Chapter 21　肾上腺　499

　一、MRI 序列 500
　二、特殊肾上腺病变 503

Chapter 22　上消化道和小肠疾病　511

　一、解剖 512
　二、MRI 技术 513
　三、上消化道病理学 515
　四、小肠病理学 519
　五、总结 526

Chapter 23　腹膜后磁共振成像　529

　一、腹膜后磁共振成像的检查序列 530
　二、病理情况 530
　三、腹部大血管 543
　四、总结 553

Chapter 24　腹壁和疝　561

　一、磁共振成像序列 562
　二、腹壁 562
　三、疝 567
　四、总结 568

Chapter 25　结肠和直肠疾病　571

　一、结肠疾病 572
　二、直肠疾病 576

Chapter 26　创伤后及术后的腹部影像 ······ 617

一、术后 MRI 应用 ······ 618

二、创伤后 MRI 的应用 ······ 635

Chapter 1
冠状动脉及心肌灌注磁共振成像概况

Coronary and Perfusion Imaging with Cardiovascular Magnetic Resonance: Current State of the Art

Amedeo Chiribiri, Markus Henningsson, Claudia Prieto, Michael Jerosch-Herold, Rene M. Botnar 著

易 妍 王 健 译

王怡宁 校

目录 CONTENTS

一、冠状动脉 CMR 的技术挑战与一般成像策略 / 2

二、临床应用 / 8

三、心肌灌注成像 / 11

四、总结与未来前景 / 13

尽管在预防和治疗方面有了显著的改善[1]，冠状动脉疾病（coronary artery disease，CAD）仍然是西方世界死亡和致残的主要病因[2]。目前诊断 CAD 的金标准是心导管检查。仅在美国，就有 16 300 000 名患者罹患 CAD，并且每年大约进行 1 000 000 例心导管介入术[2]。在这些接受介入术的患者中，高达 40% 未发现明显的冠状动脉狭窄[3]。因此，亟待一项无创检查用以直接评估冠状动脉管腔病变及狭窄情况[4]。心血管磁共振（cardiovascular magnetic resonance，CMR）可以对 CAD 患者的心肌功能、灌注和形态进行全面评估[5]。此外，磁共振血管造影（magnetic resonance angiography，MRA）可用于直接显示冠状动脉管腔，而磁共振黑血成像技术可显示冠状动脉血管壁[6]，使 CMR 成为能够在单次检查中提供所有所需诊断信息的影像技术。

此外，相同的 MRA 技术可以显示冠状静脉解剖结构，这对于心脏再同步化起搏治疗中选择起搏导线植入的最佳位置是有意义的[7,8]。

本章概述了目前冠状动脉 MRA 的最新进展和临床应用情况。

一、冠状动脉 CMR 的技术挑战与一般成像策略

冠状动脉 MRA 需要专门的技术来优化图像对比度并确保高信噪比（signal-to-noise ratio，SNR），从而保证高空间分辨率以清晰地描绘出充满血液的管腔或血管壁。由于心脏血管充分显影需要高空间分辨率，因此成像过程中所伴随的心跳和呼吸运动本身就是冠状动脉 MRA 和血管壁成像面临的主要挑战。

为了克服这个难题，标准的冠状动脉 MRA 方案包括：①心电图（electrocardiogram，ECG）门控触发用于实现心脏运动与数据采集同步；②呼吸导航用于同步/补偿呼吸运动；③成像序列本身；④自旋磁化准备预脉冲，以确保足够的图像对比度（图 1-1）。

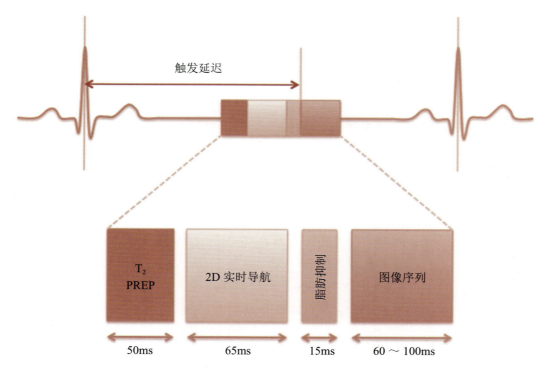

▲ 图 1-1　MRA 的脉冲序列示意图

图像采集是在心电图的 R 波触发延迟后，在心脏舒张中期进行。成像模块之前是对比增强自旋磁化准备（T₂ PREP），用于呼吸运动补偿的 2D 选择性实时导航脉冲和频率选择性脂肪抑制预脉冲（fat-suppression prepulse，FATSAT）。这些序列在每个心动周期重复进行（经许可引自 Botnar, RM 等, Circulation, 99, 3139-3148, 1999.）

Chapter 1 冠状动脉及心肌灌注磁共振成像概况
Coronary and Perfusion Imaging with Cardiovascular Magnetic Resonance: Current State of the Art

（一）心脏运动的补偿：ECG 触发

为了冻结心脏运动，数据采集必须与心动周期同步，并在心脏运动幅度最小的时期内进行[9]。静息期发生在收缩末期（R 波后 280～350 ms）和舒张中期（心房收缩前的短暂时间）。两种采集策略（收缩期或舒张期）都各有优点和缺点（表 1-1）。

表 1-1 收缩期和舒张期冠状动脉 CMR 的比较

舒张期静息期	收缩期静息期
优势	优势
较长的采集窗口（100～125ms/心搏）	对心率变异性较不敏感
血流量较高（梯度回波序列中信号较高）	静脉血管的直径更大
劣势	劣势
对心率变异性更高的敏感度	较短的采集窗口（约 50ms/心搏）

最佳的触发延迟时间和采集时间窗的长度取决于患者的心率、使用的成像序列类型、成像组织（动脉与静脉）以及其他血流动力学因素。尽管使用心率依赖性公式来确定舒张中期静息期对于许多受试者是有效的，但是可能会有相当多的受试者间变异[10]。因此，应该在冠状动脉扫描前通过自由呼吸高时间分辨率电影序列扫描快速确定相对静息期[9]。实时心律失常抑制可以剔除不规则心跳，从而可能会进一步改善冠状动脉 MRA 图像质量[11-14]。

另一个需要考虑的重要参数是静息期的持续时间。与右冠状动脉系统相比，左冠状动脉通常静息期时间相对较长。因此，整个心脏采集的时间窗长度由右冠状动脉（right coronary artery, RCA）静息期持续时间决定。

（二）呼吸运动的补偿：导航

由于呼吸引起的心脏移位可能超过 2～3cm，需要将图像采集与呼吸周期同步。高分辨率三维（3D）数据集与屏气采集不兼容。至今已测试了几种方法来减少呼吸运动对图像质量的影响。前瞻性的实时导航门控和校正技术是目前最小化呼吸运动伪影的方法[15,16]。通常在冠状动脉图像采集之前，用置于右侧膈肌穹顶上的笔形射束一维导航仪监测膈肌的头足方向运动[17]（图 1-2）。根据膈肌的位置，数据要么位于某个接收窗口内（通常为 3～5mm）被接收器接收，要么被拒绝。在后一种情况下，数据必须在随后的心动周期中重新测量。接收窗口的缩窄减少了运动伪影，但由于更多的数据被拒绝，因此延长了整体采集时间。5mm 的接收窗通常可使采集效率接近 50%[18-20]。

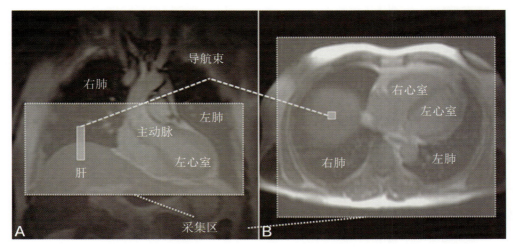

▲ 图 1-2　从冠状位（A）和轴位（B）图像确定导航位置和整个心脏成像体积

笔形射束一维导航位于右侧膈肌顶。包含整个心脏的 3D 体积数据采集在轴位平面上进行，范围自主动脉根部上方 2cm 至膈肌

为了增加接收数据的百分比，可以将成像区间位置预先适配于待测量的呼吸位置。通常，由于呼吸引起的心脏运动不如膈肌本身的运动显著，并且已经使用 0.4～0.6 的比例因子来进行最佳层面追踪。然而，在使用这些技术的情况下，呼吸引发的心脏运动常常不能通过沿着头足方向的简单平移来完全建模，并且已经显示在多达 30% 的患者中，仿射变换模型呼吸运动更准确[21,22]。

其他的推荐方法包括使用基于图像的导航仪直接跟踪心脏运动，监测心外膜脂肪运动的导航仪[23]，俯卧位扫描[24,25]，以及使用腹部或胸部束带[25,26]。

（三）冠状动脉成像

1. 序列 3D 方法需要很长的采集时间，并且最初可行性较差。Edelman[22] 和 Manning[27] 等通过二维（2D）梯度回波技术进行了首次冠状动脉血管成像。16 次心跳（单次屏息）完成一个图像层面的数据采集，患者可以在 2 次采集之间自由呼吸。导航技术的引入使得通过自由呼吸和 3D 技术采集数据成为可行。这些序列可以用全心或目标容积成像两种方式得到（表 1-2）。

目前可使用的方案包括两种：全心成像和针对血管的扫描方法，这些方法需要单独的计划程序。全心脏技术也被用于心脏静脉成像。

2. 对比度增强旋转制备 3D 采集的使用虽然能够提高 SNR 和空间分辨率，但同时也降低了血液和心肌之间的图像对比度（流入效应较小）。因此，对比增强旋转制备技术[28-30]与稳态自由进动（steady state free precession, SSFP）技术被研发出来，在成像过程中结合使用，能够保证足够的图像对比度，从而达到清晰的显示冠状动脉的目的[31]。由于具有较高的固有信噪比和血液心肌之间良好的图像对比度，对于目前 1.5T 磁共振而言，SSFP 序列要优于 T_1 加权梯度回波序列[31-33]。然而，SSFP 序列在 3T 磁共振的应用中存在重复时间较长的局限性 [更严格的特定吸收率（specific absorption rate, SAR）模型]，从而磁敏感度增加，并需要更高的翻转角以获得血液和心肌之间足够的对比度。在 3T 和更高的场强下[34]，梯度回波技术有望替代 SSFP 技术。

非对比剂增强技术通常包括脂肪抑制和 T_2 制备。频率选择性预脉冲可用于饱和来自脂肪组织的信号，从而使冠状动脉显影[22,29,30]。为了增强冠状动脉管腔和背景心肌之间的对比度，可使用 T_2 制备技术[28,29]来抑制来自心肌的信号，因为血液和心肌具有相似的 T_1 弛豫时间但不同的 T_2 弛豫时间（图 1-3）。

T_2 制备也抑制脱氧静脉血液，因此不适合用于冠状静脉成像。其他有一些用于改善血管腔与心肌之间对比度的其他技术，但尚未广泛采用[35]。

表 1-2 冠状动脉 MRA 扫描计划

全心成像	目标容积成像
轴向，矢状面或冠状面向成像体积，规划一组轴向，矢状和冠状侦察图像以包括整个心脏	右冠状动脉和左冠状动脉成像分在两个单独扫描计划中进行
优选各向同性空间分辨率以允许沿冠状血管的进程进行 3D 重新格式化	更快速扫描在低分辨率自由呼吸冠状动脉定位图像上
全面覆盖（同时采集静脉系统）	中心层面通过选择位于冠状血管路径上的三个点来定义
采集时间长	有针对性的覆盖
有限的入流效应（对比度较低，特别是梯度回波技术）	比全心的方法更短的采集时间
典型的空间分辨率：1.3mm×1.3mm×1.3mm 大小的各向同性体素	非各向同性体素，层内空间分辨率为 1mm×1mm，层厚为 2～3mm

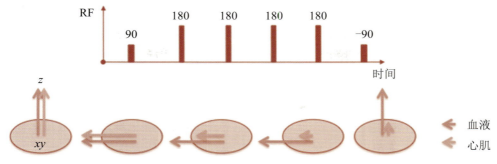

▲ 图1-3 内源性对比增强（T_2磁化准备）

T_2磁化准备可抑制具有较短T_2弛豫时间的组织（心脏肌肉、心脏静脉和心外膜脂肪），同时最小程度地影响具有较长T_2弛豫时间的组织，如动脉血。90°射频（RF）脉冲将磁化矢量从z方向翻转到xy平面。偶数个非选择性RF重聚焦脉冲使T_2制备的流动灵敏度最小化，同时允许T_2依赖性信号衰减。最后，-90° RF提升脉冲恢复z方向上的磁化（经许可引自Brittain JH, et al, Magn.Reson.Med, 33,689-696,1995.；Botnar RM, et al, Circulation, 99,3139-3148,1999.）

其中包括自旋锁定和磁化转移技术[30]。磁化转移制备不影响脱氧静脉血的信号，因此可用于冠状静脉成像[36]。血液和周围组织之间对比度的进一步提高可以通过使用对比剂来实现。

3. 对比剂 目前，通过采用细胞外[37]、血池[38-41]和与白蛋白结合力弱[42-44]的对比剂来改善冠状动脉MRA的对比噪声和图像质量。由于冠状动脉成像应该成为常规诊断缺血性心脏病或CAD的成像方案的一部分，因此对比剂的选择需要考虑到两方面的问题，即在增加管腔与心肌之间的对比度和保证延迟增强扫描钆剂在瘢痕心肌中有效存留之间的平衡。由于组织间隙的快速外渗，细胞外对比剂只允许有限的冠状动脉增强。血池内对比剂能实现血管腔与周围组织之间的最高对比度，但对于延迟强化成像可能会有限制。白蛋白结合力弱的对比剂由于在血液中的滞留时间延长及其具有较高的松弛度（可用于改善冠状动脉MRA的图像质量）[45]，同时能保持良好的延迟强化特性[46]，因此是冠状动脉和梗死心肌综合成像最理想的对比剂[45]。为了发挥对比剂对冠状动脉MRA的优势，通常采用饱和度[47]或反转预脉冲[48]代替T_2准备。在对比剂给药后，血液的T_1快速反转恢复（血液固有T_1弛豫时间=1200ms，含有对比剂的血液T_1弛豫时间=50～100ms，心肌固有T_1弛豫时间=850ms）使得冠状动脉管腔和心肌之间呈现出良好的高对比度。

4. 采集速度和分辨率的最新进展 由于更短的时间采集窗或缩短了整体数据采集时间，较为快速的图像采集速度可以降低对运动的敏感度，从而获得更好的图像质量。推荐采用以下方法来加速数据采集速度和（或）降低对运动敏感性，如使用回波平面成像实线K空间的更快编码[49,50]，使用更有效的K空间螺旋采集[51]或采用径向轨迹进行采样以获得具有更小运动敏感性K空间[52]。这些技术由于具有非共振敏感性（回波平面成像和螺旋）或信噪比损失（径向）等局限性，因而尚未得到冠状动脉MRA检查的标准认可。

最近开发的诸如敏感性编码（sensitivity encoding，SENSE）[53]或同时获取空间谐波（simultaneous acquisition of spatial harmonics，SMASH）[54]的并行成像技术已经成功实现在保持图像质量的同时缩短整体MRA采集时间。随着2D线圈阵列（例如32个通道线圈）的出现，可以应用沿层面编码和相位编码方向加速，由此进一步减少扫描时间。然而，由于信噪比的限制和重建伪影的增加，高于4的加速因子几乎难以实现[54,55]。

（四）冠状静脉成像

在过去的几十年中，心脏血管成像主要聚焦于冠状动脉上，随着心脏再同步化装置的出现，对冠状静脉走行的评估日益重要。因为对左心室CRT电极的最佳位置选择的介入前鉴定有意义，冠状静脉成像已经得到越来越多的关注。3D MR 冠状静脉血管造影图像可以被叠加到实时时间采集的 X 线图像上，为导管植入提供更好的指导[56,57]。

由于冠状静脉血氧饱和度低（导致血 T_2 值强烈降低），因此 T_2 磁化准备不适用于冠状静脉成像。目前的方法包括通过磁化转移准备进行的无对比剂平扫[36,58]或采用钆对比剂（包括血池[7,8,59]、细胞外[60]）和与白蛋白结合力弱的对比剂[61]。令人感兴趣的是，Duckett 提出的在冠状静脉 MRA 采集期间缓慢输注高弛豫度对比剂的方法，这为在对比剂重新分布后能够获得钆对比剂延迟增强图像提供了可能性[61]。

冠状静脉成像最佳采集时间窗为收缩末期，因为此时冠状静脉直径最大[36]。然而，心电图触发在心衰患者中难以施行，因为在这些患者中易发生心动过速，端坐呼吸和左心室非同步收缩，后者可导致左心室不同区域静息期不同。在上述情况下，采集参数应当调整，舒张末期数据采集可能是一种替代方法（图 1-4）。

（五）冠状血管壁成像

磁共振成像（magnetic resonance imaging, MRI）良好的软组织对比度使血管壁可视化得以实现。首先，通过 2D 脂肪饱和快速自旋回波技术获得在体冠状血管壁图像[62,63]。为了改善血液与血管壁之间的对比度，应用双反转恢复磁化准备序列以获得黑血图像[64]。

该技术的进一步发展将双反转恢复预脉冲与快速梯度回波读取技术结合起来[65]，并且最近采用螺旋[66]和径向采集轨迹[67]。临床研究证实，确诊冠心病患者往往具有相对管腔保留的外向正性重构，而 1 型糖尿病和肾功能不全患者则表现为血管壁的厚度增加[68,69]。

对于纤维性或炎性斑块的选择性成像，已经有多项采用钆对比剂进行延迟增强技术的临床前和临床研究正在开展且研究结果良好[70]。临床上批准体内应用的对比剂无论在慢性心绞痛患者[71]还是在急性冠状动脉综合征（acute coronary syndromes, ACS）患者中，可以被上述两种患者的冠状动脉斑块无特异性的摄取[72]（图 1-5）。稳定性心绞痛患者的对比剂摄取与多层螺旋 CT（multislice computed tomography, MSCT）上的钙化或混合性斑块相关，而 ACS 患者的对比剂摄取是短暂的，因此可能与炎症更为相关。

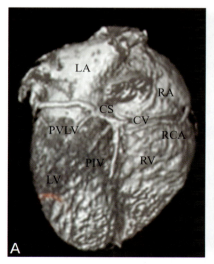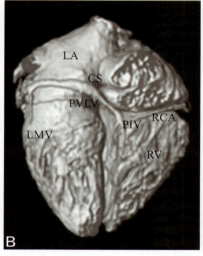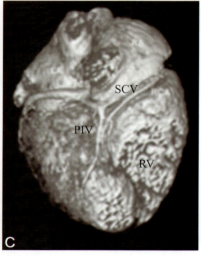

▲ 图 1-4 使用全心脏采集和血管内对比剂获得的冠状静脉 MRA

心脏静脉系统的解剖结构在冠状窦支流存在与否、相对位置和直径等方面存在广泛的个体间变异性。对于心脏静脉系统解剖变化了解以促进心脏再同步化治疗患者左心室导联最佳定位。LA. 左心房；LV. 左心室；LMV. 左边缘静脉；PIV. 后室间静脉；PVLV. 左心室后静脉；RA. 右心房；RV. 右心室；RCA. 右冠状动脉；SCV. 心脏小静脉（经许可引自 Chiribiri A，et al，Am.J.Cardiol，101,407-412,2008.）

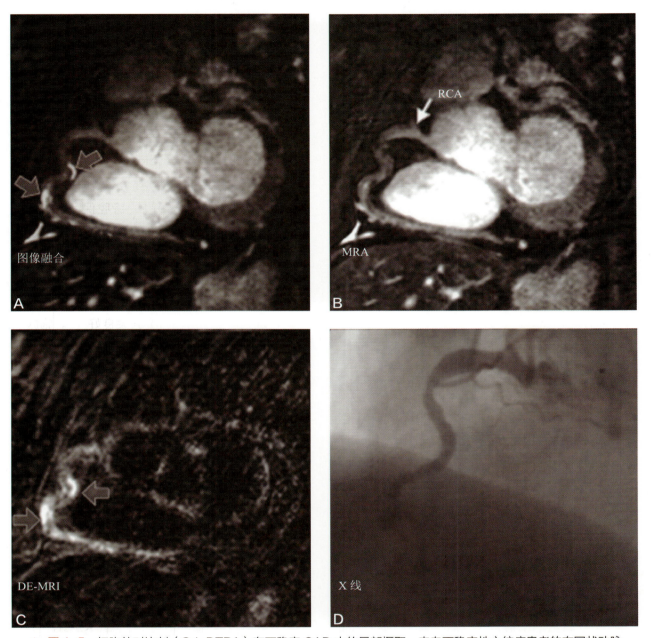

▲ 图 1-5　细胞外对比剂（Gd-DTPA）在不稳定 CAD 中的局部摄取，来自不稳定性心绞痛患者的右冠状动脉图像显示显著增强的血管壁信号的冠状动脉 MRA（A）和延迟增强（DE，B）-MRI（C）之间的图像融合。与 X 线血管造影比较（D）（经许可引自 Ibrahim T, et al, JACC Cardiovasc.Imaging, 2, 580-588, 2009.）

在实验动物模型中，已经试验了几种靶向特异性对比剂。白蛋白结合血池对比剂的积聚表明内皮细胞通透性增加和（或）新生血管形成增加[73]。氧化铁颗粒（ultrasmall particle ironoxide，USPIO）的积聚表明由于斑块内巨噬细胞的存在导致血管内皮通透性增加和血管壁炎症[74,75]。

新近开发了新型的靶向分子对比剂，其特异性作用于靶分子或细胞，使选择性地观察某些炎性标记物如细胞间黏附分子 -1（ICAM-1）、血管黏附分子 -1（VCAM-1）或基质金属蛋白酶（matrix metalloproteinase，MMP）成为可能[76,77]。

其他近期研究成果还包括纤维蛋白特异性对比剂对血栓的特异性标记[78,79]。

分子对比剂可以为提供早期动脉粥样硬化病变的特征以及评估斑块易损性提供新的可能。

（六）特殊注意事项：冠状动脉内支架

冠状动脉支架目前大规模应用于经皮血供重建患者。冠状动脉支架通常由高级不锈钢制成，在1.5T[80-85]和3T[86]磁场下引起的吸引力和局部发热可以忽略不计，已经证实患者植入该种支架后早期在1.5T磁场下行成像检查是安全的[80-82]。在美国，CYPHER™（Cordis，Miami Lakes，Florida）和Taxus® Liberté®（Boston Scientific，Natick，Massachusetts）这两种药物洗脱支架已获批准在植入后可以立即进行CMR扫描。然而，冠状动脉支架会引起局部易感性伪影和信号缺失，这会对支架旁和支架内冠状动脉完整性的评估造成影响。

二、临床应用

MRA的应用目前仅限于评估冠状动脉的异常情况（Ⅰ类适应证）和主动脉-冠状动脉旁路移植术后的桥血管（Ⅱ类适应证）。MRA用于评估自体冠状动脉尚未进入临床常规[87]。

（一）为了监测CAD所行的冠状动脉血管成像

冠状动脉主要分支的近中段常规由自由呼吸导航门控快速梯度回波技术或SSFP显示。特别是冠状动脉主要分支的近段几乎在所有受试者中都能够测量。左前降支（left anterior descending coronary artery，LAD）和右冠状动脉（right coronary artery，RCA）通常成像质量比左回旋支（left circumflex，LCX）更好，因为LCX毗邻心肌走行，且距离线圈采集中心较远。先前研究中，血管的平均显影长度分别为：LAD约50mm，RCA约80mm，LCX约为40mm[27,28,73,88-92]，且MRA测量的近段血管直径和冠状动脉造影结果就有良好一致性[93]，尽管磁共振技术正在不断发展[93]，但冠状动脉MRA的空间分辨率仍低于有创型检查冠状动脉造影，因此限制了MRA所能观察到的血管的大小。尽管存在上述的局限，冠状动脉近段的狭窄仍旧可以被MRA识别出来。在亮血（梯度回波）图像上，狭窄表现为高亮血管中出现为信号缺失（图1-6）。主要机制是因为管腔变窄，部分原因是由于狭窄处远端出现的血液湍流导致信号失相，因此与有创性影像学检查冠状动脉造影相比，冠状动脉MRA会高估病变的狭窄程度[94]。

一项评价冠状动脉MRA诊断准确性的国际多中心研究[95]显示MRA对于CAD检测具有高灵敏度（92%）和低特异性（59%）。原因在于冠状动脉MRA的相对有限的空间分辨率，这也使得其在排除左主干或三支病变（敏感性100%；阴性预测值100%）方面具有极佳的表现。同样的结论也在一系列较小型的单中心研究中得到证实，这些研究显示了MRA对于冠状动脉近段的明显的狭窄病变检出具有较好结果[26,28,96-103]。

最近有人提出将冠状动脉MRA与延迟钆对比剂增强结合起来同时使用，以排外那些前来就诊的没有心肌梗死症状的扩张型心肌病患者的缺血性因素[87]。

为了排除成年人中严重的CAD，新近的一项Meta分析对冠状动脉MRA和MSCT做了比较[104]。该项分析的结论是MSCT比MRA更精确，因此相对于心导管检查，MSCT应当是作为排外CAD首选的无创性替代方法。然而，当冠状动脉MRA扫描与其他核磁扫描整合在一起可形成全面的包含能够检测心脏功能、结构、灌注和心肌活力的临床流程，这种情况下所产生的新的价值亟待评估，故有潜力为已经确诊的或疑似的CAD患者提供更准确的评估。最近一项来自日本的全国性多中心研究证实，在1.5T下行非对比增强全心冠状动脉MRA能够无创性地检出明显的CAD，且具有高敏感性（88%）和中度特异性（72%）。在该研究中，88%的阴性预测值（negative predictive value，NPV）表明全心冠状动脉MRA可用于排除CAD[105]。值得注意的是，该MRCA多中心试验与64排MSCT多中心试验的NPV等同[106]。尤其是其对于低度预测风险患者的结果与CT相似，能够有效排除预测风险在 20% 以内的患者 CAD[107]。

（二）冠状动脉畸形和动脉瘤

冠状动脉 MRA 可准确显示冠状动脉起源及走行的异常和冠状动脉瘤，这是由于其较高的口径和处于冠状动脉近段或扩张部位好发部位所决定的。冠状动脉 MRA 还有使患者在不接触电离辐射的情况下能够做出无创可靠的诊断的优点（图 1-7）。这对于较为年轻的患者、儿童及年轻女性来说尤其重要[87,108]。

（三）冠状动脉旁路移植术

旁路移植术后桥血管的成像得益于它们具有相对固定的位置、平直和已知的走行以及与自体冠状动脉相比来说直径相对较大的特点。目前已采用自旋回波技术[109-112]和梯度回波技术来采集图像。可以应用对比剂来增强血液信号[113-115]，这使得敏感性高达 95%～100%。

桥血管成像的一个主要限制是金属夹的存在，这会由于磁敏感伪像而导致信号缺失。由于夹子通常位于桥血管和冠状动脉附近，因此产生的信号缺失通常可能导致相应的解剖结构无法评估。在专门的中心，冠状动脉 MRA 可用于识别动脉旁路血管中的冠状动脉狭窄。

（四）冠状动脉血管壁成像

通过黑血技术，目前临床应用的最新的 MRI 扫描设备可以提供冠状动脉壁的详细图像。这些技术临床应用的主要障碍是需要非常高的空间分辨率和随之相伴而来的相对长的采集时间。

血管壁可以沿横截面或血管走行路径观察。由于局部容积效应减小，横截面取向应能更准确地量化血管壁厚度，但观察的范围也有限。血管壁的长轴视图提供了更广泛的视野，评估范围约 5cm。对比剂的使用可用于选择性斑块成像观察。例如，注射细胞外对比剂后，延迟增强图像显示局灶性或弥散性的对比剂摄取和增强，可能提示斑块为纤维性的抑或是炎症性的。目前冠状动脉血管壁成像的应用仅限于研究层面，但是将来它可能成为 CAD 风险评估的一部分，并且可以用来监测患者对治疗的反应，特别是如果针对斑块的靶向药物应用于临床，那这项技术的价值则更大。

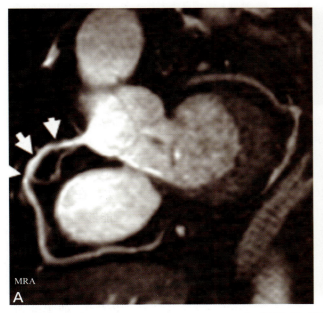
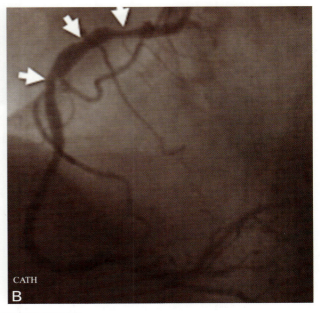

▲ 图 1-6　亮血梯度回波图像

A. 在亮血 MRA 图像上显示的冠状动脉狭窄；B. 与冠状动脉造影比较，可见 RCA 近段多个狭窄和不规则的管壁（白箭所示处）

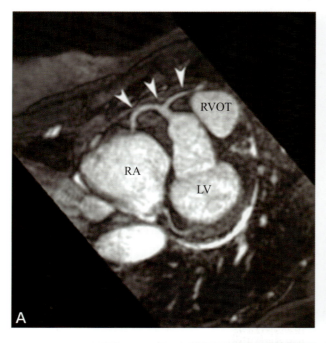 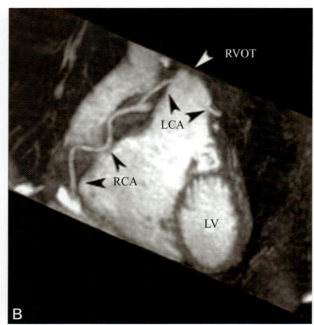
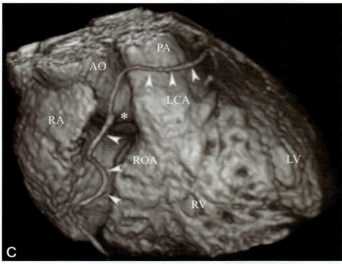 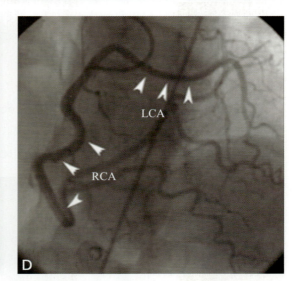

▲ 图 1-7 冠状动脉磁共振血管成像（MRA）显示冠状动脉血管起始处解剖结构

患者临床症状表现为心绞痛，T₂ 导航门控下全心成像技术显示该患者为单支冠状动脉畸形，冠状动脉起自右冠状动脉窦。A. 最大密度投影图像（MIP）显示单支冠状动脉发自右冠状动脉窦（白色箭头）；LV. 左心室；RA. 右心房；RVOT. 右心室流出道。B. MIP 图像显示右冠状动脉（RCA）及左冠状动脉（LCA）走行，跨于 RVOT 前方。C. 心脏容积重建图像显示单冠状动脉起始处（*）发自主动脉（AO），随后分出 RCA 和 LCA；PA. 肺动脉。D. 冠状动脉右前斜位造影图像显示冠状动脉树解剖形态（引自 Boffano, C. et al., Int. J. Cardiol.137, e27–e28, 2009.）

（五）冠状静脉成像

冠状静脉成像可以得到冠状静脉的解剖学情况，与心肌瘢痕信息整合在一起，可能有助于指导左心室电极的植入以达到最佳的心脏再同步化治疗（图 1-8）。早期研究表明，对比剂增强的 CMR 可用于评估冠状窦，心大静脉及各自分支的走行情况[7,8,59]。心力衰竭患者应用该技术的主要限制因素在于可能存在的左心室非同步收缩导致心脏始终存在收缩运动，这可能会导致我们通常所建议的收缩末期触发窗口不适用[36]，因此这种情况下使用舒张中期作为触发窗口可能更为有效。

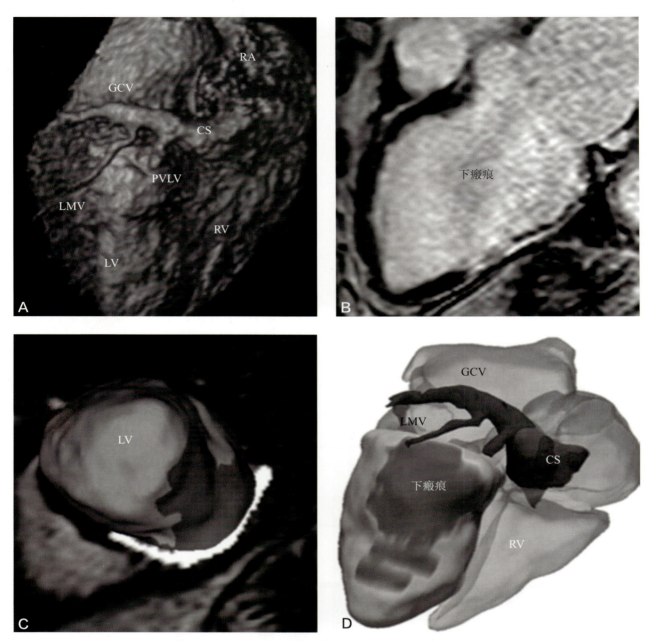

▲ 图 1-8 接受心脏再同步治疗后患者（与图 1-6 同一患者）冠状静脉及瘢痕显示

A. 心脏冠状静脉系统 3D 重建；B. 两腔心长轴图像显示延迟强化，左心室（LV）心肌下壁瘢痕；C. 在两腔心短轴图像上显示 LV 分段及瘢痕成像；D. 全心分段显示下，冠状静脉及瘢痕成像重叠显示。RA. 右心房；LMV. 左边缘静脉；RV. 右心室；LV. 左心室；GCV. 心大静脉；PVLV. 左心室后外侧静脉（引自 Duckett, S.G. et al., J. Magn. Reson. Imaging, 33, 87–95, 2011. 经许可使用）

三、心肌灌注成像

MRA 可以在冠状动脉和冠状静脉的水平很好地观察冠状动脉树，但心肌中的冠状动脉阻力血管（coronary resistance vessels）和毛细血管网由于技术所限，无法评估。直径在 10～100μm 的小动脉可以通过血管壁上的平滑肌来控制血管阻力，从而控制血液在毛细血管和小静脉中的流动。心肌血流的减少可以由于缺氧导致心肌缺血。这可能继发于供应相应心肌的冠状动脉上游狭窄，也可能由于微血管或血管平滑肌细胞功能障碍。因此心肌灌注成像的重点在于在微循环

11

水平评估心肌血流量。此外，心肌中毛细血管的密度可能也是潜在心肌缺血的原因之一。心肌灌注可以被视为患者在静息和应激状态下对心肌缺血风险的最直观的测量方法。

（一）磁共振心肌灌注成像技术

首过灌注成像是量化和评估冠状动脉微循环功能的最为广泛使用的技术。该技术依赖于团注对比剂之后，对比剂第一次通过心脏时快速采集 T_1 加权图像图像。该技术有以下几个要求：①能够在一个心动周期内完成图像的采集，以避免产生心脏运动伪影；②能够达到探测心内到心外膜梯度灌注的空间分辨率要求；③能够在对比剂通过心室腔和心肌的过程中高灵敏度地采集对比增强的图像。目前，大多数 MRI 心肌灌注成像基于心电图出发的 2D 成像方式，通过多层成像来实现心脏的覆盖。每一层 T_1 加权图像图像都需要 100～150ms 的快速单次采集 [*] 图像，层厚小于 2.5mm。通常在成像时施加翻转脉冲或饱和脉冲获取必要的 T_1WI，在随后的磁化恢复的过程中将强烈依赖于血液或心肌组织的 T_1。扫描范围应该在对比剂第一次通过开始，覆盖左心室心腔。此外，应在注射对比剂之前开始采集图像，以获得没有对比剂时的基线参考图像。通常心肌灌注研究每层需要采集 60 张图像。图 1-9 展示了 2D 多层灌注成像的常用扫描方案。

无论有或没有 SSFP，或是梯度回波与回波平面混合成像，灌注序列中的二维图像通常均采用梯度回波的采集形式[116]。在这两种情况下，MR 信号数据（即相位和频率编码的梯度回波

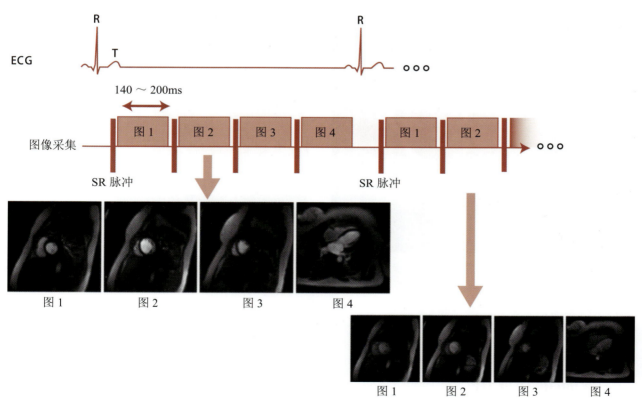

▲ 图 1-9　多层扫描，T_1 加权图像，心电门控心肌灌注显像

此示意图显示心搏约每分钟 60 次时，扫描首过灌注以及早期再循环的常见方案。窄的黑色矩形框显示采集图像之前施加磁化准备（如饱和脉冲）。灰色矩形代表二维图像采集，通常在采用成像加速的情况下每个快速梯度回波成像采集需要 150～200ms。相位编码以线性顺序进行采集，以便在采集中央 K 空间之间提供足够的恢复时间。磁化准备通常是非特定层面选择性的以避免血池中出现依赖流动的对比，而且对每层都能产生相同的 T_1 加权图像。图像显示了组合采集的三层短轴及一个四腔长轴的图像，当饱和脉冲作为磁化准备时，可以在没有明显干扰的情况下获得图像

信号）作为 K 空间数据均以笛卡尔网格线输出。如图像采用非笛卡尔数据采样，如特征采样 CT 图像[117,118]，或螺旋 K 空间轨迹[119,120] 等投影轮廓放射线形式，近年来越来越受到关注。这些非笛卡尔的采集方法不仅提供了一定的采集速度，还具有一些其他的优势，如可以避免产生在心内膜边界[122]的暗边缘伪影[121]等这些可能被认为是灌注缺陷，影响心肌灌注成像的准确性。非笛卡尔采集的缺陷是更复杂的图像重建过程。在非笛卡尔（K 空间）应用快速傅里叶变换之前，笛卡尔网格上重采样过程相对耗时。因此，螺旋和径向灌注成像对于图像采集而言需要相当长的等待时间，这导致目前不能在团注对比剂的过程中实时的对心脏进行成像。

由于心肌灌注成像覆盖范围要包含整个心脏，所以在整个心动周期期间都需要输出 2D 图像。无论是用 ECG 触发还是通过其他与心动周期相关的信号来进行触发，都需要连续采集数据图像来分析心脏的相位[118,123]。大多数心肌灌注发生在心脏舒张期间（舒张期）。如果心脏收缩期和舒张期获得的心肌灌注信号不同，这就产生问题。需要指出的是，心脏灌注成像是对整个心动周期中心肌灌注的平均估计值，也就是说，能够观察到是心脏搏动过程中的组织和血液对比的变化，而不是心动周期中特定的时间点的瞬时变化。由于每层都是在心动周期的特定阶段读取的，因此在以电影模式播放图像时，除非心电触发错误，心脏通常是静止不动的，而只有呼吸运动是保持可见的。

灌注扫描需要覆盖整个左心室，这一过程是通过多层扫描来实现的，例如使用 3～4 个短轴切面，同时结合一个长轴切面来观察心尖。3D 灌注成像作为核医学的标准，可以克服这种成像方式的局限性。对于 3D MR 心肌灌注成像，冻结心脏运动相较于 2D 多层模拟成像更具挑战性，因为 3D 整体数据采集时间决定了快门的速度，而 2D 采集则是受到每一层图像采集时间的限制。因此对于 3D 灌注成像，只能在心动周期中很短的一段时间内（舒张期）来获取部分数据，而且需要使用并行成像和稀疏采样来实现足够短的采集时间[124-126]。

（二）临床应用

在临床状况下，可以利用静息态和激发态的心肌灌注来评估检测 CAD。对于激发态的情况，通常患者需要利用药物来诱导血管舒张。除了重度狭窄（管腔狭窄超过 90%）以外，较低程度的病变仅能通过血管舒张时冠状动脉微循环阻力最小化时才能被检测到。静息条件下的灌注结果可以作为激发血管到最大舒张状态下心肌血流的情况的参考。

为了充分评估激发态的情况，使用电动注射器进行对比剂的团注，以及获得一定时间分辨率的图像都尤为重要。这是因为，心肌的强化不是依赖于心肌血流量，而是依赖于对比剂的注射速度，此外较低的时间采样也难以从视觉上检测心肌对比剂增强速度的差异。

如图 1-10 所示，MR 灌注研究主要是评估团注对比剂后首次通过时的心肌对比增强率。以电影模式显示灌注图像，可以通过比较不同心肌节段中对比剂增强的情况来进行定性评估，或基于信号 - 强度曲线来进行定量评估，甚至进行心肌灌注储备的定量评估。定量储备能力评估与量化视觉评估相比，在多支血管病变和微血管功能障碍的全局和局部的评估都具有一定的优势。次要测量指标是其他感兴趣的对比剂强化情况，对于侧支供血的心肌延迟强化需要更久的时间才能显示[127-129]。定量测量的方式受到（手动）分割图像的限制，通过图像运动矫正[130,131]，可以大大降低这些工作的难度。

四、总结与未来前景

尽管冠状动脉 MRA 的空间分辨率不如 MSCT 高，但新的冠状动脉 MRA 技术能够通过冠状动脉黑血成像，或在成像时使用非特异性或

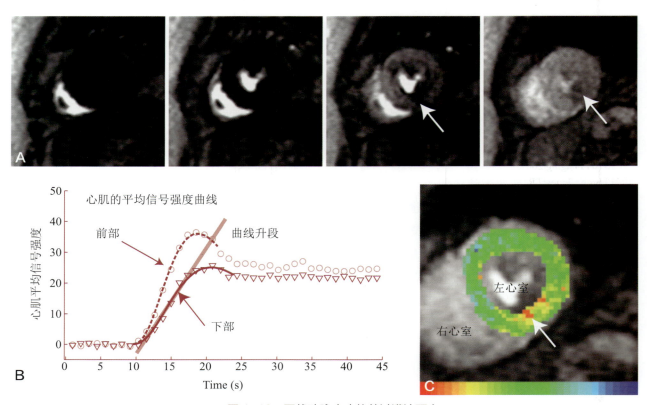

▲ 图 1-10 冠状动脉疾病的首过灌注研究

A.64 岁女性冠心病患者的最大血管舒张期间的灌注图像，描绘了 0.05mmol/kg 团注钆对比剂首次通过右心室及左心室的情况；B. 灌注成像的心前壁及下壁的时间——平均信号强度（signal intensity，SI）曲线；C. 线性编码的心肌对比增强（斜率）情况，描述 MR 灌注图像中心脏内心肌血流相对变化的情况

靶向 MR 的对比剂对于斑块负荷进行评估。目前，针对特定分子或细胞的新型造影剂正在进行临床前评估，有些已经在人体中进行过测试。此外还有一些研究在进行中，包括血栓可视化、血管内皮功能评估以及冠状动脉水肿情况评估等。

此外，运动补偿技术的不断发展将简化冠状动脉 MRA 的采集流程、提高图像质量、缩短扫描时间。

观察冠状动脉树以外的冠状动脉微血管的血液循环，可以用来预测心肌缺血的风险。通过心肌灌注成像，可以评估静息状态和负荷状态微循环的功能。虽然冠状动脉 MRA 可以用于评估斑块负荷和冠状动脉狭窄状态，但心肌灌注成像可以明确血流动力学状态以及侧支循环测存在，从而降低心外膜病变的有害影响。总而言之，这些新技术为我们带来了研究冠状动脉生理和疾病的新的角度。

参考文献

[1] Ford ES, Ajani UA, Croft JB et al. Explaining the decrease in U.S. deaths from coronary disease, 1980–2000. *New Engl J Med* 2007;356:2388–98.

[2] Roger VL, Go AS, Lloyd-Jones DM et al. Heart disease and stroke statistics—2011 update: A report from the American Heart Association. *Circulation* 2011;123:e18–e209.

[3] Patel MR, Peterson ED, Dai D et al. Low diagnostic yield of elective coronary angiography. *New Engl J Med* 2010;362:886–95.

[4] Kim WY, Danias PG, Stuber M et al. Coronary magnetic resonance angiography for the detection of coronary stenoses. *New Engl J Med* 2001;345:1863–9.

[5] Karamitsos TD, Dall'armellina E, Choudhury RP, Neubauer S. Ischemic heart disease: Comprehensive evaluation by cardiovascular magnetic resonance. *Am Heart J* 2011;162:16–30.

[6] Spuentrup E, Botnar RM. Coronary magnetic resonance imaging: Visualization of the vessel lumen and the vessel wall and molecular imaging of arteriothrombosis. *Eur Radiol* 2006;16:1–14.

[7] Chiribiri A, Kelle S, Gotze S et al. Visualization of the car-

[8] Chiribiri A, Kelle S, Kohler U et al. Magnetic resonance cardiac vein imaging: Relation to mitral valve annulus and left circumflex coronary artery. *JACC Cardiovasc Imaging* 2008;1:729–38.

[9] Kim WY, Stuber M, Kissinger KV, Andersen NT, Manning WJ, Botnar RM. Impact of bulk cardiac motion on right coronary MR angiography and vessel wall imaging. *J Magn Reson Imaging* 2001;14:383–90.

[10] Plein S, Jones TR, Ridgway JP, Sivananthan MU. Three-dimensional coronary MR angiography performed with subject-specific cardiac acquisition windows and motion-adapted respiratory gating. *AJR Am J Roentgenol* 2003;180:505–12.

[11] Jahnke C, Paetsch I, Nehrke K et al. A new approach for rapid assessment of the cardiac rest period for coronary MRA. *J Cardiovasc Magn Reson* 2005;7:395–9.

[12] Leiner T, Katsimaglis G, Yeh EN et al. Correction for heart rate variability improves coronary magnetic resonance angiography. *J Magn Reson Imaging* 2005;22:577–82.

[13] Tangcharoen T, Jahnke C, Koehler U et al. Impact of heart rate variability in patients with normal sinus rhythm on image quality in coronary magnetic angiography. *J Magn Reson Imaging* 2008;28:74–9.

[14] Ustun A, Desai M, Abd-Elmoniem KZ, Schar M, Stuber M. Automated identification of minimal myocardial motion for improved image quality on MR angiography at 3 T. *AJR Am J Roentgenol* 2007;188:W283–90.

[15] Ehman RL, Felmlee JP. Adaptive technique for high-definition MR imaging of moving structures. *Radiology* 1989;173:255–63.

[16] Nehrke K, Bornert P, Groen J, Smink J, Bock JC. On the performance and accuracy of 2D navigator pulses. *Magn Reson Imaging* 1999;17:1173–81.

[17] Wang Y, Riederer SJ, Ehman RL. Respiratory motion of the heart: Kinematics and the implications for the spatial resolution in coronary imaging. *Magn Reson Med* 1995;33:713–9.

[18] Danias PG, McConnell MV, Khasgiwala VC, Chuang ML, Edelman RR, Manning WJ. Prospective navigator correction of image position for coronary MR angiography. *Radiology* 1997;203:733–6.

[19] Danias PG, Stuber M, Botnar RM, Kissinger KV, Edelman RR, Manning WJ. Relationship between motion of coronary arteries and diaphragm during free breathing: Lessons from real-time MR imaging. *AJR Am J Roentgenol* 1999;172:1061–5.

[20] Nagel E, Bornstedt A, Schnackenburg B, Hug J, Oswald H, Fleck E. Optimization of realtime adaptive navigator correction for 3D magnetic resonance coronary angiography. *Magn Reson Med* 1999;42:408–11.

[21] Jahnke C, Nehrke K, Paetsch I et al. Improved bulk myocardial motion suppression for navigator-gated coronary magnetic resonance imaging. *J Magn Reson Imaging* 2007;26:780–6.

[22] Edelman RR, Manning WJ, Burstein D, Paulin S. Coronary arteries: Breath-hold MR angiography. *Radiology* 1991;181:641–3.

[23] Manke D, Nehrke K, Bornert P. Novel prospective respiratory motion correction approach for free-breathing coronary MR angiography using a patient-adapted affine motion model. *Magn Reson Med* 2003;50:122–31.

[24] Huber S, Bornstedt A, Schnackenburg B, Paetsch I, Fleck E, Nagel E. The impact of different positions and thoracial restrains on respiratory induced cardiac motion. *J Cardiovasc Magn Reson* 2006;8:483–8.

[25] Stuber M, Danias PG, Botnar RM, Sodickson DK, Kissinger KV, Manning WJ. Superiority of prone position in free-breathing 3D coronary MRA in patients with coronary disease. *J Magn Reson Imaging* 2001;13:185–91.

[26] Sakuma H, Ichikawa Y, Chino S, Hirano T, Makino K, Takeda K. Detection of coronary artery stenosis with whole-heart coronary magnetic resonance angiography. *J Am Coll Cardiol* 2006;48:1946–50.

[27] Manning WJ, Li W, Boyle NG, Edelman RR. Fat-suppressed breath-hold magnetic resonance coronary angiography. *Circulation* 1993;87:94–104.

[28] Botnar RM, Stuber M, Danias PG, Kissinger KV, Manning WJ. Improved coronary artery definition with T2-weighted, free-breathing, three-dimensional coronary MRA. *Circulation* 1999;99:3139–48.

[29] Brittain JH, Hu BS, Wright GA, Meyer CH, Macovski A, Nishimura DG. Coronary angiography with magnetization-prepared T2 contrast. *Magn Reson Med* 1995;33:689–96.

[30] Li D, Paschal CB, Haacke EM, Adler LP. Coronary arteries: Three-dimensional MR imaging with fat saturation and magnetization transfer contrast. *Radiology* 1993;187:401–6.

[31] Deshpande VS, Shea SM, Laub G, Simonetti OP, Finn JP, Li D. 3D magnetization-prepared true-FISP: A new technique for imaging coronary arteries. *Magn Reson Med* 2001;46:494–502.

[32] Giorgi B, Dymarkowski S, Maes F, Kouwenhoven M, Bogaert J. Improved visualization of coronary arteries using a new three-dimensional submillimeter MR coronary angiography sequence with balanced gradients. *AJR Am J Roentgenol* 2002;179:901–10.

[33] Spuentrup E, Bornert P, Botnar RM, Groen JP, Manning WJ, Stuber M. Navigator-gated free-breathing three-dimensional balanced fast field echo (TrueFISP) coronary magnetic resonance angiography. *Invest Radiol* 2002;37:637–42.

[34] Kaul MG, Stork A, Bansmann PM et al. Evaluation of balanced steady-state free precession (TrueFISP) and K-space segmented gradient echo sequences for 3D coronary MR angiography with navigator gating at 3 Tesla. *Rofo* 2004;176:1560–5.

[35] Dixon WT, Oshinski JN, Trudeau JD, Arnold BC, Pettigrew RI. Myocardial suppression in vivo by spin locking with

composite pulses. *Magn Reson Med* 1996;36:90–4.

[36] Nezafat R, Han Y, Peters DC et al. Coronary magnetic resonance vein imaging: Imaging contrast, sequence, and timing. *Magn Reson Med* 2007;58:1196–206.

[37] Regenfus M, Ropers D, Achenbach S et al. Noninvasive detection of coronary artery stenosis using contrastenhanced three-dimensional breath-hold magnetic resonance coronary angiography. *J Am Coll Cardiol* 2000;36:44–50.

[38] Huber ME, Paetsch I, Schnackenburg B et al. Performance of a new gadolinium-based intravascular contrast agent in free-breathing inversion-recovery 3D coronary MRA. *Magn Reson Med* 2003;49:115–21.

[39] Kelle S, Thouet T, Tangcharoen T et al. Whole-heart coronary magnetic resonance angiography with MS-325 (Gadofosveset). *Med Sci Monit* 2007;13:CR469–74.

[40] Li D, Dolan RP, Walovitch RC, Lauffer RB. Three-dimensional MRI of coronary arteries using an intravascular contrast agent. *Magn Reson Med* 1998;39:1014–8.

[41] Tang L, Merkle N, Schar M et al. Volume-targeted and whole-heart coronary magnetic resonance angiography using an intravascular contrast agent. *J Magn Reson Imaging* 2009;30:1191–6.

[42] Liu X, Bi X, Huang J, Jerecic R, Carr J, Li D. Contrast enhanced whole-heart coronary magnetic resonance angiography at 3.0 T: Comparison with steady-state free precession technique at 1.5 T. *Invest Radiol* 2008;43:663–8.

[43] Nassenstein K, Breuckmann F, Hunold P, Barkhausen J, Schlosser T. Magnetic resonance coronary angiography: Comparison between a Gd-BOPTA- and a Gd-DTPA-enhanced spoiled gradient-echo sequence and a non-contrast-enhanced steady-state free-precession sequence. *Acta Radiol* 2009;50:406–11.

[44] Yang Q, Li K, Liu X et al. Contrast-enhanced whole-heart coronary magnetic resonance angiography at 3.0-T: A comparative study with X-ray angiography in a single center. *J Am Coll Cardiol* 2009;54:69–76.

[45] Laurent S, Elst LV, Muller RN. Comparative study of the physicochemical properties of six clinical low molecular weight gadolinium contrast agents. *Contrast Media Mol Imaging* 2006;1:128–37.

[46] Krombach GA, Hahnen C, Lodemann KP et al. Gd-BOPTA for assessment of myocardial viability on MRI: Changes of T1 value and their impact on delayed enhancement. *Eur Radiol* 2009;19:2136–46.

[47] Goldfarb JW, Edelman RR. Coronary arteries: Breathhold, gadolinium-enhanced, three-dimensional MR angiography. *Radiology* 1998;206:830–4.

[48] Stuber M, Botnar RM, Danias PG et al. Contrast agent-enhanced, free-breathing, three-dimensional coronary magnetic resonance angiography. *J Magn Reson Imaging* 1999;10:790–9.

[49] Bhat H, Yang Q, Zuehlsdorff S, Li K, Li D. Contrast-enhanced whole-heart coronary magnetic resonance angiography at 3 T using interleaved echo planar imaging. *Invest Radiol* 2010;45:458–64.

[50] Slavin GS, Riederer SJ, Ehman RL. Two-dimensional multishot echo-planar coronary MR angiography. *Magn Reson Med* 1998;40:883–9.

[51] Bornert P, Stuber M, Botnar RM et al. Direct comparison of 3D spiral vs. Cartesian gradient-echo coronary magnetic resonance angiography. *Magn Reson Med* 2001;46:789–94.

[52] Priest AN, Bansmann PM, Mullerleile K, Adam G. Coronary vessel-wall and lumen imaging using radial k-space acquisition with MRI at 3 Tesla. *Eur Radiol* 2007;17:339–46.

[53] Pruessmann KP, Weiger M, Scheidegger MB, Boesiger P. SENSE: Sensitivity encoding for fast MRI. *Magn Reson Med* 1999;42:952–62.

[54] Sodickson DK, Manning WJ. Simultaneous acquisition of spatial harmonics (SMASH): Fast imaging with radiofrequency coil arrays. *Magn Reson Med* 1997;38:591–603.

[55] Yu J, Schar M, Vonken EJ, Kelle S, Stuber M. Improved SNR efficiency in gradient echo coronary MRA with high temporal resolution using parallel imaging. *Magn Reson Med* 2009;62:1211–20.

[56] Duckett SG, Ginks M, Shetty AK et al. Realtime fusion of cardiac magnetic resonance imaging and computed tomography venography with X-ray fluoroscopy to aid cardiac resynchronisation therapy implantation in patients with persistent left superior vena cava. *Europace* 2011;13:285–6.

[57] Duckett SG, Ginks MR, Knowles BR et al. Advanced image fusion to overlay coronary sinus anatomy with real-time fluoroscopy to facilitate left ventricular lead implantation in CRT. *Pacing Clin Electrophysiol* 2011;34:226–34.

[58] Stoeck CT, Han Y, Peters DC et al. Whole heart magnetization-prepared steady-state free precession coronary vein MRI. *J Magn Reson Imaging* 2009;29:1293–9.

[59] Rasche V, Binner L, Cavagna F et al. Whole-heart coronary vein imaging: A comparison between non-contrast-agent- and contrast-agent-enhanced visualization of the coronary venous system. *Magn Reson Med* 2007;57:1019–26.

[60] Younger JF, Plein S, Crean A, Ball SG, Greenwood JP. Visualization of coronary venous anatomy by cardio-vascular magnetic resonance. *J Cardiovasc Magn Reson* 2009;11:26.

[61] Duckett SG, Chiribiri A, Ginks MR et al. Cardiac MRI to investigate myocardial scar and coronary venous anatomy using a slow infusion of dimeglumine gadobenate in patients undergoing assessment for cardiac resynchronization therapy. *J Magn Reson Imaging* 2011;33:87–95.

[62] Botnar RM, Stuber M, Kissinger KV, Kim WY, Spuentrup E, Manning WJ. Noninvasive coronary vessel wall and plaque imaging with magnetic resonance imaging. *Circulation* 2000;102:2582–7.

[63] Fayad ZA, Fuster V, Fallon JT et al. Noninvasive in vivo human coronary artery lumen and wall imaging using black-blood magnetic resonance imaging. *Circulation* 2000;102:506–10.

[64] Edelman RR, Chien D, Kim D. Fast selective black blood MR imaging. *Radiology* 1991;181:655–60.

[65] Botnar RM, Stuber M, Lamerichs R et al. Initial experiences with in vivo right coronary artery human MR vessel wall imaging at 3 tesla. *J Cardiovasc Magn Reson* 2003;5:589–94.

[66] Botnar RM, Kim WY, Bornert P, Stuber M, Spuentrup E, Manning WJ. 3D coronary vessel wall imaging utilizing a local inversion technique with spiral image acquisition. *Magn Reson Med* 2001;46:848–54.

[67] Katoh M, Spuentrup E, Buecker A et al. MRI of coronary vessel walls using radial k-space sampling and steady-state free precession imaging. *AJR Am J Roentgenol* 2006;186:S401–6.

[68] Kim WY, Stuber M, Bornert P, Kissinger KV, Manning WJ, Botnar RM. Three-dimensional black-blood cardiac magnetic resonance coronary vessel wall imaging detects positive arterial remodeling in patients with nonsignificant coronary artery disease. *Circulation* 2002;106:296–9.

[69] Kim WY, Astrup AS, Stuber M et al. Subclinical coronary and aortic atherosclerosis detected by magnetic resonance imaging in type 1 diabetes with and without diabetic nephropathy. *Circulation* 2007;115:228–35.

[70] Kerwin WS, Zhao X, Yuan C, Hatsukami TS, Maravilla KR, Underhill HR. Contrast-enhanced MRI of carotid atherosclerosis: Dependence on contrast agent. *J Magn Reson Imaging* 2009;30:35–40.

[71] Yeon SB, Sabir A, Clouse M et al. Delayed-enhancement cardiovascular magnetic resonance coronary artery wall imaging: Comparison with multislice computed tomography and quantitative coronary angiography. *J Am Coll Cardiol* 2007;50:441–7.

[72] Ibrahim T, Makowski MR, Jankauskas A et al. Serial contrast-enhanced cardiac magnetic resonance imaging demonstrates regression of hyperenhancement within the coronary artery wall in patients after acute myocardial infarction. *JACC Cardiovasc Imaging* 2009;2:580–8.

[73] Lobbes MB, Miserus RJ, Heeneman Setal. Atherosclerosis: Contrast-enhanced MR imaging of vessel wall in rabbit model—Comparison of gadofosveset and gadopentetate dimeglumine. *Radiology* 2009;250:682–91.

[74] Kooi ME, Cappendijk VC, Cleutjens KB et al. Accumulation of ultrasmall superparamagnetic particles of iron oxide in human atherosclerotic plaques can be detected by in vivo magnetic resonance imaging. *Circulation* 2003;107:2453–8.

[75] Tang TY, Howarth SP, Miller SR et al. The ATHEROMA (Atorvastatin Therapy: Effects on Reduction of Macrophage Activity) Study. Evaluation using ultrasmall superparamagnetic iron oxide-enhanced magnetic resonance imaging in carotid disease. *J Am College Cardiol* 2009;53:2039–50.

[76] Nahrendorf M, Jaffer FA, Kelly KA et al. Noninvasive vascular cell adhesion molecule-1 imaging identifies inflammatory activation of cells in atherosclerosis. *Circulation* 2006;114:1504–11.

[77] Nahrendorf M, Keliher E, Panizzi P et al. 18F-4V for PET-CT imaging of VCAM-1 expression in atherosclerosis. *JACC Cardiovasc Imaging* 2009;2:1213–22.

[78] Botnar RM, Buecker A, Wiethoff AJ et al. In vivo magnetic resonance imaging of coronary thrombosis using a fibrin-binding molecular magnetic resonance contrast agent. *Circulation* 2004;110:1463–6.

[79] Botnar RM, Perez AS, Witte S et al. In vivo molecular imaging of acute and subacute thrombosis using a fibrin-binding magnetic resonance imaging contrast agent. *Circulation* 2004;109:2023–9.

[80] Gerber TC, Fasseas P, Lennon RJ et al. Clinical safety of magnetic resonance imaging early after coronary artery stent placement. *J Am Coll Cardiol* 2003;42:1295–8.

[81] Hug J, Nagel E, Bornstedt A, Schnackenburg B, Oswald H, Fleck E. Coronary arterial stents: Safety and artifacts during MR imaging. *Radiology* 2000;216:781–7.

[82] Kramer CM, Rogers WJ, Jr., Pakstis DL. Absence of adverse outcomes after magnetic resonance imaging early after stent placement for acute myocardial infarction: A preliminary study. *J Cardiovasc Magn Reson* 2000;2:257–61.

[83] Scott NA, Pettigrew RI. Absence of movement of coronary stents after placement in a magnetic resonance imaging field. *Am J Cardiol* 1994;73:900–1.

[84] Shellock FG, Shellock VJ. Metallic stents: Evaluation of MR imaging safety. *AJR Am J Roentgenol* 1999;173:543–7.

[85] Strohm O, Kivelitz D, Gross W et al. Safety of implantable coronary stents during 1H-magnetic resonance imaging at 1.0 and 1.5 T. *J Cardiovasc Magn Reson* 1999;1:239–45.

[86] Shellock FG, Forder JR. Drug eluting coronary stent: In vitro evaluation of magnet resonance safety at 3 Tesla. *J Cardiovasc Magn Reson* 2005;7:415–9.

[87] Hundley WG, Bluemke DA, Finn JP et al. ACCF/ACR/AHA/NASCI/SCMR 2010 expert consensus document on cardiovascular magnetic resonance: A report of the American College of Cardiology Foundation Task Force on Expert Consensus Documents. *J Am Coll Cardiol* 2010;55:2614–62.

[88] Hofman MB, Paschal CB, Li D, Haacke EM, van Rossum AC, Sprenger M. MRI of coronary arteries: 2D breathhold vs 3D respiratory-gated acquisition. *J Comput Assist Tomogr* 1995;19:56–62.

[89] Oshinski JN, Hofland L, Mukundan S, Jr., Dixon WT, Parks WJ, Pettigrew RI. Two-dimensional coronary MR angiography without breath holding. *Radiology* 1996;201:737–43.

[90] Paschal CB, Haacke EM, Adler LP. Three-dimensional MR imaging of the coronary arteries: Preliminary clinical experience. *J Magn Reson Imaging* 1993;3:491–500.

[91] Post JC, van Rossum AC, Hofman MB, Valk J, Visser CA. Three-dimensional respiratory-gated MR angiography of coronary arteries: Comparison with conventional coronary angiography. *AJR Am J Roentgenol* 1996;166:1399–404.

[92] Stuber M, Botnar RM, Danias PG et al. Double-oblique free-breathing high resolution three-dimensional coronary magnetic resonance angiography. *J Am Coll Cardiol* 1999;34:524–31.

[93] Scheidegger MB, Muller R, Boesiger P. Magnetic resonance angiography: Methods and its applications to the cor-

onary arteries. *Technol Health Care* 1994;2:255–65.

[94] Pennell DJ, Bogren HG, Keegan J, Firmin DN, Underwood SR. Assessment of coronary artery stenosis by magnetic resonance imaging. *Heart* 1996;75:127–33.

[95] Kim WY, Danias PG, Stuber M et al. Coronary magnetic resonance angiography for the detection of coronary stenoses. *N Engl J Med* 2001;345:1863–9.

[96] Bogaert J, Kuzo R, Dymarkowski S, Beckers R, Piessens J, Rademakers FE. Coronary artery imaging with real-time navigator three-dimensional turbo-field-echo MR coronary angiography: Initial experience. *Radiology* 2003;226:707–16.

[97] Dewey M, Teige F, Schnapauff D et al. Combination of free-breathing and breathhold steady-state free precession magnetic resonance angiography for detection of coronary artery stenoses. *J Magn Reson Imaging* 2006;23:674–81.

[98] Jahnke C, Paetsch I, Nehrke K et al. Rapid and complete coronary arterial tree visualization with magnetic resonance imaging: Feasibility and diagnostic performance. *Eur Heart J* 2005;26:2313–9.

[99] Jahnke C, Paetsch I, Schnackenburg B et al. Coronary MR angiography with steady-state free precession: individually adapted breath-hold technique versus free-breathing technique. *Radiology* 2004;232:669–76.

[100] Maintz D, Aepfelbacher FC, Kissinger KV et al. Coronary MR angiography: Comparison of quantitative and qualitative data from four techniques. *AJR Am J Roentgenol* 2004;182:515–21.

[101] Manning WJ, Li W, Edelman RR. A preliminary report comparing magnetic resonance coronary angiography with conventional angiography. *N Engl J Med* 1993; 328:828–32.

[102] Ozgun M, Hoffmeier A, Kouwenhoven M et al. Comparison of 3D segmented gradient-echo and steadystate free precession coronary MRI sequences in patients with coronary artery disease. *AJR Am J Roentgenol* 2005;185:103–9.

[103] Sakuma H, Ichikawa Y, Suzawa N et al. Assessment of coronary arteries with total study time of less than 30 minutes by using whole-heart coronary MR angiography. *Radiology* 2005;237:316–21.

[104] Schuetz GM, Zacharopoulou NM, Schlattmann P, Dewey M. Meta-analysis: Noninvasive coronary angiography using computed tomography versus magnetic resonance imaging. *Ann Intern Med* 2010;152:167–77.

[105] Kato S, Kitagawa K, Ishida N et al. Assessment of coronary artery disease using magnetic resonance coronary angiography: A national multicenter trial. *J Am Coll Cardiol* 2010;56:983–91.

[106] Miller JM, Rochitte CE, Dewey M et al. Diagnostic performance of coronary angiography by 64-row CT. *New Engl J Med* 2008;359:2324–36.

[107] Nagel E. Magnetic resonance coronary angiography: The condemned live longer. *J Am College Cardiol* 2010;56:992–4.

[108] Boffano C, Chiribiri A, Cesarani F. Native whole-heart coronary imaging for the identification of anomalous origin of the coronary arteries. *Int J Cardiol* 2009;137:e27–8.

[109] Galjee MA, van Rossum AC, Doesburg T, van Eenige MJ, Visser CA. Value of magnetic resonance imaging in assessing patency and function of coronary artery bypass grafts. An angiographically controlled study. *Circulation* 1996;93:660–6.

[110] Jenkins JP, Love HG, Foster CJ, Isherwood I, Rowlands DJ. Detection of coronary artery bypass graft patency as assessed by magnetic resonance imaging. *Br J Radiol* 1988;61:2–4.

[111] Rubinstein RI, Askenase AD, Thickman D, Feldman MS, Agarwal JB, Helfant RH. Magnetic resonance imaging to evaluate patency of aortocoronary bypass grafts. *Circulation* 1987;76:786–91.

[112] White RD, Caputo GR, Mark AS, Modin GW, Higgins CB. Coronary artery bypass graft patency: Noninvasive evaluation with MR imaging. *Radiology* 1987;164:681–6.

[113] Vrachliotis TG, Bis KG, Aliabadi D, Shetty AN, Safian R, Simonetti O. Contrast-enhanced breath-hold MR angiography for evaluating patency of coronary artery bypass grafts. *AJR Am J Roentgenol* 1997;168:1073–80.

[114] Wintersperger BJ, Engelmann MG, von Smekal A et al. Patency of coronary bypass grafts: Assessment with breath-hold contrast-enhanced MR angiography—Value of a non-electrocardiographically triggered technique. *Radiology* 1998;208:345–51.

[115] Wintersperger BJ, von Smekal A, Engelmann MG et al. Contrast media enhanced magnetic resonance angiography for determining patency of a coronary bypass. A comparison with coronary angiography. *Rofo* 1997;167:572–8.

[116] Wang Y, Moin K, Akinboboye O, Reichek N. Myocardial first pass perfusion: Steady-state free precession versus spoiled gradient echo and segmented echo planar imaging. *Magn Reson Med* 2005;54:1123–9.

[117] Adluru G, McGann C, Speier P, Kholmovski EG, Shaaban A, Dibella EV. Acquisition and reconstruction of undersampled radial data for myocardial perfusion magnetic resonance imaging. *J Magn Reson Imaging* 2009;29:466–73.

[118] Sharif B, Arsanjani R, Dharmakumar R, Bairey Merz CN, Berman DS, Li D. All-systolic non-ECG-gated myocardial perfusion MRI: Feasibility of multi-slice continuous first-pass imaging. *Magn Reson Med* 2015;74:1661–74.

[119] Salerno M, Sica CT, Kramer CM, Meyer CH. Optimization of spiral-based pulse sequences for first-pass myocardial perfusion imaging. *Magn Reson Med* 2011;65:1602–10.

[120] Salerno M, Taylor A, Yang Y et al. Adenosine stress cardiovascular magnetic resonance with variable-density spiral pulse sequences accurately detects coronary artery disease: initial clinical evaluation. *Circ Cardiovasc Imaging* 2014;7:639–46.

[121] Di Bella EV, Parker DL, Sinusas AJ. On the dark rim artifact in dynamic contrast-enhanced MRI myocardial per-

fusion studies. *Magn Reson Med* 2005;54:1295–9.
[122] Sharif B, Dharmakumar R, Labounty T et al. Projection imaging of myocardial perfusion: Minimizing the sub-endocardial dark-rim artifact. *J Cardiovasc Magn Reson* 2012;14 (Suppl 1):P275.
[123] DiBella EV, Chen L, Schabel MC, Adluru G, McGann CJ. Myocardial perfusion acquisition without magnetization preparation or gating. *Magn Reson Med* 2012;67:609–13.
[124] Manka R, Wissmann L, Gebker R et al. Multicenter evaluation of dynamic three-dimensional magnetic resonance myocardial perfusion imaging for the detection of coronary artery disease defined by fractional flow reserve. *Circ Cardiovasc Imaging* 2015;8:e003061.
[125] Motwani M, Kidambi A, Sourbron S et al. Quantitative three-dimensional cardiovascular magnetic resonance myocardial perfusion imaging in systole and diastole. *J Cardiovasc Magn Reson* 2014;16:19.
[126] Fair MJ, Gatehouse PD, DiBella EV, Firmin DN. A review of 3D first-pass, whole-heart, myocardial perfusion car diovascular magnetic resonance. *J Cardiovasc Magn Reson* 2015;17:68.
[127] Jerosch-Herold M, Hu XD, Murthy NS, Seethamraju RT. Time delay for arrival of MR contrast agent in collateral-dependent myocardium. *IEEE Trans Med Imaging* 2004;23:881–90.
[128] Muehling OM, Cyran C, Jerosch-Herold M et al. Quantitative magnetic resonance first-pass perfusion imaging detects collateral-dependent myocardium. *Circulation* 2005;112:2272.
[129] Muehling OM, Huber A, Cyran C et al. The delay of contrast arrival in magnetic resonance first-pass perfusion imaging: A novel non-invasive parameter detecting collateral-dependent myocardium. *Heart* 2007;93:842–7.
[130] Xue H, Guehring J, Srinivasan L et al. Evaluation of rigid and non-rigid motion compensation of cardiac perfusion MRI. *Med Image Comput Comput Assist Interv* 2008;11:35–43.
[131] Xue H, Zuehlsdorff S, Kellman P et al. Unsupervised inline analysis of cardiac perfusion MRI. *Med Image Comput Comput Assist Interv* 2009;12:741–9.

Chapter 2
心脏影像：心肌磁共振成像

Imaging of the Heart: Myocardial Imaging

Ravi S. Shah, Otavio Coelho-Filho, Ana C. Andrade, Michael Jerosch-Herold 著

代静文 译

王怡宁 校

目录　CONTENTS

一、心室功能及容积 / 22

二、区域心肌功能 / 23

三、T_1 及 T_2 加权心肌成像 / 24

四、T_2^* 加权成像 / 26

五、T_1 Mapping 及 T_2 Mapping 心肌组织定量技术 / 27

六、心肌活性 / 28

磁共振成像（MRI）现在已被认为是心脏成像的一种重要模式。这一技术有较好的软组织对比，在表征心肌组织特性方面具有多功能性，并且可以量化心肌的运动。本章旨在向读者介绍不同磁共振方法以获取心脏图像。

绝大多数临床心脏 MRI 研究开始于通过电影序列评估心室体积、心肌质量和全心室功能。因此，本章将首先介绍心脏 MRI 检查的这一重要组成部分。尽管心脏的标准磁共振电影也可以评估局部心脏功能，但是可以将一些独特的序列添加到该检查中，对区域心肌的特征进行评估。

评估心肌特性通常包括通过 T_1、T_2 和 T_2^* 加权成像进行心肌定性评估，图像所产生的软组织对比广泛用于检测心肌疾病。近年来，该领域对量化心肌组织弛豫特性的兴趣越来越浓厚，即测量并绘制弛豫时间 T_1、T_2 和 T_2^*，这克服了通过不同弛豫性质调节组织对比度的局限性。

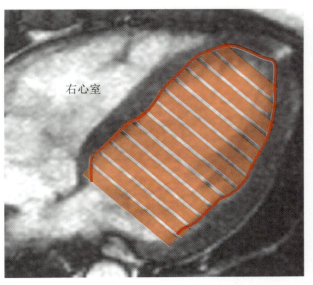

▲ 图 2-1 Simpson 法对心室容量进行量化的示意图

通过求和所有从基部到顶点覆盖左心室的短轴层面内心腔的体积，所切片不必是连续的（没有切片间隙），在这种情况下，通过从两个相邻切片的内插来估计间隙中的体积。在屏气期间获取电影 MR 图像，通常在一次屏气期间获得一个或两个层面。该图表示理想化的情况，假设患者已经暂停呼吸，使得每次电影采集心脏的位置是相同的

一、心室功能及容积

心脏磁共振（cardiovascular magnetic resonance，CMR）成像最为成熟的应用之一是对心室功能和体积的准确定量测量。左心室体积在评估预后中的重要性已得到普遍认可，许多研究证明了心肌梗死面积，左心室重塑[1-3]和进行性心室扩张[4-6]之间的关系。许多综述已阐述左心室结构和功能预后的重要性[7]，在此不再重述。在本部分，我们将重点讨论 CMR 成像技术和临床评估心室结构和功能。

鉴于心脏超声心动图（electrocardiogram，ECG）广泛用于评估心脏体积和功能，CMR 对心室体积和功能的量化方法基本上是根据超声心动图方法改编的。尽管采用了面积长度法测量左心室容积[8]，但评估左心室容积和射血分数的更常见方法是 Simpson（辛普森）法（图 2-1）。在这种方法中，采集从左心室的基底部（在二尖瓣环形水平）到心尖的短轴电影序列（具有或不具有稳态自由进动的快速梯度回波脉冲序列）。体积通过从基底段到心尖段的电影层厚和左心室心内膜容积的总和来计算。对于体积评估，乳头肌通常包括在左心室容积内。

传统上，使用心电触发的快速梯度回波（fast gradient recalled echo，FGRE）脉冲序列来实现在一个心动周期上大约 20 个相位或更多的时间分辨率。因此，图像采集只能采用节段式（segments）采集。在这里，节段（segments）指的是为每个心脏阶段采集的数据的子集。因此，图像采集分布在多个心动周期中，直到每个心动周期收集足够重建出电影的数据。在采集电影图像中，在心动周期内连续梯度回波导致心肌信号饱和，而由于不饱和的血液流入，心室腔中的血池显现为明亮的。这就是亮血的电影序列。尽管如此，在心脏功能较差的患者中，明亮血液效应消失，导致电影图像上心内膜边界的清晰度差。另外，射频脉冲的继续应用意味着它们的翻转角必须相对较低（15°～20°），所得到的信噪比有时并不

理想。

目前，稳态自由进动（steady-state free precession, SSFP）电影序列已被用于进行心脏电影成像，其可获得更高的信噪比，更短的采集时间和更清楚的心内膜边界[9]。（这里应该指出的是，通过并行采集技术获得较高的信噪比为加速图像采集留下了更多技术空间，这种技术使用多个接收线圈与接收器来加速图像采集。）然而，一些大规模研究显示，利用传统的 FGRE 成像技术，SSFP 和 FGRE 其结果存在一些差异[10]。通常，使用 SSFP 方法测得的左心室容积更高，左心室质量更低[11]。这可能与 SSFP 图像中心内膜边界更明确有关，也就是说，观察到明亮的血池信号直至达到真正的心肌边界。

与区域长度方法或视觉评估不同，连续层面的采集可以对左心室体积、射血分数和舒张末期心肌质量（如果同时勾画心外膜和心内膜边界）进行可重复的及精确的定量评估，而无须假设腔体几何形状[12,13]。使用该技术已经为右心室容积和左心室容积以及射血分数制订了正常的范围，并且已发表文献表明，这种方法高度可重复，且比 ECG 更精确[14]，甚至可以使得使用左心室体积或功能作为研究终点的研究所纳入的样本量更小[15]。左心室质量评估也采用类似的方式进行，以 Simpson 法计算从基底到心尖心内膜和心外膜之间的区域体积（大多数情况下除外乳头肌）。心肌体积乘以 1.02 g/ml（心肌的近似密度），从而获得左心室心肌质量。

在某些疾病或病理生理状态，如肺动脉高压、心力衰竭和先天性心脏病中，右心室结构的量化评估十分重要。由于 CMR 基于断层成像平面，隐私是评估右心室形态、结构和功能的金标准。尽管右心室（RV）长轴成像的精确度已经得到提高[16]，但目前右心室成像仍然依赖于短轴图像，短轴图像范围通常从肺动脉瓣到心尖区域。

CMR 作为量化心脏体积和功能的金标准是基于研究结果。其中一项有趣的研究对比了体内与死后离体心脏容积及射血分数。Rehr 等采用乳胶浇灌心脏的模型，研究显示 CMR 测量的容积与实际解剖容积间具有相当高的相关性（系数 0.997）[17]。左心室质量和右心室质量测量结果也进行了相应的解剖学验证[18,19]，体外标本与 CMR 测量的心室质量之间也具有极好的相关性。CMR 的精确度提高（相较于心电图或核医学）可以有效地减少临床研究需要纳入的样本量，一项研究显示，心室形态的 CMR 评估相较于 ECG 评估研究，其样本量减少了 10 倍以上[20]。

许多研究都应用 CMR 成像对不同疾病（包括心肌梗死后的心脏瓣膜病和心力衰竭）中心脏质量、功能和体积进行定量评估。重要的是，CMR 可以根据不同的临床情况调整扫描参数及序列，包括心肌梗死面积评估、心肌灌注和 T_2 心肌特性，以进一步评价心肌功能降低的区域。本章在此不展开论述。

几项基于人群的研究（例如动脉粥样硬化的多种族研究）采用无对比剂 CMR 对全心和区域功能进行量化，从而在更大的患者人群中揭示了疾病生理学及机制[21-24]。此外，最近的研究（例如英国生物银行）开始将生物标志物和大数据方法结合起来评估局部心肌表型、质量和功能，作为研究疾病生理的手段。这些研究提示，CMR 可以结合这些方法用以阐明心肌生物学与临床结果之间的关系。

二、区域心肌功能

除了左心室和右心室整体功能的量化之外，CMR 对于评估区域功能障碍和亚临床功能障碍非常有效。包括将 CMR 用于评估区域心肌组织亚临床重塑。区域性心肌功能障碍的预后价值可能高于整体心肌功能，尤其是在疾病的临床前期（如高血压、肥胖和糖尿病）（MESA REF）。作为心脏功能领域最开始的评估方法，ECG 已经建立了评估心肌区域功能的技术，包括区域室壁厚度（收缩和舒张期）、室壁增厚，以及使用斑点追踪技术显示心肌应变和应变率。CMR 也采用了类似的方法，利用心肌运动（标记、相位对比[25]和区域心肌增厚）来检查评估功能。在本部分中，我们将描述用于获取心肌标记图像的方法以及从这些方法获得的一些参数。此外，读者还可以阅读近期的综述，详细了解该领域的历史和当前最新技术[26]。

目前，量化区域心肌功能技术有多种[26]。最初的方法是利用磁化空间调制方案（complementary spatial modulation of magnetization，CSPAMM）在心动周期开始时在心肌中铺设网格标记线，随后通过成像来追踪这些网格内的心肌变形[27,28]。标记线（例如，平行线或网格图案）在心动周期开始、电影读出之前，利用射频脉冲和梯度脉冲的组合通过饱和磁化来产生生成。图 2-2 显示了一个示例。标记线按 5～10mm 进行顺序分割，这有效地定义了可以从标记的 MR 图像计算所得应变图的空间分辨率。通过平行成像，潜在的图像空间分辨率可以达到 1～2mm，且随心肌中追踪标记线移动的时间分辨率接近 20～50ms。这一方法已经成功适用于多种图像读出技术（例如，回波平面成像、SSFP 和 GRE）来获取标记图像。通常通过对短轴（或长轴）电影进行采集标记，从而在心动周期的过程中量化心肌的区域应变和应变率。标记网格线的衰减取决于心肌 T_1 弛豫。因此，标记的电影成像通常在对比剂之前进行（以利用更长的 T_1 弛豫时间，即在心动周期上减慢标记线的衰减）。

图像标记分析依赖于网格线的正确识别，并在心动周期期间随时间跟踪这些标记线。通常，获取四组电影标记图像用于分析，包括长轴（四腔心）和三个短轴切片（基底段、中间段和心尖段），用于评估区域 LV 功能。从短轴图像评估周向和径向应变，而从长轴图像（例如，围绕左心室长轴旋转的径向长轴视图）评估纵向应变。多种专有的分析软件可获得周向、径向和纵向应变分量，应变率和更高阶参数（例如，扭转）。组织标记已被广泛应用于心肌疾病的评估，包括衰老[29]、RV 功能[30]、冠心病[31]、心肌病和失同步[32]。然而，定量应变成像的临床应用受限于相对大量的后处理程序，对于训练有素的观察者来说，目前每层电影所需时间已经减少到 2～3min。

未来信噪比和自动化控制台分析的提升将改善 CMR 区域心肌功能的临床可译性并将其整合作为临床 CMR 检查不可或缺的组成部分。

三、T_1 及 T_2 加权心肌成像

T_2 弛豫时间常数是指由初始射频产生的横向磁化的衰减。对于 T_2 测量，横向磁化被重新聚焦成自旋回波，使得衰减速率与磁场不均匀性无关，这导致相位相干性的损失。自旋回波由初始 90°射频脉冲产生，随后进行单个（常规自旋回波）或多个 180°脉冲重新聚焦。初始 90°射频脉冲与自旋回波产生之间的时间延迟称为回波时间（echo time，TE）。此外，重复 90°激励脉冲和自旋回波间的时间间隔为重复时间（repetition time，TR），这对于 T_1 加权图像是重要的。一系列由 TE 间隔的 180°脉冲可以产生多个自旋回波。由所得回波幅度的衰减定义 T_2 弛豫时间。当射频脉冲停止时，即在回波链的末端，1H 旋转以由 T_1 弛豫时间确定的速率，即纵向磁化，沿静磁场返回其原始方向。最初由第一个 90°脉冲转换成横向的磁化矢量随后以 T_1 弛豫速率恢复。（实际上，T_1 和 T_2 弛豫过程并行发生，但是在回波序列生成期间的 T_1 效应可以忽略，因为 T_2 与 T_1 相比通常较短）。如果在完全弛豫之前再次产生自旋回波，所得到的图像将获得 T_1 加权，即，来自这种图像中的不同组织类型的信号将反映组织的 T_1。

MRI 利用 T_1 和 T_2（或 T_2^*）弛豫的差异来产生不同软组织之间的对比。在 ECG 门控自旋回波成像中，TE 决定 T_2 对比，且自旋回波读取 TR（如在 90°脉冲之间）决定 T_1 加权。通过减小 TR 来增加 T_1 加权，保持较短的 TE 以避免 T_2 加权的影响。在 T_1 加权自旋回波图像上，脂肪为明亮（高）信号，而心肌具有相对低的

信号。对于常规心脏自旋回波成像，短 TR 对应于一个 R-R 间隔，而长 TR 对应于两个或三个 R-R 间隔。利用长 TR 和长 TE 获得 T_2 加权。T_2 加权自旋回波图像用于水肿成像，因为液体含量的增加使 T_2 延长。

在心脏自旋回波成像中，来自血池的明亮信号可产生相当多的心肌上重影。由于血池的信号强度通常不是特别重要，因此人们倾向于抑制来自血池的信号，从而产生所谓的 T_1 或 T_2 加权的黑血自旋回波序列。其中之一是具有双反转恢复抑制的黑血自旋回波成像[33]。双反转准备非层面选择性反转脉冲应用于要成像的整个体积，紧接着为层面选择性反转脉冲，主要用于恢复心肌的信号。这意味着有效地心肌磁化经历 360°

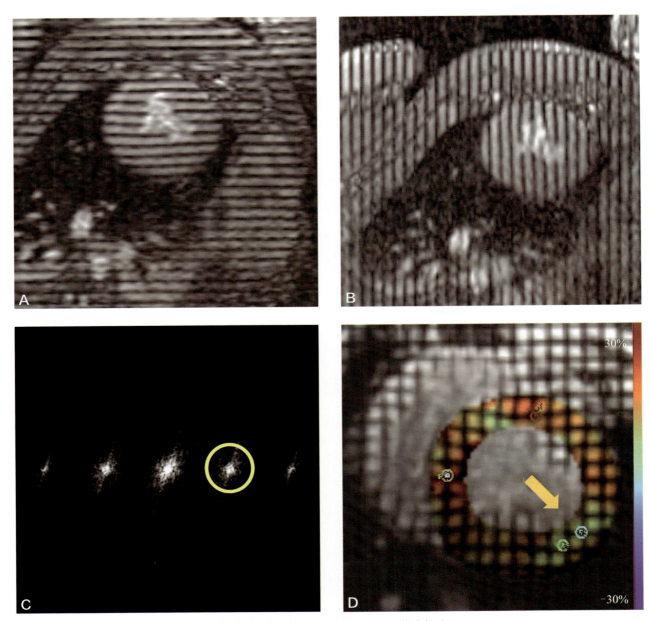

▲ 图 2-2　标记线在量化区域心肌功能中的应用

在心电图 R- 波之后立即施加磁化的空间调制，使用电影梯度回波脉冲序列采集具有（A）水平和（B）垂直标记线的 MR 图像；C. 由图像中的图案周期性生成的平行标记线，可以产生傅里叶变换图像中的特征峰及其谐波，并利用其进行标记线变形的半自动定量检测。可以使用从图像到图像的谐波峰值（黄色圆圈）位置和相位的变化来量化标记线变形；D. 显示了（A）和（B）的叠加图像上的心肌应变图。其可以由磁化的空间调制直接获得标记的网格图案

旋转（即恢复到其原始状态），而血液经历了反转，除了在图像获得的时间内该层面的自旋已移出该平面。自旋回波读出的时间，与其反转恢复期间的血液磁化矢量过零时间一致。该延迟时间称为反转时间（inversion time，TI）。在实际扫描中，在 ECG 上的 R 波之后延迟触发双反转准备脉冲，并且在 400～600ms 之后产生自旋回波，使得它们落入舒张期。自旋回波序列通过多个 180° 脉冲重新聚焦，称为回波链长度，在每个心搏期间获得多行 K 空间，每个自旋回波填充一行 K 空间。回波链长度为 10～20 个回波，通常允许在单次屏气中采集 1～2 个层面，尽管它会受到 T_2 加权的影响。对于 T_1 加权自旋回波成像，通过在回波链早期得到图像特征决定图像对比度，T_2 加权影响较小。（对于熟悉 K 空间概念的读者来说，这可以是等效状态，因为在回波序列的早期获得了中心 K 空间线。）

双反转恢复自旋回波成像的常见挑战是由于心脏运动（其不能通过 180° 聚焦脉冲补偿）导致的心肌信号损失。成像结构可移出该层面，使得其不会经历第二反转脉冲。这通常通过增加层面选择脉冲的厚度来弥补。通过在自旋回波序列之前添加第三反转脉冲或通过抑制具有脂肪分子的共振频率的信号来进行压脂成像。除抑制血液信号外，通常还应用脂肪饱和技术，以增加正常和水肿心肌之间的对比度。

双反转恢复 T_2 加权黑血成像已被用于显示心肌梗死后缺血危险区域并识别心肌水肿和炎症。（图 2-3 示例为急性胸痛患者）T_2 加权快速自旋回波或梯度回波技术已被用于显示由于缺血引起的心肌水肿程度[34]。在急性冠状动脉综合征的临床应用已经显示出不错的结果，尽管心肌对比度可能受到诸如心脏的线圈灵敏度变化之类的外来因素的影响。因此，T_2 加权快速自旋回波成像优选体线圈用于射频传输和信号接收，而不使用表面线圈，即使这可能导致较低的信噪比。

Cury 及其同事对 62 名急诊胸痛患者进行了评估，发现加入 T_2 加权成像显示心肌水肿有利于急性冠状动脉疾病与慢性冠状动脉疾病的鉴别[32]。T_2 加权技术将诊断急性冠状动脉综合征的阳性预测值从 55% 提高到 85%。在急性心肌梗死后，心肌重塑持续数月，并且由冠状动脉血流状态、持续缺血、侧支形成和梗死位置决定。因此，新型 CMR 技术有望能够探索心肌不同生理状态，并探讨除了总梗死面积、危险面积和左心室功能之外具有预后价值的参数。

四、T_2^* 加权成像

T_2^* 加权图像可以用梯度回波序列获得，并可用于评估心肌铁含量。铁过载会导致组织的信号丢失。铁沉积会引起局部磁场不均匀，导致这些沉积物周围的水质子更快地失去相位一致性。这种效应取决于组织铁浓度。T_2^* 加权图像由单次屏气多梯度回波技术获得。在 2～18ms 内多个 TE 下获得单层短轴切面。并在室间隔绘制感兴趣区域（region of intrest，ROI）以测量该处各 TE 时间点的信号强度。绘制 TE 信号强度衰减曲线，并从中计算 T_2^*。

CMR 测量的心肌 T_2^* 时间（以 ms 为单位）与心肌中的铁沉积量成反比。在 1.5T 磁共振上，心肌 T_2^* 小于 20ms 被认为是异常的并且存在铁过载的可能，且心肌 T_2^* 小于 10ms 表示严重的铁过载。铁过载可导致心力衰竭和死亡。然而，使用螯合疗法可以达到很好的治疗效果，改善左心室功能障碍。较短的 T_2^* 时间与左心室功能障碍和心力衰竭恶化有关[35,36]。Anderson 及其同事的研究可心肌 T_2^* 的阈值，低于该阈值提示未确诊心力衰竭患者可能是由于铁过载引起的心功能不全[37]。一些研究表明，T_2^* CMR 成像可用于监测正在接受螯合治疗的患者的治疗反应[38-40]。最近一项针对 650 名患者的多中心研究显示，47% 1 年内发生心力衰竭患者、14% 的心律失常患者其心脏 T_2^* < 6ms[41]。其他研究也表明，心脏 T_2^* 测量是

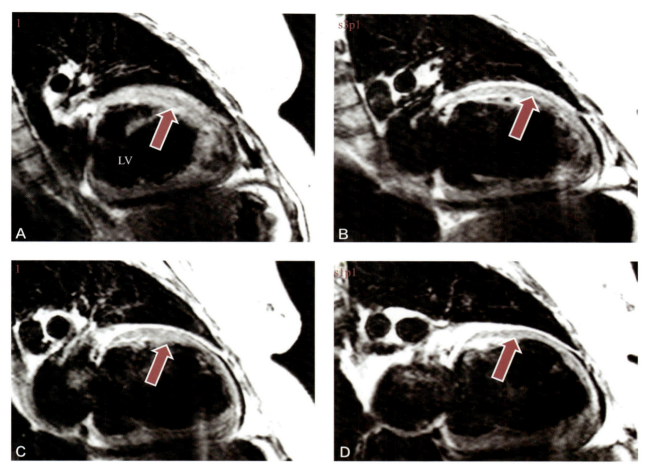

▲ 图 2-3 突发呼吸急促和胸痛的 26 岁女性急诊患者，四个平行长轴左心室（LV）自旋回波黑血 T_2 加权图像

利用这种技术，血池的信号被抑制以避免心肌的重影伪影，并突出心肌内信号强度差异。黑血序列是通过连续层面选择性和非层面选择性反转脉冲的组合实现的，其对心肌没有效应，只是图像获取时血池中的信号被反转。通过调整反转脉冲和图像采集之间的时间使血池中的磁化矢量为零

可重复的，并且是较强的临床结果预测因子。这种非侵入性技术不仅是研究新螯合疗法疗效的工具，而且应该应用于所有接受长期输血治疗的患者评估。CMR 已成为该患者群体初步诊断和随访评估的有效工具。

T_2 或 T_2^* 成像也可用于评估心肌的氧合状态，因为脱氧血红蛋白的增加将导致 T_2 和 T_2^* 信号减低。对于 T_2 或 T_2^* 加权成像，静息状态携带的信息很少。然而，如果 T_2/T_2^* 加权成像也在应激期间进行（通常是药理学诱导的应激，如使用多巴胺等正性肌力药），则可以评估 T_2/T_2^* 加权信号的相对变化。基线和应激之间的这种血氧水平依赖性（blood oxygen level dependent，BOLD）对比度变化已被证明可用于鉴别心肌缺血。

五、T_1 Mapping 及 T_2 Mapping 心肌组织定量技术

虽然 T_1 或 T_2 加权心肌成像已证明对心肌表征非常有用，但所得图像一般只能进行定性评估，而信号强度的细微差异，如由于心肌水肿引起的 T_2 信号升高，可能会忽略，或者存在其他混淆效应，也会影响心肌信号强度。例如，表面线圈的灵敏度随着心脏的体积而变化，可能导致 T_2 加权图像上与水肿无关的信号变化。而过去几年有助于量化心肌 T_1 和 T_2 参数的 T_1 和 T_2 Mapping（定量成像）技术开始逐渐被研究。

T_1 Mapping 在注射细胞外造影剂之前和之后通过血液和心肌的 T_1 量化计算心肌细胞外

容积（extracellular volume，ECV）。随着细胞间质空间中结缔组织的沉积ECV随之升高。ECV已被证明是反映心肌弥漫性纤维化积聚较为敏感的指标。同样，淀粉样蛋白的沉积也可以使得ECV显著增加，可作为心肌延迟强化弥漫分布的患者定量指标。在心脏淀粉样变性患者中，该疾病对全心心肌均有累及，使得LGE中缺乏正常心肌的对比，而T_1 Mapping提取出的ECV可作为评估心肌淀粉样蛋白沉积的客观定量参数。在不注射对比剂的情况下也可以评估心肌T_1参数，即所谓的平扫T_1（native T_1）。已证明其对心肌水肿非常敏感[42]，水肿可以延长T_1，而心肌铁的存在可以导致T_1缩短[43]。

T_1图像是通过反转脉冲之后获取的一系列图像得到的。使用最广泛的技术为单次梯度回波读数和反转后稳态自由序列在每个采样时间进行读取，因为这种类型的图像获取对反转恢复影响较小[44]。因此，可以在反转脉冲之后获取多个图像，并且可以通过信号强度和反转之后的时间（TI）拟合函数来计算真实T_1。在反转脉冲之后读出信号强度的方法最初是在MR成像时代之前由Look和Locker引入的[45]。该技术后来适用于MR成像，最近修改为心脏T_1成像以在心动周期的同一时相内在反转脉冲（TI）之后的不同时间获取图像，修改的Look-Locker成像首字母缩略词为MOLLI[46]。由于所有具有不同TI时间的图像都是在心动周期的同一时相获得的，因此心脏看起来是静止的，这使得为MOLLI图像中的每个像素位置映射T_1相对明确[47]。由此产生的高分辨率T_1 Mapping对各种心肌病变研究产生了重大影响。

T_2或T_2^* Mapping也可用类似的方法通过生成具有不同有效TE权重的一系列图像获得。且这些参数图近乎只反映T_2/T_2^*的变化，其大大改善了组织病理学导致的T_2或T_2^*改变的评估，如铁过载。根据现有的研究经验和结果认为，这对于疑似铁过量患者的心肌组织特征评估是十分重要的[48,49]。

ECV的定性评估可以在疾病研究、疾病进展、预后和治疗方面提供有价值信息。不同疾病如梗死、心肌炎、肥厚性和扩张性心肌病、心脏淀粉样变性、全身性红斑狼疮或人类免疫缺陷病毒等全身性疾病的心脏受累，其心肌间质纤维化的程度也不同[50]。

无创的磁共振取样分析与解剖病理学分析同样可靠，并且可以获得只有通过尸检才能取得而活检无法获得的区域。某些区域的组织活检可能导致假阴性结果，而T_1 Mapping允许对整个心肌进行可重复的评估[51]。

六、心肌活性

心肌存活率降低与心肌细胞膜的破坏相关。通过常用的细胞外钆对比剂，MRI可以用来评估急性心肌梗死中细胞膜完整性的破坏。心肌细胞在健康心肌中占心肌组织体积的＞70%。在存活的心肌中，钆对比剂多被排出，但随着心肌细胞膜完整性的破坏，在心肌中对比剂含量增加。

LGE成像可以突出显示相对于存活心肌的异常钆对比度分布增加的区域[52]。增强后心肌对比剂分布的差异可以由心肌T_1对比度差异得到。在反转恢复期间，心肌磁化位于从倒置状态恢复到平衡状态期间的某一点，其纵向磁化矢量分量，即可以产生图像信号的分量为零。如果在该特定时间点获取成像数据，则纵向磁化穿过零点的任何组织都是黑色的。在无活性的心肌组织中，由于对比剂分布增加，T_1弛豫将更短，或者换句话说，每体素体积内的对比剂累积增加。通过反转恢复使正常心肌的信号受到抑制，非存活心肌可以具有更高的信号强度。

对于LGE成像，仍需要克服一些成像难点：①图像对比度应主要为T_1加权，对心脏运动的敏感度尽可能小，以便用较高的空间分辨率以准确地评估透壁的梗死灶；②图像数据只能在反转恢复后的一个较小的时间窗内获得，此时正常心肌的纵向磁化为零。Simonetti及其同事研究了一

种非常有效的 T_1 加权成像技术——分段梯度回波成像技术以满足这些要求[53]。术语"分段"在这里指的是以分段方式获取图像数据，即图像数据的获取分布在多个心跳上。每次读出图像数据之前是非层面选择性反转脉冲，且由操作者调整反转恢复之后读取图像的时间，以抑制正常心肌中的信号。图 2-4 说明了该技术。由于想要在心动周期的相对静止的期间（例如，舒张早期）获取图像数据，该技术允许设定图像采集的触发延迟时间，以及反转脉冲之后的 TI 时间。当 TI 改变时，反转脉冲的时间相对于图像获取时间会发生改变，而心动周期内图像获取的时间则未发生改变。

为了保证用于使正常心肌中的信号抑制的最佳 TI，通常在注射对比剂后和 LGE 成像之前用 TI Scout 序列以快速确定准确的 TI 值。这本质上是一种电影技术，与反转脉冲相结合，使得每个图像对应于不同的 TI。它是在单次屏气时间内获得的，与 LGE 技术相反，LGE 技术通常仅在屏气持续时间内针对单个 TI 值获取图像。随后采用 TI Scout 序列确认的正常心肌抑制最佳 TI 采集 LGE 图像。

在注射对比剂后获得 LGE 图像的最佳延迟最初认为为 20min，但随着该技术的广泛应用，至少在急性心肌梗死中，LGE 成像最早可以在注射对比剂后约 5min 就可以采集。

采用 TI 以抑制正常心肌中的信号似乎并不适用于检测不存活心肌。然而，由于 LGE 成像通常在心脏检查将近结束时进行，当心脏的电影成像完成后，可以认为运动正常的心肌节段至少可用作正常心肌的参考区域。电影成像对于 LGE 成像有用的另一个原因，是帮助判断心肌梗死区域内膜边界，因增强的心肌组织和血池的信号一样明亮；在平扫电影上，在梗死区域心内膜边界较为清晰的描绘，从而为确定心肌梗死或瘢痕的透壁范围。

LGE 成像是梗死心肌组织范围的可靠定量技术[54]。Kim 及其同事研究表明，LGE 技术可以判断梗死心肌的跨壁程度，并可区分可逆性和不可逆性心肌损伤，不受静息时室壁运动、梗死的年龄或再灌注状态的影响[52,55]。

在一项具有里程碑意义的冠状动脉疾病患

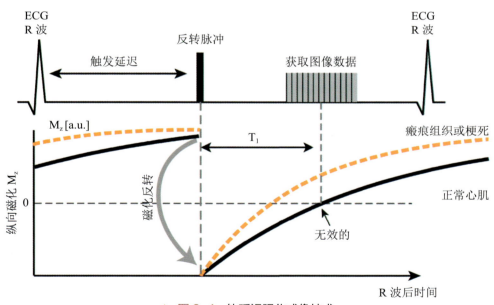

▲ 图 2-4　钆延迟强化成像技术

钆延迟强化成像的技术是基于反转脉冲，并在已设定好的特定时间后采集图像数据。通常每隔一次心搏重复该脉冲序列块以获取整个图像。在磁化反转之后，图像数据的采集时间与正常心肌中的纵向磁化矢量过零点一致。梗死的心肌或心肌瘢痕具有较短的 T_1，并且当获取图像时正常心肌磁化已经通过零点，使得这些区域在所得图像中看起来是明亮的。触发延迟的选择，可以在心动周期相对静止的阶段获取图像

者研究中，冠状动脉血供重建成功后，局部心肌收缩力改善与血供重建术前LGE的透壁程度成反比[54]。此外，LGE的透壁范围可以准确预测心力衰竭患者β受体阻断药治疗后左心室功能的改善[56]。在另一项研究中，Orn等[57]发现CMR瘢痕大小的评估是急性心肌梗死患者射血分数和左心室容量以及心力衰竭的最有价值的独立预测因子。

参考文献

[1] Pfeffer, M.A. and E. Braunwald, Ventricular remodeling after myocardial infarction. Experimental observations and clinical implications. *Circulation*, 1990. 81(4): 1161–72.

[2] Chareonthaitawee, P. et al., Relation of initial infarct size to extent of left ventricular remodeling in the year after acute myocardial infarction. *J Am Coll Cardiol*, 1995. 25(3): 567–73.

[3] Van Gilst, W.H. et al., Which patient benefits from early angiotensin-converting enzyme inhibition after myocardial infarction? Results of one-year serial echocardiographic follow-up from the Captopril and Thrombolysis Study (CATS). *J Am Coll Cardiol*, 1996. 28(1): 114–21.

[4] Douglas, P.S. et al., Left ventricular shape, afterload and survival in idiopathic dilated cardiomyopathy. *J Am Coll Cardiol*, 1989. 13(2): 311–5.

[5] Konstam, M.A. et al., Effects of the angiotensin converting enzyme inhibitor enalapril on the long-term progression of left ventricular dysfunction in patients with heart failure. SOLVD Investigators. *Circulation*, 1992. 86(2): 431–8.

[6] Konstam, M.A. et al., Effects of the angiotensin converting enzyme inhibitor enalapril on the long-term progression of left ventricular dilatation in patients with asymptomatic systolic dysfunction. SOLVD (Studies of Left Ventricular Dysfunction) Investigators. *Circulation*, 1993. 88(5 Pt 1): 2277–83.

[7] Heckbert, S.R. et al., Traditional cardiovascular risk factors in relation to left ventricular mass, volume, and systolic function by cardiac magnetic resonance imaging: the Multiethnic Study of Atherosclerosis. *J Am Coll Cardiol*, 2006. 48(11): 2285–92.

[8] Lawson, M.A. et al., Accuracy of biplane long-axis left ventricular volume determined by cine magnetic resonance imaging in patients with regional and global dysfunction. *Am J Cardiol*, 1996. 77(12): 1098–104.

[9] Thiele, H. et al., Functional cardiac MR imaging with steady-state free precession (SSFP) significantly improves endocardial border delineation without contrast agents. *J Magn Reson Imaging*, 2001. 14(4): 362–7.

[10] Malayeri, A.A. et al., Cardiac cine MRI: Quantification of the relationship between fast gradient echo and steady-state free precession for determination of myocardial mass and volumes. *J Magn Reson Imaging*, 2008. 28(1): 60–6.

[11] Moon, J.C. et al., Breath-hold FLASH and FISP cardiovascular MR imaging: Left ventricular volume differences and reproducibility. *Radiology*, 2002. 223(3): 789–97.

[12] Longmore, D.B. et al., Dimensional accuracy of magnetic resonance in studies of the heart. *Lancet*, 1985. 1(8442): 1360–2.

[13] Maceira, A.M. et al., Normalized left ventricular systolic and diastolic function by steady state free precession cardiovascular magnetic resonance. *J Cardiovasc Magn Reson*, 2006. 8(3): 417–26.

[14] Grothues, F. et al., Comparison of interstudy reproducibility of cardiovascular magnetic resonance with two-dimensional echocardiography in normal subjects and in patients with heart failure or left ventricular hypertrophy. *Am J Cardiol*, 2002. 90(1): 29–34.

[15] Bellenger, N.G. et al., Reduction in sample size for studies of remodeling in heart failure by the use of cardiovascular magnetic resonance. *J Cardiovasc Magn Reson*, 2000. 2(4): 271–8.

[16] Alfakih, K. et al., Comparison of right ventricular volume measurements between axial and short axis orientation using steady-state free precession magnetic resonance imaging. *J Magn Reson Imaging*, 2003. 18(1): 25–32.

[17] Rehr, R.B. et al., Left ventricular volumes measured by MR imaging. *Radiology*, 1985. 156(3): 717–9.

[18] Katz, J. et al., Estimation of human myocardial mass with MR imaging. *Radiology*, 1988. 169(2): 495–8.

[19] Katz, J. et al., Estimation of right ventricular mass in normal subjects and in patients with primary pulmonary hypertension by nuclear magnetic resonance imaging. *J Am Coll Cardiol*, 1993. 21(6): 1475–81.

[20] Bottini, P.B. et al., Magnetic resonance imaging compared to echocardiography to assess left ventricular mass in the hypertensive patient. *Am J Hypertens*, 1995. 8(3): 221–8.

[21] Chahal, H. et al., Obesity and right ventricular structure and function: The MESA-Right Ventricle Study. *Chest*, 2012. 141(2): 388–95.

[22] Yan, R.T. et al., Regional left ventricular myocardial dysfunction as a predictor of incident cardiovascular events MESA (multi-ethnic study of atherosclerosis). *J Am Coll Cardiol*, 2011. 57(17): 1735–44.

[23] Rosen, B.D. et al., Reduction in regional myocardial function is associated with concentric left ventricular remodeling: Multi-ethnic study of atherosclerosis. *J Am College Cardiol*, 2004. 43(5): 221A–221A.

[24] Rosen, B.D. et al., Left ventricular concentric remodeling is associated with decreased global and regional systolic function: The Multi-Ethnic Study of Atherosclerosis. *Circulation*, 2005. 112(7): 984–91.

[25] Pelc, L.R. et al., Evaluation of myocardial motion tracking with cine-phase contrast magnetic resonance imaging. *Invest*

[26] Ibrahim el, S.H., Myocardial tagging by cardiovascular magnetic resonance: Evolution of techniques—Pulse sequences, analysis algorithms, and applications. *J Cardiovasc Magn Reson*, 2011. 13: 36.

[27] Axel, L. and L. Dougherty, MR imaging of motion with spatial modulation of magnetization. *Radiology*, 1989. 171(3): 841–5.

[28] Zerhouni, E.A. et al., Human heart: Tagging with MR imaging—A method for noninvasive assessment of myocardial motion. *Radiology*, 1988. 169(1): 59–63.

[29] Fonseca, C.G. et al., Aging alters patterns of regional nonuniformity in LV strain relaxation: A 3-D MR tissue tagging study. *Am J Physiol Heart Circ Physiol*, 2003. 285(2): H621–30.

[30] Haber, I., D.N. Metaxas, and L. Axel, Three-dimensional motion reconstruction and analysis of the right ventricle using tagged MRI. *Med Image Anal*, 2000. 4(4): 335–55.

[31] Kraitchman, D.L. et al., Quantitative ischemia detection during cardiac magnetic resonance stress testing by use of FastHARP. *Circulation*, 2003. 107(15): 2025–30.

[32] Curry, C.W. et al., Mechanical dyssynchrony in dilated cardiomyopathy with intraventricular conduction delay as depicted by 3D tagged magnetic resonance imaging. *Circulation*, 2000. 101(1): E2.

[33] Simonetti, O.P. et al., "Black blood" T2-weighted inversion-recovery MR imaging of the heart. *Radiology*, 1996. 199(1): 49–57.

[34] Aletras, A.H. et al., Retrospective determination of the area at risk for reperfused acute myocardial infarction with T2-weighted cardiac magnetic resonance imaging: Histopathological and displacement encoding with stimulated echoes (DENSE) functional validations. *Circulation*, 2006. 113(15): 1865–70.

[35] Westwood, M. et al., A single breath-hold multiecho T2* cardiovascular magnetic resonance technique for diagnosis of myocardial iron overload. *J Magn Reson Imaging*, 2003. 18(1): 33–9.

[36] Tanner, M.A. et al., Myocardial iron loading in patients with thalassemia major on deferoxamine chelation. *J Cardiovasc Magn Reson*, 2006. 8(3): 543–7.

[37] Anderson, L.J. et al., Cardiovascular T2-star (T2*) magnetic resonance for the early diagnosis of myocardial iron overload. *Eur Heart J*, 2001. 22(23): 2171–9.

[38] Mavrogeni, S.I. et al., A comparison of magnetic resonance imaging and cardiac biopsy in the evaluation of heart iron overload in patients with beta-thalassemia major. *Eur J Haematol*, 2005. 75(3): 241–7.

[39] Westwood, M.A. et al., Myocardial biopsy and T2* magnetic resonance in heart failure due to thalassaemia. *Br J Haematol*, 2005. 128(1): 2.

[40] Westwood, M.A. et al., Left ventricular diastolic function compared with T2* cardiovascular magnetic resonance for early detection of myocardial iron overload in thalassemia major. *J Magn Reson Imaging*, 2005. 22(2): 229–33.

[41] Kirk, P. et al., Cardiac T2* magnetic resonance for prediction of cardiac complications in thalassemia major. *Circulation*, 2009. 120(20): 1961–8.

[42] Ferreira, V.M. et al., Non-contrast T1-mapping detects acute myocardial edema with high diagnostic accuracy: A comparison to T2-weighted cardiovascular magnetic resonance. *J Cardiovasc Magn Reson*, 2012. 14: 42.

[43] Sado, D.M. et al., Noncontrast myocardial T mapping using cardiovascular magnetic resonance for iron over-load. *J Magn Reson Imaging*, 2014. 41: 1505–1511.

[44] Scheffler, K. and J. Hennig, T(1) quantification with inversion recovery TrueFISP. *Magn Reson Med*, 2001. 45(4): 720–3.

[45] Look, D. and D. Locker, Time saving in measurement of NMR and EPR relaxation times. *Rev Sci Instrum*, 1970. 41: 250–251.

[46] Messroghli, D.R. et al., Modified Look-Locker inversion recovery (MOLLI) for high-resolution T1 mapping of the heart. *Magn Reson Med*, 2004. 52(1): 141–6.

[47] Messroghli, D.R. et al., Myocardial T1 mapping: Application to patients with acute and chronic myocardial infarction. *Magn Reson Med*, 2007. 58(1): 34–40.

[48] Baksi, A.J. and D.J. Pennell, T2* imaging of the heart: Methods, applications, and outcomes. *Top Magn Reson Imaging*, 2014. 23(1): 13–20.

[49] Pennell, D.J. et al., Cardiovascular function and treatment in beta-thalassemia major: A consensus statement from the American Heart Association. *Circulation*, 2013. 128(3): 281–308.

[50] Ferreira, V.M. et al., Myocardial tissue characterization by magnetic resonance imaging: Novel applications of T1 and T2 mapping. *J Thorac Imaging*, 2014. 29(3): 147–54.

[51] Flett, A.S. et al., Equilibrium contrast cardiovascular magnetic resonance for the measurement of diffuse myocardial fibrosis: Preliminary validation in humans. *Circulation*, 2010. 122(2): 138–44.

[52] Kim, R.J. et al., Relationship of MRI delayed contrast enhancement to irreversible injury, infarct age, and contractile function. *Circulation*, 1999. 100(19): 1992–2002.

[53] Simonetti, O.P. et al., An improved MR imaging technique for the visualization of myocardial infarction. *Radiology*, 2001. 218(1): 215–23.

[54] Kim, R.J. et al., The use of contrast-enhanced magnetic resonance imaging to identify reversible myocardial dysfunction. *N Engl J Med*, 2000. 343(20): 1445–53.

[55] Kim, R.J. et al., Myocardial Gd-DTPA kinetics determine MRI contrast enhancement and reflect the extent and severity of myocardial injury after acute reperfused infarction. *Circulation*, 1996. 94(12): 3318–26.

[56] Bello, D. et al., Gadolinium cardiovascular magnetic resonance predicts reversible myocardial dysfunction and remodeling in patients with heart failure undergoing beta-blocker therapy. *Circulation*, 2003. 108(16): 1945–53.

[57] Orn, S. et al., Effect of left ventricular scar size, location, and transmurality on left ventricular remodeling with healed myocardial infarction. *Am J Cardiol*, 2007. 99(8): 1109–14.

Chapter 3
心包疾病的 CT 和 MR 成像

Computed Topography/Magnetic Resonance Imaging of Pericardial Disease

Marco Francone, Giorgia Giustini,
Gianluca De Rubeis, Iacopo Carbone,
Nicola Galea 著

赵 蕾 译

王怡宁 校

目录 CONTENTS

一、心包解剖和生理学 / 34
二、CT 和 MR 成像技术 / 35
三、先天性疾病 / 37

由于对心包病变的复杂病理生理学过程理解不断加深，以及无创成像技术的发展和广泛应用，该技术可对心包疾病的功能和形态学改变进行综合准确评估，因此临床越来越重视心包病变。

心包疾病包括多种先天性和获得性疾病，临床表现各异，可能影响双心室功能进而影响患者的治疗和预后。

除了心包原发病变外，"一切疾病都会导致心包病变"，这强调了在日常临床实践中，心包经常继发受累，不同器官和全身状况，包括感染性、自身免疫性、肿瘤性疾病和医源性过程（如心脏手术或放疗后的并发症）都可累及心包[1,2]。

尽管心包的宏观和微观结构相对简单，但心包在心脏生理学中起着复杂的作用，它通过结合机械牵拉和锚定功能参与调节心室的顺应性。心包协助最大限度减少心室扩张，通过产生液体和表面活性剂来保护心脏，并限制心脏在纵隔的移位[1,3]。

临床表现典型的心包疾病用常规诊断方法可以直接确诊[4,5]（如急性心包炎在直立位时因为心包间相互摩擦会出现胸痛加剧），然而有相当一部分不具有典型临床表现的心包疾病，需要通过二线影像检查如 CT 和 MR 来确诊及辅助患者治疗[6]。

常规经胸超声心动图的准确性在很多情况下会受到影响，例如声窗欠佳（肥胖者，严重慢性阻塞性肺疾病或骨骼畸形者），且超声心动图对少量心包积液或高蛋白含量渗出物的评估有一定困难[4,6,7]。

MR/CT 有助于识别疑诊肿瘤性疾病的心包浸润，其高分辨率结合大视野成像能够更好地描述疾病的病变过程。

对疑诊各种类型的缩窄性心包炎（CP），MR 也有辅助诊断价值，比如评价心包不厚但有限制性心室功能障碍的病例，以及进行心包缩窄和限制性心肌病（RC）的鉴别[8,9]。

综上，随着技术的不断发展，包括从心脏 MR 实时成像到 MDCT 高时间分辨率和功能成像技术，CT 和 MR 广泛应用于不同心包病变的诊断中。

一、心包解剖和生理学

心包是一层菲薄的弹性膜，覆盖在心脏和大血管的周围（图 3-1），宏观上分为两层：内层为浆膜层（脏层心包或心外膜）和外层为纤维层（壁层心包）[10-12]。

浆膜层是一个完整的囊性结构，内可充填 15～50ml 不等的血浆超滤液，并通过松散的心外膜结缔组织和一系列间皮细胞与心脏分开。围绕心包的脂肪组织分为两部分：浆膜下脂肪和心外膜脂肪（后者由于其旁分泌功能和生理作用更为重要）。浆膜下脂肪可见于正常体重人群中，主要分布在房间隔和房室沟，在肥胖人群中更常见[13]。

与内脏脂肪类似，肥胖者心外膜脂肪厚度增加，可直接影响冠状动脉粥样硬化的发生，因为没有纤维层阻止游离脂肪酸和调节动脉血栓形

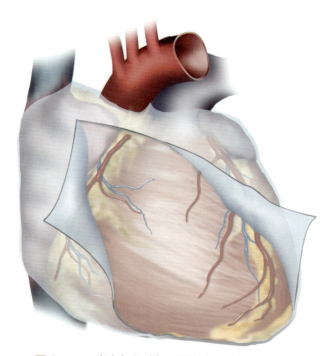

▲ 图 3-1 正常心包部分切开的解剖示意图
脏层心包紧密毗邻心外膜（由 Sapienza 大学 Bettina Conti 提供）

成的脂肪因子扩散到其下方的冠状动脉中[13-15]。

在解剖学上，右心室周围分布的心外膜脂肪比左心室多3～4倍[13]，尤其是右心室游离壁周围[13-15]，使得脏层心包与心肌组织形成更好的天然对比，在 CT 和 MR 图像上有利于其解剖结构显示。

外层（纤维心包）与心外膜紧贴，并向主动脉根部方向延伸，与颈深筋膜延续；纤维心包通过韧带附着在胸骨和膈肌上，防止心脏移位并保护心脏免受邻近结构的损伤。

当外科手术切开时，心包的纤维收缩会产生机械应力，主要作用于右心室和心房这类薄壁结构，与心腔的病理性过度扩张相反（如存在慢性大量积液），并直接影响腔内舒张压。

心包相对无弹性，这是维持心室同步运动的必要条件，以均衡两个心室的收缩与舒张，可见于缩窄性心包炎或心脏压塞等病理情况［见"三（二）"和"三（三）"］[10,16]。

心包的另一个特性是其生理性收缩，使心脏能够适应胸膜和胸腔内压力[2,8,17]，心包在胸膜腔和心腔之间充当传感器，直接将胸内呼吸变化传递给心脏。这一现象可见于生理性吸气过程中，吸气时，由于胸膜 - 心包相互作用，胸膜压力下降，静脉回流和右心充盈增加，从而直接增加右心室的前负荷和射血。

浆膜心包在两套复杂的连接管道周围形成两个主要反折：前者覆盖上下腔静脉和右肺静脉，后者覆盖左肺静脉。这些反折界定了两个囊袋状结构，称为斜窦和横窦，包括多个心包隐窝，形成所谓的心包储备容量，在液体含量增多的情况下优先积聚于此[11,18]。

横窦位于大动脉、左心房和上腔静脉之间，是一个线形的虚拟腔，在 CT-MR 检查中有时候可能被错认为主动脉局灶夹层 / 血栓或病理性淋巴结肿大[11]。斜窦位于左心房后面，呈 J 形[2,11,12]。

如前所述，心包有三个主要功能。

机械性：维持心室顺应性，限制心室过度扩张；心包内液体可以保护心脏免受拉伸，并产生一些生理性压力。心包在右心室与左心室的生理性互相作用中起关键作用，称为心室耦联，在正常负荷条件下，左心室舒张压稍高于右心室压，故室间隔轻微右凸。一些心包疾病可能会影响心室间的相互作用，例如在心包顺应性或压力改变的情况下，右心室舒张压高于左心室，室间隔会变平直或左凸。心包还调节着心脏和胸膜之间的压力，正常情况下，吸气时右心室充盈压增加。这种重要的生理特征对于鉴别 CP（缩窄性心包炎）和 RC（限制型心肌病）至关重要。

膜性：保护心脏不受其他邻近器官病变的感染，如肺部、外伤以及邻近器官的肿瘤浸润。

韧带：将心脏固定在纵隔腔内，以防止间接被动过度运动。

二、CT 和 MR 成像技术

大多数情况下，CT 和 MR 成像可清晰显示心包，表现为平行于心肌的细线状结构，周围环绕心外膜脂肪（图 3-2）。

心包在右心室游离壁显示清晰，因为其周围有较多的脂肪组织，在左心室外侧壁和后壁通常不可见（或不明显）[2,12,19]。

正常心包可在 MR 和 CT 测量厚度，分别在 1.2～1.7mm[20-22] 和（2.0±0.4）mm[23]，较病理结果均高估厚度[24]，可能由于空间和时间分辨率的限度，MR 和 CT 不能完全区分心包膜和其内液体成分[25]。

心包在 CT 上显示为一层高密度结构，与周围低密度脂肪形成良好天然对比，使用或不使用造影剂都很容易检测到该结构；增强后，心包轻度强化，可能是由于壁层心包中存在小的毛细血管[22,26]。

为显示心包病变，CT 扫描通常采用高分辨容积采集（即层厚＜ 3mm），可很好勾勒出心包[19,27]，使用心电门控或触发技术有助于最大限度地减少心脏运动伪影，并改善对上纵隔水平心包窦和心包隐窝的显示，避免误诊为淋巴结肿大和其他纵隔或肺门疾病[18,27]。

回顾性心电门控 MDCT 扫描图像可动态观察缩窄性心包炎的室间隔摆动[22,28,29]，评价心包病变对室间隔运动和形态的影响，但扫描辐射剂量大；因此在这种情况下，应优先选用 MRI 或超声心动图。

尽管 CT 组织分辨率较低，不利于心包层与液体的区分，且相对有创（电离辐射和碘造影剂）并无法提供功能信息，但 CT 的优点是扫描时间短，能较好显示心包轮廓，并且对于检测心包钙化（CP 的典型特征）或出血的灵敏度高，出血在紧急情况下可危及生命。

在出现可疑继发性心包受累的情况下（如转移性或全身性疾病），应优先选择 CT，一次性全身扫描（包含肺实质）可更快更好诊断。

心脏 MR 是评价心包病变的理想无创成像技术，将心包的形态和组织特征与功能信息相结合，有助于评价心包病变对心室充盈特别是舒张功能和心室耦连的影响。

优选用于心包成像的 MR 技术是黑血 T_1 加

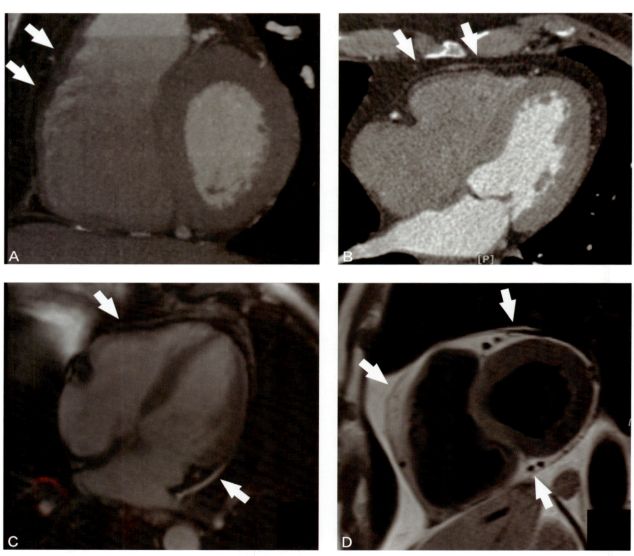

▲ 图 3-2　正常心包

双源 CT 对比增强成像 1.0mm 准直短轴（A）和水平长轴（B）图像。心包在右室游离壁旁脂肪衬托下可清晰显示（箭）。水平长轴自由稳态进动（SSFP）电影 MR 图像（C）由于化学位移伪影的作用，在水脂界面间形成黑线（也称作黑边伪影），因此当存在少量心包积液时可清晰显示心包结构。在黑血 T_1 加权快速自旋回波短轴 MR 图像中（D），心包显示为曲线状低信号结构（箭），由于心包内存在少量液体，周围环绕脂肪组织时心包可清晰显示

权 ECG-门控快速自旋回波序列，通常采用小视野和饱和带以减少相位展开伪影，心包显示为由高信号纵隔和心外膜脂肪以及中等信号心肌环绕的低信号带。

T_2 加权自旋回波形态学成像与三反转恢复黑血序列相结合，抑制脂肪和血流的信号，可用于检测心包炎时的心包水肿和（或）积液[25,30]。

平衡稳态自由进动（SSFP）序列可进行功能成像，定量测量整体和局部心室功能，也可用于心包移动的评估，提供心包僵硬度的相关信息并评价其对舒张期充盈的潜在影响。

cine-SSFP 图像的数据也可以与信号标记的 cine-MR 序列结合，整个心动周期标记信号在心包/心肌界面持续出现，有助于识别增厚的心包对心肌的纤维化粘连[31]。

疑诊缩窄性心包炎时，可以采用另一种 MR 功能成像方法——实时非触发成像，使用 SSFP 并行采集技术，时间分辨率高，可评估呼吸对室间隔运动的影响[8,17]。

采用快速自旋回波（TSE）或反转恢复序列的增强 T_1 加权成像，心包炎时炎症心包会出现强化，间接提示活动性炎症，还可区分心包炎和心肌炎的不同成分（如液性还是层状）[32]（图 3-3）。

当怀疑有心包占位时，推荐使用顺磁性对比剂，以检测心肌是否受累（如可疑心包心肌炎时）。

最后，必须使用速度编码 cine MRI（VENC）或相位对比成像，通过测量房室瓣和肺静脉和（或）体静脉的流速、流入模式可用于评估心包病变对舒张功能的影响[33-35]。

三、先天性疾病

（一）心包囊肿和憩室

心包囊肿和憩室是罕见的先天性疾病，发病率为 1/100 000，占全部纵隔囊肿的 13%～17%[36]。

先天性心包囊肿是胚胎发生时体腔起源的良性单房性肿块[37]，多见于无临床症状的个体在做胸部 X 线检查或经胸超声心动图检查中偶然发现，心包囊肿的症状一般是由邻近结构的压迫引起[1]。

心包囊肿在 CT 和 MR 上表现为内含透明液体的囊袋状结构，无分隔或壁结节，常位于右心膈角（30%），左心膈角（20%）[38]，直接附着于心包或少数情况下经蒂与心包相连（图 3-3 和图 3-4）。

心包憩室是心包的局灶性向外膨出，特点是与心包腔直接相通，与心包囊肿不同，憩室的大小会随体位改变而变化[18,36]。

（二）心包缺如

先天性心包缺如是一种比较罕见的心包发育不全，由于在胚胎发生过程中，供应形成胸膜心包皱襞的主静脉过早萎缩导致心包膜发育停滞。缺如大小，从小孔到完全缺如，可能由血管发生变性的时间决定[39,40]。大多数心包缺如无症状，于手术或尸检中偶然发现[39]，但也可伴有胸痛、呼吸困难、心律失常、晕厥，甚至合并心脏嵌顿疝而猝死[41]。

心包部分缺如主要位于心脏左侧，但也可位于心包的任何位置。心包缺如可合并其他先天性心脏异常，如房间隔或室间隔缺损、动脉导管未闭、主动脉瓣二叶畸形、膈疝或肺部畸形[39]。

在胸片上，心脏结构以及肺实质的移位可导致心影和主动脉结左移（左侧心包缺损），而此时气管居中。

在胸部 X 线检查后，可进一步行（CT/MR）断层扫描，尽管左心侧心包经常显示不良，而这恰好是心包缺损最常见位置，这一定程度上限制了 CT 和 MR 对心包缺如的诊断。

因此，一般需要根据心包缺如的间接征象来确定诊断，包括心脏在胸腔内左移或通过缺如处向外疝出（部分心包缺如时），并根据位置的变化及电影图像上心尖运动的增加进行诊断[42-44]。

心包积液 当脏层内产生的液体增多或心脏淋巴和静脉引流阻塞时，就出现心包积液。很多局部和系统性疾病均可引起心包积液，包括心力衰竭、肿瘤性疾病、炎症、肝肾功能不全、外伤和心肌梗死[1-3]。

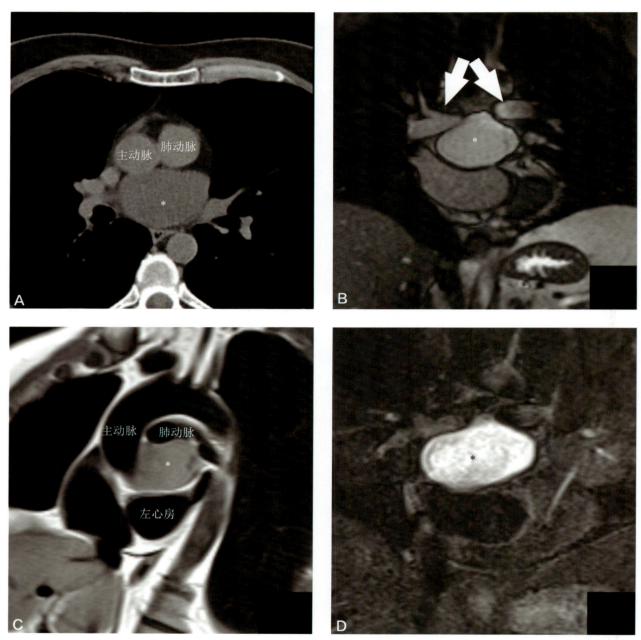

▲ 图 3-3 典型的横窦心包囊肿

轴位平扫 CT（A）和冠状位 bSSFP 电影 MR（B）图像显示，在肺动脉主干及其主要分支（箭），升主动脉和左心房之间的纵隔内可见一边缘锐利的椭圆形囊性结构（*）。囊肿呈低密度（CT值：7HU），经 CT 扫描壁无增厚（A）。SSFP 电影 MR（B）有助于确定薄而规则的边缘，并排除血凝块或任何血细胞成分的存在。在自旋回波 T_1 加权序列（C）中呈低信号，在冠状位 STIR T_2 加权序列（D）中呈高信号，提示为液性成分

作为一种快速、应用广泛、价格相对低廉的诊断工具，经胸超声心动图是检测心包积液和准确诊断大多数病例的首选影像学方法。然而，超声心动图在声窗不佳的患者或局灶性少量积液的患者中应用受限[6,16]；此外，超声通常无法评价心包厚度，尤其是可疑合并炎症时评价明显受限[16]。

CT 和 MR 对证实心包积液的存在、测量积液量、分析成分特征（漏出液与渗出液）、检测心包炎症、评估其血流动力学对心室充盈的影响，以及最终指导心包穿刺术都具有很高的准确性（图 3-5 和图 3-6）。

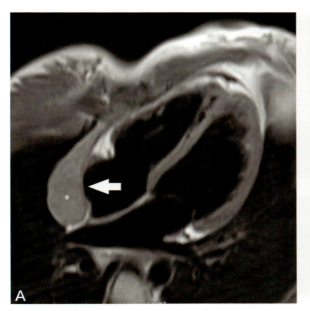
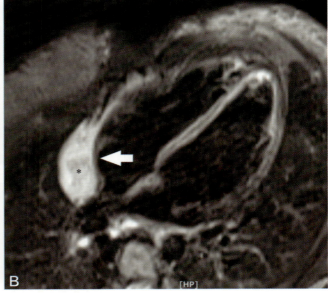

▲ 图 3-4 先天性囊肿

TSE T_1 加权（A）和 STIR T_2 加权（B）图像显示在心房侧壁水平（箭）的心包腔内见一囊性长条结构（*）。信号特征与不均匀的微粒样成分一致

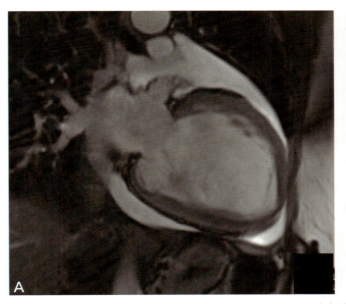
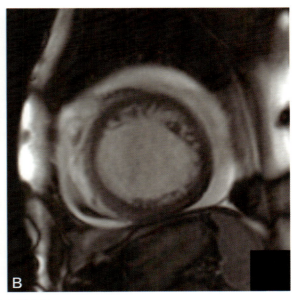

▲ 图 3-5 心包渗出性积液

在纵向（A）和轴向（B）长轴位上采集的平衡稳态自由进动电影 MR 图像显示扩张型心肌病患者有大量的心包渗出性积液。大量心包积液逐渐缓慢地积聚使心包腔拉伸、顺应性增加，但不增加心包压力

排除引起积液的可能原因，包括心包炎到肿瘤性病变，或者在超声心动图中观察到复杂不均匀回声渗出物时[5]，通常都需要进行 CT 和 MR 成像。

这两种方法均可准确评估心包宽度，甚至可检测恰好积聚在那些解剖隐窝中，通常超声无法评价的极少量液体（最多 10~40ml，代表生理血浆超滤液[45,46]），如在右心房的后基底壁或斜窦内。

CT 和 MR 可以半定量测量积液的量。右心室前的心包间隙大于 5mm 至少相当于中度积液（即 100~500ml）或采用一种类似测量心室容积的方法，即基于多层手动勾画积液轮廓容积法[47]。

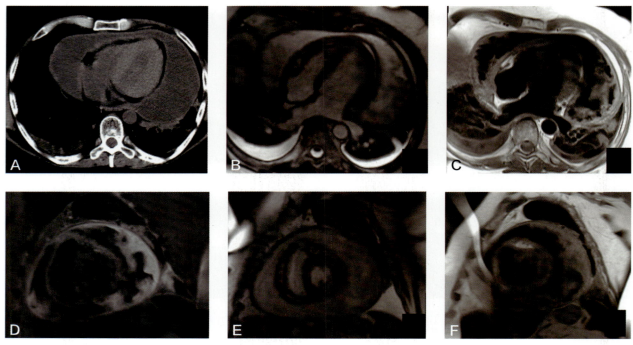

▲ 图 3-6　心包积液

轴位平扫 CT 图像（A）显示一例骨髓再生障碍患者的大量心包积液（1100～1200 ml），其内成分呈低 - 中度密度（15～25HU）。bSSFP 电影 MR（B、E）和黑血 TSE T_1 加权（C、F）图像分别在长轴和短轴图像上显示出不均匀的液体聚集混合成分，提示渗出性来源。请注意，心电门控短时反转恢复（STIR）T_2 加权序列（D）对描述心包积液成分并非十分有用，因心脏搏动易产生血流伪影，特别是在大量积液时。也可检测到双侧少量胸腔积液

一般来说，心包腔充满了 25～30ml 液体并且其内呈负压状态，引起心室偶联（ventricular coupling）现象。积液使心包内压增加，阻碍静脉回流，引起心脏血流动力学紊乱。

对液体密度 / 信号强度的分析也可以鉴别漏出液和渗出液。然而，由于渗出物的性质极易变化、心脏运动相关伪影和周围脂肪组织的存在（图 3-6），也会影响对液体成分的判断的可靠性。

当高密度的积液出现时，心包积血或脓性渗出液在 MDCT 上很容易发现。与心包积血、脓性渗出液或以不均匀低密度为特征的乳糜心包积液不同，典型心包积液表现为水样密度；在心包积气或化脓性厌氧菌感染的患者中，心包脏层内也可出现气 - 液平面[22]。

相比于高蛋白性渗出液 T_1 和 T_2 弛豫时间不同程度的缩短，漏出液在 MR 成像中表现出一种特异的均匀 T_1 加权低信号和 T_2 加权高信号。曾接受主动脉 / 心脏手术，有外伤、肿瘤、结核病史或心肌梗死后综合征（Dressler 综合征）病史的患者可发现心包积血，其特点是 T_1 加权图像呈高信号，电影 SSFP 图像呈不均匀低信号[19,25,26]。

然而，值得注意的是，由于水的非层流运动和心包周围脂 - 液分界面水平化学位移伪影的存在，在 MR（主要是 T_1 加权序列）上液体的信号强度可能有所不同[2,12,26]。亮血动态电影 MR 成像通常能识别心包内的成分，例如显示纤维束或凝血[25]。

最后，CT/MR 成像的核心功能是能够准确地评估心包层的厚度和组成成分，从而能够鉴别单纯的心包积液、炎性渗出性心包炎或恶性心包疾病[12]。

（三）心脏压塞

渗出对舒张功能的影响在很大程度上取决于心包腔的机械特征，即心包腔通常使整个心室的

舒张末期跨壁压力均衡化，而对心室充盈没有显著影响。

一般来说，心包的弹性特性可耐受储存大量液体（高达 1000 ml）[48]，特别是缓慢累积时（图 3-6）。然而，当心包积液迅速大量增加，心包内压力增加时，可以克服心包的拉伸能力，导致心腔受压，舒张期充盈障碍，室间隔反向运动，心输出量突然减少，随后出现低血压、心动过速，并进展为心源性休克[49]（图 3-7 和图 3-8）。

这种情况称为心脏压塞，其血流动力学可能形成危及生命的情况，必须迅速诊断，然后紧急治疗[71]。

心脏压塞所致机械功能障碍的一个征象是一旦心包内压超过腔内压，右心室舒张功能衰竭，随后出现腔静脉扩张，下腔静脉系统和肝静脉舒张期反向扩张，并且由于心室间依赖性增加，二尖瓣和三尖瓣流入的呼吸变异增加[5,50]。

心脏压塞可由多种原因引起，包括创伤、炎症、主动脉夹层、心包腔肿瘤侵犯、急性心肌梗死和心脏手术[49,50]。

临床表现（急性或慢性）取决于液体的绝对容量、积液的增长速度和心包的弹性，因此，迅速出现 200～250 ml 的心包积液可能是致命的，而缓慢积累的 2L 可无症状，没有血流动力学改变。

因为需要快速获得形态学和功能信息以确定诊断，所以经胸超声心动图是评估心脏血流动力学损害的一线方法；然而，CT 和 MR 特别适用于血流动力学稳定的压塞类型，CT 和 MR 高分辨率和组织学定性优势可能有助于描述液体成分（或其他成分，如空气）（图 3-9）。

此外，心脏压塞应区别于渗出性缩窄性心包炎（CP），后者是由心包的病理性非顺应性引起的，而不是由积液本身引起的。

1. 急性及慢性心包炎　术语急性和慢性心包炎（炎性心包炎）是不同病理性和病原性疾病的临床表现，包含特发性到感染性和自身免疫性疾病、心肌梗死后、放疗后反应和副肿瘤综合征[16]。

除外发病率在 30%～85% 的特发性心包炎，心包炎症最常见的病因是病毒感染（柯萨奇 A 和 B 病毒，艾柯病毒，腮腺炎病毒，巨细胞病毒，单纯疱疹病毒，带状疱疹病毒，腺病毒和 EB

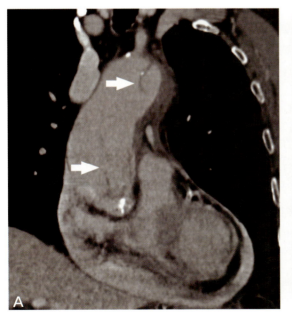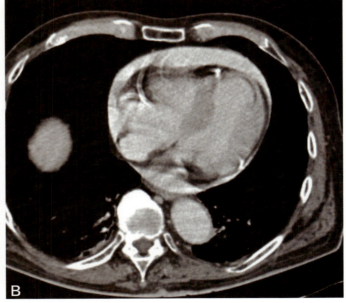

▲ 图 3-7　主动脉夹层破裂所致急性心脏压塞

冠状位（A）和轴向（B）增强 CT 图像显示升主动脉内膜片延伸至主动脉弓（箭），符合 Stanford A 型主动脉夹层，大量高密度的心包积液符合充血性心包积液表现。患者在 CT 血管造影检查后立即死亡（由意大利罗马的 G. F. Gualdi 医生，C. Valentini 医生提供）

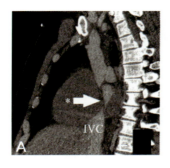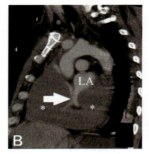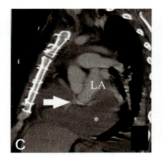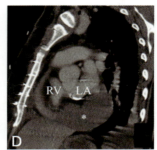
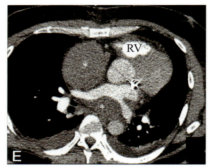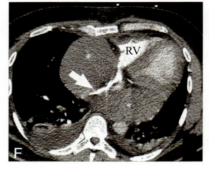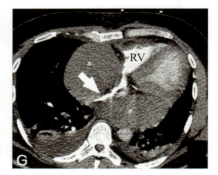

▲ 图 3-8　心包血肿引起心脏压塞

重建斜矢状位（A～D）和轴位（E～G）的增强 CT 图像显示，1 例 53 岁的男性患者在最近（4d 前）做了心脏二尖瓣置换术，表现为进行性加重的呼吸困难、缺氧、高碳酸血症以及内脏和外周充血的迹象（如足部水肿和颈静脉怒张），显示出大量的心包低密度液体积聚（*）。心包血肿位于心脏基底部，压迫上腔静脉、下腔静脉（IVC）、右心房（RV，箭）和左心房（LA），导致严重的静脉系统回流障碍和右心室舒张期充盈受限，表现为右心房体积缩小

病毒），然后是细菌和结核性感染性疾病；非传染性病因（一般为自身免疫性疾病，如类风湿关节炎、系统性红斑狼疮和进行性系统性硬化），心肌梗死和放射治疗是心包炎的另外两种并不罕见的病因[16,51]。

最近，发达国家报道的结核相关性心包炎病例越来越多，已引起广泛关注，人口流动或与人体免疫缺陷病毒感染有关是其主要原因[52-55]（图 3-10）。

心包炎的其他主要病因包括乳腺癌和纵隔肿瘤放射治疗后的医源性创伤后心包炎和心脏介入如心脏手术，经皮冠状动脉介入治疗，起搏器植入和导管消融术后[56]。

由心肌梗死相关性炎症所致的直接心外膜增殖（心外膜心包炎）（图 3-11），约 10% 的透壁性急性心肌梗死患者出现梗死后心包炎[57]。

梗死后心包炎应与晚期梗死后心包炎（或 Dressler 综合征）在临床上有所区别，晚期梗死后心包炎代表的是罕见的自身免疫过程，其与梗死的发生时间关系不大（梗死后 2～3 周），不同于梗死后心包炎（心梗后立即发生）。

急性心包炎的典型表现为急性胸痛，心包摩擦音和心电图上广泛的 ST 段抬高及病理性 Q 波缺失，占急诊科就诊的主诉急性胸痛患者的约 5%，也是胸痛三联 CTA 检查的主要鉴别诊断之一[58-60]（图 3-7）。

由于病理基质不同，影像结果包括从单纯的液性渗出到由于蛋白质渗出而变为脓性渗出，进而导致心脏压塞或进展为心包缩窄的各种表现。

还有一种称为干性心包炎（或心包炎干燥症），即纯粹的心包炎症而没有液体渗出，其病理特征为纤维蛋白性炎性渗出物，产生典型心包摩擦音[61]。

在急性情况下，炎症过程的特征在于形成高度血管化的肉芽组织及心包出现液体，在 CT 上表现为弥漫性和不规则的心包线性增厚，包括液性和纤维蛋白炎性成分[32]。

如前所述，在这种情况下 CT 成像的局限性在于区分小渗漏与心包增厚的能力有限[5]。

Chapter 3 心包疾病的 CT 和 MR 成像
Computed Topography/Magnetic Resonance Imaging of Pericardial Disease

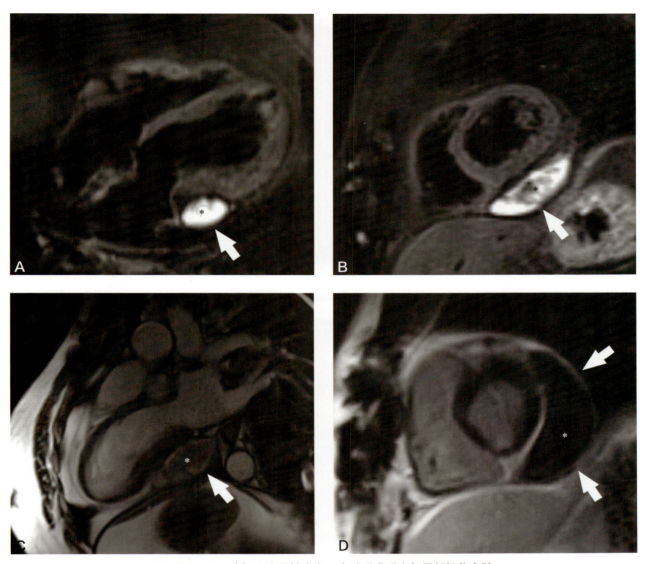

▲ 图 3-9 1 例 74 岁男性患者，心脏手术后心包局部机化血肿

CMR 图像显示卵圆形心包积液（*）轻度压迫左心室下壁，其特征是 T_2 加权 STIR（A、B）呈不均匀高信号，SSFP 图像（C）呈中等信号。CE-IR T_1 加权短轴图像（D）显示低信号液体成分，邻近心包层增厚并有强化（箭）

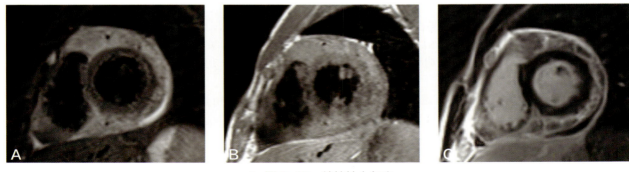

▲ 图 3-10 结核性心包炎

T_2 加权 STIR 序列（A）和 T_1 加权 TSE 黑血序列（B）的短轴层面可见大量心包积液：信号不均匀的固液混合成分，T_1 和 T_2 加权序列均为干酪样高信号。相应的 LGE（C）短轴层面可见心包膜增厚，特别是脏层心包增厚，以及组织渗出物内部的粘连成分、纤维束的不规则条索状强化

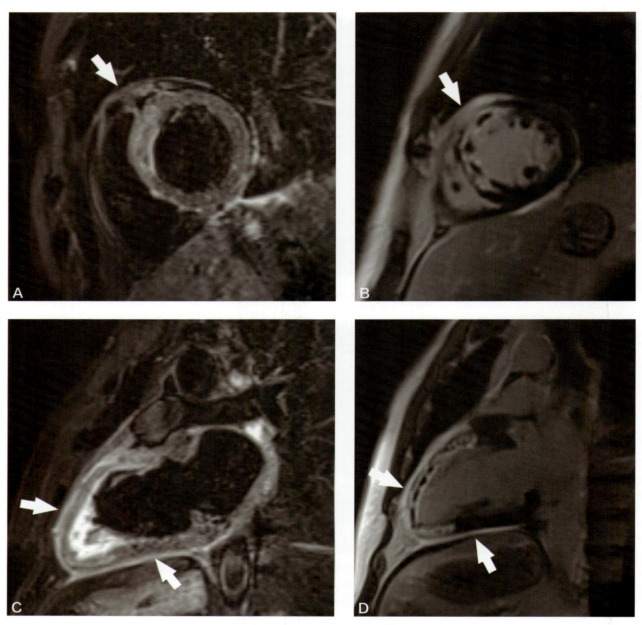

▲ 图 3-11　心外膜心包炎

近期左心室前壁大片梗死的 65 岁患者，早期心肌梗死后心包炎。T_2 加权 STIR 序列的短轴层面（A）和垂直长轴层面（C）图像和相应的 LGE 短轴层面（B）和垂直长轴层面（D）图像显示累及室间隔，左心室前壁和心尖部的大量透壁性急性心肌梗死，心肌内出血区域（T_2 加权 STIR 序列）和微血管阻塞（LGE 序列）。在 T_2 加权 STIR 序列（A、C）可见整个心包增厚的水肿信号，对应了 LGE 的明显强化（B、D），反映了心包炎症的活动期（箭）

超声心动图仍然是诊断的首选，通常足以支持患者的临床处置；然而，在某些情况下，使用断层成像可能为发现病理特征或指导诊断或治疗提供额外信息（心包穿刺或心包活检）。

急性 / 活动期心包炎的 MR 特征包括：脏层心包弥漫性水肿，T_2 加权短时间反转恢复（STIR）序列图像上表现为高信号，通常伴随 TSE 的 T_1 加权和 SSFP 电影序列图像上显示的不同程度的积液和不规则的心包增厚（图 3-12）。

活动性炎症的特征还包括一定程度的心包强化，例如各种报道中出现的单纯急性心包炎和临床反复发作的慢性心包炎患者，在 T_1 加权 TSE 或反转恢复序列可见心包延迟强化[23,32,62]（图 3-13）。

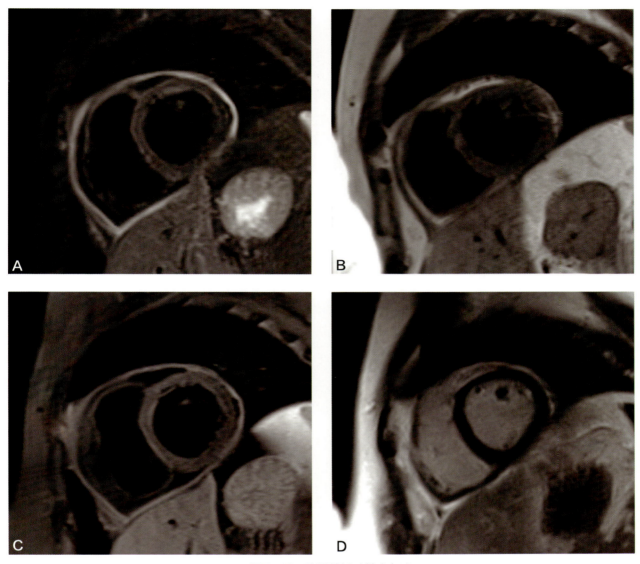

▲ 图 3-12 弥漫性活动性心包炎

短轴层面上 STIR 自旋回波 T_2 加权序列（A）和非增强的 TSE T_1 加权黑血序列（B）很好地显示了病毒性心包炎的弥漫性心包增厚。心电门控下的 T_1 加权脂肪抑制 TSE 增强序列的相应短轴层面图像（C）显示，对比剂注入后整个心包明显均匀强化，这反映了炎症活动性，而传统的延迟强化技术（D）对心包强化和心外膜脂肪组织的区分较差

此外，MR 增强成像可以评估炎症侵犯周围脂肪和邻近心肌组织的范围[12]。

急性心包炎在大多数病例中没有后遗症，可能最终留下晚期纤维性或纤维肉芽肿性残余粘连[61]。然而，尽管患者通常对非甾体抗炎药物反应良好，但在某些情况下，它可以发展为慢性硬化性心包炎，通常伴有广泛的渐进性成纤维细胞增殖和胶原沉积，最终导致增厚的纤维化心包限制心脏收缩（CP）。

慢性纤维化心包炎在 CT 和 MR 影像上表现为局灶性心包膜不表现为心包局部不强化或广泛心包增厚，常常表现为局灶性粘连引起的包裹性积液[32,61]。

如前所述，MR 标记技术可以发现心包粘连的存在，表现为整个心动周期内心包与心肌之间的标记信号持续存在[31]。

最后，正电子发射断层扫描（PET）/CT 的优势在于，存在复杂心包炎的情况下，由于能够检测到心包膜或心包液中的代谢活动，所以可以区分感染性或恶性病变与纯粹的炎性病变[23,63]。

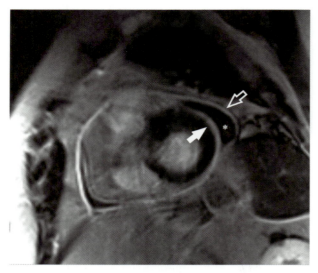

▲ 图 3-13 弥漫性活动性心包炎

CE-IR T_1 加权图像的短轴层面显示由少量心包积液（*）分隔的壁层和脏层（白箭）心包的弥漫性增厚和强化。强化是活动性炎症的特征

2. 心包心肌炎（或心肌心包炎） 心包炎通常伴有不同程度的心肌炎（反之亦然），这是心外膜直接播散导致（反之亦然）的炎症过程，并且因为它们的共同病原体，主要是心脏相关病毒。

通常心包心肌炎或心肌心包炎两个术语可以互换使用，分别用于强调其中一种的主要临床和病理表现，两者程度相同的情况很少[64]。例如，心肌心包炎主要指与心肌炎症较轻的心包炎，而心包心肌炎则以心肌炎综合征为主要表现[51]。

心肌心包炎的检出与临床关系密切，是心包炎患者的不良预后因子，通常需要住院治疗和全面的病因学检查[12,53,64,65]。

当出现非典型 ECG 变化（如新发心律失常、窦性心动过速和 Q-T 间期延长）与一过性的节段性和全心室壁运动异常并且心肌酶升高时，可以怀疑急性心包炎的心肌受累。

这种情况下，超声心动图的作用有限，主要是因为许多心肌受累不严重或者即使心肌炎较严重的患者都可能超声心动检查结果正常，或者只表现出非特异性征象和各种不典型表现[66]。

在这种情况下，尽管可以显示急性心肌炎时的心外膜延迟强化，且与 MR 征象相关，CT 的诊断作用也是有限的[67]。

因为可以同时评估结构和功能，心脏 MR 已成为无创评估心肌炎的标准[7,68-70]。急性心肌炎伴有心包炎症时，T_2 加权 STIR 序列上通常可见心肌中层至心外膜的明显延迟强化并伴有局灶性水肿和不同程度的局部功能障碍[7,68-70]（图 3-14）。

3. 缩窄性心包炎 缩窄性心包炎（CP）的主要特征是在心脏周围形成厚的，无弹性纤维或钙化纤维囊，并且阻碍双心室的生理学舒张，伴有逐渐进展的舒张功能障碍[1]。

心包纤维化通常是过度愈合的结果，可能继发于任何形式的急性炎症，形成厚的瘢痕组织，导致心包腔全部或大部分闭塞，充满渗出物/脓性物质[1,54,61]。

这种情况下也常见钙沉积，并可能由于慢性炎症刺激而导致心包硬化（图 3-15）。

引起心包缩窄的疾病谱随着时间的推移逐渐从单纯的感染性疾病（特别是结核病）变为以放疗和术后并发症为最常见病因[71,72]。

急性病毒性或特发性心包炎后出现缩窄性心包炎的风险很低（< 0.5%），但在化脓性心包炎中相对常见，慢性病程伴较多心包积液时更易出现[72,73]。

临床症状通常是由于心室充盈受损，严重的舒张功能障碍和右心衰竭导致的，首发症状为内脏和外周充血（如下肢水肿、腹水和颈静脉怒张），随后症状向心性发展，例如呼吸困难、咳嗽和乏力[16,61]。

CP 通常是一种慢性过程，随着时间推移慢慢进展，通常起病几年后才有临床症状；然而，亚急性（少于 1 年），甚至急性（几天）类型也可以导致 CP，如广泛的心脏压塞或进行外科手术（在心包引流术）后，导致的带状纤维粘连的局灶性瘢痕[16,61]。

慢性 CP 的心包组织通常以纤维结缔组织为主，伴少量炎症细胞，而急性和亚急性 CP 在组织学上以炎症细胞为主，伴少量的结缔组织[61,72]。

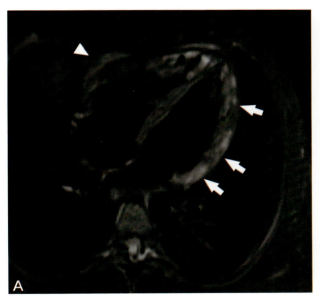
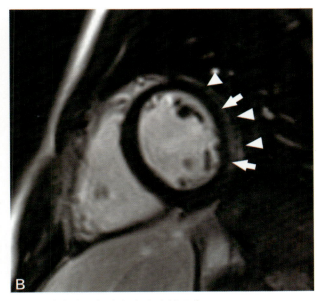

▲ 图 3-14　54 岁女性急性心包心肌炎患者,伴胸痛和轻度左心室功能不全

STIR T_2 加权序列的短轴图像（A）可见左心室侧壁心外膜下的心肌斑片状水肿,与 LGE T_1 加权序列（B）增厚的心外膜内带状心肌强化区域相匹配。在 STIR T_2 加权序列上可见近右心室游离壁处的局限性心包增厚（A,箭）,LGE T_1 加权序列上可见左心室侧壁的局限性心包增厚（B,箭）。左心室心肌活检证实了心肌炎症

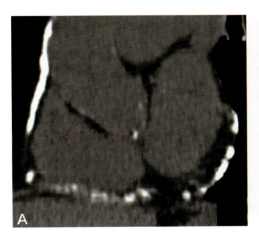
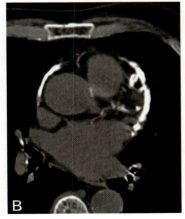
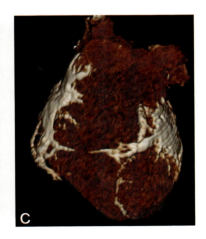

▲ 图 3-15　心包钙化

上图患者没有特异性的心脏疾病病史,在 CT 钙化积分扫描中检测到广泛的心包钙化。CT 平扫的短轴（A）和轴位（B）图像可见增厚和严重钙化的心包。CT 容积再现三维重建（C）图像能最好地展现心包钙化的范围

尽管对心包缩窄的复杂血流动力学理解不断加深,无创诊断方法也取得了一定进展,但诊断 CP 仍然有一定困难,特别是需要与限制性心肌病(RC)和其他病因(包括右心衰竭和限制性疾病)导致的系统性静脉淤血鉴别,以及症状不典型时。

RC 和 CP 的鉴别诊断尤其困难,因为限制性心肌病和缩窄性心包炎的病理生理学的特征均为舒张功能受损且临床症状一致[71,74]。

这两种疾病最根本的区别是 CP 手术可治愈,而 RC 主要为心肌舒张功能障碍和顺应性降低,因此治疗很大程度上是姑息性的,且预后不良[16,75]。

由于早期 CP 心包切除术后预后良好,临床上应该尽早明确诊断,在广泛钙化和明显心肌受累的情况下心包切除术效果较差[71,74,76]。

由于没有单一成像方法可以鉴别 CP 的所有病因,因此应针对不同患者采用个性化的成像方法[16,77,78]。

4. 形态异常 局灶性或弥漫性的心包增厚（>4 mm）是缩窄性心包炎的典型形态学征象，通常在右心室游离壁和前房室沟处更为明显，心包形态不规则，常表现为一定程度的钙化（图3-16）。

Young PM 等[23]在一项与手术相关的回顾性分析中发现，无钙化的缩窄性心包炎患者平均心包厚度为（4.6±2.1）cm，而出现钙化的缩窄性心包炎患者平均心包厚度增加到（9.2±7.0）cm。

据报道，心包厚度 > 6 mm 对诊断心包缩窄具有很高的特异性；在 4～6 mm 时，结合典型的临床症状也可以诊断；而当心包厚度小于 2mm 时，基本可以排除缩窄性心包炎的可能[4,54,79]。

然而最近有研究证明，无论钙化是否出现，组织学上的纤维化几乎总是存在的（96%）。在心包缩窄的患者中，最大心包厚度的可能有很大差异（1～17mm；平均值4mm），它只与心脏收缩程度有微弱的相关性，高达20%的患者心包厚度表现正常（<2 mm）[16,54,80]。

没有弥漫性（甚至局灶性）的心包增厚并不能排除心包缩窄的出现；先前的研究表明，正常厚度但质地僵硬的心包也可能是造成严重心脏舒张功能障碍的原因[8,80]。

因此，在患者有心包限制症状但无心包增厚证据支持的情况下，强烈推荐使用心脏磁共振进行功能评估[8,80]。此外，一些学者提出，长期的慢性炎症导致心包变薄是向终末期不可逆的纤维性心包炎演变的特征[81-83]。

心脏 CT 是一种可以很好地发现钙化的检查，它甚至可以识别微小的钙化灶，而广泛的钙化可能会被 MR 漏诊[12,22,29,45]。

在有心包缩窄症状的患者，多达50%的患者出现了心包钙化，存在钙化通常可以排除限制性心肌病[4,22,84]。

尽管心包钙化是结核性心包炎的典型表现，但大约28%经组织学证实的缩窄性心包炎患者在排除结核后也可出现钙化[76]。因此，钙化应该被认为是慢性炎症的非特异性反应。

在术前评估心包手术时，术前 CT 检查可用于详细描述心包增厚程度和钙化的存在及位置，从而更好地实现手术方案的制订和手术风险的分层[26]。

在磁共振成像中，增厚的纤维化和（或）钙化的心包在 T_1、T_2 加权成像及电影成像上信号较低，容易与积液区分。

正常情况下室间隔可以呈弯曲或平直的形态，或可能由于跨室间隔充盈压力升高而向左弯曲。

额外的间接心包缩窄征象包括腔静脉和肝静脉系统的扩张，单侧或双侧心房增大（尤其是左侧）以及由增厚的心包直接压迫引起的心室管状形态。

MR 也可观察到双侧胸腔积液和腹水。在很多情况下并不能看到缩窄性心包炎的典型形态学特征，需要结合临床数据和功能评价，使诊断更加具有挑战性[74,80]。

一些局限性的、发生在关键位置以及浆膜层增厚引起的心包缩窄可以导致严重的血流动力学障碍，如发生部位靠近右侧房室沟处。在这种情况下，通过横断面成像模式全面评估心包线是非常有帮助的[2,9,25]，MR 的标记技术可能特别有助于直接识别心包的局灶性粘连。

对比注射钆剂后，处于终末期慢性纤维化的缩窄性心包炎不会出现明显的对比增强，而心包的强化则提示残余炎症的存在[32,83]。

持续性慢性炎症活动的存在与缩窄性心包炎对抗炎治疗有可逆或短暂的反应有关。在此临床背景下，MR 增强显像有助于鉴别具有残留活动性炎症的患者，这些患者可以通过药物治疗获益，而无须进行心包切除术[81-83]。

最后，还存在一种隐匿性心包炎（或容量衰竭型缩窄性心包炎）[25]，其在一般情况下缺乏临床症状和血流动力学表现，而仅在静脉回流增加的情况下出现临床症状，如深吸气或剧烈运动时。因此使用类似于 Valsalva 动作的动态操作辅助影像诊断检查可能有助于诊断这种潜在的疾病，并显示与右心室流入增加相关的舒张功能改变[17,25]。

Chapter 3 心包疾病的 CT 和 MR 成像
Computed Topography/Magnetic Resonance Imaging of Pericardial Disease

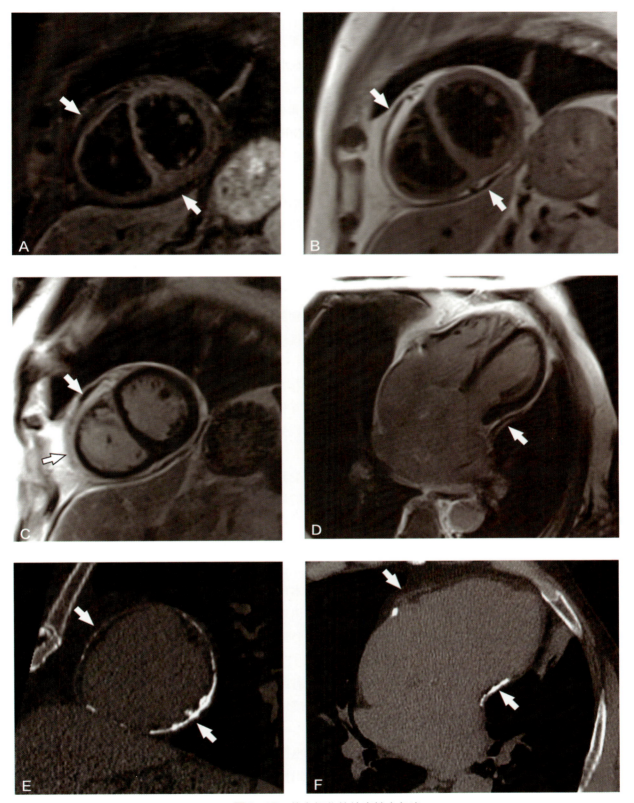

▲ 图 3-16 伴有钙化的缩窄性心包炎

在心电门控下 STIR T_2 加权成像（A）和 TSE T_1 加权成像（B）的短轴图像可见心包不规则弥漫增厚及室间隔平直，主要累及心室基底段（箭）。在 LGE 短轴（C）和水平长轴（D）图像中，增厚的非钙化心包层的强化与心外膜及其邻近的心包脂肪组织很难区分。自旋回波序列 T_1 加权的短轴图像（B）显示位于心脏下方的异常心包的范围（箭）。矢状位（E）和轴位（F）的 CT 图像可见钙化

5. 功能异常　缩窄性心包炎的功能异常的原因是解剖上心包缩窄引起的，主要是由于舒张期双心室扩张受阻，充血速度加快所致。

实际上，增厚的心包提高了心室的耦联，引起心室容积/压力关系增加，并导致舒张压的上升，且在所有心腔内几乎均等增加。

由充盈压力增加产生的影响在室间隔水平上表现得尤为明显。由于跨室间隔充盈压力升高，在舒张期早期出现间隔壁向左侧异常摆动。这种现象也被称为室间隔矛盾运动，是鉴别缩窄性心包炎与限制性心肌病的一个典型特征[8,9]。

缩窄性心包炎的另一个相关征象是呼吸过程中心腔内压力与胸腔内压力关系的分离，这是Hatle等最先发现的[85]，它会使正常呼吸过程中心腔内压力隔离。在深吸气时，如果心脏被增厚的心包完全包裹住，胸腔内气压的下降不会影响到心腔内的高压，从而引起肺静脉回流减少，最终导致左心室充盈受限；相反，心脏的收缩功能通常不会减低。

值得注意的是，以上这些重要的功能和血流动力学特征都可以通过经胸超声心动图和心导管检查来检测，它们在临床应用中都是可靠且广泛使用的检查方法[75,86]。

心脏CT在评估与缩窄性心包炎相关的功能改变方面的作用非常有限，尽管在理论上，使用高时间分辨率的回顾性心电门控技术对室间隔的运动进行动态评估是可行的[28]。

心脏MR对评估缩窄性心包炎相关功能学改变的作用更为全面，通过综合应用平衡稳态进动电影成像（cine-SSFP）、相位对比、磁共振实时电影成像（real-time cine-MR imaging）和磁共振标记序列，可以识别上述心包缩窄所引起的大部分功能异常特点。

应用cine-SSFP成像技术描述室间隔矛盾运动在文献中已得到广泛证实，其与超声心动图相比具有更好的图像对比度分辨率[9]。

Giorgi等[9]采用常规cine-SSFP屏气技术发现，大多数缩窄性心包炎的患者在舒张早期室间隔呈平直或反曲状改变。这一现象在基底段水平上更为明显，其特征是在心动周期中室间隔呈S形改变，而在限制性心肌病患者中不存在。

缩窄性心包炎的患者与健康的受试者相比，典型的舒张期三尖瓣早期波比在速度编码的cine-MR序列上降低，且a波（代表心房充盈）减低或消失[87]。

在下腔静脉水平也可以出现收缩期前向血流的减少甚至逆转，并可能与病理生理上的限制性改变所导致早期舒张前向血流增加有关。

呼吸对室间隔运动的影响可以通过实时磁共振技术进行评估，这种技术可以利用SSFP非触发电影磁共振成像技术结合并行采集技术，识别缩窄性心包炎患者舒张中早期室间隔的呼吸摆动[8,17]。

在正常情况下，左、右心室之间正压梯度的存在使室间隔凸向右心室侧，由于胸膜-心包相互作用使压力平衡的原因，正常受试者的这种结构受呼吸活动的影响最小。

而在缩窄性心包炎患者中，右心室向外扩张受到病变心包的限制，导致右心室压力突然增加，随后引起室间隔向左移位，呈平直或反曲状改变。

Francone通过实时屏气技术对缩窄性心包炎、限制性心肌病和炎性心包炎[8]患者进行研究，最先提出了呼吸活动对室间隔运动和构型的影响。本研究结果显示，缩窄性心包炎患者在舒张早期出现典型的室间隔平坦化或反曲，在深吸气开始时最明显，在舒张晚期迅速消失（图3-17）。

这一现象在限制性心肌病患者中并不存在，有助于两者的鉴别，尤其是在心包厚度正常或轻度增厚的情况下。

心包的活动度和僵硬度也可以通过传统的心电图门控标记的磁共振电影序列来评估，它可以识别脏层与壁层心包之间的局灶性纤维化粘连，表现为在心动周期中持续显示的线状影[31]。

（四）心包肿物

不同类型的心包肿物包括囊肿、血肿、复杂的

Chapter 3 心包疾病的 CT 和 MR 成像
Computed Topography/Magnetic Resonance Imaging of Pericardial Disease

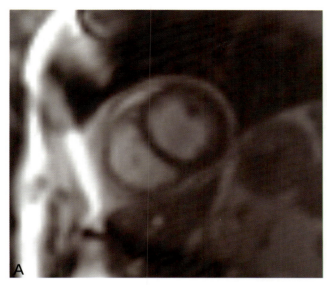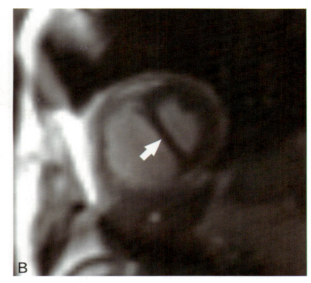

▲ 图 3-17　缩窄性心包炎（与图 3-13 为同一病例）

实时 cine-SSFP 的短轴图像显示呼气末（A）及吸气时（B），室间隔反曲（箭），这是由于右心室迅速充盈而没有相应心包膨胀补偿所致

组织渗出液和发生于心包的原发及继发恶性肿瘤。

肿物通常在超声心动图初检或者在胸部 X 线或 CT 检查中偶然发现，需要 CT 和 MR 成像技术来进一步评估。横断面成像可以区分真正的心包肿物和所谓的伪肿物；准确界定病变的位置、范围及其与周围结构的关系；提供一定程度的组织学特征。

通过 CT 和 MRI 检查，组织血肿、囊性肿物或假性肿物通常可以很好地与肿瘤进行区分（图 3-3 和图 3-9）。在经胸超声心动图检查时，即使是有经验的操作者，大量的心外膜脂肪也可能被误诊为心包肿物，而通过 MR 脂肪饱和序列或 CT 成像则很容易被鉴别。

假性室壁瘤的发生是由于心肌破裂引起心包积血被增厚的心包所覆盖[88]。

原发性心包肿瘤性疾病极为罕见，而已有报道高达 10%～12% 的已知肿瘤患者会发生心包的继发累及[89,90]。

积液量的持续变化这一特点可能有助于心包肿物的诊断，且与病灶实性成分的大小不成比例，常常是血性的，因此在 CMR 的 T_1 和 T_2 加权成像序列上表现为不均匀的富含蛋白成分的高信号，在 CT 平扫中表现为较高的密度（图 3-18）。

心包良性肿瘤如纤维瘤、畸胎瘤、血管瘤和脂肪瘤总体来讲极其罕见的。

原发肿瘤多为恶性，包括间皮瘤、肉瘤、脂肪肉瘤和淋巴瘤（图 3-19）。恶性间皮瘤是最常见的原发性肿瘤，占所有心包肿瘤的 50%，通常以心包内结节或团块状病灶伴心包积液为特征[91,92]。

心包的转移肿瘤可以由附近解剖结构如肺、纵隔（淋巴瘤）或心肌（血管肉瘤）的肿瘤直接侵袭而发生；也可以通过血液播散（最常见的是恶性黑色素瘤、淋巴瘤和乳腺肿瘤）或腔静脉蔓延（侵犯右心腔，通常是肾细胞或肝细胞癌）（图 3-20）。

原发病灶侵犯心肌引起脏层或壁层的心包局部连续性中断是提示恶性肿瘤的典型征象，在右心室游离壁的水平上很容易被发现。

有时可以观察到脏层心包的直接侵犯，例如原发性血管肉瘤，它通常起源于右心房，迅速浸润生长并导致大量的心包积液。壁层心包常被肺门周围的原发侵袭性肿瘤侵犯。

虽然 CT 和 MRI 对诊断可以提供大量的信息，但对大多数心包肿瘤仍然需要进行活检和组织病理学分析，以明确诊断[92]。

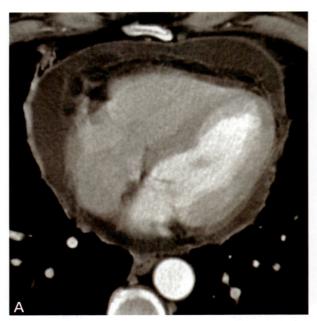 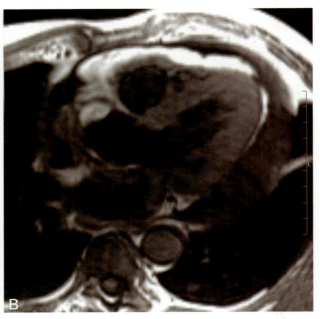

▲ 图 3-18　心包间皮瘤

增强 CT 轴位图像（A）和黑血 TSE T_1 加权成像（B）图像显示，心包弥漫性强化，伴增厚软组织结节和含血液成分的中等量心包积液。行心包穿刺术进行细胞学分析诊断为原发性恶性心包间皮瘤

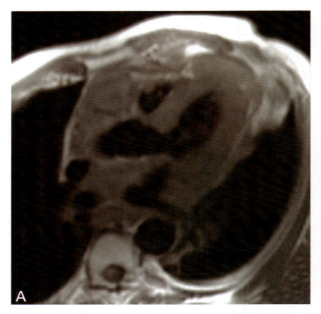 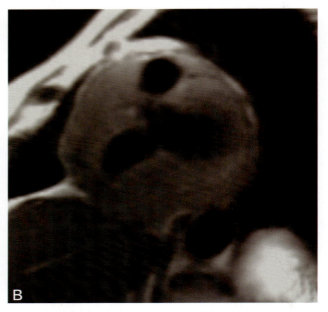

▲ 图 3-19　原发非霍奇金淋巴瘤

非增强的黑血 T_1 加权成像在长轴（A）和短轴（B）上显示心包弥漫性重度增厚，软组织界限不清，侵犯心外膜脂肪间隙并完全包裹心腔

Chapter 3　心包疾病的 CT 和 MR 成像
Computed Topography/Magnetic Resonance Imaging of Pericardial Disease

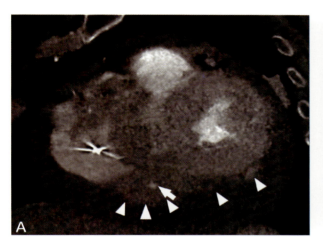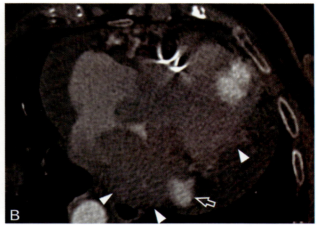

▲ 图 3-20　肾细胞癌患者心包的转移

心电门控 CT 增强在心脏短轴重建（A）和轴位（B）的图像显示后降支（箭）周围有大量浸润性软组织影（箭头），弥漫侵犯心包和右心室腔。病理组织沿心包生长扩散，覆盖左心室下外侧壁，浸润并导致冠状静脉窦的狭窄（空心箭）。此外可见中量心包积液和右心室电极

参考文献

[1] Spodick DH. *The Pericardium: A Comprehensive Textbook.* New York: Marcel Dekker, Inc., 1997.

[2] Francone M, Dymarkowski S, Kalantzi M, Bogaert J. Magnetic resonance imaging in the evaluation of the pericardium: A pictorial essay. *La Radiologia medica* 2005;109:64–74; quiz 75–76.

[3] Ivens EL, Munt BI, Moss RR. Pericardial disease: What the general cardiologist needs to know. *Heart* 2007;93:993–1000.

[4] Maisch B, Seferovic PM, Ristic AD et al. Guidelines on the diagnosis and management of pericardial diseases executive summary; The Task force on the diagnosis and management of pericardial diseases of the European Society of Cardiology. *European Heart Journal* 2004;25:587–610.

[5] Verhaert D, Gabriel RS, Johnston D, Lytle BW, Desai MY, Klein AL. The role of multimodality imaging in the management of pericardial disease. *Circulation: Cardiovascular Imaging* 2010;3:333–343.

[6] Imazio M, Spodick DH, Brucato A, Trinchero R, Adler Y. Controversial issues in the management of pericardial diseases. *Circulation* 2010;121:916–928.

[7] Pennell DJ, Sechtem UP, Higgins CB et al. Clinical indications for cardiovascular magnetic resonance (CMR): Consensus Panel report. *European Heart Journal* 2004;25:1940–1965.

[8] Francone M, Dymarkowski S, Kalantzi M, Rademakers FE, Bogaert J. Assessment of ventricular coupling with realtime cine MRI and its value to differentiate constrictive pericarditis from restrictive cardiomyopathy. *European Radiology* 2006;16:944–951.

[9] Giorgi B, Mollet NR, Dymarkowski S, Rademakers FE, Bogaert J. Clinically suspected constrictive pericarditis: MR imaging assessment of ventricular septal motion and configuration in patients and healthy subjects. *Radiology* 2003;228:417–424.

[10] Spodick DH. Macrophysiology, microphysiology, and anatomy of the pericardium: A synopsis. *American Heart Journal* 1992;124:1046–1051.

[11] Groell R, Schaffler GJ, Rienmueller R. Pericardial sinuses and recesses: Findings at electrocardiographically triggered electron-beam CT. *Radiology* 1999;212:69–73.

[12] Bogaert J, Francone M. Pericardial disease: Value of CT and MR imaging. *Radiology* 2013;267:340–356.

[13] Rabkin SW. Epicardial fat: Properties, function and relationship to obesity. Obesity reviews : An official journal of the International Association for the *Study of Obesity* 2007;8:253–261.

[14] Iacobellis G, Corradi D, Sharma AM. Epicardial adipose tissue: Anatomic, biomolecular and clinical relationships with the heart. *Nature Clinical Practice Cardiovascular Medicine* 2005;2:536–543.

[15] Sacks HS, Fain JN. Human epicardial adipose tissue: A review. *American Heart Journal* 2007;153:907–917.

[16] Troughton RW, Asher CR, Klein AL. Pericarditis. *Lancet* 2004;363:717–727.

[17] Francone M, Dymarkowski S, Kalantzi M, Bogaert J. Real-time cine MRI of ventricular septal motion: A novel approach to assess ventricular coupling. *Journal of Magnetic Resonance Imaging: JMRI* 2005;21:305–309.

[18] Truong MT, Erasmus JJ, Gladish GW et al. Anatomy of pericardial recesses on multidetector CT: Implications for oncologic imaging. *AJR American Journal of Roentgenology* 2003;181:1109–1113.

[19] Wang ZJ, Reddy GP, Gotway MB, Yeh BM, Hetts SW, Higgins

CB. CT and MR imaging of pericardialdis ease. *RadioGraphics: A Review Publication of the Radiological Society of North America, Inc* 2003;23(Spec. No.): S167–S180.

[20] Sechtem U, Tscholakoff D, Higgins CB. MRI of the normal pericardium. *AJR American Journal of Roentgenology* 1986;147:239–244.

[21] Bogaert J, Duerinckx AJ. Appearance of the normal pericardium on coronary MR angiograms. *Journal of Magnetic Resonance Imaging: JMRI* 1995;5:579–587.

[22] O'Leary SM, Williams PL, Williams MP et al. Imaging the pericardium: Appearances on ECG-gated 64-detec tor row cardiac computed tomography. *The British Journal of Radiology* 2010;83:194–205.

[23] Young PM, Glockner JF, Williamson EE et al. MR imaging findings in 76 consecutive surgically proven cases of pericardial disease with CT and pathologic correlation. *The International Journal of Cardiovascular Imaging* 2012;28:1099–1109.

[24] Ferrans VJ IT, Roberts WC. Anatomy of the pericardium. In: Reddy PS LD, Shaver JA, eds., *Pericardial Disease*. New York: Raven, 1982: pp. 77–92.

[25] Bogaert J, Francone M. Cardiovascular magnetic resonance in pericardial diseases. *Journal of Cardiovascular Magnetic Resonance: Official Journal of the Society for Cardiovascular Magnetic Resonance* 2009;11:14.

[26] Yared K, Baggish AL, Picard MH, Hoffmann U, Hung J. Multimodality imaging of pericardial diseases. *JACC Cardiovascular Imaging* 2010;3:650–660.

[27] Kodama F, Fultz PJ, Wandtke JC. Comparing thin section and thick-section CT of pericardial sinuses and recesses. *AJR American Journal of Roentgenology* 2003;181:1101–1108.

[28] Ghersin E, Lessick J, Litmanovich D et al. Septal bounce in constrictive pericarditis. Diagnosis and dynamic evaluation with multidetector CT. *Journal of Computer Assisted Tomography* 2004;28:676–678.

[29] Belgour A, Christiaens LP, Varroud-Vial N, Vialle R, Tasu JP. Chronic pericarditis: CT and MR imaging features. *Journal de radiologie* 2010;91:615–622.

[30] Francone M, Carbone I, Agati L et al. Utility of T2-weighted short-tau inversion recovery (STIR) sequences in cardiac MRI: An overview of clinical applications in ischaemic and non-ischaemic heart disease. *La radiologia medica* 2011;116:32–46.

[31] Kojima S, Yamada N, Goto Y. Diagnosis of constrictive pericarditis by tagged cine magnetic resonance imaging. *The New England Journal of Medicine* 1999;341:373–374.

[32] Taylor AM, Dymarkowski S, Verbeken EK, Bogaert A. Detection of pericardial inflammation with lateenhancement cardiac magnetic resonance imaging: Initial results. *European Radiology* 2006;16:569–574.

[33] Rademakers FE, Bogaert J. Cardiac dysfunction in heart failure with normal ejection fraction: MRI measurements. *Progress in Cardiovascular Diseases* 2006;49:215–227.

[34] Paelinck BP, Lamb HJ, Bax JJ, Van der Wall EE, de Roos A. Assessment of diastolic function by cardiovascular magnetic resonance. *American Heart Journal* 2002;144:198–205.

[35] Mohiaddin RH, Wann SL, Underwood R, Firmin DN, Rees S, Longmore DB. Vena caval flow: Assessment with cine MR velocity mapping. *Radiology* 1990;177:537–541.

[36] Akiba T, Marushima H, Masubuchi M, Kobayashi S, Morikawa T. Small symptomatic pericardial diverticula treated by video-assisted thoracic surgical resection. *Annals of Thoracic and Cardiovascular Surgery: Official Journal of the Association of Thoracic and Cardiovascular Surgeons of Asia* 2009;15:123–125.

[37] Feigin DS, Fenoglio JJ, McAllister HA, Madewell JE. Pericardial cysts. A radiologic-pathologic correlation and review. *Radiology* 1977;125:15–20.

[38] Jeung MY, Gasser B, Gangi A et al. Imaging of cystic masses of the mediastinum. *RadioGraphics: A Review Publication of the Radiological Society of North America, Inc* 2002;22(Spec. No.):S79–S93.

[39] Drury NE, De Silva RJ, Hall RM, Large SR. Congenital defects of the pericardium. *The Annals of Thoracic Surgery* 2007;83:1552–1553.

[40] Yamano T, Sawada T, Sakamoto K, Nakamura T, Azuma A, Nakagawa M. Magnetic resonance imaging differentiated partial from complete absence of the left pericardium in a case of leftward displacement of the heart. *Circulation Journal: Official Journal of the Japanese Circulation Society* 2004;68:385–388.

[41] Peebles CR, Shambrook JS, Harden SP. Pericardial disease—Anatomy and function. *The British Journal of Radiology* 2011;84(Spec. No. 3):S324–S337.

[42] Scheuermann-Freestone M, Orchard E, Francis J et al. Images in cardiovascular medicine. Partial congenital absence of the pericardium. *Circulation* 2007;116:e126–e129.

[43] Psychidis-Papakyritsis P, de Roos A, Kroft LJ. Functional MRI of congenital absence of the pericardium. *AJR American Journal of Roentgenology* 2007;189:W312–W314.

[44] Abbas AE, Appleton CP, Liu PT, Sweeney JP. Congenital absence of the pericardium: Case presentation and review of literature. *International Journal of Cardiology* 2005;98:21–25.

[45] Ovchinnikov VI. Computerized tomography of pericardial diseases. *Vestnik rentgenologii i radiologii* 1996:10–15.

[46] Mulvagh SL, Rokey R, Vick GW, 3rd, Johnston DL. Usefulness of nuclear magnetic resonance imaging for evaluation of pericardial effusions, and comparison with two-dimensional echocardiography. *The American Journal of Cardiology* 1989;64:1002–1009.

[47] Frank H, Globits S. Magnetic resonance imaging evaluation of myocardial and pericardial disease. *Journal of Magnetic Resonance Imaging: JMRI* 1999;10:617–626.

[48] Breen JF. Imaging of the pericardium. *Journal of Thoracic Imaging* 2001;16:47–54.

[49] Spodick DH. Acute cardiac tamponade. *The New England Journal of Medicine* 2003;349:684–690.

[50] Restrepo CS, Lemos DF, Lemos JA et al. Imaging findings in cardiac tamponade with emphasis on CT. *RadioGraphics: A Review Publication of the Radiological Society of North America, Inc* 2007;27:1595–1610.

[51] Imazio M, Trinchero R. Myopericarditis: Etiology, management, and prognosis. *International Journal of Cardiology* 2008;127:17–26.

[52] Restrepo CS, Diethelm L, Lemos JA et al. Cardiovascular complications of human immunodeficiency virus infection. *RadioGraphics: A Review Publication of the Radiological Society of North America, Inc* 2006;26:213–231.

[53] Little WC, Freeman GL. Pericardial disease. *Circulation* 2006;113:1622–1632.

[54] Oh KY, Shimizu M, Edwards WD, Tazelaar HD, Danielson GK. Surgical pathology of the parietal pericardium: A study of 344 cases (1993-1999). *Cardiovascular Pathology: The Official Journal of the Society for Cardiovascular Pathology* 2001;10:157–168.

[55] Syed FF, Ntsekhe M, Gumedze F, Badri M, Mayosi BM. Myopericarditis in tuberculous pericardial effusion: Prevalence, predictors and outcome. *Heart* 2014;100:135–139.

[56] Imazio M, Brucato A, Derosa FG et al. Aetiological diagnosis in acute and recurrent pericarditis: When and how. *Journal of Cardiovascular Medicine* 2009;10:217–230.

[57] Doulaptsis C, Cazacu A, Dymarkowski S, Goetschalckx K, Bogaert J. Epistenocardiac pericarditis. *Hellenic Journal of Cardiology: HJC = Hellenike kardiologike epitheo rese* 2013;54:466–468.

[58] Halpern EJ. Triple-rule-out CT angiography for evaluation of acute chest pain and possible acute coronary syndrome. *Radiology* 2009;252:332–345.

[59] Takakuwa KM, Halpern EJ, Shofer FS. A time and imaging cost analysis of low-risk ED observation patients: A conservative 64-section computed tomography coronary angiography "triple rule-out" compared to nuclear stress test strategy. *The American Journal of Emergency Medicine* 2011;29:187–195.

[60] Frauenfelder T, Appenzeller P, Karlo C et al. Triple rule-out CT in the emergency department: Protocols and spectrum of imaging findings. *European Radiology* 2009;19:789–799.

[61] Spodick DH. Pericarditis, pericardial effusion, cardiac tamponade, and constriction. *Critical Care Clinics* 1989;5:455–476.

[62] Yelgec NS, Dymarkowski S, Ganame J, Bogaert J. Value of MRI in patients with a clinical suspicion of acute myocarditis. *European Radiology* 2007;17:2211–2217.

[63] Strobel K, Schuler R, Genoni M. Visualization of pericarditis with fluoro-deoxy-glucose-positron emission tomography/computed tomography. *European Heart Journal* 2008;29:1212.

[64] Spodick DH. Risk prediction in pericarditis: Who to keep in hospital? *Heart* 2008;94:398–399.

[65] Lange RA, Hillis LD. Clinical practice. Acute pericarditis. *The New England Journal of Medicine* 2004;351:2195–2202.

[66] Pinamonti B, Alberti E, Cigalotto A et al. Echocardiographic findings in myocarditis. *The American Journal of Cardiology* 1988;62:285–291.

[67] Brett NJ, Strugnell WE, Slaughter RE. Acute myocarditis demonstrated on CT coronary angiography with MRI correlation. *Circulation Cardiovascular Imaging* 2011;4: e5–e6.

[68] Friedrich MG, Sechtem U, Schulz-Menger J et al. Cardiovascular magnetic resonance in myocarditis: A JACC White Paper. *Journal of the American College of Cardiology* 2009;53:1475–1487.

[69] Hundley WG, Bluemke DA, Finn JP et al. ACCF/ACR/AHA/NASCI/SCMR 2010 expert consensus document on cardiovascular magnetic resonance: A report of the American College of Cardiology Foundation Task Force on Expert Consensus Documents. *Journal of the American College of Cardiology* 2010;55:2614–2662.

[70] Francone M, Chimenti C, Galea N et al. CMR sensitivity varies with clinical presentation and extent of cell necrosis in biopsy-proven acute myocarditis. *JACC Cardiovascular Imaging* 2014;7:254–263.

[71] Bertog SC, Thambidorai SK, Parakh K et al. Constrictive pericarditis: Etiology and cause-specific survival after pericardiectomy. *Journal of the American College of Cardiology* 2004;43:1445–1452.

[72] Cameron J, Oesterle SN, Baldwin JC, Hancock EW. The etiologic spectrum of constrictive pericarditis. *American Heart journal* 1987;113:354–360.

[73] Imazio M, Brucato A, Maestroni S et al. Risk of constrictive pericarditis after acute pericarditis. *Circulation* 2011;124:1270–1275.

[74] Schwefer M, Aschenbach R, Heidemann J, Mey C, Lapp H. Constrictive pericarditis, still a diagnostic challenge: Comprehensive review of clinical management. *European Journal of Cardio-Thoracic Surgery: Official Journal of the European Association for Cardio-Thoracic Surgery* 2009;36:502–510.

[75] Nishimura RA. Constrictive pericarditis in the modern era: A diagnostic dilemma. *Heart* 2001;86:619–623.

[76] Ling LH, Oh JK, Breen JF et al. Calcific constrictive pericarditis: Is it still with us? *Annals of Internal Medicine* 2000;132:444–450.

[77] DeValeria PA, Baumgartner WA, Casale AS et al. Current indications, risks, and outcome after pericardiectomy. *The Annals of Thoracic Surgery* 1991;52:219–224.

[78] Uchida T, Bando K, Minatoya K, Sasako Y, Kobayashi J, Kitamura S. Pericardiectomy for constrictive pericarditis using the harmonic scalpel. *The Annals of Thoracic Surgery* 2001;72:924–925.

[79] Soulen RL, Stark DD, Higgins CB. Magnetic resonance imaging of constrictive pericardial disease. *The American Journal of Cardiology* 1985;55:480–484.

[80] Talreja DR, Edwards WD, Danielson GK et al. Constrictive pericarditis in 26 patients with histologically normal pericar-

dial thickness. *Circulation* 2003;108:1852–1857.
[81] Zurick AO, Bolen MA, Kwon DH et al. Pericardial delayed hyperenhancement with CMR imaging in patients with constrictive pericarditis undergoing surgical pericardiectomy: A case series with histopathological correlation. *JACC Cardiovascular Imaging* 2011;4:1180–1191.
[82] Haley JH, Tajik AJ, Danielson GK, Schaff HV, Mulvagh SL, Oh JK. Transient constrictive pericarditis: Causes and natural history. *Journal of the American College of Cardiology* 2004;43:271–275.
[83] Feng D, Glockner J, Kim K et al. Cardiac magnetic resonance imaging pericardial late gadolinium enhancement and elevated inflammatory markers can predict the reversibility of constrictive pericarditis after anti inflammatory medical therapy: A pilot study. *Circulation* 2011;124:1830–1837.
[84] Masui T, Finck S, Higgins CB. Constrictive pericarditis and restrictive cardiomyopathy: Evaluation with MR imaging. *Radiology* 1992;182:369–373.
[85] Hatle LK, Appleton CP, Popp RL. Differentiation of constrictive pericarditis and restrictive cardiomyopathy by Doppler echocardiography. *Circulation* 1989;79:357–370.
[86] Rajagopalan N, Garcia MJ, Rodriguez L et al. Comparison of new Doppler echocardiographic methods to differentiate constrictive pericardial heart disease and restrictive cardiomyopathy. *The American Journal of Cardiology* 2001;87:86–94.
[87] Bauner K, Horng A, Schmitz C, Reiser M, Huber A. New observations from MR velocity-encoded flow measurements concerning diastolic function in constrictive pericarditis. *European Radiology* 2010;20:1831–1840.
[88] Mangia M, Madeo A, Conti B, Galea N. Giant left ventricular pseudoaneurysm following coronary artery bypass graft surgery. *European Journal of Cardio-Thoracic Surgery: Official Journal of the European Association for Cardio-Thoracic Surgery* 2012;41:e21.
[89] Meleca MJ, Hoit BD. Previously unrecognized intrapericardial hematoma leading to refractory abdominal ascites. *Chest* 1995;108:1747–1748.
[90] Brown DL, Ivey TD. Giant organized pericardial hematoma producing constrictive pericarditis: A case report and review of the literature. *The Journal of Trauma* 1996;41:558–560.
[91] Hoffmann U, Globits S, Frank H. Cardiac and paracardiac masses. Current opinion on diagnostic evaluation by magnetic resonance imaging. *European Heart journal* 1998;19:553–563.
[92] Grebenc ML, Rosado de Christenson ML, Burke AP, Green CE, Galvin JR. Primary cardiac and pericardial neoplasms: Radiologic-pathologic correlation. *RadioGraphics: A Review Publication of the Radiological Society of North America, Inc* 2000;20:1073–1103; quiz 1110–1111, 1112.

Chapter 4
头颈部血管成像

Vascular Imaging of the Head and Neck

Miguel Trelles，Tobias Saam 著

李 潇 王 悦 译

王怡宁 校

目录 CONTENTS

一、血管解剖结构 / 58

二、弓上动脉病变 / 62

三、总结 / 87

一、血管解剖结构

磁共振成像（MRI）通过常规平面成像、对比剂增强磁共振血管成像（magnetic resonance angiography, MRA）以及平扫 MRA 可以很好地显示血管解剖结构。传统血管造影更适用于显示小血管，如血管炎的评估，以及介入治疗。图 4-1A 容积再现图像展示最常见的主动脉及其分支走行：左位主动脉弓，主动脉发出右头臂干、左颈总动脉和左锁骨下动脉，双侧锁骨下动脉发出双侧椎动脉。图 4-1B 和 C 展示常见变异，包括牛型主动脉弓（图 4-1B），即双侧颈总动脉共干（其实是误称，牛的解剖并非如此）；右锁骨下动脉由主动脉弓左侧发出（图 4-1C），又称迷走动脉。后者可能引起食管受压，在透视下也可观察到。此类患者可伴右锁骨下动脉起始处扩张，称为 Kommerell 憩室。主动脉弓的重要变异包括右位主动脉弓伴镜像分支，可能与发绀型先天性心脏病相关；以及右位主动脉弓伴左锁骨下动脉变异，虽然与先天性心脏病相关性不及前者那么密切，但血管环压迫气管或食管会引起吸气相喉鸣、喘息、呼吸困难、咳嗽、吞咽困难和反复呼吸道感染等症状[1]。

颈总动脉于 $C_3 \sim C_4$ 水平在颈动脉球部分为颈外动脉和颈内动脉。如后文所述，颈动脉球部是粥样硬化好发部位。颈外动脉依次发出甲状腺上动脉、咽升动脉、舌动脉、面动脉、枕动脉、耳后动脉、颞浅动脉和上颌动脉，对初学者来说很难掌握。为了便于记忆，可以借助顺口溜"她总是喜欢朋友更甚于爸爸、姐姐和妈妈（SALFOPSM）"[2]。图 4-2 展示了颈外动脉主要分支。

颈内动脉可分为 7 段（$C_1 \sim C_7$）[3]：颈段（因其无分支，易与颈外动脉鉴别）、岩段、破裂孔段、海绵窦段、床突段（在此穿过硬膜进入颅内）、眼段和交通段。MRA 可见的第一根分支为眼动脉（眼段）。小分支，如颈鼓动脉、翼管动脉、脑膜垂体干、下侧干以及前床突动脉等，正常情况下在 MRA 上很难看到（图 4-3）。

颅外和颅内循环间有多重吻合通路[4]。当栓塞发生在颅外循环时，这些交通支可为颅内循环

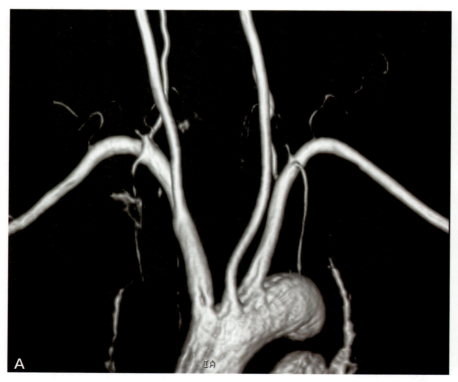
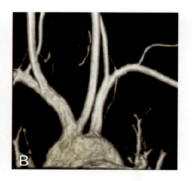
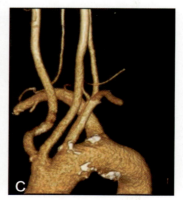

▲ 图 4-1 计算机断层血管成像（computed tomography angiography, CTA）
容积再现图像显示正常主动脉弓（A）、牛型主动脉弓（B）和右锁骨下动脉（C）变异

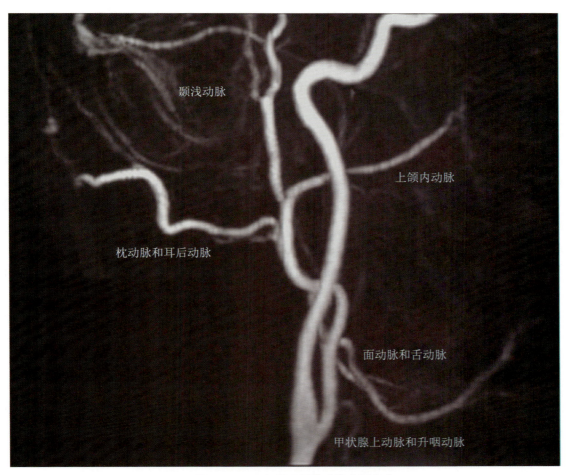

▲ 图 4-2　MRA 显示颈外动脉主要分支

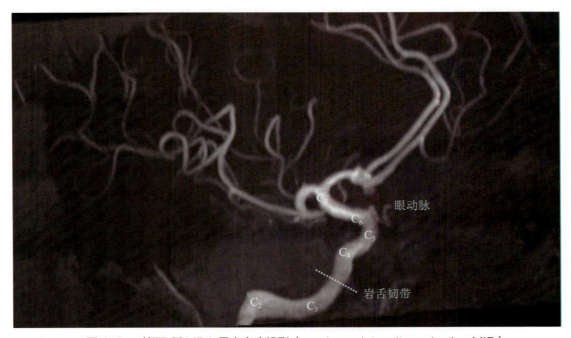

▲ 图 4-3　时间飞跃 MRA 最大密度投影（maximum intensit yprojection,MIP）

侧位像显示颈内动脉颅内段：C_1. 颈段（未显示）；C_2. 岩段；C_3. 破裂孔段；C_4. 海绵窦段；C_5. 床突段；C_6. 眼段；C_7. 交通段

供血，因而具有重要的临床意义。同样的，当颅内循环阻塞时，这些交通支可为其提供侧支循环。

Willis 环是指颅底的一组吻合动脉系统，由双侧颈内动脉和基底动脉远端分支，即双侧大脑前动脉（anterior cerebral arteries, ACA）A_1 段、前交通动脉（anterior communicating artery, AComm）、双侧后交通动脉（posterior communicating artery, PComm）和基底动脉末端构成动脉环或五边形（图 4-4）。当单侧甚至双侧血管狭窄时，可通过侧支循环保证大脑供血而避免生命危险。常见的解剖学变异包括节段性发育不全及动脉环不完整，拥有完整 Willis 环的人群占比不到 50%[5,6]。

椎动脉一般由锁骨下动脉发出，分为4段。V_1 段，走行于颈长肌和前斜角肌之间；V_2 段，依次穿过 C_6 ~ C_2 横突孔；V_3 段，穿过 C_1 横突孔，绕过后关节突进入脊柱管；V_4 段，穿过硬膜，与对侧椎动脉交通构成基底动脉。解剖变异包括起始于主动脉弓，或较为罕见地起始于颈总动脉[7]。重要的分支包括脊髓前动脉、小脑后下动脉（postero-inferior cerebellar arptery, PICA）。基底动脉发出小脑前下动脉（anterior inferior cerebellar artery, AICA）、小脑上动脉（superior cerebellar artery, SCA）、脑桥穿支动脉，终止于大脑后动脉（posterior cerebral artery, PCA）。

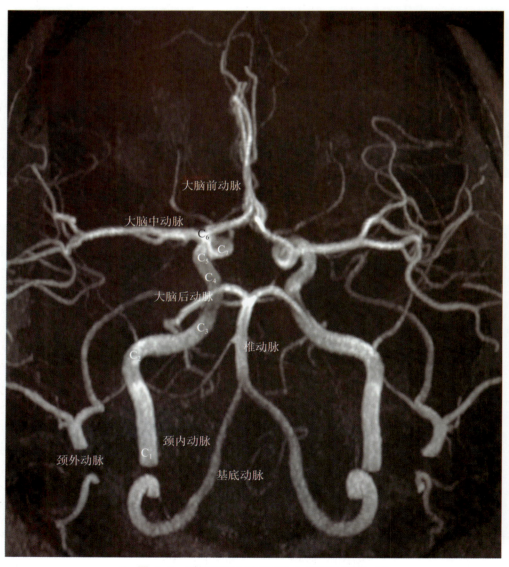

▲ 图 4-4　时间飞跃 MRAMIP 上位相示 Willis 环
右侧标注了主要组成动脉和颈内动脉

Percheron动脉为一种解剖学上的变异，起源于PCA近端可能为双侧内侧丘脑供血[8]。

（一）血管壁组织学

血管壁由内膜、中膜和外膜三层构成。最里层为内膜，由血管内皮和薄层结缔组织支撑组成。中膜由不同比例的平滑肌细胞和弹力组织组成。弹性动脉弹力组织比例最高，而肌性动脉平滑肌比例最高。中膜和内膜间有一层连续的弹力组织，即内弹力膜。外膜由纤维结缔组织组成，可与血管周围的脏器间质结缔组织相延续。外膜也可有大量的弹性纤维。不同的动脉、小动脉、毛细血管、小静脉和静脉以及不同部位的血管具有不同的成分。

（二）血管成像

血管腔内支架植入手术的发展需要对血管狭窄部位、受累长度以及基于直径、面积或血流情况所测定的血管狭窄程度等许多数据的精准测算[9]。利用时间飞跃（time-of-flight, TOF）和相位对比MRA等平扫或增强技术可以显示血管腔情况；利用黑血成像可以显示血管壁；利用相位对比成像可以分析血流速度。应根据研究对象和预期效果来选择特定的扫描序列。下面简要介绍几种常用技术。

1. TOF MRA TOF MRA是通过显示流动血来实现血管成像的平扫技术。简单来说，通过成像平面的血流未受射频脉冲的影响而无纵向磁化衰减，因此在梯度回波序列上呈T_1高信号。TOF成像利用短重复时间（repetition time, TR）和大翻转角进一步弱化背景（静态）组织信号而优化血流信号。需要注意的是，TOF是基于T_1加权的成像，高铁血红蛋白和脂肪也呈高信号。TOF成像可一次采集获得一幅图像（2D）或一系列图像（3D）。后者更为推荐，可减少图像间由于运动产生的空间误配准，甚至可利用更短的回波时间（echo time, TE）减弱背景信号和伪影。此外，高场强下信噪比也能进一步改善。

主要的缺点是，狭窄或分支附近的复杂血流容易产生信号缺失，从而引起过轻、过重评价或误诊。总体来说，3D TOF操作方便、应用广泛，是颅内血管无创评价的理想一线检查。

2. 对比剂增强MRA 增强MRA分别在对比剂注射前和血管内对比剂浓度最高时采集图像，利用类似CTA的高压单次快注和对比剂追踪触发方法。序列扫描时间把控十分重要，最终成像效果取决于K空间中心填充时的血管内钆浓度，而非序列扫描中点的浓度。增强MRA比TOF MRA空间分辨率更高、血流相关伪影更少，但需要注射对比剂并承担相关风险，一般用于颈动脉球部、主动脉及其他分支狭窄的评估[10]。

动态、高时间分辨率增强MRA是一种对比剂单次快注超速3D成像新技术。扫描过程中仅填充K空间中心及周边部分，其余部分则由多个时间点的数据重建而得，因而大大减少了单位体积扫描时间。该技术可用于颅内或颅外血管畸形、动静脉瘘的初次或随访无创评估[11,12]，当然DSA仍是金标准。

3. 相位对比MRA 相位对比MRA可以分析成像层面的血流速度。通过磁场梯度的血流由于局部磁场的不同而进动速度不同，并产生相位偏移。相位偏移最终取决于血流途经距离，而后者取决于血流速度。若血管横截面已知，便可计算血流速度和压力差。相位对比MRA不仅可用于血流评估，在中枢神经系统中，还可用于导水管或枕骨大孔狭窄时脑脊液流动的评估[13]。

（三）黑血成像

血管病变常起始于血管壁，而前述成像方法以显示管腔为主，对血管疾病的诊断和鉴别诊断价值有限。增强扫描可以区别血管壁的炎性和非炎性病变，对诊断和治疗非常重要。大多数MRA技术致力于获得血管腔高信号而压低背景信号；而黑血成像相反，通过压低管腔信号来显示血管壁、避免流入或搏动伪影。进一步地，通过压脂可以更好地显示出血、水肿或炎症。该技术利用扫描过程中血液持续流动的特性，借助一系列反转脉冲可以实现成像（图 4-5）。颈部冠状位图像（图 4-5A），动脉显示为红色。初始非选择性射频脉冲（图 4-5B）激发平面内包括组织和血流在内的所有自旋。灰色为被激发区域。层面选择性反转射频脉冲（图 4-5C）将选定区域内的自旋反转。高亮区域为接受两种脉冲的组织（图 4-5D）。短暂的停顿后，激发的血流流出选定区域，被反转的血流替代。只有接受两种脉冲的静态组织被显像，动态血流由于未被编码而不显影。

二、弓上动脉病变

头颈部可发生多种血管性疾病，临床表现多种多样，如头痛、脑病、癫痫、头晕和视觉障碍等，其中失明、短暂性缺血发作和卒中的发病率和死亡率很高[14]。常见炎性病变包括中枢神经系统

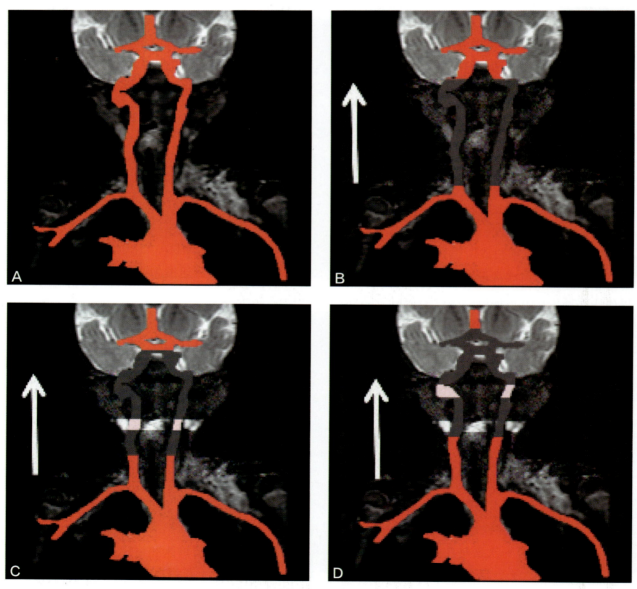

▲ 图 4-5 黑血成像

A. 颈部冠状位图像，红色为主要动脉；B. 初始非选择性射频脉冲激发平面内包括组织和血流在内的所有自旋。灰色为被激发区域；C. 层面选择性反转射频脉冲将选定区域内的自旋反转。高亮区域为接受两种脉冲的组织；D. 短暂的停顿后，激发的血流流出选定区域，被反转的血流替代。只有接受两种脉冲的静态组织被显像，动态血流由于未被编码而不显影

动脉炎、大动脉炎、巨细胞动脉炎和颈动脉周围炎等，非炎性病变如肌纤维发育不良、可逆性血管收缩综合征和 CADASIL 综合征等。动脉粥样硬化是一类慢性炎性疾病，但兼具炎性和非炎性病变的特点。此外，任何血管壁异常都可能继发夹层或动脉瘤形成。颅内小动脉瘤将在第 24 章讨论。

（一）动脉粥样硬化

1. 颈动脉球部粥样硬化 动脉粥样硬化以胆固醇等脂质在血管壁内膜的慢性沉积为特点，脂质聚结形成粥样斑块时可引起动脉壁内膜周围的炎症反应。图 4-6 展示了粥样斑块不同发展阶段的组织学切片。斑块钙化、融入血管壁重塑之后血管腔大致正常是最好的临床结局（图 4-6）[15]。粥样斑块也可向腔内生长、压迫管腔导致进行性狭窄。如果这一过程足够慢，侧支循环形成并足以保证远端血流灌注。但斑块表面也可能破裂并释放促血栓成分（图 4-6），继而引起远端栓塞性卒中和（或）原位梗阻性狭窄伴远端灌注压减低。根据侧支循环的情况（以及 Willis 环的开放程度），可表现为分水岭卒中或区域性梗死。根据 TOAST 分类，17%～20% 的缺血性卒中归咎于大血管粥样硬化，其中 80%～90% 由斑块破裂导致，10%～20% 由血管重度狭窄或闭塞导致；25% 归咎于小血管疾病；15%～27% 归咎于心源性栓塞；35% 未定论，并有一定比例源于非狭窄性斑块破裂 [16-19]。

常规血管腔成像方法只能诊断管腔狭窄，而黑血成像可以详细分析斑块成分和形态。NASCET 标准计算颈内动脉最狭窄节段和远端正常节段的狭窄百分比，与未来卒中事件具有相关性 [20]，是评价血栓栓塞事件风险和治疗（内膜剥脱术）指征的金标准（图 4-7）。需要注意，同样的公式用面积计算狭窄程度会比用直径计算更准确。增强 MRA 是观察颈动脉球狭窄的常用方法 [10]。

高分辨率 MRI 可以识别动脉粥样硬化的不同时期，包括斑块并发症，有助于动脉粥样硬化疾病的评估。Cai 等 [21] 基于动脉粥样硬化不同时期的 AHA 病理分型，提出改良的 AHA MRI 分型（表 4-1）。同一血管都可能有不同部位不同类别的病灶，以最严重的类别为准。斑块并发症包括斑块内出血、纤维帽破裂和附壁血栓，归为 AHA VI（AHA LT:VI）型病灶，是独立于管腔狭窄的卒中危险因素 [22,23]。

表 4-2 总结了不同斑块成分的 MRI 信号特点。正常血管壁以及病灶的纤维成分可有强化。脂质坏死核（lipid-rich necrotic core, LR-NC）在

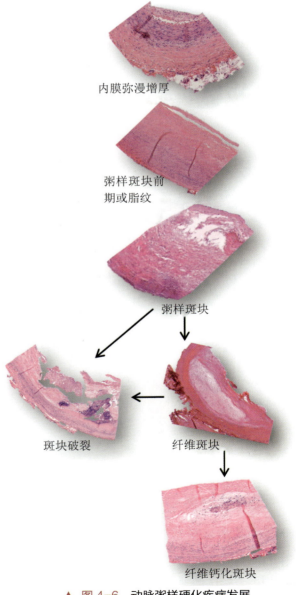

▲ 图 4-6 动脉粥样硬化疾病发展

表 4-1　基于 MRI 的动脉粥样硬化斑块管壁成分改良 AHA 分型

传统 AHA 病理分型	改良 AHA MRI 分型
Ⅰ型：早期病变伴泡沫细胞	Ⅰ～Ⅱ型：血管壁厚度基本正常，无钙化
Ⅱ型：脂纹伴多层泡沫细胞	
Ⅲ型：粥样斑块前病变伴细胞外脂滴	Ⅲ型：内膜弥漫增厚，或偏心小斑块不伴钙化
Ⅳ型：粥样斑块伴细胞外脂核	Ⅳ～Ⅴ型：斑块伴脂核或坏死核，周围伴纤维组织，可伴钙化
Ⅴ型：纤维斑块	
Ⅵ型：复杂斑块伴血栓形成、出血或纤维帽破裂	Ⅵ型：复杂斑块伴血栓形成、出血或纤维帽破裂
Ⅶ型：钙化斑块	Ⅶ型：钙化斑块
Ⅷ型：纤维斑块不伴脂核	Ⅷ型：纤维斑块不伴脂核，可伴小钙化

引自 Cai J M et al., Circulation, 106（11），1368–1373, 2002.

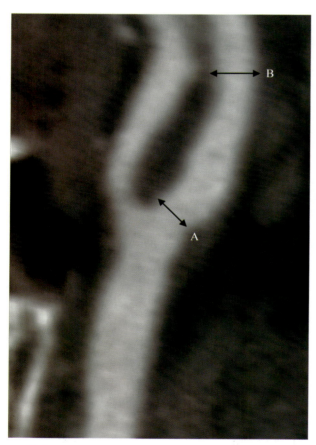

▲ 图 4-7　NASCET 标准测量狭窄程度 =（B-A）/B
A. 最狭窄处直径；B. 狭窄远端正常血管直径

表 4-2　斑块成分 MRI 信号特点

	TOF	T_1	PD	T_2	强化
正常	o	o	o	o	-/ 轻度
粥样斑块前病变	o	o	o	o	-/ 轻度
粥样斑块	o/+	o/+	-	-	无
1 型出血	+	+	-/o	-/o	无
2 型出血	+	+	+	+	无
钙化	-	-			无

高分辨率黑血 MRI T_1、T_2 压脂加权相上均呈等信号，增强呈低信号，可与周围纤维成分清楚鉴别。LR-NC 伴出血在 TOF 和 T_1 加权像均呈高信号；T_2 信号取决于出血的期别，细胞内高铁血红蛋白呈低信号（1 型或早期亚急性出血），而细胞外高铁血红蛋白呈高信号（2 型或晚期亚急性出血）[24]。钙化在所有序列上均呈低信号，不伴周围强化。

正常血管（AHA LT：Ⅰ～Ⅱ）管壁较薄（图 4-8）。粥样斑块前病变（AHA LT：Ⅲ）可见血管壁弥漫或局部轻度增厚（3～4mm），不伴脂质坏死核（图 4-9）。粥样斑块（AHA LT：Ⅳ～Ⅴ）可见不同成分信号的脂质坏死核，但大致与血管壁等信号（图 4-10，白色箭头），无强化是其与纤维组织的主要鉴别依据（图 4-10F，箭头）。CT 可以显示软斑块成分（图 4-10A，黑箭头），虽然较大的软斑块更有可能是复杂斑块[25]，但并不能准确鉴别 AHA LT：Ⅳ～Ⅴ 和 Ⅵ。

复杂斑块（AHA LT：Ⅵ）的特点为伴出血、

Chapter 4 头颈部血管成像
Vascular Imaging of the Head and Neck

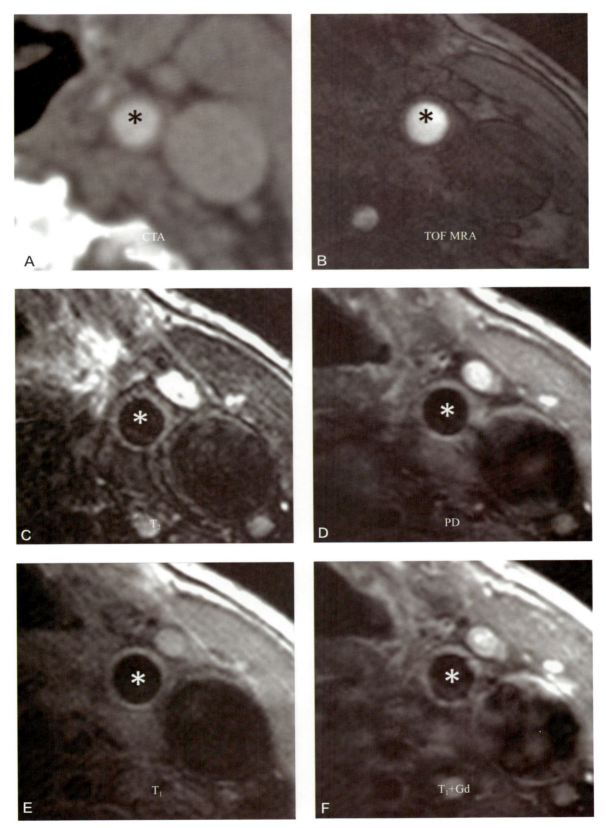

▲ 图 4-8 55 岁患者，无症状

CTA 轴位（A）、TOF MRA（B）和高分辨率压脂黑血 T_2 加权（C）、质子像（D）、T_1 加权（E）、增强（F）图像显示左颈总动脉远端血管壁厚度正常伴正常轻度强化

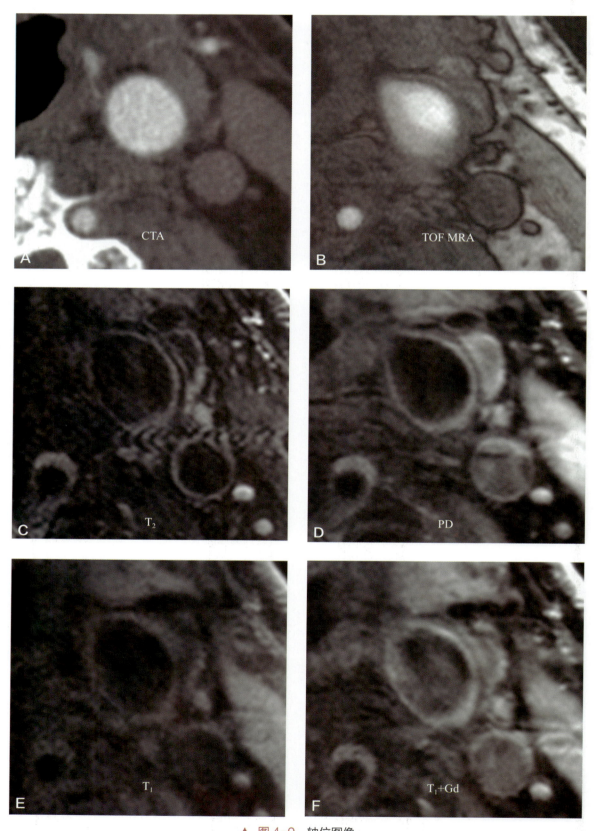

▲ 图 4-9 轴位图像

显示左侧颈总动脉分支处略近端血流动力学 5 点钟方向内膜轻度增厚

Chapter 4 头颈部血管成像
Vascular Imaging of the Head and Neck

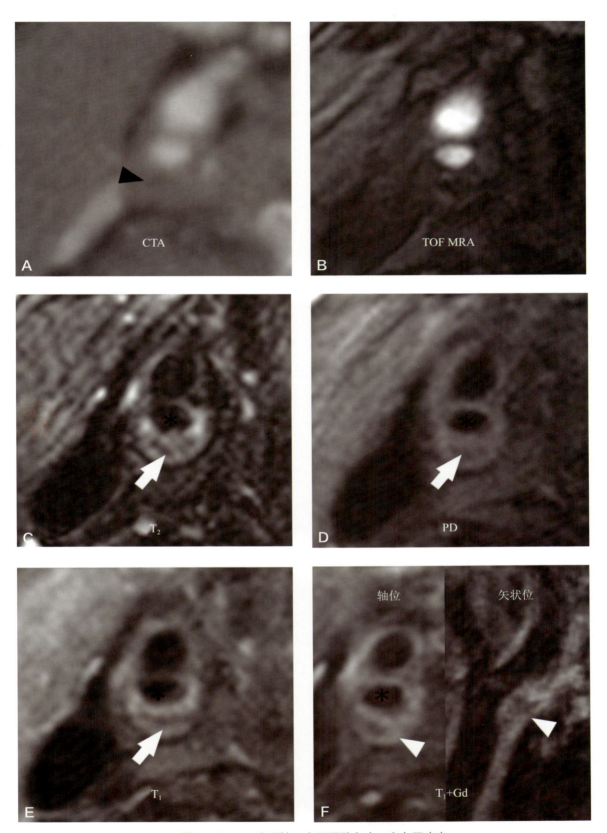

▲ 图 4-10 54 岁男性，高胆固醇血症、高血压病史

右侧颈总动脉分支处管壁增厚较大粥样斑块，CT 值减低（A，黑色箭头），MRI 平扫各序列呈低信号（C～E，白箭），周围伴 T_2 高信号和轻度强化（F，箭头）

易促血栓形成的表面缺损（纤维帽破裂）或血栓。出血呈平扫 T_1 高信号；而 T_2 加权像或质子像可呈低、中等或略高信号，取决于出血时间和成分。图 4-11 显示软斑块内 TOF 和 T_1（白色箭）高信号、无强化成分，提示出血。血栓表现为附壁薄层高信号，可有强化。图 4-12 显示血栓呈 T_2 高信号伴强化，管腔几乎完全闭塞（*）。纤维帽破裂可表现为：①TOF 和（或）T_1 增强图像上低信号帽缺失；②管腔表面不规则；③TOF MRA 上管腔和管壁间连续高信号。理想情况下三者皆备才能诊断。图 4-13（白色箭头）和图 4-14 显示出血性斑块和血管腔之间低信号纤维帽破裂。

钙化斑块（AHA LT：Ⅶ）在 MRI 上较难观察。大多数斑块或多或少伴有钙化，需要对每一处病灶进行评估，以病变最重的节段为准。图 4-15 显示钙化斑块在 CTA 上易见，但在 MRI 上呈低信号而较难发现。钙化容易与管腔或脂质坏死核混淆，鉴别需要结合亮血和黑血图像。在 T_1 加权图像上（图 4-15E），附壁低信号区易被误认为是管腔的一部分；而在质子和 T_2 加权图像上（图 4-15C、D），表现类似脂质坏死核或粥样斑块。如果有条件，最好结合 CTA 和 TOF 图像诊断。

纤维斑块（AHA LT：Ⅷ）在颈动脉较少见，表现为血管壁环周增厚伴斑块纤维化，进而引起重度狭窄或闭塞（图 4-16）。纤维斑块见于动脉粥样硬化进程的晚期，多由于慢性炎性反应伴瘢痕形成导致，常伴钙化和狭窄管腔环周轻度强化。

颈动脉狭窄的治疗取决于血管狭窄程度以及患者症状、性别和其他危险因素，不同国家地区的指南不同。根据 NASCET 标准，70% 以上狭窄可选择颈动脉内膜剥脱术或支架植入，非狭窄性的复杂斑块以药物治疗为主。

2. 颅内动脉粥样硬化 动脉粥样硬化是可累及所有血管床的系统性疾病。颅内动脉受累可无症状，也可引起狭窄、闭塞或栓塞。短暂性脑缺血发作或卒中是主要的终点事件，血管性痴呆在老年化西方国家的发病率逐渐升高。颅内动脉粥样硬化占卒中的 5%~10%[18]，在亚洲人群更为常见，同时也是复发性卒中的危险因素。大脑中动脉狭窄相关卒中的发生机制可能包括原位血栓形成、血管源性栓塞、穿支动脉闭塞和低灌注等[26]。

TOF MRA 具有快速、无创的优点，是颅内血管的首选筛查方法。在高场强下，信噪比和空间分辨率还能有所提高。主要的缺点是对小血管和狭窄远端的慢血流显示欠佳，容易过判狭窄程度。因此，TOF MRA 检出的异常需要结合增强 MRA、CTA 或 DSA 进一步检查，特别是在拟行介入操作前，诊断差异极大程度影响治疗方案时。

高分辨率黑血 MRI 可以显示颅内血管斑块，表现为管壁局部偏心不规则增厚伴管腔狭窄。斑块的强化程度与斑块稳定性和缺血事件相关[27]。图 4-17 黑血图像显示左侧大脑中动脉粥样硬化斑块可见强化，提示斑块不稳定。受分辨率所限，目前尚不能显示粥样斑块和出血等斑块并发症[28]。与其他部位的血管不同，颅内动脉缺乏滋养血管，其动脉粥样硬化进程的研究成果有限[29]。

颅内动脉粥样硬化的治疗仍存在争议，最近的研究认为积极的药物治疗优于血管成形术或支架植入[30]。

脑负荷试验是评估大脑通过自主调节机制维持正常血流能力的新技术[31]。类似心脏负荷试验，通过给予刺激物诱发血管舒张，增加正常血管供血区域的血流灌注，导致狭窄动脉的盗血现象或血管扩张减低，从而引起狭窄区域的灌注减少。负荷药物可用颅内血管扩张药如二氧化碳或乙酰唑胺[32]，成像方法可用灌注 MRI 或 BOLD（见第 1 章和第 7 章）。负荷前后的结果对比反映了大脑血流储备情况，有助于预测未来缺血事件风险并指导治疗，但是否能普遍应用于临床还未可知。

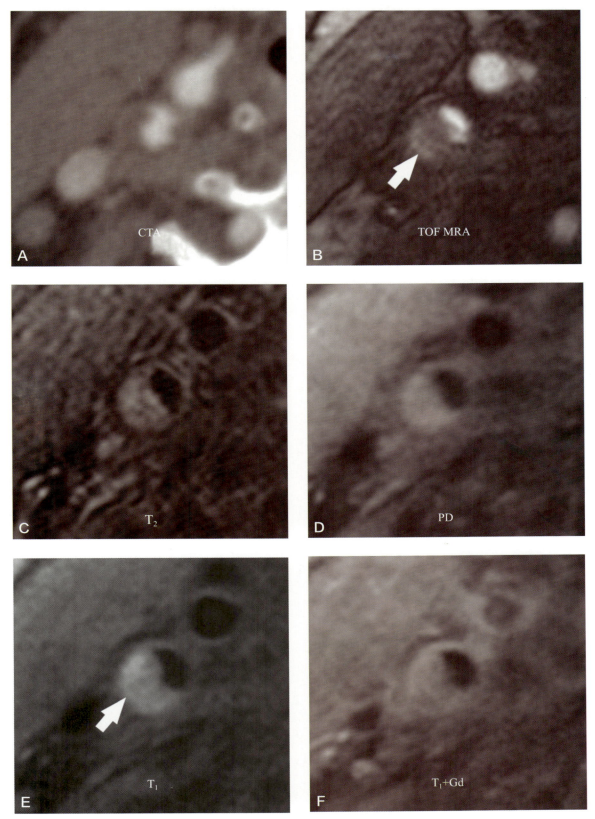

▲ 图 4-11　64 岁男性，右侧前循环卒中

轴位图像显示右侧颈总动脉分支处远端软斑块。CTA 可见斑块溃疡（矢状位重建更清晰）。TOF 和 T_1 加权图像可见斑块内高信号无强化成分（B、E，箭），提示脂质坏死核内出血，符合 AHA：Ⅵ型斑块

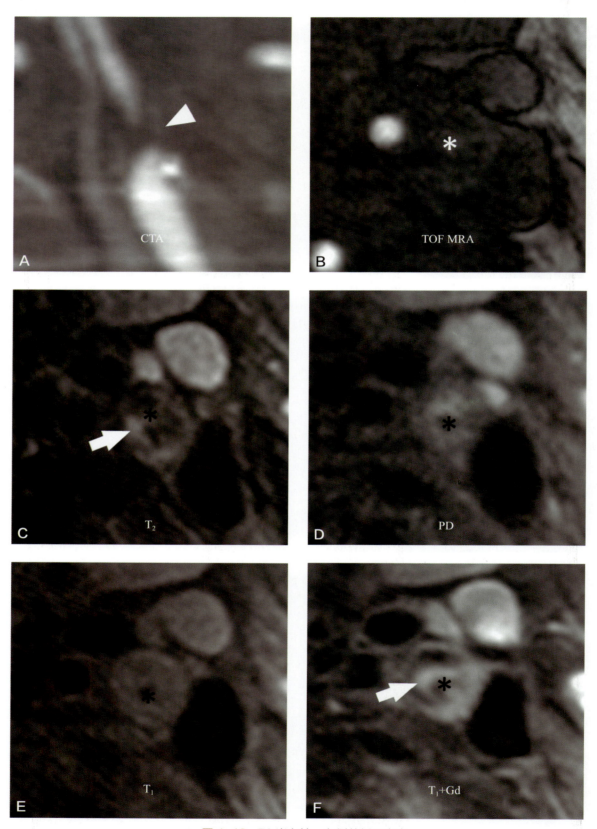

▲ 图 4-12 78 岁女性，左侧前循环卒中

CTA 矢状位图像显示左侧颈内动脉近端管腔几乎完全闭塞，腔内充盈缺损（箭头）。MRI 显示管腔几乎完全闭塞（*），腔内 T_2 高信号伴强化（C、F，白箭），提示附壁血栓形成

Chapter 4 头颈部血管成像
Vascular Imaging of the Head and Neck

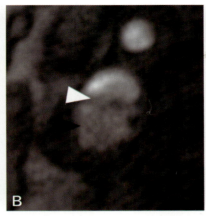
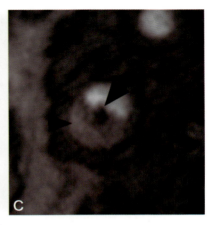

▲ 图 4-13　67 岁男性，右侧前循环 TIA

连续 TOF MRI 轴位图像显示斑块内出血呈血管壁高信号区（黑箭头）。颈内动脉近端可见完整纤维低信号带（A，白箭），远端纤维带破裂（B，白色箭头），更远端可见湍流（C，黑箭）

（二）非炎性病变

1. 肌纤维发育不良　肌纤维发育不良是一种少见的、通常无明显表现的、非炎性、非粥样硬化改变的中、小动脉病变。好发于女性，发病年龄一般在 20—40 岁。最常累及肾动脉（60%～75%），其次为颈动脉（25%～30%）。实际上，肌纤维发育不良可见于所有血管。具体致病机制目前尚不清楚，可能与遗传、环境、激素水平及吸烟等多因素相关。主要按照肌纤维发育不良的具体位置进行分类[33]。1 型，即中层肌纤维发育不良，最为常见（85%），主要累及中等动脉。图 4-18 显示了该型的典型表现，长节段血管多发狭窄、扩张交替出现，即所谓的"串珠状"改变。2 型，即内膜肌纤维发育不良，仅见于不到 10% 的患者。典型表现为局灶性的向心性狭窄。也可以表现为长节段的血管光滑变窄，易误诊为大动脉炎，尤其是 Takayasu 动脉炎。3 型，即外膜增生，是最少见的，血流动力学占不到 5%。血管形态不规则增加了动脉瘤、狭窄、夹层、动静脉瘘或栓塞形成的危险因素[34]。

任一型颈动脉肌纤维发育不良都很少见于颈总动脉起始处及双侧颈动脉分叉前，血管中段更容易发病，尤其是 C_1～C_2 段。与血管炎的鉴别点在于：向心性的管壁狭窄、强化，黑血图像显示血管周水肿。

治疗方案取决于狭窄的位置、狭窄程度，是否出现动脉瘤及病程、症状、年龄、并发症。可以选择抗血小板治疗、抗凝治疗、经皮血管成形术或外科手术[35]。目前尚无关于治疗方案、药物等的随机对照试验结果，主要依靠"经验"性治疗[36]。

2. 动脉夹层　动脉夹层主要是指内膜撕裂，血液从撕裂口处流入由内膜及外膜形成的假腔内。假腔可以不断扩张、挤压真腔甚至闭塞，导致远端灌注减低；或者不断挤压外膜，形成动脉瘤样的外凸影，被称作"夹层动脉瘤"，这会对周围组织造成占位效应如神经受压，也容易形成栓塞。并且，夹层处血栓形成堵塞，可导致远端缺血[36]。

具体病理生理学机制目前尚不明确，但是基础疾病如结缔组织病，遗传因素，环境因素如外伤、感染、血管炎性改变等是部分患者的危险因素或致病因素[37]。

近年来，动脉夹层被认为可导致 TIA 或卒中，可自发或见于外伤后。虽然自发的夹层较为少见，却是 < 50 岁患者卒中的重要原因[38]。所有颈髓受伤累及横突孔的患者都不能除外椎动脉夹层。

影像学表现包括长节段管腔狭窄，"串珠状"改变、T_1 压脂像假腔内或血管壁上高铁血红蛋白形成的高信号。最近的研究表明，局限

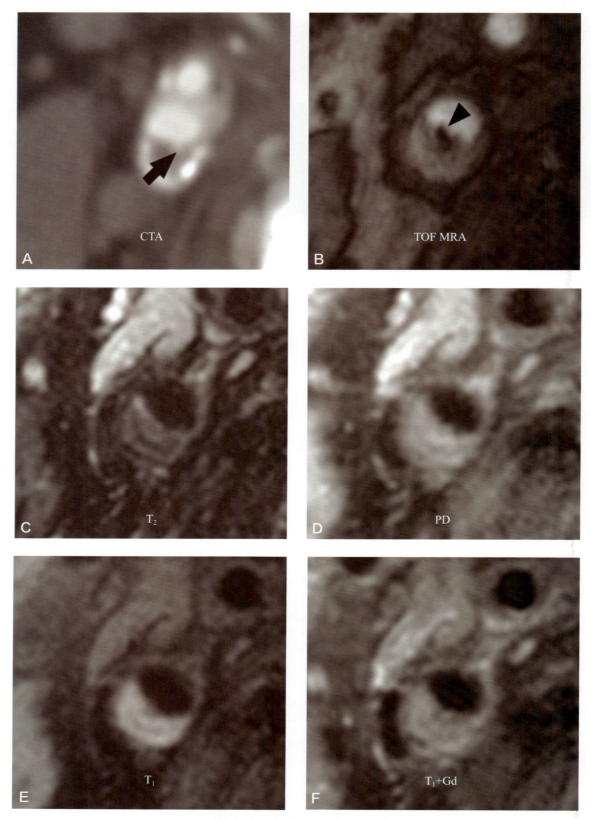

▲ 图 4-14 与图 4-13 为同一患者

CTA 示右侧颈总动脉分支处略远端 7 点钟方向结构欠规则（A，黑箭；可为管腔不规则或钙化）。TOF MRA（B，黑箭头）可见湍流伪影，质子像（D）无光晕，不符合钙化。同时，T_1 加权图像和 TOF 可见斑块内出血

Chapter 4 头颈部血管成像
Vascular Imaging of the Head and Neck

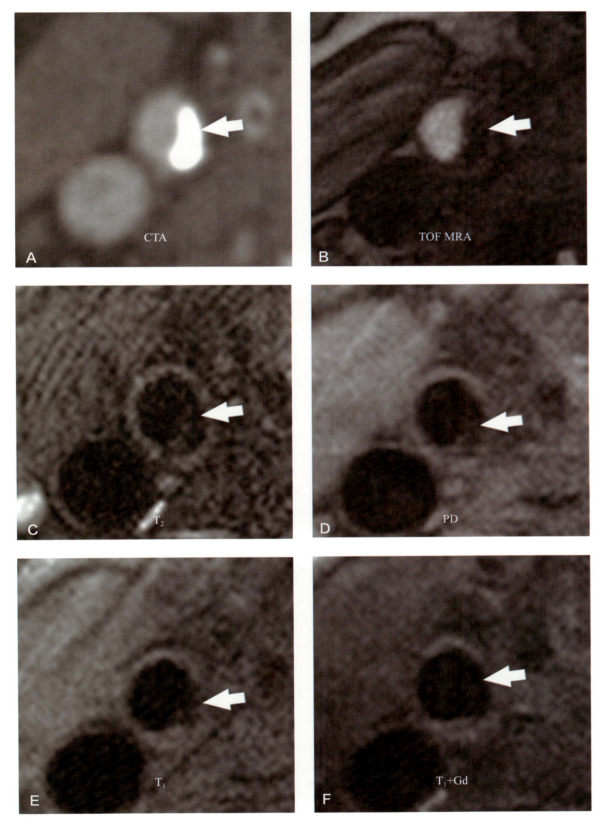

▲ 图 4-15 67 岁男性，糖尿病病史

CTA 上易见右侧颈内动脉近端钙化斑块（A，白箭）。而在 MRI 上各序列呈低信号（B～F），需结合亮血和黑血序列才能准确诊断

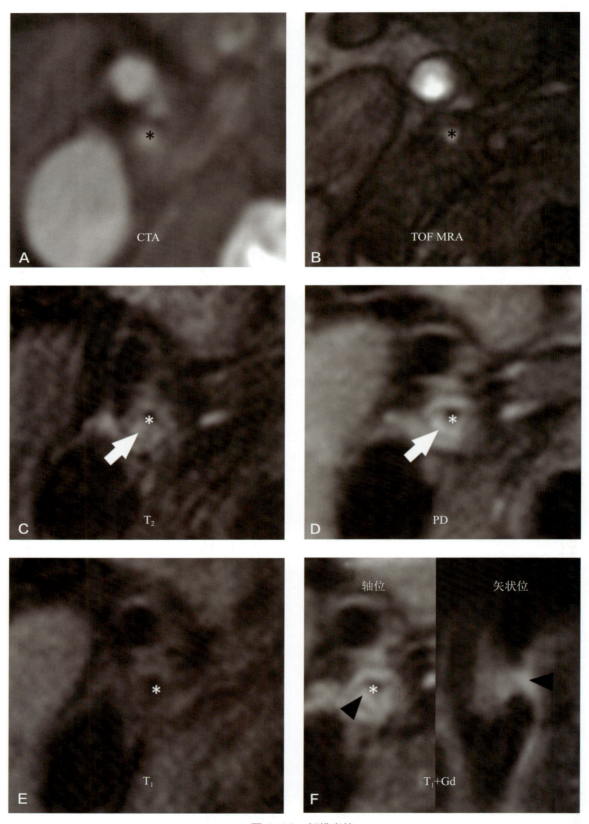

▲ 图 4-16 纤维斑块

管腔环周狭窄（*），伴 7 点钟方向管壁 T_2 和质子像高信号（白箭）及强化（黑箭头），提示疏松的纤维间质或血栓

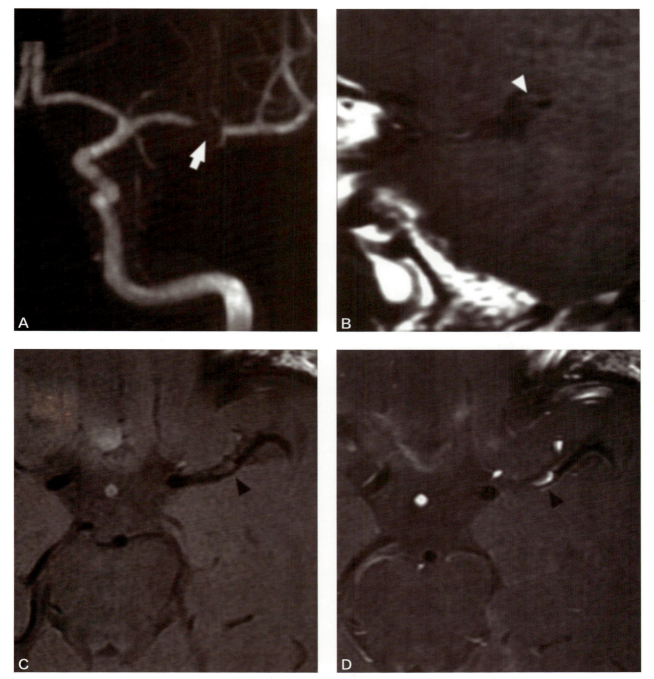

▲ 图 4-17 颅内动脉粥样硬化

A.TOFMRA 最大密度投影图像显示左侧大脑中动脉局部狭窄（白箭）；B. 矢状位 T_1 FLAIR 图像显示前上侧管壁偏心增厚（白色箭头）；轴位 T_1 黑血 FLAIR 平扫（C）和增强（D）显示管壁增厚处斑块强化（黑箭头），提示斑块不稳定（由 Dr. D. Mikulis 提供；引自 Swartz RH, Bhuta SS, Farb RI et al. Intracranial arterial wall imaging using high-resolution 3-tesla contrast-enhanced MRI. Neurology. 2009;72:627–634.）

性强化是夹层的一个常见表现[37]。在 TOF MRA 图上，一定要注意鉴别假腔内高铁血红蛋白的高信号，这极易被误诊为正常血流高信号（图 4-19）。图 4-20 显示了右侧颈内动脉长节段闭塞，以及血管壁的 T_1 高信号（红箭），代表假腔内血栓。夹层动脉瘤向外突出后与动脉瘤形态相似，也都会对周围结构产生占位效应。

治疗方案仍有争议，主要是根据临床表现、

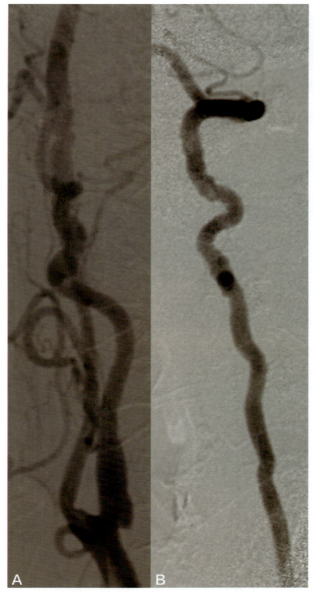

▲ 图 4-18 肌纤维发育不良

两例伴有血管长节段多发狭窄及扩长，即"串珠状"改变的患者，分别为 1 型 ICA（A）和椎动脉肌纤维发育不良（B）

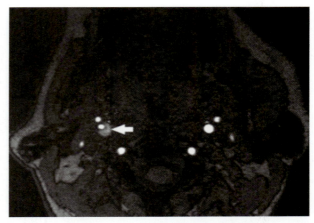

▲ 图 4-19 上颈部 TOF 血管成像

显示右侧颈内动脉自发夹层，可见假腔血管壁 T_1 高信号，MIP 图上易被误诊为血流信号

患者基础情况综合考虑，可进行保守治疗、抗凝治疗或者支架置入[39,40]。

3. 可逆性血管收缩综合征 可逆性血管收缩综合征（reversible cerebral vasoconstriction syndrome, RCVS）也叫 Call-Fleming 综合征，是一种以雷击样头痛、一过性多发脑血管收缩、局灶性神经症状、伴或不伴卒中为表现的少见综合征。诊断主要是排除其他常见病因，如动脉瘤破裂、血管炎及数周内临床症状自行缓解、影像学征象自行消失等。大脑凸面蛛网膜下腔出血是常见表现，当见到此征象时，影像诊断者应考虑该病的可能。导致颅内血管收缩的机制尚不明确，但某些药物被认为是诱发因素[41,42]。女性发病较男性多见。

初次影像学检查经常只能发现大脑凸面蛛网膜下腔积血[43]。MRI 可以发现分水岭区缺血表现。TOF MRA 得到的 Willis 环是一线的非有创性检查，但所有病变仍需经 DSA 证实。血管造影图上"香肠-细线"征或"串珠状"改变是诊断标志。主要需要与中枢神经系统血管炎鉴别，但难以通过血管腔内成像鉴别。近期研究报道认为，黑血图像上血管壁高强化有助于与中枢神经系统血管炎相鉴别[44]。临床病史及实验室检查有助于两者鉴别。新近发展的颅内血管黑血成像结合临床病史及实验室检查有助于诊断。

图 4-21 显示了 1 例伴有大脑凸面出血的典型 RCVS 患者，FLAIR 上分水岭区异常信号提示缺血性改变。图 4-22 显示了 DSA 证实颈内动脉远端、双侧大脑中动脉、双侧大脑前动脉轻中度收缩。1 个月后随诊图像显示血管收缩已缓解。

治疗方案尚有争议，可以确定的是，这是一种自限性病变。血管内注射钙通道阻滞药如尼莫地平、硝苯地平、维拉帕米以及血管成形术也不同程度有效[45,46]。

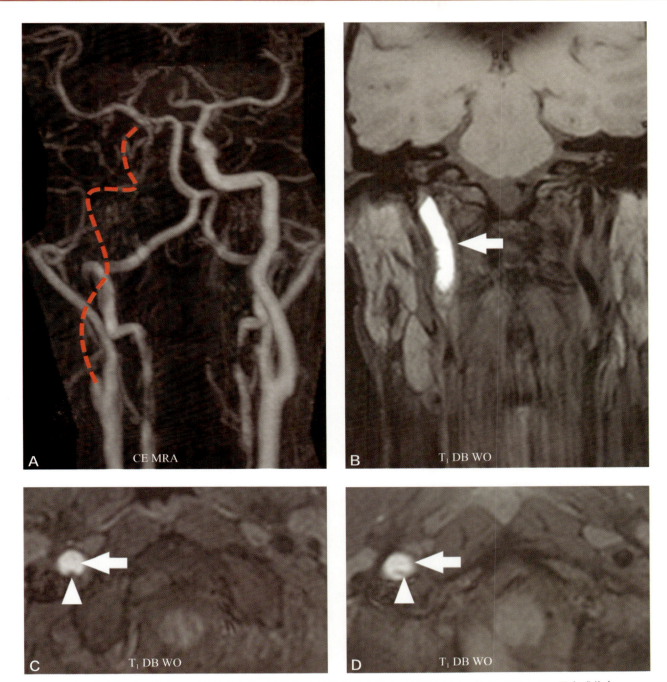

▲ 图 4-20 26 岁女性，增强后血管减影 MRAMIP（CEMRA：增强 MRA，T_1DBWO，T_1 黑血成像）
A. 显示右侧颈内动脉长节段狭窄，虚线代表的是未显影血管走行；B～D. 血管壁 T_1 高信号（白箭）代表假腔内血栓；C、D. 轴位图像上高信号呈半月形。黑血图上真腔表现为一个小黑点（C～D，箭头）

4. CADASIL 综合征 伴皮质下梗死及宾斯旺格病的常染色体显性遗传性脑动脉病（cerebral autosomal dominant arteriopathy with subcortical infarcts and leukoencephalopathy, CADASIL）是导致成年人卒中及血管性痴呆最常见的遗传因素。以偏头痛、TIA、缺血性卒中、抑郁、渐进性痴呆以及发展至行走困难、死亡为特征。平均发病年龄在 40—60 岁。从确诊到死亡平均持续时间为 23 年。

MRI 上异常影像学表现常早于临床症状，因此有助于临床医师早期诊断。最重要的影像学征象是比随年龄增长导致退行性变更明显的

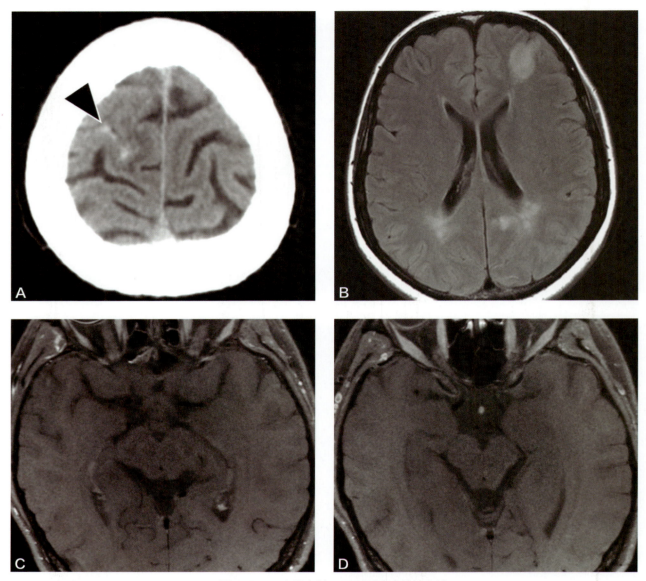

▲ 图 4-21 51 岁女性，因剧烈头痛就诊急诊

A. 平扫头 CT 显示大脑凸面血肿（箭头）；B. 轴位 FLAIR 上多发异常信号显示分水岭区缺血性改变；C、D. 颅底黑血增强图像未见明显异常强化

弥漫性白质病变，并且不伴有脱髓鞘病变的典型表现。诊断主要依靠排除其他更为常见的白质病变以及渐进性病程。颞叶前部、额叶上部白质（图 4-23A、B）和外囊受累是特征性表现[47]。病变初期，皮质下 μ 纤维不被累及。梯度回波成像或磁敏感成像（susceptibility weighted imaging，SWI）可发现多发微出血灶[48]。病变后期由于铁沉积（图 4-23C）可出现皮质下 T_2 低信号及 FLAIR 异常信号[49]。尽管这些表现有助于诊断，但无一是 CADASIL 的特征性表现。影像诊断医师的作用主要在于提示临床医师考虑该病的可能性，尤其对于年轻的、无明确其他诊断的患者。

图 4-24 显示了病变在长达 15 年时间的发展变化。到目前为止，没有任何疗法可以延缓病变发展。

（三）炎性病变

1. 中枢神经系统血管炎　中枢神经系统（central nervous system，CNS）血管炎是一种异质性炎性改变，首先累及柔脑膜及脑实质血管、

Chapter 4　头颈部血管成像
Vascular Imaging of the Head and Neck

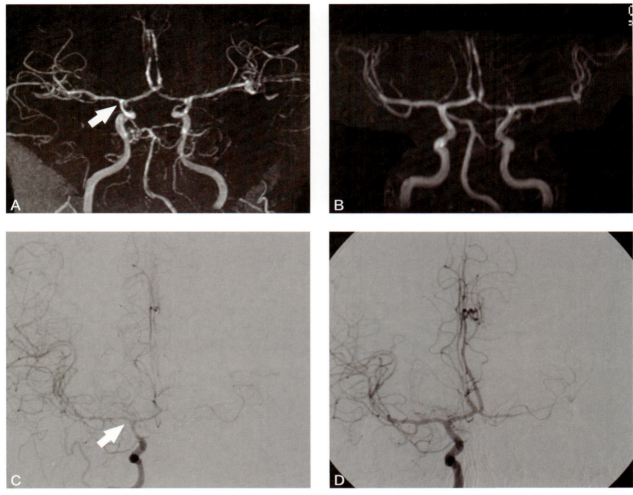

▲ 图 4-22　可逆性血管收缩综合征

患者的 TORMRA 图像显示 Willis 环（A、B）和右侧颈内动脉 DSA（C、D）症状发作急性期（A、C）和缓解后（B、D）。初次发病时双侧颈内动脉远端、双侧大脑中动脉、双侧大脑前动脉血管收缩（白箭）。1 个月后症状缓解后随诊图像显示血管管径正常

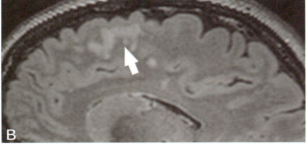

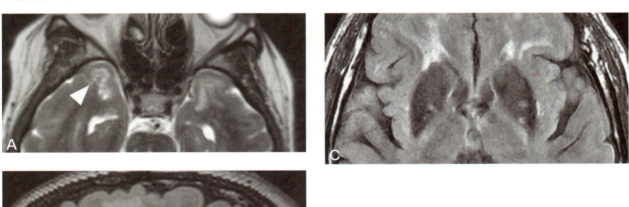

▲ 图 4-23　52 岁女性，伴有渐进性痴呆

T_2（A）和 FLAIR（B、C）显示颞叶前部（A，箭头）、额叶上部（B，白箭）白质内多发高信号。T_2 及 FLAIR（C）显示的皮质下低信号是由于铁沉积导致，是病变晚期的典型表现

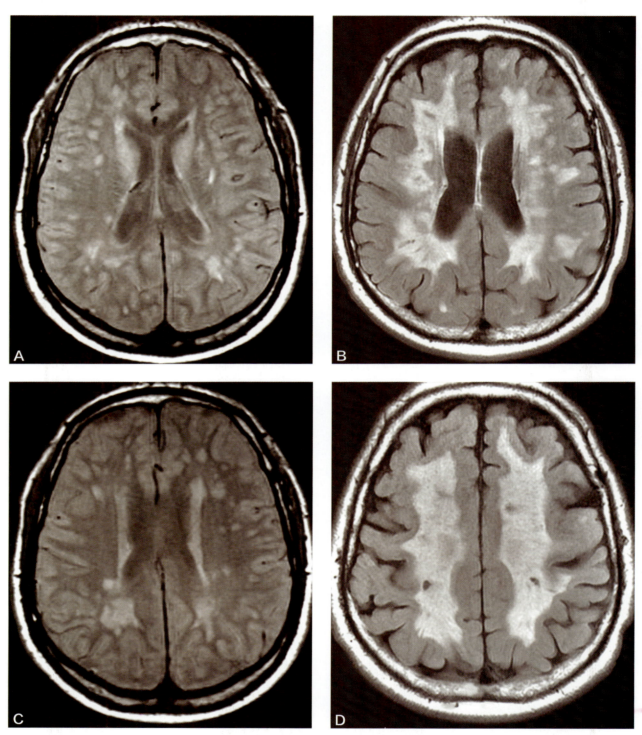

▲ 图 4-24 1 例 45 岁女性的 FLAIR 图像

1 例 45 岁女性在 1997 年的初次轴位 FLAIR 图像（A、C），显示多发皮质下卒中，远多于年龄相关退行性变所致改变。早期病变不累及皮质下 μ 纤维。2012 年随诊图像（B、D），此时患者 60 岁，可见多发连续性病变伴囊变，且累及 μ 纤维脊髓及柔脑膜。由于临床病史、实验室检查及病理特征与其他病变多有重叠，因此分类困难、存在争议。最核心的病理组织学表现是血管壁的炎性改变。只累及 CNS 的血管炎被称为原发性中枢神经系统血管炎（primary CNS vasculitis，PCNSV）。继发性的血管炎可由其他自身免疫性疾病或其他多因素如感染、恶性病变、电离辐射、药物及自身免疫性疾病导致。PCNSV、系统性红斑狼疮、多结节性血管炎、巨细胞动脉炎及干燥综合征等是最常见的导致中枢神经系统血管炎的自身免疫性疾病[50]。

最常见的临床表现有卒中、宾斯旺格病、癫痫。依靠临床、实验室检查及影像学资料综合诊断。很多病例都需要活检来证实，因为症状及影像表现多无特异性[51]。免疫抑制药是治疗的核心。

不同病因引起的病变影像表现并不特异，均表现为受累血管区脑实质缺血性改变，往往是多根血管重叠供血区。少数血管，初次 CT 检查可发现大脑凸面蛛网膜下腔出血。

常规 MRI 检查无特异性表现，但是皮质及皮质下白质病变及基底节区受累等不呈明显血管分布表现时高度提示改变。T_2/FLAIR 对病变的显示更为敏感。GRE 和 SWI 序列可发现多发微小出血灶或蛛网膜下腔出血。也可表现为斑片状脑实质强化、局限性或线状强化，但是亚急性期梗死也可强化，难以明确鉴别。

血管多发不规则狭窄、扩张呈"串珠状"表现是最特征的影像学征象。血管壁的炎性改变增加了形成夹层、梭形动脉瘤等的危险。轴位图像上，血管壁增厚是一种微小改变，有时可以发现。

该病主要是以广泛的临床症状为表现，影像诊断医师的主要任务是发现责任血管、并提醒临床医师鉴别诊断时考虑该病。MRA 虽然是一种很好的影像学手段，但是不能用来诊断或除外血管炎，因为它不具备诊断小血管狭窄或扩张的空间分辨率。尽管 CTA 空间分辨率较高，但所有怀疑血管炎的患者，最终仍需进行 DSA 检查以确诊。

黑血 MRI 是新出现的诊断血管炎很有潜力的影像学方法，可以显示血管壁、向心性管壁狭窄，以及更重要的是显示增强后强化提示活动性炎性改变[52]。图 4-25 显示急性左侧脑梗死，颈内动脉远端、大脑前动脉 A1 段、大脑中动脉 M1 段以及 Willis 环后部多发血管壁增强后强化，经免疫抑制药治疗后，症状不再加重。该患者不伴有中枢神经系统以外的其他症状，最终经验性的诊断为 PCNSV。但是黑血 MRI 对颅内大、中等血管的显示价值仍有限。

2. 巨细胞动脉炎　巨细胞动脉炎是一种累及大、中血管的肉芽肿性血管炎。最常累及颞上动脉，其次可累及主动脉一级、二级分支包括锁骨下动脉、腋动脉、颞浅动脉、睫后动脉、椎动脉[53]。但其实所有血管均可受累。常见表现有头痛、头皮触痛、下颌关节运动障碍及全身炎症性改变，颈部血管及颅内血管受累可有卒中表现。最严重的并发症是动脉受累后无痛性失明。

诊断主要依靠临床及实验室检查，颞动脉活检是金标准[54]。对于不典型患者，常需要进行超声或 MRI 检查，因为进行有创性活检操作前需要证实血管受累。常规 T_2 图像即可发现血管壁增厚。高分辨黑血 MRI 可以显示血管壁增厚及强化，也称为"靶征"[55,56]。图 4-26 左侧颞叶黑血 MRI 显示 1 例经活检证实巨细胞动脉炎的患者左侧颞浅动脉管壁增厚，T_2 信号增高伴强化。系统化激素治疗是最主要的治疗方法。

3. 大动脉炎　大动脉炎是一种累及大血管的慢性肉芽肿性改变，可累及主动脉及其主要分支。病程特点呈三峰表现，早期系统性炎症时多表现为全身症状，中间可有多发血管受累，比如血管痛，晚期表现为血管狭窄、闭塞[57]。晚期表现可有大动脉炎的特征性表现"无脉"期。症状主要与受累血管有关。

超声、CT 或 MRI 等可显示血管壁增厚和炎性改变。早期血管造影可呈阴性表现，晚期所有影像学均可发现血管狭窄。MRI 可以通过评价血管壁增厚、强化以及水敏感序列高信号，即"靶征"来监测病变发展。在血管闭塞期也就是病变晚期，对比剂增强 CTA 或 MRA 可无创评价血管狭窄的程度和范围，侧支循环形成即其他并发症如血管栓塞、少见的动脉瘤形成或夹层[58]。尽管 DSA 是诊断金标准，但由于是有创操作，目前主要用于特定患者的治疗策略。

图 4-27 显示主动脉弓大动脉炎，左侧颈总动脉、左锁骨下动脉完全闭塞，主动脉弓管及邻近大血管壁明显增厚伴强化。图 4-28 显示活检证实的左侧椎动脉大动脉炎，管壁明显增厚、强化，管腔狭窄。

治疗主要依靠免疫抑制药，有时也会同时口服糖皮质激素。为了治疗并发症或保证远端血供时可行外科手术或血管内操作[59]。

4. 颈动脉周围炎 颈动脉周围炎是一种特发性的颈动脉分叉区疼痛、压痛、触痛及同侧颈部疼痛综合征[60]。尽管是临床诊断，很多疾病都可有类似表现，比如血管炎、肌纤维发育不良、复杂动脉粥样硬化伴动脉瘤或夹层，以及其他非

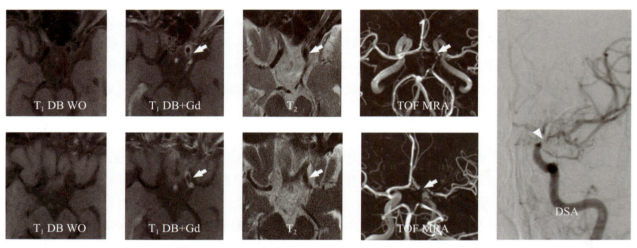

▲ 图 4-25　60 岁女性，左侧前循环卒中（T₁DBWO，T₁ 黑血平扫，T₁DB+Gd，T₁ 黑血增强）
黑血 MRI 显示颈内动脉远端、大脑前动脉及大脑中动脉近端管壁增厚、狭窄，提示 CNS 血管炎（白箭）。所有这些表现均经 DSA 证实（箭头）。经激素治疗后，症状不再进展

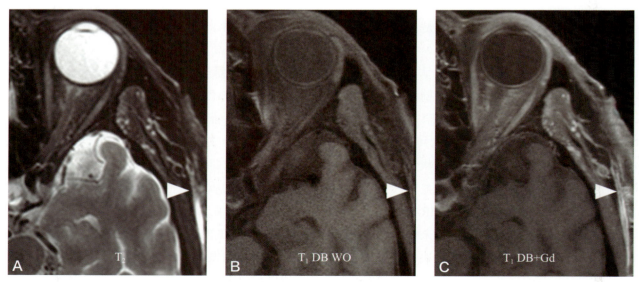

▲ 图 4-26　77 岁男性，头痛及左侧颞叶触痛（T₁DBWO，T₁ 黑血平扫，T₁DB+Gd，T₁ 黑血增强）
A. 轴位黑血 MRI 图像上左侧颞叶多发 T₂ 高信号提示血管水肿；B、C. 左侧颞动脉（箭头）增强后强化。活检证实为巨细胞动脉炎并行激素治疗

血管源性病如淋巴结炎、脊柱退行性变、涎腺炎等[61]。影像学可通过显示颈动脉管壁增厚、水肿的炎性改变以辅助诊断及除外其他混杂病变。颈动脉球部高分辨 MRI 成像可显示无名动脉管壁增厚和强化，通常是局灶性、偏心性，也可以是环周病变[62]。狭窄并不常见[63,64]。也可见到 T_2 信号增高，一般认为是炎性相关水肿导致。图 4-29 显示了典型的颈动脉周围炎，表现为局灶性的管壁强化，激素治疗后部分缓解。

（四）不明原因病变

Moyamoya 病和 Moyamoya 综合征

Moyamoya 病是一种以颈内动脉颅内段及近端分支渐进性狭窄伴颈内动脉末端、皮质区、柔脑膜及供应硬脑膜及颅骨的颈外动脉多发分支小血管形成侧支循环的特发性脑血管闭塞性病变。根据定义，Moyamoya 病是双侧病变，虽然可无明显症状[65]。少数患者病变可累及后循环[66]。主要好发于 5 岁左右的儿童及 40 岁左右的成人。

患者多表现为典型血管病变，尚未见报道其他病变合并 Moyamoya 病。当颅内动脉狭窄、闭塞伴局部多发侧支循环继发于动脉粥样硬化、唐氏综合征、神经纤维瘤病、镰状细胞贫血等病变时，称为 Moyamoya 综合征。

临床症状主要与两种病理生理基础相关：渐进性狭窄及易于破裂的侧支循环。颈内动脉远端、大脑前动脉、中动脉近端渐进性狭窄以及难以代偿的侧支循环引起灌注减低，导致脑实质缺血，引发卒中，TIA 或其他缺血性症状，比如神经功能不全，恶心/呕吐，眩晕，甚至癫痫[66]。易于

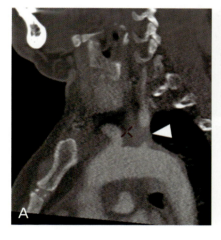

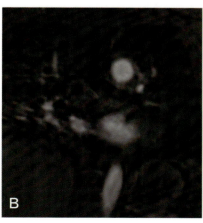

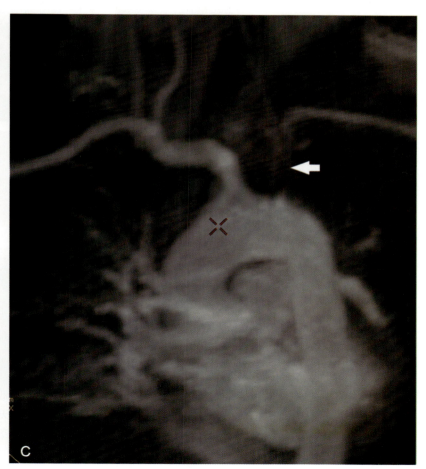

▲ 图 4-27　21 岁女性大动脉炎患者

A. 斜位重建 CTA 显示胸主动脉管壁增厚，左侧颈总动脉近端（白色箭头）完全闭塞；B. 冠位增强后 MRI 显示主动脉弓管壁增厚伴多发强化；C. 相应的 MRA 显示左侧颈总动脉即左侧锁骨下动脉（白箭）完全闭塞

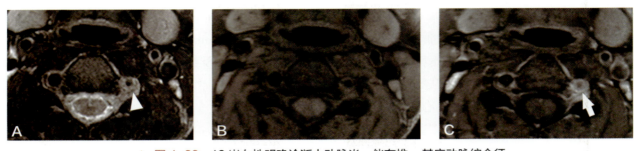

▲ 图 4-28 19 岁女性明确诊断大动脉炎，伴有椎-基底动脉综合征

MRI 显示左侧椎动脉管壁明显增厚，管腔狭窄，T_2 信号增高提示水肿（A，白色箭头），增强后可见强化（C，白箭）

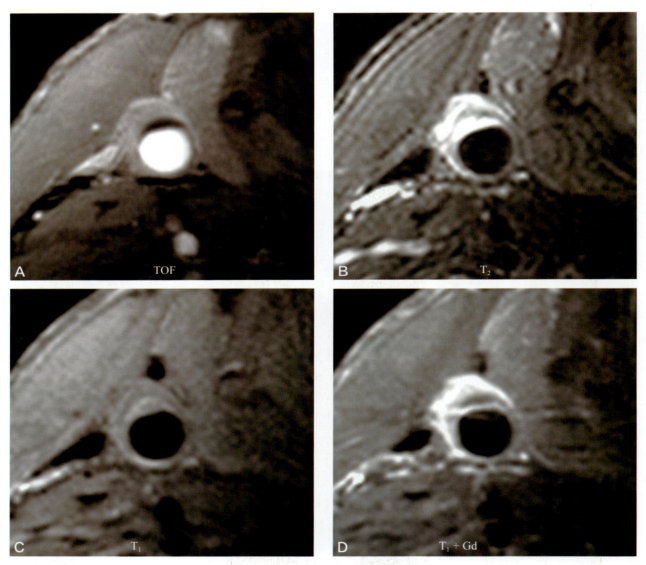

▲ 图 4-29 44 岁男性，右侧颈痛 8 天

TOF（A）及高分辨黑血 MRI（B～D）显示右侧颈动脉分叉下方血管壁 12 点钟方向的局限性增厚，伴有 T_2 信号增高（B），周围强化（C、D）。血管未见明显狭窄

破裂的侧支循环网更易诱发微出血或大出血，或经硬脑膜侧支血管扩张引起的头痛[66,67]。由于血管床受累程度不同，狭窄进展速度不同，以及受累缺血的皮质位置不同，患者的表现较为多样。但后循环，包括大脑后动脉一般不受累。

图4-30显示了3条最基本的侧支循环：起自穿支动脉的基底节区侧支循环（橙色），起自大脑后动脉的柔脑膜侧支循环（蓝色）以及起自颈外动脉经硬脑膜的侧支循环（绿色）。影像学上这些血管看起来就像喷出的烟雾一样，即"烟雾征"（日语为moyamoya）[68]，代表了多发混杂小血管（图4-31C和图4-32E、F）。MRI上表现为颈内动脉远端流空效应减少，以及继发于侧支循环形成的有近端线状信号、基底节区、丘脑流空信号。

在增强MRI上，侧支循环可表现为柔脑膜区多发异常线状强化，经硬脑膜侧支循环可表现为邻近大脑凸面的柔脑膜强化，被称作"常春藤征"（图4-31C）[69]。磁敏感成像及梯度回波可更好显示实质内侧支循环（即"毛刷征"），被认为可以作为评价病变进展分级的一个方法[70]。

病变分期最早是Suzuki和Takaku在1969年提出[65]，早期表现为颈内动脉远端狭窄（Ⅰ期），渐进性狭窄加重伴病变周围多发侧支循环形成，呈烟雾状（Ⅱ期），血管进一步狭窄，烟雾状侧支血管进一步增多（Ⅲ期），侧支血管无法满足灌注需求出现缺血性症状，出现颅外侧支循环（Ⅳ期），颈内动脉进一步狭窄，颅内侧支血管的烟雾状改变减少，颅外侧支循环增加（Ⅴ期），Ⅵ期特征性表现为颅内主要动脉完全闭塞，依靠侧支循环供血，烟雾征消失。随病变进展，由灌注减低导致的缺血性症状、多发易破裂侧支循环导致出血性并发症等相关症状发生的可能性增加。

除了诊断病变和评估进展，影像学的另一个重要作用在于评估并发症，比如卒中、出血等。并且这些微弱的侧支血管易形成动脉瘤或夹层[71]。极少数病变，也可并发动静脉瘘。目前尚不明确获得性动静脉瘘是否与血管生成障碍之间存在某种病理生理关系，或只是巧合[72]。

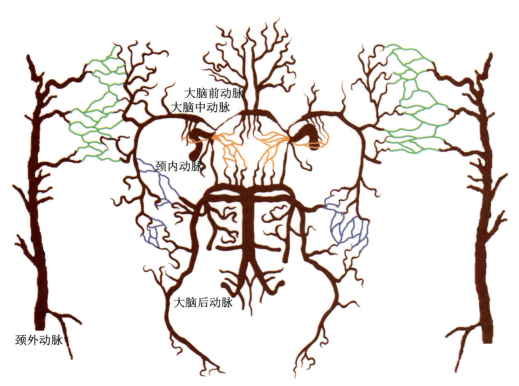

▲ 图 4-30　Moyamoya 病侧支循环的示意图

起自穿支动脉的基底节区侧支循环标为橙色，起自大脑后动脉柔脑膜区的侧支循环标为蓝色，起自颈外动脉、经硬脑膜的侧支循环标为绿色

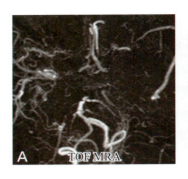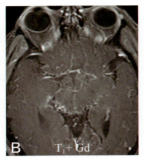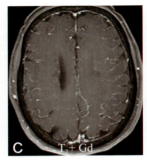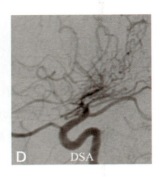

▲ 图 4-31 Moyamoya 病变

A. 轴位 TOR MRA MIP 图显示双侧颈内动脉远端闭塞，周围多发线状异常信号代表多发小血管形成侧支循环；B. 轴位增强 T_1 显示多发线状异常强化对应于基底节区及柔脑膜多发侧支循环；C. 常青藤征，经大脑皮质增强 T_1 轴位图像显示柔脑膜多发迂曲线状强化影，代表来自硬脑膜内动脉的多发侧支循环；D. 经右侧颈内动脉注射 DSA 成像证实颈内动脉远端完全闭塞伴烟雾征

　　Moyamoya 综合征的治疗主要是针对基础疾病。治疗方案目前仍存争议，且没有任何方案能阻止病变进展。目前的治疗方案多侧重于增加受累区灌注，以减少缺血性或出血性卒中[73]。内科治疗包括抗血小板、抗凝疗法，行血管再通术仍是最根本的治疗方案。两种方法较为常用：直接再通，将颈外动脉分支比如颞浅动脉通过颅骨微小钻孔，与颈内动脉直接吻合；间接再通，将颈外动脉供血区的组织连同其内的血管残端直接与大脑接触，这些血管向内生长，以向邻近大脑

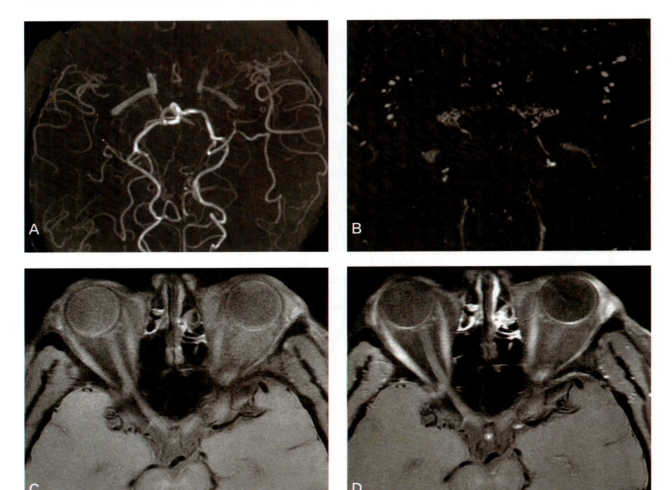

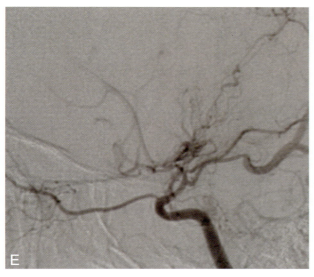
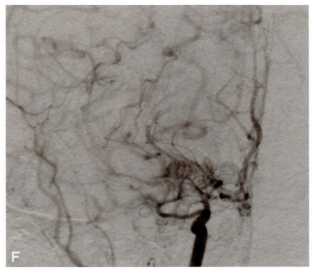

▲ 图 4-32　15 岁男性，耳鸣 2～3 年

TOF MRA MIP（A）及轴位图像（B）显示双侧颈内动脉远端狭窄，颅底复杂的侧支循环血管网。高分辨黑血 MRI（C、D）图像未发现提示活动性炎性改变的异常强化。DSA（E、F）证实颈内动脉远端狭窄及对应于多发侧支循环的典型的烟雾征

皮质供血。两种方法各有其优缺点，临床上常将两种方法结合应用[74]。

三、总结

传统血管腔成像方法如 CTA 及常规 MRA 被优化来显示血管腔，力求达到与 DSA 结果一致。新近出现的技术，可以将血管壁可视化和成像，而且能进一步反映累及血管壁的疾病过程的特点。该领域内的两个主要突破性进展包括能够鉴别颈动脉球部的斑块成分和形态，以及能够通过评估增强图像及向心性管壁增厚的方法来鉴别血管狭窄的病因是炎性还是非炎性。表 4-3 总结了常见的动脉病变的临床病史及典型影像学表现。未来的发展方向包括：①寻找动脉粥样硬化的生物标志物，来发现斑块内出血，纤维帽变薄、破裂等以识别出卒中风险性增加的患者；②进一步评价非狭窄性血管病变，以期早期诊断并进一步加深我们对血管病变的整体认知；③进一步提高空间分辨率以评估更为细小的血管及血管远端病变。

表 4-3 常见动脉病变的临床表现及影像特点总结

	动脉粥样硬化	肌纤维发育不良	夹层	可逆性血管收缩综合征	CADASIL	CNS 血管炎	巨细胞动脉炎	大动脉炎	颈动脉周围炎	烟雾病
病史	>50岁，随年龄增加发病率增高，TIA，卒中，同侧大脑半球反复卒中	20—40岁，女性	极少见于65岁以后，40—45岁为高峰期，可自发形成或继发于外伤后	严重的雷击样头痛，局灶性神经症状，自行缓解，排除性诊断	40—60岁，遗传因素导致的早发性血管性痴呆	异质性脑疾病，可有卒中，宾斯旺格病，癫痫	>50岁，头痛，头皮痛，触痛，下颌关节僵硬，系统性炎性表现	<40岁，女性，无脉	颈动脉分叉区周围触痛，压痛，同侧颈部疼痛	双峰（5岁和40岁），头痛，卒中，TIA，局灶性神经症状，微出血或大出血
位置	颈动脉球，颅内，椎动脉分叉处	60%～75%，肾动脉，25%～30%，颈动脉	颈内动脉，椎动脉长节段区	所有颅内血管均可累及，可累及单个节段，整根血管或多根血管	弥漫白质病变，好发于额叶前部及额叶上部，皮质下白质及外囊区	所有颅内血管均可累及，可累及单个节段，整根血管或多根血管	颞叶上部，少见于主动脉主要分支，睫后动脉，椎动脉	主动脉及其主要分支	颈动脉球部	颈内动脉远端，大脑前动脉，大脑后动脉近端
形态	偏心性短节段多发狭窄	长节段多发狭窄及扩张	管腔内血肿，呈半月形	管腔不同程度狭窄	小血管及毛细血管受累	血管不同程度狭窄及扩张	长节段向心性狭窄，管径狭窄	长节段向心性狭窄，管径狭窄	偏心或环，周性管壁水肿	不伴有管壁增厚的管腔狭窄
典型影像表现	动化区无强化，寻找提示复杂斑块的征象	串珠征	T1压脂像管腔内半月形高信号	"香肠-细线征"或串珠征	弥漫性白质病变，范围远超过年龄相应的退行性变	串珠征	靶征	靶征	增强后偏心性或环周性强化	狭窄伴多发侧支循环形成（血管造影见烟雾征，MRI上见常春藤征或毛刷征）
狭窄	不同程度	+，伴有管腔扩张	>70%，随时间发展病变减小	+++	—	+++，伴有管腔扩张	不同程度	不同程度	不常见	+++
黑血MR管壁强化	—	无	+	—	—	++	++	++	+++	—
管壁水肿	无	无	+	—	—	++	++	++	+++	—

参考文献

[1] Humphrey C, Duncan K, Fletcher S. Decade of experience with vascular rings at a single institution. *Pediatrics*. 2006;117(5):e903–e908.

[2] Yousem DM, Grossman RI. *Neuroradiology : The Requisites*. 3rd ed. Philadelphia, PA: Mosby/Elsevier, 2010.

[3] Bouthillier A, van Loveren HR, Keller JT. Segments of the internal carotid artery: A new classification. *Neurosurgery*. 1996;38(3):425–432; discussion 32–33.

[4] Liebeskind DS. Collateral circulation. Stroke. 2003;34(9):2279–2284.

[5] Riggs HE, Rupp C. Variation in form of circle of Willis. The relation of the variations to collateral circulation: Anatomic analysis. *Arch Neurol*. 1963;8:8–14.

[6] Eftekhar B, Dadmehr M, Ansari S, Ghodsi M, Nazparvar B, Ketabchi E. Are the distributions of variations of circle of Willis different in different populations?—Results of an anatomical study and review of literature. *BMC Neurol*. 2006;6:22.

[7] Chen CJ, Wang LJ, Wong YC. Abnormal origin of the vertebral artery from the common carotid artery. *AJNR Am J Neuroradiol*. 1998;19(8):1414–1416.

[8] Lazzaro NA, Wright B, Castillo M et al. Artery of percheron infarction: Imaging patterns and clinical spectrum. *AJNR Am J Neuroradiol*. 2010;31(7):1283–1289.

[9] Finlay A, Johnson M, Forbes TL. Surgically relevant aortic arch mapping using computed tomography. *Ann Vasc Surg*. 2012;26(4):483–490.

[10] Lim RP, Shapiro M, Wang EY et al. 3D time-resolved MR angiography (MRA) of the carotid arteries with time-resolved imaging with stochastic trajectories: Comparison with 3D contrast-enhanced Bolus-Chase MRA and 3D time-of-flight MRA. *AJNR Am J Neuroradiol*. 2008;29(10):1847–1854.

[11] Meckel S, Maier M, Ruiz DS et al. MR angiography of dural arteriovenous fistulas: Diagnosis and follow-up after treatment using a time-resolved 3D contrast-enhanced technique. *AJNR Am J Neuroradiol*. 2007;28(5):877–884.

[12] Kramer U, Ernemann U, Fenchel M et al. Pretreatment evaluation of peripheral vascular malformations using low-dose contrast-enhanced time-resolved 3D MR angiography: Initial results in 22 patients. *AJR Am J Roentgenol*. 2011;196(3):702–711.

[13] Alperin N, Ranganathan S, Bagci AM et al. MRI evidence of impaired CSF homeostasis in obesity-associated idiopathic intracranial hypertension. *AJNR Am J Neuroradiol*. 2013;34(1):29–34.

[14] Birnbaum J, Hellmann DB. Primary angiitis of the central nervous system. *Arch Neurol*. 2009;66(6):704–709.

[15] Varnava AM, Mills PG, Davies MJ. Relationship between coronary artery remodeling and plaque vulnerability. *Circulation*. 2002;105(8):939–943.

[16] Kolominsky-Rabas PL, Weber M, Gefeller O, Neundoerfer B, Heuschmann PU. Epidemiology of ischemic stroke subtypes according to TOAST criteria: Incidence, recurrence, and long-term survival in isch emic stroke subtypes: A population-based study. *Stroke*. 2001;32(12):2735–2740.

[17] Kizer JR. Evaluation of the patient with unexplained stroke. *Coron Artery Dis*. 2008;19(7):535–540.

[18] Sacco RL, Kargman DE, Gu Q, Zamanillo MC. Race-ethnicity and determinants of intracranial atherosclerotic cerebral infarction. The Northern Manhattan Stroke Study. *Stroke*. 1995;26(1):14–20.

[19] Freilinger TM, Schindler A, Schmidt C et al. Prevalence of nonstenosing, complicated atherosclerotic plaques in cryptogenic stroke. *JACC Cardiovasc Imaging*. 2012;5(4):397–405.

[20] Clinical alert: Benefit of carotid endarterectomy for patients with high-grade stenosis of the internal carotid artery. National Institute of Neurological Disorders and Stroke Stroke and Trauma Division. North American Symptomatic Carotid Endarterectomy Trial (NASCET) investigators. *Stroke*. 1991;22(6):816–817.

[21] Cai JM, Hatsukami TS, Ferguson MS, Small R, Polissar NL, Yuan C. Classification of human carotid atherosclerotic lesions with in vivo multicontrast magnetic resonance imaging. *Circulation*. 2002;106(11):1368–1373.

[22] Saam T, Hetterich H, Hoffmann V et al. Meta-analysis and systematic review of the predictive value of carotid plaque hemorrhage on cerebrovascular events by magnetic resonance imaging. *J Am Coll Cardiol*. 2013; 62(12):1081–1091.

[23] Gupta A, Baradaran H, Schweitzer AD et al. Carotid plaque MRI and stroke risk: A systematic review and meta-analysis. *Stroke*. 2013;44(11):3071–3077.

[24] Underhill HR, Yuan C, Terry JG et al. Differences in carotid arterial morphology and composition between individuals with and without obstructive coronary artery disease: A cardiovascular magnetic resonance study. *J Cardiovasc Magn Reson*. 2008;10:31.

[25] Trelles M, Eberhardt KM, Buchholz M et al. CTA for screening of complicated atherosclerotic carotid plaque—American Heart Association Type Ⅵ lesions as defined by MRI. *AJNR Am J Neuroradiol*. 2013;34(12):2331–7.

[26] Wong KS, Gao S, Chan YL et al. Mechanisms of acute cerebral infarctions in patients with middle cere bral artery stenosis: A diffusion-weighted imaging and microemboli monitoring study. *Ann Neurol*. 2002;52(1):74–81.

[27] Swartz RH, Bhuta SS, Farb RI et al. Intracranial arterial wall imaging using high-resolution 3-tesla contrast- enhanced MRI. *Neurology*. 2009;72(7):627–634.

[28] Turan TN, Bonilha L, Morgan PS, Adams RJ, Chimowitz MI. Intraplaque hemorrhage in symptomatic intracranial atherosclerotic disease. *J Neuroimaging*. 2011;21(2):e159–e161.

[29] Portanova A, Hakakian N, Mikulis DJ, Virmani R, Abdalla WM, Wasserman BA. Intracranial vasa vasorum: Insights and implications for imaging. *Radiology*. 2013;267(3):667–679.

[30] Chimowitz MI, Lynn MJ, Derdeyn CP et al. Stenting versus aggressive medical therapy for intracranial arterial stenosis. *N Engl J Med*. 2011;365(11):993–1003.

[31] Vagal AS, Leach JL, Fernandez-Ulloa M, Zuccarello M. The acetazolamide challenge: Techniques and applications in the evaluation of chronic cerebral ischemia. *AJNR Am J Neuroradiol*. 2009;30(5):876–884.

[32] Gambhir S, Inao S, Tadokoro M et al. Comparison of vasodilatory effect of carbon dioxide inhalation and intravenous acetazolamide on brain vasculature using positron emission tomography. *Neurol Res*. 1997;19(2):139–144.

[33] Harrison EG, Jr., McCormack LJ. Pathologic classification of renal arterial disease in renovascular hypertension. *Mayo Clin Proc*. 1971;46(3):161–167.

[34] Slovut DP, Olin JW. Fibromuscular dysplasia. *N Engl J Med*. 2004;350(18):1862–1871.

[35] Begelman SM, Olin JW. Fibromuscular dysplasia. *Curr Opin Rheumatol*. 2000;12(1):41–47.

[36] Lucas C, Moulin T, Deplanque D, Tatu L, Chavot D. Stroke patterns of internal carotid artery dissection in 40 patients. *Stroke*. 1998;29(12):2646–2648.

[37] Pfefferkorn T, Saam T, Rominger A et al. Vessel wall inflammation in spontaneous cervical artery dissection: A prospective, observational positron emission tomography, computed tomography, and magnetic resonance imaging study. *Stroke*. 2011;42(6):1563–1568.

[38] Ducrocq X, Lacour JC, Debouverie M, Bracard S, Girard F, Weber M. Cerebral ischemic accidents in young subjects. A prospective study of 296 patients aged 16 to 45 years. *Rev Neurol (Paris)*. 1999;155(8):575–582.

[39] Norris JW. Extracranial arterial dissection: Anti coagulation is the treatment of choice: For. *Stroke*. 2005;36(9):2041–2042.

[40] Lyrer PA. Extracranial arterial dissection: Anticoagulation is the treatment of choice: Against. *Stroke*. 2005;36(9):2042–2043.

[41] Meschia JF, Malkoff MD, Biller J. Reversible segmental cerebral arterial vasospasm and cerebral infarction: Possible association with excessive use of sumatriptan and Midrin. *Arch Neurol*. 1998;55(5):712–714.

[42] Singhal AB, Caviness VS, Begleiter AF, Mark EJ, Rordorf G, Koroshetz WJ. Cerebral vasoconstriction and stroke after use of serotonergic drugs. *Neurology*. 2002;58(1):130–133.

[43] Ducros A, Fiedler U, Porcher R, Boukobza M, Stapf C, Bousser MG. Hemorrhagic manifestations of reversible cerebral vasoconstriction syndrome: Frequency, features, and risk factors. *Stroke*. 2010;41(11):2505–2511.

[44] Mandell DM, Matouk CC, Farb RI et al. Vessel wall MRI to differentiate between reversible cerebral vasoconstriction syndrome and central nervous system vasculitis: Preliminary results. *Stroke*. 2012;43(3):860–862.

[45] Sattar A, Manousakis G, Jensen MB. Systematic review of reversible cerebral vasoconstriction syndrome. *Expert Rev Cardiovasc Ther*. 2010;8(10):1417–1421.

[46] Farid H, Tatum JK, Wong C, Halbach VV, Hetts SW. Reversible cerebral vasoconstriction syndrome: Treatment with combined intra-arterial verapamil infusion and intracranial angioplasty. *AJNR Am J Neuroradiol*. 2011;32(10):E184–E187.

[47] Auer DP, Putz B, Gossl C, Elbel G, Gasser T, Dichgans M. Differential lesion patterns in CADASIL and sporadic subcortical arteriosclerotic encephalopathy: MR imaging study with statistical parametric group comparison. *Radiology*. 2001;218(2):443–451.

[48] Dichgans M, Holtmannspotter M, Herzog J, Peters N, Bergmann M, Yousry TA. Cerebral microbleeds in CADASIL: A gradient-echo magnetic resonance imaging and autopsy study. *Stroke*. 2002;33(1):67–71.

[49] Liem MK, Lesnik Oberstein SA, Versluis MJ et al. 7 T MRI reveals diffuse iron deposition in putamen and caudate nucleus in CADASIL. *J Neurol Neurosurg Psychiatry*. 2012;83(12):1180–1185.

[50] Fieschi C, Rasura M, Anzini A, Beccia M. Central nervous system vasculitis. *J Neurol Sci*. 1998;153(2):159–171.

[51] Marsh EB, Zeiler SR, Levy M, Llinas RH, Urrutia VC. Diagnosing CNS vasculitis: The case against empiric treatment. *Neurologist*. 2012;18(4):233–238.

[52] Saam T, Habs M, Pollatos O et al. High-resolution black-blood contrast-enhanced T1 weighted images for the diagnosis and follow-up of intracranial arteritis. *Br J Radiol*. 2010;83(993):e182–e184.

[53] Kale N, Eggenberger E. Diagnosis and management of giant cell arteritis: A review. *Curr Opin Ophthalmol*. 2010;21(6):417–422.

[54] Borchers AT, Gershwin ME. Giant cell arteritis: A review of classification, pathophysiology, geoepidemiology and treatment. *Autoimmun Rev*. 2012;11(6–7):A544–A554.

[55] Saam T, Habs M, Cyran CC et al. New aspects of MRI for diagnostics of large vessel vasculitis and primary angiitis of the central nervous system. *Radiologe*. 2010;50(10):861–871.

[56] Bley TA, Uhl M, Carew J et al. Diagnostic value of high-resolution MR imaging in giant cell arteritis. *AJNR Am J Neuroradiol*. 2007;28(9):1722–1727.

[57] Miller DV, Maleszewski JJ. The pathology of large-vessel vasculitides. *Clin Exp Rheumatol*. 2011;29(1 Suppl. 64):S92–S98.

[58] Khalife T, Alsac JM, Lambert M et al. Diagnosis and surgical treatment of a Takayasu disease on an abdominal aortic dissection. *Ann Vasc Surg*. 2011;25(4):556.e1–556.e5.

[59] Sparks SR, Chock A, Seslar S, Bergan JJ, Owens EL. Surgical treatment of Takayasu's arteritis: Case report and literature review. *Ann Vasc Surg*. 2000;14(2):125–129.

[60] Roseman DM. Carotidynia. A distinct syndrome. *Arch Otolaryngol*. 1967;85(1):81–84.

[61] Schaumberg J, Eckert B, Michels P. Carotidynia: Magnetic resonance imaging and ultrasonographic imaging of a self-limiting disease. *Clin Neuroradiol*. 2011;21(2):91–94.

[62] Comacchio F, Bottin R, Brescia G et al. Carotidynia: New aspects of a controversial entity. *Acta Otorhinolaryngol Ital*. 2012;32(4):266–269.

[63] da Rocha AJ, Tokura EH, Romualdo AP, Fatio M, Gama

HP. Imaging contribution for the diagnosis of carotidynia. *J Headache Pain*. 2009;10(2):125–127.

[64] Burton BS, Syms MJ, Petermann GW, Burgess LP. MR imaging of patients with carotidynia. *AJNR Am J Neuroradiol*. 2000;21(4):766–769.

[65] Suzuki J, Takaku A. Cerebrovascular "moyamoya" disease. Disease showing abnormal net-like vessels in base of brain. *Arch Neurol*. 1969;20(3):288–299.

[66] Scott RM, Smith ER. Moyamoya disease and moyamoya syndrome. *N Engl J Med*. 2009;360(12):1226–1237.

[67] Sun W, Yuan C, Liu W et al. Asymptomatic cerebral microbleeds in adult patients with moyamoya disease: A prospective cohort study with 2 years of follow-up. *Cerebrovasc Dis*. 2013;35(5):469–475.

[68] Ortiz-Neira CL. The puff of smoke sign. *Radiology*. 2008;247(3):910–911.

[69] Yoon HK, Shin HJ, Chang YW. "Ivy sign" in childhood moyamoya disease: Depiction on FLAIR and contrast-enhanced T1-weighted MR images. *Radiology*. 2002;223(2):384–389.

[70] Horie N, Morikawa M, Nozaki A, Hayashi K, Suyama K, Nagata I. "Brush Sign" on susceptibility-weighted MR imaging indicates the severity of moyamoya disease. *AJNR Am J Neuroradiol*. 2011;32(9):1697–1702.

[71] Nagamine Y, Takahashi S, Sonobe M. Multiple intra cranial aneurysms associated with moyamoya disease. Case report. *J Neurosurg*. 1981;54(5):673–676.

[72] Nakashima T, Nakayama N, Furuichi M, Kokuzawa J, Murakawa T, Sakai N. Arteriovenous malformation in association with moyamoya disease. Report of two cases. *Neurosurg Focus*. 1998;5(5):e6.

[73] Ikezaki K. Rational approach to treatment of moyamoya disease in childhood. *J Child Neurol*. 2000;15(5):350–356.

[74] Fung LW, Thompson D, Ganesan V. Revascularisation surgery for paediatric moyamoya: A review of the literature. *Childs Nerv Syst*. 2005;21(5):358–364.

Chapter 5
主动脉和内脏血管磁共振成像

Magnetic Resonance Imaging: Aorta and Splanchnic Vessels

Christopher J. François 著

王 芬 译

邱健星 校

目录 CONTENTS

一、MR 血管成像技术 / 94

二、主动脉 / 99

三、内脏动脉 / 102

四、总结 / 106

由于硬件和成像技术的进步，磁共振血管成像（magnetic resonance angiography，MRA）在临床上越来越多地被应用于已知或可疑心血管疾病患者的检查中。这一观点随着公众对CT血管成像（CT angiography，CTA）中电离辐射和肾毒性造影剂认识的增强变得尤为正确。本章将简要回顾对比增强MR血管成像（contrast enchanced-MRA，CE-MRA）和非对比增强MR血管成像（noncontrast enchanced-MRA，NCE-MRA）技术的最新进展。随后将更详细地介绍CE-MRA和NCE-MRA在评估主动脉和内脏血管疾病中的应用。

一、MR血管成像技术

（一）对比增强MR血管成像（CE-MRA）

与NCE-MRA技术相比，CE-MRA扫描时间更短，视野（FOV）更广（图5-1），因此CE-MRA更常用。此外，CE-MRA技术在很大程度上克服了血液流动伪影和血管脉动伪影。以钆为基础的造影剂（GBCA）可用来增加脉管系统与周围软组织的信号对比。CE-MRA可以采用静态的三维CE-MRA序列或者时间分辨CE-MRA序列进行扫描。静态CE-MRA，即当感兴趣区的血管达到最大程度增强时开始采集图像，可采用团注跟踪方法实时检测或者采用试注射对比剂的方法进行实现。时间分辨CE-MRA，则不需要特定的图像采集时间，就像数字减影血管造影一样，在通过感兴趣的血管进行对比的整个过程中获取多个3D CE-MRA数据集，确保在感兴趣的血管最高增强时至少获取一组数据集。

出于对采集时间、空间分辨率及时间分辨率的综合评估，静态3D CE-MRA相对于时间分辨CE-MRA技术具有更高的时间和空间分辨率，在并行采集成像技术中尤其如此。另一方面，时间分辨CE-MRA较静态3D CE-MRA提供了更多的血流动态信息。

1. 静态3D CE-MRA 高空间分辨CE-MRA基于三维扰相梯度回波序列。在钆对比增强扫描中感兴趣区血管达最高强化时进行采集，填充K空间中心区域。利用现有的序列，胸和腹部CE-MRA的空间分辨率通常为≤1.5mm各向同性。因此CE-MRA可以用来勾画各种心血管疾病患者小而复杂的解剖结构（图5-2）。此外，在

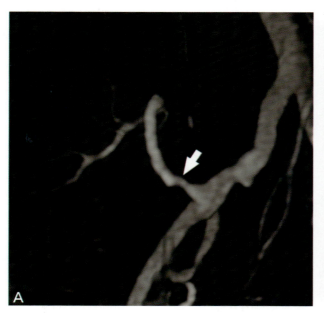 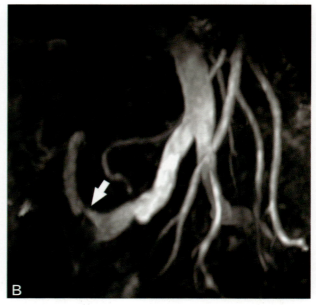

▲ 图5-1 CE-MRA和NCE-MRA对比

右髂窝肾移植的CE-MRA（A）和NCE-MRA（B）图像。这两种技术都清楚地显示了移植肾动脉的严重狭窄（箭）。然而，CE-MRA的采集时间小于20s，而NCE-MRA的采集时间大于3min

相同时间内，图像加速采集方法可以比非加速方法获得更大的成像范围。因此，现在可以对整个胸部或胸部和腹部进行高分辨率 3D CE-MRA 图像的采集（图 5-3）。

单剂量细胞外 GBCA（0.1mmol/kg）通常足以满足大多数 CE-MRA 的扫描应用。GBCA 采用 18～22 号标准导管于静脉内（最好是肘前静脉）注射。导管的大小、患者静脉的质量和采集时间将影响 GBCA 的注射速度（0.5～4.0ml/s）。感兴趣区强化较高时获得的是较低的 K 空间频率。这是因为 K 空间的中心主要是图像信号的增强，而较高的 K 空间频率则可获得较高的图像清晰度（图 5-4）。小剂量 GBCA 的测试团注可用于确定感兴趣血管到达增强峰值的时间，当峰值出现在 K 空间中心时进行采集，或者采用实时团注追踪技术当对比剂到达感兴趣血管时开始采集图像。当时间设定不合理时会出现伪影，包括低信噪比、边缘模糊、截断伪影[1]。

大多数 CE-MRA 的 GBCA 分布于细胞外间隙，但在某些血管扫描应用中，当试图达到血管与周围软组织的最大对比度时，这会带来一些问题。这时使用血管内 GBCA，可以延长扫描

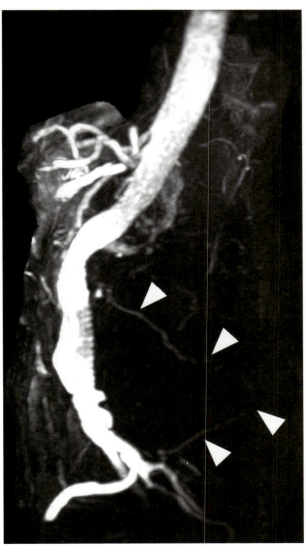

▲ 图 5-2 腹主动脉瘤腔内修复术 Ⅱ 型内漏的高分辨率 3D CEMRA 图像
采集的高空间分辨率的图像中可以清楚地看到滋养血管（箭头）

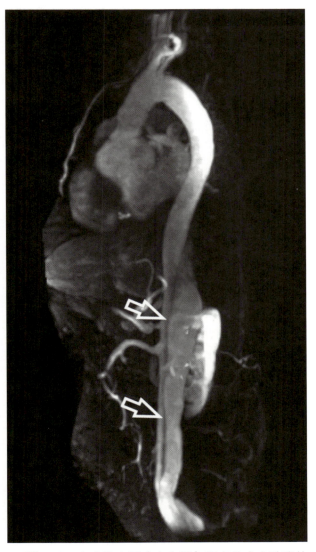

▲ 图 5-3 主动脉夹层（空心箭）患者的全主动脉的 3D CEMRA 图像
采用并行采集技术，在静脉给药 0.1mmol/kg，钆贝葡胺获取时间 18s（Multithance®，Bracco.）

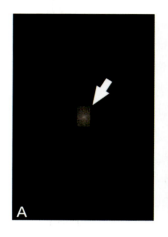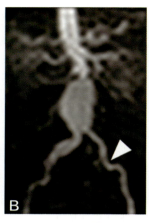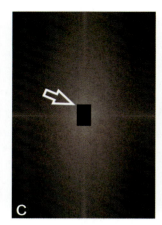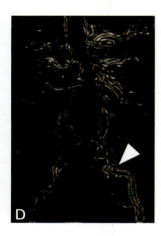

▲ 图 5-4　腹主动脉 CE-MRA

当仅使用中心 10% 的 K 空间数据（A）来重建图像（B）时，可以清晰地描述血管，但血管边缘是模糊的（箭头）。当去除中心 10% 的 K 空间数据（C）时，得到的图像（D）在血管内没有什么信号，但边缘清晰（箭头）

时间，以提高空间分辨率和对比度分辨率。钆磷维塞三钠是一种蛋白质结合的血管内造影剂，已被批准用于评估腹主动脉 - 髂动脉闭塞性疾病[2]，这种蛋白结合延长了该对比剂在血管内的半衰期；此外，相对于其他 GBCA，该对比剂具有更高的弛豫[3]。因此，获得相同的成像质量时，钆磷维塞三钠对比增强 MRA 的成像范围要小于其他 GBCA[4,5]。高空间分辨率 CE-MRA 图像可以利用血管内 GBCA 在稳定状态下采集数据。由于在对比剂首次通过循环系统时，对组织的增强可以忽略，因此在自由呼吸时可以进行稳态成像。由于成像速度快，也不用担心在对比剂首次通过时周围组织增强而产生的伪影，因此可以在自由呼吸模式下进行稳态成像[6]。

在胸部三维 CE-MRA 的应用中，为了优化升主动脉的图像质量，需要对心脏运动进行补偿。应用心电图触发仅在舒张期采集图像（图 5-5）。由于数据是在舒张期获取的，所以 ECG 触发的 CE-MRA 技术比非 ECG 触发的 CE-MRA 技术成像时间要长，因此，扫描时视场（FOV）通常仅限于主动脉，以确保在一次屏气时获得。

由于信噪比（signal-to-noise ratio，SNR）与场强呈正比，因此在较高场强（≥ 3T）下扫描更有利于 CE-MRA 成像。3T 场强下的信噪比约为 1.5T 时的 2 倍。与在低场强下相比，在相同或更好的图像质量下，较高场强下增加的 SNR 可用

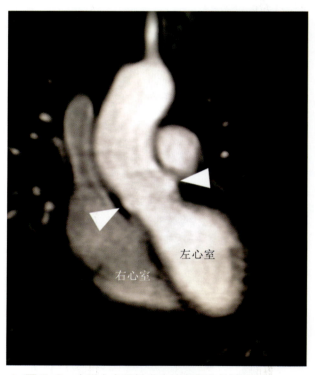

▲ 图 5-5　应用心电图触发来控制采集的图像

在主动脉瓣根部瘤或升主动脉瘤患者中使用心电门控触发的 3D CE-MRA 成像，以减少心脏运动产生的伪影。上图中可清晰地显示锐利的主动脉根部（箭头）

于减少扫描时间和（或）提高空间分辨率[7]。另一个在高场强下进行 CE-MRA 成像的优势是可以使用较小剂量的 GBCA[8-11]，这是由于不同场强下 GBCA 的缩短效应不同，场强越大，增强血管与周围组织之间的对比度越大。

然而，由于场强较大，基于 3T 磁共振的 CE-

MRA 同样存在挑战和局限性。3TCE-MRA 更容易受到射频磁场不均匀性的影响。由于磁场不均匀性导致的信号强度的增加或降低，可以通过多线圈发射线圈来抑制涡流[12]或者应用新的三维射频脉冲技术[13]来减轻。在 3T 场强下进行 CE-MRA 扫描时，可由于磁场不均匀性导致的比吸收率（specific absorption ratio，SAR）的增加。SAR 是射频脉冲传递给组织能量的近似，与主磁场强度的平方成正比。假设所有参数相等，同一序列在 3T 场强下的 SAR 较 1.5T 场强下增加 4 倍[14]。因此，需要对脉冲序列、采集技术及硬件设计进行修改，以确保扫描在 SAR 允许的范围内进行。

2. 时间分辨 CE-MRA 如前所述，相对于静态 3D CE-MRA，时间分辨 CE-MRA 的优点在于：由于在对比剂通过心血管系统时连续进行采集，因此不需要对采集时间点进行精确定时。为了获得高时间分辨率的 CE-MRA，人们提出了多种加速图像采集的方法。这可以通过三维、非对称 K 空间欠采集成像以及切片编码方向上较厚的层厚来实现[15]。然而，层厚的增加导致多平面重构受到限制。因此为了获得较高的空间分辨率，必须采用其他欠采集 K 空间方法。总之，较高空间频率的 K 空间采集频率降低[16-19]，而较低的 K 空间频率则更频繁的被采集更新，来增加图像中血管的对比度（图 5-6）。通过频繁更新 K 空间的中心，并在多幅图像之间共享 K 空间的较高频率，可以生成高时间分辨率和高空间分辨率的图像。通过从使用 GBCA 后图像中减去在 GBCA 使用之前的初始图像，就可以生成类似于数字减影血管造影的纯血管信号的图像。

（二）非对比增强 MR 血管成像（NCE-MRA）

主动脉和内脏血管成像的 NCE-MRA 由于采集时间长以及心脏和呼吸运动伪影而受到限制。然而，软件和硬件的升级重新引起了研究者对 NCE-MRA 的兴趣，特别是对禁止使用 GBCA 存在禁忌证的患者。有数据显示肾源性系统性纤维化的进展与肾功能降低的患者需进行 GBCA 相关检查的情况[20-22]是增加 NCE-MRA 使用的主要推动力。GBCA 的其他禁忌证包括对 GBCA 过敏、妊娠和静脉状况不良。时间飞跃 MRA 是临床上用于宫颈和颅内研究的常规序列，其诊断能力可

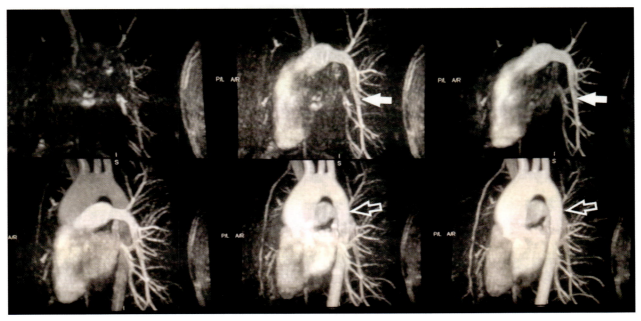

▲ 图 5-6 时间分辨 CE-MRA

图像显示了对比剂通过胸部循环的动态过程。正如预期的那样，肺动脉（空心箭）的增强比主动脉（白箭）更早

与 CTA 和数字减影血管造影相媲美[23,24]。然而，时间飞跃 MRA 在胸部的使用是非常有限的。这里将主要对用于主动脉和内脏血管成像的两种 NCE-MRA 序列进行讲述。

1. 三维平衡稳态自由进动（3D bSSFP）

三维平衡稳态自由进动（3D bSSFP）序列是主要用于胸部和腹部的 NCE-MRA，这是由于 3D bSSFP 序列本身具有较高的血池信号强度，且其信号相对独立[25]。3D bSSFP 序列的图像对比度由组织的 T_2 和 T_1 特征共同决定，从而产生高的血池信号。利用 3D bSSFP NCE-MRA 技术获得的图像动脉和静脉均为高信号（图 5-7）。对于主动脉成像[26-29]来说，这不是一个问题，因为它的体积较大，获得的信号也较高。

实际上，3D bSSFP NCE-MRA 可以用来可靠地测量疑诊或确诊有主动脉瘤的患者的主动脉横径，甚至可能获得比 CE-MRA 技术更好的主动脉根部图像[26]。3D bSSFP NCE-MRA 也被广泛用于评估肾脏和肠系膜血管（图 5-1B）。

3D bSSFP 序列是在自由呼吸的过程中获取的，使用呼吸补偿或导航呼吸触发以提高空间分辨率和扫描覆盖范围。3D bSSFP NCE-MRA 也通过心电触发来采集舒张期的数据，从而使心脏运动伪影最小化。与其他应用中的 bSSFP 序列一样，3D bSSFP NCE-MRA 容易受磁场不均匀性的影响，在肺 - 软组织界面以及金属器件和植入物附近，容易导致图像质量下降。

2. 四维血流成像（4D-Flow MRI）

相位对比法（phase-contrast，PC）MRA 的信号强度与成像视野中流动质子的速度成正比，与扫描方案中选择的速度编码成正比。时间分辨、心电图触发、二维血流敏感 MRI 经常用于心脏 MRI 研究，以量化通过大血管和心脏瓣膜的血流[30,31]。血流敏感相位对比 MRA 同样可以用于 NCE-MRA 成像（图 5-8），这是通过在三个方向上均施加血流敏感的相位编码梯度，采用三维采集方式实现的[32]。使用三维相位对比法（3D PC）进行 NCE-MRA 扫描时，因忽略了血流的实时

信息，所获得的图像代表了获取期间血管内的平均流量。将时间和流向数据添加到解剖信息中后，通常称为四维（4D）血流磁共振成像（三个方向速度编码时间，以及三个空间维数）[33]。使用并行成像[34]或三维径向欠采样[35]进行大量数据采集加速以缩短 4D 血流磁共振成像的扫描时间，增加其临床可用性。除了用于 NCE-MRA，4D 血流磁共振成像还可用于定量描述心血管疾病的各种血流动力学参数。

由于 4D-Flow MRI 的分析是预先确定成像体积中包含的血管的数量进行的，因此简化了血流定量[36]。除了量化血流速度和容积外，4D-Flow MRI 数据还可以得到更复杂的血流动力学参数，这些参数可以诊断或分析的严重程度。初步研究表明，使用 4D-Flow MRI 可以用来评估心血管疾病患者血流模式的变化（图 5-9），以及这些血流

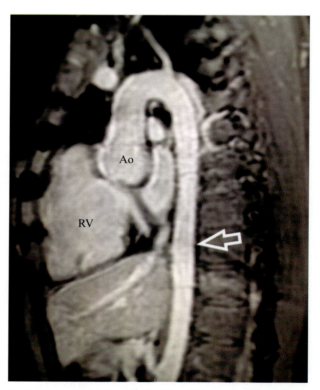

▲ 图 5-7 3D bSSFP NCE-MRA 技术获得的高信号动脉和静脉图像

15 岁法洛四联症患者修复术后，自由呼吸、心电门控触发的 3D bSSFP NCE-MRA 矢状位图像，清晰显示了心血管解剖，包括右心室（RV）、升主动脉（Ao）以及降主动脉（空心箭）

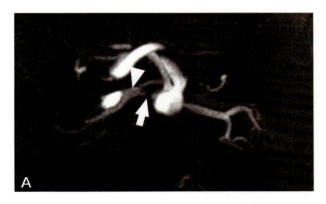

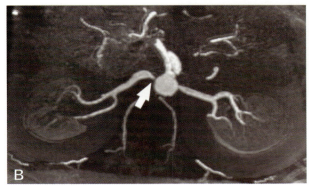

▲ 图 5-8 3D PC NEC-MRA 图像

A.3D PC NEC-MRA 图像显示严重的右肾动脉狭窄（箭头），狭窄右肾动脉远端信号因血流缓慢而减弱（箭）；B.3D CE-MRA 证实右肾动脉重度狭窄

模式的变化与剪切力[33,34]、血流速度[33]、压力梯度[37-41]之间的关系。

二、主动脉

（一）急性主动脉综合征

急性主动脉综合征是一组具有相似临床表现的主动脉病变，包括穿透性动脉硬化性溃疡（penetrating atherosclerotic ulcer, PAU）、壁内血肿（aorta intramural hematoma, IMH）和主动脉夹层（aortic dissection, AD）。常见的临床表现是急性的剧烈胸背痛，其他常见的临床表现有呼吸困难、出汗，当累及腹部血管时可出现腹痛。常见诱因包括高血压、马方综合征、主动脉瓣二叶瓣畸形或其他导致主动脉壁薄弱的病变。三种诱因的急性主动脉综合征均表现为一层或多层主动脉壁的破裂。壁内血肿表现为主动脉壁中膜

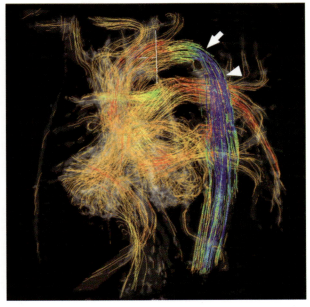

▲ 图 5-9 4D-Flow MRI 评估血流模式的变化

主动脉缩窄（箭）患者胸循环的 4D-Flow MRI 图像。曲线的颜色编码为整个心脏周期的平均速度，橙色和黄色表示较低的速度，蓝色表示较高的速度。缩窄远端（箭头）有较高的血流速度

出血，内膜或外膜没有破裂[42]。主动脉夹层表现为内膜撕裂，主动脉壁的损伤沿主动脉的长轴延伸，并局限于中膜内，主动脉外膜完整，当发生主动脉夹层破裂时外膜破裂。穿透性动脉硬化性溃疡累及动脉的内膜及中膜，邻近动脉可见粥样硬化斑块[43]。

对于怀疑有急性主动脉夹层的患者需要及时做出准确的诊断。因此，CTA 是首选的检查方法，准确率接近 100%。对于对碘化造影剂过敏的患者，在没有时间进行药物治疗的情况下，MRA 也是确定患者是否有主动脉夹层的可靠方法[44,45]。一般来说，MRA 更常用于主动脉夹层患者的随访，特别是年轻患者或肾功能不全的患者。

前面提到的 CE-MRA 和 NCE-MRA 都可用于急性主动脉综合征的诊断，由于 CE-MRA 技术成像速度快，因此可作为急性病例的首选；CE-MRA 和 NCE-MRA 均可用于后期的随访。先前发表的关于 MRA 诊断主动脉夹层的报道中，已经成功地使用了多种不同剂量的 GBCA 和在不同注射速率下进行扫描。MRA 诊断主动脉夹层的

敏感性和特异性在 90%～100%。

MRA 诊断主动脉夹层的标准与 CTA 类似。主动脉夹层的解剖特点是沿主动脉长轴延伸的移位的内膜分离真假腔（图 5-10）。观察到撕裂的内膜更有助于主动脉夹层的诊断。内膜瓣的存在和累及长度有助于区分主动脉夹层与其他原因导致的急性主动脉综合征（壁内血肿和穿透性动脉粥样硬化性溃疡）。MRA 在急性主动脉综合征诊断中的作用是评估夹层的位置和范围、内膜撕裂的位置（图 5-11）、腔的相对充盈情况和主动脉的横径。时间分辨 CE-MRA 有助于区分缓慢充盈的假腔和血栓形成的假腔（图 5-12）。

（二）主动脉瘤

主动脉瘤通常没有临床症状，而是在 X 线、超声心动图、超声和 CT 检查中偶然被发现。超声心动图和超声可以对胸主动脉和腹主动脉的轻

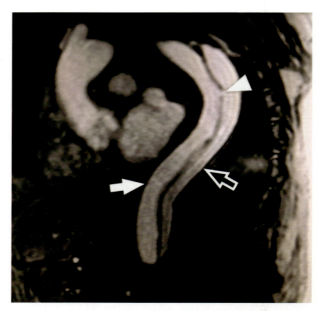

▲ 图 5-11　胸部降主动脉夹层的 CE-MRA 图像
可以看到位于前方的真腔（白箭）、位于后方的假腔（空心箭），以及撕裂的内膜口（箭头）

度扩张进行随访。此外，有证据支持使用超声检查可对 65 岁以上有吸烟史的男性进行腹主动脉瘤（abdominal aortic aneurysms，AAA）筛查。然而相对于 CTA 和 MRA，超声心动图和超声检查往往会低估主动脉瘤的大小。肥胖或者其他导致声窗显影差的患者，超声心动图和超声检查并不能很好地评估，对于此类患者 CTA 和 MRA 能更好地评估主动脉瘤的大小及范围[46]，尤其是对于准备行腔内修复术的主动脉迂曲或复杂主动脉瘤的患者。

主动脉瘤的持续增大，有导致主动脉夹层或破裂的风险，其发生与主动脉瘤大小有直接关系。胸主动脉瘤最大直径大于 5～6cm 时可进行修复治疗，对于有潜在结缔组织病的患者可尽早治疗。腹主动脉瘤通常在直径大于 5.5cm 时进行治疗。升主动脉瘤的修复通常选择开放式手术治疗。降主动脉瘤、胸-腹主动脉瘤及腹主动脉瘤往往选择血管腔内置入支架治疗。修复路径的选择基于多种因素，最重要的是动脉瘤的位置及范围。

CTA 和 MRA 在确定动脉瘤的大小和范围方面有相似的结果[47]。CE-MRA、NCE-MRA 可对已知主动脉瘤患者进行随访。较新的 3D CE-

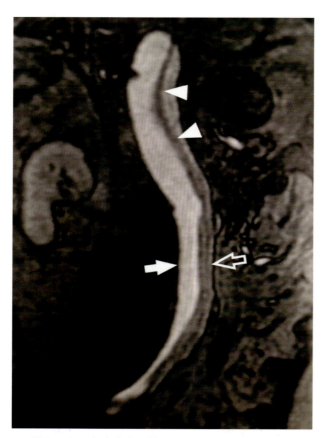

▲ 图 5-10　主动脉夹层的 CE-MRA 图像
可以看到薄薄的移位的内膜片（箭头）分隔真腔（白箭）和假腔（空心箭）

Chapter 5　主动脉和内脏血管磁共振成像
Magnetic Resonance Imaging: Aorta and Splanchnic Vessels

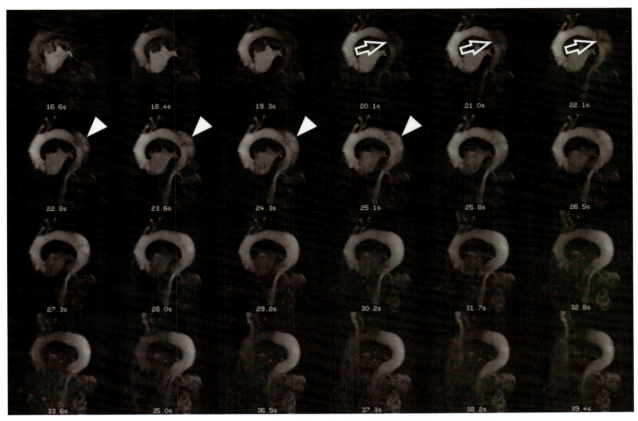

▲ 图 5-12　陈旧性胸主动脉夹层患者的时间分辨 CE-MRA 图像
真腔（空心箭）比假腔（箭头）强化早

MRA 检查方法能够在短时间内对整个胸部和腹部进行成像，因此更适用于随访。与 CTA 相比，MRA 避免了肾毒性造影剂的使用和电离辐射的接触。

　　动脉瘤是指大于 50% 正常主动脉横径的局限性或弥漫性主动脉扩张。从主动脉壁向外延伸的动脉瘤称为囊状动脉瘤（图 5-13），导致血管周向扩张的动脉瘤称为梭形动脉瘤（图 5-14）。动脉瘤也可以根据血管壁的完整性来描述。在真性动脉瘤中，血管壁的三层都是完整的，而假动脉瘤（或假性动脉瘤）则有内膜和部分中膜的破裂。由于血管壁的破裂，假性动脉瘤比真正的动脉瘤更不稳定，需要更紧急的修复治疗。

　　由于胸主动脉瘤与腹主动脉瘤之间存在关联，因此对确诊有腹主动脉瘤的患者评估胸主动脉是非常重要的。女性和老年患者胸主动脉瘤与腹主动脉瘤的相关性高于男性和年轻患者。

　　大的主动脉瘤可因血流缓慢而形成腔内血栓。

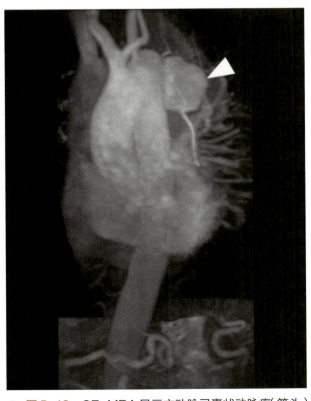

▲ 图 5-13　CE-MRA 显示主动脉弓囊状动脉瘤（箭头）

101

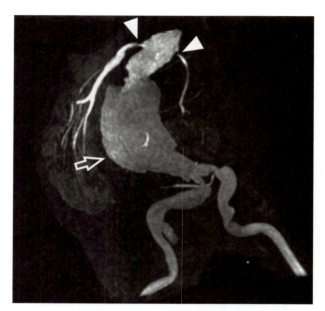

▲ 图 5-14　CE-MRA 显示腹主动脉瘤梭形主动脉瘤（空心箭）

由于双肾动脉狭窄（箭头）导致肾功能不全，CE-MRA 检查显示

法检测到血管厚度的变化。因此，MRA 和 MRI 被用于观察由受累血管供血的远端器官的继发改变。

由于不同的 MRA 成像序列可获得不同的组织对比，因此同其他成像方法相比 MRI 通常更适于检测主动脉炎的血管受累。NCE-MRA 和 CE-MRA 序列都可用于评估血管壁厚度和活动性炎症的存在。炎症活动性征象包括血管壁强化和水肿（图 5-15）。经过治疗，这些变化可迅速消失[51]。因此，在主动脉炎开始治疗之前或之后尽快扫描至关重要。另外，MRA 可用于评估疾病活动或评估对治疗的反应。巨细胞动脉炎和 Takayasu 动脉炎患者都有发生狭窄和动脉瘤的危险（图 5-16）。

巨细胞性动脉炎常累及头颈部动脉，对巨细胞性动脉炎患者头颈部 MRI 和 MRA 是至关重要的。这种联合检查方法可以帮助患者和医务人员了解这种系统性血管炎的累及范围及其活动性。

因此，主动脉横径应从主动脉外壁到主动脉外壁进行测量。当动脉瘤内有血栓时，重建或最大密度投影往往低估主动脉的真实大小。

（三）大动脉炎

目前根据累及血管的大小将系统性血管炎分为小动脉炎、中动脉炎和大动脉炎[48]。MRA 主要用于大血管病变的诊断和随访，而对中动脉炎的诊断和随访价值有限。大血管的炎症包括巨细胞性动脉炎和 Takayasu 动脉炎。中等血管炎包括多动脉炎、结节性动脉炎和川崎病。MRA 在评估小血管炎-肉芽肿性多发性血管炎、Churg-Strauss 血管炎、显微镜下血管炎和与免疫复合物相关的小血管炎方面的作用有限。非感染性大动脉炎也可能是其他全身炎症疾病的组成部分，如类风湿关节炎、结节病、多软骨炎、脊柱关节炎和 Behcet 病。

由于 MRA 在中小血管患者评价中的作用较有限，本节将重点介绍 MRA 在大血管炎诊断中的应用。高分辨率 MRA 可以显示受累大血管内壁的炎性改变[49,50]。中、小血管由于血管太小，无

三、内脏动脉

（一）肠系膜动脉

尽管肠系膜缺血并不常见，但急性肠系膜缺血具有很高的发病率及死亡率。肠系膜缺血的体征和症状是非特异性的，因此临床上诊断困难，继而导致更严重的并发症。引起急性腹痛的原因很多，包括血管源性的和非血管源性的。而慢性肠系膜缺血则主要表现为体重减轻和餐后腹痛。

急性腹痛患者的首选影像学检查方法是腹部 X 线片，但在出现肠梗阻之前，这些检查都是非特异性的和不敏感的[52]。CTA 因其可操作性和扫描快速的特点，因此对可疑急性肠系膜缺血的患者其使用条件相对较宽。CTA 作为急性肠系膜缺血患者的首选检查方法，能很好地显示缺血肠壁的变化[53]。

研究表明，MRA 对肠系膜血管狭窄和闭塞的诊断具有较高的敏感性和特异性[54]，但由于其扫描时间长、可用性低以及对肠系膜缺血继发征象的敏感性低，因此在急性肠系膜缺血的急性

Chapter 5　主动脉和内脏血管磁共振成像
Magnetic Resonance Imaging: Aorta and Splanchnic Vessels

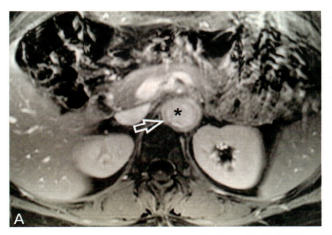 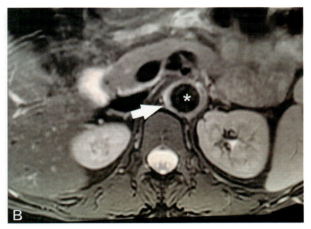

▲ 图 5-15　39 岁女性的大动脉炎累及腹主动脉（*）图像

A. T_1 加权快速扰相梯度回波获得的图像，给药后，显示主动脉壁环周增厚（空心箭）；B. 压脂 T_2 加权图像显示增厚的血管壁伴高信号（白箭），提示血管壁的炎性水肿

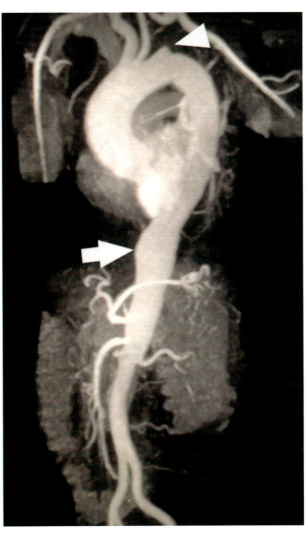

▲ 图 5-16　Takayasu 动脉炎患者的 CE-MRA 图像

CE-MRA 显示 Takayasu 动脉炎患者出现梭形胸腹主动脉瘤（长箭），左锁骨下动脉闭塞（箭头）

诊断和治疗中的作用非常有限[55,56]。对于有 CTA 禁忌证的患者，相对于 CT 平扫，CE-MRA 可以显示缺血肠管的血管结构（图 5-17）。

如前所述，餐后腹痛和体重减轻是慢性肠系膜缺血患者最常见的症状。在老年患者中，通常继发于动脉粥样硬化性疾病。在年轻患者中，较少见的引起慢性肠系膜缺血的病因包括纤维肌肉发育不良、血管炎和中弓状韧带综合征。

MRA 诊断腹腔干动脉和肠系膜上动脉狭窄的准确率与 CTA 相似，大于 90%，可观察到包括腹腔干近端和肠系膜上动脉狭窄或闭塞的征象（图 5-18）[54]。在非闭塞性肠系膜动脉狭窄的情况下，利用增加饮食来检测肠系膜血流量对于其诊断可能非常有益[52,57]。在健康人群中，饭后流经胃肠道的血流量通常会加倍。然而，在肠系膜缺血患者中，通过肠系膜血管的血流量增加要少得多。

对于怀疑为中弓状韧带综合征的患者，进行动态 MRA 成像以评价中弓状韧带对腹腔干动脉压迫的影响是非常重要的。呼气时腹腔干受压，吸气时受压减轻，同时伴有慢性肠系膜缺血的表现，可以做出中弓韧带综合征的诊断（图 5-19）。

（二）肾血管病变

高血压是一种常见的疾病，发病率随着年龄的增加而增加。超过 90% 的高血压患者为原发性

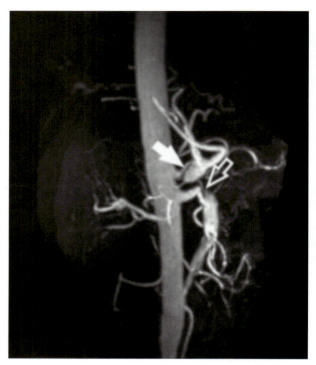

▲ 图 5-17 CE-MRA 显示缺血肠管的血管结构

节段性动脉中膜溶解（segmental arterial mediolysis, SAM），病变累及腹腔干（白箭）及肠系膜上动脉（空心箭）由于存在碘对比剂禁忌证而行 CE-MRA 检查

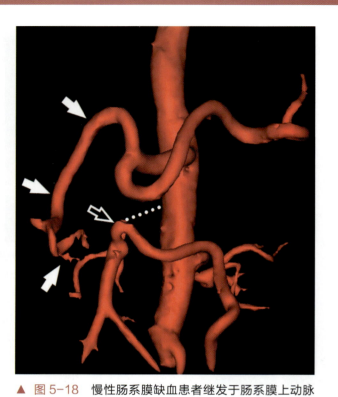

▲ 图 5-18 慢性肠系膜缺血患者继发于肠系膜上动脉闭塞的 MRA 图像（虚线）

远端见由胃十二指肠动脉（白箭）及胰十二指肠动脉（空心箭）开放形成的侧支循环

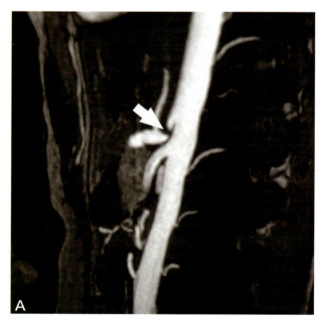

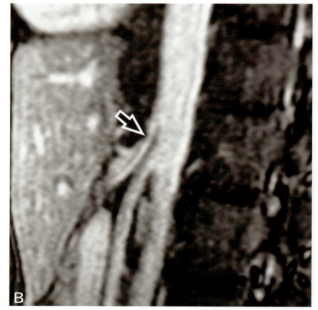

▲ 图 5-19 29 岁慢性肠系膜缺血患者

继发于中弓韧带综合征的慢性肠系膜缺血的 29 岁患者。腹腔干在呼气时几乎完全闭塞（A，白箭）、在吸气时表现为轻度狭窄（B，空心箭）

高血压，病因不明，原因可能是遗传、肥胖、饮食不良或运动不足。继发性高血压是指高血压的症状与另一种疾病有关。继发性高血压的病因很多，包括肾动脉狭窄（renal artery stenosis，RAS）。对于腹部有瘀伤、血压迅速上升、高血压发病年龄超过 50 岁，或者对医疗管理无效的患者应怀疑有无肾源性高血压的可能[58]。50 岁以上 RAS 患者最常见的原因是慢性动脉粥样硬化，急性 RAS 以及继发于血管炎或炎性肌纤维发育不良的 RAS 并不常见。其他原因包括血管炎、纤维肌发育不良和神经纤维瘤病（图 5-20），更常见于 30 岁以下的患者[58]。

多普勒超声由于其低成本和可行性，仍然是疑诊 RAS 的患者首选的检查方法[59]。然而，多普勒超声不能完全排除 RAS 的其他病因。对于多普勒超声阳性或高度怀疑 RAS 的患者，可行 CTA 及 MRA 检查。由于继发性高血压患者的肾动能经常受损或者有受损的风险，MRA 是避免使用肾毒性造影剂的首选检查方法。

肾动脉 MRA 安全准确，适用于所有没有 MRI 禁忌证的患者。MRA 检查的敏感性高于 95%、特异性高于 85%。在临床工作中，CE-MRA（图 5-1A、图 5-20 和图 5-21）[60] 及 NCE-MRA（图 5-1B 和图 5-22）[25,61-63] 具有相近的准确性。RAS 诊断的直接征象是 MRA 图像上显示的肾动脉的解剖学狭窄（图 5-1 和图 5-14），继发征象包括延迟强化（图 5-21）或者相对于对侧正常肾脏的萎缩。对于中、重度狭窄，单凭解剖难以确定狭窄的血流动力学意义，本章前面描述的 PC MRA 技术可以有助于识别狭窄远端的湍流增加或血流加速（图 5-8），其结果将证实血流动力学意义重大的病变。最近的研究数据表明，新兴的 4D-flow MRI 能够准确地量化狭窄处的压力梯度，而且是无创的。

MRA 可以发现或者排除近端肾动脉的狭窄，但是对于较小的肾动脉分支的评估可能因其体积较小而受到限制。例如，对纤维肌肉发育不良[64] 的患者，MRA 可能难以发现多病灶的狭窄和扩张[65]。在这些情况下，应考虑进行 CTA 检查。此外，CTA 也适用于评估已经接受 RAS 血管内治疗的患者肾动脉支架的通畅程度。

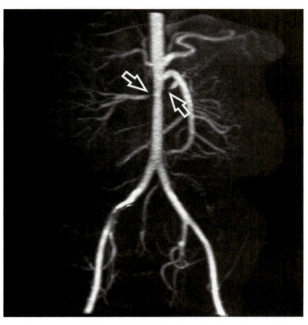

▲ 图 5-20　继发于神经纤维瘤病的双侧肾动脉狭窄（空心箭）

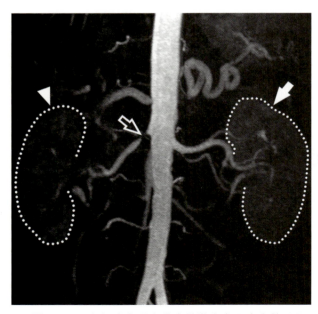

▲ 图 5-21　右肾动脉重度狭窄继发高血压患者的 CE-MRA 图像（空心箭）
与左肾实质（白箭）相比，右肾实质（箭头）可见延迟强化

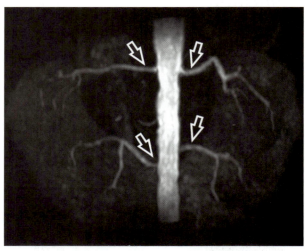

▲ 图 5-22　四支肾动脉的 NCE-MRA 图像

NCE-MRA 图像中显示了四支肾动脉（空心箭），利用血流反转恢复准备 3D bSSFP 技术，实现了主动脉和肾动脉的高质量显像。反转恢复准备脉冲用于抵消来自周围软组织和静脉的信号

四、总结

硬件和软件的改进大大提高了评估胸腹心血管疾病的 CE-MRA 和 NCE-MRA 的图像质量。主要进展包括以下几个方面：①加速图像采集方法以扩大视野或时间分辨 CE-MRA 的时间分辨率；②更高的磁场强度以改善血管信号和血管与周围软组织之间的对比；③对基于 3D bSSFP 和 PC 采集的更高空间分辨率和更快的 NCE-MRA 方法。尽管超出了本章的范围，4D-flowMR 成像技术因为它们能够提供精细的解剖细节和广泛的血流动力学参数在心血管疾病患者未来的评估和管理方面有很大的潜力。

尽管 MRA 在急性主动脉综合征或急性肠系膜缺血等急性心血管病变的评估中所起的作用有限，但 MRA 具有空间分辨率高、获取时间快、安全性高等优点，在慢性心血管疾病的临床治疗中起着不可或缺的作用。年轻的患者，尤其是对于主动脉瘤、慢性主动脉夹层、慢性肠系膜缺血和 RAS 的检出及随访均有帮助。

参考文献

[1] Maki JH, Prince MR, Londy FJ, Chenevert TL. The effects of time varying intravascular signal intensity and k-space acquisition order on three-dimensional MR angiography image quality. *J Magn Reson Imaging* 1996;6(4):642–651.

[2] Rapp JH, Wolff SD, Quinn SF et al. Aortoiliac occlusive disease in patients with known or suspected peripheral vascular disease: Safety and efficacy of gadofosveset- enhanced MR angiography—Multicenter comparative phase III study. *Radiology* 2005;236(1):71–78.

[3] Rohrer M, Bauer H, Mintorovitch J, Requardt M, Weinmann HJ. Comparison of magnetic properties of MRI contrast media solutions at different magnetic field strengths. *Invest Radiol* 2005;40(11):715–724.

[4] Klessen C, Hein PA, Huppertz A et al. First-pass whole-body magnetic resonance angiography (MRA) using the blood-pool contrast medium gadofosveset trisodium: Comparison to gadopentetate dimeglumine. *Invest Radiol* 2007;42(9):659–664.

[5] Maki JH, Wang M, Wilson GJ, Shutske MG, Leiner T. Highly accelerated first-pass contrast-enhanced magnetic resonance angiography of the peripheral vasculature: Comparison of gadofosveset trisodium with gadopentetate dimeglumine contrast agents. *J Magn Reson Imaging* 2009;30(5):1085–1092.

[6] Naehle CP, Kaestner M, Muller A et al. First-pass and steady-state MR angiography of thoracic vasculature in children and adolescents. *JACC Cardiovasc Imaging* 2010;3(5):504–513.

[7] Nael K, Fenchel M, Krishnam M, Finn JP, Laub G, Ruehm SG. 3.0 Tesla high spatial resolution contrast enhanced magnetic resonance angiography (CE-MRA) of the pulmonary circulation: Initial experience with a 32-channel phased array coil using a high relaxivity contrast agent. *Invest Radiol* 2007;42(6):392–398.

[8] Huang BY, Castillo M. Neurovascular imaging at 1.5 tesla versus 3.0 tesla. *Magn Reson Imaging Clin N Am* 2009;17(1):29–46.

[9] Tomasian A, Salamon N, Lohan DG, Jalili M, Villablanca JP, Finn JP. Supraaortic arteries: Contrast material dose reduction at 3.0-T high-spatial-resolu tion MR angiography—Feasibility study. *Radiology* 2008;249(3):980–990.

[10] Habibi R, Krishnam MS, Lohan DG et al. High-spatial resolution lower extremity MR angiography at 3.0 T: Contrast agent dose comparison study. *Radiology* 2008;248(2):680–692.

[11] Attenberger UI, Michaely HJ, Wintersperger BJ et al. Three-dimensional contrast-enhanced magnetic-reso nance angiography of the renal arteries: Interindividual comparison of 0.2 mmol/kg gadobutrol at 1.5 T and 0.1 mmol/kg gadobenate dimeglumine at 3.0 T. *Eur Radiol* 2008;18(6):1260–1268.

[12] Vaughan JT, Adriany G, Snyder CJ et al. Efficient high-frequency body coil for high-field MRI. *Magn Reson Med* 2004;52(4):851–859.

[13] Saekho S, Yip CY, Noll DC, Boada FE, Stenger VA. Fast-kz three-dimensional tailored radiofrequency pulse for reduced

[14] Barth MM, Smith MP, Pedrosa I, Lenkinski RE, Rofsky NM. Body MR imaging at 3.0 T: Understanding the opportunities and challenges. *RadioGraphics* 2007;27(5):1445–1462; discussion 1462–1464.

[15] Finn JP, Baskaran V, Carr JC et al. Thorax: Low-dose contrast-enhanced three-dimensional MR angiography with subsecond temporal resolution—Initial results. *Radiology* 2002;224(3):896–904.

[16] van Vaals JJ, Brummer ME, Dixon WT et al. "Keyhole" method for accelerating imaging of contrast agent uptake. *J Magn Reson Imaging* 1993;3(4):671–675.

[17] Korosec FR, Frayne R, Grist TM, Mistretta CA. Time-resolved contrast-enhanced 3D MR angiography. *Magn Reson Med* 1996;36(3):345–351.

[18] Lim RP, Shapiro M, Wang EY et al. 3D time-resolved MR angiography (MRA) of the carotid arteries with time-resolved imaging with stochastic trajectories: Comparison with 3D contrast-enhanced Bolus-Chase MRA and 3D time-of-flight MRA. *AJNR Am J Neuroradiol* 2008;29(10):1847–1854.

[19] Haider CR, Hu HH, Campeau NG, Huston J, 3rd, Riederer SJ. 3D high temporal and spatial resolution contrast-enhanced MR angiography of the whole brain. *Magn Reson Med* 2008;60(3):749–760.

[20] Perazella MA. Advanced kidney disease, gadolinium and nephrogenic systemic fibrosis: The perfect storm. *Curr Opin Nephrol Hypertens* 2009;18(6):519–525.

[21] Perazella MA, Rodby RA. Gadolinium-induced nephrogenic systemic fibrosis in patients with kidney disease. *Am J Med* 2007;120(7):561–562.

[22] Sadowski EA, Bennett LK, Chan MR et al. Nephrogenic systemic fibrosis: Risk factors and incidence estimation. *Radiology* 2007;243(1):148–157.

[23] Provenzale JM, Sarikaya B. Comparison of test performance characteristics of MRI, MR angiography, and CT angiography in the diagnosis of carotid and vertebral artery dissection: A review of the medical literature. *AJR Am J Roentgenol* 2009;193(4):1167–1174.

[24] Buhk JH, Kallenberg K, Mohr A, Dechent P, Knauth M. Evaluation of angiographic computed tomography in the follow-up after endovascular treatment of cerebral aneurysms—A comparative study with DSA and TOF-MRA. *Eur Radiol* 2009;19(2):430–436.

[25] Miyazaki M, Lee VS. Nonenhanced MR angiography. *Radiology* 2008;248(1):20–43.

[26] Francois CJ, Tuite D, Deshpande V, Jerecic R, Weale P, Carr JC. Unenhanced MR angiography of the thoracic aorta: Initial clinical evaluation. *AJR Am J Roentgenol* 2008;190(4):902–906.

[27] Francois CJ, Tuite D, Deshpande V, Jerecic R, Weale P, Carr JC. Pulmonary vein imaging with unenhanced three-dimensional balanced steady-state free precession MR angiography: Initial clinical evaluation. *Radiology* 2009;250(3):932–939.

[28] Krishnam MS, Tomasian A, Malik S, Desphande V, Laub G, Ruehm SG. Image quality and diagnostic accuracy of unenhanced SSFP MR angiography compared with conventional contrast-enhanced MR angiography for the assessment of thoracic aortic diseases. *Eur Radiol* 2010;20(6):1311–1320.

[29] Pasqua AD, Barcudi S, Leonardi B, Clemente D, Colajacomo M, Sanders SP. Comparison of contrast and noncontrast magnetic resonance angiography for quantitative analy- sis of thoracic arteries in young patients with congenital heart defects. *Ann Pediatr Cardiol* 2011;4(1):36–40.

[30] Pelc NJ, Herfkens RJ, Shimakawa A, Enzmann DR. Phase contrast cine magnetic resonance imaging. *Magn Reson Q* 1991;7(4):229–254.

[31] Chai P, Mohiaddin R. How we perform cardiovascular magnetic resonance flow assessment using phase-contrast velocity mapping. *J Cardiovasc Magn Reson* 2005;7(4):705–716.

[32] Pelc NJ, Bernstein MA, Shimakawa A, Glover GH. Encoding strategies for three-direction phase-contrast MR imaging of flow. *J Magn Reson Imaging* 1991;1(4):405–413.

[33] Markl M, Frydrychowicz A, Kozerke S, Hope M, Wieben O. 4D flow MRI. *J Magn Reson Imaging* 2012;36(5):1015–1036.

[34] Markl M, Harloff A, Bley TA et al. Time-resolved 3D MR velocity mapping at 3T: Improved navigator-gated assessment of vascular anatomy and blood flow. *J Magn Reson Imaging* 2007;25(4):824–831.

[35] Gu T, Korosec FR, Block WF et al. PC VIPR: A high-speed 3D phase-contrast method for flow quantification and high-resolution angiography. *AJNR Am J Neuroradiol* 2005;26(4):743–749.

[36] Stalder AF, Russe MF, Frydrychowicz A, Bock J, Hennig J, Markl M. Quantitative 2D and 3D phase contrast MRI: Optimized analysis of blood flow and vessel wall parameters. *Magn Reson Med* 2008;60(5):1218–1231.

[37] Lum DP, Johnson KM, Paul RK et al. Transstenotic pressure gradients: Measurement in swine—Retrospectively ECG-gated 3D phase-contrast MR angiography versus endovascular pressure-sensing guidewires. *Radiology* 2007;245(3):751–760.

[38] Turk AS, Johnson KM, Lum D et al. Physiologic and anatomic assessment of a canine carotid artery stenosis model utilizing phase contrast with vastly undersam pled isotropic projection imaging. *AJNR Am J Neuroradiol* 2007;28(1):111–115.

[39] Bley TA, Johnson KM, Francois CJ et al. Noninvasive assessment of transstenotic pressure gradients in porcine renal artery stenoses by using vastly undersampled phase-contrast MR angiography. *Radiology* 2011;261(1):266–273.

[40] Tyszka JM, Laidlaw DH, Asa JW, Silverman JM. Three-dimensional, time-resolved (4D) relative pressure mapping using magnetic resonance imaging. *J Magn Reson Imaging* 2000;12(2):321–329.

[41] Bock J, Frydrychowicz A, Lorenz R et al. In vivo noninva-

sive 4D pressure difference mapping in the human aorta: Phantom comparison and application in healthy volunteers and patients. *Magn Reson Med* 2011;66(4):1079–1088.

[42] Evangelista A, Mukherjee D, Mehta RH et al. Acute intramural hematoma of the aorta: A mystery in evolution. *Circulation* 2005;111(8):1063–1070.

[43] Hayashi H, Matsuoka Y, Sakamoto I et al. Penetrating atherosclerotic ulcer of the aorta: Imaging features and disease concept. *RadioGraphics* 2000;20(4):995–1005.

[44] Klem I, Heitner JF, Shah DJ et al. Improved detection of coronary artery disease by stress perfusion cardiovascular magnetic resonance with the use of delayed enhancement infarction imaging. *J Am Coll Cardiol* 2006;47(8):1630–1638.

[45] Panting JR, Norell MS, Baker C, Nicholson AA. Feasibility, accuracy and safety of magnetic resonance imaging in acute aortic dissection. *Clin Radiol* 1995;50(7):455–458.

[46] Desjardins B, Dill KE, Flamm SD et al. ACR Appropriateness Criteria((R)) pulsatile abdominal mass, suspected abdominal aortic aneurysm. *Int J Cardiovasc Imaging* 2013;29(1):177–183.

[47] Atar E, Belenky A, Hadad M, Ranany E, Baytner S, Bachar GN. MR angiography for abdominal and thoracic aortic aneurysms: Assessment before endovascular repair in patients with impaired renal function. *AJR Am J Roentgenol* 2006;186(2):386–393.

[48] Gornik HL, Creager MA. Aortitis. *Circulation* 2008;117(23):3039–3051.

[49] Bley TA, Uhl M, Venhoff N, Thoden J, Langer M, Markl M. 3-T MRI reveals cranial and thoracic inflammatory changes in giant cell arteritis. *Clin Rheumatol* 2007;26(3):448–450.

[50] Bley TA, Uhl M, Carew J et al. Diagnostic value of high-resolution MR imaging in giant cell arteritis. *AJNR Am J Neuroradiol* 2007;28(9):1722–1727.

[51] Bley TA, Ness T, Warnatz K et al. Influence of corticosteroid treatment on MRI findings in giant cell arteritis. *Clin Rheumatol* 2007;26(9):1541–1543.

[52] Burkart DJ, Johnson CD, Reading CC, Ehman RL. MR measurements of mesenteric venous flow: Prospective evaluation in healthy volunteers and patients with suspected chronic mesenteric ischemia. *Radiology* 1995;194(3):801–806.

[53] Bowersox JC, Zwolak RM, Walsh DB et al. Duplex ultrasonography in the diagnosis of celiac and mesenteric artery occlusive disease. *J Vasc Surg* 1991;14(6):780–786; discussion 786–788.

[54] Meaney JF, Prince MR, Nostrant TT, Stanley JC. Gadolinium-enhanced MR angiography of visceral arteries in patients with suspected chronic mesenteric ischemia. *J Magn Reson Imaging* 1997;7(1):171–176.

[55] Shih MC, Angle JF, Leung DA et al. CTA and MRA in mesenteric ischemia: Part 2, Normal findings and complications after surgical and endovascular treatment. *AJR Am J Roentgenol* 2007;188(2):462–471.

[56] Shih MC, Hagspiel KD. CTA and MRA in mesenteric ischemia: Part 1, Role in diagnosis and differential diagnosis. *AJR Am J Roentgenol* 2007;188(2):452–461.

[57] Li KC, Hopkins KL, Dalman RL, Song CK. Simultaneous measurement of flow in the superior mesenteric vein and artery with cine phase-contrast MR imaging: Value in diagnosis of chronic mesenteric ischemia. Work in progress. *Radiology* 1995;194(2):327–330.

[58] Safian RD, Textor SC. Renal-Artery Stenosis. *N Engl J Med* 2001;344(6):431–442.

[59] De Cobelli F, Venturini M, Vanzulli A et al. Renal arterial stenosis: Prospective comparison of color Doppler US and breath-hold, three-dimensional, dynamic, gadolinium-enhanced MR angiography. *Radiology* 2000;214(2):373–380.

[60] Vasbinder GBC, Nelemans PJ, Kessels AGH et al. Accuracy of computed tomographic angiography and magnetic resonance angiography for diagnosing renal artery stenosis. *Ann Intern Med* 2004;141(9):674–682.

[61] Maki JH, Wilson GJ, Eubank WB, Glickerman DJ, Pipavath S, Hoogeveen RM. Steady-state free precession MRA of the renal arteries: Breath-hold and navigator-gated techniques vs. CE-MRA. *J Magn Reson Imaging* 2007;26(4):966–973.

[62] Wyttenbach R, Braghetti A, Wyss M et al. Renal artery assessment with nonenhanced steady-state free precession versus contrast-enhanced MR angiography. *Radiology* 2007;245(1):186–195.

[63] Spuentrup E, Manning WJ, Bornert P, Kissinger KV, Botnar RM, Stuber M. Renal arteries: Navigator-gated balanced fast field-echo projection MR angiography with aortic spin labeling: Initial experience. *Radiology* 2002;225(2):589–596.

[64] Slovut DP, Olin JW. Fibromuscular dysplasia. *N Engl J Med* 2004;350(18):1862–1871.

[65] Willoteaux S, Faivre-Pierret M, Moranne O et al. Fibromuscular dysplasia of the main renal arteries: Comparison of contrast-enhanced MR angiography with digital subtraction angiography. *Radiology* 2006;241(3):922–929.

Chapter 6
周围血管磁共振成像

Peripheral Magnetic Resonance Angiography

Michele Anzidei, Beatrice Sacconi, Beatrice Cavallo Marincola, Pierleone Lucatelli, Alessandro Napoli, Mario Bezzi, Carlo Catalano 著

王 健 译

王怡宁 校

目录 CONTENTS

一、磁共振技术 / 110

二、无对比剂 MRA：飞行时间序列和稳态自由运动序列 / 110

三、对比剂增强 MRA / 111

四、时间分辨或四维 MRA / 111

五、上肢血管疾病病理学 / 112

六、动脉粥样硬化 / 112

七、急性动脉闭塞 / 112

八、雷诺现象 / 112

九、胸廓出口综合征 / 113

十、血液透析管 / 113

十一、上肢动脉瘤 / 113

十二、锁骨下动脉盗血综合征 / 114

十三、下肢血管疾病病理学 / 114

磁共振血管成像（MRA）包含了多项技术，包括飞行时间（time of fly，TOF）、相位对比血管成像技术等无对比剂血管成像技术和利用钆螯合剂作为对比剂的增强技术。其中，无对比剂技术利用血液流动的特性产生亮血信号。但这些技术往往非常耗时，而且会过分评估狭窄，尤其当血管走行曲折或存在异常血流时，这种情况尤为明显。

对比剂增强的 MRA 是流动相关成像技术的有力替代方案，相较于无对比剂 MRA 需要以分钟计算，对比剂增强 MRA 只需几秒即可完成图像采集。其基本原理是利用顺磁性对比材料缩短血液的 T_1 弛豫时间来实现血管和背景之间的对比。

然而对比剂增强 MRA 的最大挑战之一，是推注对比剂的最佳时机选择和限制静脉显影对图像的污染。在外周肢体血管成像中，推注对比剂的时间特别具有挑战性。对比剂推注时机的测试和推注对比剂追踪技术，因小血管可能被流入效应遮盖，而受到一定的限制。

一、磁共振技术

1. 上肢成像时患者摆位要点

（1）患者仰卧位进入磁体，手臂置于身体两侧。如果仅需对前臂或手进行成像，则推荐采用超人体位（superman position）。

（2）尽可能采用多通道相阵线圈或肢体线圈，高密度线圈应放置在感兴趣区。

（3）对比剂需通过对侧手臂注入。

（4）脱去任何含金属的衣服。

2. 下肢成像时患者摆位要点

（1）患者仰卧位进入磁体，足先进，下肢尽可能并拢并微微内旋。

（2）采用腹部或肢体的多通道相阵线圈。

（3）静脉注射对比剂。

（4）脱去任何含有金属的衣服。

二、无对比剂 MRA：飞行时间序列和稳态自由运动序列

飞行时间（TOF）序列是最常用的无对比剂 MRA 最常用的序列之一，常用于对比剂不耐受的患者以及血液透析患者造瘘管的评估。

二维（2D）和三维（3D）血管 TOF 技术可以通过快速射频（radio frequency, RF）脉冲在每个切面中饱和背景信号区分血管内静止的组织和运动的质子。新鲜流入的血液具有大量的自旋信号而未接收任何快速 RF 信号，所以血管呈现为非常明亮的信号，而静止的组织信号几乎完全被抑制。TOF 序列使用梯度回波（gradient-echo, GRE）序列族，利用很小的翻转角可以产生一系列的 RF 脉冲。如果我们选择垂直于血管的角度进行成像，那么我们就可以使得信号最大化。利用 TOF 技术最大的优势之一是只需施加不同的饱和带，就可以选择性的对动脉或静脉进行成像。

TOF 技术也存一些缺陷，采集时间偏长，而且对于狭窄或血管分叉处产生的湍流比较敏感[1,2]（表 6-1 和表 6-2）。

稳态自由进动（steady-state free-precession, SSFP）序列可以在不适用钆（Gd）对比剂的情况下快速产生亮血图像。事实上，SSFP 技术可以在非常短的重复时间（TR）（3ms）和大翻转角的条件下，在不到 1s 的时间内生成 2D 图像。正因如此，单次 SSFP 不需要屏气，且使用该序列可以应用于主动脉、肾动脉、颈动脉、外周动脉成像等多种临床场景。

表 6-1　上肢 TOF 序列技术参数

MRI 参数	值
TR（ms）	11
TE（ms）	6.9
FoV（mm）	450×450
层厚（mm）	5
矩阵	384×384
采集时间（s）	135

表 6-2 下肢 TOF 序列技术参数

MRI 参数	值
TR（ms）	30
TE（ms）	3.9
FoV（mm）	180×140
层厚（mm）	1
矩阵	256×224
采集时间（s）	5

三、对比剂增强 MRA

与利用 TOF 技术成像的 MRA 不同，对比剂增强 MRA 不是依靠血流，而是依靠静脉注射钆螯合剂来缩短血液 T_1 值。这可以大大增快采集时间。对比剂注射后需要精确的在动脉期采集以减少静脉的污染。快速插值 3D 采集允许近似各向同性采集，以改善复杂血管条件下的成像。这些序列并不依赖血流动力学状态。最小流量相关伪影可以实现高时间和空间分辨率。根据造影剂推注的时机可以实现动脉或静脉成像。钙化、金属器件、支架及高浓度钆对比剂引起的 T_2^* 效应可能影响图像质量[1-5]（表 6-3 和表 6-4）。

以下为该方案要点：冠状定位器；冠状平面上 GRE 3D 遮罩；MR 荧光镜技术实现可视化对比剂流量（在胸主动脉水平采集多个低分辨率图像）；获取冠状面上的 GRE 3D 序列图像（与遮罩相同）；处理减影图像。

四、时间分辨或四维 MRA

利用诸如对比动力学的时间分辨成像（TRICKS）技术可以实现高时间分辨率的同时，不损失空间信息。在注射对比剂之前采集获得初始遮罩，可用于对比剂增强后数据的减去。在对比剂注射后在多个时间点多次重复该序列获得多个时间点的血管系统的快照。这就能够使得小的病变血管或侧支血管逐渐显示。同时，在低剂量对比剂（<0.1mmol/kg）的情况下获得形态学和动力学的信息[6-12]（表 6-5）。

这些序列可以与 GRE 3D 序列形成混合方案（hybrid protocol），该方案适用于搭桥手术或糖尿病等肢体血流不对称的患者。这项技术还可以显示 GRE 3D 技术无法显示的细小血管（图 6-1）。

以下为该方案要点：第一次团注对比剂（8～10ml）可以对于远端血管（小腿和足）进行时间分辨 MRA 成像；第二次团注对比剂（10～15ml）可以用于腹部和大腿血管进行常规 GRE 3D 成像。

表 6-3 上肢三维 T_1WI 梯度回波的技术参数

MRI 参数	值
TR（ms）	3.5
TE（ms）	1.2
FoV（mm）	140×180
层厚（mm）	1
矩阵	384×384
采集时间（s）	14

表 6-4 下肢三维 T_1WI 梯度回波的技术参数

	腹 部	大 腿	小 腿
TE（ms）	3	3	3
FoV（mm）	0.9	0.9	1.4
层厚（mm）	1.4	1.4	1.2
矩阵	384×384	384×384	512×512
采集时间（s）	15	16	21

表 6-5 下肢三维 T_1WI 梯度回波的技术参数

	Twist（西门子）	Tricks（GE）	4D-Trak（Philips）
TR（ms）	2.7	5.5	2.2
TE（ms）	1.1	1.2	0.9
翻转角	20°	30°	15°
层厚	1.8	1.8	1.1
矩阵	384×384	384×384	224×178

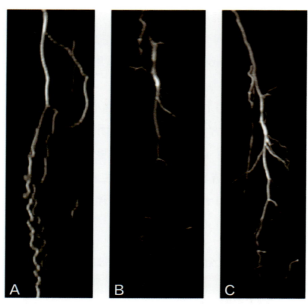

▲ 图 6-1　74 岁男性，左侧股前动脉闭塞
A. 飞行时间（TOF）序列显示血管闭塞以及股深动脉侧支血管开放，以及由于各向非同性体素造成一些阶梯伪影；
B. 稳态自由进动（SSFP）序列显示静脉血管残留信号；
C. 对比剂增强 MRA（CE-MRA）可以证实以上两种未增强技术的效果

五、上肢血管疾病病理学

手部和上肢血管异常包括多种疾病，包括从急性肢体缺血疾病到慢性致残疾病等。虽然不如下肢血管疾病常见，但其人群发病率也达到了 10%。

为了获得较好的成像效果，应该根据特定的临床问题和症状量身定制方案。如果怀疑锁骨下动脉盗血综合征，可以使用颈部 2D TOF 序列（5~6 节段），将饱和带放置在成像区域的上方，然后可评估椎动脉内血流的流动方向。除此之外，2D 相位对比或时间分辨成像也可以达到相似的成像效果。

如果怀疑血管炎，则推荐使用脂肪抑制的 T_2 加权图像序列，如反转恢复快速自旋回波序列，可以通过增强后的 T_1 加权图像 GRE 序列来检查血管壁疾病。

如果怀疑胸廓出口综合征，则应在扫描过程中保持患者手臂呈抬起状态。如果脉管系统确实存在异常压迫，则应放下手臂之后，再次进行 MRA 检查。

六、动脉粥样硬化

上肢动脉粥样硬化远不如下肢常见，上肢动脉粥样硬化病变可能涉及无名动脉及锁骨下动脉起源处。当动脉狭窄或者闭塞时可能导致上肢运动障碍及上肢缺血，但可能因侧支血管的存在而并无症状产生。有症状的患者可以接受各种手术，如颈动脉 - 锁骨下旁路手术或锁骨下动脉转位手术。在这些情况下，MR 可以用于评估移植物的位置，吻合口状态，管腔通畅程度以及潜在再狭窄可能。

在 MR 图像报告中，需要严格遵守以下模式：定位和描述病变，评估狭窄程度；在血管闭塞存在时，需要描述侧支血管；描述病变上方和下方解剖学异常和血管状况（包括口径和血管管壁状况）；评估手臂血液循环（包括血流不对称性）和其他较小病变的存在；注意非血管异常情况的表现。

七、急性动脉闭塞

上肢动脉闭塞性疾病可表现为局部或全身性的疾病。动脉疾病的表现因病因而异。影响头臂动脉血管的疾病包括动脉粥样硬化、动脉炎、先天发育异常、外伤和肌肉发育不良。在美国，动脉粥样硬化是锁骨下动脉狭窄的最常见原因；在美国以外，大动脉炎则更为常见。腋动脉和肱动脉是最常见受累部位。1/3 外周动脉栓塞发生在上肢，可产生急性动脉闭塞。胸部和乳腺的放射治疗也可能诱发锁骨下动脉疾病。急性动脉闭塞的常见原因如下：栓塞、急性血栓形成、动脉痉挛、压迫、夹层。

报告应包括与动脉粥样硬化疾病相同的要点，需要注意的是，在急性血栓形成时，无侧支循环血管形成。

八、雷诺现象

雷诺现象是一种血管痉挛性疾病，可导致手指、脚趾和其他部位的变色。雷诺现象包括可产生特发性现象的雷诺病（也称为原发性雷诺现象）和雷诺综合征。雷诺综合征大致分类如下。

1. 原发性雷诺现象，是由于某些调节因素异常引起的功能性微血管病，最常见的是由于诸如系统性红斑狼疮等结缔组织病引起。

2. 继发性雷诺现象，由于诸如胸廓出口综合征等压迫性疾病引起。

当考虑到小血管疾病时，由于评估效力有限，但 MRI 可被用来排除其他诊断，如大血管的压迫等（图 6-2）。

九、胸廓出口综合征

动作引起的胸廓出口通道中神经、动脉压迫可以引起胸廓出口综合征，静脉受压情况较为少见。胸廓出口综合征的诊断基于临床评估的结果，如进行各种动作时（包括手臂太高）可以重复患者的症状。胸廓出口或颈 - 胸 - 肱交界处，包括三个狭小的空间，包括斜角肌间隙、肋锁骨间隙、胸小肌间隙，从颈椎和纵隔延伸至胸小肌下部边界为神经血管压迫的潜在部位（表 6-6）。

表 6-6　胸廓出口综合征的主要病因

一般情况	特定病理学
肌肉和骨骼的异常	颈肋或细长的 C_7 横突 外生骨疣或第 1 肋、锁骨的肿瘤 第 1 肋或锁骨的多余愈伤组织
软组织异常	纤维带 先天性肌肉异常
获得性软组织异常	创伤后纤维瘢痕 手术后纤维瘢痕
姿势易感类型	肌肉支持力羸弱

虽然诊断一般是临床性的，但 MR 和 CT 可以用来：定位压迫位置；明确病因和所涉及的结构；评估压迫的程度。

CT 能够充分明确血管压迫的情况，但对于臂丛分支的详细分析较为困难，应使用 MR 来进行评估[13]。

十、血液透析管

血液透析需要功能良好的血管通路，以能够允许充足的血液流动，来获得足够的清除率和透析剂量。中心静脉插管并随后通过手术建立动静脉瘘管或移植物可以获得使用时间更久的通路。上腔静脉瘘通常通过桡动脉或肱动脉与邻近贵要静脉、头静脉或肘正中静脉行端侧吻合术形成。血液透析的并发症包括静脉狭窄、血栓形成、感染和动脉瘤等，罕见并发症为动脉盗血综合征。现已证明 MR 是可以用来准确进行血液透析管的解剖和功能综合评估以及相关并发症的评估。它可以非侵入性地进行监测并早期发现可以通过血管成形术进行治疗的血管狭窄，从而大大减少继发性的血栓形成的频率[14-17]。

十一、上肢动脉瘤

动脉瘤是血管壁上的局部球状隆起。真性动

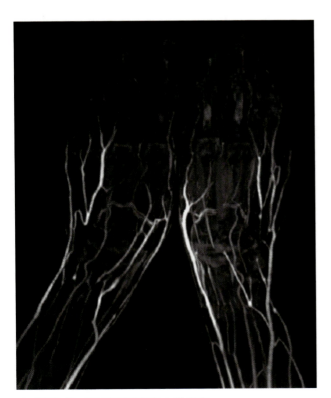

▲ 图 6-2　52 岁雷诺现象女性患者
在平衡期获得 CE-MRA 图像，显示双侧手指动脉渐进性管腔缩小

脉瘤可见动脉壁的所有三层结构（内膜、中膜和外膜），其成因包括动脉粥样硬化、梅毒和先天性动脉瘤。假性动脉瘤或假动脉瘤是由于血液从动脉或静脉泄漏，但被周围组织限制在血管周围。形成的这个充满血液的空腔最终会充分凝血（形成血凝块）来封闭泄漏的部分及周围撕裂的组织。假性动脉瘤可由以下原因产生，包括刀或子弹形成的动脉穿刺伤、冠状动脉造影或血管成形术等手术操作、动脉注射操作等[18]。动脉瘤也可以根据其大小和形状来进行分类，其外形可以为囊状或梭形。动脉瘤的形状和特定的疾病并无关系。囊状动脉瘤的形状通常为球形，它的形成仅涉及血管壁的一部分，它的直径大小从 5cm 到 20cm 不等，并且它们通常部分或完全被血栓填充。梭形动脉瘤的直径和长度都不相同（表 6-7）。

表 6-7 动脉瘤的主要病因

受累血管	受累节段	病 因
锁骨下动脉	斜角肌前段	动脉粥样硬化微粒形成
锁骨下动脉	远段	狭窄后创伤
腋动脉		创伤
桡动脉和尺动脉		慢性创伤

在 MR 图像报告中，需要严格遵守以下模式：描述动脉瘤的位置、大小和纵向延伸的范围；描述动脉瘤中血栓形成的位置（中心性/偏心性）；描述动脉瘤上方与下方距正常血管的距离；确定动脉瘤破裂或闭塞的位置；描述动脉瘤与周围血管和非血管结构的关系。

十二、锁骨下动脉盗血综合征

锁骨下动脉盗血综合征是由左侧锁骨下动脉或邻近同侧椎动脉起源的头臂干主干闭塞或严重狭窄所致。随着上肢对血液供应的需求增加（头部活动及肌肉的压力），血流从椎 - 基底系统转移或被盗，并随后通过同侧椎动脉内的逆行绕过手臂。锁骨下动脉的狭窄和闭塞最常见于动脉粥样硬化性疾病，其鉴别诊断包括创伤、血管炎、动脉夹层和先天异常。锁骨下动脉盗血对左侧锁骨下动脉影响比右侧多 3 倍。在此病患者中，MR 和 CT 可以用来确定近端锁骨下动脉的狭窄或梗阻，并提供狭窄处长度的信息，并可通过椎动脉评估同侧再灌注情况（图 6-3）。

十三、下肢血管疾病病理学

（一）动脉粥样硬化

动脉粥样硬化性疾病是外周动脉疾病的主要病因，主要由于血管狭窄和闭塞引起相应血管供血区动脉供血减少。早期临床上主要表现为运动过程中小腿后部慢性痉挛和酸痛，该病晚期常见症状急剧恶化。外周动脉闭塞性疾病（peripheral artery occlusive disease，PAOD）是该病最严重的进展表现。其主要危险因素包括年龄、男性、吸烟、糖尿病和血脂异常[7,19]。

从放射学角度来看，目前外周动脉疾病治疗的指南根据病变范围和潜在手术治疗方式或血管内治疗方式进行分类。动脉粥样硬化性病变可重新分为流入病变（涉及主动脉和髂动脉病变）和

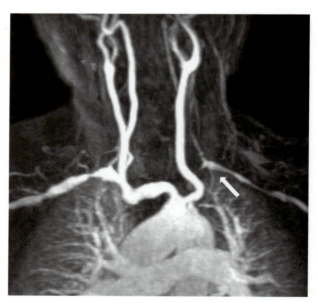

▲ 图 6-3　67 岁男性，左上肢痉挛
CE-MRA 图像显示左侧锁骨下动脉严重狭窄（箭）；血流从同侧椎 - 基底动脉系统转移

流出性病变（涉及股动脉和腘动脉）。在这些部位，动脉粥样硬化病变使用四点量表分类[20]。

1. 应优先采用血管内方式治疗的病变。
2. 血管内治疗能够得到良好疗效，而手术治疗获益有限的病变。
3. 手术治疗能够取得良好疗效，而血管内治疗获益有限的病变。
4. 应优先采用手术方式治疗的病变。

在治疗过程中，成像能够诊断狭窄和对治疗计划进行量化和定位，例如分析血管解剖和选择更有效的治疗方法。

在 MR 图像报告中，需要严格遵守以下模式：①定位病变，评估狭窄程度；②如果为闭塞病变，注意描述侧支循环；③注意描述病变血管解剖学异常（包括管腔和管壁的情况）；④评估肢体循环状态（包括血流不对称性）以及其他同时存在的较小病变；⑤注意非血管病变。

外周血管阻塞性病变的介入和外科治疗包括经皮腔内血管成形术、溶栓治疗、旁路和支架置入，随着血管成形术技术的提高和改进，血管内治疗已经成为外科手术治疗的有效替代方法。

MRA 对于外周血管疾病的治疗后评估十分有效。

经皮血管腔内成形术为一线治疗技术，治疗后进行成像可以确定支架的再狭窄。然而，多种血管支架在 MR 扫描期间均会产生扫描伪影，因此使用 CT 通常是首选的治疗后检查。治疗后的早期并发症包括出血和远端血管栓塞。MR 可以显示血肿和出血的部位，而且 MR 可以有助于识别远端栓塞（绝大多数可以与治疗前检查的结果进行对比），可以清晰显示先前正常的远端血管分支消失。

远期并发症主要包括由于粥样硬化疾病进展和内膜增生引起的假性动脉瘤和支架闭塞/再狭窄。

内膜切除术为沿血管内膜将粥样硬化斑块切除，但其治疗后再狭窄的发生十分频繁。手术搭桥是从阻塞物上方向阻塞远端放置移植物，虽然这种情况可能发生各种并发症，但这种治疗方式最为可靠。早期并发症包括血肿、皮下水肿、淋巴管囊肿，所有这些并发症通常都存在液体的封闭，可以在 MRA 上呈现流体信号。血管内或者移植物内产生血栓、血液或血凝块可以使得信号改变。在 MR 图像上，当信号混杂时，高度提示管腔阻塞的发生。当吻合口或沿移植物走行出现液体伴随周围出现气体及软组织肿胀时，可以诊断移植物感染[21,22]。

晚期并发症包括继发的移植物狭窄闭塞，狭窄可以发生在吻合口处或移植物中间区域。移植物狭窄表现与原生血管狭窄表现在 MR 上类似。由于外界的压迫、扭转或远端及近端的疾病进展，在移植物中也可以形成狭窄或血栓。其他并发症包括假性动脉瘤形成和吻合口裂开，其主要危险因素表现为移植血管张力过大。在 MR 上，假性动脉瘤可能会被误认为吻合口附近的局灶溢出。即使能够及时诊断，但主动脉瘘发生时也是死亡率极高的危及生命的并发症（图 6-4 至图 6-6）。

（二）下肢动脉瘤

腘动脉诊断动脉瘤的管径比的界值为 > 0.7，股动脉为 > 1.5。

真性动脉瘤主要与粥样硬化疾病相关，常发

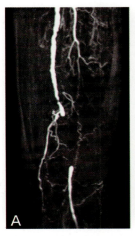
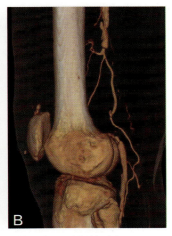

▲ 图 6-4　79 岁男性，左下肢急性跛行
A.CE-MRA 显示远段股前动脉和近段腘动脉闭塞；B. 外周血管 CTA 立体渲染图像绘制证实了 MRI 结果，同时显示出了股浅动脉的侧支循环形成远端血供重建

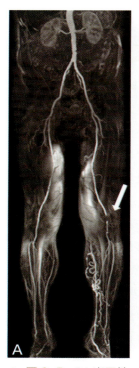
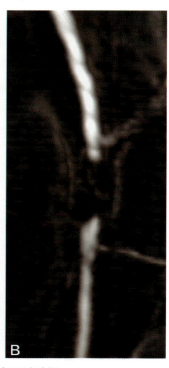

▲ 图 6-5　81 岁男性，左下肢跛行
A.CE-MRA 的最大密度投影图像显示左侧关节上腘动脉节段性阻塞（箭）；B. 局部放大图像确认先前结果

生于腘动脉区。假性动脉瘤主要与创伤（常见为医源性）或感染相关动脉缺陷。

报告需包括以下内容：描述动脉瘤的位置、大小和延伸长度；描述动脉瘤的血栓形成的位置（中心性/偏心性）；描述动脉瘤上方和下方正常血管的距离；发现早期破裂或闭塞的征象；描述动脉瘤与周围血管和非血管结构的关系。

在动脉瘤较大时，MR 可以通过增加对比剂及增打给药和扫描之间的时间来取得更好的效果。但事实上，动脉瘤的附近血流可能非常湍急，可能造成对比剂稀释[5,9,23]（图 6-7）。

（三）压迫综合征

腘动脉压迫综合征（popliteal artery entrapment syndrome, PAES），是一种继发于腘动脉与腓肠肌发育异常导致腘动脉的偏离和压迫，在较罕见的情况也可能继发于异常纤维带或腘肌的存在。PAES 存在 4 种基本的解剖异常。

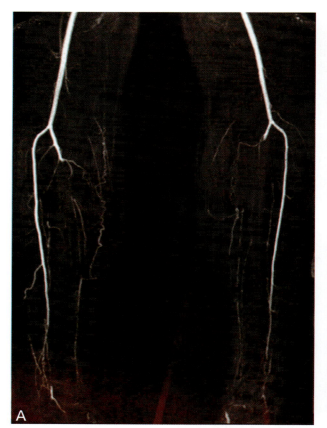

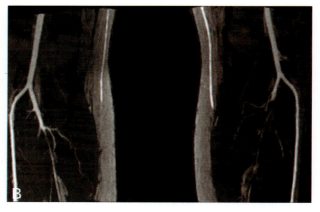

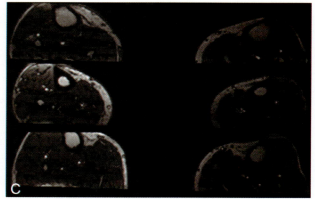

▲ 图 6-6　78 岁男性，双侧急性跛行及足部溃疡
A.CE-MRA 显示双侧胫腓干闭塞；B、C. 平衡期采集的轴向重建图像可获得与高分辨序列一致的结果

Chapter 6 周围血管磁共振成像
Peripheral Magnetic Resonance Angiography

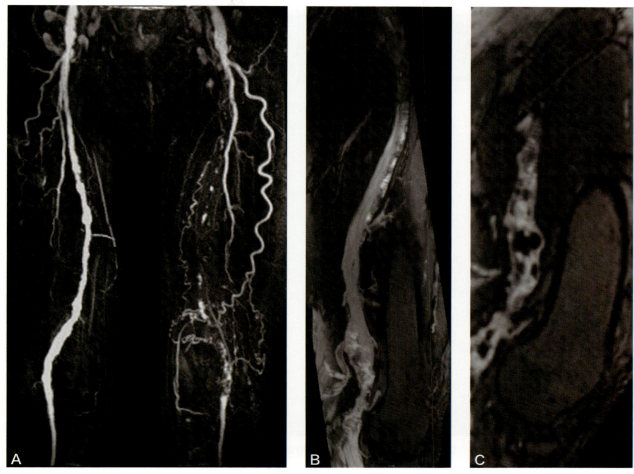

▲ 图 6-7 74 岁男性，双侧跛行

A.CE-MRA 显示双侧股浅动脉和腘动脉节段增粗，以及股浅动脉远段及腘动脉近段血栓形成；B、C. 在平衡期高分辨序列图像可获得一致结果

因患者年龄较小，通常可以采用压力 MR（stress MR），分别在静息状态和脚背绷直的压迫状态进行扫描，以得到有意义的结果[5,9,23]。

（四）血管夹层

外周动脉夹层通常是腹主动脉夹层的延伸。有时也可以观察到由于局部穿刺引起的股动脉的局灶夹层。

除了常规的扫描方案以外，怀疑本病时，还需要在注射对比剂之前扫描 T_1WI 和 T_2WI 序列，来寻找可能发现的血管内膜片（图 6-8）。

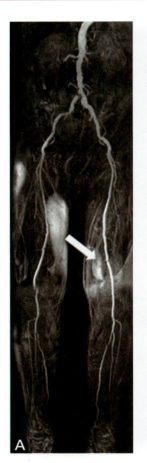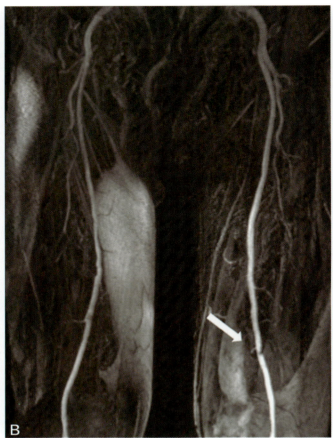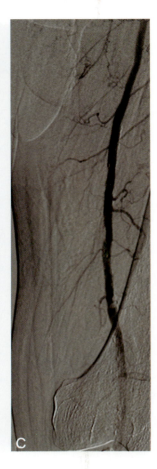

▲ 图 6-8　68 岁男性

A.CE-MRA 示左侧股浅动脉局灶夹层（箭）；B. 局部放大图像确认先前结果；C. 同一患者股动脉造影结果

参考文献

[1] Lee VS. *Cardiovascular MRI: Physical Principles to Practical Protocols*. Philadelphia, PA: Lippincott Williams &Wilkins, 2006; p. 14.

[2] Krinsky G, Rofsky NM. MR angiography of the aortic arch vessels and upper extremities. *Magn Reson Imaging Clin N Am* 1998; 6(2): 269–292.

[3] Prince MR, Yucel EK, Kaufman JA, Harrison DC, Geller SC. Dynamic gadolinium-enhanced three-dimensional abdominal MR arteriography. *J Magn Reson Imaging* 1993; 3(6): 877–881.

[4] Lee VS, Lee HM, Rofsky NM. Magnetic resonance angiography of the hand: A review. *Invest Radiol* 1998; 33(9): 687–698.

[5] Demondion X, Herbinet P, Van Sint Jan S, Boutry N, Chanteot C, Cotten A. Imaging assessment of thoracic outlet syndrome. *RadioGraphics* 2006; 26: 1735–1750.

[6] Korosec FR, Frayne R, Grist TM, Mistretta CA. Time-resolved contrast-enhanced 3D MR angiography. *Magn Reson Med* 1996; 36(3): 345–351.

[7] Van Rijswijk CS, van der Linden E, van der Woude HJ, van Baalen JM, Bloem JL. Value of dynamic contrast-enhanced MR imaging in diagnosing and classifying peripheral vascular malformations. *AJR Am J Roentgenol* 2002; 178(5): 1181–1187.

[8] Konez O, Burrows PE. Magnetic resonance of vascular anomalies. *Magn Reson Imaging Clin N Am* 2002; 10(2): 363–388, vii.

[9] Connell DA, Koulouris G, Thorn DA, Potter HG. Contrast-enhanced MR angiography of the hand. *RadioGraphics* 2002; 22(3): 583–599.

[10] Choe YH, Han BK, Koh EM, Kim DK, Do YS, Lee WR. Takayasu's arteritis: Assessment of disease activity with contrast-enhanced MR imaging. *AJR Am J Roentgenol* 2000; 175(2): 505–511.

[11] Herborn CU, Goyen M, Lauenstein TC, Debatin JF, Ruehm SG, Kroger K. Comprehensive time-resolved MRI of peripheral vascular malformations. *AJR Am J Roentgenol* 2003; 181(3): 729–735.

[12] Shah DJ, Brown B, Kim RJ, Grizzard JD. Magnetic resonance evaluation of peripheral arterial disease. *Cardiol Clin* 2007; 25(1): 185–212.

[13] Demondion X, Herbinet P, Van Sint Jan S. et al. Stenosis detection in forearm hemodialysis arteriovenous fistulae

by multiphase contrast-enhanced magnetic resonance angiography: Preliminary experience. *J Magn Reson Imaging* 2003; 17(1): 54–64.

[14] Zhang J, Hecht EM, Maldonado T, Lee VS. Time-resolved 3D MR angiography with parallel imaging for evaluation of hemodialysis fistulas and grafts: Initial experience. *AJR Am J Roentgenol* 2006; 186(5): 1436–1442.

[15] Fayad L, Hazirolan T, Bluemke D, Mitchell S. Vascular malformations in the extremities: Emphasis on MR imaging features that guide treatment options. *Skeletal Radiol* 2006; 35(3): 127–137.

[16] Norgren L, Hiatt WR, Dormandy JA. et al. Intersociety consensus for the management of peripheral arterial disease. *Int Angiol* 2007; 26(2): 81–157.

[17] Cavagna E, D'Andrea P, Schiavon F, Tarroni G. Failing hemodialysis arteriovenous fistula and percutaneous treatment: Imaging with CT, MRI and digital subtraction angiography. *Cardovasc Intervent Radiol* 2000; 23: 262–265.

[18] Chaudhry N, Salhab KF. Hand, upper extremity vascular injury. *Emedicine* 2003; http://www.emedicine.com/plastic/topic461.htm. Accessed August 3, 2006.

[19] Prince MR, Narasimham DL, Stanley JC. et al. Breath-hold gadolinium-enhanced MR angiography of the abdominal aorta and its major branches. *Radiology* 1995; 197(3): 785–792.

[20] Ichihashi S, Higashiura W, Itoh H, Sakaguchi S, Nishimine K, Kichikwa K. Long-term outcomes for systematic primary stent placement in complex iliac artery occlusive disease classified according to Trans-Atlantic Inter-Society Consensus (TASC)-II. *J Vasc Surg* 2011; 53(4): 992–999.

[21] Ye W, Liu CW, Ricco JB, Mani K, Zeng R, Jiang J. Early and late outcomes of percutaneous treatment of Trans-Atlantic Inter-Society Consensus class C and D aortoiliac lesions. *J Vasc Surg* 2011; 53(6): 1728–1737.

[22] Sultan S, Hynes N. Five-year Irish trial of CLI patients with TASC II type C/D lesions undergoing subintimal angioplasty or bypass surgery based on plaque echolucency. *J Endovasc Ther* 2009; 16(3): 270–283.

[23] Lee VS, Martin DJ, Krinsky GA, Rofsky NM. Gadolinium-enhanced MR angiography: Artifacts and pitfalls. *AJR Am J Roentgenol* 2000; 175(1): 197–205.

Chapter 7
磁共振静脉成像

Magnetic Resonance Venography

Simon Gabriel, Chun Kit Shiu, Stefan G.Ruehm 著

林 路 张大明 译

王怡宁 校

目录 CONTENTS

一、MRV 技术简介 / 122

二、无对比剂增强序列 / 123

三、临床应用 / 132

磁共振静脉成像（magnetic resonance venography, MRV）已经成为一种经临床验证的评价静脉系统的可靠、有效成像方法。本章论述的大多数技术被同时应用于动脉和静脉系统成像[1]。与动脉成像相比，由于静脉血流速较慢且信号较均一，MRV 在成像技术上的要求较低。本章将阐述 MRV 的原理、技术和当前临床应用。

一、MRV 技术简介

磁共振成像显示血流的能力和其特有的高软组织对比度使其在某些特定情况下，成为能够切实解决临床问题的一线影像诊断工具。

MRV 技术大体上可分为无对比剂增强与对比剂增强两大类（表 7-1）。无对比剂增强 MRV 应用的序列包括自旋回波（spin-echo, SE）/ 快速自旋回波（fast spin-echo, FSE）、传统时间飞跃（time-of-fly, TOF）、相位对比（phase contrast, PC）、平衡稳态自由进动（balanced steady-state free precession, bSSFP）、磁敏感加权成像（susceptibility-weighted imaging, SWI）、信号靶向交替射频（radio frequency, RF）和非流动依赖弛豫强化，以及直接血栓成像（表 7-2）。对比剂增强 MRV 序列包括时间分辨 MRV 和传统定时 MRV（表 7-3）。尽管存在 MRI 扫描仪厂商、平台及对比剂的技术差异，MRV 的成像基础是一致的。表 7-1 总结了本章讨论的不同 MRV 技术。表 7-2 和表 7-3 总结了不同厂商对常规应用序列不同的命名。

与传统无对比剂增强技术相比，对比剂增强技术可以得到更高的图像分辨率和对比噪声比，更快的成像速度，且非血流依赖，故更受青睐。在大多数单位中，当患者存在如肾功能不全等钆对比剂禁忌证时，会使用无对比剂增强技术或其他替代成像方法。我们倾向使用一种具有不同白蛋白结合度的钆对比剂，其在血管中具有更长的半衰期，从而增强 T_1 缩短效应提高血管信号。有时候在有钆对比剂禁忌证的患者中，我们会使用一类新兴的不含钆对比剂——超微氧化铁颗粒（ultrasmall iron-oxide particles, USPIO）。

表 7-1 磁共振静脉成像的常用技术

	主要特征	优 势	限 制
无对比剂增强技术			
TOF	垂直位血流成像，可选择饱和带，梯度回波（GRE）为基础	一线非增强序列，常用于脑部	扫描时间长，平行位血流饱和伪影
相位对比	信号依赖于流动血液的自旋相位变化	定量测量血流速度，包括经狭窄梯度	扫描时间长，需预估血流速度以准确设定扫描参数
T_1-3D GRE	三维直接血栓成像	非增强，直接显示血栓	依赖血栓的 T_1 缩短，准确性有限
SWI	顺磁性脱氧血红蛋白的频移	信号不依赖于血流	高场强有益
SSFP	血液固有的信号	高信噪比，快速，稳健，运动伪影少	对血流方向不敏感，受磁场不均一性影响，易产生非共振伪影特别在高场系统（3T）
对比剂增强技术			
CE 3D MRV	三维，对比剂依赖	高空间分辨率，用途广，快速，稳健	对比剂禁忌证（需静脉注射）
直接 MRV	直接下游静脉成像	选择性显示静脉，对比剂用量少，血管对比强	显示的静脉区域有限，需进行受累静脉的注射

表 7-2 不同厂商对通用无对比剂增强序列的命名

	GE	西门子	东芝	飞利浦	日立
SE/FSE	SE/FSE	SE/TSE	SE/FSE	SE/TSE	SE/FSE
TOF	TOF	TOF	TOF	Inflow MRA	TOF
PC	PC	PC	PC	PC	VNEC
bSSFP	FIESTA	True FISP	True SSFP	Balanced FFE	BASG（balanced SARGE）
SWI	SWAN	SWI	Flow-sensitive black blood（FSBB）	Venous bold	BSI

SE. 自旋回波；FSE. 快速自旋回波；TOF. 时间飞跃；PC. 相位对比；bSSFP. 平衡稳态自由进动；SWI. 磁敏感加权成像

表 7-3 不同厂商对通用对比剂增强序列的命名

	GE	Siemens	Toshiba	Phillips	Hitachi
时间分辨磁共振血管成像	TRICKS（time-resolved imaging of contrast kinetics，对比剂动态时间分辨成像）	TWIST（time-resolved angiography with interleaved stochastic trajectories，时间分辨交错随机轨迹血管成像）	Freeze frame/DRKS	4D TRAK（time-resolved angiography using keyhole，时间分辨锁孔血管成像）	TRAQ
传统定时血管成像	Smart prep；fluoro triggered MRA	Care bolus	Visual prep	Bolus trak	FLUTE

二、无对比剂增强序列

（一）自旋回波和快速自旋回波

SE 和 FSE 序列常被用于心脏成像并被称为"黑血"成像技术，由于快速的血流产生流空信号，血管腔内呈黑色/低信号。在感兴趣血管节段近端应用预饱和脉冲，可以更有效消除流动的自旋信号，保留静止组织的自旋信号。黑血成像中的血管内高信号可能与湍流、层面内血液流动时间延长，血流速度慢等因素相关[2]。为解决传统黑血技术的内在技术限制，更加稳健的序列设计被提出[3]。

传统黑血成像适用于评价血管壁和血管周围组织的形态，尤其在同时采集压脂和非压脂图像的情况下。但是当前传统的 SE 和 FSE 技术在评价静脉腔内病变中存在限制。

（二）时间飞跃

TOF MRV 使用短重复时间（repetition time, TR）梯度回波脉冲序列以加强血流信号。静止组织的信号被抑制，自成像层面外流入的血流未暴露于脉冲，故完整保留纵向弛豫。进入成像层面后，纵向弛豫被激发脉冲翻转至横向平面而产生高信号。二维（2D）或三维（3D）TOF 成像在技术上均可行。2D 成像通过顺序逐层激发获取每一薄层图像。3D 成像中，一定体积的组织被同时激发，之后被分割成多层。2D TOF 适用于静脉成像，因为其可以检测慢速血流，覆盖范围大并且对 T_1 效应敏感[4]。2D TOF 成像的劣势包括分辨率受限、平行位血流饱和和潜在呼吸伪影。

当血流在成像平面中时间过长而接受多次脉冲激发时，由于自旋饱和产生信号丢失。这种效应见于方向平行于成像平面的血管。

动脉和静脉在 TOF 成像中通常均为高信号。特定方向的血流信号可以通过使用血流预饱和带饱和（图 7-1），从而消除感兴趣区内特定方向的血流信号。对静脉磁共振成像，饱和带置于检查解剖区域的近端。以此得到选择性 TOF 静脉成像。

TOF 成像中，使用更长的 TR 时间可以使数量更多的弛豫自旋进入成像平面，增强血流信号，但延长扫描时间。回波时间（echo time，TE）要短，TE 时间设为 8ms（在 1.5T 系统中）可以使水和脂肪的信号不同相以达成脂肪抑制。

合适的翻转角度选择同时与扫描层面方向和检查血管的轴线相关。对纵向/平行位血流 20°～25°的翻转角较为合理，对横向/垂直位血流可选择 45°翻转角。需要注意：降低翻转角造成平行位血流饱和降低，需要更多射频脉冲达到纵向磁化平衡。翻转角过大可能造成静脉信号饱和，但翻转角过小可能造成强噪声。

为提高最大密度投影（maximum intensity projection，MIP）的图像重建质量，层面分割需要连续甚至有所重叠以减弱阶梯状重建伪影（图 7-1D）。

（三）相位对比 MRV

PC 成像基于移动质子的相位差别。双极磁场梯度的应用造成移动的质子自旋获得与静止质子自旋不同的相位（相位偏移）。一个正极梯度跟着一个负极梯度产生双极梯度，方向相反的梯度造成流动血液的相位偏移，而静止组织不产生净相位差。通常使用减影成像时静止质子自旋信号最小，而移动质子自旋的磁化被增强[5]。PC 成像产生的流速图中，体素对应的强度值与特定血流方向的实际血流速度呈正比。每个血流体素中测得的相位差与初始方向的流速变化和速度编码时间（ΔT）直接相关。通常应用 2D 技术进行 PC-MRV 成像（图 7-2）。3D 序列曾用于颅内静脉成像，但在当前应用有限，因为与其他成像技术相比其图像质量欠佳。

信号强度依赖于相位偏移量：信号越亮或越暗，相位偏移越大。对流动的敏感性可以通过变量速度编码值（velocity encoding value，VENC）调节，其决定可测量的最大流速。合理的 VENC 应当高于预测的最大流速约 25%。如果 VENC 过低，产生混淆伪影/卷折伪影；如果 VENC 过高，对慢

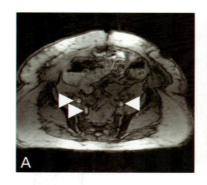
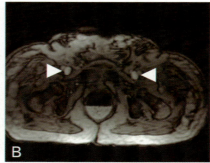
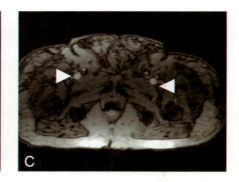
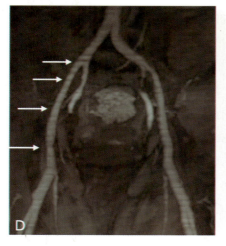
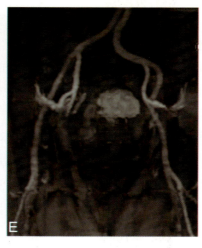

▲ 图 7-1　TOF：盆腔静脉 2D TOF MRV

A～C. 于盆腔连续逐层激发，设置近端预饱和带以消除动脉血流信号，仅静脉血（箭头）呈高信号；静脉横轴位图（D）和动脉横轴位图（E）（未展示）的冠状位 MIP 重建图像，请注意水平条带（白箭）为自旋饱和伪影

速血流的敏感性和流速的定量测量准确性下降。对静脉成像通常推荐设定小于 20cm/s 的 VENC。血流的定量测量由软件计算，要求操作者人工绘制感兴趣血管每个相位的轮廓，并需放射科医师复核。自由呼吸 PC-MRV 被证明是一种可用于无创测量肝脏血流的技术，与超声多普勒相比变异性小、可重复性高[6]。

（四）直接血栓成像

与多数成像技术通过流空效应或对比剂充盈缺损显示血栓不同，MR 直接血栓成像使用 T_1-3D 梯度回波（gradient-echo，GRE）序列在抑制的背景中显示血栓[7]（图 7-3B 和图 7-6F）。在血栓形成的过程中，栓子 T_1 值减低代表正铁血红蛋白的产生，其含有具强顺磁性的三价铁。血栓中的高信号首发于外周端，随时间延长逐渐向心扩展。除去血栓本身产生的高信号，应用反转恢复脉冲去除未凝固血液的信号进一步增强血栓与周围血液的对比。通过选择性水分子射频激发可以在 T_1 加权图像中进一步去除背景中的脂肪信号。在临床怀疑深静脉血栓（deep venous thrombosis，DVT）的患者中，磁共振直接血栓成像可以准确发现急性 DVT[8]。由于经过约 6 个月的时间后，血栓 T_1 信号趋于正常，该方法可能较超声更好地发现新发 DVT[9]。

（五）磁敏感加权成像

SWI 是一种高分辨 3D GRE 序列，结合幅度和相位信号以得到对组织磁敏感性差别高敏感性的成像方法[10,11]。

在 SWI 中，脱氧血红蛋白、含铁血黄素、铁蛋白及钙均可产生低信号。在静脉中，脱氧血红蛋白引起幅度图中 T_2^* 相关信号的缺失及相位图中因磁敏感差异造成的相位偏移。在动脉中，TOF 效应及 T_2^* 效应的缺失造成管腔内高信号。

硬脑膜动静脉瘘的软脑膜静脉引流反向与高发病率和死亡率相关。治疗前/后的随访研究均证实，以数字减影血管成像为参照，颅内静脉的 SWI 高信号均可以准确发现硬脑膜动静脉瘘患者的软脑膜静脉引流反向[12,13]。此外，SWI 可以证明静脉充血的缓解，从而有助于对治疗后脑循环

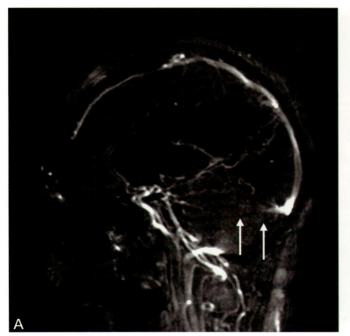
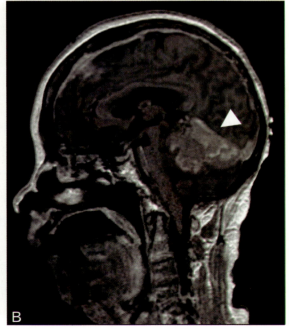

▲ 图 7-2 2D PC MRV（VENC=10cm/s）
A. 正中矢状位颅内静脉的速度编码幅度图成像显示直窦（箭）未充盈；B. 对比剂增强 MRI 显示其继发于脑膜瘤侵犯（箭头）

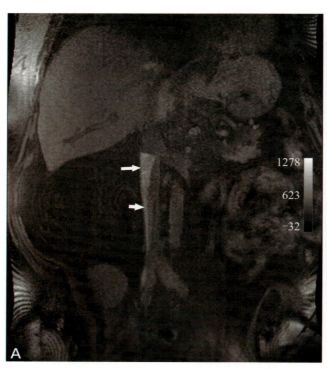 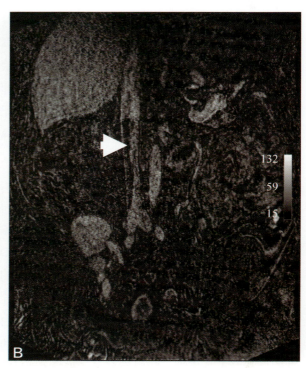

▲ 图 7-3 冠状位压脂 T_1 梯度回波序列（FLASH）图像

A. 示自下腔静脉至右侧髂内静脉的血栓呈高信号（箭）；B. 对应间接减影 CE MRV 图像（示血栓表现为低信号充盈缺损（箭头）

改善的评价[13]。因此，SWI 可能替代被作为软脑膜静脉引流反向诊断和评估"金标准"的传统血管造影（图 7-4）。

由于 3D GER 序列对呼吸伪影敏感，SWI 首先被用于颅内成像，但近期研究显示 2D SWI 亦可应用于腹部成像[14]。

（六）平衡稳态自由进动

bSSFP［FIESTA（GE）；True FISP（Siemens）］是一种在动脉和静脉中均得到高信号的亮血技术，被广泛应用于心脏电影成像。

bSSFP 为采用快速 GRE 脉冲的序列，使纵向和横向磁化维持在一种平衡态，赋予的静相位为零。信号强度与 T_2/T_1 成比例，长 T_2 和短 T_2 组织均可成高信号。数据可 2D 采集，亦可应用呼吸导航 3D 采集。bSSFP 采集时间短，尤其与如 TOF 等无对比剂增强 MRV 技术相比。bSSFP 被证明可有效进行肺静脉[15]（图 7-5）、胸部中心静脉[16]，以及门静脉[17]成像。

（七）信号靶向交替射频和非流动依赖弛豫强化

信号靶向交替射频和非流动依赖弛豫强化（signal targeting using alternative radiofrequency and flow-independent relaxation enhancement，STARFIRE）是一种无对比剂增强的非血流依赖磁共振血管成像（MRA）新技术，可同时抑制脂肪和肌肉背景。和 bSSFP 相同，STARFIRE 技术在动脉和静脉中均产生高信号，但是其可通过同时抑制脂肪和肌肉背景进行外周小动静脉的成像。

该技术通过 T_1 依赖机制压脂；使用线性相位编码顺序和大翻转角激发的 bSSFP 脉冲序列抑制肌肉信号。为选择性增强静脉信号，每 50ms 对流入血流应用一系列空间选择性预饱和射频脉冲。该技术可对大感兴趣区成像，受磁场不均一性影响较小。在小样本患者的定性分析中，STARFIRE 和对比剂增强 3D MRA 具有相似的图像质量稳定性和浅表静脉结构显示能力，两者均优于 2D TOF[18]。

Chapter 7 磁共振静脉成像
Magnetic Resonance Venography

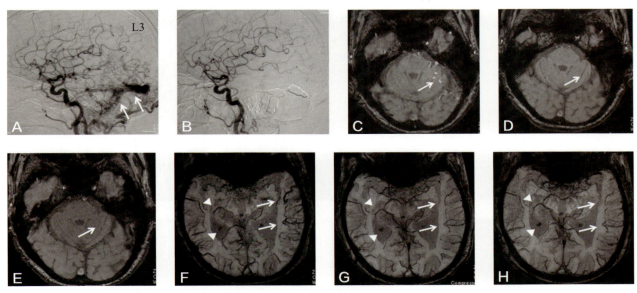

▲ 图 7-4 76 岁耳鸣女患者

A. 术前左侧颈总动脉侧位血管造影显示 Cognard Ⅱ a+b 型动静脉瘘（箭）累及左侧横窦及乙状窦，左侧颞部静脉淤血严重；B. 治疗后即时左侧颈总动脉侧位血管造影显示瘘完全闭合；C~E. 治疗前（C）至横窦栓塞治疗后 12 个月（E）的磁敏感加权磁共振成像，治疗前（C，箭）的静脉高信号在治疗后 3 个月（D，箭）和 12 个月（E，箭）的图像中消失；F~H. 治疗前（F）至横窦栓塞治疗后 12 个月（H）的磁敏感加权静脉成像，治疗前左侧颞叶呈静脉淤血表现（F，箭），治疗后 12 个月恢复正常（H，箭）；对应右侧颞叶静脉管径在治疗前后无显著变化（F~H，箭头）

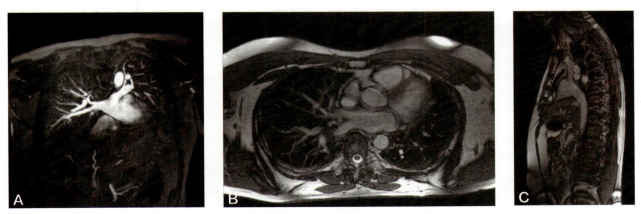

▲ 图 7-5 传统肺静脉回流：使用对比剂增强（A）和 bSSFP（B 和 C）技术的 MR 肺静脉成像

A. 高分辨 3D MRV 清楚显示肺静脉解剖并可行多平面重建进行准确测量；同一患者的轴位（B）和矢状位（C）2D bSSFP 图像，清晰显示右上、右下肺静脉

（八）三维对比剂增强 MRV 技术

为了克服无对比剂增强序列分辨率较低和采集时间较长的局限性，提倡应用对比剂增强 3D MRV（CE MRV）作为评价静脉系统的主要技术（图 7-6 和图 7-7）。

CE MRV 使用与对比剂增强磁共振动脉成像基本相同的技术，区别为在增强静脉期或平衡期采集图像。CE MRV 亦可使用时间分辨技术。对比剂注射可应用直接法或间接法。间接法为经非目标外周静脉注入对比剂，于平衡早期采集图像；由于对比剂到达扫描静脉区域常明显稀释，通常需要使用较高浓度剂量的对比剂，其优势为无须目标静脉上游血管的直接穿刺。

减影技术常被用于改善强化血管的图像对比噪声比（图 7-6E）。减影需要同时采集增强前本

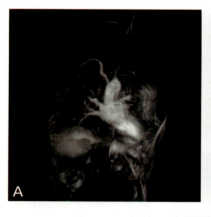
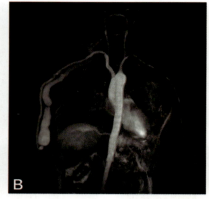
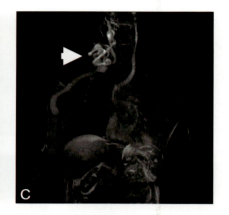
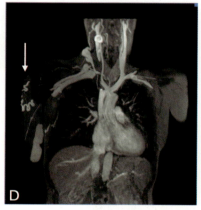
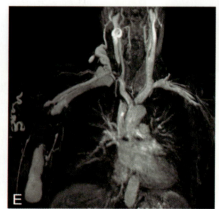

▲ 图 7-6 CEMRV 用于评价静脉系统

A～C. 早、中、晚期时间分辨图像示右侧头臂动静脉间瘘形成，伴静脉瘤形成与右侧无名静脉、颈内静脉及锁骨下静脉近段闭塞，右侧颈外静脉发出多支侧支血管（箭头）；D. 高分辨对比剂增强 MRA MIP 图像（层厚 17.8mm）确认右侧无名静脉、颈内静脉及锁骨下静脉近段闭塞伴右上肢侧支循环形成（箭）；E. 融合无对比剂增强本底和增强平衡期图像的减影图，与（D）图相比肌肉和软组织信号减低

底图像和增强后图像。在胸部和腹部，呼吸运动可能造成减影图像误匹配的伪影。

直接法 MRV 需要将稀释对比剂自感兴趣血管上游持续注入，可以类似传统静脉血管造影对浅表和深静脉系统进行全面显示。与间接法相比，直接注射技术可以少量对比剂得到局部的高信噪比。通常应用 1:10～20 的稀释因子（对比剂：盐水），以避免 T_2 缩短效应造成血管腔内明显低信号。增强前本底采集后，通常以约 1ml/s 的速度缓慢注入稀释对比剂行 3D 图像数据采集。可重复扫描动态观察对阻塞静脉行功能评价（图 7-8）[19]。

为提高信噪比和分辨率扫描需应用体表线圈。推荐采集参数设置短 TR 和 TE 值及 30°～40° 的翻转角。采集期间，需持续应用对比剂以避免采集 K 空间中心数据时对比剂浓度波动造成的伪影，持续注射对比剂还可以保证在存在静脉闭塞时侧支静脉的充盈。

（九）时间分辨 MRV

时间分辨 MRV 为一个较新的概念，是对预设区域的快速动态成像，同时提供解剖和血流信息。对比剂注射期间的快速图像采集获得高时间分辨率，但同时牺牲空间分辨率。时间分辨 MRV 得益于并行采集、K 空间采集重排序、K 空间加速填充技术以及新的图像重建算法。实时采集每帧图像需 1～6s。该技术在评价血管畸形[20]（图 7-6、图 7-9 和图 7-10）、静脉反流[21]，以及同时累及动静脉的复杂先天心血管疾病中很有帮助。时间分辨成像所需的对比剂用量约减少为传统 CE MRV 用量的 1/10。

Chapter 7 磁共振静脉成像
Magnetic Resonance Venography

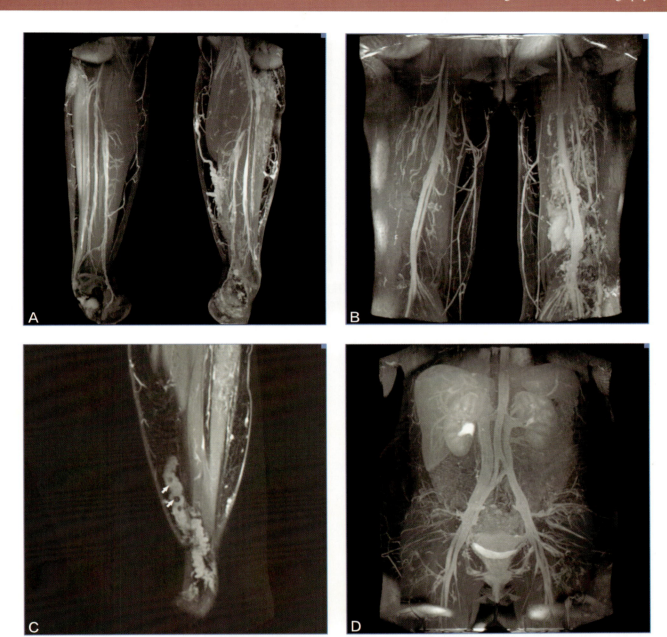

▲ 图 7-7　Klippel Trenaunay 患者静脉注入 0.05mmol/kg 钆（Ablavar）后的高空间分辨 3D MRV
A、B. 增强后压脂 3D GRE 图像示自足部至大腿上段广泛静脉畸形形成并浸润肌肉，左侧下肢皮下脂肪层内见多发曲张静脉，伴多发血栓形成（C，箭头）；D. 最大密度投影图示双下腔静脉

（十）对比剂

1. 细胞外钆对比剂　细胞外钆对比剂最常应用于 CE MRV 和对比剂增强磁共振动脉成像（contrast-enhanced magnetic resonance angiography，CEMRA）。与碘对比剂相比，此种细胞外对比剂安全性更高。现今共有 9 种含钆对比剂获 FDA 批准应用于 MRI，其中两种具有应用于 MR 血管成像的特别批准（表 7-4）。需注意其中任何一种均未获得静脉成像的特别批准，因此 MRV 为其超适应证应用。此类对比剂从毛细血管渗入组织间质的速度相对较快，因此随时间推移血管强化减弱而背景信号增高。通过回顾时间分辨 MRV 不同时相的动态图像，可能有助于寻找合适的成像时间点。与血池对比剂相比，细胞外钆对比剂的优势是较高的安全性和较低的价格。

2. 血池对比剂　血池对比剂代表了与细胞

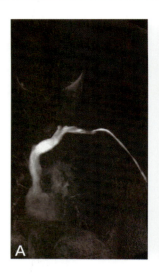 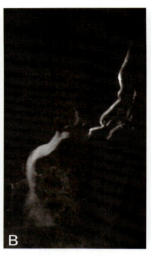 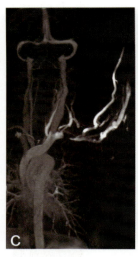 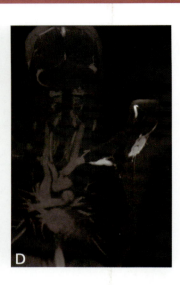

▲ 图 7-8　直接时间分辨 MRV

A. 左上肢中立位直接静脉注射 2ml Ablavar 后未见明显静脉狭窄；B. 左上肢外展位再次注入 2ml Ablavar 后于静脉早期成像见锁骨下静脉中段明显狭窄伴局部侧支开放；C. 其平衡期时间分辨图像示大量侧支循环形成，未见充盈缺损或血栓形成；D. 高分辨平衡期图像验证了直接时间分辨 MRV 的发现

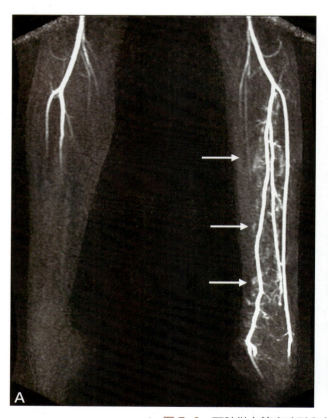 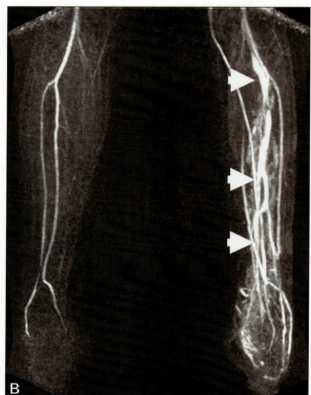

▲ 图 7-9　下肢微血管瘘畸形患者的动态对比剂增强 MR 血管成像

静脉注射 1ml 钆对比剂后，应用交错随机轨迹时间分辨血管成像（TWIST）对下肢微血管瘘畸形患者的动态对比剂增强 MR 血管成像。A. 在时间分辨图像中，左腿血液循环呈高动力，于动脉早期强化，可见多发微血管瘘造成的交通（箭）；B. 左侧小腿见引流深静脉扩张、早显（箭头）

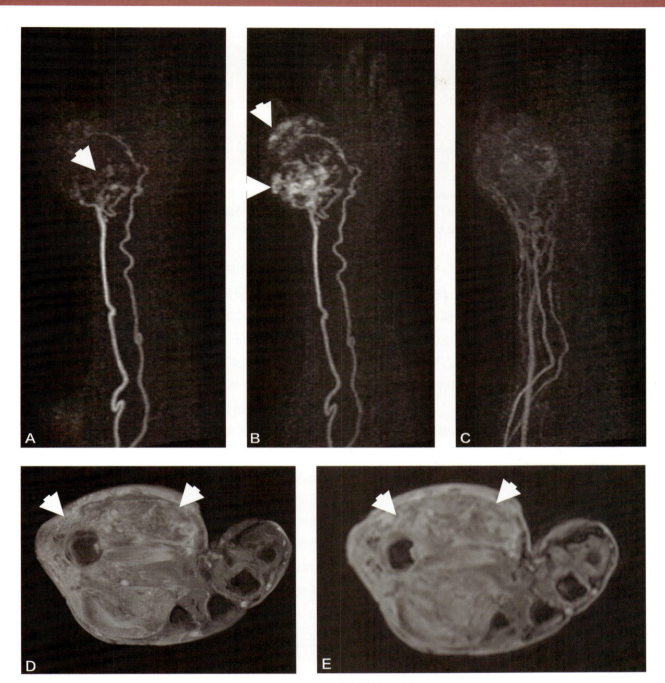

▲ 图 7-10　巨大血管畸形成像

A、B. 早期时间分辨图像显示桡动脉、尺动脉供血的巨大血管畸形（箭头）；C. 略晚期时间分辨图示主要通过桡静脉引流；T_1 FLASH 2D 横轴位图（D）和对比剂后 T_1 压脂 VIBE 图（E）清晰显示动静脉畸形与手掌侧及左外侧肌肉和软组织关系密切（箭头）

外对比剂相比血管内分布时间更长的新一代对比剂。血池对比剂包括超微超顺磁性氧化铁颗粒、含钆大分子、具有可逆强血浆蛋白结合力的含钆小分子等多种化合物[22,23]。

钆磷维塞三钠（Ablavar）是现今唯一经 FDA 批准的血池对比剂。FDA 批准钆磷维塞三钠静脉内应用于 MR 血管成像，评价已知或怀疑外周血管疾病成人的主动脉 - 髂动脉闭塞性疾病（FDA 网站，http://www.fda.gov/Drugs, accessed 1/15/2014）。应用钆磷维塞三钠于 MRV 为超适应证应用，但是我们的经验证实其在显示小血管及慢速或复杂血流上具有优势[23]。钆磷

表 7-4 FDA 批准的 MR 血管成像用对比剂

化学名	商品名	公司	C（molar）（mmol/ml）	MW（g/mol）	批准适应证	初始排泄	分布
钆贝酸二葡甲胺	MultiHance®	Bracco	0.5	1058	肾/主动脉-髂动脉-股动脉闭塞疾病	肾	细胞外
钆磷维塞三钠	Ablavar	Bayer health care	0.25	957	主动脉-髂动脉闭塞疾病	肾	血池对比剂/血管内

FDA 批准的 9 种含钆对比剂（gadolinium-based contrast agents, GBCAs）：①钆特酸葡甲胺（Dotarem®）；②钆双胺（Omniscan）；③钆贝酸盐（MultiHance）；④钆喷酸葡胺（Magnevist）；⑤钆特醇（ProHance®）；⑥钆膦维司（Ablavar，曾用名 Vasovist）；⑦钆弗塞胺（OptiMARK™）；⑧钆塞酸二钠（Eovist®）；⑨钆布醇（Gadavist®）

维塞三钠与白蛋白非共价结合并经肾脏排泄。钆磷维塞三钠与白蛋白的可逆结合使得其与传统细胞外对比剂相比钆用量显著降低，并增加钆的顺磁效应[23]。钆磷维塞三钠在 1.0T 磁场下的弛豫率为钆喷酸-二乙烯三胺五乙酸（DTPA）的 6～10 倍[24]。这种对比剂可同时应用于首过效应和稳态成像。

3. 技术的陷阱和限制 当静脉成像要求同时包括视野中的侧支静脉时可能很有挑战性，比如显示血栓形成后的改变，因此可能需要具有一定层厚的 3D 容积成像。

使用 CE MRV 的传统血栓成像依赖于血管腔内低信号充盈缺损反映血栓。MIP 图像中血栓周围的高信号可能遮蔽中心的充盈缺损或血栓。TOF MRV 中，如果静脉血倾斜流入采集层面，饱和效应可能造成血管内信号降低，在 MIP 重建中被解读为血栓。因此必须仔细查看原始图像，不能仅依赖 MIP 重建图像评估静脉系统中血栓。

在图像采集过程中，一些患者的静脉可能存在显著的呼吸相关变化。如果使用血流敏感 TOF MRV，当采集中心部分于呼气期静脉血流显著减低时获取，静脉可能表现为低信号。这种情况时，需要于屏气时采集数据。

对于传统 CE MRV，在静脉完全闭塞时，扫描时间间隔可能并不适于显示侧支静脉及闭塞以远的静脉重构。为克服此困难，需要在注射对比剂期间及短时间后采集多组数据。如果采集的图像不满足要求，需尝试增加对比剂总用量和延长注射时间。在间接传统定时 MRV 中，应使用 3D 采集使 K 空间采集中心与对比剂团注的静脉期相吻合。如果采集时间不合适，可能产生边缘或环状伪影。

血管内金属装置或电极（支架、腔静脉滤器或起搏器电极）可能在大多数 MRI 序列中造成局部磁敏感伪影限制血管腔的观察（图 7-11 和图 7-12）。当高分辨对比剂增强图像无法用于诊断时，时间分辨图像通常有助于对支架通畅性的评价。评价是否存在局部静脉侧支以及支架近端及远端对比剂流的多时相图像，可以推测支架的通畅性。但大多数时候，支架腔内内膜增生程度和管腔直径的测量是明显受限的。作为替代，单侧或双侧肢体直接 MRV 可能获得更有诊断意义的图像。在这些困难情况下，CT 静脉成像和彩超可能更有帮助。

三、临床应用

MRV 有大量的临床应用，是一项一线检查技术，或者可以作为超声或 CT 的补充检查方法。下文（一）将会阐述相关的解剖、成像技术和临床应用。

（一）上肢和胸部循环静脉

1. 解剖 上腔静脉（superior vena cava, SVC）是一条主要的全身性静脉，长度较短（约 7cm）但直径较宽；负责将膈肌上方结构（除了肺和心脏）的无氧血液回流至右心房。左右头臂

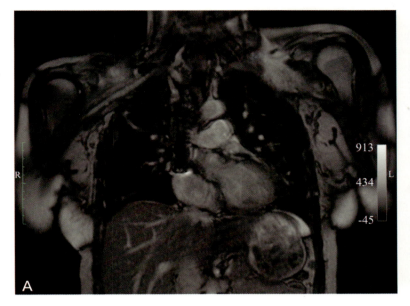
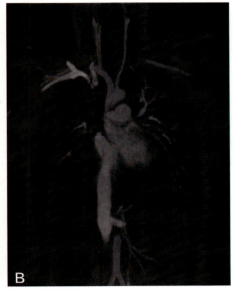
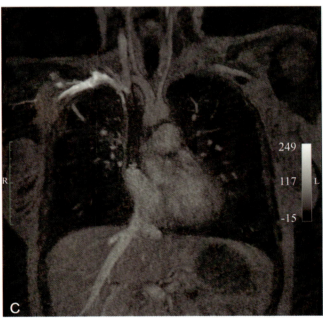
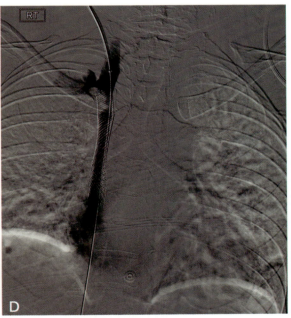

▲ 图 7-11　上腔静脉支架：37 岁纵隔内纤维化女性患者，既往上腔静脉狭窄支架置入后

A.true FISP 冠状位图像内上腔静脉支架周围见明显磁敏感伪影；B. 冠状位 10mm MIP 图显示上腔静脉支架局部磁敏感伪影造成低信号，右侧无名静脉呈高信号；C.CEMRA 源图像显示支架内管腔较清晰；D.DSA 显示右侧无名静脉及上腔静脉内支架通畅

静脉（亦称为无名静脉）汇合形成 SVC。SVC 的近段位于上纵隔右侧、右侧第 1 肋软骨水平。SVC 的下段被心包包绕。后方在第 2 肋软骨水平紧邻心包包绕处，奇静脉跨越右肺根部汇入 SVC 的后方。SVC 的终点位于上腔静脉孔，位于中纵隔第 3 肋软骨水平，与右心房相延续。

SVC 及双侧头臂静脉是上纵隔的主要全身性静脉，通过双侧锁骨下静脉、颈内静脉引流双上肢及头颈部静脉回流至右心房。左侧的头臂静脉长度是右侧的 2 倍，因为它需要从左侧跨越至右侧，在主动脉弓主要分支的起始处前方经过汇入 SVC。在右侧头臂干静脉起始处，右侧颈内静脉及右侧锁骨下静脉汇合，此外右侧淋巴管在此处汇入。相似的，在左侧头臂干静脉起始处，左

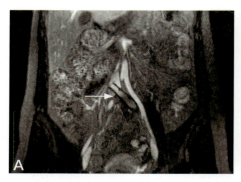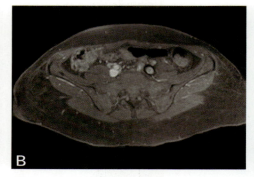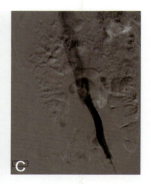

▲ 图 7-12　髂外静脉镍钛支架

A. 左侧髂总静脉内支架，近端至下腔静脉（箭）远端至左侧髂外静脉，支架磁敏感伪影轻微，管腔通畅；B. 增强后 T_1 压脂 vibe 图像显示左侧髂外静脉通畅的支架内腔，与数字减影静脉成像（C）结果相符，镍钛合金材质的支架在 MRI 中有特别优势

侧颈内静脉及左侧锁骨下静脉汇合，同时胸导管在此处汇入。

锁骨下静脉延续至第 1 肋水平并被称为腋静脉，腋静脉再向远端延续为上肢的贵要静脉。头静脉属于浅静脉系统，汇入腋静脉。

2. 成像技术　CE MRV 非常适合这一解剖部位的成像。最常用的为间接法成像。可以通过肘正中静脉单次注射对比剂或者使用 3D 数据库联合采集平衡期图像（图 7-6 和图 7-13）。间接法尤其适用于动脉和静脉图像信息都需要的患者（例如显示透析造瘘的吻合口）。

直接法成像较少应用，其在肾损伤（因为可以减少对比剂用量）、透析分流术、透析造瘘或者长期中心静脉置管的患者中具有优势。为了同时显示双侧的腋静脉、锁骨下静脉和头臂静脉及 SVC，需要同时在左右上肢注射对比剂。使用 2 个高压注射器，每个配有 2 个装有稀释对比剂的套筒，协调进行注射。目标是 2 个高压注射器的第 1 个套筒内对比剂在大致相同的时间内注射完。在第 2 个套筒内的对比剂注射完一半时开始采集图像。

由于胸部和上肢静脉走行的方向多变，2D TOF 和 MRV 的图像数据必须在不同的平面进行采集，以保证扫描平面与静脉垂直。这意味着大部分图像必须为轴位采集，2D TOF 的采集会非常耗时。

3. 临床应用　MRV 可以用于诊断 SVC 综合征、Paget-Schroetter 综合征、中心静脉血栓、可能累及血管的纵隔畸形和评价解剖变异（图 7-8 和图 7-14）。MRV 还可以用于随诊 DVT 患者短期或长期治疗后改变。无对比剂 MRV 和对比剂增强 MRV 均适用于上述临床情况。

SVC 综合征是指任何阻碍血流流入 SVC 的临床情况。SVC 综合征可能是用于血栓或者外压引起静脉狭窄或闭塞所致。SVC 综合征的临床表现为头颈部、上肢水肿、静脉充血或肿胀。在 20 世纪 80 年代，最常见的引起 SVC 综合征的是恶性疾病，85% 的 SVC 综合征是由恶性疾病造成，多由于恶性疾病外压或浸润 SVC 引起[25]。目前，由于血管腔内治疗装置临床应用的增长，恶性疾病尽管仍是 SVC 综合征的主要病因（占 60%），但是 40% 的病例是由于良性疾病导致[26]。良性病因包括纵隔纤维化和继发于中心静脉置管或经静脉的起搏器电线的血栓。

锁骨下静脉梗阻可能是胸廓出口综合征（thoracic outlet syndrome，TOS）的部分表现。TOS 是由于颈胸部锁骨下动脉、锁骨下静脉、臂丛受压或者上述三者均受压所致。压迫可能是由于异常的第 1 肋、C_7 横突较长、肌肉异常、短斜角肌、外生骨疣和血管由肌肉内穿行所导致[27]。为除外动脉性 TOS，我们使用 Ablavar 进行了外展位和中立位的时间分辨率的 MRA 和高清对比剂增强的 MRV（图 7-8A、B）。

永久左侧 SVC（persistent left SVC，PLSVC）是最常见的先天胸部静脉发育异常，发病率为 0.3%～0.5%[28]。在大多数病例中，左侧和

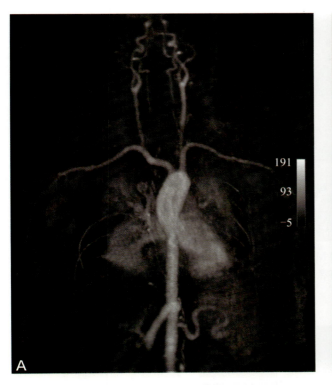

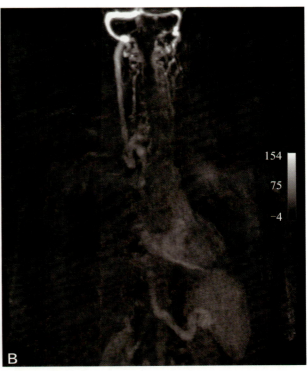

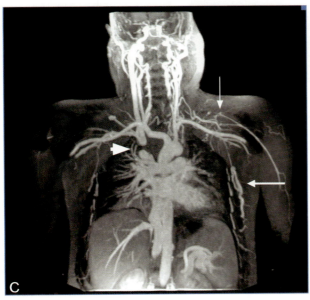

▲ 图 7-13　间接法对比剂增强 MRV 显示胸部中心静脉
在经静脉注射 1ml 钆对比剂后，使用 TWIST 进行动态 CE MRA 扫描。冠状位采集动脉期（A）和静脉期（B）图像；B. 所示左侧颈内静脉未显影；C. 显示在静脉追加注射 10ml 钆对比剂后进行高空间分辨率的 3D MRV 扫描。动脉和静脉系统均显影；左侧颈内静脉、无名静脉、腋静脉、锁骨下静脉闭塞；左肩和左侧上胸部有大量的侧支静脉（箭）；右侧无名静脉亦闭塞（箭头）

右侧 SVC 均存在。40% 的 PLSVC 患者伴有心脏发育异常[28]。左侧 SVC 多通过冠状窦回流至右心房（图 7-15），偶尔可见左侧 SVC 回流至左心房，从而导致右向左分流。

（二）下肢和下腔静脉

1. 解剖　下腔静脉（inferior vena cava，IVC）始于 L_5 椎体水平前方，由双侧髂静脉汇合而成。IVC 位于中位平面右侧 2.5cm，低于主动脉的分叉和右髂总动脉的近端部分。IVC 沿着 $L_3 \sim L_5$ 椎体的右侧、右侧腰大肌的前方走行。IVC 在 T_8 椎体水平由膈肌的腔静脉孔出腹腔，在进入胸腔后，汇入右心房。下腔静脉的腹腔部分收集了来自下肢肌腹盆部非门静脉系统的无氧静脉血。

IVC 发育异常的发病率不到 1%，在合并有其他心血管发育异常的人群中，发病率略高[29]。

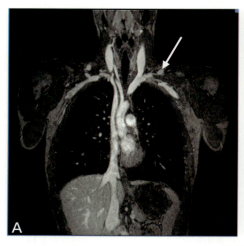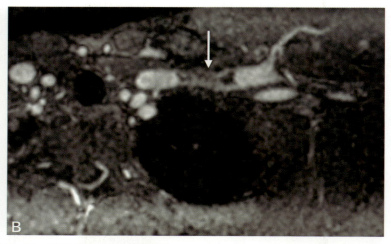

▲ 图 7-14　3D MRV 评价解剖变异

3D MRV 的冠状位（A）和斜轴位（B）重建图像显示，胸廓出口处左侧锁骨下静脉存在重度狭窄血栓（箭），周围无侧支静脉形成，符合 Paget-Schroetter 综合征表现

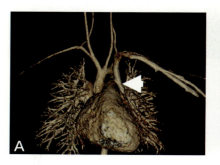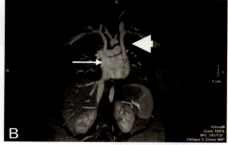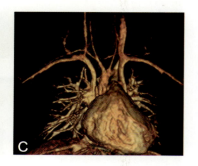

▲ 图 7-15　左侧 SVC

A. 通过左侧上肢静脉注射对比剂（箭头），对动脉早期进行 3D 容积重建，显示出左侧 SVC；B. 斜冠状位显示 LSVC 汇入冠状窦（箭头），最终汇入右心房（箭）；C. 右侧 SVC 在平衡期也显示了出来，通过 3D 容积重建显示右侧 SVC 和永久左侧 SVC

IVC 发育异常包括左侧 IVC、双 IVC（图 7-7D）、非对称的 IVC 延续（图 7-16）、左肾静脉环绕主动脉、肾下段 IVC 缺如和整个 IVC 缺如。在这些发育异常中，左侧 IVC 是最常见的，发病率为 0.2%~0.5%[30]。左侧 IVC 多在左肾静脉水平截止，在这个水平横跨主动脉与右肾静脉汇合形成正常的右侧肾上段 IVC。

下肢静脉可以被分为表浅静脉和深部静脉系统。深静脉通常与主要的下肢动脉伴行。下肢主要的深静脉系统包括股静脉、股深静脉、腘静脉、胫前静脉、胫后静脉和腓静脉。这些静脉在小腿水平成对出现。

大隐静脉是人体最长的静脉。它沿着足背背弓上行至胫骨内侧、大腿内侧并汇合成股静脉。小隐静脉沿着足背外侧向后外侧走行至腓肠肌，汇入腘静脉。表浅静脉在 DVT 患者中是重要的侧支静脉通路。

2. 成像技术　在 GRE 技术问世不久，TOF MRV 成为评价盆腔及下肢静脉 DVT 的首选 MR 技术[31-33]。TOF 静脉造影术可以准确地评价股静脉及小腿静脉的 DVT；但是，其在盆腔的应用仍受到限制，原因在之前已经提到过，包括成像时扫描平面需要与静脉走行垂直、可能存在呼吸运动伪影。同理，TOF MRV 不适合评价静脉曲张或者复杂的血栓后改变。

对比剂增强 3D MRV 克服了 TOF 静脉造影术的固有限制。传统的 CE MRA 具有快速高分辨率成像的优势，扫描时可以不进行屏气。此外，通过注射稀释的顺磁性对比剂进行间接法MRV可以显影所有静脉，不受血管走行及静脉流速的影响。小的穿支和表浅静脉可能血流速度较慢甚至存在反流，但均可清晰显影。

总之，间接法CE MRV由于其在空间分辨率、图像重建和数据采集时间方面的优势被广泛认为是标准的成像技术。

3. 临床应用 IVC和下肢静脉的MRV可以用来评价继发于内源性或外源性的静脉梗阻（图7-17），评估先天解剖变异，或者用来在术前或介入治疗前进行静脉解剖显示及尺寸测量。

IVC和盆腔静脉明显的血栓形成造成的血流动力学改变可以导致多发侧支静脉形成。在单侧髂静脉血栓（图7-18）或闭塞时，血液可以通过骶骨、直肠、子宫、膀胱或者前列腺静脉丛的侧支静脉引流。IVC完全的栓塞或闭塞可能会导致血液通过侧支静脉引流回半奇或奇静脉，侧支静脉的位置可以位于上腹部静脉、胸上腹部静脉或者椎体静脉丛最终回流至SVC。

无对比剂的MRV在"二"中介绍过，可以显示IVC和盆腔、下肢静脉的基本的解剖变异或病理改变。尽管传统的静脉造影术作为诊断DVT的金标准被广泛接受，但是由于多普勒超声便宜易行，现在许多机构仍将其作为一线技术广泛应用。值得注意的是，MRV检出单纯DVT的频率（图7-19）高于超声或者传统的提升静脉造影术[34]。

由于MRV软组织分辨率高并且可以进行增强检查（图7-20和图7-21），其在鉴别静脉血栓或肿瘤血栓之间具有优势，尤其是肾静脉或IVC。MRV在鉴别血栓组成[35]，尤其是增强特点上很有优势，通常来说瘤栓会呈现不同程度的强化，但是血栓不强化。因此，MRV对于肾细胞癌分期非常重要，适用于疑似肾静脉血栓的评价。

在进行下肢高分辨率MRV时，应使用直接法成像，通过双足静脉注射稀释的对比剂。直接法MRV对于准确显示下肢深浅静脉的形态、血栓后改变及静脉曲张非常可靠有效[19]。

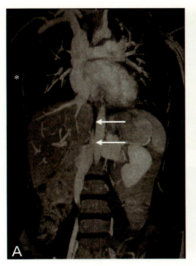
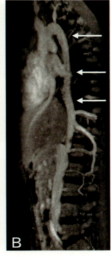

▲ 图7-16 胸腹部3D MRV

A.冠状图像显示肝段IVC中断（箭），伴随肝上重构的静脉回流至右心房；B.矢状位显示肝下IVC（箭）非对称的回流至SVC。注意肋间静脉增粗（A，星号）

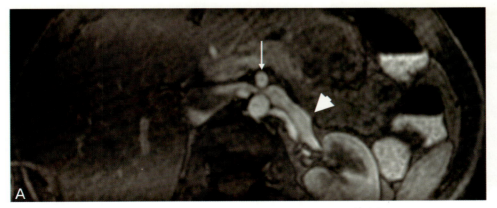
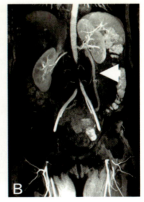

▲ 图7-17 胡桃夹综合征

A.患者为血尿患者，腹部的高分辨率3D MRV显示左肾静脉受到肠系膜上动脉（箭）外源性压迫，近端左肾静脉扩张（箭头）；B.厚层MIP图像显示左侧肾上腺静脉扩张（箭头）

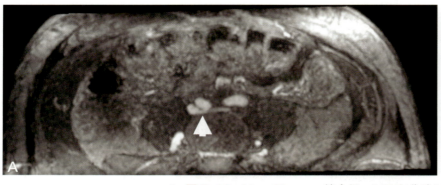
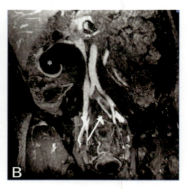

▲ 图 7-18 May-Thurner 综合征：IVC 和盆腔 MRV

A. 近端左侧髂总静脉受右侧髂总动脉重度外源性压迫（箭头）；B. 伴远端扩张及腔内血栓（箭），符合表现；通过多普勒超声发现血栓（未显示），并偶然发现肾积水（*）

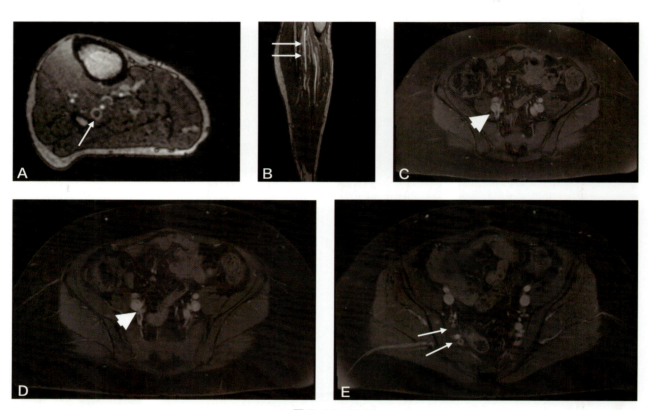

▲ 图 7-19 DVT

高分辨率 3D MRV 的轴位（A）和冠状位（B）重建。在腓静脉显示腔内充盈缺损（箭），符合血栓的影像表现；C～E. 轴位 T_1 FLASH 2D 图像显示右侧髂内静脉（箭头）及其远端分支（箭）内充盈缺损；与之相比，左侧髂内静脉分支通畅

4. 门静脉、肝静脉和肠系膜静脉 MRI/MRV 可以用来评价门静脉和肝静脉解剖，评价静脉血栓或闭塞（图 7-20 和图 7-22），作为肝移植术患者术前和（或）术后评价。这项技术也可以用于评价局部肿瘤播散，这在胰腺癌、肝癌分期、肝移植前治疗方案确定、移植后吻合口评价都非常重要（图 7-20）。目前已被证明，3D CEMR 门静脉造影术在评价门静脉通畅程度及门静脉高压患者血栓检出方面与数字减影血管造影术一样有效[36]。

5. 肺静脉系统 使用传统 CE MRV 在心房颤动患者 RF 治疗前后评价肺静脉已经被广泛认可（图 7-5）。在大多数情况下，附加的心脏 MRI 可以显示延迟强化，用以评价心肌瘢痕。如果患者存在 MRI 或钆对比剂应用的绝对或相对禁

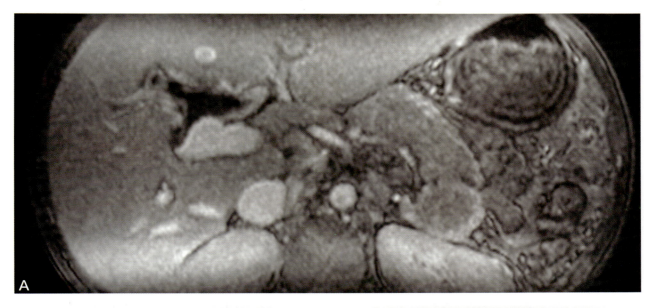
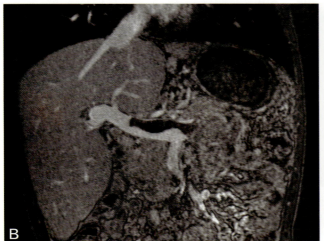
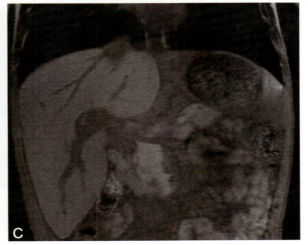

▲ 图 7-20　门静脉血栓

A. 轴位 CEMRA 显示右前、右后门静脉及汇合处均存在血栓；B. 在肝外门静脉主干、脾静脉断端（脾脏手术切除）存在非闭塞性的血栓；C. T_1 FLASH 2D 强化前图像在 CEMRA 相应的血栓部位显示轻度不均匀 T_1 高信号

忌证，可以使用无对比剂 MRV 技术。

作为无对比剂技术，bSSFP 成像提供了非常好的信号对比度及信噪比。为了评价心脏周围的静脉结构，更推荐使用带有心脏门控的 3D SSFP 技术。Francois 等进行的一项研究显示，CE MRA 和 bSSFP 相比，在显示肺静脉变异及肺静脉开口处测量方面没有显著差异[37]。此外，bSSFP 对于显示非血管结构更具优势。包括评价左心房与食管之间的距离与关系，以防在 RF 消融时造成严重并发症心房食管瘘。Francois 等使用 3D SSFP 扫描发现 4 例食管裂孔疝、2 例肺结节 / 肿物、1 例支气管囊肿和 2 例淋巴结肿大，这些在 CEMRA 中均未发现[37]。该技术主要的缺点是与 CEMRA 相比，扫描时间较长。

6. 未来的优势　含钆的对比剂在某些情况是禁忌证，包括 4 或 5 级慢性肾病患者［肾小球滤过率 < 30ml/（min·1.73m²）］、急性肾损伤和肝功能不全的肝肾移植的受体，可能会造成肾源性系统性纤维化（nephrogenic systematic fibrosing, NSF)[38,39]。尽管 NSF 并不常见，但是一旦出现，临床症状会很重乃至导致死亡。无对比剂 MRV 技术可以为无法使用钆对比剂的患者提供另一个

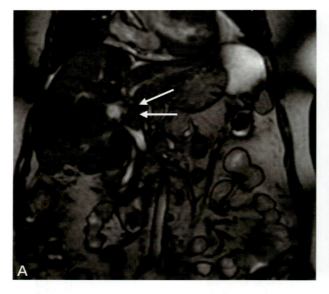
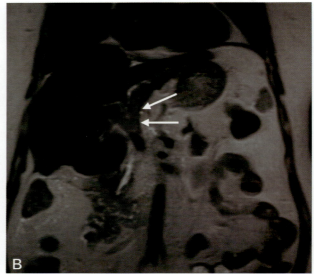
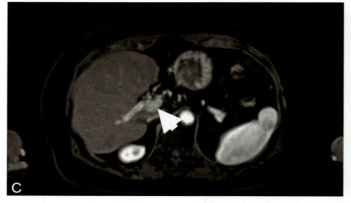
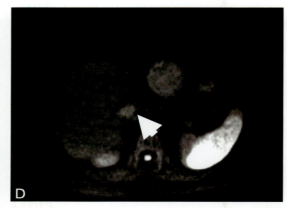

▲ 图 7-21　肝细胞肝癌术后

A. 患者门静脉冠状位稳定进动快速成像（trufi）；B. T₂半傅里叶采集单次涡轮自旋回波（haste）成像。在门静脉左支移行至门静脉主干的水平存在栓子（箭）；C. 栓子（箭头）在增强的 CE MRA 上出现强化；D. 在弥散加权成像上扩散受限，与瘤栓的特点相符

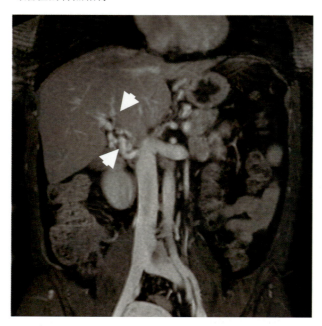

选择。但是，一般情况下，首先增强检查，因为其分辨率高、扫描速度快、可以进行 3D 重建，同时，还可以提供更高的组织定性。

超小超顺磁的氧化铁粒子（ultrasmall superparamagntic iron oxide, USPIO）可能可以在肾损伤的患者中代替传统的含钆对比剂[40]。在大量的铁氧化物纳米颗粒中，纳米氧化铁似乎是 Gd 的安全替代物，并且已被认为是肾损伤患者进行血管成像中的对比剂[40]。纳米氧化铁（Feraheme™；

◀ 图 7-22　腹部对比剂增强 3D MRV 检查

1 例特发性门静脉血栓的患者进行腹部对比剂增强 3D MRV 检查；图像显示肝外门静脉完全闭塞，肝门区伴有广泛的门静脉侧支循环（海绵样变性，箭头）

AMAG Pharmaceuticals，Inc.，Cambridge，MA）是一种经静脉注射的碳水化合物涂层的超顺磁性氧化铁纳米粒子，其在 2009 年被美国食品药品监督管理局批准作为治疗慢性肾病造成的贫血的静脉铁替代治疗药物。它 T_1 弛豫时间长，不经过肾脏排泄。对于血管成像，纳米氧化铁可以作为血池对比剂注射，作为 MRA 及动态 MR 的团剂注射。此外，它的血浆半衰期很长，可以有较大的瞬时窗口进行静脉平衡期高分辨率成像（图 7-23 和图 7-24）。

另一个可能的应用前景为使用靶向的对比剂通过 MRV 进行血凝块成像。这些特殊的含钆对比剂可能可以弥补平扫 MR 技术或者作为 CE MRV 技术的替代方法。Flacke 等提到一种配体导向、脂质包裹的全氟化碳液体纳米颗粒具有高

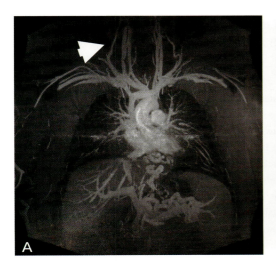
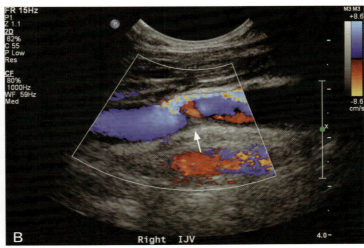
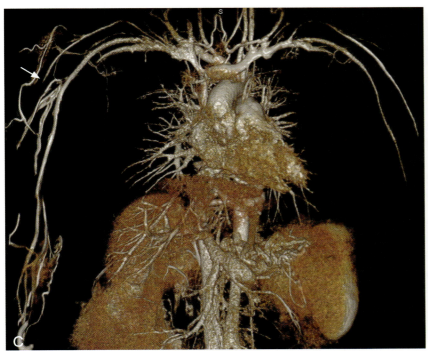
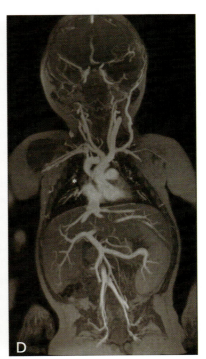

▲ 图 7-23 终末期肾衰竭

A. 在 1 例 39 岁终末期肾衰竭患者中注射了 15ml 纳米氧化铁之后通过后处理得到的 46mm 的薄层 MIP 图像；患者存在中度的右下 IJ 狭窄（箭头）；B. 彩色多普勒超声（箭）显示由隔膜造成；C. 在 3D 容积重建上显示右侧头臂静脉在中段闭塞（箭）；D. 1 例 3 岁的终末期肾衰竭患者进行的平衡期全身 3D MRV。注射总量 1.6ml 的纳米氧化铁，可发现右侧颈内静脉、SVC 在汇入右心房处闭塞（星号）

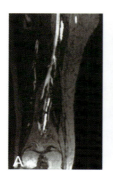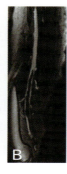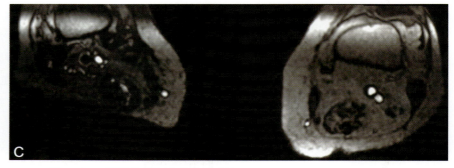

▲ 图 7-24 肾损伤伴坏疽的血管成像

FH2：1 例 93 岁老年女性伴有肾损伤及右足第 4 趾坏疽。使用 6.5ml 纳米氧化铁（Feraheme, AMAG Pharmaceutricals, Waltham, MA）进行血管成像；A～C. 冠状位、矢状位和轴位平衡期右大腿重建图像显示右侧股静脉远段及腘静脉闭塞性血栓伴有局部侧支静脉形成

亲和力、长半衰期并携带高负荷的 Gd-DTPA，对于纤维蛋白的检出敏感性很高[41]。在 1.5T 场强下，该对比剂可以在体外和体内检出血管内 500nm 的血凝块。尽管十多年前即有血凝块靶向的对比剂成像技术的相关论文，但是至今这些对比剂均没有通过实验性的临床前阶段。

参考文献

［1］Spitzer, CE (2009) Progress in MR imaging of the venous system. *Perspect Vasc Surg Endovasc Ther* 21(2):105–116

［2］Bradley WG Jr, Waluch V, Lai KS et al. (1984) The appearance of rapidly flowing blood on magnetic resonance images. *AJR Am J Roentgenol* 143(6):1167–1174

［3］Liu CY, Bley TA, Wieben O et al. (2010) Flow-independent T2-prepared inversion recovery black-blood MR imaging. *J Magn Reson Imaging* 31(1):248–254

［4］Butty S, Hagspiel KD, Leung DA et al. (2002) Body MR venography. *Radiol Clin North Am* 40(4):899–919

［5］Constantinesco A, Mallet JJ, Bonmartin A et al. (1984) Spatial or flow velocity phase encoding gradients in NMR imaging. *Magn Reson Imaging* 2(4):335–340

［6］Yzet T, Bouzerar R, Allart JD et al. (2010) Hepatic vascular flow measurements by phase contrast MRI and Doppler echography: A comparative and reproducibility study. *J Magn Reson Imaging* 31(3):579–588

［7］Kelly J, Hunt BJ, Moody A et al. (2003) Magnetic resonance direct thrombus imaging: A novel technique for imaging venous thromboemboli. *Thromb Haemost* 89(5):773–782

［8］Fraser DG, Moody AR, Morgan PS et al. (2002) Diagnosis of lower-limb deep venous thrombosis: A prospective blinded study of magnetic resonance direct thrombus imaging. *Ann Intern Med* 136(2):89–98

［9］Westerbeek RE, Van Rooden CJ, Tan M et al. (2008) Magnetic resonance direct thrombus imaging of the evolution of acute deep vein thrombosis of the leg. *J Thromb Haemost* 6(7):1087–1092

［10］Haacke EM, Mittal S, Wu Z et al. (2009) Susceptibility-weighted imaging: Technical aspects and clinical applications, part 1. *AJNR Am J Neuroradiol* 30(1):19–30

［11］Mittal S, Wu Z, Neelavalli J, Haacke EM (2009) Susceptibility- weighted imaging: Technical aspects and clinical applications, part 2. *AJNR Am J Neuroradiol* 30(2):232–252

［12］Letourneau-Guillon L, Krings T (2012) Simultaneous arteriovenous shunting and venous congestion identification in dural arteriovenous fistulas using susceptibility-weighted imaging: Initial experience. *AJNR Am J Neuroradiol* 33:301–307

［13］Nakagawa I, Taoka T, Wada T (2013) The use of susceptibility-weighted imaging as an indicator of retrograde leptomeningeal venous drainage and venous congestion with dural arteriovenous fistula: Diagnosis and follow-up after treatment. *Neurosurgery* 72:47–55

［14］Dai Y, Zeng M, Li R et al. (2011) Improving detection of siderotic nodules in cirrhotic liver with a multi-breath-hold susceptibility-weighted imaging technique. *J Magn Reson Imaging* 34(2):318–325

［15］Krishnam MS, Tomasian A, Malik S et al. (2009) Three-dimensional imaging of pulmonary veins by a novel steady-state free-precession magnetic resonance angiography technique without the use of intravenous contrast agent: Initial experience. *Invest Radiol* 44(8):447–453

［16］Tomasian A, Lohan DG, Laub G et al. (2008) Noncontrast 3D steady state free precession magnetic resonance angiography of the thoracic central veins using nonselective radiofrequency excitation over a large field of view: Initial experience. *Invest Radiol* 43(5):306–313

［17］Wilson MW, LaBerge JM, Kerlan RK et al. (2002) MR portal venography: Preliminary results of fast acquisition without contrast material or breath holding. *Acad Radiol* 9(10):1179–1184

[18] Edelman RR, Koktzoglou I (2009) Unenhanced flow- independent MR venography by using signal targeting alternative radiofrequency and flow-independent relaxation enhancement. *Radiology* 250(1):236–245

[19] Ruehm SG, Zimny K, Debatin JF (2001) Direct contrast-enhanced 3D MR venography. *Eur Radiol* 11(1):102–112

[20] Herborn CU, Goyen M, Lauenstein TC (2003) Comprehensive time-resolved MRI of peripheral vascular malformations. *AJR Am J Roentgenol* 181(3):729–735

[21] Dick EA, Burnett C, Anstee A (2010) Time-resolved imaging of contrast kinetics three-dimensional (3D) magnetic resonance venography in patients with pelvic congestion syndrome. *Br J Radiol* 83(994):882–887

[22] Bellin MF, Van Der Molen AJ (2008) Extracellular gadolinium-based contrast media: An overview. *Eur J Radiol* 66(2):160–167

[23] Bremerich J, Bilecen D, Reimer P (2007) MR angiography with blood pool contrast agents. *Eur Radiol* 17(12):3017–3024

[24] Lauffer RB, Parmelee DJ, Dunham SU (1998) MS-325: Albumin-targeted contrast agent for MR angiography. *Radiology* 207(2):529–38

[25] Schraufnagel DE, Hill R, Leech JA et al. (1981) Superior vena caval obstruction: Is it a medical emergency? *Am J Med* 70:1169–1174

[26] Rice TW, Rodriguez RM, Light RW (2006) The superior vena cava syndrome: Clinical characteristics and evolving etiology. *Medicine (Baltimore)* 85(1):37–42

[27] Aralasmak A, Cevikol C, Karaali K et al. (2012) MRI findings in thoracic outlet syndrome. *Skeletal Radiol* 41(11):1365–1374

[28] Goyal SK, Punnam SR, Verma G et al. (2008) Persistent left superior vena cava: A case report and review of literature. *Cardiovasc Ultrasound* 10;6:50

[29] Gayer G, Luboshitz J, Hertz M et al. (2003) Congenital anomalies of the inferior vena cava revealed on CT in patients with deep vein thrombosis. *AJR Am J Roentgenol* 180(3):729–732

[30] Bass JE, Redwine MD, Kramer LA (2010) Spectrum of congenital anomalies of the inferior vena cava: crosssectional imaging findings. *RadioGraphics* 20(3):639–652

[31] Lanzer P, Gross GM, Keller FS et al. (1991) Sequential 2D inflow venography: Initial clinical observations. *Magn Reson Med* 19:470–476

[32] Spritzer CE, Sostman HD, Wilkes DC et al. (1990) Deep venous thrombosis: Experience with gradient echo MR imaging in 66 patients. *Radiology* 177:235–241

[33] Erdman WA, Weinreb JC, Cohen JM et al. (1986) Venous thrombosis: Clinical and experimental MR imaging. *Radiology* 161:233–238

[34] Spritzer CE, Arata MA, Freed KS (2001) Isolated pelvic deep venous thrombosis: Relative frequency as detected with MR imaging. *Radiology* 219(2):521–525

[35] Engelbrecht M, Akin O, Dixit D et al. (2011) Bland and tumor thrombi in abdominal malignancies: Magnetic resonance imaging assessment in a large oncologic patient population. *Abdom Imaging* 36(1):62–68

[36] Kreft B, Strunk H, Flacke S et al. (2000) Detection of thrombosis in the portal venous system: Comparison of contrast-enhanced MR angiography with intra-arterial digital subtraction angiography. *Radiology* 216(1):86–92

[37] François CJ, Tuite D, Deshpande V et al. (2009) Pulmonary vein imaging with unenhanced three-dimensional balanced steady-state free precession MR angiography: Initial clinical evaluation. *Radiology* 250(3):932–939

[38] Cowper SE, Robin HS, Steinberg SM et al. (2000) Scleromyxoedema-like cutaneous diseases in renal-dialysis patients. *Lancet*. 356(9234):1000–1001

[39] Rydahl C, Thomsen HS, Marckmann P et al. (2008) High prevalence of nephrogenic systemic fibrosis in chronic renal failure patients exposed to gadodiamide, a gadolinium-containing magnetic resonance contrast agent. *Invest Radiol*. 43(2):141–144

[40] Neuwelt EA, Hamilton BE, Varallyay CG et al. (2009) Ultrasmall superparamagnetic iron oxides (USPIOs): A future alternative magnetic resonance (MR) contrast agent for patients at risk for nephrogenic systemic fibrosis (NSF)? *Kidney In* 75:465–474.

[41] Flacke S, Fischer S, Scott MJ et al. (2001) Novel MRI contrast agent for molecular imaging of fibrin: Implication for detecting vulnerable plaques. *Circulation* 104:1280–1285

Chapter 8
血管畸形

Vascular Malformations

Michele Anzidei, Beatrice Sacconi, Beatrice Cavallo Marincola, Pierleone Lucatelli, Alessandro Napoli, Mario Bezzi, Carlo Catalano 著

杨洁瑾 译

邱健星 校

目录 CONTENTS

一、分类 / 146
二、影像 / 148
三、治疗 / 154
四、总结 / 156

血管畸形包括一系列疾病，可累及人体各个器官，在成人和儿童中都有较高的发病率，甚至可以导致死亡。由于血管畸形的类型会导致治疗策略有所不同，因此混乱的学术名词和影像指南可能导致临床错误的诊断和治疗[1]。针对血管异常已经提出多种分类系统。

在1982年，Mulliken和Glowacki提出了最为广泛接受的分类。这种生物学分类是基于细胞更替速度、组织学特点、自然病程和体格检查[2]，将血管异常分为血管瘤和血管畸形。血管瘤是婴幼儿及儿童时期的良性血管肿瘤，包括细胞增殖和畸形生长，可分为早期的快速增生期和晚期的退化期。血管畸形由发育不良的血管管道引起，并呈现正常内皮循环，且不会因儿童生长而退化[2-4]。

1993年，Jackon等[5]提出了血管畸形的影像学分类，基于血流动力学，根据这个分类，我们能将其分为低流量畸形和高流量畸形。

1996年，通过国际血管异常学会（International Society for the Study of Vascular Anomalies, ISSVA）这些体统被广泛接受[6]。血管异常被分为血管肿瘤（以初期的血管瘤最为常见）和血管畸形两类。血管畸形再根据流量动力学分为低流量畸形（静脉畸形、淋巴管畸形、毛细血管畸形、毛细血管-静脉畸形和毛细血管-淋巴管-静脉畸形）和高流量畸形[动静脉畸形（arteriovenous malformation，AVMs）和动静脉瘘（arteriovenous fistulae，AVFs）]。任何包括动脉的血管畸形都被认为是高流量，相反，那些不包含动脉的血管畸形为低流量血管畸形。血管异常的分类、主要临床表现及其磁共振影像特点总结见表8-1。

一、分类

血管畸形为先天异常，出生携带，但不一定明显。血管畸形随儿童一起长大，不会出现退化。青春期或妊娠时身体激素变化或者血栓、感染、创伤和不完全的治疗，都可能导致血管畸形的恶变[4]。不像血管瘤，它们可能呈浸润性，并累及多个组织平面。

表8-1 血管畸形的特点

血管异常	临床特点	形态学特点	MR特点
血管肿瘤			
血管瘤	出现于胚胎第1周；生长迅速	草莓样、温暖、搏动的肿块	增殖期：边界清晰，分叶状肿块，呈T_1加权图像低信号、T_2加权图像高信号，自旋回波图像中呈流空信号，早期均匀强化退化期：脂肪替代，低强化
低流量血管畸形			
静脉	出现在儿童期或青少年时期	蓝色、柔软、不可压迫、不能流动的肿块	分叶状、内含分隔的肿块，没有占位效应、静脉石及液液平，无流空信号，在T_1加权图像呈低信号，T_2加权图像呈高信号，增强扫描可见逐渐强化
淋巴管	发生在儿童，随儿童长大，不会退化	边界平滑，不可压缩的胶状肿块	分叶状、内含分隔的肿块，没有占位效应、静脉石及液液平，无流空信号，在T_1加权图像呈低信号，T_2加权图像呈高信号，增强扫描可见逐渐强化。大囊型可有边缘强化，微囊型没有明显强化
毛细血管	发生在儿童，随儿童长大，不会退化	皮肤红色	皮肤增厚病灶
高流量血管畸形			
动静脉畸形	发生在儿童，随儿童长大，不会退化	红色温暖、有搏动的肿块	没有明确的肿块，可见增宽的供血动脉和引流静脉；血管流空；增强扫描可见早期增强供血动脉，病灶短路至引流静脉

Chapter 8 血管畸形
Vascular Malformations

血管畸形可被分为高流量和低流量。基于流量动力学的分类对于外科手术和影像引导下治疗有着重要的意义。

复杂多发的畸形可见于 Klippel–Trénaunay 综合征、Sturge–Weber 综合征、Parkes Weber 综合征、Blue Rubber Bleb 综合征、Proteus 综合征和 Maffucci 综合征[3]。

1. 低流量血管畸形

（1）静脉畸形：静脉畸形是最常见的周围血管畸形[7-9]，常见于头颈部（40%）、躯干（20%）、四肢（40%），这些占了几乎 2/3 的血管畸形[7,10]。

静脉畸形是由异常的静脉网络构成的低流量畸形[9]，由或大或小的发育不良、后毛细静脉，无平滑肌的薄壁血管腔和数量不等的基质、血栓、静脉石组成。发育不良的静脉通道通常通过狭窄的支流与相邻的生理静脉相连[7]。血管壁肌肉异常可能是这些病变逐渐扩大的原因[9,11]。

静脉畸形在出生时即出现，但患者通常在儿童晚期或成人早期出现症状。其临床表现取决于病变的深度和范围。皮肤和皮下静脉畸形表现为浅蓝色、柔软、易于压迫的非流动性肿块[7,12]，其特征是随着 Valsalva（瓦氏）动作和特定位置而扩大，并且随着肢体抬高和局部压迫而减压。静脉畸形可浸润穿透组织全层并侵入多个邻近组织（脂肪、肌肉、肌腱和骨骼），导致疼痛、运动障碍和骨骼畸形[7,13]。

静脉畸形或静脉淋巴畸形可出现于多种不同的综合征。蓝色橡胶疱疹综合征（Blue Rubber Bleb nevus syndrome）是一种家族性疾病，以进行性多发性皮肤、肌肉骨骼和胃肠静脉畸形为特点。患者可能因慢性出血、肠套叠或胃肠道静脉畸形扭转而出现慢性失血和间歇性小肠梗阻[3,13]。变形杆菌综合征可表现为皮肤和内脏淋巴 - 静脉畸形，多发皮下错构瘤、色素痣、偏身肥大、手足过度生长、骨外生骨疣和脂肪瘤[4,13]。Maffucci 综合征包括弥漫性软骨瘤病，可累及手和脚的指骨，并伴有多种静脉或淋巴管畸形[3]。

（2）淋巴管畸形：淋巴管畸形是仅次于静脉畸形的第二大常见的血管畸形[14]，通常位于颈部（70%～80%），特别是在颈后三角，腋窝（20%），很少位于四肢[4,15]。

淋巴管畸形是内衬有内皮细胞的充满乳糜液的囊肿[4,6]。它们是由于隔离的淋巴囊无法与外周引流通道相通所产生的[15]。这些畸形可分为微囊型（在实性成分背景中多发的直径小于 2mm 的囊肿）和大囊型（形态可变的较大的囊肿）[4]。淋巴管畸形通常与其他血管畸形相关[16]。

大多数淋巴管畸形通常在 2 岁前即可发现，表现为边界光整的软组织密度胶状肿物。

（3）毛细血管畸形：有 0.3% 的儿童出生时患有毛细血管畸形[4]，表现出局部皮肤红色改变。它们主要位于头颈部[17]。毛细血管畸形是皮肤管腔较细的薄壁血管的先天性扩张。虽然毛细血管畸形通常与真皮或黏膜相关，但它们也可能是某些更为复杂的、异常的特征表现，如 Sturge-Weber、Klippel-Trénaunay 和 Parkes Weber 综合征[4,17]；这些患者的症状是更严重的相关畸形所导致的[2,7]。

Sturge-Weber 综合征包括头面部三叉神经分布区单侧的毛细血管畸形，伴有同侧软脑膜畸形、脑萎缩，邻近大脑皮质的钙化和脉络膜畸形[3,13]。

Klippel-Trénaunay 综合征即先天性静脉畸形肢体肥大综合征，涉及肢体过度生长相关的躯干和四肢的毛细血管静脉畸形，包括皮肤毛细血管畸形伴有肢体肥大，可伴有动静脉畸形、先天性静脉曲张。

（4）淋巴管静脉畸形：毛细血管静脉畸形是由发育不良的毛细血管和扩大的毛细血管后血管腔隙形成的低流量畸形。

2. 高流量血管畸形
高流量血管畸形约占四肢畸形的 10%，包括动静脉畸形和动静脉瘘。高流量病灶也包括在增殖期的婴儿血管瘤。

动静脉瘘是动脉和静脉由单一的管道相连，而动静脉畸形是由供血动脉、引流静脉和与之相连的发育不良的血管腔，其缺乏正常的毛细血管床。

147

（1）动静脉畸形：动静脉畸形在出生时已经存在，病变处于静止状态[17]，但直到儿童期或成年期才常常变得明显。与其他血管畸形一样，它们通常随着儿童的生长发育按比例增大，可受青春期或妊娠期间的激素变化[13]、血栓形成、感染或创伤等因素影像，导致生长加快[7]。

由于病变的高血流，其表现为红色、搏动、温暖的肿块，带有刺激，可能导致骨骼过度生长、动脉窃血现象和皮肤缺血。病灶在后期可能会出现溃疡和出血。

（2）动静脉瘘：先天性动静脉瘘好发于头颈部，不同于获得性动静脉瘘，通常由医源性或外伤所致的穿透伤导致。MRI 在自旋回波序列上显示动脉和静脉成分均表现为流空信号，在梯度回波（gradient-echo，GRE）图像上表现为没有明确边界的高信号灶[16]。慢性继发性动静脉瘘影像学表现可类似于动静脉畸形，因为动静脉畸形的供血动脉可有更强的血流，同时也可见远端引流静脉的增宽[18]。

二、影像

评价病灶的特征需要利用多种影像形式，这些特征包括病灶大小、流速、流向、相关的周围结构（血管、肌肉、神经、骨骼、皮肤）和病灶成分。

（一）普通 X 线

普通 X 线摄影在血管病变的诊断和分类中只占很小的一部分，但它可有效提供有关骨和关节受累的信息。骨质侵蚀、骨质硬化改变、骨膜反应和病理性骨折均表明骨受累。

（二）超声

超声检查是一种必不可少的非侵入性工具，广泛用于检查浅表血管病变。彩色多普勒成像可对动脉和静脉进行实时分析和流速的测量。它是监测接受治疗的患者的重要方法，但对于干扰性空气或骨骼附近的深部病变，超声检查只能做有限的评估。

（三）CT

静脉对比增强计算机断层扫描（computed tomography，CT）可用于评估血管畸形。多排螺旋 CT 是评估病变的强化程度、钙化或血栓形成、远端径流（当病变位于四肢时）和伴随病变的有效手段。CT 的高时间分辨率和空间分辨率有利于评估血管病变（图 8-1 和图 8-2）。

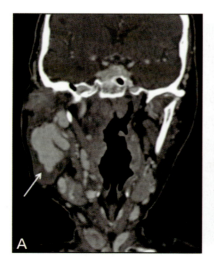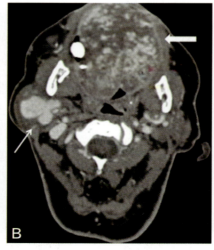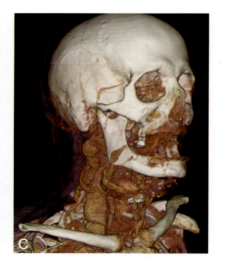

▲ 图 8-1　28 岁男性的血管病变

冠状位图像（A）、轴位图像（B）、容积重建图像（C）。CT 扫描静脉期显示右颧部的大动静脉畸形，其弥漫累及腮腺（细箭）和舌头（粗箭）

由于 CT 有电离辐射，并且提供的血流信息较少，因此在评估血管畸形方面 MRI 已逐步取代 CT。但是，CT 可以清楚地显示静脉石及部分脂肪成分，同时评估可能伴随血管异常的骨过度生长或溶解。此外，CT 可用于不能镇静及禁用 MRI 的患者，故 CT 检查依然在血管畸形的诊断中起到重要作用。

（四）MR

MRI 是对血管异常分类最有价值的影像学检查[19]。它能帮助人们获取血管病变的范围及病灶与邻近结构间解剖关系的信息[3]，从而为治疗计划提供重要信息。

线圈的选择取决于病变的大小和位置，但通常应选择覆盖整个病变的最小线圈。如果病变可触及或可见，通常需在临床感兴趣区域上放置皮肤标记。

基本的序列集如下：SE 或快速 SE T_1 加权成像、脂肪抑制快速 SE T_2 加权成像或短时间反转恢复（short time inversion recovery，STIR）成像和 3D 动态时间分辨 MR 血管造影（magnetic resonance angiography，MRA）。

利用 SE 或快速 SE T_1 加权成像可对基本解剖进行评估。脂肪抑制快速 SE T_2 加权成像或 STIR 成像用于评估病变的范围（图 8-3）。

对血管异常的综合评估需要对相关血管进行功能分析。为此，动态时间分辨 MRA 已成为必不可少的工具。通过该技术可获取具有高时间分辨率和空间分辨率的图像。这些序列可每 2 秒采集一个 3D 数据集。这种高时间分辨率能够：①区别供血动脉与引流静脉，并检测早期静脉分流；②获取关于造影剂到达时间的信息（定义为血管开始增强和对比剂在静脉内达到最高浓度的间隔时间）和流向；③减少运动伪影[4,13]（图 8-4）。

因此，动态时间分辨 MRA 能够对血管畸形的结构和血流动力学特性进行良好描述[17]，获取关于供血动脉和引流静脉的重要数据，这对于治疗计划的制订是至关重要的[20]。该技术已被证明可以区分低流量和高流量的血管畸形[17,21]。这些序列在团注对比剂后立即开始，以便实时观察对比剂通过病变的血管床。背景减影和最大强度投影（maximum intensity projection，MIP）重建生成用于功能图像评估的类透视 MRA 数据集。

最后，在对比剂给药后 3min，在对比剂循环的平衡阶段获得经过修改的 3D T_1 加权高分辨率序列，以获得详细的血管图并描绘病灶内形成的血栓（图 8-5）。

在某些情况下，可以使用 GRE T_2^* 加权图像来发现钙化或含铁血黄素以及高流量血管。在 GRE 图像上，血管中信号缺乏代表低流量畸形[3,22]，

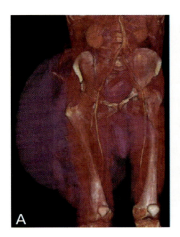
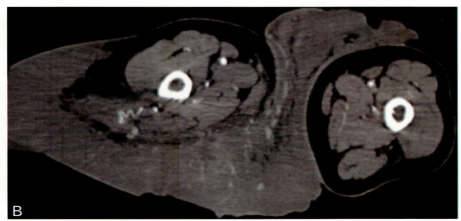

▲ 图 8-2 37 岁男性的血管病变

VR 图像（A）和轴位图像（B）。动脉期 CT 扫描显示臀肌区较大的动静脉畸形，皮下软组织弥漫性增厚，局部小血管充盈显影

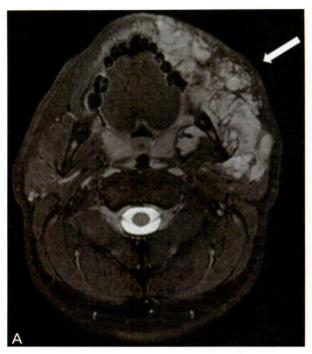 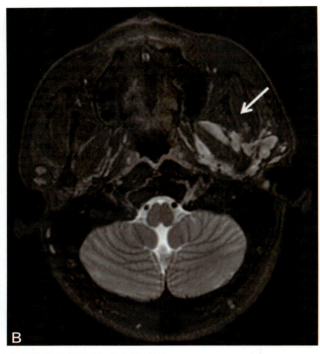

▲ 图 8-3 STIR 序列轴位 T₂ 加权图像用于评估病变的扩展

A.23 岁女性，STIR 序列轴位 T₂ 加权图像显示左颧骨区域的静脉畸形（粗箭）；B.18 岁男性，STIR 序列轴位 T₂ 加权像显示左腮腺的静脉畸形，累及翼状肌（细箭）

而高流量血管具有高信号强度。

为了便于分析对比度增强的 MRA 的图像，可在必要时使用减法以及 3D 重建技术，包括多平面重组、MIP 和 VR 技术。

1. 低流量血管畸形 MR 特点 就治疗决策而言，识别病变是否为低流量血管畸形比确定病变是否主要是静脉、淋巴或毛细血管更为重要[7,20,21,23]。低流量畸形的诊断是基于 SE 图像上缺乏流空信号。少数情况下，低信号条纹、间隔、血栓或静脉石在横截面图像上表现可类似于信号流空。此时对比增强和 GRE 图像可帮助区分这些低信号与血管腔内流空信号。静脉石和钙化通常在所有脉冲序列均表现为低信号，而与高流量相关的信号流空增强可见强化，并且在 GRE 图像上显示为高信号。

静脉畸形通常易于分辨，T_1 加权图像上信号病灶呈中等至低信号，T_2 加权像和 STIR 图像呈高信号。当病灶内出血或蛋白质含量较高时，病灶内可出现液 - 液平面。

在血栓形成或出血的情况下，可以在 T_1 加权图像上观察到病灶内信号不均匀。鉴定静脉畸形的最佳线索是发现静脉石[17]的存在，表现为各个序列均为小的低信号灶（图 8-6 和图 8-7）。

脂肪抑制的 T_2 加权图像和 STIR 图像已被证明能够精确地确定静脉畸形的范围[3,13]。

静脉畸形的特征在于缺乏动脉和早期静脉增强，并且没有粗大的供血血管及动静脉分流。它们通常表现出对比剂的缓慢逐渐填充，在静脉期上显示迂曲血管，表现为特征性的结节状强化[20]。低流量血管畸形，主要是静脉畸形，对比剂浓度增高时间约为 90s，明显高于高流量 AVM[23]。低流量静脉畸形在延迟期 T_1 加权图像上通常表现为弥漫强化[4]（图 8-8）。

描述畸形与深静脉系统之间的关系对于制订治疗计划有重要的意义，因为血管畸形可增加深静脉血栓形成的风险。延迟对比增强序列可用于发现血管畸形和深静脉系统的关系[4]。缺乏明显的静脉引流并在 MR 图像中边界清晰的病灶已被证实是经皮硬化治疗后预后良好的预测因子[17,24,25]。

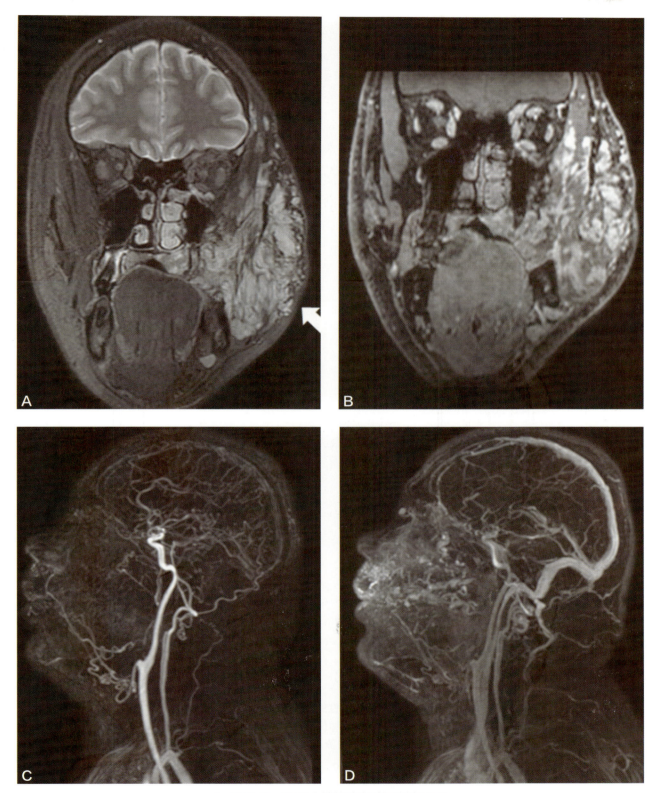

▲ 图 8-4　23 岁女性的动态时间分辨 MRA

MR 图像显示累及左颧部的巨大血管畸形；动态时间分辨图像能够涉及血管的功能；病变由面动脉的分支供血，经颈内静脉的分支引流。A. 冠状位 STIR 序列 T_2 加权像显示左颧部的畸形（箭）；B. 冠状增强 3D T_1 加权高分辨率序列；C～D. 动态时间分辨 MRA（动脉和静脉期）

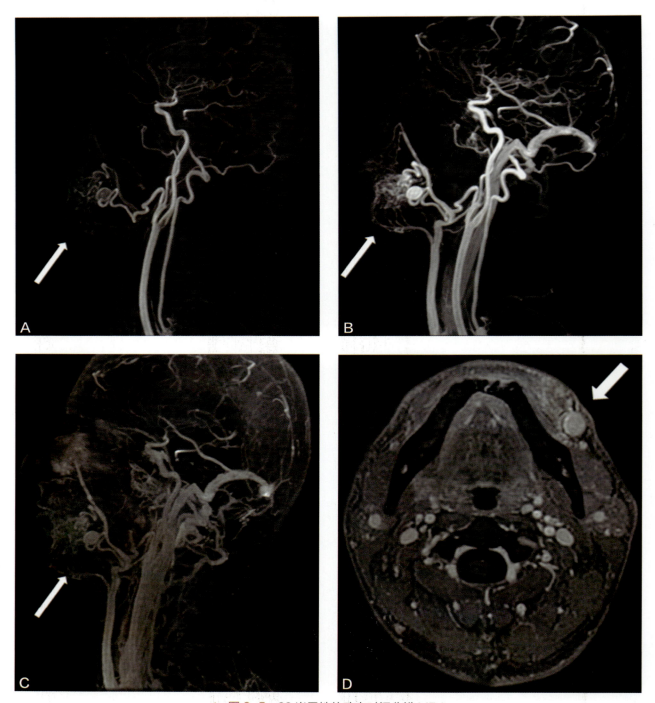

▲ 图 8-5 22 岁男性的动态时间分辨 MRA

动态时间分辨 MRA（动脉、静脉和延迟期）（A～D）及轴位增强 3D T_1 加权高分辨率图像（D）显示下颌区偏左侧的 AVM（箭）。动态时间分辨图像可以正确描绘畸形结构和血流动力学特性

尽管静脉畸形可能与周围水肿或纤维脂肪性基质有关，但它们很少出现肿块[13,23]。因此，对于具有不寻常临床和影像学特征的病变应通过活组织检查评估[23]。

淋巴管畸形通常表现为分叶状、边界清晰的肿块，T_1 加权图像上呈中等至低信号，T_2 加权和 STIR 图像上呈高信号，病灶内常见液-液平面。淋巴管畸形具有穿透性，可浸润脂肪层，并累及多个组织[4,13]。

微囊型淋巴管畸形通常无明显强化[4]，而

Chapter 8 血管畸形
Vascular Malformations

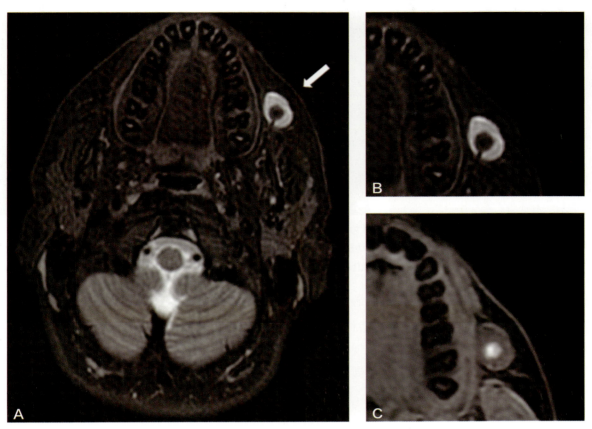

▲ 图 8-6 29 岁女性，左颧部血管畸形

STIR 序列 T$_2$ 加权像（A～B）、FS 序列轴位 T$_1$ 加权像（C），示左颧部血管畸形（箭）。MR 图像显示出血表现为 T$_2$ 加权像低信号、T$_1$ 加权像高信号

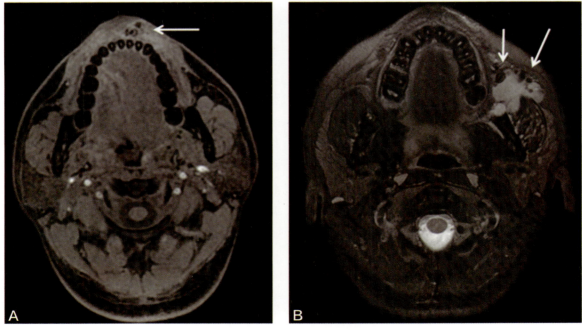

▲ 图 8-7 静脉石 MR 图像

A.33 岁女性，轴位 T$_1$ 加权 FS 序列；B.24 岁女性，轴位 T$_2$ 加权 STIR 序列。MR 图像显示静脉石在 T$_1$ 和 T$_2$ 加权像上均为低信号（箭）

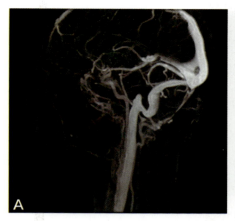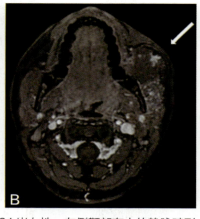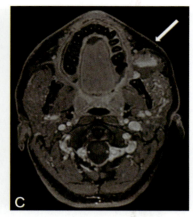

▲ 图 8-8　24 岁女性，左侧颧部有大的静脉畸形（箭）

A. 注射对比剂后，轴位动态时间分辨 MRA（动脉期）；B～C. 延迟 3D T_1 加权高分辨率序列。动态时间分辨序列显示动脉期及门静脉期病变无强化；延迟期 3D T_1 加权序列显示了对比剂逐渐灌注和迂曲血管的特征性结节状强化

大囊型淋巴管畸形可见病灶边缘和间隔强化，对比增强囊性结构无对比剂填充[4,7]。少数情况下，微囊型淋巴管畸形或淋巴静脉畸形可表现为弥漫增强，这是由于微囊型淋巴管畸形中小囊肿的隔膜强化或混合畸形中的静脉成分的强化。这种表现可能使其与静脉畸形难以区分[7,10]。

毛细血管畸形可在临床上做出诊断，通常不需要行 MRI。毛细血管畸形的 MRI 表现较为隐蔽，皮肤增厚或皮下软组织增厚可能是唯一的表现[4,7,26]。MRI 可用于评估可能的相关潜在疾病。

毛细血管 - 静脉畸形影像表现与静脉畸形无明显区别。动态对比增强 MRI 可用于区分毛细血管 - 静脉畸形和静脉畸形，因为毛细血管 - 静脉畸形通常表现为早期均匀增强，而静脉畸形仅见延迟强化[4,27]。

2. 高流量血管畸形的 MR　AVM 的 MRI 表现包括高流量蛇形增粗的供血动脉和引流静脉，这些在 SE 图像上表现为流空信号或在 GRE 图像上表现为高信号，缺乏清晰边界的肿块。病变的骨内浸润可表现为 T_1 加权图像上骨髓信号强度的降低[17]。T_1 加权图像上的高信号区域可能代表出血、血管内血栓形成或流动相关增强的区域[28]。

钆剂对比增强检查可用于评估供血动脉和引流静脉。注射对比剂后，对比剂浓度上升时间为 5～10s，使用时间分辨动态 3D MRA，可以很好地评估 AVM，通常表现为静脉早期对比剂填充（图 8-9）。

三、治疗

婴儿血管瘤倾向于自发消失；因此通常不需要治疗。但是，应该治疗血管畸形以防止永久性功能及容貌损害。治疗策略通常由多个治疗方案组成，取决于血流动力学的畸形分类，包括微创和外科手术干预。

AVM 的治疗可以是外科手术、血管内和（或）经皮的。

通常，由于病变定位和出血风险较高，须避免外科手术（尽管可以行放射线切除）。

对于低流量血管畸形，选择的治疗方法是经皮硬化疗法；对于高流量病变，可选择经动脉栓塞[3,4,15]，有时栓塞后须行手术切除。经皮硬化疗法对高流量病变无效，因为输注的药物会迅速从病灶中冲走[4]。高流量型血管畸形通常需要更多步骤进行治疗，因为在随访期间经常观察到从病灶中生出新的供血血管（新血管生成）。

经皮治疗包括直接穿刺病灶和注射 95% 的乙醇或 2% 的甲氧基硬脂酸（泡沫或液体）；治疗使用的针为不同口径的。在进行硬化之前，必须进行数字减影血管造影以研究病灶真正的引流静脉；治疗必须直接针对病灶进行对比剂注射，避免栓

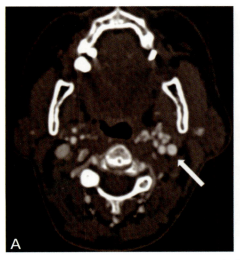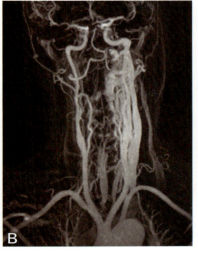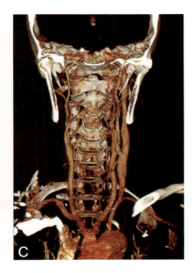

▲ 图 8-9　45 岁男性，左颈部 AVM

A. 轴位 CT 静脉期图像；B. 动态时间分辨 MRA（MIP）；C. 容积重现图像。CT 和 MR 图像显示左颈部 AVM。与对侧血管（箭）相比，可见左侧颈内静脉的早期强化

塞剂的全身扩散。

通常通过股动脉进行血管内栓塞，通过使用 Onyx®、聚乙烯醇颗粒或氰基丙烯酸酯，对病灶供血动脉进行选择性或甚至超选择性栓塞。术后并发症表现为疼痛、水肿、肿胀、皮肤溃疡以及非目标血管栓塞（图 8-10）。

治疗后表现

MRI 是评估治疗结果和建立长期管理策略的极好工具[29]。在随访期间采用的成像方式在技术方面与术前无差异。

1. 静脉畸形　乙醇引起内皮几乎瞬间剥脱、强烈的炎症反应，以及畸形血栓形成均与明显的肿胀有关[17]。在接下来的几周内，病灶纤维化，并可观察到畸形逐渐缩小。长达数月的随诊是必要的，以评估硬化疗法后的治疗反应，让短暂的炎症反应逐渐消失[9]。

在 MRI 中，硬化疗法后的静脉畸形在 T_1 和 T_2 加权图像上表现为混杂信号[9]。治疗后即刻行 MRI 显示治疗区域以及沿着肌间隔在 T_2 加权和 STIR 图像上呈高信号[30]。根据我们的经验，治疗后畸形的高信号可持续长达 3 个月，但在肌间隔不再出现[30]。

在 MRA 中，治疗病灶的中央部分没有强化，

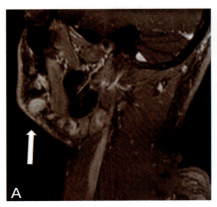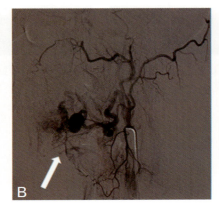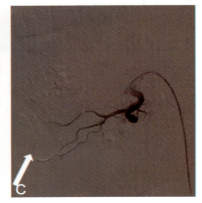

▲ 图 8-10　22 岁的男性，下颌部偏左侧可见 AVM（箭）

A. 矢状位对比增强 3D T_1 加权序列；B～C. 栓塞前后的血管造影图像。注意，在手术结束时，其供血动脉（面动脉分支）畸形几乎完全消失

病灶周围可由于反应性充血而强化[30]。这种增强已经在动脉期图像上看到。3个月后，增强通常消失仅留下瘢痕，在 T_1 加权图像和非增强的 STIR 图像上表现为低信号[30]。病变的通常逐渐缩小[30]（图 8-11）。

在畸形广泛的情况下，尽管进行了多次治疗，但仍难以检测治疗效果[30]。因此，钆对比增强成像可用于证明畸形的残余灌注并指导其他治疗[9]。

2. 动脉畸形和动静脉畸形 为了完全根除高血管畸形的病灶，必须更改治疗策略，因为任何不完全治疗都可能刺激病灶更活跃的生长[17]。经动脉栓塞后，血管畸形病灶内常见血栓形成；MRA 可显示出分流的减少或消失，伴有静脉系统早期强化的减少或缺失。早期治疗后须再次评估，任何剩余的畸形都必须在第二阶段进行治疗。在使用铁磁性弹簧圈进行栓塞的情况下，MR 图像中存在伪影，可能掩盖其附近的残余血管畸形[30]（图 8-12 和图 8-13）。

四、总结

血管畸形是罕见但重要的疾病，通常需要积极治疗，影像学检查在其诊断中起重要作用。MRI 已成为评估这些病变的卓越成像方式。对比增强 MRA，尤其是动态时间分辨 MRA，可提供关于血管异常的血流动力学信息，从而有助于病变的分类。此外，MRI 是评估治疗效果和制订长期管理策略的极好工具。

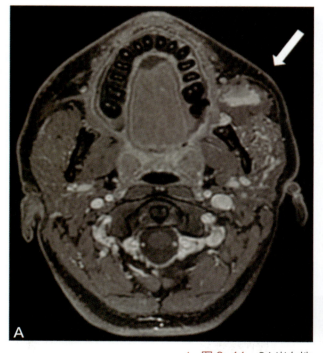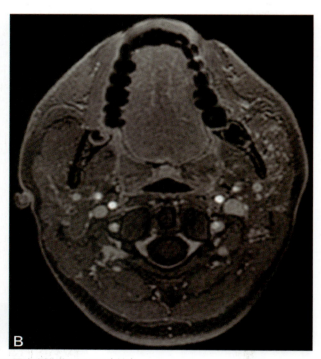

▲ 图 8-11 24 岁女性，可见左侧颧部 AVM（箭）
在硬化疗法之前（A）和之后（B）的轴位对比增强 3D T_1 加权图像。畸形几乎完全消失，延迟期未见强化

Chapter 8 血管畸形
Vascular Malformations

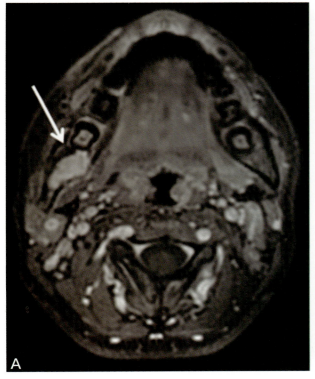
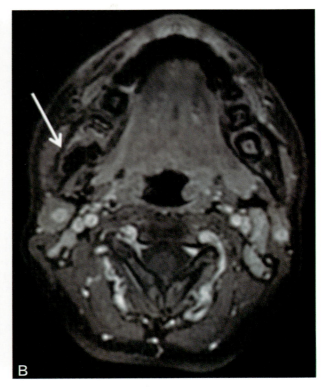

▲ 图 8-12 42 岁的女性，患有右半颌部的 AVM（箭）
栓塞前（A）和栓塞后（B），轴位对比增强 3D T_1 加权图像。治疗后病变完全无强化

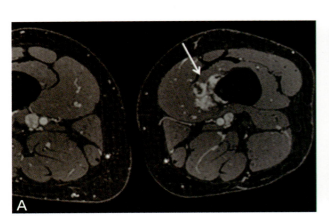
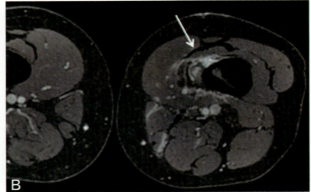

▲ 图 8-13 25 岁女性，左膝血管畸形（箭）
栓塞术前（A）和栓塞术后（B），轴位对比增强 3D T_1 加权图像。手术后病变可见体积减小和强化减低

参考文献

[1] Hand JL, Frieden IJ. Vascular birthmarks of infancy: Resolving nosologic confusion. *Am J Med Genet* 2002;108(4):257–264.

[2] Mulliken JB, Glowacki J. Hemangiomas and vascular malformations in infants and children: A classification based on endothelial characteristics. *Plast Reconstr Surg* 1982;69(3):412–422.

[3] Dubois J, Alison M. Vascular anomalies: What a radiologist needs to know. *Pediatr Radiol* 2010;40(6): 895–905.

[4] Moukaddam H, Pollak J, Haims AH. MRI characteristics and classification of peripheral vascular malformations and tumors. *Skeletal Radiol* 2009;38(6):535–547.

[5] Jackson IT, Carreño R, Potparic Z, Hussain K. Hemangiomas, vascular malformations, and lymphovenous malformations: Classification and methods of treatment. *Plast Reconstr Surg* 1993;91(7): 1216–1230.

[6] Enjolras O. Classification and management of the various superficial vascular anomalies: Hemangiomas and vascular malformations. *J Dermatol* 1997;24(11):701–710.

[7] Fayad LM, Hazirolan T, Bluemke D, Mitchell S. Vascular malformations in the extremities: Emphasis on MR imaging features that guide treatment options. *Skeletal Radiol* 2006;35(3):127–137.

[8] Breugem CC, Maas M, Reekers JA, van der Horst CM. Use of magnetic resonance imaging for the evaluation of vascular malformations of the lower extremity. *Plast Reconstr Surg* 2001;108(4):870–877.

[9] Dubois J, Soulez G, Oliva VL, Berthiaume MJ, Lapierre C, Therasse E. Soft-tissue venous malformations in adult patients: Imaging and therapeutic issues. *RadioGraphics* 2001;21(6):1519–1531.

[10] Laor T, Burrows PE. Congenital anomalies and vascular birthmarks of the lower extremities. *Magn Reson Imaging Clin N Am* 1998;6(3):497–519.

[11] Mulliken JB, Fishman SJ, Burrows PE. Vascular anomalies. *Curr Probl Surg* 2000;37(8):517–584.

[12] Rak KM, Yakes WF, Ray RL et al. MR imaging of symptomatic peripheral vascular malformations. *AJR Am J Roentgenol* 1992;159(1):107–112.

[13] Donnelly LF, Adams DM, Bisset GS 3rd. Vascular malformations and hemangiomas: A practical approach in a multidisciplinary clinic. *AJR Am J Roentgenol* 2000;174(3):597–608.

[14] Marler JJ, Mulliken JB. Current management of hemangiomas and vascular malformations. *Clin Plast Surg* 2005;32(1):99–116.

[15] Dubois J, Garel L. Imaging and therapeutic approach of hemangiomas and vascular malformations in the pediatric age group. *Pediatr Radiol* 1999;29 (12):879–893.

[16] Navarro OM, Laffan EE, Ngan BY. Pediatric soft-tissue tumors and pseudotumors: MR imaging features with pathologic correlation. I. Imaging approach, pseudotumors, vascular lesions, and adipocytic tumors. *RadioGraphics* 2009;29(3):887–906.

[17] Ernemann U, Kramer U, Miller S et al. Current concepts in the classification, diagnosis and treatment of vascular anomalies. *Eur J Radiol* 2010;75(1):2–11.

[18] Lawdahl RB, Routh WD, Vitek JJ, McDowell HA, Gross GM, Keller FS. Chronic arteriovenous fistulas masquerading as arteriovenous malformations: Diagnostic considerations and therapeutic implications. *Radiology* 1989;170(3 Pt. 2):1011–1015.

[19] Hyodoh H, Hori M, Akiba H, Tamakawa M, Hyodoh K, Hareyama M. Peripheral vascular malformations: Imaging, treatment approaches, and therapeutic issues. *RadioGraphics* 2005;25(suppl. 1): S159–S171.

[20] Herborn CU, Goyen M, Lauenstein TC, Debatin JF, Ruehm SG, Kröger K. Comprehensive time-resolved MRI of peripheral vascular malformations. *AJR Am J Roentgenol* 2003;181(3):729–735.

[21] Ohgiya Y, Hashimoto T, Gokan T et al. Dynamic MRI for distinguishing high-flow from low-flow peripheral vascular malformations. *AJR Am J Roentgenol* 2005; 185(5):1131–1137.

[22] Siegel MJ. Magnetic resonance imaging of musculoskeletal soft tissue masses. *Radiol Clin North Am* 2001;39(4):701–720.

[23] Dobson MJ, Hartley RW, Ashleigh R, Watson Y, Hawnaur JM. MR angiography and MR imaging of symptomatic vascular malformations. *Clin Radiol* 1997;52(8):595–602.

[24] Goyal M, Causer PA, Armstrong D. Venous vascular malformations in pediatric patients: Comparison of results of alcohol sclerotherapy with proposed MR imaging classification. *Radiology* 2002;223(3): 639–644.

[25] Yun WS, Kim YW, Lee KB et al. Predictors of response to percutaneous ethanol sclerotherapy (PES) in patients with venous malformations: Analysis of patient self-assessment and imaging. *J Vasc Surg* 2009;50(3):581–589.

[26] Breugem CC, Maas M, van der Horst CM. Magnetic resonance imaging findings of vascular malformations of the lower extremity. *Plast Reconstr Surg* 2001;108(4):878–884.

[27] Van Rijswijk CS, van der Linden E, van der Woude HJ, van Baalen JM, Bloem JL. Value of dynamic contrast-enhanced MR imaging in diagnosing and classifying peripheral vascular malformations. *AJR Am J Roentgenol* 2002;178(5):1181–1187.

[28] Abernethy LJ. Classification and imaging of vascular malformations in children. *Eur Radiol* 2003; 13(11):2483–2497.

[29] Lee BB, Choe YH, Ahn JM et al. The new role of magnetic resonance imaging in the contemporary diagnosis of venous malformation: Can it replace angiography? *J Am Coll Surg* 2004;198(4):549–558.

[30] Hagspiel K, Stevens P, Leung D et al. Vascular malformations of the body: Treatment follow-up using MRI and 3D gadolinium-enhanced MRA. In: CIRSE 2002. Abstracts of the annual meeting and postgradu ate course of the Cardiovascular and Interventional Radiological Society of Europe and the 4th Joint Meeting with the European Society of Cardiac Radiology (ESCR). Lucern, Switzerland, October 5–9, 2002. *Cardiovasc Intervent Radiol* 2002;25(suppl. 2):S77–S265.

Chapter 9
4D 血流成像

Four-Dimensional Flow Imaging

Sergio Uribe, Israel Valverde, Pablo Bächler 著

曹 剑 代静文 译

王怡宁 校

目录 CONTENTS

一、4D 血流磁共振成像 / 160
二、4D 血流成像的潜在临床应用 / 166
三、先天性心脏病 4D 血流成像 / 168
四、4D 血流成像的展望 / 176

欲获得心脏和血管的速度图像通常采用相位对比技术。在这个序列中，采用流动编码梯度将磁化矢量的流速编码转化为图像中的相位[1]。最常见的流动编码梯度是双极速度编码梯度（图9-1）。

双极梯度的施加决定了流动敏感的方向。这可以单独添加到三个逻辑轴中的任意一个（层面选择、频率编码或相位编码）中，也可以同时添加到两个或更多个逻辑轴，以实现沿任意轴的流动敏感性。

由于双极梯度下的净面积为零，因此静态自旋不会产生相位累积。然而，对于移动的自旋，例如血流，引入自旋的相位与每个双极梯度的速度和面积成正比。

速度编码梯度以其混叠速度参数为特征，通常表示为 VENC。根据定义，当沿梯度方向的速度分量等于 ±VENC 时，所得相差为 ±π，如公式 9.1 所示。

$$\text{VENC} = \frac{\pi}{\gamma A_g \tau} \quad (9.1)$$

由于 MR 图像包含对相位的其他贡献因素（例如，B_0 不均匀），相位对比成像利用相同的成像参数获得两组完整的图像数据，除了在双极梯度。这两幅图像的相位或复合值都是按像素减影的。减影过程突出血流同时抑制不需要的相位变化和背景静止组织。常用两种不同的减影：复差重建和相位差重建。

复差重建通过从两组数据集中减去复杂数据来完成此方法的结果是一个量级数值，因此像素强度值与血流速度成正比。这种重建方法也被称为相位对比血管造影，它可以用于获得脑动静脉血管造影。这种重建的主要问题是不提供方向性或定量的信息。

相位差重建也被称为速度图或相位速度图，通常用来描述血流的方向及量化血管净流速。相位差重建在成像域进行。每对数据集通过傅里叶变换成两个独立的复合图像。从这两个图像中计算出角度差或相位差（Δφ），流速计算见公式9.02。

$$v = \left(\frac{\Delta\varphi}{\pi}\right)\text{VENC} \quad (9.2)$$

VENC 是速度编码参数。

由于相位差重建的动态范围是 [-π，π]，所以只能在 |v| ≤ VENC 时可靠地反映流动方向，除非采用相位展开算法[2]。

一、4D 血流磁共振成像

血流编码梯度的轴决定了敏感方向。此信息可以添加到三个逻辑轴中的任意一个（层面选择、频率编码或相位编码）单独或同时实现沿任意轴的流动敏感性。当沿 3 个逻辑轴连续应用流动编码梯度时，可以在 3 个正交方向测量血流速度。这种技术被称为三维相位对比磁共振成像。当三维速度编码应用于三维体积时（图 9-2）或 4D 血流 MRI[1,3,4]。

在下面的章节中，我们将回顾关于采集和 4D 血流数据量化的技术进展。随后我们将总结文献报道的 4D 血流成像 MRI 的一些潜在临床应用。最后以我们对 4D 血流成像 MRI 的未来展望来结束这一章。

（一）4D 血流成像技术概览：图像采集、可视化工具和数据量化方法

在 3D 成像体中获得 3D 速度信息所需收集的数据量很大。根据视野的大小以及空间和时间分辨率，扫描时间从 5～20min 不等。这意味着 4D 血流成像的采集不能在一次屏气中进行。因此需采用扫描时间最小化的方法获取数据集。此外，这些采集技术需要结合呼吸运动校正算法。

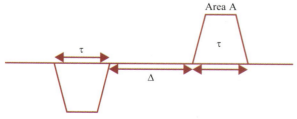

▲ 图 9-1 双极梯度用于编码速度信息

静态自旋不获得任何净相；然而，运动自旋获得一个与梯度面积成比例的净相位

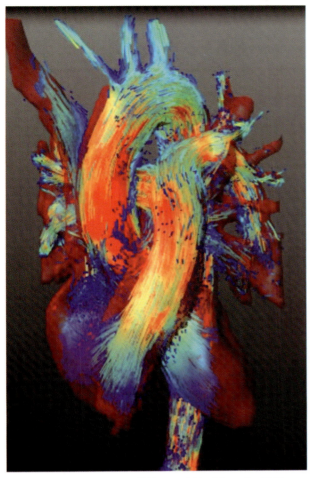

▲ 图 9-2 心脏和大血管的 4D 血流成像 MRI 示例

获取 4D 血流成像数据集的标准方法采用分段梯度回波序列。需要在几次心跳中收集 Ny×Nz 条 K 空间线，其中 Ny 和 Nz 分别为相位和层面编码方向的 K 空间线的数量。为完成 3D 采集，总共需要采集 Ny×Nz/N_{LS} 次心跳，其中 N_{LS} 是每段的 K 空间线数量。为了在三维空间中实现速度编码，每段中的每条 K 空间线都需要被采集几次。

有几种方法可以获得三维速度编码[3]。一种方法是在每个方向进行 1 次成对测量，包括 1 次流动补偿和 1 次流动编码，最终在 3 个方向进行 6 次测量获得三维流动编码[1,3,5]。这种方法被称为六点法。更有效的方法被称为四点采集法。其中一种包括 4 次连续的采集，即 1 次流动补偿和 3 次双极梯度施加于两个轴上的采集（图 9-3）。还有一些其他方法采用了平衡四点法[3,6,7]。无论采用何种编码策略，4D 血流成像都需要获取一张解剖图像和三张各方向流速编码的图像。

目前，四点法是对 4D 血流成像数据进行编码的最有效的技术。但是该方法需要相当于原先 4 倍的 TR，限制了其时间分辨率。在每段采集中，只能获取一条 K 空间线的情况下，最小 TR 取决于速度编码参数 VENC，该参数与双极梯度的强度和持续时间有关。较低的 VENC 需要较强的梯度和（或）更长的持续时间，由此会导致更低的时间分辨率。另一方面，设置较高的 VENC 所需的梯度较弱，允许更高的时间分辨率。然而，将 VENC 设置过高可能会影响慢血流测量的准确性，如静脉血流。

在接下来的章节中，我们将回顾 4D 血流成像的不同采样和采集策略，以及控制呼吸运动伪影的呼吸运动补偿方法。

（二）采集和采样策略

采用传统的三维笛卡尔采样方法[4,6,8]，可以进行 4D 血流成像量数据采集。这种方法的优点是可直接重建每个数据集；然而，缺点是扫描时间往往很长，限制了空间分辨率。

另一种方法是采用欠采样的三维径向轨迹，又称为大范围欠采样各向同性投射重建（PC-VIPR）[9]。这种方法可以减少扫描时间和（或）提高 4D 血流成像采集的空间分辨率。K 空间轨道由穿越 K 空间中心的多个投影组成。该方法的优点是在球形大 FOV 上提供了各向同性的高空间分辨率。该序列可用于小血管的血流动力学研究，如脑动脉瘤。该序列还可用于需要大 FOV 的情形，如全心和大血管[10-13]，以及研究肝脏血流等[14]应用。

堆叠螺旋轨迹[15]也被用于有效地采样 K 空间和获得 4D 血流成像数据，可以相对于笛卡尔成像方法减少 2～3 倍的扫描时间。但是，对失谐效应和轨迹误差的精确校正是获取高质量图像的必要前提。

并行成像技术也被用于加速 4D 血流成像数

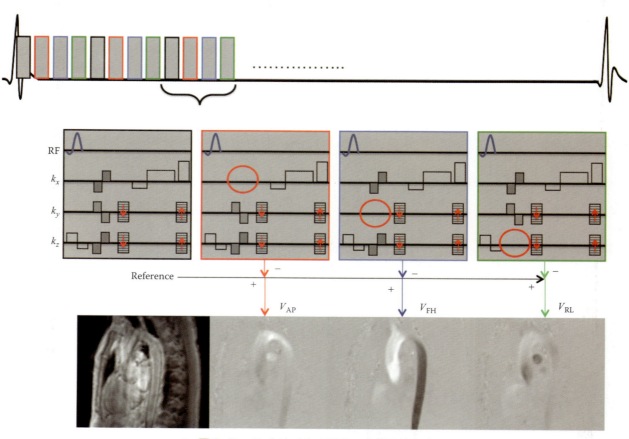

▲ 图9-3 4D 血流成像序列的四点获取法示意图

采集包括一个流量补偿图像（参考图像）以及随后三次采集。在后者中双极梯度只施加于两个轴。通过从参考图像中分别减去后面 3 次采集的图像，可以获得编码 3 个不同方向的速度图像。V_{AP}、V_{FH} 和 V_{RL} 代表了前后、脚头和右左方向的速度

据的获取。加速系数在 3 以内，使用 GRAPPA[16] 或 SENSE[17] 采集的结果与全采样图像一致性较好。然而，更高的欠采样系数会使图像质量下降，并低估流动速度[17]。除并行成像外，有些方法还利用了时空相关性或流动数据的稀疏性来取得更高的欠采样系数。以下参考资料可供有兴趣的读者查阅[18-24]。

（三）呼吸补偿技术

为避免不准确的速度测量，必须使用呼吸运动补偿技术，特别在胸腹部检查中。呼吸绑带和呼吸导航回波是最标准的技术，可以用于 4D 血流成像的采集。两种方法均通过测量横膈膜的位置来间接（绑带）或直接（导航回波）的实现门控采集。采集时常会预设呼气窗口，用于接收或拒绝数据。多数情况下扫描效率在 40%～60%，

因此使用这种方法会延长扫描时间。K 空间重排列算法也会用于采集 4D 血流成像数据集，以提高门控采集下的效率[25]。

虽然呼吸绑带和导航回波是各 MR 厂商应用最广泛的技术，但也有一些缺点。从绑带上获得的呼吸位置可能不准确，可重复性低，难以得到横膈膜在毫米内的运动。另一方面呼吸导航回波干扰了采集，扰乱了平稳状态并可能产生伪影。此外，添加一个或多个导航回波所需的时间限制了 4D 血流成像采集的时间分辨率，导航回波插入在心动周期开始和（或）结束时[25]都有明显的缺点，例如影响对舒张功能和逆行流量的评估[26]。

为了克服这些局限性，提出了自呼吸导航回波技术。这些方法在获取 K 空间数据时，允许在整个心跳周期内采样 4D 血流成像数据且不会或仅

少量增加额外的时间。两种主要策略是获取 K 空间中心点或 K 空间中心线。在这两种情况下，呼吸信号都被作为采集门控。K 空间中心点提供整个成像对象的 MR 信号，因此它的幅值是由心动周期和呼吸运动调节的。另一方面，K 空间中心线的 1D 傅里叶变换是对整个成像体的 1D 投影，由此可以获得成像对象的运动。一个利用 K 空间中心门控采集 4D 血流成像数据的例子可参考[27]。这两种方法的一个共同问题是可能在含大量脂肪组织的患者中失效。脂肪的高信号与 K 空间中心相关性更高，因此可能掩盖呼吸运动。

有一些更前沿的方法可对二维和三维动态和电影成像做回顾性运动修正，从导航回波，绑带和（或）相同的 K 空间数据中获取多个信号。然而，尚未报道这些方法在 4D 血流成像方面的应用情况。

（四）可视化方法

4D 血流成像所采集的数据是带有时间精度的速度向量（Vx、Vy 和 Vz）和幅值数据的三维成像体。有几个软件可量化和展示这些数据，如 GTFlow（Gyrotools, Zurich, Switzerland）[28],EnSight（CEI Inc., Apex, NC）[29]和 Mediframe（University of Karlsruhe, Karlsruhe, Germany）[30]。速度数据可以在每个速度编码方向的图像中可视化。例如，图 9-4 显示了 1 张解剖图像和另外 3 张，前后、右左、足头方向的流动编码图像。后 3 张图片中的信号强度表示血流在每个特定方向的速度。

速度数据也可在某个截面内被描绘成向量场形式，可用流线型或微粒轨迹的形式展示。通过选择一个感兴趣的平面，这个平面的速度可以被表示为向量（图 9-5）。这种方式适合于对局部流动模式的精细分析，如螺旋方向[30]，以及识别涡流[31,32]。

流线是在心动周期特定时相内的假想的线条，与局部速度场平行（图 9-5）[33]。它们提供了流速向量场的三维透视；然而，流线是一种静态的展示，并不一定显示血液沿着心脏循环的路径。

微粒轨迹是假想的微粒随时间运动的路线[34]。通过选择感兴趣的平面并在特定的心跳时相释放假想微粒，可以追踪微粒在心动周期内的轨迹（图 9-6）。它们更真实地代表了血流的路径。

（五）血流的回顾性量化

在离线回顾核磁影像时，通常会发现在数据采集过程中没有被描述或怀疑的诊断。因此，在 MRI 扫描过程中没有包含所需的 2D PC-MRI 序列，无法取得相应信息。不过 4D 血流成像允许离线任意选择平面重建，而不受预先获取的 2D PC-MRI 的限制。我们将在"四"中再次提到这个话题。

（六）血流数据量化的新方法

几项半定量研究用 4D 血流成像描述了心脏和大血管中正常和异常的血流模式。血流数据可

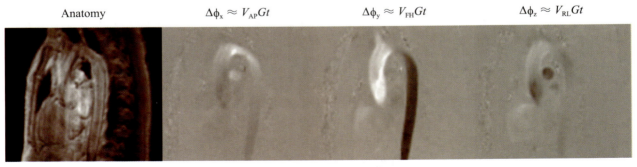

▲ 图 9-4　从 4D 血流成像扫描获得的原始图像

分别为 1 张解剖图像和 3 个方向的流动编码图像。流动编码图像的强度表示每个特定方向的流速（AP. 前 - 后；FH. 脚 - 头；RL. 右 - 左）

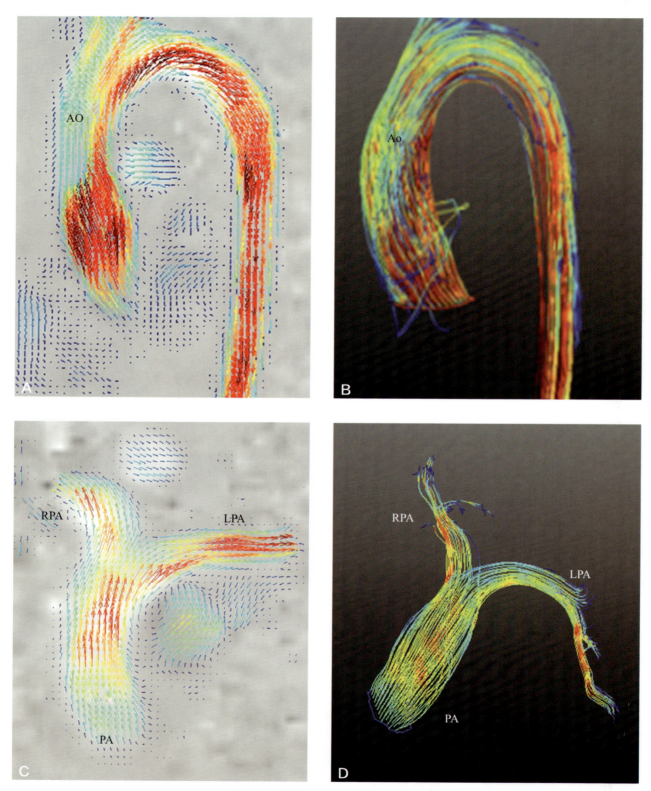

▲ 图 9-5 速度的可视化方法：向量与流线

A 和 C. 显示主动脉和肺动脉（PA）、右肺动脉（RPA）和左肺动脉（LPA）分支中速度的向量场，B 和 D. 为同一血管的流线型表示

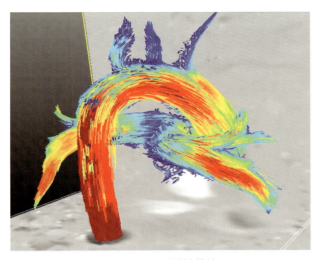

▲ 图 9-6　微粒轨迹

利用主动脉和肺动脉中某一特定心跳间期的微粒轨迹来表示 4D 血流成像数据

视化后处理方法的多样性和一次扫描获取 3D 流速矢量场的能力，使 4D 血流成像可以提供多种疾病的血流动力学详细描述，如主动脉病、肺动脉高压、心力衰竭、颅内动脉瘤或某些先天性心脏病。在这些疾病中的一些主要发现将在"三"中讨论。

除了半定量分析外，还可以利用 4D 血流成像获得各种定量的血流动力学指标。在以下章节中我们将讨论这些血流动力学指标，重点关注它们在临床实践中的潜在效用。

1. 管壁剪切力　在长直血管中的非脉动血流，血流的流动在血管中心最快，在靠近管壁的地方最慢。因流体速度假定满足抛物面剖面，称为层流[35]。这种现象是由血流内部和血流与管壁之间的摩擦导致的。由此产生了一种由血流施加给内皮的摩擦力，即所谓的管壁剪切应力（wall shear stress，WSS）。WSS 的强度取决于从血管壁到血管中心的流速梯度。靠近管壁的流速梯度被称为管壁剪切率，并可通过 4D 血流成像估计 WSS。然而由于有限的时空分辨率、图像分割误差和部分容积效应，MRI 得到的 WSS 通常被低估[36,37]。尽管 WSS 的绝对值可能不准确，但其相对测量可能有助于识别血管内异常血流动

力学应力的区域。高的 WSS 值会促使脑动脉瘤形成[38,39]，变化的 WSS 已被证明在动脉粥样硬化形成和斑块破裂中起着重要作用[40]。另外据推测，WSS 异常区域可能会加速动脉瘤的进展或破裂[41]。

2. 脉搏波速度　脉搏波速度（pulse wave velocity，PWV）反映了血管的刚度，并被公认为测定动脉刚度的最简单、无侵入性、稳定和可重复的方法[42]。PWV 是指脉搏波在已知血管距离上沿着血管（通常是动脉）传播的速度[43]。该指标可用多普勒超声进行计算，但磁共振成像也有一些优点，因为其测量不像超声受到几何形态假设的限制，并可对感兴趣区域进行分析[37,44]。已有结果表明 4D 血流成像 MRI 对 PWV 的量化与传统的 2D PC-MRI 测量结果有很好的相关性[45,46]，并可在具有曲折解剖结构的血管中提供更准确的估计。颈动脉 - 股骨 PWV 和主动脉 PWV 是心血管事件结局的有效预测因子[42]。此外，PWV 可预测某些疾病的进展，比如马方综合征患者的主动脉扩张[47]。

3. 血流分配　微粒轨迹或路径主要用于动态血流的可视化。但它们也可能提供与血流分配有关的有价值的量化信息。由于从某一特定的血管中释放出的微粒轨迹可以在时间上向前和向后跟踪，因此有可能确定此处的血流流向何处或来自何处。这可以用来确定流向分支血管的血流分配，特别是经历了复杂的保守治疗手术后的先天性心脏病患者（如 Fontan 手术或其他双进双出口连接），在这种情形下传统方法无法分离每个血管的血流供给[48,49]。此外，微粒轨迹已被用来对心室内的各种子成分进行分类[50]，这可能有助于早期识别和监测心脏功能障碍[见三（一）]。需要注意的是，当有脉冲血流时流线型表示不应用于这些目的，因为它们只反映给定时刻处的血流场[37,51]。

4. 能量耗散　能量耗散也可以通过 4D 血流成像 MRI 进行非侵入性评估。它被定义为血管间总传输能量的差，例如在肺动脉分支和肺主动脉之间[52]。这一定量指标可为比较先天性心脏病患者不同保守治疗方案的疗效提供新的视角。

5. 湍流 湍流血流的特征是时间和空间上快速随机的血流速度,与正常心血管系统有序的典型层流形成鲜明对比。但这些不规则和快速的波动并不表现为 4D 血流成像量计算出的体素内速度均值[43]。尽管如此,信号的大小仍可用来衡量体素内速度分布的标准差[53,54],其与湍流动能有关,是衡量湍流强度的独立变量。一些研究证明了其与参考方法的良好一致性[55]。由于湍流被认为在血栓形成和动脉粥样硬化的发病机制中起作用[56,57],湍流的成像可能有助于早期识别有风险的血管区域。

6. 压力梯度 压力梯度可用于评估血管或瓣膜狭窄的严重程度。压力导丝是目前压力梯度估计的金标准,但这是一种侵入性手术。4D 血流成像 MRI 提供了利用 Navier-Stokes 方程精确测量局部压力差的可能性。从 4D 血流成像数据获得的速度向量场能够生成 3D 压力图[58]。然而,这种方法的主要局限性是基于非湍流假设,这使得该技术的价值在血管狭窄区域大为下降,因为狭窄处通常伴有湍流。尽管如此,心脏内的湍流通常很小,在此情形下 4D 血流成像是一项很有前景的压力成像技术[37]。

7. 偏心血流 正如前面提到的,血流速度的假设为在一个长直血管内呈抛物面分布的非脉动血流,血管中心具有最高流速。虽然升主动脉的血流是脉冲式的,但它通常呈现出一个近似抛物面的速度剖面,在血管的中心速度最高。有趣的是,瓣膜和血管疾病可能在许多情况下改变这个速度分布,导致外周高速的偏心流动。正常速度分布剖面的这种变化可以通过升主动脉的 4D 血流成像 MRI 进行量化,方法有两种:测量相对于血管中心线的收缩期血流位移[59]和测量左心室流出和主动脉根之间偏心血流的角度[60]。有假说认为血流偏心可能导致二叶式主动脉瓣畸形(bicuspid aortic valve,BAV),患者的主动脉扩张,尽管偏心血流也可能是这类人群主动脉扩张的结果。

8. 涡量和旋度 涡量被定义为绕血管中心线正交轴向旋转或涡旋的运动[43]。与之相对应的,旋度的定义是绕血管中心线轴向的旋转运动,即生理血流方向上形成了一种螺旋状的流动模式[43]。虽然之前的大部分研究都对涡量和旋度进行了半定量的分析,但由 4D 血流成像数据[32,61-63]可进一步量化这两个指标。螺旋式血流在主动脉和肺动脉中是一种正常的生理现象,被认为可以防止动脉粥样硬化的发生[64]。

二、4D 血流成像的潜在临床应用

(一)心力衰竭

心力衰竭是一种复杂的临床综合征,可由心室充盈或搏出血液的任何结构或功能障碍引起[65]。心力衰竭患者,特别是舒张功能障碍的患者,经常出现心脏内血流异常。其中一些异常可以用 4D 血流成像来量化。例如流经左心室或右心室的血液可以通过微粒轨迹将其分成 4 种不同的功能成分:①直接血流,指在一次心跳中进、出的血液;②保留的流入,即进入但不流出的血液;③延迟喷射血流,即开始在里面而在随后的心跳流出;④残余体积,至少在心室中停留 2 次心脏循环[50]。用 4D 血流成像区分这 4 种血流成分表明,在心力衰竭患者中,直接血流的百分比以及舒张末期直接血流的动能均降低,导致左心室排出相同血流的工作负荷增加[50]。

这些低效率心内血流的独特标志物可以帮助识别疾病早期的患者,监测治疗效果,并且在舒张-收缩有障碍的情况下影响治疗的起搏策略或目标心率[37]。

(二)瓣膜疾病

4D 血流成像可以在单次 MR 采集下,准确地评估采集范围内的所有心脏瓣膜异常情况[66]。此外,心脏瓣膜在心脏循环过程中运动明显,使用容积 4D-血流数据进行回顾性的 3D 瓣膜跟踪运动修正可以减轻这种影响,可以比 2D PC-MRI 提供更好的评估结果[67,68]。与标准 2D PC-MRI

相比，4D 血流成像的这些优点可能有助于临床实践中对瓣膜疾病的血流动力学评估。

（三）主动脉夹层

Stanford B 型主动脉夹层通常由内科治疗。目前临床对存在夹层并发症的患者放置覆膜支架，并发症包括终末器官缺血、动脉瘤形成或者主动脉破裂。尽管如此，一些患者在疾病的晚期出现假性动脉瘤扩张，这是一种严重的并发症[69]。影像在这些患者的随访中起着关键作用，因为主动脉的直径和假腔内血栓的数量可以用来进行主动脉破裂的风险分层，以及筛选需要血管内治疗的患者[70,71]。

有人认为血流动力学参数，如血流模型、流量和流速，可能在假腔扩张和动脉瘤形成中发挥作用[72,73]。4D 血流成像可以在体量化这些血流动力学参数，这些信息有助于在主动脉扩张发生之前，识别那些早期血管内治疗可能获益的患者[74]。

（四）肺动脉高压

肺动脉高压定义为静息状态下平均肺动脉压大于 25mmHg[75]。尽管诊断肺动脉高压的标准是右心导管造影，但我们可以从 4D 血流成像中无创性地获得预测因子。当 4D 血流成像检测到主肺动脉的血流涡流时，可以确定有明显的肺动脉高压，并且具有很好的敏感性和特异性[76]（图 9-7）。此外，4D 血流可以提供肺动脉的平均流速和最小肺动脉面积，这些参数在 PC-MRI 中显示了最佳诊断性能[77]。这些流动特征的可视化和量化对于指导医疗治疗和评估治疗反应可能是有用的，而其他成像方式是不可行的。

（五）慢性肝病：肝和门静脉血流

肝硬化是一种常见且严重的疾病，可导致肝脏血流异常。多普勒超声是目前评价肝硬化、门静脉高压症或肝移植患者门静脉血流动力学变化的无创性标准手段。然而，多普勒超声有缺点，如较差的声窗、操作者依赖性和观察者间的重复性差。肝脏和门静脉血流的 4D 血流 MRI 分析是可行的，并且可以克服超声的这些限制[14,78]，但是仍然存在一些不足。主要因为肝和门静脉流的复杂性，3 个感兴趣的血管床（肝动脉门静脉流入和肝静脉引流）具有明显不同的速度分布，这使得 4D 血流成像具有挑战性[79]。双 VENC 编码可能是一种解决办法，可同时准确测量门静脉和肝动脉血流速度，避免混叠形成[22]并在所有这些血管中实现高的速度 - 噪声比。

（六）神经血管应用

4D 血流成像在神经领域最令人兴奋的发现或许是与中风相关。升主动脉和主动脉弓的斑块是栓塞性卒中的一个相关原因[80,81]。复杂主动脉斑块在降主动脉近端发生率最高，但仅在严重主动脉瓣关闭不全导致血流逆行和斑块破裂这两种情况同时发生时，这些斑块才被认为是栓塞性卒中的来源[82]。尽管如此，4D 血流成像显示复杂降主动脉斑块逆行栓塞在动脉粥样硬化患者中很常见，并且可以到达主动脉弓上方所有动脉，这表明降主动脉斑块应该被认为是新的卒中栓塞源，即使不合并主动脉瓣关闭不全[26,83,84]（图 9-8）。这一机制已被证明是隐源性卒中亚组患者中脑梗死的唯一可能来源。

4D 血流成像在颅内动脉瘤应用亦有相关研究[85,86]，发现了具有涡流形成的复杂血流模型。此外，4D 血流成像可识别变化的管壁剪切应力（wall shear stress, WSS）或量化的动脉瘤内压力梯度，这两个变量均可导致动脉瘤进展或破裂[10,41]。尽管 4D 血流成像可以提供一些证据来识别有动脉瘤生长或破裂风险的患者，但需要大量的队列研究以及长期随访来证实这一假设。

（七）其他应用

有研究使用 4D 血流成像来分析其他血管，如颈动脉[87,88]、肾动脉[11,89]和下肢动脉[90]。在

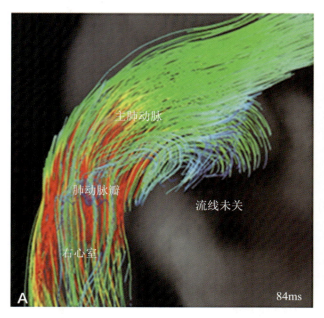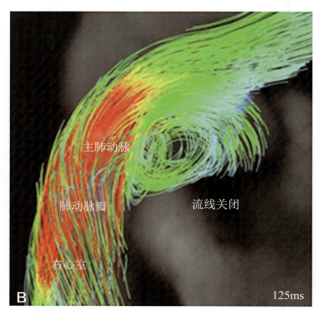
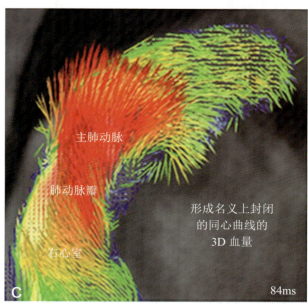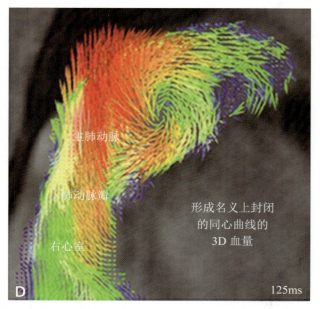

▲ 图 9-7　右心室流出道在心跳不同周期（A～D）的典型流动模式（经许可引自 Reiter, U.et al., PLoS ONE, 8, e82212, 2013.doi:10.1371/journal.pone.008221.）

颈动脉中，4D 血流成像可作为评估血流介导的动脉粥样硬化和斑块进展的个体风险的有价值的技术。在肾动脉中，通过非增强 MR 血管成像，4D 血流成像可提供形态学评价以及功能信息如跨狭窄的压力梯度。

三、先天性心脏病 4D 血流成像

在当前的临床实践中，心血管磁共振由于是一种无创、无电离辐射、不受声窗限制的技术，越来越多地被应用于先天性心脏病患者。结合病理解剖的精确描述以及使用 4D 血流成像的精确性和可重复的血流定量的能力，心血管 MR 成为这些患者的全面的成像技术。

（一）4D 血流成像在先天性心脏病中的优势

1. 时间效率　2D PC-MRI 的量化需要获取

Chapter 9　4D 血流成像
Four-Dimensional Flow Imaging

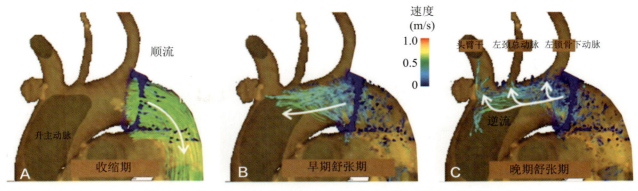

▲ 图 9-8　应用 4D 血流成像技术在体测量和显示近端降主动脉三维血流

主动脉粥样硬化患者主动脉硬度增加导致舒张期逆向血流，如来自近端降主动脉（DAo）发射平面的时间分辨 3D 路径线所示。舒张期逆行血流清晰地到达所有 3 条脑供血动脉，并可能为 DAo 中具有高危斑块的卒中患者提供先前被忽视的逆行栓塞机制（经许可引自 Markl, M. et al., J. Magn. Reson. Imaging, 36, 1015, 2012, doi: 10.1002/jmri.23632.）

感兴趣的每个心血管结构的垂直平面。由于心血管结构的异常排列和复杂的空间取向，2D PC-MRI 在先天性心脏病患者中尤其具有挑战性[91]。不同血流的量化需要为每个感兴趣的结构进行规划和进行 2D PC-MRI 采集。当前用于图像规划的方法，例如实时或交互式定位[91,92]，存在空间分辨率低的问题，并且可能无法识别小的或狭窄的结构。因此，如果需要对多个血管进行检查，例如多级分流的情况，可能导致扫描时间延长。为了缩短扫描时间，2D PC-MRI 可以通过屏气完成，单次屏气时间 10～15s。然而，自由呼吸 2D PC-MRI 是更符合生理性，通常需要 2～3min。此外，患病者和年幼者可能很难屏住呼吸。因此，2D PC-MRI 采集很难规划，并且可能为了获得最佳垂直平面而需要多次采集，这可能导致扫描时间延长。儿童 MR 扫描的成本会变得更高，因为通常是在全身麻醉下进行的。

4D 血流成像采集与单次 2D PC-MRI 采集相比，需要更长的扫描时间。然而，它具有一定的时间效率优势。例如，全心和大血管的 4D 血流成像[27]是一个易于规划的序列。其 FOV 的几何结构是一个简单的容积盒，覆盖心脏和大血管即可。因此，对复杂的心血管解剖，操作者不需要专业知识就可以完成。对数据进行离线分析，可以从单次 MR 扫描所得图像中评估所有感兴趣的血管（图 9-9）。此外，失真和未对齐的结构的血流评估可由其他高分辨率心血管 MR 图像引导，例如三维稳态自由进动或黑血序列。在房间隔缺损和部分肺静脉异常回流组成的多节段分流的病例中，已经显示了这一时间效率的优势。这种情况下，自由呼吸状态下需要 6 个 2D PC-MRI 序列，与单个 4D 流采集相比，需要更长的扫描时间[93]。

2. 回顾性分析　正如我们已经提到的，在心血管 MR 图像的后处理期间可能会有新的发现，这在先天性心脏病情况下尤其常见。由于 2D PC-MRI 扫描的局限性，如果在采集时没有定位，这些临床相关的血流评估将不能进行，或者患者需要重新预约再次进行扫描。如在半 Fontan 循环情况下，体循环到肺循环的侧支血管可能在 MR 扫描过程中不被注意，因而常规 2D PC-MRI 无法显示和评估。与 2D PC-MRI 不同的是，4D 血流成像中包含相关血管的所有血流信息。有文献报道，如有新的发现可随时对血管进行回顾性分析[94]。

3. 不同血流源的个体定量　分流是心室和血管之间的异常交通，因此，分流的血液来自正常的循环系统回路。肺循环与体循环的血流量分别以 Qp 和 Qs 表示，两者的比值即 Qp:Qs 反映分流的方向（从左到右或从右到左）和严重性。这些信息对随访和治疗措施选择有很大帮助。2D PC-MRI 可以通过分别对主肺动脉和主动脉成像来解决这个问题[95]。另一方面，在多节段分流的情况下，例如，异常肺静脉回流和房间隔缺损，

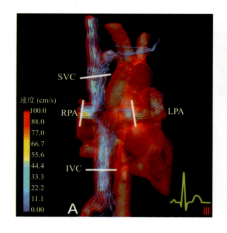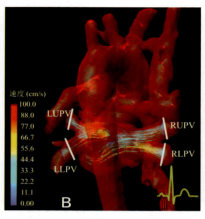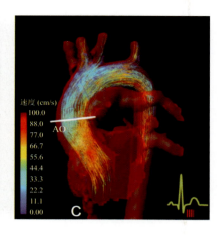

▲ 图 9-9

A～C. 展示了在单心室先心病患者中获得的单次 4D 血流成像影像，可以提供多种血流测量结果，而无需进行多次 2D PC-MRI 图像采集。AO. 主动脉；IVC. 下腔静脉；LLPV. 左下肺静脉；LPA. 左肺动脉；LUPV. 左上肺静脉；RLPV. 右下肺静脉；RPA. 右肺动脉；RUPV. 右上肺静脉（经许可引自 Valverde, I. et al., J. Cardiovasc. Magn. Reson., 14, 25, 2012, doi: 10.1186/1532-429X-14-25.）

各分流源的定量对于分流手术的选择很重要，有助于评估手术修复的风险。如果通过常规 2D PC-MRI 来进行评估，由于本身技术的局限性，需要通过多次 2D PC-MRI 扫描来完成。

研究证实，4D 血流成像是对总分流流量有贡献的各血流源进行定量的精确工具，例如弯刀综合征和房间隔缺损的情况[96]。所描述的不同血流源的定量也是流量测量精度的一个很好的内部验证。例如，肺血流量可以表示为肺动脉血流或肺静脉回流[93]。

（二）先天性心脏病的应用

1. 主动脉 4D 血流成像有助于了解主动脉的血流动力学，以及血流异常与疾病进展的关系。

（1）主动脉瓣：人群中先天性二叶式主动脉瓣畸形（bicuspid aortic valve，BAV）发生率约 1.3%，而主动脉缩窄患者中这一畸形发生率约 85%[97]。大约 1/3 的患者会出现主动脉反流[98]。传统 MRI 利用梯度回波电影序列可以显示主动脉狭窄收缩期低信号流束和舒张期反流束，并且可以利用 2D PC-MRI 进行净流量和反流分数的定量。这些患者血流变化与主动脉瘤的相关性尚不清楚。既往对动静脉透析瘘近端桡动脉的研究表明，超生理血流动力学导致血管尺寸增加[99]，研究结论支持 BAV 患者近端主动脉血流动力学负荷增加可能导致主动脉扩张的理论[100]。Hope 等[101] 报道了 BAV 患者升主动脉在收缩期中段血流的两个离散嵌套螺旋（图 9-10），表明血流动力学负荷增加，这可能导致动脉瘤形成[102]。4D 血流成像评价显示收缩期血流螺旋样改变，伴有收缩期偏心喷射流，导致升主动脉特定区域的局灶性 WSS。这些位置与随时间发展而发生动脉瘤的位置一致。因此，4D 血流成像可能有助于确定这些患者有发生主动脉瘤甚至进展破裂的风险。

（2）主动脉缩窄：主动脉缩窄是一种先天性狭窄，几乎总是发生在动脉导管与降主动脉交界处。可以利用 PC-MRI 评估跨狭窄的压力梯度。前文提到的 2D PC-MRI 中平面对准和平面放置的缺陷，可以通过对 4D 血流成像中狭窄后射流的分析来解决。除了可以对侧支血流进行定量分析之外，4D 血流成像能够对缩窄下游甚至缩窄上游的血流模式的改变进行分析[103]。主动脉缩窄修补术后动脉瘤的发生，与手术操作方式[104]、初次修补时的患者年龄[105] 以及血流动力学的改变均相关[106]。根据文献，WSS 的改变可以影响内皮功能，出现心血管重塑的危险区域，这可能导致主动脉瘤和动脉粥样硬化的发生[56]。Frydrychowicz 等[107] 研究揭示了主动脉缩窄术后

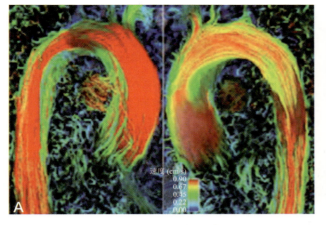
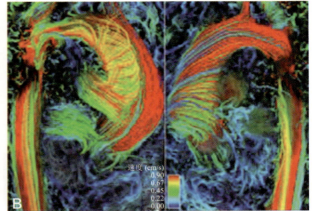
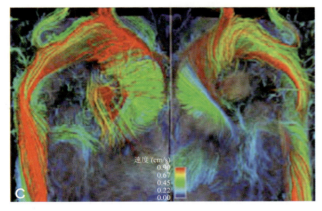

▲ 图 9-10 不同心跳周期阶段时 BAV 患者升主动脉的典型流动模式

（引自 Hope,M.D.et al.,J.Cardiovasc.Magn.Reson.,11,P184,2009,doi:10.1186/1532-429X-11-S1-P184.）

动脉瘤发生相关血流动力学的多样性。他们认为血流模式可以预测疾病的严重程度，并可能与动脉瘤的形状有关（图 9-11）。

2. Fallot 四联症 Fallot 四联症是最常见的发绀型先天性心脏病。手术修补后整体预后良好；然而，在多数患者中，修补可引起慢性肺血反流，这与右心室扩张和功能障碍、低运动耐受性、严重心律失常倾向以及心源性猝死有关[108]。

如前所述，单次扫描的 4D 血流成像对个体血流定量不仅可用于评估肺血反流的程度，而且可用于评估残余肺动脉狭窄情况下两根肺动脉之间的流量比。这个有价值的信息可以作为评估血管内介入治疗的额外的解剖参数。收缩期峰值速度升高和主动脉的异常涡流已被证实，并可能为这类人群提供一个新的危险分层参数[109]。

3. 肺静脉狭窄 肺静脉狭窄可以是先天性的，如完全异常肺静脉回流（total anomalous pulmonary venous return,TAPVR）[110]，或者获得性的，如心血管外科手术后[111]，或房颤射频消融术后[112]。目前，心导管造影术被认为是评估肺静脉解剖结构的金标准，但有创且具有 X 线依赖性。传统的心血管 MRI 受到空间分辨率的限制，因此小的肺静脉结构会被忽视。另外，目前的 2D PC-MRI 技术难以显示狭窄的结构中的湍流。经食管超声心动图[112]可以提供这些血流信息，但是对于儿童，需在全身麻醉后进行操作。Valverde 等[113]认为心血管 MR 是评估这种状况的完备手段，因为它可以提供术后肺静脉狭窄全面的解剖学和 4D 血流信息。4D 血流成像与经食管超声心动图相一致，能够对常规经食管超声心动图无法评估的远端肺静脉进行评估。更重要的是，4D 血流成像还可以对肺静脉血流定量（图 9-12）。

4. 心血管分流 先天性心脏病患者分流量的定量及肺（Qp）、体循环（Qs）流量比 Qp:QS 是临床决策和随访的重要参数。如前所述，2D PC-MRI 可以提供净流量比，但有时难以识别不同来源的分流量。4D 血流成像可描述和定量心房、心室、动脉导管未闭、主肺动脉窗和部分肺静脉反流的分流。

（1）房间隔缺损和肺静脉回流异常：房间隔缺损是成年人最常见的分流病变，占所有先天性心脏病的30%。房间隔缺损可能与部分肺静脉回流异常有关，导致较大的左向右分流。这可能增加发展为肺动脉高压的风险，因此外科手术的计划不仅应包括精确的解剖学描绘，而且应评估分流的不同来源。Valverde 等研究表明，4D 血流成像能够准确评估先天性心脏病多节段三尖瓣前左向右分流[93]，单次成像可以对分流的不同来源进行精确的个体量化（图 9-13）。在流量测量精度和时间效率的内

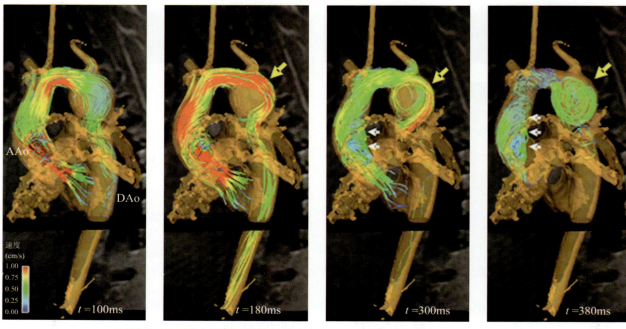

▲ 图 9-11　降主动脉近端主动脉瘤患者，不同心跳周期时胸主动脉血流模型
（经许可引自 Frydrychowicz, A. et al., J.Cardiovasc.Magn.Reson., 10, 30, 2008, doi:10.1186/1532-429X-10-30.）

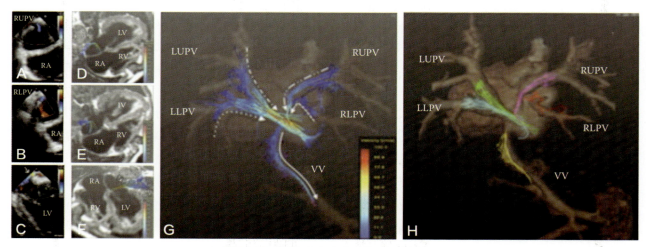

▲ 图 9-12　肺静脉血流定量的 4D 血流成像

患者诊断为右下肺静脉（RLPV）狭窄，左肺静脉汇合处出现高速多普勒（2.4m/s）。然而，经食管超声心动图（A～F）不能进一步描绘更远处的肺静脉（PV），但是在 4D 血流成像中可以显示（G、H）。LA. 左心房；LLPV. 左下肺静脉；LUPV. 左上肺静脉；LV. 左心室；RA. 右心房；RV. 右心室；VV. 垂直静脉（经许可引自 Valverde, I. et al., J. Am. Coll. Cardiol., 58, e3, 2011.）

部验证方面，也显示出优于目前 2D PC-MRI 的优势。

（2）动脉导管未闭：未闭的动脉导管是左第六主动脉弓的末端。使用超声心动图和常规 MRI 可以很容易地诊断。然而，人们对其血流动力学知之甚少。最近，Frydrychowicz 等用 Eisenmenger 的生理学方法全面地描述了大的动脉导管未闭血流模式的时间和空间分布[114]。

（3）室间隔缺损：基于净速度测量和平面成像的方法，如多普勒超声，在描述心腔内血流的时变三维特征方面并不令人满意。Bolger 等用 4D 血流成像描述并定量了正常左心室内血流各组分的体积、分布和时间变化[115]。对 1 例室间隔缺损患者的 4D 血流成像研究表明，在收缩早期，左心室颗粒穿过室间隔缺损并充满主肺动脉，导致早期肺动脉溢流和收缩压峰值。在收缩后期，由于肺动脉压力的增加，来自左心室的血流直接进入主动脉[29]。

（4）主肺动脉窗：Wong 等通过回顾性分析，展示了 4D 血流成像在主动脉窗方面的应用[116]。由于异常的血流模式，使用传统的 2D PC-MRI 进行分析是困难的（见 Wong 等文献[116] 中图 1），而使用 4D 血流成像可以准确地量化任何感兴趣平面内的分流。

5. 侧支循环的量化

（1）主动脉 - 肺动脉侧支循环：在分期 Fontan 手术缓解单心室心脏生理状态后，由于动脉低氧血症，经常观察到体循环到肺循环的侧支循环的发生。这与 Fontan 手术后胸腔积液变多以及死亡率增加相关，但其对长期预后的影响尚待研究[117]。先前利用传统的 2D PC-MRI 对几个单独侧支的血流进行研究[117]。这种小血管网络连接到毛细血管前肺血管，导致肺血流增加。在这种情况下，肺灌注的血流量大于肺动脉的供血量。4D 血流成像可以通过测量肺静脉回流来评估肺灌注，并且还提供关于右肺和左肺之间流量分布的信息[118]。

（2）静脉 - 静脉侧支循环：在单心室畸形生理学缓解后的患者中，静脉 - 静脉侧支循环的存在也是常见的。它们通常与颈静脉相连并回流到左心房，增加三尖瓣前血流量，但对肺氧合没有贡献。在肺灌注分析的后处理分析中，这些血管可以被识别和排除[94]。

（3）主动脉缩窄中的侧支循环：在血流动力学改变明显的主动脉缩窄的情况下，从肋间动脉和其他侧支通道发展出侧支循环，绕过主动脉缩窄将上半身与降主动脉相连。评估这些侧支循环对于外科计划很重要，因为它是缩窄严重程度的间接标志。在侧支血流显著的情况下，可以通过单独主动脉阻断来进行外科修复，因为侧支可确保适当的血流到下肢。否则，需要其他手术技术。因此，明确降主动脉从近侧到远侧增加的血流量，是对身体下部的侧支血流的直接测量[119]。

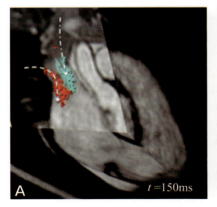 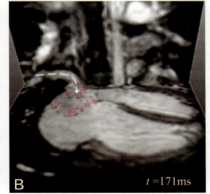 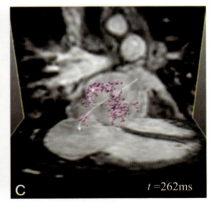

▲ 图 9-13 不同来源的微粒有助于评估不同血流源对分流的贡献

A. 从右上肺静脉释放的微粒（RUPV，红色）清楚地显示了左向右的分流，因为 RUPV 中的微粒与来自上腔静脉的微粒混合，进入右心房；B. 从右下肺静脉（深紫红色）释放出的微粒进入右心房；C. 左肺静脉释放的微粒（粉红色）击中房间隔，但其中一些通过房间隔缺损流至右心房（经许可引自 Valverde, I. et al., Pediatr. Cardiol., 31, 1244, 2010. doi: 10.1007/s00246-010-9782-x.）

与多次 2D PC-MRI 扫描相比，单次 4D 血流成像可以充分评估侧支血流[103]。

6. 单心室心脏生理学

（1）阶段二：Glenn 术 / 双向腔静脉 - 肺动脉吻合术。功能性单心室姑息术即 Glenn 术或腔静脉肺动脉吻合术是 Fontan 手术完成的前一阶段。由于没有有效的泵力来迫使血液进入肺，所以最佳的重建吻合应该避免任何狭窄，这些狭窄会导致能量损失，从而引起上腔静脉上游的压力升高，可能导致其中 1/3 的患者经肺压力梯度升高和静脉 - 静脉侧支的形成。这样的静脉 - 静脉侧支通道可能导致严重的体循环稀释。不幸的是，由于其直径纤细和解剖的变异性，识别分流和更重要的分流的量化是具有挑战性的。在选择一个半心室修补术时，4D 血流成像分析的血流模型使我们能够评估右心室和 Glenn 分流之间的竞争。Uribe 等发现，当出现严重的肺血反流时，存在不对称的血流分布和低效率（图 9-14），因为大部分来自上腔静脉的血流被吸入了右心室而不是流入肺动脉[49]。

（2）阶段三：Fontan 术 / 全腔静脉 - 肺动脉吻合术。Fontan 手术完成了单个功能性心室从平行循环到串联循环的转换。Fontan 手术预后的预测因素包括：解剖学（肺动脉大小和重建的主动脉弓）、心室大小和功能、侧支的存在以及重要的血流动力学和效率。一项 4D 血流成像研究显示，

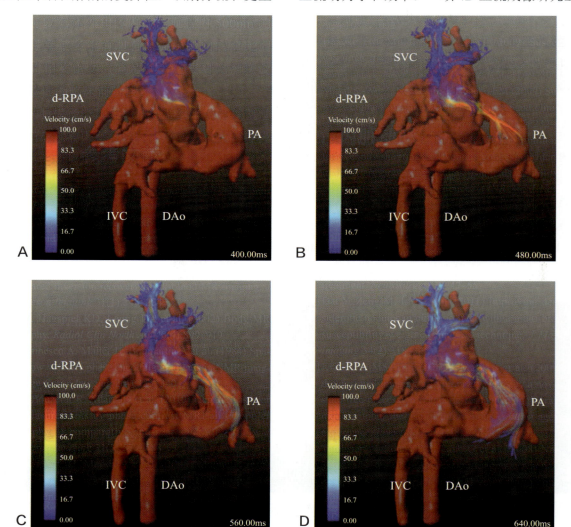

▲ 图 9-14　1 例半心室修补术患者 4D 血流成像

图像显示来自上腔静脉的血流进入右肺动脉和主肺动脉而不是右肺。A～D. 显示了心脏循环期间不同时间点的血流动力学（经许可引自 Uribe, S. et al., Pediatr. Cardiol., 2012, doi: 10.1007/s00246-012-0288-6.）

回顾性分析可以量化那些意料外的胸部血管，如半奇静脉可能会导致窃血低氧综合征（图9-15）。

4D血流成像还可以提供关于Fontan手术患者腔静脉对双侧肺动脉贡献血流的新发现。最近Bächler等验证了流量贡献的评估可以通过使用微粒轨迹来进行[48,120]（图9-16和图9-17）。从上腔静脉和下腔静脉到右肺动脉和左肺动脉的血流分布不均匀可能导致肺动脉静脉畸形的发生，因此4D血流成像可能给这个患者群体带来新的发现。其潜在的临床应用是显而易见的：识别有发生肺动静脉畸形风险的患者，以及帮助腔静脉肺动脉通路修改后Fontan循环患者的随访，以恢复更平衡的血流分布。

（三）4D血流成像和心血管模型

计算流体动力学（computational fluid dynamics，CFD）是一种通过求解运动方程来确定流体流动特性的技术。在心血管疾病领域，它已被应用于了解血流动力学和流动障碍对动脉粥样硬化、动脉瘤破裂和几种先天性心脏病的影响[121]。求解流体流动方程需要预先确定一定的初始条件。用4D血流成像实现数值模拟的一大优点是可以利用患者特定的血流动力学信息，从而计算受试者特定的相对压力和导出其他的参数。无创MR评价心血管的几何形态和血流速度对于利用有限元计算求解方程有重要价值。4D血流成像和CFD的结合可以用于改进这两种方法，这有助于增强对

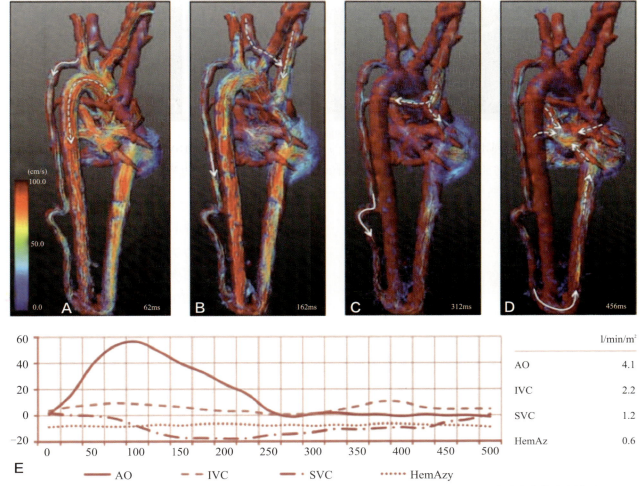

▲ 图9-15 4D血流成像能够识别和定量患者在半Fontan手术后的头－足方向顺流的半奇静脉血流量

A～D. 显示心脏循环中的血流动力学；E. 显示了主动脉（AO）、下腔静脉（IVC）、上腔静脉（SVC）和半奇静脉中的流量曲线和定量（经许可引自 Valverde, I. et al., Cardiol. Young, 1, 4, 2012.）

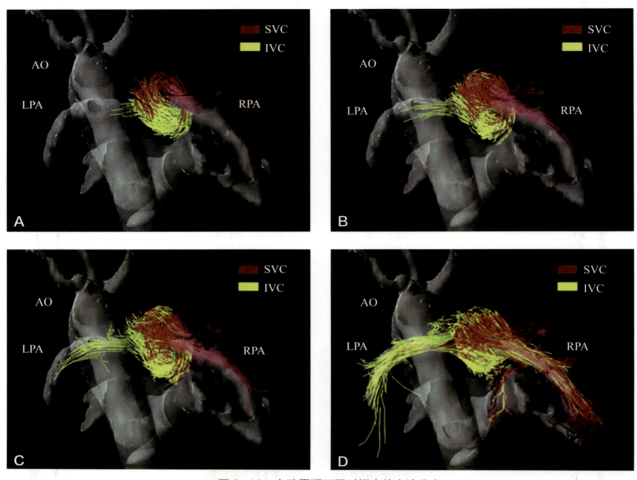

▲ 图 9-16 心动周期不同时间点的血流分布

从上腔静脉和下腔静脉（分别是 SVC 和 IVC，红色和黄色）发射微粒轨迹可以量化从每条静脉流入肺动脉的血流。A～D. 显示在心动周期不同时间点的血流分布，AO. 主动脉；IVC. 下腔静脉；LPA. 左肺动脉；RPA. 右肺动脉；SVC. 上腔静脉（经许可引自 Bachler, P. et al., J. Thorac. Cardiovasc., 2012.）

在体血流的评估和理解[122]。

四、4D 血流成像的展望

4D 血流成像提供了惊人的数据，从中获取对心血管系统新的理解。数据采集的进步使得扫描时间大大缩短，并且有助于获得没有呼吸运动伪影的 4D 血流数据。数据的可视化和评估仍然是难题；然而至少对于研究而言，从这些数据中能够提取的信息量考虑是值得做的。尽管有新的软件，我们仍然需要更多的自动处理方法，虽然这在复杂的心血管结构情况（如先天性心脏病）下可能难以实现。

4D 血流成像使我们能够理解基本的正常的血流模式，这是理解不同的心血管病理和疾病如何改变正常血流动力学的首要步骤。我们对于理解各种主动脉和肺部疾病以及健康志愿者的血流模式已经做出了很大的努力[32,76,109,123]。

4D 血流成像不仅提供了血流模式，而且提供了心血管定量参数，为临床应用提供了新的影像生物标志物。例如，最近的研究显示了狭窄后区域的 WSS 改变[124] 可能有助于血管重塑[40]。Morbiducci 等[31] 提出了螺旋血流定量分析模型，更好地理解了螺距和扭转对血流的作用。这些研究可能有助于检测血流模型中的异常，这对诊断[124-126]、预后[107] 和治疗[127-130] 是有帮助的。4D 血流成像的压力图已经在体模和一些患者中得到证实；然而，需要进一步的研究来证实其在

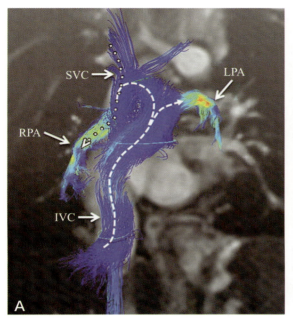 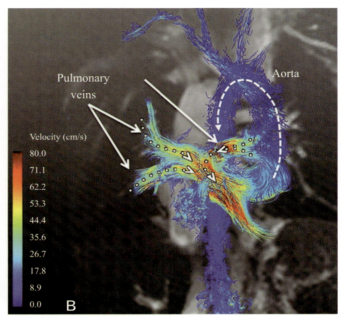

▲ 图 9-17　1 例心外全腔静脉肺动脉连接患者的微粒轨迹

Fontan 循环（A）、肺静脉回流和主动脉血流（B）。注意，在（A）中，从下腔静脉（IVC）向右肺动脉和左肺动脉（RPA 和 LPA）分流，并且优势血流是从上腔静脉（SVC）流向 RPA［经许可引自 Bächler, P. et al., Radiology（Internet）, 1, 14, 2013. doi: 10.1148/radiol.12120778.］

心血管疾病特别是在先天性心脏病患者中应用的价值[58]。

新的成像技术，如 4D 血流成像，是探索血流动力学、生物力学和心血管重构知识新领域的关键，这可能有助于早期发现一些心血管疾病患者的病理生理改变。

参考文献

[1] Moran PR. A flow velocity zeugmatographic interlace for NMR imaging in humans. *Magn. Reson. Imaging* 1982;1:197–203. doi: 10.1016/0730-725X(82)90170-9.

[2] Liang ZP. A model-based method for phase unwrapping. *IEEE Trans. Med. Imaging* 1996;15:893–897.

[3] Pelc NJ, Shimakawa A, Bernstein MA. Encoding strategies for three-direction phase-contrast MR imaging of flow. *J. Magn. Reson. Imaging* 1991;1:405–413.

[4] Markl M, Chan FP, Alley MT et al. Time-resolved three-dimensional phase-contrast MRI. *J. Magn. Reson. Imaging* 2003;17:499–506. doi: 10.1002/jmri.10272.

[5] Dumoulin CL, Souza SP, Walker MF, Wagle W. Three dimensional phase contrast angiography. *Magn. Reson. Med.* 1989;9:139–149. doi: 10.1002/mrm.1910090117.

[6] Bernstein M, Shimakawa A, Pelc N. Minimizing TE in moment-nulled or flow-encoded two- and three-dimensional gradient-echo imaging. *J. Magn. Reson. Imaging* 1992;Sep–Oct:583–588.

[7] Johnson KM, Markl M. Improved SNR in phase contrast velocimetry with five-point balanced flow encoding. *Magn. Reson. Med.* 2010;63:349–355. doi: 10.1002/ mrm.22202.

[8] Wigström L, Sjöqvist L, Wranne B. Temporally resolved 3D phase-contrast imaging. *Magn. Reson. Med.* 1996;36:800–803.

[9] Gu T, Korosec FR, Block WF, Fain SB, Turk Q, Lum D, Zhou Y, Grist TM, Haughton V, Mistretta CA. PC VIPR: A high-speed 3D phase-contrast method for flow quantification and high-resolution angiography. *AJNR Am. J. Neuroradiol.* 2005;26:743–749. doi: 26/4/743 [pii].

[10] Moftakhar R, Aagaard-Kienitz B, Johnson K, Turski PA, Turk AS, Niemann DB, Consigny D, Grinde J, Wieben O, Mistretta CA. Noninvasive measurement of intra-aneurysmal pressure and flow pattern using phase contrast with vastly undersampled isotropic projection imaging. *AJNR Am. J. Neuroradiol.* 2007;28:1710–1714. doi: 10.3174/ ajnr. A0648.

[11] François CJ, Lum DP, Johnson KM, Landgraf BR, Bley TA, Reeder SB, Schiebler ML, Grist TM, Wieben O. Renal arteries: Isotropic, high-spatial-resolution, unenhanced MR angiography with three-dimensional radial phase contrast. *Radiology* 2011;258:254–260. doi: 10.1148/ radiol.10100443.

[12] Turk AS, Johnson KM, Lum D, Niemann D, Aagaard-Kienitz B, Consigny D, Grinde J, Turski P, Haughton V, Mistretta C. Physiologic and anatomic assessment of a ca-

nine carotid artery stenosis model utilizing phase contrast with vastly undersampled isotropic projection imaging. *AJNR Am. J. Neuroradiol.* 2007;28:111–115.

[13] Jiang J, Strother C, Johnson K, Baker S, Consigny D, Wieben O, Zagzebski J. Comparison of blood velocity measurements between ultrasound Doppler and accelerated phase-contrast MR angiography in small arteries with disturbed flow. *Phys Med Biol.* 2011 Mar 21;56(6):1755–1773. doi: 10.1088/0031-9155/56/6/015.

[14] Frydrychowicz A, Landgraf BR, Niespodzany E, Verma RW, Roldán-Alzate A, Johnson KM, Wieben O, Reeder SB. Four-dimensional velocity mapping of the hepatic and splanchnic vasculature with radial sampling at 3 tesla: A feasibility study in portal hypertension. *J. Magn. Reson. Imaging* 2011;34:577–584. doi: 10.1002/jmri.22712.

[15] Pike GB, Meyer CH, Brosnan TJ, Pelc NJ. Magnetic resonance velocity imaging using a fast spiral phase contrast sequence. *Magn. Reson. Med.* 1994;32:476–483.

[16] Griswold MA, Jakob PM, Heidemann RM, Nittka M, Jellus V, Wang J, Kiefer B, Haase A. Generalized autocalibrating partially parallel acquisitions (GRAPPA). *Magn. Reson. Med.* 2002;47:1202–1210. doi: 10.1002/mrm.10171.

[17] Peng H-H, Bauer S, Huang T-Y, Chung H-W, Hennig J, Jung B, Markl M. Optimized parallel imaging for dynamic PC-MRI with multidirectional velocity encoding. *Magn. Reson. Med.* 2010;64:472–480. doi: 10.1002/mrm.22432.

[18] Giese D, Schaeffter T, Kozerke S. Highly undersampled phase-contrast flow measurements using compartment-based k-t principal component analysis. *Magn. Reson. Med.* 2013;69:434–443. doi: 10.1002/mrm.24273.

[19] Knobloch V, Boesiger P, Kozerke S. Sparsity transform k-t principal component analysis for accelerating cine three-dimensional flow measurements. *Magn. Reson. Med.* 2012;63:53–63. doi: 10.1002/mrm.24431.

[20] Kwak Y, Nam S, Akçakaya M, Basha TA, Goddu B, Manning WJ, Tarokh V, Nezafat R. Accelerated aortic flow assessment with compressed sensing with and without use of the sparsity of the complex difference image. *Magn. Reson. Med.* 2012;000:1–8. doi: 10.1002/mrm.24514.

[21] Jung B, Stalder AF, Bauer S, Markl M. On the undersampling strategies to accelerate time-resolved 3D imaging using k-t-GRAPPA. *Magn. Reson. Med.* 2011;66:966–975. doi: 10.1002/mrm.22875.

[22] Nett EJ, Johnson KM, Frydrychowicz A, Del Rio AM, Schrauben E, Francois CJ, Wieben O. Four-dimensional phase contrast MRI with accelerated dual velocity encoding. *J. Magn. Reson. Imaging* 2012;35:1462–1471. doi: 10.1002/jmri.23588.

[23] Carlsson M, Töger J, Kanski M, Bloch K, Ståhlberg F, Heiberg E, Arheden H. Quantification and visualization of cardiovascular 4D velocity mapping accelerated with parallel imaging or k-t BLAST: Head to head comparison and validation at 1.5 T and 3 T. *J. Cardiovasc. Magn. Reson.* 2011;13:55. doi: 10.1186/1532-429X-13-55.

[24] Hsiao A, Lustig M, Alley MT, Murphy M, Chan FP, Herfkens RJ, Vasanawala SS. Rapid pediatric cardiac assessment of flow and ventricular volume with compressed sensing parallel imaging volumetric cine phase-contrast MRI. *AJR Am. J. Roentgenol.* 2012;198:W250–W259. doi: 10.2214/AJR.11.6969.

[25] Markl M, Harloff A, Bley TA, Zaitsev M, Jung B, Weigang E, Langer M, Hennig J, Frydrychowicz A. Time-resolved 3D MR velocity mapping at 3T: Improved navigator-gated assessment of vascular anatomy and blood flow. *J. Magn. Reson. Imaging* 2007;25:824–831. doi: 10.1002/jmri.20871.

[26] Harloff A, Strecker C, Frydrychowicz AP, Dudler P, Hetzel A, Geibel A, Kollum M, Weiller C, Hennig J, Markl M. Plaques in the descending aorta: A new risk factor for stroke? Visualization of potential embolization pathways by 4D MRI. *J. Magn. Reson. Imaging* 2007;26:1651–1655. doi: 10.1055/s-2007-987599.

[27] Uribe S, Beerbaum P, Sørensen TS, Rasmusson A, Razavi R, Schaeffter T. Four-dimensional (4D) flow of the whole heart and great vessels using real-time respiratory self-gating. *Magn. Reson. Med.* 2009;62:984–992. doi: 10.1002/mrm.22090.

[28] Stadlbauer A, van der Riet W, Crelier G, Salomonowitz E. Accelerated time-resolved three-dimensional MR velocity mapping of blood flow patterns in the aorta using SENSE and k-t BLAST. *Eur. J. Radiol.* 2010;75:e15–e21. doi: 10.1016/j.ejrad.2009.06.009.

[29] Hope TA, Herfkens RJ. Imaging of the thoracic aorta with time-resolved three-dimensional phase-contrast MRI: A review. *Semin. Thorac. Cardiovasc. Surg.* 2008;20:358–364. doi: 10.1053/j.semtcvs.2008.11.013.

[30] Unterhinninghofen R, Ley S, Ley-Zaporozhan J, von Tengg-Kobligk H, Bock M, Kauczor H-U, Szabó G, Dillmann R. Concepts for visualization of multidirectional phase-contrast MRI of the heart and large thoracic vessels. *Acad. Radiol.* 2008;15:361–369. doi: 10.1016/j.acra.2007.11.012.

[31] Morbiducci U, Ponzini R, Rizzo G, Cadioli M, Esposito A, De Cobelli F, Del Maschio A, Montevecchi FM, Redaelli A. In vivo quantification of helical blood flow in human aorta by time-resolved three-dimensional cine phase contrast magnetic resonance imaging. *Ann. Biomed. Eng.* 2009;37:516–531. doi: 10.1007/s10439-008-9609-6.

[32] Bächler P, Pinochet N, Sotelo J, Crelier G, Irarrazaval P, Tejos C, Uribe S. Assessment of normal flow patterns in the pulmonary circulation by using 4D magnetic resonance velocity mapping. *Magn. Reson. Imaging* 2013 Feb;31(2):178–188. doi: 10.1016/j.mri.2012.06.036.

[33] Buonocore MH. Visualizing blood flow patterns using streamlines, arrows, and particle paths. *Magn. Reson. Med.* 1998;40:210–226. doi: 10.1002/mrm.1910400207.

[34] Wigström L, Ebbers T, Fyrenius A, Karlsson M, Engvall J, Wranne B, Bolger AF. Particle trace visualization of intracardiac flow using time-resolved 3D phase contrast MRI. *Magn. Reson. Med.* 1999;41:793–799. doi: 10.1002/(SICI)1522-

[35] Shaaban A, Duerinckx A. Wall shear stress and early atherosclerosis: A review. *AJR Am. J. Roentgenol.* 2000;174:1657–1665.

[36] Petersson S, Dyverfeldt P, Ebbers T. Assessment of the accuracy of MRI wall shear stress estimation using numerical simulations. *J. Magn. Reson. Imaging* 2012;36:128–38. doi: 10.1002/jmri.23610.

[37] Hope MD, Sedlic T, Dyverfeldt P. Cardiothoracic magnetic resonance flow imaging. *J. Thorac. Imaging* 2013;28:217–230. doi: 10.1097/RTI.0b013e31829192a1.

[38] Chalouhi N, Hoh B, Hasan D. Review of cerebral aneurysm formation, growth, and rupture. *Stroke* 44:3613–3622.

[39] Meng H, Wang Z, Hoi Y, Gao L, Metaxa E, Swartz DD, Kolega J. Complex hemodynamics at the apex of an arterial bifurcation induces vascular remodeling resembling cerebral aneurysm initiation. *Stroke* 2007;38:1924–1931. doi: 10.1161/STROKEAHA.106.481234.

[40] Cheng C, Tempel D, van Haperen R, van der Baan A, Grosveld F, Daemen MJAP, Krams R, de Crom R. Atherosclerotic lesion size and vulnerability are determined by patterns of fluid shear stress. *Circulation* 2006;113:2744–2753. doi: 10.1161/CIRCULATIONAHA.105.590018.

[41] Boussel L, Rayz V, McCulloch C, Martin A, Acevedo-Bolton G, Lawton M, Higashida R, Smith WS, Young WL, Saloner D. Aneurysm growth occurs at region of low wall shear stress: Patient-specific correlation of hemodynamics and growth in a longitudinal study. *Stroke* 2008;39:2997–3002. doi: 10.1161/STROKEAHA.108.521617.

[42] Laurent S, Cockcroft J, Van Bortel L, Boutouyrie P, Giannattasio C, Hayoz D, Pannier B, Vlachopoulos C, Wilkinson I, Struijker-Boudier H. Expert consensus document on arterial stiffness: Methodological issues and clinical applications. *Eur. Heart J.* 2006;27:2588–2605. doi: 10.1093/eurheartj/ehl254.

[43] Markl M, Kilner PJ, Ebbers T. Comprehensive 4D velocity mapping of the heart and great vessels by cardiovascular magnetic resonance. *J. Cardiovasc. Magn. Reson.* 2011;13:7. doi: 10.1186/1532-429X-13-7.

[44] Mohiaddin RH, Firmin DN, Longmore DB. Age-related changes of human aortic flow wave velocity measured non-invasively by magnetic resonance imaging. *J. Appl. Physiol.* 1993;74:492–497. doi: 10.1161/01.CIR.0000069826.36125.B4.

[45] Wentland AL, Wieben O, François CJ, Boncyk C, Munoz Del Rio A, Johnson KM, Grist TM, Frydrychowicz A. Aortic pulse wave velocity measurements with under-sampled 4D flow-sensitive MRI: Comparison with 2D and algorithm determination. *J. Magn. Reson. Imaging* 2013;37:853–859. doi: 10.1002/jmri.23877.

[46] Markl M, Wallis W, Brendecke S, Simon J, Frydrychowicz A, Harloff A. Estimation of global aortic pulse wave velocity by flow-sensitive 4D MRI. *Magn. Reson. Med.* 2010;63:1575–1582. doi: 10.1002/mrm.22353.

[47] Nollen GJ, Groenink M, Tijssen JGP, Van Der Wall EE, Mulder BJM. Aortic stiffness and diameter predict progressive aortic dilatation in patients with Marfan syndrome. *Eur. Heart J.* 2004;25:1146–1152. doi: 10.1016/j.ehj.2004.04.033.

[48] Bachler P, Valverde I, Uribe S. Quantification of caval flow contribution to the lungs in vivo after total cavopulmunary connection with 4-dimensional flow magnetic resonance imaging. *J. Thorac. Cardiovasc.* 2012 Mar;143(3):742–743. doi: 10.1016/j.jtcvs.2011.11.003.

[49] Uribe S, Bächler P, Valverde I, Crelier GR, Beerbaum P, Tejos C, Irarrazaval P. Hemodynamic assessment in patients with one-and-a-half ventricle repair revealed by four-dimensional flow magnetic resonance imaging. *Pediatr. Cardiol.* 2013 Feb;34(2):447–451. doi: 10.1007/s00246-012-0288-6.

[50] Eriksson J, Carlhäll CJ, Dyverfeldt P, Engvall J, Bolger AF, Ebbers T. Semi-automatic quantification of 4D left ventricular blood flow. *J. Cardiovasc. Magn. Reson.* 2010;12:9. doi: 10.1186/1532-429X-12-9.

[51] Bogren H, Buonocore M. Helical-shaped streamlines do not represent helical flow. *Radiology* 2010 Dec;257(3):895–896; author reply 896. doi: 10.1148/radiol.101298.

[52] Lee N, Taylor MD, Hor KN, Banerjee RK. Non-invasive evaluation of energy loss in the pulmonary arteries using 4D phase contrast MR measurement: A proof of concept. *Biomed. Eng. Online* 2013;12:93. doi: 10.1186/1475-925X-12-93.

[53] Dyverfeldt P, Gårdhagen R, Sigfridsson A, Karlsson M, Ebbers T. On MRI turbulence quantification. *Magn. Reson. Imaging* 2009;27:913–922. doi: 10.1016/j.mri.2009.05.004.

[54] Dyverfeldt P, Sigfridsson A, Kvitting J-PE, Ebbers T. Quantification of intravoxel velocity standard deviation and turbulence intensity by generalizing phase-contrast MRI. *Magn. Reson. Med.* 2006;56:850–858. doi: 10.1002/mrm.21022.

[55] Petersson S, Dyverfeldt P, Gårdhagen R, Karlsson M, Ebbers T. Simulation of phase contrast MRI of turbulent flow. *Magn. Reson. Med.* 2010;64:1039–1046. doi: 10.1002/mrm.22494.

[56] Malek AM, Alper SL, Izumo S. Hemodynamic shear stress and its role in atherosclerosis. *JAMA* 1999;282:2035–2042. doi: 10.1001/jama.282.21.2035.

[57] Stein PD, Sabbah HN. Measured turbulence and its effect on thrombus formation. *Circ. Res.* 1974;35:608–614. doi: 10.1161/01.RES.35.4.608.

[58] Tyszka JM, Laidlaw DH, Asa JW, Silverman JM. Three-dimensional, time-resolved (4D) relative pressure mapping using magnetic resonance imaging. *J. Magn. Reson. Imaging* 2000;12:321–329. doi: 10.1002/1522-2586(200008)12:2<321::AID-JMRI15> 3.0.CO;2-2 [pii].

[59] Sigovan M, Hope MD, Dyverfeldt P, Saloner D. Comparison of four-dimensional flow parameters for quantification of flow eccentricity in the ascending aorta. *J. Magn. Reson. Imaging* 2011;34:1226–30. doi: 10.1002/jmri.22800.

[60] Den Reijer PM, Sallee D, van der Velden P et al. Hemodynamic predictors of aortic dilatation in bicuspid aortic valve by velocity-encoded cardiovascular magnetic resonance. *J. Cardiovasc. Magn. Reson.* 2010;12:4. doi: 10.1186/1532-429X-12-4.

[61] Morbiducci U, Ponzini R, Rizzo G, Cadioli M, Esposito A, Montevecchi FM, Redaelli A. Mechanistic insight into the physiological relevance of helical blood flow in the human aorta: An in vivo study. *Biomech. Model. Mechanobiol.* 2011;10:339–355. doi: 10.1007/s10237-010-0238-2.

[62] Lorenz R, Bock J, Barker AJ, von Knobelsdorff- Brenkenhoff F, Wallis W, Korvink JG, Bissell MM, Schulz-Menger J, Markl M. 4D flow magnetic resonance imaging in bicuspid aortic valve disease demonstrates altered distribution of aortic blood flow helicity. *Magn. Reson. Med.* 2013;00:1–12. doi: 10.1002/ mrm.24802.

[63] Wong KKL, Tu J, Kelso RM, Worthley SG, Sanders P, Mazumdar J, Abbott D. Cardiac flow component analysis. *Med. Eng. Phys.* 2010;32:174–188. doi: 10.1016/j. medengphy.2009.11.007.

[64] Liu X, Pu F, Fan Y, Deng X, Li D, Li S. A numerical study on the flow of blood and the transport of LDL in the human aorta: The physiological significance of the helical flow in the aortic arch. *Am. J. Physiol. Heart Circ. Physiol.* 2009;297:H163–H170. doi: 10.1152/ajpheart.00266.2009.

[65] Yancy CW, Jessup M, Bozkurt B et al. 2013 ACCF/AHA guideline for the management of heart failure: A report of the American College of Cardiology Foundation/ American Heart Association Task Force on Practice Guidelines. *J. Am. Coll. Cardiol.* 2013;62:e147–e239. doi: 10.1016/j.jacc.2013.05.019.

[66] Roes SD, Hammer S, van der Geest RJ, Marsan NA, Bax JJ, Lamb HJ, Reiber JHC, de Roos A, Westenberg JJM. Flow assessment through four heart valves simultaneously using 3-dimensional 3-directional velocity-encoded magnetic resonance imaging with retrospective valve tracking in healthy volunteers and patients with valvular regurgitation. *Invest. Radiol.* 2009;44:669–675. doi: 10.1097/RLI.0b013e3181ae99b5.

[67] Van der Hulst AE, Westenberg JJM, Kroft LJM, Bax JJ, Blom NA, de Roos A, Roest AAW. Tetralogy of Fallot: 3D velocity-encoded MR imaging for evaluation of right ventricular valve flow and diastolic function in patients after correction. *Radiology* 2010;256:724–734. doi: 10.1148/ radiol.10092269.

[68] Westenberg JJM, Danilouchkine MG, Doornbos J, Bax JJ, van der Geest RJ, Labadie G, Lamb HJ, Versteegh MIM, de Roos A, Reiber JHC. Accurate and reproducible mitral valvular blood flow measurement with three-directional velocity-encoded magnetic resonance imaging. *J. Cardiovasc. Magn. Reson.* 2004;6:767–776. doi: 10.1081/JCMR-200036108.

[69] Song J-M, Kim S-D, Kim J-H, Kim M-J, Kang D-H, Seo JB, Lim T-H, Lee JW, Song M-G, Song J-K. Long-term predictors of descending aorta aneurysmal change in patients with aortic dissection. *J. Am. Coll. Cardiol.* 2007;50:799–804. doi: 10.1016/j.jacc.2007.03.064.

[70] Tsai TT, Evangelista A, Nienaber CA et al. Partial thrombosis of the false lumen in patients with acute type B aortic dissection. *N. Engl. J. Med.* 2007;357:349–359. doi: 10.1056/NEJMoa063232.

[71] Svensson LG, Kouchoukos NT, Miller DC et al. Expert consensus document on the treatment of descending thoracic aortic disease using endovascular stent-grafts. *Ann. Thorac. Surg.* 2008; 85:S1–S41. doi: 10.1016/j. athoracsur.2007.10.099.

[72] Tse KM, Chiu P, Lee HP, Ho P. Investigation of hemo- dynamics in the development of dissecting aneurysm within patient-specific dissecting aneurismal aortas using computational fluid dynamics (CFD) simulations. *J. Biomech.* 2011;44:827–836. doi: 10.1016/j. jbiomech.2010.12.014.

[73] Cheng Z, Tan FPP, Riga CV, Bicknell CD, Hamady MS, Gibbs RGJ, Wood NB, Xu XY. Analysis of flow patterns in a patient-specific aortic dissection model. *J. Biomech. Eng.* 2010;132:051007. doi: 10.1115/1.4000964.

[74] Clough RE, Waltham M, Giese D, Taylor PR, Schaeffter T. A new imaging method for assessment of aortic dissection using four-dimensional phase contrast magnetic resonance imaging. *J. Vasc. Surg.* 2012;55:914–923. doi: 10.1016/j. jvs.2011.11.005.

[75] McLaughlin V V, Archer SL, Badesch DB et al. ACCF/AHA 2009 expert consensus document on pulmonary hypertension: A report of the American College of Cardiology Foundation Task Force on Expert Consensus Documents and the American Heart Association: Developed in collaboration with the American College. *Circulation* 2009;119:2250–2294.

[76] Reiter G, Reiter U, Kovacs G, Kainz B, Schmidt K, Maier R, Olschewski H, Rienmueller R. Magnetic resonance- derived 3-dimensional blood flow patterns in the main pulmonary artery as a marker of pulmonary hypertension and a measure of elevated mean pulmonary arterial pressure. *Circ. Cardiovasc. Imaging* 2008;1(1):23–30. doi: 10.1161/CIRCIMAGING.108.780247.

[77] Sanz J, Kuschnir P, Rius T, Salguero R, Sulica R, Einstein AJ, Dellegrottaglie S, Fuster V, Rajagopalan S, Poon M. Pulmonary arterial hypertension: Noninvasive detection with phase-contrast MR imaging. *Radiology* 2007;243:70–79. doi: 10.1148/radiol.2431060477.

[78] Stankovic Z, Csatari Z, Deibert P, Euringer W, Blanke P, Kreisel W, Abdullah Zadeh Z, Kallfass F, Langer M, Markl M. Normal and altered three-dimensional portal venous hemodynamics in patients with liver cirrhosis. *Radiology* 2012;262:862–873. doi: 10.1148/ radiol.11110127.

[79] Markl M, Frydrychowicz A, Kozerke S, Hope M, Wieben O. 4D flow MRI. *J. Magn. Reson. Imaging* 2012;36:1015–1036. doi: 10.1002/jmri.23632.

[80] Sen S, Hinderliter A, Sen PK, Simmons J, Beck J, Of-

fenbacher S, Ohman EM, Oppenheimer SM. Aortic arch atheroma progression and recurrent vascular events in patients with stroke or transient ischemic attack. *Circulation* 2007;116:928–935. doi: 10.1161/ CIRCULATIONAHA.106.671727.

[81] Amarenco P, Cohen A, Tzourio C, Bertrand B, Hommel M, Besson G, Chauvel C, Touboul PJ, Bousser MG. Atherosclerotic disease of the aortic arch and the risk of ischemic stroke. *N. Engl. J. Med.* 1994;331:1474–1479. doi: 10.1056/NEJM199412013312202.

[82] Kronzon I. Aortic atherosclerotic disease and stroke. *Circulation* 2006;114:63–75. doi: 10.1161/ CIRCULATIONAHA.105.593418.

[83] Harloff A, Simon J, Brendecke S et al. Complex plaques in the proximal descending aorta: An underestimated embolic source of stroke. *Stroke* 2010;41:1145–1150. doi: 10.1161/STROKEAHA.109.577775.

[84] Harloff A, Strecker C, Dudler P et al. Retrograde embolism from the descending aorta: Visualization by multidirectional 3D velocity mapping in cryptogenic stroke. *Stroke* 2009;40(4):1505–1508. doi: 10.1161/ STROKEAHA.108.530030.

[85] Hope TA, Hope MD, Purcell DD, von Morze C, Vigneron DB, Alley MT, Dillon WP. Evaluation of intracranial stenoses and aneurysms with accelerated 4D flow. *Magn. Reson. Imaging* 2010;28:41–46. doi: 10.1016/j. mri.2009.05.042.

[86] Meckel S, Stalder AF, Santini F, Radü E-W, Rüfenacht DA, Markl M, Wetzel SG. In vivo visualization and analysis of 3-D hemodynamics in cerebral aneurysms with flow-sensitized 4-D MR imaging at 3 T. *Neuroradiol.* 2008;50(6):473–484. doi: 10.1007/s00234-008-0367-9.

[87] Markl M, Wegent F, Zech T, Bauer S, Strecker C, Schumacher M, Weiller C, Hennig J, Harloff A. In vivo wall shear stress distribution in the carotid artery: Effect of bifurcation geometry, internal carotid artery stenosis, and recanalization therapy. *Circ. Cardiovasc. Imaging* 2010;3:647–655. doi: 10.1161/ CIRCIMAGING.110.958504.

[88] Harloff A, Albrecht F, Spreer J et al. 3D blood flow characteristics in the carotid artery bifurcation assessed by flow-sensitive 4D MRI at 3T. *Magn. Reson. Med.* 2009;61:65–74. doi: 10.1002/mrm.21774.

[89] Bley TA, Johnson KM, Francois CJ, Reeder SB, Schiebler ML, R. Landgraf B, Consigny D, Grist TM, Wieben O. Noninvasive assessment of transstenotic pressure gradients in porcine renal artery stenoses by using vastly undersampled phase-contrast MR angiography. *Radiology* 2011;261:266–273. doi: 10.1148/ radiol.11101175.

[90] Frydrychowicz A, Winterer JT, Zaitsev M, Jung B, Hennig J, Langer M, Markl M. Visualization of iliac and proximal femoral artery hemodynamics using time-resolved 3D phase contrast MRI at 3T. *J. Magn. Reson. Imaging* 2007;25:1085–1092. doi: 10.1002/ jmri.20900.

[91] Boegaert J, Dymarkowski S, Taylor AM, Muthurangu V eds. Cardiovascular MRI planes and segmentations. In *Clinical Cardiac MRI*: With Interactive CD-ROM. Berlin: New York: Springer; 2005, p. 549.

[92] Lee VS, Resnick D, Bundy JM, Simonetti OP, Lee P, Weinreb JC. Cardiac function: MR evaluation in one breath hold with real-time true fast imaging with steady-state precession. *Radiology* 2002;222:835–842. doi: 10.1148/radiol.2223011156.

[93] Valverde I, Simpson J, Schaeffter T, Beerbaum P. 4D phase-contrast flow cardiovascular magnetic resonance: Comprehensive quantification and visualization of flow dynamics in atrial septal defect and partial anomalous pulmonary venous return. *Pediatr. Cardiol.* 2010;31:1244–1248. doi: 10.1007/s00246-010-9782-x.

[94] Valverde I, Rachel C, Kuehne T, Beerbaum P. Comprehensive four-dimensional phase-contrast flow assessment in hemi-Fontan circulation: Systemic-to-pulmonary collateral flow quantification. *Cardiol. Young* 2011;21:116–119. doi: 10.1017/S1047951110001575.

[95] Beerbaum P, Körperich H, Barth P, Esdorn H, Gieseke J, Meyer H. Noninvasive quantification of left-to-right shunt in pediatric patients: Phase-contrast cine magnetic resonance imaging compared with invasive oximetry. *Circulation* 2001;103:2476–2482. doi: 10.1161/01. CIR.103.20.2476.

[96] Frydrychowicz A, Landgraf B, Wieben O, François CJ. Images in Cardiovascular Medicine. Scimitar syndrome: Added value by isotropic flow-sensitive four dimensional magnetic resonance imaging with PC-VIPR (phase-contrast vastly undersampled isotropic projection reconstruction). *Circulation* 2010;121:e434–e436.

[97] Hoffman JIE, Kaplan S. The incidence of congenital heart disease. *J. Am. Coll. Cardiol.* 2002;39:1890–1900.

[98] Fenoglio JJ, McAllister HA, DeCastro CM, Davia JE, Cheitlin MD. Congenital bicuspid aortic valve after age 20. *Am. J. Cardiol.* 1977;39:164–169. doi: 10.1016/ S0002-9149(77)80186-0.

[99] Girerd X, London G, Boutouyrie P, Mourad JJ, Safar M, Laurent S. Remodeling of the radial artery in response to a chronic increase in shear stress. *Hypertension* 1996;27:799–803. doi: 10.1161/01.HYP.27.3.799.

[100] Davies RR, Kaple RK, Mandapati D, Gallo A, Botta DM, Elefteriades JA, Coady MA. Natural history of ascending aortic aneurysms in the setting of an unreplaced bicuspid aortic valve. *Ann. Thorac. Surg.* 2007;83:1338–1344. doi: 10.1016/j.athoracsur.2006.10.074.

[101] Hope MD, Meadows AK, Hope TA, Ordovas KG, Saloner D, Reddy GP, Alley MT, Higgins CB. 4D flow evaluation of abnormal flow patterns with bicuspid aortic valve. *J. Cardiovasc. Magn. Reson.* 2009;11:P184. doi: 10.1186/1532-429X-11-S1-P184.

[102] Hope MD, Meadows AK, Hope TA, Ordovas KG, Reddy GP, Alley MT, Higgins CB. Images in cardiovascular medicine. Evaluation of bicuspid aortic valve and aortic coarctation with 4D flow magnetic resonance imaging. *Circulation* 2008;117:2818–2819. doi: 10.1161/ CIRCU-

[103] Hope MD, Meadows AK, Hope TA, Ordovas KG, Saloner D, Reddy GP, Alley MT, Higgins CB. Clinical evaluation of aortic coarctation with 4D flow MR imaging. *J. Magn. Reson. Imaging* 2010;31:711–718. doi: 10.1002/jmri.22083.

[104] Martin RS 3rd, Edwards WH J, JM J, Edwards WH S, JL M. Ruptured abdominal aortic aneurysm: A 25-year experience and analysis of recent cases. *Am. Surg.* 1988;54:539–543.

[105] De Divitiis M, Pilla C, Kattenhorn M, Zadinello M, Donald A, Leeson P, Wallace S, Redington A, Deanfield JE. Vascular dysfunction after repair of coarctation of the aorta: Impact of early surgery. *Circulation* 2001 Sep;104(-12Suppl1):I165–I170. doi: 10.1161/hc37t1.094900.

[106] Von Kodolitsch Y, Aydin MA, Koschyk DH et al. Predictors of aneurysmal formation after surgical correction of aortic coarctation. *J. Am. Coll. Cardiol.* 2002;39:617–624. doi: 10.1016/S1062-1458(02)00754-7.

[107] Frydrychowicz A, Arnold R, Hirtler D, Schlensak C, Stalder AF, Hennig J, Langer M, Markl M. Multidirectional flow analysis by cardiovascular magnetic resonance in aneurysm development following repair of aortic coarctation. *J. Cardiovasc. Magn. Reson.* 2008;10:30. doi: 10.1186/1532-429X-10-30.

[108] Gatzoulis MA, Balaji S, Webber SA et al. Risk factors for arrhythmia and sudden cardiac death late after repair of tetralogy of Fallot: A multicentre study. 2000;356(9234):975–981. doi: 10.1016/S0140-6736(00)02714-8.

[109] Francois CJ, Srinivasan S, Schiebler ML, Reeder SB, Niespodzany E, Landgraf BR, Wieben O, Frydrychowicz A. 4D cardiovascular magnetic resonance velocity mapping of alterations of right heart flow patterns and main pulmonary artery hemodynamics in tetralogy of Fallot. *J. Cardiovasc. Magn. Reson.* 2012;14:16. doi: 10.1186/1532-429X-14-16.

[110] Holt DB, Moller JH, Larson S, Johnson MC. Primary pulmonary vein stenosis. *Am. J. Cardiol.* 2007;99:568–572. doi: 10.1016/j.amjcard.2006.09.100.

[111] Hancock Friesen CL, Zurakowski D, Thiagarajan RR, Forbess JM, del Nido PJ, Mayer JE, Jonas RA. Total anomalous pulmonary venous connection: An analysis of current management strategies in a single institution. *Ann. Thorac. Surg.* 2005;79:596–606; discussion 596–606. doi: 10.1016/j.athoracsur.2004.07.005.

[112] Sigurdsson G, Troughton RW, Xu XF, Salazar HP, Wazni OM, Grimm RA, White RD, Natale A, Klein AL. Detection of pulmonary vein stenosis by transesophageal echocardiography: Comparison with multicletector computed tomography. *Am. Heart J.* 2007;153:800–806.

[113] Valverde I, Miller O, Beerbaum P, Greil G. Imaging of pulmonary vein stenosis using multidimensional phase contrast magnetic resonance imaging (4 Dimensional flow). *J. Am. Coll. Cardiol.* 2011;58:e3.

[114] Frydrychowicz A, Bley TA, Dittrich S, Hennig J, Langer M, Markl M. Visualization of vascular hemodynamics in a case of a large patent ductus arteriosus using flow sensitive 3D CMR at 3T. *J. Cardiovasc. Magn. Reson.* 2007;9:585–587. doi: 772835820.

[115] Bolger AF, Heiberg E, Karlsson M, Wigström L, Engvall J, Sigfridsson A, Ebbers T, Kvitting J-PE, Carlhäll CJ, Wranne B. Transit of blood flow through the human left ventricle mapped by cardiovascular magnetic resonance. *J. Cardiovasc. Magn. Reson.* 2007;9:741–747. doi: 10.1080/10976640701544530.

[116] Wong J, Marthur S, Giese D, Pushparajah K, Schaeffter T, Razavi R. Analysis of aortopulmonary window using cardiac magnetic resonance imaging. *Circulation* 2012;126:e228–e229.

[117] Grosse-Wortmann L, Al-Otay A, Yoo S-J. Aortopulmonary collaterals after bidirectional cavopulmonary connection or Fontan completion: Quantification with MRI. *Circ. Cardiovasc. Imaging* 2009;2:219–225. doi: 10.1161/CIRCIMAGING.108.834192.

[118] Valverde I, Nordmeyer S, Uribe S, Greil G, Berger F, Kuehne T, Beerbaum P. Systemic-to-pulmonary collateral flow in patients with palliated univentricular heart physiology: Measurement using cardiovascular magnetic resonance 4D velocity acquisition. *J. Cardiovasc. Magn. Reson.* 2012;14:25. doi: 10.1186/1532-429X-14-25.

[119] Steffens JC, Bourne MW, Sakuma H, O'Sullivan M, Higgins CB. Quantification of collateral blood flow in coarctation of the aorta by velocity encoded cine magnetic resonance imaging. *Circulation* 1994;90:937–943. doi: 10.1161/01.CIR.90.2.937.

[120] Bächler P, Valverde I, Pinochet N, Nordmeyer S, Kuehne T, Crelier G, Tejos C, Irarrazaval P, Beerbaum P, Uribe S. Caval blood flow distribution in patients with Fontan circulation: Quantification by using particle traces from 4D flow MR imaging. *Radiology* 2013;267(1):67–75. doi: 10.1148/radiol.12120778.

[121] DeCampli WM, Argueta-Morales IR, Divo E, Kassab AJ. Computational fluid dynamics in congenital heart disease. *Cardiol. Young* 2012;22:800–808.

[122] Wittek A, Nielsen PMF, Miller K eds. Patient specific hemodynamics: Combined 4D flow-sensitive MRI and CFD. In *Computational Biomechanics for Medicine*. New York: Springer; 2011, pp. 27–38.

[123] Hope TA, Markl M, Wigström L, Alley MT, Miller DC, Herfkens RJ. Comparison of flow patterns in ascending aortic aneurysms and volunteers using four-dimensional magnetic resonance velocity mapping. *J. Magn. Reson. Imaging* 2007;26:1471–1479. doi: 10.1002/jmri.21082.

[124] Frydrychowicz A, Berger A, Russe MF et al. (2008). Time-resolved magnetic resonance angiography and flow-sensitive 4-dimensional magnetic resonance imaging at 3 Tesla for blood flow and wall shear stress analysis. *J. Thorac. Cardiovasc. Surg.* 2008;136:400–407. doi: 10.1016/j.jtcvs.2008.02.062.

[125] Frydrychowicz A, Harloff A, Jung B, Zaitsev M, Weigang E, Bley TA, Langer M, Hennig J, Markl M. Time-resolved, 3-dimensional magnetic resonance flow analysis at 3 T: Visualization of normal and pathological aortic vascular hemodynamics. *J. Comput. Assist. Tomogr.* 31:9–15.

[126] Frydrychowicz A, Weigang E, Langer M, Markl M. Flow-sensitive 3D magnetic resonance imaging reveals complex blood flow alterations in aortic Dacron graft repair. *Interact. Cardiovasc. Thorac. Surg.* 2006;5:340–2.

[127] Fogel MA, Weinberg PM, Hoydu AK, Hubbard AM, Rychik J, Jacobs ML, Fellows KE, Haselgrove J. Effect of surgical reconstruction on flow profiles in the aorta using magnetic resonance blood tagging. *Ann. Thorac. Surg.* 1997;63(6):1691–1700. doi: 10.1016/S0003-4975(97)00330-5.

[128] Frydrychowicz A, Arnold R, Harloff A, Schlensak C, Hennig J, Langer M, Markl M. Images in cardiovascular medicine. In vivo 3-dimensional flow connectivity mapping after extracardiac total cavopulmonary connection. *Circulation* 2008;118:e16–e17.

[129] Reiter U, Reiter G, Kovacs G et al. Evaluation of elevated mean pulmonary arterial pressure based on magnetic resonance 4D velocity mapping: Comparison of visualization techniques. *PLoS ONE* 2013;8(12):e82212. doi:10.1371/journal.pone.008221.

[130] Valverde I, Razishankar A, Miller O, Razavi R. Hemiazygos vein "steal hypoxic-sindrome" after hemi-Fontan operation: Comprehensive four-dimensional flow magnetic resonance imaging. *Cardiol. Young* 2012;22(4):481–484. doi: 10.1017/S1047951112000248.

Chapter 10
气管、支气管及肺部磁共振成像

Magnetic Resonance Imaging for Trachea, Bronchi, and Lung

Yoshiharu Ohno 著

徐晓莉 译

宋 伟 校

目录 CONTENTS

一、肺磁共振成像的影响因素 / 186

二、气管 MRI / 186

三、气道病变支气管及细支气管磁共振成像 / 187

四、肺部 MRI / 190

五、总结 / 201

当磁共振成像（MRI）初步投入使用时，许多研究者对此新技术产生兴趣，包括头部、胸部及其他部位MRI。因此，自20世纪80年代至90年代初，许多物理学家及放射学家曾尝试应用MRI评估不同肺疾病及纵隔、胸膜、心脏疾病。然而，由于MR成像系统、序列及其他应用条件在当时十分简陋、受限，在一定检查时间内无法获取满意的图像质量，因此尚且无法认为MRI可替代CT、肺血管造影及核医学等检查。直到2000年，MRI才开始应用于一些简单的临床适应证。

但21世纪以来，许多基础、临床研究者报道了MRI多种技术进展，包括序列、扫描仪及线圈的技术进步，平行采集成像的技术改进，对比剂应用及后处理技术的发展，尤其在肺部MRI方面，这是MRI成像更具挑战性的领域之一。因此，肺部最先进的MRI检查有可能在肺部/心肺疾病的患者管理中起替代或补充性作用。此外，随着1.5T及3T MR成像系统不断发展，肺部MRI检查不仅可提供形态学信息，还可提供功能性、生理性及生理病理性信息。因此，本章着重介绍MRI近年来在肺部几种重要疾病的应用进展，以期指导当前及未来临床实践中MRI的应用。希望读者进一步了解20世纪以来肺部MRI的进展，从而利用这些信息指导自身临床实践。

一、肺磁共振成像的影响因素

应用于临床的常规MRI是基于质子磁共振成像，主要依赖于水分子的氢核质子信号。常规质子MRI中，氢原子核旋转是在MR扫描仪较大的静态磁场内以1核/百万的速率优先排列。由于肺内物理密度低及质子密度低导致的肺实质信号微弱，肺部MR成像困难。此外，大量气-肺组织交界面造成肺磁化率极度不均[1-6]。尽管气体交换是必需的，但气体-软组织交界面产生较大磁场梯度，造成肺内MR信号失相位并迅速衰减。另外，肺内T_2^*值非常短，范围为$0.9 \sim 2.2ms$[5,6]。基于上述难题及解决的必要性，目前认为肺部MRI是MRI乃至放射学更具挑战性的领域之一。

作为这一新学术、临床研究领域的第一步，尽管肺组织T_2^*值较短，肺部MRI最近仍被证实是可行的。应用20世纪90年代之后发展的几项新技术，使肺部MR成像成为可能，例如超极化惰性气体MRI，对比剂的应用，超短回波时间（echo time，TE）、投影重建技术的快速自旋回波（spin-echo，SE）或梯度回波（gradient-echo，GRE）序列的应用，即在自由感应衰减的过程中获取数据，心电/呼吸触发快速MRI序列的应用以及抑制脂肪、血液信号的新技术等[5-12]。

二、气管MRI

肿瘤侵犯气管是甲状腺癌患者的主要死因，气管MRI主要用于检出甲状腺癌所引起的气管受侵[13]。据报道，甲状腺癌侵犯气管的发生率为$1\% \sim 13\%$[14,15]，对于无气管受侵的甲状腺癌患者而言，手术切除肿瘤是其主要的治疗方案[16]。因此，一旦发现肿瘤侵犯气管，甲状腺癌患者的手术计划则会完全改变[17,18]，术前影像学评估气管有无受侵、肿瘤侵犯气管的程度，将有利于临床制订手术方案及预测预后。

目前，气管腔内肿物是诊断肿瘤侵犯气管的唯一可靠影像学征象，病变侵犯气管浅表层仅在外科医师术中探查时才能被发现[17-19]。但是，过去10年中，一些研究者已尝试探究MRI在评估甲状腺癌患者气管、周围器官及喉返神经受累中的应用价值[20-22]。

其中一项研究[21]结果表明，正常气管表现为马蹄形或环形结构，气管中心与脊柱中线的距离小于4mm。MRI平扫图像上，正常气管信号、黏膜厚度及气管后壁膜厚度与尸检气管类似。气管外膜很薄，难以在MR图像上显示，但有时可观察到气管软骨与甲状腺间不完整的脂肪层。在T_2加权快速SE序列图像上，80%以上正常患者可见到低信号马蹄形的气管，低于 15% 的患者可见气管软骨局部高信号影。增强 T_1 加权 SE 图像中，气管黏膜及甲状腺表现为中度 - 明显强化，但气管软骨、软骨间膜及气管后壁膜无明显强化，由此可容易区分气管环与其他结构。

另一方面，此研究发现平扫 T_1 加权快速 SE 序列图像上可见 48% 的甲状腺癌呈高信号、43% 呈等信号及 9% 呈低信号，T_2 加权 SE 序列图像上分别约 85%、9%、6%。此外，增强扫描 T_1 加权快速 SE 序列示 80% 以上的甲状腺癌呈明显强化（84%），其他为中等强化（11%）或轻度强化（5%）。比较两组伴、不伴气管受累的甲状腺癌的影像学表现，发现气管轴位最大径及位移距离、气管软骨内软组织影、肿瘤侵犯气管后壁膜、气管腔内肿物在两组均有统计学差异。另外，两组患者气管变形及肿瘤周长范围有明显差异。气管软骨内软组织影、气管腔内肿物及气管肿瘤周长范围≥ 180° 认为是气管受侵的显著预测因素，诊断敏感性为 43% ～ 100%，特异性 84% ～ 100%，准确性 81% ～ 90%（图 10-1）。此外，另有研究表明，不论受累器官肿瘤大小，气管腔内肿瘤、气管壁受侵、气管结构受肿瘤推移以及气管旁脂肪层消失均可作为颈动脉及气管软骨受侵的形态学诊断标准，其诊断准确性高于肿瘤外周侵犯程度这一标准。另外，对于气管和食管受侵，诊断准确性是相反的。因此，气管 MRI 可以作为临床常规中甲状腺癌患者良好的预测因素。

三、气道病变支气管及细支气管磁共振成像

（一）囊性纤维化

囊性纤维化（cysticfibrosis，CF）是一种气道疾病，致病原因为 CFTR 基因突变，CF 是欧美国家人群中最常见的、致死性的遗传性疾病之一。由于治疗手段不断进展，CF 患者的生存期已明显提升，影像学检查评估对于 CF 患者的成功治疗至关重要。因此，目前认为 CT 是评估气道及肺实质形态学改变的金标准[23-26]，但在过去 10 年中，MRI 被推荐为评估 CF 的新技术。

尽管 MRI 空间分辨率低于 CT，但其优势在于可利用增强 T_1、T_2 加权快速 SE 图像有效区分不同组织结构及其对比增强的差异[27]。在定量评估 CF 患者方面，MR 评估支气管扩张的准确度取决于支气管水平、直径、管壁厚度、管壁信号及支气管腔内信号。一般情况下，MRI 可显示中央支气管及中央支气管扩张。但第 3 ～ 4 级正常的周围支气管显示较差，其支气管壁增厚的显示程度取决于支气管径大小及信号[27]。T_2 加权快速 SE 图像上支气管壁的高信号代表水肿，可能由急性炎性反应所致。此外，压脂 / 不压脂增强 T_1 加权 MR 图像上，支气管壁增厚伴强化与炎性反应相关。另外，T_2 加权快速 SE 序列可清晰显示支气管内黏液栓，可达小气道水平，由于黏液栓不强化，很容易与增厚的支气管壁区分[27]。气 - 液平表现为高信号，提示急性感染。但支气管内气 -

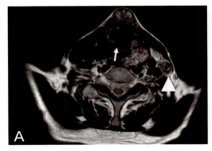 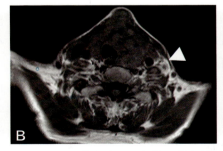 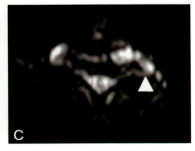

▲ 图 10-1　74 岁男性，甲状腺癌侵及气管、伴左侧颈淋巴结转移

可见甲状腺左叶及峡部肿块影。A.T_2 加权快速 SE 图像示病变呈不均匀等 / 高信号，气管软骨信号消失（箭）；B.T_1 加权快速 SE 图像呈均匀低信号，颈部淋巴结（箭头）呈高信号；C.DWI 呈不均匀低 / 高信号，颈部淋巴结（箭头）呈高信号。患者手术标本病理证实气管受侵及左颈部淋巴结转移的诊断

液平与部分性黏液栓、明显增厚的支气管壁很难鉴别。

MRI除了可显示支气管病变，还可显示肺实变，后者是CF患者的一个重要表现，多为肺泡内充满炎性物质所致，在T_2加权快速SE图像上呈高信号。与CT相似，MRI可显示支气管气相，表现为肺实变内沿细支气管走行的低信号影[27,28]。随着疾病进展，肺段或肺叶被完全破坏，可由T_1、T_2加权快速SE序列或传统/薄层CT评估。

与CT相比[29-33]，MRI在评价CF方面缺乏专门的评分系统及定量参数。因此，在临床中，MRI视觉评估对CF患者至关重要，应用改良Brody[32]或Bhalla/Helbich评分系统[29,31,34]，可使MRI、CT评分相一致。部分研究已经证实了这些评分系统在MRI及CT临床评估中的可行性[34]。

除了应用传统MRI外，CF患者还可应用功能性MRI，如增强灌注MRI、氧增强MRI、超极化惰性气体MRI，以鉴别肺实质内区域性功能改变。CF患者区域性通气缺损可引起局部肺灌注变化，为缺氧性血管收缩或组织破坏引起的反射性改变。增强灌注MRI是一种质子MRI技术，其评价的CF患者肺灌注缺损与肺组织的破坏程度呈良好的相关性。此外，增强灌注MRI定量化分析区域灌注的视觉差异，可用于监测治疗反应[27]。

另外一种质子MRI技术是氧增强MRI，基于100%氧分子的顺磁性特点，可用作评估肺通气的对比剂[35]。将这种技术应用于CF患者，100%氧吸入后，可观察到由局部通气灌注不均引起的不均匀的信号改变[36]。质子MRI可用于形态学及功能性评价，具备评估CF疾病严重程度及治疗反应的潜能，因此可用于辅助CT及核医学检查。

（二）哮喘

哮喘是肺部慢性炎性疾病，主要累及中、小气道。哮喘的发病机制为气道平滑肌增厚、炎性细胞浸润、结缔组织沉积（上皮下纤维化）、血管改变及黏液腺增生所引起的气道壁增厚。因此，有假说认为，由于哮喘的发病机制包括气道高反应、黏液分泌过多、平滑肌增生及上皮下纤维化，CT上气道壁及肺密度的定量评估可能有助于评价疾病严重程度及治疗疗效。哮喘的症状通常与上述病理生理改变所引起的不同程度气道阻塞有关，而超极化惰性气体MRI可以显示这些致病改变，在过去10年已得到广泛验证。

另一方面，尚未发现传统质子MRI在哮喘方面的应用价值。因此质子加权MRI未用于评估哮喘，直到2011年证实了氧增强MRI在评价哮喘方面的价值[37]。研究者将氧增强MRI直接与定量CT相比，发现两者在评价哮喘患者肺功能受损及临床分期方面作用等同[37]。随着进一步临床评估、改进及软件的开发，氧增强MRI有望成为一种替代性的MR检查用于评估哮喘。

（三）慢性阻塞性肺疾病

据美国胸科协会/欧洲呼吸协会共识及慢性阻塞性肺疾病指南的全球倡议，由炎症、瘢痕引起的小气道狭窄和黏液分泌引起的小气道腔的阻塞是气道内气流受限的主要病理改变，这种气流受限在慢性阻塞性肺疾病（chronic obstructive pulmonary disease，COPD）患者中是不完全可逆的。气流受限是由小气道内异常炎症反应及肺实质破坏所引起。在过去几十年中，许多研究认为小气道是引起COPD患者气流受限的最重要的原因。肺实质破坏（如肺气肿）是一个明确的致病因素，但其程度因人而异。薄层CT最常用于评估COPD严重程度，在临床及科研中，几种商用或专有软件及视觉评分系统现已用于COPD的CT评估[38-43]。与薄层CT相比，传统质子MRI在评估COPD形态学改变方面作用有限。有研究认为，传统质子MRI评估COPD时，由于肺组织受损、血容量减少、肺过度充气及低氧性血管收缩可引起T_1/T_2加权MRI上低信号，肺气肿的程度理论上等于MRI肺内异常低信号的区域[44]。但相对于CT，MRI在应用上更有难度，因此临

Chapter 10　气管、支气管及肺部磁共振成像
Magnetic Resonance Imaging for Trachea, Bronchi, and Lung

床上不会常规应用传统质子 MRI 评价或诊断肺气肿。

与传统质子 MRI 不同，几种肺功能 MRI 技术现用于评价 COPD，例如超极化惰性气体 MRI、动态增强灌注 MRI、氧增强 MRI、呼吸运动评估的动态 MRI 及超短回波时间质子 MRI。尽管应用超极化惰性气体 MRI 的研究已经产生的阳性结果，但由于政策限制，这项技术无法应用到世界范围，因此研究者们仍在努力探究质子 MRI 技术在评估 COPD 方面的应用价值。

在临床可行性方面，这些质子 MRI 技术、动态增强灌注 MRI 或时间分辨率（4D）MR 血管造影已在临床常规应用中证实有效，包括定量、定性评估由肺实质破坏引起局部肺灌注差异以及肺气肿的严重程度[45-48]。COPD 患者肺气肿通常表现为不均匀的肺实质信号减低（图 10-2）。此外，动态增强灌注 MRI 可定量评估 COPD，与健康志愿者相比，COPD 患者的平均肺血流量（mean pulmonary blood flow，PBF）、平均通过时间（mean transit time，MTT）、平均肺血容量（mean pulmonary blood volume，PBV）明显弥漫不均匀减低[45-48]。如果这一技术用于预测术后肺功能，动态增强灌注 MRI 则有替代定性定量评估的薄层 CT 和核医学检查的潜能，后者包括灌注扫描、灌注单光子发射计算机断层成像（perfusion single-photon emission tomography，SPECT）及灌注 SPECT/CT[49-51]。

尽管相对于动态增强灌注 MRI，氧增强 MRI 在临床上较难获得，但它是一种无须校正即可应用于临床的 MR 成像方法。氧增强 MRI 的潜在生理机制可能不同于超极化惰性气体 MRI，前者可提供基于通气、灌注及肺泡至毛细血管床的氧气转换的区域性信息[52-58]。2001 年以来，已经有几项研究评估了氧增强 MRI 在评价 COPD 及肺气肿方面的效能，并将其与薄层 CT 定量评估肺功能的检查进行了比较[52-57]。与健康志愿者相比，氧增强 MRI 示 COPD 患者的氧强化程度不均匀减低。这些研究证实，氧增强 MRI 中氧强化程度与第 1 秒用力呼气容积（forced expiratory volume in one second，FEV_1）、FEV_1/用力肺活量（FEV_1/forced vital capacity，FEV_1/FVC）、肺一氧化碳弥散功能（diffusing capacity of the lungs for carbon monoxide，DL_{CO}）及 / 或 DLCO 与肺泡容量比值（diffusing capacity divided by the alveolar volume，DLCO/VA）有明显良好的相关性。此外，氧增强 MRI 有较好的 COPD 临床分期的潜能，在这方面优于定量薄层 CT[52,53,56]。因此，在临床常规评估肺功能受损及临床分期方面，定量氧增强 MRI 至少与定量薄层 CT 等效[56]。此外，对动态氧增强 MRI 信号强度 - 时间进程曲线进行详细分析，可获得气流受限依赖性、氧气转换依赖性参数以及薄层 CT 可提供的气道、肺实质受损程度的定量评估[55,57]。另外，氧增强 MRI 有评价肺部分切除患者的潜能，评价效果等同于薄层 CT 和核医学检查[58]。

呼吸运动评估动态 MRI 是一项更加简便可行的质子 MRI 技术，但对临床评估 COPD 作用不大。几位研究者评价了此项技术在评估横膈及

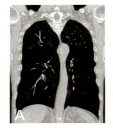
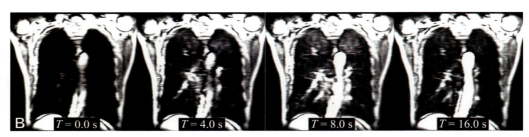

▲ 图 10-2　72 岁男性，慢性阻塞性肺病

A. 薄层 CT 冠状位多平面重建图示双肺气肿，表现为不均匀分布的低密度区，主要位于双肺下叶；B.3T 时间分辨率增强 MRI 血管造影（从左到右为对比剂注射后不同时间点的图像）示肺实质内强化不均。双下肺野，尤其是左下肺野强化程度较双上肺野减低。双肺强化程度和分布与肺气肿的程度相关

胸壁运动、肺气肿患者肺体积或形态学变化以及肺部分切除患者肺体积改变中的作用[59-65]。结果发现,呼吸运动评估参数与肺功能参数明显相关,临床上,这项技术还可检测到膈肌矛盾运动或肺部分切除患者的靶病灶[59-65]。尽管呼吸运动评估动态 MRI 还可评价肺、胸壁及膈肌运动引起的 COPD 患者肺功能的变化,但还需进一步研究证实此项肺功能成像技术的实际意义及其对 COPD 患者的临床价值。

近期,临床常规中的体部 MRI 检查设备逐渐由 1.5T 转变到应用 3T。因此,3T MR 系统的定量 T_2^* 序列作为一种具有超短回波时间的新的质子 MR 成像技术,被提倡用于评估吸烟相关的 COPD 患者肺实质形态学改变[28,66-68]。肺组织、PBF 的减少以及肺气肿、空气潴留引起的气体-软组织交界面不均匀增多、增大,可影响肺实质 T_2^* 值。在一项研究中,平均 T_2^* 值及 CT 肺功能容积、气道壁厚度与总气道横截面积之比(ratio of wall area to total airway area,WA%)与肺功能检查指标、临床分期呈明显相关[67]。此外,与不患 COPD 的吸烟人群相比,COPD 患者肺 T_2^* 值依肺功能受损及临床分期的不同而不均匀减低[67,68]。因此认为在评估吸烟 COPD 患者的肺功能受损及临床分期方面,超短回波时间 T_2^*MRI 成像的定量评估作用等效于定量薄层 CT[67,68]。但是,未来尚需进一步研究证实这种 MR 新技术在临床常规管理 COPD 患者中是否等效于薄层 CT。

四、肺部 MRI

(一)肺结节

胸部平片及 CT 检查经常可检出肺结节。绝大部分检出的肺结节(90%)是因不相关的诊断性检查于胸片(chest radio-grams,CXRs)上偶然发现[69,70]。此外,全国范围的肺癌筛查试验及以往报道的 CT 肺癌筛查结果推动了临床管理肺结节的需要[70]。临床常规中,CT 是最常用于诊断的检查方式,正电子发射断层显像(positron emission tomography,PET)或 ^{18}F-脱氧葡萄糖 PET/CT(fluorodeoxyglucose,FDG-PET/CT)扫描次之,是需要进一步影像学评估肺结节时所做的检查[71-74]。另外,传统质子 MRI 可能有助于肺结节的诊断。

既往的研究报道[75-83],基于病变特殊的 MRI 表现,T_2 加权、平扫或增强 T_1 加权 SE 序列或快速 SE 序列图像可用于诊断支气管囊肿、结核球、含黏液的肿瘤、错构瘤以及曲霉菌球。但许多肺结节 T_1 加权成像呈低或中等信号,T_2 加权成像呈稍高信号,包括肺癌、肺转移瘤及低级别恶性肿瘤。此外,肺部良恶性结节或肿块间有明显重叠的弛豫时间,使其难以用于鉴别肺部良恶性结节[81-83]。

为了克服弛豫时间评估的局限性,引入了短反转时间反转恢复(short inversion time inversion recovery,STIR)快速 SE 成像和弥散加权 MRI(diffusion-weighted MRI,DWI),相对于其他 SE 或快速 SE 成像序列而言,STIR 快速 SE 成像和 DWI 在平扫 MRI 评估肺结节方面有更好的应用前景[84-87]。STIR 快速 SE 成像的相关研究证实了其定量评估的能力,鉴别肺部良恶性结节的敏感性、特异性及准确性可分别达 83.3%、60.6% 及 74.5%,明显优于平扫 T_1、T_2 加权快速 SE 成像[84]。DWI 是另一个有发展前景的平扫 MR 成像方法(图 10-4 和图 10-5)[85-87]。理论上,DWI 可评估组织内水分子的扩散性,以 ADC(apparent diffusion coefficient)值的方式反映组织内的细胞水平、灌注、组织结构破坏、细胞外间隙及其他变量。最大 b 值范围为 500~1000s/mm² 的条件下,ADC 值定量、定性鉴别肺部良恶性结节的敏感性为 70.0%~88.9%,特异性 61.1%~97.0%[85-87],DWI 的敏感性(97.0%)要明显高于 FDG-PET/CT(79.0%)[85]。此外,研究发现,当采用病变与脊髓信号比值这一参数而非 ADC 值鉴别肺结节良恶性时,敏感性、特异性及准确性可分别达 83.3%、90.0%、85.7%,其准确性明显高于

ADC 值（50.0%）[87]。尽管此研究的样本量有限，但仍认为其研究结果是有价值的。目前认为这些平扫 MRI 技术至少与 FDG-PET 或 PET/CT 等效，未来有望用于肺良恶性结节的鉴别诊断。

在过去 20 年中，动态增强 MRI 用于探究其鉴别肺部良恶性结节，或鉴别需要进一步干预、治疗的结节和仅需要随诊的结节方面的效能（图 10-3 和图 10-4）[83,88-98]。研究结果发现，动态增强 MRI 至少与动态增强 CT、FDG-PET 或 PET/CT 等效[83,97,98]。这些研究应用不同的动态 MR 技术鉴别肺部良恶性结节，敏感性达 94%～100%，特异性 70%～96%，准确性超过 94%[88-98]。此外，据一项 meta 分析报道，动态增强 CT、动态增强 MRI 和 FDG-PET 的诊断效能无明显差异[98]。因此，在鉴别肺部结节方面，动态 MRI 可补充或替代动态增强 CT、FDG-PET 和（或）PET/CT。但需要注意的是，MRI 在应用方面存在一定缺陷，如无法用于体内有植入装置的患者、幽闭恐惧症者、肾功能障碍患者等。

（二）肺癌

肺癌是世界上最常见的癌症，高居男女性死亡率的首位[99]。目前，非小细胞肺癌（non-small cell lung cancer，NSCLC）占所有肺癌类型的 80%，其早期发现可手术治愈[100]。但大部分 NSCLC 患者发病之时即为晚期，无法行手术治疗[101-103]。小细胞肺癌占所有肺癌类型的 13%～20%[104]，依据 Veterans 管理肺癌研究组的两期法分期，而并非肿瘤、淋巴结及转移（tumor, lymph node and metastasis，TNM）分期。无论用哪一种肺癌分期方法，CT、PET 及 PET/CT 等影像学检查方法都被认为是重要的治疗前评估

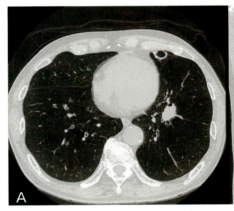
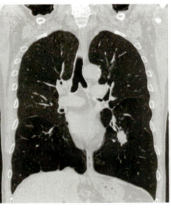
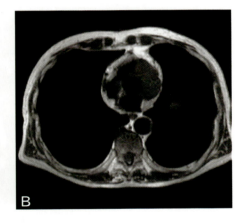
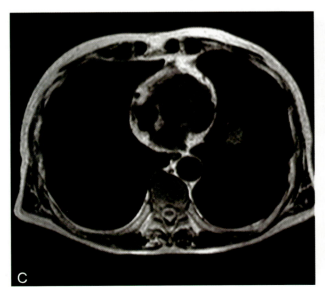
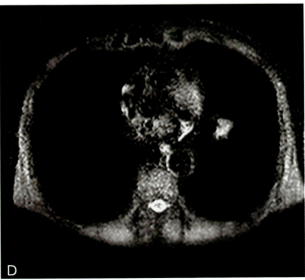

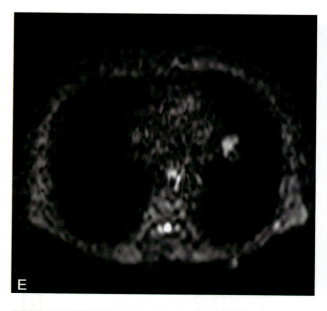
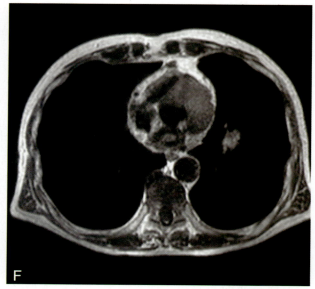
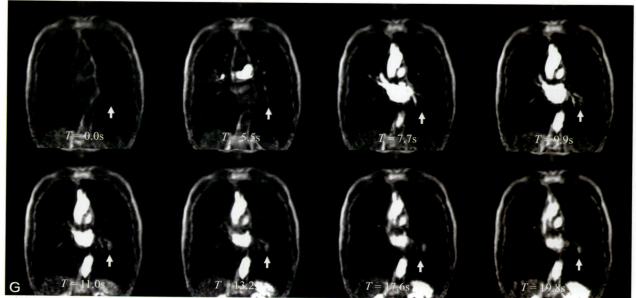

▲ 图 10-3　78 岁男性，侵袭性肺腺癌

A. 薄层 CT 和 MPR 图像肺窗示左肺下叶直径 20mm 的结节。病理诊断为侵袭性肺腺癌；B. 平扫黑血 T_1 加权快速 SE 图像示结节呈均匀低信号；C. 平扫黑血 T_2 加权快速 SE 图像示结节呈均匀等信号；D. 黑血 STIR 快速 SE 图像示结节呈高信号。结节 / 肌肉信号比值为 1.7，结节诊断为恶性。STIR 快速 SE 图像诊断结节为真阳性；E.DWI 示结节呈高信号。ADC 值为 $0.9×10^{-3}mm^2/s$。ADC 值诊断结节为真阳性；F. 钆对比剂注入后，增强黑血 T_1 加权快速 SE 图像上，结节呈均匀强化；G. 超短 TE（T：注入对比剂后的时间点）动态增强 T_1 加权 GRE 成像示，9.9s 后结节开始出现明显强化，血供主要来自体循环。平均相对强化比值及增强斜率分别为 0.6/s、0.2/s。此每项参数评价结节均为真阳性

手段。相对于 CT、FDG-PET 及 PET/CT，1991 年研究者们提出，MRI 临床用途有限，与 CT 相比，MRI 可多平面扫描，并且肿瘤与纵隔或胸壁软组织对比度更高，因此其在鉴别纵隔及胸壁侵犯方面可能会更有价值[105]。但近年来 MR 扫描系统的不断发展，脉冲序列的改进或更新以及对比剂的有效利用，使临床评估肺癌 TNM 分期的准确性进一步提高[81-83]。

1. T 因素评估　许多外科医师认为轻微侵犯纵隔脂肪的病变是可切除的[106]，因此临床

医师术前需明确肿瘤轻微侵犯（T_3 期）或真正侵犯（T_4 期）纵隔。大量研究[57-66,81-83,105-115]表明，螺旋或非螺旋 CT 评估纵隔受侵的敏感性为 38% ～ 84%，特异性为 40% ～ 94%。尽管 PET 或 PET/CT 常规用于评估临床肺癌分期，但很少有关于 PET 或 PET/CT 评估 T 分期的研究。影像诊断肿瘤研究组（RDOG）[105]应用非心电/呼吸门控 T_1、T_2 加权 SE 成像评估肿瘤 T 分期，发现

在鉴别 T_3 ～ T_4 与 T_1 ～ T_2 肿瘤方面，MRI 的诊断效能（敏感性，56.0%；特异性，80.0%）与传统 CT（敏感性，63.0%；特异性，84.0%）无明显差异[105]。但在无心电/呼吸门控的情况下，T_1、T_2 加权 SE 图像可见到运动伪影，因而会影响心包或纵隔侵犯的清晰显示。应用心电/呼吸门控及快速 MR 序列后，提高了 T_1、T_2 加权 SE 或快速 SE 图像上肿瘤侵犯心包（T_3）或心脏（T_4）

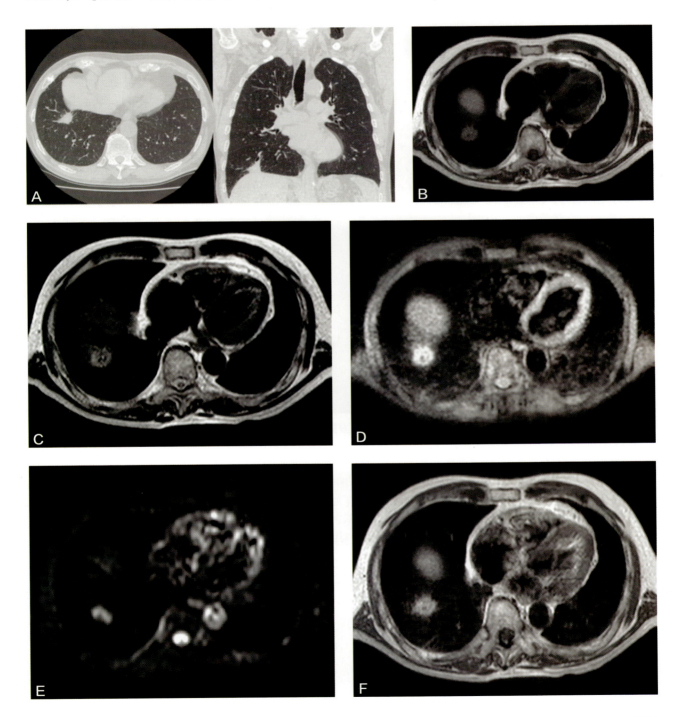

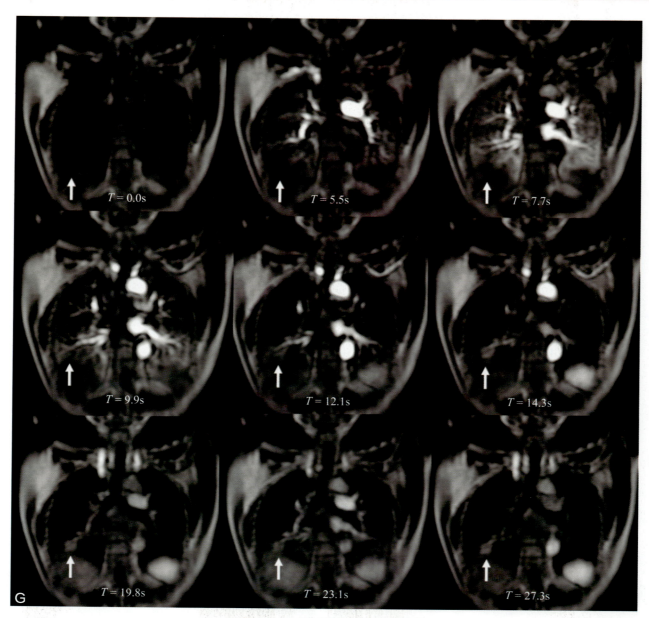

▲ 图 10-4　80 岁男性，机化性肺炎

A. 薄层 CT 及 MPR 图像肺窗示右肺下叶直径约 23mm 的结节。病理诊断为机化性肺炎；B. 平扫黑血 T_1 加权快速 SE 图像上，结节呈低信号，内见更低信号；C. 平扫黑血 T_2 加权快速 SE 图像上，结节呈中等、低信号；D. 黑血 STIR 快速 SE 图像上，结节呈高信号。结节与肌肉信号比值为 1.8。STIR 快速 SE 图像诊断结节为假阳性；E.DWI 示结节呈高信号。ADC 值为 $0.85×10^{-3}mm^2/s$。ADC 值诊断结节为假阳性；F 增强黑血 T_1 加权快速 SE 图像上，钆对比剂注入后，结节呈相对均匀强化；G. 动态增强 T_1 加权 GRE 序列伴超短 TE（T：注入对比剂后的时间）图像示，12.1s 后结节明显强化，血供来自体循环。平均相对强化比值及强化斜率分别为 0.4/s、0.03/s。平均相对强化比值诊断结节为假阳性，强化斜率诊断结节为真阴性

的显示程度，诊断效能明显提高。由于传统平扫 MRI 相对于 CT 具备多平面扫描及良好软组织对比度的优势，MRI 除了可评估纵隔受侵之外，还被推荐用于胸壁受侵的评估[81-83,105,115-120]。在显示肿瘤与胸壁结构的解剖关系方面，CT 冠矢状位重建图优于轴位图像，Padovani 等提出，静脉内注入对比剂可进一步提高诊断效能[118]。此外，应用 STIR 快速 SE 成像时，在胸壁的压脂信号中可见肺癌病变为高信号，由此可明确胸壁内肿瘤的大小（图 10-5）[81-83]。

快速 GRE 非心电门控或心电门控增强 MR 血管造影序列推荐用于评估心血管或纵隔肿瘤

Chapter 10　气管、支气管及肺部磁共振成像
Magnetic Resonance Imaging for Trachea, Bronchi, and Lung

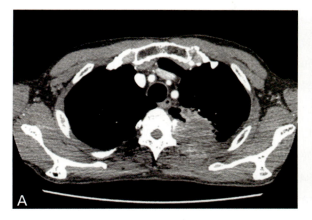
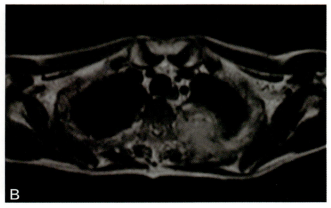
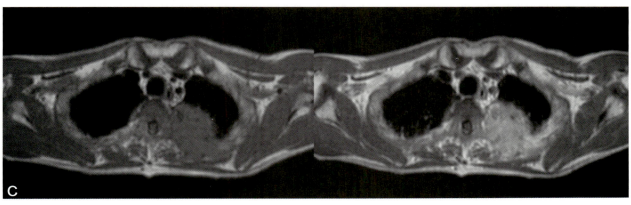
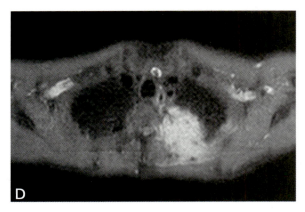

▲ 图 10-5　61 岁女性，肺鳞癌侵犯胸壁

A. 尽管薄层增强 CT 上可见胸壁及脊柱受侵，怀疑病变为肺尖部肺癌，但 CT 图像上伪影严重、肿瘤与胸壁间对比度较低，使细节显示欠清；B. 黑血 T_2 加权快速 SE 序列示肿瘤呈高信号。尽管可清晰显示胸壁受侵，但脊柱受侵显示不清；C. 从左到右分别为平扫、增强黑血 T_1 加权快速 SE 图像。平扫黑血 T_1 加权快速 SE 图像可清晰显示胸壁、脊柱肿瘤侵犯以及原发肿瘤呈低信号。尽管增强黑血 T_1 加权快速 SE 图像示肿瘤明显强化，但胸壁及脊柱受侵的显示程度并无提高；D. 黑血 STIR 快速 SE 图像示原发肿瘤及胸壁、脊柱受侵均呈明显高信号。另外可清晰显示左椎弓根受侵

侵犯[121,122]。心电门控增强 MR 血管造影检出纵隔或肺门肿瘤侵犯的敏感性、特异性及准确性分别 78%～90%、73%～87%、75%～88%，均高于增强 CT 及传统心电 - 呼吸门控 T_1 加权 SE 成像[122]。因此，认为增强 MR 血管造影可以提高 T 分期评估的准确性，进而促进胸部 MR 检查在这方面的应用。

另一种有助于 T 分期的 MR 技术是动态电影 MRI，它可在呼吸状态下评估肿瘤沿邻近胸膜运动的情况。一项应用此技术的研究发现，肿瘤侵犯胸壁时会被固定在胸壁上，而未侵犯胸壁时，则会沿着胸膜自由移动[123]。此研究中，动态电影 MRI 检出胸壁受侵的敏感性、特异性及准确性分别为 100%、70% 及 76%，而传统 CT 及 MRI 则为 80%、65% 及 68%[123]。因此，动态电影 MRI 联合静态 MRI 将有助于评估肿瘤侵犯胸壁。

2. N 分期评估　CT 是肺癌分期中常用的无创性检查方法，转移性淋巴结的诊断是基于肿大淋巴结的短径做出的。来自 RDOG 和 Leuven 肺

癌组（Leuven Lung Cancer Group，LLCG）的两篇主要论文报道了CT评估N分期的诊断效能，敏感性为52%～69%，特异性为69%～71%[105,124-130]。基于上述结果，研究者认为在评估肺癌N分期时应用传统的纵隔镜活检较为可靠。

自20世纪90年代以来，基于肿瘤葡萄糖代谢增高或肿瘤细胞增殖的生化机制，FDG-PET用于鉴别转移和非转移性淋巴结[131-143]。但在继发性肿瘤、感染及炎性病变中，葡萄糖代谢也会升高。此外，PET的空间分辨率要低于CT及MR。因此，在过去10年中，研究者认为FDG-PET或PET/CT在显示转移及非转移性淋巴结方面有很大重叠，其诊断效能有限[131-143]。

传统T_1、T_2加权SE或快速SE成像评估肺癌N分期（即鉴别淋巴结转移或非转移）的标准是淋巴结的大小，与CT标准相似。RDOG的一项研究直接比较了MRI和CT的诊断效能，发现MRI唯一的优势在于可获得淋巴结多平面图像，但在主肺动脉窗、隆突下等区域淋巴结轴位图像显示欠佳。该研究进一步表示，传统MRI和CT在肺癌N分期中的诊断效能无明显差异。

为提高MRI评估N分期的效能，2002年以来发表的多项研究探索了心电/呼吸触发传统或黑血STIR快速SE成像的临床价值，证实其优于增强CT、FDG-PET、PET/CT及其他MR序列[144-149]。通过与0.9%生理盐水体模（淋巴结-盐水比）或肌肉（淋巴结-肌肉比）比较，这些新序列可用于定量评估淋巴结信号[144-146,149]。此外，通过视觉上比较淋巴结与肌肉或原发肿瘤的信号差异，可鉴别转移与非转移性淋巴结，研究表明，此种方法的诊断效能要优于其他方法[144-149]。这些研究中，应用STIR快速SE成像定量定性评估淋巴结转移的敏感性、特异性及准确性分别为83.7%～100.0%、75.0%～93.1%及86.0%～92.2%，均等于或高于增强CT、FDG-PET及PET/CT。将STIR快速SE序列应用于肺癌患者胸部MR检查中，MRI在鉴别转移与非转移性淋巴结中的效能较其他检查方式进一步提高。此外，当这种技术与FDG-PET/CT联合应用（特异性：96.9%，准确性：90.3%）时，每位患者的诊断效能均较FDG-PET/CT（特异性：65.6%，准确性：81.7%）有所提高[148]。

近期，DWI作为另一种MR技术应用于淋巴结转移的诊断[149-152]。DWI定性定量评估的敏感性、特异性及准确性分别为77.4%～80.0%、84.4%～97.0%和89.0%～95.0%，均等于或高于FDG-PET或PET/CT[149-152]。但目前DWI图像是无心电/呼吸门控的SE平面回波成像，图像质量常因心肺运动及磁敏感伪影而受损，因此DWI检出小转移灶或转移淋巴结的能力有限，与FDG-PET/CT类似。一项前瞻性研究比较了STIR快速SE图像与DWI、FDG-PET/CT在鉴别转移、非转移性淋巴结的效能，发现STIR快速SE图像（定量敏感性：82.8%，定性敏感性：77.4%，定量准确性：86.8%）诊断的敏感性和准确性要明显高于DWI（分别为74.2%、71.0%及84.4%）和FDG-PET/CT（定量敏感性：74.2%）[149]。

STIR快速SE成像是一个简单的序列，可轻松纳入临床常规扫描中，类似于压脂序列伴T_1、T_2扫描对比。此外，另一个既往报道且成功应用的STIR快速SE序列是心电-呼吸触发传统或黑血T_1加权STIR快速SE成像。在STIR快速SE图像上，转移性淋巴结表现为高信号，非转移性淋巴结为低信号（图10-6和图10-7）。因此，基于上述结果，STIR快速SE成像相较于其他MR技术可能更有效，可应用于开胸手术及纵隔镜淋巴结活检前、术后及放化疗前对肿瘤的精确病程性TNM分期。此外，在临床中，STIR快速SE成像有望在NSCLC患者N分期方面对FDG-PET或PET/CT起替代或补充作用。

3. M分期评估 肿瘤转移性病变检出是影响肺癌患者管理及预后的重要因素之一。约40%的初诊肺癌患者在就诊时可检出胸外转移[153,154]，因此，临床医师通常认为，胸内病变及胸外转移的准确诊断有助于肺癌患者的准确治疗及管理。术前指南中推荐胸片、全身CT、头MRI、骨扫描、

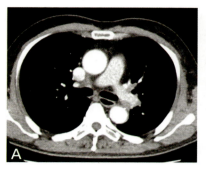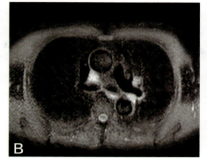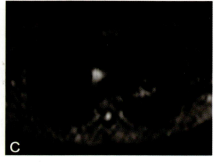

▲ 图 10-6　77 岁男性，侵袭性肺腺癌伴纵隔及肺门淋巴结转移（N3 期）

A. 增强 CT 示左肺门及纵隔淋巴结短径＜ 9mm。所有淋巴结均评为非转移性病灶，该病例淋巴结评为假阴性；B. 黑血 STIR 快速 SE 图像清晰显示所有淋巴结呈高信号。所有淋巴结诊断为转移性，正确评为 N3 期；C.DWI 示左肺门及右下气管旁淋巴结呈高信号，隆突下淋巴结由于伪影干扰无法准确评估。所有高信号淋巴结均正确诊断为转移性淋巴结，隆突下淋巴结评为假阴性。但 DWI 将此病例正确评为 N3 期，此病例评为真阳性

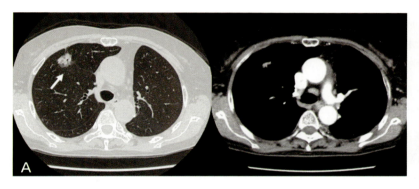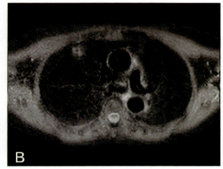

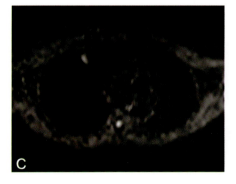

▲ 图 10-7　75 岁女性，侵袭性肺腺癌，纵隔无淋巴结转移（N0 期）

该患者因左肺侵袭性腺癌于 7 年前行手术切除治疗。A. 从左到右分别为薄层 CT 肺窗及增强 CT。薄层 CT 示右肺上叶部分实性结节，诊断为侵袭性肺腺癌。增强 CT 示右下气管旁淋巴结短径为 11mm。该病例诊断为 N2 期，淋巴结评为假阳性；B. 黑血 STIR 快速 SE 图像示原发病变呈高信号，右下气管旁淋巴结呈低信号。该病例诊断为 N0 期，淋巴结评为真阴性；C. DWI 示原发病灶呈明显高信号，右下气管旁淋巴结因伪影显示不清。这一意外发现的病变诊断为 N0 期，评为真阴性。DWI 显示淋巴结受限被认为是目前 DWI 序列成像的主要缺陷之一

临床症状及肿瘤标志物作为监测肿瘤转移的指标[155-157]。此外，几位研究者认为，除头 MRI 外，全身 FDG-PET 或 PET/CT 是评估可疑 NSCLC 胸外转移的更有效的工具，而非传统检查中的 CT、骨扫描[135,136,138,140,141]。

近期，有研究者建议应用全身 MRI 检出转移性病变，利用移床技术、全身线圈、具有平行成像能力的多阵列线圈以及多种新的快速 MR 序列，可实现全身 MR 成像。这种联合技术现认为是一种简单、性价比高的影像学检查，可于 1.5T 或 3T 设备上扫描，不仅适用于肺癌患者，还可用于其他恶性肿瘤患者（图 10-8）[147,158-161]。此外，全身 DWI 认为是肿瘤患者全身 MR 检查中有应用前景的新方法[159-161]。在评估肿瘤 M 分期中，将全身 MRI 与 FDG-PET 或 PET/CT 相比，发现前者伴或不伴 DWI 的诊断效能（敏感性：52.0%～80.0%，特异性：74.3%～94.0%，准确性：80.0%～87.7%）等于或明显高于后两者（敏感性：48.0%～80.0%；特异性：74.3%～96.0%，准确性：73.3%～88.2%）[147,158-161]。尽管如此，应慎重考虑全身 MR 检查中应用全身 DWI 所存在的

缺陷。当仅应用全身 DWI 时，患者的特异性（87.7%）和准确性（84.3%）均明显低于 FDG-PET/CT（特异性：94.5%，准确性：90.4%）[159]。同一研究表明，全身 MRI 联合 DWI 的诊断准确性（87.8%）与 FDG-PET/CT 无明显差异，但全身 MRI 不伴 DWI 的诊断准确性（85.8%）要明显低于 FDG-PET/CT。由此说明，全身 MRI 联合 DWI 在评估 NSCLC 患者 M 分期方面准确性同 FDG-PET/CT 相似。因此，为提高 NSCLC 患者 M 分期的准确性，建议全身 MR 检查中加入全身 DWI 序列[159]。

除此之外，研究发现，当应用全身 MRI 评估 NSCLC 患者术后复发情况时[162]，新的增强 T_1 加权 3D 高分辨 GRE 序列联合双压脂射频（radiofrequency，RF）脉冲技术会比以往应用的增强 T_1 加权 GRE 序列更有效，前者可在临床常规中对全身 PET/CT 起补充作用。该研究表明，全身 MRI 应用了双压脂 RF 脉冲技术的增强 T_1 加权 3D 高分辨 GRE 序列后，诊断特异性（100%）和准确性（95.5%）要明显高于 FDG-PET/CT（特异性：93.6%，P=0.02；准确性：89.6%，P=0.01）及传统影像学检查（特异性：92.7%，P=0.01；准确性：91.0%，P=0.03），但既往应用增强 T_1 加权 GRE 序列的全身 MRI 诊断特异性（100%）同样高于 FDG-PET/CT（P=0.02）及传统影像学检查（P=0.01）。由此表明，全身 MRI 联合 DWI 及新的增强 T_1 加权 GRE 序列同 FDG-PET 或 PET/CT 一样，可能有助于临床中肺癌患者的管理，可促进世界范围内癌症中心或癌症研究中心的应用。

（三）间质性肺疾病

官方美国胸科协会/欧洲呼吸协会更新了国际多学科间质性肺疾病（interstitial lung disease，ILD）分类的新标准[163]。该声明指出，临床、血清学、薄层 CT 及病理学诊断可能有助于鉴别特发性间质性肺炎与结缔组织病相关的其他 ILD[163]。临床常规中，薄层 CT、肺功能检查及血清学标志物常用于 ILD 诊断、严重程度评估及治疗疗效评价。除薄层 CT 外，MRI 也可用于评估 ILD，但临床中应用的传统 T_1、T_2 加权及质子密度 SE 序列对肺实质结构及 ILD 病变显示能力较差，因此很少应用。

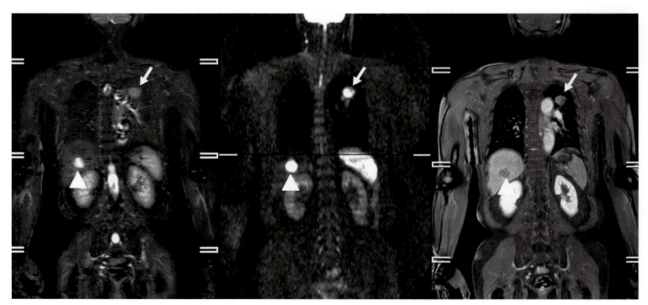

▲ 图 10-8　63 岁男性，侵袭性肺腺癌伴肝脏转移

从左向右分别为 STIR 快速 SE 序列、DWI、增强 T_1 加权高分辨各向同性体积检查（THRIVE）成像。STIR 快速 SE 图像和 DWI 图像上，原发病灶（箭）及肝脏转移灶（箭头）呈高、更高信号，该病例评为Ⅳ期。增强 THIRVE 图像上，原发病灶呈明显强化（箭）。另外，肝内肿物呈环形低信号（箭头）。据病灶强化方式很容易诊断为肝转移，同样评为Ⅳ期

1999 年以来，MR 技术的不断进展为肺实质成像打开了新局面，包括 MR 成像系统的发展，更新更快 MR 序列，应用半傅里叶采集技术，采用某种平行成像及射频脉冲技术提高肺内图像对比度及信噪比[164]。基于上述新技术，多位研究者分别应用更短回波时间三维（3D）屏气 GRE 成像[165]、选择性衰减反转恢复脉冲或三重反转黑血脉冲的 T_2 加权快速 SE 成像[166,167]、二维平衡稳态自由进动成像[168]、增强 T_1 加权 GRE 成像[169,170] 及动态增强 T_1 加权快速 GER 成像[167] 序列评估了 ILD 形态学改变。此外，近期有研究者发现，MRI 3D 径向超短 TE 脉冲序列在显示肺实质结构方面要更优于以往报道的质子 MRI 成像序列[171]。

与薄层 CT 和常规 MRI 用于评估肺形态学改变相比，自 2007 年以来氧增强 MRI[172, 173] 和超短 TE 肺 MRI[174] 用于质子肺功能 MRI 成像。据报道，氧增强 MRI 在评估区域性肺通气、肺泡-毛细血管氧分子交换、每个呼吸循环的氧摄取及气流受限方面有良好的应用潜能[52-58]。此外，在结缔组织病相关 ILD 患者中，氧增强 MRI 的区域氧强化值及超短 TE 肺 MRI 的定量 T_2^* 值等效于薄层 CT 肺功能受损评估，并与血清标志物反映的疾病严重程度有很好的相关性[173,174]。因此，有望在临床常规中应用上述 MRI 技术评估 ILD 患者肺形态学及功能学，从而发挥更高的影像学价值，但仍需进一步临床评价。

（四）除肺栓塞及肺高压外的肺血管性疾病

过去几十年中，MRI 被推荐用于评估急慢性肺栓塞及原发性、继发性肺高压。这类疾病在第 13 章中有详细介绍，本章着重介绍肺动静脉畸形和肺隔离症。

（五）肺动静脉畸形或瘘（肺 AVM 或 AVF）

肺动静脉畸形（pulmonary arteriovenous malformation，AVM）或动静脉瘘（pulmonary arteriovenous fistula，AVF）是指肺动静脉分支经薄壁动脉瘤样结构的异常沟通[175]。20 世纪 80 年代早期，由于栓塞治疗无须切除肺实质即可减少脑栓塞和脓肿的发生率，因而被用于治疗大部分肺 AVM 或 AVF 患者[175-178]。单排或多排螺旋 CT 的出现，使准确评估肺 AVM 或 AVF 的治疗疗效成为可能，CT 可在血管水平评价病变形态学改变，随着技术的进一步发展，可在一次检查中同时评估肺循环及体循环血管的情况[179-182]。

2002 年发表的一项研究表明，肺 AVM 均有动脉瘤囊、供血动脉及引流静脉的结构，CT 血管造影、时间分辨率增强 MR 血管造影及肺血管造影对≥ 3cm 的肺 AVM 的检出效能、测量结果是相似的[183]。另外有研究针对评价治疗后随诊，发现 58.4%（7/12）的治疗后 AVM 体积有缩小，病变内残留少许对比剂，增强灌注 MRI 可看到残留灶内支气管动脉-肺动脉侧支血流[183]。因此，时间分辨率增强 MR 血管造影和增强灌注 MRI 之类的质子 MRI，可以作为管理肺 AVM 和 AVF 的新技术。

（六）肺隔离症

肺隔离症是一种相对罕见，但临床特征显著的先天性支气管肺前肠发育畸形，其包含一系列结构异常：肺气道、肺动脉血供、肺实质及静脉引流。依据病变不同形态学亚型，静脉可回流至肺静脉或体部静脉。尽管多种影像学技术可应用于肺隔离症的诊断，包括常规胸片、增强 CT、MDCT 血管造影、核医学检查、支气管镜检查、超声及 MRI，但临床常规中，肺隔离症确诊需要靠传统或数字减影血管造影检查。自从传统或时间分辨率增强 MR 血管造影应用以来[185-188]，研究者们发现质子 MRI 同样可用于临床评估肺隔离症（图 10-9）。因此，MRI 有望在评估肺隔离症中广泛应用。另外，随着 MRI 时间、空间分辨率的进一步提高，MRI 在未来有可能同传统或数字减影血管造影一样，发挥确诊的重要作用。

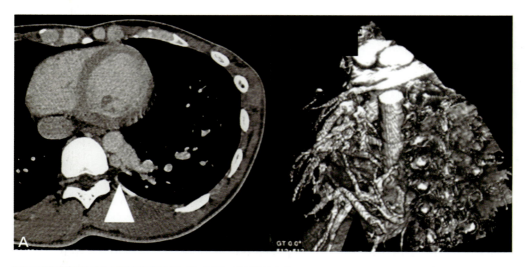
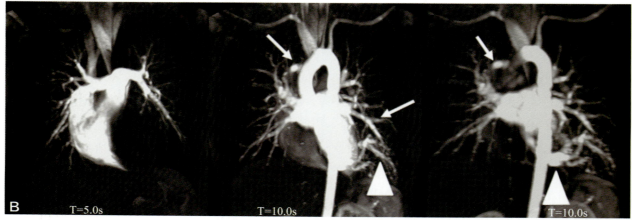
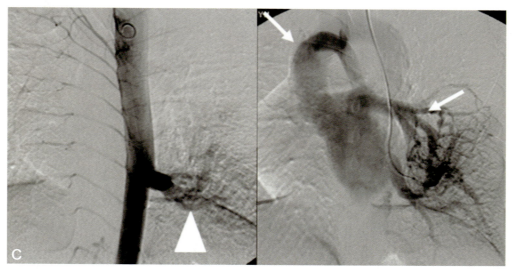

▲ 图 10-9 23 岁男性，肺隔离症

A.（从左向右分别为增强 CT、3D CT 血管造影）增强 CT 和 3D CT 血管造影示胸主动脉起源的异常动脉（白箭头）；B.［从左向右分别为时间分辨率 MR 血管造影检查对比剂注入后 5s、10s 的最大密度投影（MIPs）及 10s 的薄 MIP 图］MIP 图示肺动脉期的灌注缺损（5.0s MIP 图）、胸主动脉起源的异常动脉（箭头）及肺静脉期和体循环动脉期（10.0s MIP 图）的肺隔离症病变。此外，10.0s MIP 图上均可见异常动脉、肺及奇静脉（箭）间的异常沟通。这些征象与主动脉造影所示相一致；C.（从左向右分别为主动脉血管造影，选择性异常动脉血管造影）主动脉血管造影可清晰显示起源于胸主动脉的异常动脉（箭头）。选择性血管造影示异常动脉、肺及奇静脉（箭）间的异常沟通

五、总结

本章回顾了当前最先进的质子 MR 技术在各种颈胸部疾病中对气管、支气管及肺实质的评估价值。目前，实现先进的 MR 设备、快速成像及平行成像技术 MR 新序列的常规应用从而获得新对比标准，有 / 无对比剂的超高分辨率以及 MRI 定性定量分析已成为可能。此外，近期发表的文献证实了 MRI 对气管、支气管及肺实质疾病的潜在应用优势。但仍需要进一步的方案优化、更多的临床试验及高级统计分析工具来明确 MRI 的真正价值。另外，既往及目前的研究结果表明，MRI 在胸部疾病的形态学诊断中起补充性作用，或对某些检查可发挥替代作用，未来需进一步研究来证实 MRI 在临床常规中的应用价值。

参考文献

[1] Ailion DC, Case TA, Blatter DD et al. (1984) Application of NMR spin imaging to the study of lungs. *Bull Magn Reson* 6: 130–139.

[2] Case TA, Durney CH, Ailion DC, Cutillo AG, Morris AH (1987) A mathematical model of diamagnetic line broadening in lung tissue and similar heterogenous systems: Calculations and measurements. *J Magn Reson* 73: 304–314.

[3] Bergin CJ, Pauly JM, Macovski A (1991) Lung parenchyma: Projection reconstruction MR imaging. *Radiology* 179: 777–781.

[4] Cutillo AG, Ganesan K, Ailion DC et al. (1991) Alveolar air–tissue interface and nuclear magnetic resonance behavior of lung. *J Appl Physiol* 70: 2145–2154.

[5] Bergin CJ, Glover GH, Pauly JM (1991) Lung parenchyma: Magnetic susceptibility in MR imaging. *Radiology* 180: 845–848.

[6] Hatabu H, Alsop DC, Listerud J, Bonnet M, Gefter WB (1999) T2* and proton density measurement of normal human lung parenchyma using submillisecond echo time gradient echo magnetic resonance imaging. *Eur J Radiol* 29: 245–252.

[7] Mayo JR, MacKay A, Muller NL (1992) MR imaging of the lungs: Value of short TE spin-echo pulse sequences. *AJR Am J Roentgenol* 159: 951–956.

[8] Alsop DC, Hatabu H, Bonnet M, Listerud J, Gefter W (1995) Multi-slice, breathhold imaging of the lung with submillisecond echo times. *Magn Reson Med* 33: 678–682.

[9] Yamashita Y, Yokoyama T, Tomiguchi S, Takahashi M, Ando M (1999) MR imaging of focal lung lesions: Elimination of flow and motion artifact by breath-hold ECG-gated and black-blood techniques on T2-weighted turbo SE and STIR sequences. *J Magn Reson Imaging* 9: 691–698.

[10] Biederer J, Reuter M, Both M et al. (2002) Analysis of artefacts and detail resolution of lung MRI with breathhold T1-weighted gradient-echo and T2-weighted fast spin-echo sequences with respiratory triggering. *Eur Radiol* 12: 378–384.

[11] Bruegel M, Gaa J, Woertler K et al. (2007) MRI of the lung: Value of different turbo spin-echo, single-shot turbo spin echo, and 3D gradient-echo pulse sequences for the detection of pulmonary metastases. *J Magn Reson Imaging* 25: 73–81.

[12] Yi CA, Jeon TY, Lee KS et al. (2007) 3-T MRI: Usefulness for evaluating primary lung cancer and small nodules in lobes not containing primary tumors. *AJR Am J Roentgenol* 189: 386–392.

[13] Tollefsen HR, DeCosse JJ, Hutter RVP (1964) Papillary carcinoma of the thyroid: A clinical and pathological study of 70 fatal cases. *Cancer* 17: 1035–1044.

[14] Cody HS 3rd, Shah JP (1981) Locally invasive, well differentiated thyroid cancer. 22 years' experience at Memorial Sloan-Kettering Cancer Center. *Am J Surg* 142: 480–483.

[15] Park CS, Suh KW, Min JS (1993) Cartilage-shaving procedure for the control of tracheal cartilage invasion by thyroid carcinoma. *Head Neck* 15: 289–291.

[16] Clark OH, Levin K, Zeng QH, Greenspan FS, Siperstein A (1988) Thyroid cancer: The cases for total thyroidectomy. *Eur J Cancer Clin Oncol* 24: 305–313.

[17] Ishihara T, Kikuchi K, Ikeda T et al. (1978) Resection of thyroid carcinoma infiltrating the trachea. *Thorax* 33: 378–386.

[18] Nakao K, Miyata M, Izukura M, Monden Y, Maeda M, Kawashima Y (1984) Radical operation for thyroid carcinoma invading the trachea. *Arch Surg* 119: 1046–1049.

[19] Ozaki O, Sugino K, Mimura T, Ito K (1995) Surgery for patients with thyroid carcinoma invading the trachea: Circumferential sleeve resection followed by end-to-end anastomosis. *Surgery* 117: 268–271.

[20] Takashima S, Takayama F, Wang Q et al. (2000) Differentiated thyroid carcinomas. Prediction of tumor invasion with MR imaging. *Acta Radiol* 41: 377–383.

[21] Wang JC, Takashima S, Takayama F et al. (2001) Tracheal invasion by thyroid carcinoma: Prediction using MR imaging. *AJR Am J Roentgenol* 177: 929–936.

[22] Takashima S, Takayama F, Wang J, Kobayashi S, Kadoya M (2003) Using MR imaging to predict invasion of the recurrent laryngeal nerve by thyroid carcinoma. *AJR Am J Roentgenol* 180: 37–42.

[23] Davis SD, Fordham LA, Brody AS et al. (2007) Computed tomography reflects lower airway inflammation and tracks changes in early cystic fibrosis. *Am J Respir Crit Care Med* 175: 943–950.

[24] Davis SD, Brody AS, Emond MJ et al. (2007) Endpoints for

clinical trials in young children with cystic fibrosis. *Proc Am Thorac Soc* 4: 418–430.

[25] Sly PD, Brennan S, Gangell C et al. (2009) Lung disease at diagnosis in infants with cystic fibrosis detected by newborn screening. *Am J Respir Crit Care Med* 180: 146–152.

[26] Tiddens HA (2006) Chest computed tomography scans should be considered as a routine investigation in cystic fibrosis. *Paediatr Respir Rev* 7: 202–208.

[27] Eichinger M, Heussel CP, Kauczor HU, Tiddens H, Puderbach M (2010) Computed tomography and magnetic resonance imaging in cystic fibrosis lung disease. *J Magn Reson Imaging* 32: 1370–1378.

[28] Ohno Y, Koyama H, Yoshikawa T et al. (2011) Pulmonary magnetic resonance imaging for airway diseases. *J Thorac Imaging* 26: 301–316.

[29] Bhalla M, Turcios N, Aponte V et al. (1991) Cystic fibrosis: Scoring system with thin-section CT. *Radiology* 179: 783–788.

[30] Santamaria F, Grillo G, Guidi G et al. (1998) Cystic fibrosis: When should high-resolution computed tomography of the chest be obtained? *Pediatrics* 101: 908–913.

[31] Helbich TH, Heinz-Peer G, Eichler I et al. (1999) Cystic fibrosis: CT assessment of lung involvement in children and adults. *Radiology* 213: 537–544.

[32] Brody AS, Kosorok MR, Li Z et al. (2006) Reproducibility of a scoring system for computed tomography scanning in cystic fibrosis. *J Thorac Imaging* 21: 14–21.

[33] De Jong PA, Tiddens HA (2007) Cystic fibrosis specific computed tomography scoring. *Proc Am Thorac Soc* 4: 338–342.

[34] Puderbach M, Eichinger M, Haeselbarth J et al. (2007) Assessment of morphological MRI for pulmonary changes in cystic fibrosis (CF) patients: Comparison to thin-section CT and chest x-ray. *Invest Radiol* 42: 715–725.

[35] Edelman RR, Hatabu H, Tadamura E et al. (1996) Noninvasive assessment of regional ventilation in the human lung using oxygen-enhanced magnetic resonance imaging. *Nature Med* 2: 1236–1239.

[36] Jakob PM, Wang T, Schultz G, Hebestreit H, Hebestreit A, Hahn D (2004) Assessment of human pulmonary function using oxygen-enhanced T(1) imaging in patients with cystic fibrosis. *Magn Reson Med* 51: 1009–1016.

[37] Ohno Y, Koyama H, Matsumoto K et al. (2011) Oxygen enhanced MRI vs. quantitatively assessed thin-section CT: Pulmonary functional loss assessment and clinical stage classification of asthmatics. *Eur J Radiol* 77: 85–91.

[38] Mishima M, Oku Y, Kawakami K et al. (1997) Quantitative assessment of the spatial distribution of low attenuation areas on X-ray CT using texture analysis in patients with chronic pulmonary emphysema. *Front Med Biol Eng* 8: 19–34.

[39] Madani A, Keyzer C, Gevenois PA (2001) Quantitative computed tomography assessment of lung structure and function in pulmonary emphysema. *Eur Respir J* 18: 720–730.

[40] Goldin JG (2004) Quantitative CT of emphysema and the airways. *J Thorac Imaging* 19: 235–240.

[41] Coxson HO, Rogers RM (2005) Quantitative computed tomography of chronic obstructive pulmonary disease. *Acad Radiol* 12: 1457–1463.

[42] Hoffman EA, Simon BA, McLennan G (2006) State of the Art. A structural and functional assessment of the lung via multidetector-row computed tomography: Phenotyping chronic obstructive pulmonary disease. *Proc Am Thorac Soc* 3: 519–532.

[43] Matsuoka S, Yamashiro T, Washko GR, Kurihara Y, Nakajima Y, Hatabu H (2010) Quantitative CT assessment of chronic obstructive pulmonary disease. *RadioGraphics* 30: 55–66.

[44] Bankier AA, O'Donnell CR, Mai VM et al. (2004) Impact of lung volume on MR signal intensity changes of the lung parenchyma. *J Magn Reson Imaging* 20: 961–966.

[45] Ohno Y, Hatabu H, Murase K et al. (2004) Quantitative assessment of regional pulmonary perfusion in the entire lung using three-dimensional ultrafast dynamic contrast enhanced magnetic resonance imaging: Preliminary experience in 40 subjects. *J Magn Reson Imaging* 20: 353–365.

[46] Morino S, Toba T, Araki M et al. (2006) Noninvasive assessment of pulmonary emphysema using dynamic contrast enhanced magnetic resonance imaging. *Exp Lung Res* 32: 55–67.

[47] Jang YM, Oh YM, Seo JB et al. (2008) Quantitatively assessed dynamic contrast-enhanced magnetic resonance imaging in patients with chronic obstructive pulmonary disease: Correlation of perfusion parameters with pulmonary function test and quantitative computed tomography. *Invest Radiol* 43: 403–410.

[48] Sergiacomi G, Bolacchi F, Cadioli M et al. (2010) Combined pulmonary fibrosis and emphysema: 3D time-resolved MR angiographic evaluation of pulmonary arterial mean transit time and time to peak enhancement. *Radiology* 254: 601–608.

[49] Ohno Y, Hatabu H, Higashino T et al. (2004) Dynamic perfusion MRI versus perfusion scintigraphy: Prediction of postoperative lung function in patients with lung cancer. *AJR Am J Roentgenol*. 182: 73–78.

[50] Ohno Y, Koyama H, Nogami M et al. (2007) Postoperative lung function in lung cancer patients: Comparative analysis of predictive capability of MRI, CT, and SPECT. *AJR Am J Roentgenol*. 189: 400–408.

[51] Ohno Y, Koyama H, Nogami M et al. (2011) State-of-the art radiological techniques improve the assessment of postoperative lung function in patients with non-small cell lung cancer. *Eur J Radiol* 77: 97–104.

[52] Ohno Y, Hatabu H, Takenaka D et al. (2001) Oxygen enhanced MR ventilation imaging of the lung: Preliminary clinical experience in 25 subjects. *AJR Am J Roentgenol* 177: 185–194.

[53] Ohno Y, Hatabu H, Takenaka D, Van Cauteren M, Fujii M, Sugimura K (2002) Dynamic oxygen-enhanced MRI reflects

diffusing capacity of the lung. *Magn Reson Med* 47: 1139–1144.

[54] Ohno Y, Hatabu H, Higashino T et al. (2005) Oxygen enhanced MR imaging: Correlation with postsurgical lung function in patients with lung cancer. *Radiology* 236: 704–711.

[55] Ohno Y, Koyama H, Nogami M et al. (2008) Dynamic oxygen-enhanced MRI versus quantitative CT: Pulmonary functional loss assessment and clinical stage classification of smoking-related COPD. *AJR Am J Roentgenol* 190: W93–W99.

[56] Ohno Y, Iwasawa T, Seo JB et al. (2008) Oxygen-enhanced magnetic resonance imaging versus computed tomography: Multicenter study for clinical stage classification of smoking-related chronic obstructive pulmonary disease. *Am J Respir Crit Care Med.* 177: 1095–1102.

[57] Ohno Y, Koyama H, Yoshikawa T et al. (2012) Comparison of capability of dynamic O2-enhanced MRI and quantitative thin-section MDCT to assess COPD in smokers. *Eur J Radiol* 81: 1068–1075.

[58] Ohno Y, Nishio M, Koyama H et al. (2012) Oxygen-enhanced MRI, thin-section MDCT, and perfusion SPECT/CT: Comparison of clinical implications to patient care for lung volume reduction surgery. *AJR Am J Roentgenol.* 199: 794–802.

[59] Qanadli SD, Orvoen-Frija E, Lacombe P, Di Paola R, Bittoun J, Frija G (1999) Estimation of gas and tissue lung volumes by MRI: Functional approach of lung imaging. *J Comput Assist Tomogr* 23: 743–748.

[60] Suga K, Tsukuda T, Awaya H et al. (1999) Impaired respiratory mechanics in pulmonary emphysema: Evaluation with dynamic breathing MRI. *J Magn Reson Imaging* 10: 510–520.

[61] Suga K, Tsukuda T, Awaya H, Matsunaga N, Sugi K, Esato K (2000) Interactions of regional respiratory mechanics and pulmonary ventilatory impairment in pulmonary emphysema: Assessment with dynamic MRI and xenon 133 single-photon emission CT. *Chest* 117: 1646–1655.

[62] Iwasawa T, Yoshiike Y, Saito K, Kagei S, Gotoh T, Matsubara S (2000) Paradoxical motion of the hemidiaphragm in patients with emphysema. *J Thorac Imaging* 15: 191–195.

[63] Iwasawa T, Kagei S, Gotoh T et al. (2002) Magnetic resonance analysis of abnormal diaphragmatic motion in patients with emphysema. *Eur Respir J.* 19: 225–231.

[64] Iwasawa T, Takahashi H, Ogura T et al. (2011) Influence of the distribution of emphysema on diaphragmatic motion in patients with chronic obstructive pulmonary disease. *Jpn J Radiol* 29: 256–264.

[65] Shibata H, Iwasawa T, Gotoh T et al. (2012) Automatic tracking of the respiratory motion of lung parenchyma on dynamic magnetic resonance imaging: Comparison with pulmonary function tests in patients with chronic obstructive pulmonary disease. *J Thorac Imaging* 27: 387–392.

[66] Takahashi M, Togao O, Obara M et al. (2010) Ultra-short echo time (UTE) MR imaging of the lung: Comparison between normal and emphysematous lungs in mutant mice. *J Magn Reson Imaging* 32: 326–333.

[67] Ohno Y, Koyama H, Yoshikawa T et al. (2011) T2* measurements of 3-T MRI with ultrashort TEs: Capabilities of pulmonary function assessment and clinical stage classification in smokers. *AJR Am J Roentgenol* 197: W279–W285.

[68] Ohno Y, Nishio M, Koyama H et al. (2014) Pulmonary 3 T MRI with ultrashort TEs: Influence of ultrashort echo time interval on pulmonary functional and clinical stage assessments of smokers. *J Magn Reson Imaging* 39: 988–997.

[69] Ost D, Fein AM, Feinsilver SH (2003) Clinical practice. The solitary pulmonary nodule. *N Engl J Med* 348: 2535–2542.

[70] National Lung Screening Trial Research Team, Aberle DR, Adams AM, Berg CD et al. (2011) Reduced lung cancer mortality with low-dose computed tomographic screening. *N Engl J Med* 365: 395–409.

[71] Patz EF Jr, Lowe VJ, Hoffman JM et al. (1993) Focal pulmonary abnormalities: Evaluation with F-18 fluorode oxyglucose PET scanning. *Radiology* 188: 487–490.

[72] Dewan NA, Gupta NC, Redepenning LS, Phalen JJ, Frick MP (1993) Diagnostic efficacy of PET-FDG imaging in solitary pulmonary nodules. Potential role in evaluation and management. *Chest* 104: 997–1002.

[73] Croft DR, Trapp J, Kernstine K et al. (2002) FDG-PET imaging and the diagnosis of non-small cell lung cancer in a region of high histoplasmosis prevalence. *Lung Cancer* 36: 297–301.

[74] Chun EJ, Lee HJ, Kang WJ et al. (2009) Differentiation between malignancy and inflammation in pulmonary groundglass nodules: The feasibility of integrated (18) F-FDG PET/CT. *Lung Cancer* 65: 180–186.

[75] Sakai F, Sone S, Maruyama A et al. (1992) Thin-rim enhancement in Gd-DTPA-enhanced magnetic resonance images of tuberculoma: A new finding of potential differential diagnostic importance. *J Thorac Imaging* 7: 64–69.

[76] Sakai F, Sone S, Kiyono K et al. (1994) MR of pulmonary hamartoma: Pathologic correlation. *J Thorac Imaging* 9: 51–55.

[77] Fujimoto K, Meno S, Nishimura H et al. (1994) Aspergilloma within cavitary lung cancer: MR imaging findings. *AJR Am J Roentgenol* 163: 565–567.

[78] Blum U, Windfuhr M, Buitrago-Tellez C et al. (1994) Invasive pulmonary aspergillosis. MRI, CT, and plain radiographic findings and their contribution for early diagnosis. *Chest* 106: 1156–1161.

[79] Chung MH, Lee HG, Kwon SS et al. (2000) MR imaging of solitary pulmonary lesion: Emphasis on tuberculomas and comparison with tumors. *J Magn Reson Imaging* 11: 629–637.

[80] Gaeta M, Vinci S, Minutoli F et al. (2002) CT and MRI findings of mucin-containing tumors and pseudotumors of the thorax: Pictorial review. *Eur Radiol* 12: 181–189.

[81] Ohno Y, Sugimura K, Hatabu H (2002) MR imaging of lung

cancer. *Eur J Radiol* 44: 172–181.
[82] Sieren JC, Ohno Y, Koyama H, Sugimura K, McLennan G (2010) Recent technological and application developments in computed tomography and magnetic resonance imaging for improved pulmonary nodule detection and lung cancer staging. *J Magn Reson Imaging* 32: 1353–1369.
[83] Koyama H, Ohno Y, Seki S (2013) Magnetic resonance imaging for lung cancer. *J Thorac Imaging* 28: 138–150.
[84] Koyama H, Ohno Y, Kono A et al. (2008) Quantitative and qualitative assessment of non-contrast-enhanced pulmonary MR imaging for management of pulmonary nodules in 161 subjects. *Eur Radiol* 18: 2120–2131.
[85] Mori T, Nomori H, Ikeda K et al. (2008) Diffusion-weighted magnetic resonance imaging for diagnosing malignant pulmonary nodules/masses: Comparison with positron emission tomography. *J Thorac Oncol* 3: 358–364.
[86] Satoh S, Kitazume Y, Ohdama S, Kimula Y, Taura S, Endo Y (2008) Can malignant and benign pulmonary nodules be differentiated with diffusion-weighted MRI? *AJR Am J Roentgenol* 191: 464–470.
[87] Uto T, Takehara Y, Nakamura Y et al. (2009) Higher sensitivity and specificity for diffusion-weighted imaging of malignant lung lesions without apparent diffusion coefficient quantification. *Radiology* 252: 247–254.
[88] Kono M, Adachi S, Kusumoto M, Sakai E (1993) Clinical utility of Gd-DTPA-enhanced magnetic resonance imaging in lung cancer. *J Thorac Imaging* 8: 18–26.
[89] Kusumoto M, Kono M, Adachi S et al. (1994) Gadopentetate-dimeglumine-enhanced magnetic resonance imaging for lung nodules. Differentiation of lung cancer and tuberculoma. *Invest Radiol* 29: S255–S256.
[90] Guckel C, Schnabel K, Deimling M, Steinbrich W (1996) Solitary pulmonary nodules: MR evaluation of enhancement patterns with contrast-enhanced dynamic snapshot gradient-echo imaging. *Radiology* 200: 681–686.
[91] Ohno Y, Hatabu H, Takenaka D, Adachi S, Kono M, Sugimura K (2002) Solitary pulmonary nodules: Potential role of dynamic MR imaging in management initial experience. *Radiology* 224: 503–511.
[92] Fujimoto K, Abe T, Muller NL et al. (2003) Small peripheral pulmonary carcinomas evaluated with dynamic MR imaging: Correlation with tumor vascularity and prognosis. *Radiology* 227: 786–793.
[93] Ohno Y, Hatabu H, Takenaka D et al. (2004) Dynamic MR imaging: Value of differentiating subtypes of peripheral small adenocarcinoma of the lung. *Eur J Radiol* 52: 144–150.
[94] Schaefer JF, Vollmar J, Schick F et al. (2004) Solitary pulmo-nary nodules: Dynamic contrast-enhanced MR imaging-perfusion differences in malignant and benign lesions. *Radiology* 232: 544–553.
[95] Schaefer JF, Schneider V, Vollmar J et al. (2006) Solitary pulmonary nodules: Association between signal characteristics in dynamic contrast enhanced MRI and tumor angiogenesis. *Lung Cancer* 53: 39–49.
[96] Kono R, Fujimoto K, Terasaki H et al. (2007) Dynamic MRI of solitary pulmonary nodules: Comparison of enhancement patterns of malignant and benign small peripheral lung lesions. *AJR Am J Roentgenol* 188: 26–36.
[97] Ohno Y, Koyama H, Takenaka D et al. (2008) Dynamic MRI, dynamic multidetector-row computed tomography (MDCT), and coregistered 2-[fluorine-18]-fluoro-2-deoxy d-glucose-positron emission tomography (FDG-PET)/CT: Comparative study of capability for management of pulmonary nodules. *J Magn Reson Imaging* 27: 1284–1295.
[98] Cronin P, Dwamena BA, Kelly AM, Carlos RC (2008) Solitary pulmonary nodules: Meta-analytic comparison of cross-sectional imaging modalities for diagnosis of malignancy. *Radiology* 246: 772–782.
[99] Parkin DM, Bray F, Ferlay J, Pisani P (2005) Global cancer statistics, 2002. *CA Cancer J Clin* 55: 74–108.
[100] Melamed MR, Flehinger BJ, Zaman MB (1987) Impact of early detection on the clinical course of lung cancer. *Surg Clin North Am* 67: 909–924.
[101] Geddes DM (1979) The natural history of lung cancer: A review based on rates of tumour growth. *Br J Dis Chest* 73: 1–17.
[102] Spiro SG, Silvestri GA (2005) One hundred years of lung cancer. *Am J Respir Crit Care Med* 172: 523–529.
[103] Nahmias C, Hanna WT, Wahl LM et al. (2007) Time course of early response to chemotherapy in non–small cell lung can cer patients with 18F-FDG PET/CT. *J Nucl Med* 48: 744–751.
[104] Allen MS, Darling GE, Pechet TT et al.; ACOSOG Z0030 Study Group (2006) Morbidity and mortality of major pulmonary resections in patients with early-stage lung cancer: Initial results of the randomized, prospective ACOSOG Z0030 trial. *Ann Thorac Surg* 81: 1013–1019.
[105] Webb WR, Gatsonis C, Zerhouni EA et al. (1991) CT and MR imaging in staging non-small cell bronchogenic carcinoma: Report of the Radiologic Diagnostic Oncology Group. *Radiology* 178: 705–713.
[106] Baron RL, Levitt RG, Sagel SS, White MJ, Roper CL, Marbarger JP (1982) Computed tomography in the preoperative evaluation of bronchogenic carcinoma. *Radiology* 145: 727–732.
[107] Martini N, Heelan R, Westcott J et al. (1985) Comparative merits of conventional, computed tomographic, and magnetic resonance imaging in assessing mediastinal involvement in surgically confirmed lung carcinoma. *J Thorac Cardiovasc Surg* 90: 639–648.
[108] Rendina EA, Bognolo DA, Mineo TC et al. (1987) Compu- ted tomography for the evaluation of intrathoracic inva- sion by lung cancer. *J Thorac Cardiovasc Surg* 94: 57–63.
[109] Quint LE, Glazer GM, Orringer MB (1987) Central lung masses: Prediction with CT of need for pneumonectomy versus lobectomy. *Radiology* 165: 735–738.

[110] Glazer HS, Kaiser LR, Anderson DJ et al. (1989) Indeterminate mediastinal invasion in bronchogenic carcinoma: CT evaluation. *Radiology* 173: 37–42.

[111] Herman SJ, Winton TL, Weisbrod GL, Towers MJ, Mentzer SJ (1994) Mediastinal invasion by bronchogenic carcinoma: CT signs. *Radiology* 190: 841–846.

[112] White PG, Adams H, Crane MD, Butchart EG (1994) Preoperative staging of carcinoma of the bronchus: Can computed tomographic scanning reliably identify stage III tumours? *Thorax* 49: 951–957.

[113] Takahashi M, Shimoyama K, Murata K et al. (1997) Hilar and mediastinal invasion of bronchogenic carcinoma: Evaluation by thin-section electron-beam computed tomography. *J Thorac Imaging* 12: 195–199.

[114] Quint LE, Francis IR (1999) Radiologic staging of lung cancer. *J Thorac Imaging* 14: 235–246.

[115] Higashino T, Ohno Y, Takenaka D et al. (2005) Thin section multiplanar reformats from multidetector-row CT data: Utility for assessment of regional tumor extent in non-small cell lung cancer. *Eur J Radiol* 56: 48–55.

[116] Rapoport S, Blair DN, McCarthy SM, Desser TS, Hammers LW, Sostman HD (1988) Brachial plexus: Correlation of MR imaging with CT and pathologic findings. *Radiology* 167: 161–165.

[117] Heelan RT, Demas BE, Caravelli JF et al. (1989) Superior sulcus tumors: CT and MR imaging. *Radiology* 170: 637–641.

[118] Padovani B, Mouroux J, Seksik L et al. (1993) Chest wall invasion by bronchogenic carcinoma: Evaluation with MR imaging. *Radiology* 187: 33–38.

[119] Bonomo L, Ciccotosto C, Guidotti A, Storto ML (1996) Lung cancer staging: The role of computed tomography and magnetic resonance imaging. *Eur J Radiol* 23: 35–45.

[120] Freundlich IM, Chasen MH, Varma DG (1996) Magnetic resonance imaging of pulmonary apical tumors. *J Thorac Imaging* 11: 210–222.

[121] Takahashi K, Furuse M, Hanaoka H et al. (2000) Pulmonary vein and left atrial invasion by lung cancer: Assessment by breath-hold gadolinium-enhanced three-dimensional MR angiography. *J Comput Assist Tomogr* 24: 557–561.

[122] Ohno Y, Adachi S, Motoyama A et al. (2001) Multiphase ECG-triggered 3D contrast-enhanced MR angiography: Utility for evaluation of hilar and mediastinal invasion of bronchogenic carcinoma. *J Magn Reson Imaging* 13: 215–224.

[123] Sakai S, Murayama S, Murakami J, Hashiguchi N, Masuda K (1997) Bronchogenic carcinoma invasion of the chest wall: Evaluation with dynamic cine MRI during breathing. *J Comput Assist Tomogr* 21: 595–600.

[124] Glazer GM, Orringer MB, Gross BH, Quint LE (1984) The mediastinum in non-small cell lung cancer: CT-surgical correlation. *AJR Am J Roentgenol* 142: 1101–1105.

[125] Glazer GM, Gross BH, Aisen AM, Quint LE, Francis IR, Orringer MB (1985) Imaging of the pulmonary hilum: A prospective comparative study in patients with lung cancer. *AJR Am J Roentgenol* 145: 245–248.

[126] Musset D, Grenier P, Carette MF et al. (1986) Primary lung cancer staging: Prospective comparative study of MR imaging with CT. *Radiology* 160: 607–611.

[127] Poon PY, Bronskill MJ, Henkelman RM et al. (1987) Mediastinal lymph node metastases from bronchogenic carcinoma: Detection with MR imaging and CT. *Radiology* 162: 651–656.

[128] Laurent F, Drouillard J, Dorcier F et al. (1988) Bronchogenic carcinoma staging: CT versus MR imaging. Assessment with surgery. *Eur J Cardiothorac Surg* 2: 31–36.

[129] McLoud TC, Bourgouin PM, Greenberg RW et al. (1992) Bronchogenic carcinoma: Analysis of staging in the mediastinum with CT by correlative lymph node mapping and sampling. *Radiology* 182: 319–323.

[130] Dillemans B, Deneffe G, Verschakelen J, Decramer M (1994) Value of computed tomography and mediastinoscopy in preoperative evaluation of mediastinal nodes in non-small cell lung cancer. A study of 569 patients. *Eur J Cardiothorac Surg* 8: 37–42.

[131] Wahl RL, Quint LE, Greenough RL, Meyer CR, White RI, Orringer MB (1994) Staging of mediastinal non-small cell lung cancer with FDG PET, CT, and fusion images: Preliminary prospective evaluation. *Radiology* 191: 371–377.

[132] Patz EF, Jr., Lowe VJ, Goodman PC, Herndon J (1995) Thoracic nodal staging with PET imaging with 18FDG in patients with bronchogenic carcinoma. *Chest* 108: 1617–1621.

[133] Boiselle PM, Patz EF, Jr., Vining DJ, Weissleder R, Shepard JA, McLoud TC (1998) Imaging of mediastinal lymph nodes: CT, MR, and FDG PET. *RadioGraphics* 18: 1061–1069.

[134] Gupta NC, Graeber GM, Bishop HA (2000) Comparative efficacy of positron emission tomography with fluorodeoxyglucose in evaluation of small (<1 cm), intermediate (1 to 3 cm), and large (>3 cm) lymph node lesions. *Chest* 117: 773–778.

[135] Marom EM, Erasmus JJ, Patz EF (2000) Lung cancer and positron emission tomography with fluorodeoxyglucose. *Lung Cancer* 28: 187–202.

[136] Vansteenkiste JF (2002) Imaging in lung cancer: Positron emission tomography scan. *Eur Respir J Suppl* 35: S49–S60.

[137] Antoch G, Stattaus J, Nemat AT et al. (2003) Non-small cell lung cancer: Dual-modality PET/CT in preoperative staging. *Radiology* 229: 526–533.

[138] Acker MR, Burrell SC (2005) Utility of 18F-FDG PET in evaluating cancers of lung. *J Nucl Med Technol* 33: 69–74.

[139] Kim BT, Lee KS, Shim SS et al. (2006) Stage T1 non-small cell lung cancer: Preoperative mediastinal nodal stag-ing with integrated FDG PET/CT—A prospective study. *Radiology* 241: 501–509.

[140] Bruzzi JF, Munden RF (2006) PET/CT imaging of lung

[141] Kligerman S, Digumarthy S (2009) Staging of non-small cell lung cancer using integrated PET/CT. *AJR Am J Roentgenol* 193: 1203–1211.

[142] Billé A, Pelosi E, Skanjeti A et al. (2009) Preoperative intrathoracic lymph node staging in patients with non small-cell lung cancer: Accuracy of integrated positron emission tomography and computed tomography. *Eur J Cardiothorac Surg* 36: 440–445.

[143] Fischer B, Lassen U, Mortensen J et al. (2009) Preoperative staging of lung cancer with combined PET-CT. *N Engl J Med* 361: 32–39.

[144] Takenaka D, Ohno Y, Hatabu H et al. (2002) Differentiation of metastatic versus non-metastatic mediastinal lymph nodes in patients with non-small cell lung cancer using respiratory-triggered short inversion time inversion recovery (STIR) turbo spin-echo MR imaging. *Eur J Radiol* 44: 216–224.

[145] Ohno Y, Hatabu H, Takenaka D et al. (2004) Metastases in mediastinal and hilar lymph nodes in patients with non-small cell lung cancer: Quantitative and qualitative assessment with STIR turbo spin-echo MR imaging. *Radiology* 231: 872–879.

[146] Ohno Y, Koyama H, Nogami M et al. (2007) STIR turbo SE MR imaging vs. coregistered FDG-PET/CT: Quantitative and qualitative assessment of N-stage in non-small-cell lung cancer patients. *J Magn Reson Imaging* 26: 1071–1080.

[147] Yi CA, Shin KM, Lee KS et al. (2008) Non-small cell lung cancer staging: Efficacy comparison of integrated PET/CT versus 3.0-T whole-body MR imaging. *Radiology* 248: 632–642.

[148] Morikawa M, Demura Y, Ishizaki T et al. (2009) The effectiveness of 18F-FDG PET/CT combined with STIR MRI for diagnosing nodal involvement in the thorax. *J Nucl Med* 50: 81–87.

[149] Ohno Y, Koyama H, Yoshikawa T et al. (2011) N stage disease in patients with non-small cell lung cancer: Efficacy of quantitative and qualitative assessment with STIR turbo spin-echo imaging, diffusion-weighted MR imaging, and fluorodeoxyglucose PET/CT. *Radiology* 261: 605–615.

[150] Nomori H, Mori T, Ikeda K et al. (2008) Diffusion weighted magnetic resonance imaging can be used in place of positron emission tomography for N staging of non-small cell lung cancer with fewer false-positive results. *J Thorac Cardiovasc Surg* 135: 816–822.

[151] Hasegawa I, Boiselle PM, Kuwabara K, Sawafuji M, Sugiura H (2008) Mediastinal lymph nodes in patients with non-small cell lung cancer: Preliminary experience with diffusion-weighted MR imaging. *J Thorac Imaging* 23: 157–161.

[152] Pauls S, Schmidt SA, Juchems MS et al. (2012) Diffusion weighted MR imaging in comparison to integrated [^{18}F]-FDG PET/CT for N-staging in patients with lung cancer. *Eur J Radiol* 81: 178–182.

[153] Quint LE, Tummala S, Brisson LJ et al. (1996) Distribution of distant metastases from newly diagnosed non-small cell lung cancer. *Ann Thorac Surg* 62: 246–250.

[154] Pantel K, Izbicki J, Passlick B et al. (1996) Frequency and prognostic significance of isolated tumour cells in bone marrow of patients with non-small-cell lung cancer without overt metastases. *Lancet* 347: 649–653.

[155] Silvestri GA, Gould MK, Margolis ML et al.; American College of Chest Physicians (2007) Noninvasive staging of non-small cell lung cancer: ACCP evidenced-based clinical practice guidelines (2nd edition). *Chest* 132(3 Suppl.): 178S–201S.

[156] Simon GR, Turrisi A; American College of Chest Physicians (2007) Management of small cell lung cancer: ACCP evidence-based clinical practice guidelines (2nd edition). *Chest* 132: S324–S339.

[157] Samson DJ, Seidenfeld J, Simon GR et al.; American College of Chest Physicians (2007) Evidence for management of small cell lung cancer: ACCP evidence-based clinical practice guidelines (2nd edition). *Chest* 132: S314–S323.

[158] Ohno Y, Koyama H, Nogami M et al. (2007) Whole-body MR imaging vs. FDG-PET: Comparison of accuracy of M-stage diagnosis for lung cancer patients. *J Magn Reson Imaging* 26: 498–509.

[159] Ohno Y, Koyama H, Onishi Y et al. (2008) Non-small cell lung cancer: Whole-body MR examination for M-stage assessment–utility for whole-body diffusion-weighted imaging compared with integrated FDG PET/CT. *Radiology* 248: 643–654.

[160] Takenaka D, Ohno Y, Matsumoto K et al. (2009) Detection of bone metastases in non-small cell lung cancer patients: Comparison of whole-body diffusion-weighted imaging (DWI), whole-body MR imaging without and with DWI, whole-body FDG-PET/CT, and bone scintigraphy. *J Magn Reson Imaging* 30: 298–308.

[161] Sommer G, Wiese M, Winter L et al. (2012) Preoperative staging of non-small-cell lung cancer: Comparison of whole-body diffusion-weighted magnetic resonance imaging and 18F-fluorodeoxyglucose-positron emission tomography/computed tomography. *Eur Radiol* 22: 2859–2867.

[162] Ohno Y, Nishio M, Koyama H et al. (2013) Comparison of the utility of whole-body MRI with and without contrast-enhanced Quick 3D and double RF fat suppression techniques, conventional whole-body MRI, PET/CT and conventional examination for assessment of recurrence in NSCLC patients. *Eur J Radiol* 82: 2018–2027.

[163] Travis WD, Costabel U, Hansell DM et al.; ATS/ERS Committee on Idiopathic Interstitial Pneumonias (2013) An official American Thoracic Society/European Respiratory Society statement: Update of the international multidisciplinary classification of the idiopathic interstitial pneumonias. *Am J Respir Crit Care Med* 188: 733–748.

[164] Puderbach M, Hintze C, Ley S, Eichinger M, Kauczor HU,

Biederer J (2007) MR imaging of the chest: A practical approach at 1.5T. *Eur J Radiol* 64: 345–355.

[165] Biederer J, Both M, Graessner J et al. (2003) Lung morphology: Fast MR imaging assessment with a volumetric interpolated breath-hold technique: Initial experience with patients. *Radiology* 226: 242–249.

[166] Lutterbey G, Grohé C, Gieseke J (2007) Initial experience with lung-MRI at 3.0T: Comparison with CT and clinical data in the evaluation of interstitial lung disease activity. *Eur J Radiol* 61: 256–261.

[167] Yi CA, Lee KS, Han J, Chung MP, Chung MJ, Shin KM (2008) 3-T MRI for differentiating inflammation and fibrosis-predominant lesions of usual and nonspecific interstitial pneumonia: Comparison study with pathologic correlation. *AJR Am J Roentgenol* 190: 878–885.

[168] Rajaram S, Swift AJ, Capener D et al. (2012) Lung morphology assessment with balanced steady-state free precession MR imaging compared with CT. *Radiology* 263: 569–577.

[169] Semelka RC, Cem Balci N, Wilber KP et al. (2000) Breath-hold 3D gradient-echo MR imaging of the lung parenchyma: Evaluation of reproducibility of image quality in normals and preliminary observations in patients with disease. *J Magn Reson Imaging* 11: 195–200.

[170] Karabulut N, Martin DR, Yang M, Tallaksen RJ (2002) MR imaging of the chest using a contrast-enhanced breath-hold modified three-dimensional gradient-echo technique: Comparison with two-dimensional gradient-echo technique and multidetector CT. *AJR Am J Roentgenol* 179: 1225–1233.

[171] Johnson KM, Fain SB, Schiebler ML, Nagle S (2013) Optimized 3D ultrashort echo time pulmonary MRI. *Magn Reson Med* 70: 1241–1250.

[172] Molinari F, Eichinger M, Risse F et al. Navigator-triggered oxygen-enhanced MRI with simultaneous cardiac and respiratory synchronization for the assessment of interstitial lung disease. *J Magn Reson Imaging* 26: 1523–1529.

[173] Ohno Y, Nishio M, Koyama H et al. (2014) Oxygen enhanced MRI for patients with connective tissue diseases: Comparison with thin-section CT of capability for pulmonary functional and disease severity assessment. *Eur J Radiol* 83: 391–397.

[174] Ohno Y, Nishio M, Koyama H et al. (2013) Pulmonary MR imaging with ultra-short TEs: Utility for disease severity assessment of connective tissue disease patients. *Eur J Radiol* 82: 1359–1365.

[175] White RI Jr, Pollak JS, Wirth JA (1996) Pulmonary arteriovenous malformations: Diagnosis and transcatheter embolotherapy. *J Vasc Interv Radiol* 7: 787–804.

[176] Terry PB, Barth KH, Kaufman SL et al. (1980) Balloon embolization for treatment of pulmonary arteriovenous fistulas. *N Engl J Med* 302: 1189–1190.

[177] White RI Jr., Lynch-Nyhan A, Terry P et al. (1988) Pulmonary arteriovenous malformations: Techniques and long-term outcome of embolotherapy. *Radiology* 69: 663–669.

[178] Hartnell GG, Jackson JE, Allison DJ (1990) Coil embolization of pulmonary arteriovenous malformations. *Cardiovasc Intervent Radiol* 13: 347–350.

[179] Remy J, Remy-Jardin M, Wattinne L, Deffontaines C (1992) Pulmonary arteriovenous malformations: Evaluation with CT of the chest before and after treatment. *Radiology* 182: 809–816.

[180] Remy J, Remy-Jardin M, Giraud F, Wattinne L (1994) Angio architecture of pulmonary arteriovenous malformations: Clinical utility of three-dimensional helical CT. *Radiology* 191: 657–664.

[181] Remy-Jardin M, Dumont P, Brillet PY, Dupuis P, Duhamel A, Remy J (2006) Pulmonary arteriovenous malformations treated with embolotherapy: Helical CT evaluation of long-term effectiveness after 2-21-year fol low-up. *Radiology* 239: 576–585.

[182] Brillet PY, Dumont P, Bouaziz N et al. (2007) Pulmonary arteriovenous malformation treated with embolotherapy: Systemic collateral supply at multidetector CT angiography after 2-20-year follow-up. *Radiology* 242: 267–276.

[183] Ohno Y, Hatabu H, Takenaka D, Adachi S, Hirota S, Sugimura K (2002) Contrast-enhanced MR perfusion imaging and MR angiography: Utility for management of pulmonary arteriovenous malformations for embolo therapy. *Eur J Radiol* 41: 136–146.

[184] Naidich DP, Rumancik WM, Lefleur RS, Estioko MR, Brown SM (1987) Intralobar pulmonary sequestration: MR evaluation. *J Comput Assist Tomogr* 11: 31–33.

[185] Au VW, Chan JK, Chan FL (1999) Pulmonary sequestration diagnosed by contrast enhanced three-dimensional MR angiography. *Br J Radiol* 72: 709–711.

[186] Lehnhardt S, Winterer JT, Uhrmeister P, Herget G, Laubenberger J (2002) Pulmonary sequestration: Demonstration of blood supply with 2D and 3D MR angiography. *Eur J Radiol* 44: 28–32.

[187] Sancak T, Cangir AK, Atasoy C, Ozdemir N (2003) The role of contrast enhanced three-dimensional MR angiography in pulmonary sequestration. *Interact Cardiovasc Thorac Surg* 2: 480–482.

[188] Epelman M, Kreiger PA, Servaes S, Victoria T, Hellinger JC (2010) Current imaging of prenatally diagnosed congenital lung lesions. *Semin Ultrasound CT MR* 31: 141–157.

Chapter 11
磁共振成像在肺部的临床应用

Clinical Magnetic Resonance Imaging Applications for the Lung

Mark O. Wielpütz, Jim M. Wild, Grzegorz Bauman, Edwin J.R. van Beek, Jürgen Biederer 著

隋 昕 译

宋 伟 校

目录 CONTENTS

一、肺部磁共振成像的物理学特点（从磁共振扫描仪角度）/ 210

二、肺部 MR 序列 / 217

三、现有技术的临床应用 / 223

近年来，磁共振成像（MRI）逐渐应用于肺部疾病的临床诊断。胸片和 CT 是标准化、全面的三维肺部成像技术，继胸片和 CT 后，MRI 在应用于一些特殊肺部病例时，逐渐被认为是一种可选择的、补充的影像学方法。一旦广泛应用，对于应严格避免暴露于电离辐射的人群，包括儿童、孕妇和需要长时间反复随访的患者，MRI 可显著降低辐射剂量和治疗负担，它可能成为常规影像学检查方法。

MRI 在一次检查中结合了结构和功能成像，并且有可能在不久的将来提供代谢分子成像信息。MRI 在肺形态学的关键技术是检测组织和液体中质子即 ^1H 的自旋共振信号。基本脉冲序列可以被肺和血管系统中的生理过程激活。它可反复多次测量评估胸腔内脏器和大血管的运动过程，例如肺膨胀、血液流动等。MRI 在心脏的应用很好地体现了 MR 的优势。随着近期技术的进步，MRI 有望克服其主要缺陷，即质子密度低和由于空气 - 组织界面处信号减低导致的磁敏感伪影。针对特定临床需求（结节检测，肺炎和肺栓塞）采用一系列脉冲序列，并测试了图像质量和诊断准确性的稳定性和可重复性。吸入气体超极化氦 -3 和氙 -129，也可产生磁共振信号，代替氢质子 MRI 成像，提供组织结构成像信息。

尽管 MRI 有上述优势，但是目前 MRI 仍存在各种不足限制其临床广泛应用，包括 MRI 检查时间过长，缺乏标准化的、统一的、满足临床需求的定制序列，缺乏有经验的放射科医师和临床相关医师。由于新用户在自己的平台上难以完成合适的扫描序列，本章拟说明：①是解释通过 MR 获得肺部图像的物理挑战。现有技术方面，MRI 脉冲序列、射频（radio frequency，RF）线圈和肺部 MRI 成像所需的肺实质和脉管系统概述，参见"二"；②说明可实施且有效的、适用于特定临床需求的，而非特定的供应商、目前最先进的 MRI 序列，参见"三"；③解释当前肺部 MRI 在临床应用中的优缺点，参见"四"；④概述肺部 MRI 的临床发展前景。本章基于 3 篇已经发表的综述，并进一步扩展到近期出版的有关肺 MRI 的文献[1-3]。有关肺部功能成像、肺栓塞的检查和肺灌注成像请参阅第 13 章。

一、肺部磁共振成像的物理学特点（从磁共振扫描仪角度）

肺实质的物理学特征与身体其他组织，如肝脏和脑组织，有很大不同[1]；从 MR 成像的角度来看，肺部两个重要特征是低质子密度和肺组织、空气间的磁敏感性不同。在健康人的肺组织中，组织密度为 $0.1 \sim 0.2 g/cm^3$，仅为其他组织的 1/10。由于 MR 信号与组织质子密度成正比，即使在完美的成像条件下（即忽略弛豫效应），邻近组织的 MR 信号比肺组织的 MR 信号高 5 ~ 10 倍。低信噪比（signal-noise ratio，SNR）为质子 MRI 显示肺部微结构带来极大挑战：为了增加 SNR，可采用信号平均技术，但是增加了图像采集时间，不利于临床应用。通过使用扩大的体素尺寸可以增加 SNR，但是，部分容积效应会导致较小的病变如肺野外周部的肺转移病变漏诊。空气中的氧气是顺磁性的，组织是反磁性的，导致肺 - 空气界面处的磁化率差异（$\Delta \chi = 8ppm$）。在每个组织界面处，磁化率差异形成静态局部场梯度。由气道和肺泡在肺中形成多个微观表面，多小于 2 ~ 5mm 成像体素，产生高度不均匀的局部磁性梯度。这些微观梯度导致梯度回波（gradient recalled echo，GRE）成像中出现快速去相位，该信号衰减通常用表观横向弛豫时间 T_2^* 描述，其在 $B_0=1.5T$ 时可缩短至 2ms 或更短。因此，肺 MRI 的 GRE 序列非常具有挑战性，需要短回波时间（TE<1 ~ 2ms）的脉冲序列。磁场不均匀性随着 B_0 的增加而增长，如果应用 3T 磁共振检查需要更短的 T_2^*，约 0.5ms[4]。由于需要缩短 TE，通常无法实性从 1.5T 到 3T 对 SNR 增长的预期。使用相同的脉冲序列，只有采用更强的梯度系统才能实现更短的 TE，但目前的 3T MR 通常使用与高端 1.5T 相同的梯度单位。

B_0=0.5T 或更低的低场 MRI 对肺部在磁性不均匀性方面具有潜在优势[4]，并且有希望应用低场 MRI 代替非电离的胸部 X 线检查[5]。但是低场强 MRI 需要信号平均技术来提高信噪比，导致成像时间延长，不利于临床应用。

因此，本章所示的方法主要是基于 1.5T 场强，因为它代表了肺部 MRI 的现有和可实现的最佳场强。

这里概述的大多数成像方法通常屏气时间小于 20s。屏气可于呼气末，亦可于深吸气末期。肺组织膨胀的状态有一定作用，呼气时肺实质的信号强度更高[6,7]。在呼气相，肺实质的质子密度增加，并且随着空气排出，体积磁化率差异减小。另一方面，深吸气相的成像可以提供更暗的背景，有利于提高肺血管或结节之间的对比噪声。

为了在呼吸期间获取特定时相的可靠图像（如深吸气相），可以使用肺量计触发和呼吸门控。在 MRI 中使用外部硬件或肺自身 MR 信号获取与肺的呼吸状态成比例的信号，可以将图像采集同步到呼吸循环中。MR 制造商通常为此提供了气动波纹管，当然 MR 兼容的呼吸速度描记器也有上述功能[8]。

导航回波可通过 MRI 直接测量呼吸运动。应用特定的 90°～180° 自旋回波激励或笔形束测量与膈肌基底部垂直的 MR 信号。亚秒导航扫描被整合到成像序列中以提供运动信息。因此，监测膈肌运动可用于在自由呼吸期间回顾性的门控[9]。只要采集时间与膈肌运动相比较快，导航信号也可以从自由呼吸的非门控二维（2D）肺图像中获取。还可采用最初为心脏成像设定的自导航序列[10]获取运动信息。额外的快速信号且没有空间编码的信号变化，易于并入其他成像序列。自导航器信号反映了与呼吸运动相关的肺信号的周期性变化，用于对采集数据进行回顾性分类。

（一）肺部图像的采集技术

1. 肺部并行采集成像　在 1.5T 的场强下，MR 的大体线圈提供相对均匀的发射场，在肺 FOV 上提供均匀的翻转角。在 3T 磁共振场强下，RF 波长较短导致胸腔内的翻转角不均匀。原则上，体线圈可以用作肺成像的接收线圈，但是使用专门针对胸部 MRI 优化的局部接收线圈可显著提高 SNR。通常，胸部 MR 线圈包括前、后两部分，前部为柔性部分，后部为嵌入患者检查床的部分。线圈阵列由 2～16 个线圈单元组成，具体取决于接收通道的数量。线圈单元排列成行和列，以便实现并行采集在各个方向上快速获取图像。

并行采集成像方法[11,12]利用空间线圈阵列的敏感性通过加速因子 R 获取图像（参阅第 1 章）。如果线圈单元的敏感度在空间上是离散的，则每个线圈阵列已具有 MR 固有空间信号编码。并行采集在肺部 MRI 检查中至关重要，可实现快速采集图像，减少屏气时间，提高时间分辨率。尤其在单次激发快速自旋回波（single shot fast spin echo，SSFSE）序列中，可缩短回波链长度[13]和相关的 K 空间滤波器，从而减少模糊效应。在 3T 磁场中，并行采集可降低 SSFSE 序列的射频特定吸收率（specific absorptionrate，SAR），缩短回波时间[14]。

然而，应谨慎使用并行采集序列，因为并行采集提高检查速度是以降低 SNR 为代价：SNR 随着 R 增加而降低，并且 g 因子噪声增大而进一步降低 SNR。由于肺实质 SNR 较低，在心脏成像中使用较高的加速因子 R>4，无法获得肺部成像。多元素的线圈对于肺的并行成像不是必需的（即使它们有助于增加局部 SNR），加速因子 R≈2，在相位编码或层厚选择/编码方向是合适的。并行采集成像的重要细节是线圈敏感性的校准，确定用于图像重建的线圈的敏感性。由于呼吸运动，优选具有整合或自动校准的方法［例如，一般性自动校准并行采集（general－ized autocalibrating partially parallel acquisition，GRAPPA）、敏感度编码技术（sensitivity encoding，SENSE）和可变的容积加速（FLEX）］。由于校准信息与成像数据在空间上不匹配，单独的敏感性扫描的序列容易产生伪影。

2. 脉冲序列 现代MR系统配备梯度系统，梯度强度为40mT/m或更高，压摆率超过200mT/（m·ms），达到1～3mm的空间分辨率，需要使用短回波时间TE＜1.5ms的GRE序列。在1.5T时，可获得纤维化和肺实质密度的图像。应用并行采集成像方法使得三种基本序列可应用于肺部成像，它们均具有短TE、采集时间短的共同特征[11]。它们可以在有或没有呼吸门控下使用，因此在自由呼吸或屏气时均可获得图像。

3. 毁损GRE 毁损GRE序列[快速低角度拍摄（fast low angle shot，FLASH）、变质梯度反弹回波成像（spoiled phase gradient echo，SPGR）和快速回波（fast field echo，FFE）]在概念上是最简单的脉冲成像序列，在临床广泛应用。本质上，该序列以低角度RF脉冲（α＜90°）激发后获得GRE，在数据获取后破坏剩余的磁化。该序列为固有T_2^*加权，取决于TR和α，可获得额外的自旋密度加权或T_1加权。由于肺T_2^*值较短，需要使用1ms或更短的TE获得肺实质信号。此外，需要施加非常低的角度α＜10°，应用相对长但是最小化的T_1加权序列获得肺实质图像（在1.5T时为1300ms）。在频率编码方向上使用非对称回波（约30%）和部分傅里叶重建，带宽＞60kHz，可满足TE约为1ms。

该序列在肺部MRI广泛应用，可获得解剖成像，获得有或无脂肪抑制的2D和3D图像。首先，无脂肪抑制的非对比增强图像，以便检出纵隔脂肪包围的淋巴结。注射后T_1-缩短对比剂[例如，Gadolinium-DTPA（Gd-DTPA）]应用脂肪抑制技术，使淋巴结在纵隔脂肪的抑制背景中显示出来[15]。GRE序列联合并行采集成像方法和（或）切片内插技术[例如，体积内插屏气检查（volume interpolated breath-holdexamination，VIBE）]能够在屏气时快速获得层厚5mm全肺的图像。低分辨率的动态重复采集提供了一种强有力的胸壁运动评估方法，用于研究动态肺容积[16]，放疗中的肿瘤运动[17]和反常的膈肌运动。

由于高翻转角度可抑制非增强区的信号，所以具有短TR和高α的重T_1加权3D毁损GRE序列是肺中任何对比度增强结构成像的基础。肺MR血管造影和灌注成像的序列参数将在"二（二）"中讨论。

4. 平衡稳态自由进动 平衡稳态自由进动（flow-sensitive dephasing magnetization preparation，bSSFP）序列[稳态进动的真正快速成像序列（true fast imaging with steady state precession，TrueFISP）、稳态采集的快速成像序列（fast imaging employing steady state acquisition，FIESTA）和屏气快速编码（BFE）]在结构上与毁损GRE序列相似；但它不会破坏而是在每个TR间隔结束时重新聚焦横向磁化，可更有效地利用磁化强度。通过交替相位RF脉冲（即反复翻转磁化），在每个TR内，所有梯度失相被重新聚焦（平衡）达到高度相干的稳态。与毁损GRE序列相比，横向相干的传播导致更复杂的对比度行为，并且对于短TR，对比度与T_2/T_1成正比例。这些序列使用较大的翻转角（约70°），使MR信号更强，SAR值更大。对于更高的TR值，bSSFP序列易受非共振和场不均匀性的影响，出现带状伪影，出现一些暗带。快速bSSFP序列已在心脏MRI中广泛应用，也可应用于肺部成像。bSSFP序列与毁损GRE序列相似，采用短TE和TR，适合在屏气的时间窗内快速成像。通常使用100kHz的高带宽最大化磁化回收并最小化TR，减小非共振带状伪像的大小。例如，最近出现了TR＜1ms的超快SSFP[18]。固有的T_2/T_1对比度使其与长T_2序列[19]相比，有利于血液和黏液成像。此外，多层或3D bSSFP序列应用于快速和无对比剂的肺血管成像[20]和最近刚证实的膈肌门控的超短径3D bSSFP序列[21]。

5. 单次快速自旋回波（RARE/HASTE和Turbo FSE） SSFSE序列或弛豫增强快速采集（rapid acquisition with relaxation enhancement，RARE）序列[RARE/半傅里叶采集单发涡轮自

旋回波（half-Fourior acquisition single-shot turbo spin echo，HASTE）和涡轮快速自旋回波（turbo fast spin echo，Turbo FSE）][22] 使用自旋回波（与使用 GRE 的 FLASH 和 bSSFP 相比），在概念上与以往的成像序列不同。为了使自旋回波采集适合于快速成像，通过第一自旋回波的重复聚焦产生一系列自旋回波。从而，K 空间中的所有线都在单个回波串中获得。SSFSE 序列有利于肺成像，因为 180°脉冲序列重新聚焦在任何场不均匀性上，使得图像变为 T_2 加权。T_2 加权的程度由中心 K 空间线的回波时间（有效 TE）决定，可通过选择不同的 K 空间采样模式调整。肺实质 T_2 的回声时间（1.5T 时约 40ms）仍然适合肺成像。与梯度回波序列所需的亚毫秒回波时间相比，长 TE 更容易实现。但是，内部回声间距约为 4ms，192 个相位编码的典型回波链仍然为 192×4ms = 768ms。在回波链的后期 T_2 衰减将导致信号减弱。相位编码方向上的 T_2 衰减还导致 K 空间中的滤波效果，使图像模糊。可通过半傅里叶编码，矩形 FOV 选择组合（例如，在轴位上选择前后方向上相位编码）和平行成像，减少测量的 K 空间行数。SSFSE 回波链中的大量 180°脉冲也导致大量的能量沉积（高 SAR 水平），SAR 随着场强而增加，使得 SSFSE 难以在 3T 上使用。

另一种降低相位编码方向上的模糊效应是 K 空间的分割，不是所有 K 空间线都在一个回波链中获得，只对一小部分 N 进行采样，并且重复采集 N 次以覆盖整个 K 空间。K 空间分割显著延长了采集时间，为了获得 1mm 或更好的空间分辨率，不配合的患者需要呼吸触发采集。SSFSE 序列可以与磁化准备模块组合，如脂肪饱和度，反转恢复，或扩散加权，以增加图像对比度。

6. 超短回波时间成像 最初由 Bergin 等[23]提出对肺实质成像，采用超短回波时间（ultra short echo time,UTE）序列，使径向 K 空间采样回波时间缩短至低于 1ms。当 100μs 或更短的 TE 时，肺实质的短 T_2^* 不是约束，并且可以获得对肺实质敏感的 MR 图像。二维 UTE 序列[23]需要 2 倍 RF 脉冲，导致采集时间加倍，才可达到层厚的需求。此外，在频率编码方向上肺实质 T_2^* 信号衰减引入 K 空间滤波器（类似于 SSFSE 成像中的相位编码方向），限制了其空间分辨率。分辨率远低于标称分辨率。然而，UTE 成像有望应用于肺部 MRI，质子密度对比成像类似于胸部 CT。最近，自由呼吸、呼吸门控 3D 扫描可改善肺实质的图像质量[24]。该序列有应用于肺部破坏性病变的潜力，如肺气肿，以往 MRI 序列尚无法做到。

（二）对比度增强

钆对比剂

通过静脉注射缩短 T_1 弛豫时间的对比剂（如 Gd-DTPA），经屏气的重 T_1 加权 3D GRE 序列，可获得高质量的肺血管成像。高分辨率 3D 肺部 MR 血管造影的首选脉冲序列是损毁 GRE 序列（FLASH、SPGR 和 FFE），具有尽可能短的 TR 和 TE 以及高读出带宽。适度的并行采集成像可提高屏气状态下的空间分辨率。

对于成年患者，典型的成像参数为冠状 3D 数据集 TR = 2.5～3ms，TE = 1.0～1.5ms，α= 30°～40°，矩阵：40×192×256 和 FOV：460mm。中心椭圆相位编码[25]，扫描采集从峰值增强开始，确保最大 SNR 和动静脉期的最佳分离。常用的对比剂用量为 0.2mmol/kg 体重 Gd-DTPA，20ml 盐水冲洗，注射速度为 5ml/s。从注射造影剂到开始采集的时间，可团注对比剂优化对比剂用量为 1ml。或者，可使用具有视图共享时间分辨 3D 采集，例如对比动力学的时间分辨成像（time resolved imaging of contrast kinetics,TRICKS）/ 交错随机轨迹的时间分辨率血管成像（time-resolved imaging with interleaved stochastic trajectories,TWIST）序列[26]，额外显示动静脉走行区域的血流动力学，区域灌注缺损和心脏分流（图 11-1）。使用 TRICKS，K 空间数据在连续数据间共享，会导致较小的时间插值伪影，因此，TRICKS 数据在快速信号变化时（例如，在团注到达期间）谨慎使用（图 11-1）。

可通过使用上述时间分辨的低空间分辨率序列来获得定量 T_1 加权灌注图像。这里，常规的成像参数是 TR = 2.0～2.5ms，TE = 0.8～1.0ms，α= 30°～40°，矩阵：32×96×128，以及 FOV：460mm。利用每个 3D 数据集优于 1 s 的时间分辨率，该技术可产生血流动力学曲线和区域血流量，血容积和通过时间的参数图。同样，并行采集成像和视图共享可以增强时间分辨率。对比剂用量应小于肺血管造影所需的剂量。例如，0.05 ml/kg Gd-BT-DO3A + 20 ml 盐水以 5 ml/s 冲洗，可显示患者肺部的血管病变。如果需要肺血容量（pulmonary blood volume，PBV），血流量和通过时间的完全定量图，则需要采用去卷积模型在较大动脉中测量的动脉输入函数（arterial input function，AIF）。因此，仍然需要较弱的剂量以显示对比剂浓度和 T_1 加权引起的 AIF 信号改变间的线性关系[27]（图 11-2）。

（三）先进技术

1. 氧增强的 ^{1}H-MRI 当受试者吸入纯氧而不是室内空气时，顺磁氧会缩短肺部血液，血浆和组织的 T_1 弛豫时间。这种 T_1 缩短导致信号增强，可使用固有通气和灌注加权的参数图量化。已经提出了通气和灌注成像方法：半定量的且利用反转恢复 HASTE 序列。2D HASTE 使用短回波时间显示肺实质；然而，在数采集据前，应用非选择性反转脉冲，随后采用反转延迟 TI 在 HASTE 图像上增加 T_1 的图像的对比度。应该使用整体反转脉冲而不是选择层面的脉冲以避免血液的磁化流入效应[28]。选择 TI，使吸入室内空气时肺血管床灌注的信号为空（在 1.5T 下，肺实质 T_1 为 1100～1300ms[29]，TI = 0.69×T_1 = 700～900ms）。通过紧密贴合的面罩给予纯氧降低肺血浆和组织的平均 T_1，并在 IR-HASTE 图像中显示信号增强[30]。该技术隐含了通气和灌注加权，因此间接显示了肺功能。T_1 映射应用 IR-HASTE 使用反转脉冲可以定量更为准确，但会产生一系列低翻转角 FLASH 图像（Look-Locker

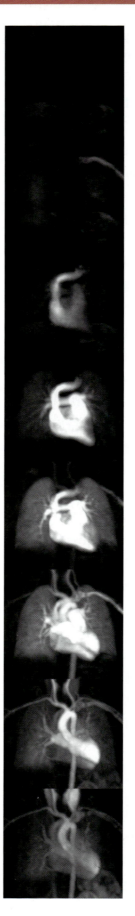

◀ 图 11-1 视图共享的时间分辨灌注成像

理论上，肺灌注通过时间分辨梯度回波序列成像，具有低空间分辨率，通过联合并行成像和视图共享，调整到整个肺容积 1.5s 高时间分辨率。因此，在静脉团注对比剂时，可获得一系列的肺部可测量图像。该图像显示了对比剂首次通过右心、肺、左心和体循环。每第二次采集的系列图像作为最大强度投影的减影

序列)[31]，可定量测量肺组织/血浆氧分压（pO₂）。在吸氧前后测量，通过自动门控技术和可变形注册可缩短采集时间和减少患者的运动伪影[32]（图 11-3）。

2. 非对比增强通气和灌注成像 研究肺功能的另一种方法傅里叶分解（Fouier decompo

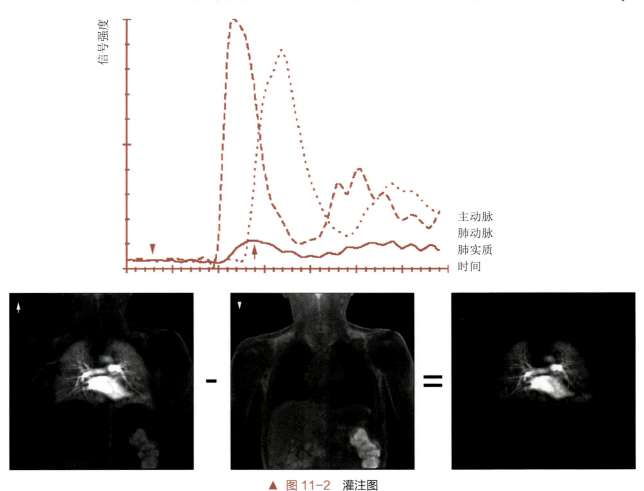

▲ 图 11-2 灌注图

应用四维动态增强灌注图行视觉评估，推荐建立减影灌注图。增强后肺实质强化最强的时间点图（白色箭头）与增强前肺实质图（白箭）相减。请注意，这种方法忽略了动态评估肺实质信号的变化，动态评估肺实质信号变化有助于区分延迟灌注区域和完全灌注缺损

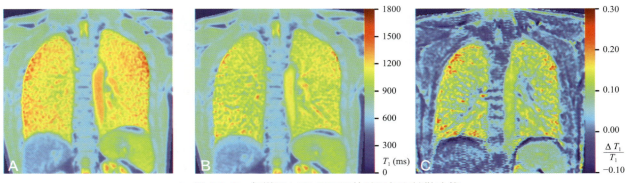

▲ 图 11-3 氧增强 MRI 用于评估肺通气和扩散功能

应用径向自门控反转恢复多梯度回波序列测量健康志愿者的 T_1 组织学特征。显示呼气加权图像。A. 受试者首先呼吸室内空气；B. 通过面罩补充纯 O_2，随后在通气肺区域由于肺泡和组织溶解 O_2 使 T_1 下降；C. 精确的可变形配准可创建减影图，显示 O_2 的 T_1 弛豫时间变化。注意，肺静脉在 T_1 弛豫中没有显示出差异（由德国海德堡的 Dipl.-Phys.Simon Triphan 提供）

sition, FD) MRI 技术评估肺灌注和通气功能, 无电离辐射, 无须静脉注射或吸入造影剂[33]。FD MRI 方法是在 1.5T 临床 MR 扫描仪上开发的, 在自由呼吸下应用时间分辨率为亚毫秒回波采样的 2D bSSFP 成像。随后采用非刚性图像配准校正呼吸和心脏运动, 可跟踪由呼吸所致的肺实质收缩和心脏搏动所致的肺血流信号变化。像素傅里叶分析可用于分离频率和空间分辨以产生通气和灌注加权图像。FD MRI 在 10min 内可完成覆盖整个肺容积的多层采集, 适用于临床常规检查。它对患者的依从性要求低并且不依赖任何触发技术。

以往的研究证明了 FD MRI 的可行性, 并通过健康志愿者中证实了可重复性[34]。该技术经过临床的金标准——单光子发射计算机断层扫描 (single-photon emission computed tomography, SPECT) /CT、完善的动态对比增强 (dynamic contrast enhanced, DCE) MRI 和 ³He-MRI 证实[35,36]。FD MRI 首先应用于囊性纤维化 (cysticfibrosis, CF) 人群中, 证实与 DCE MRI 技术有良好的相关性[37,38]。最近的一项研究显示了 FD MRI 应用于非小细胞肺癌患者术前评估肺灌注的可行性[39]。此外, 提出了图像后处理的扩展, 允许量化灌注加权图像[40]。FD MRI 还有望在将来应用于急性肺栓塞的形态学和功能学评估, 在自由呼吸模式下完成非对比增强的 MR 检查需要 10~15min (图 11-4)。

(四) 用其他核素对肺进行成像

MRI 对其他细胞核如 ³He、¹³C、¹⁹F、²³Na、³¹P 和 ¹²⁹Xe 的磁共振很敏感。尤其是 ³He 和 ¹²⁹Xe 气态元素, 它们可作为吸入造影剂直接显示肺通气气流, 气体扩散和气体交换。与 ¹H 比较时, 气态的低自旋密度和这些核的固有较弱的 MR 信号需要使用超极化过程增强信号来成像。通过使用激光光学泵技术, 使 ³He 和 ¹²⁹Xe 的极化达到 20%~60% 的水平, 吸入气体 (<1L) 就可满足常规临床成像。除了制备气体所需的定制极化系统外, 还需要额外的专用发射/接收 RF 线圈, 调节到 ³He 或 ¹²⁹Xe 共振频率; 然而, 这种硬件是可购买的, 并且比 MRI 扫描仪要便宜。

迄今为止, 临床工作上吸入气体 MRI 集中在吸入 ³He, 并且该技术已被证实对可视化和量化区域肺通气非常敏感, 可在单个屏气中通过毁损 GRE 序列和 SSFP 序列获得高 SNR 的肺通气图像, 实现 2D 和 3D 容积成像, 各向同性像素可达 3~4mm。³He 通气 MRI 可早于肺功能检查, CT 或 ¹H-MRI, 发现早期肺阻塞性病变和通气异质性病变, 如囊性纤维化 (CF) (图 11-5)[41,42]、哮喘[43] 和慢性阻塞性肺病 (chronic obstructive pulmonary diseases, COPD)[44,45]。

通过呼吸 ¹H 的获得的结构信息[46], 可同时定量分析气体通气图像和评估增强灌注, 以评估局部肺通气-灌注情况[47]。³He 通气成像可用于评估 CF[48,49]、哮喘[50,51]、COPD 患者治疗前后

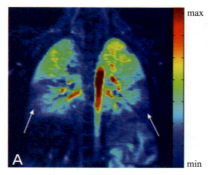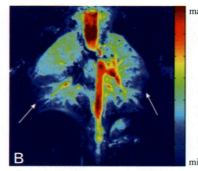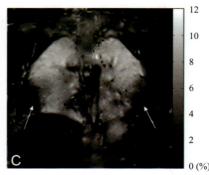

▲ 图 11-4 傅里叶分解可同时评估通气和灌注

A. 5 岁男性囊性纤维化患者, FD-MRI 冠状位图像, 彩色编码的动态对比增强 MRI 显示两肺下叶的灌注异常 (白箭); B. 显示在非对比灌注加权 FD MRI 中可见相同区域的灌注减低; C. 通气加权 FD-MRI 显示在呼吸间匹配肺部低灌注区与肺部相应区域信号成比例减低, 反映了通气减低和随之导致的缺氧血管收缩的区域

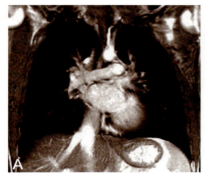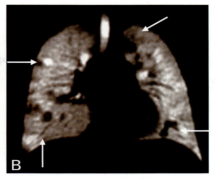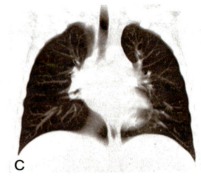

▲ 图 11-5　8 岁的囊性纤维化患儿的 ^{3}He-MRI 的通气成像

A. 是常规肺功能形态学成像，采用 ^{1}H-MRI 2D bSSFP 序列；C. 为 CT 图像，均未显示气道或肺实质的病变；B. 在 ^{3}He-MRI（箭）上，可早期显示通气不均匀性征象

肺通气的局部变化，该方法的灵敏度、安全性和可重复性都很高，可用于新疗法的评估。

气道中气体动态流动的快速成像，可评估 COPD 和哮喘患者的局部空气潴留和侧支通气[52,53]。肺中气体的扩散性也可以用表观扩散系数测量，可在非侵入性的方式下，测量肺泡和腺泡的平均长度。可早期检测出肺气肿的变化，有利于观察肺部病变的发展，具有重要的临床意义[54,55]。

尽管 ^{3}He 通气 MRI 联合 CT 和肺活量测定已经在多个中心研究中应用，但 ^{3}He 通气 MRI 的临床应用仍受气体摄取的限制[56]。然而，为了增加气体极化水平、提高图像质量，更廉价的 ^{129}Xe 有望用于临床肺通气成像，但还需要更大规模的临床研究[57,58]。有趣的是 Xe 在肺组织和血液中的溶解度，对肺间质性病变（interstitial lung disease，ILD），如特发性肺纤维化[59-61]，患者体内气体交换途径和肺微观结构的变化非常敏感。

二、肺部 MR 序列

（一）临床放射科医师的期望

现在各个公司的标准化 1.5 T 磁共振扫描机提供的肺部 MRI 基本序列应满足大多数临床预期的肺部问题[15]，可通过附加序列和静脉团注对比剂完成特定的临床应用，如恶性肿瘤的分期，评估肺血管病变和肺灌注。应避免使用复杂的序列、避免延长采集时间，例如 ECG 触发或呼吸门控。应容易解决临床的基本问题，例如患者不能屏住呼吸或幼儿配合不佳等。先进的 MRI 设备的投入、维护和人员的运行成本较高，在 MR 室的检查时间是行 MR 检查的关键。如将 MRI 应用于检出急性肺栓塞等紧急情况，则需快速有效的流程，以便缩短 MR 检查时间[3,38]。根据现有标准，要求在磁共振室内 15min 完成基本序列或紧急检查[3,15]。除基本序列、协议序列（例如增强序列，动态增强 MRI 和可视化呼吸运动）应少于 15min。肺 MRI 具有软组织对比度高和功能成像的优势。已发表的文章中对供应商特定序列的首字母缩略词均有论著，大多数序列在其他供应商的平台上都有对应的序列[2,3]。肺 MR 成像中，病变的命名仍使用临床常规应用的胸部 X 线和 CT 的 Fleischner 命名法[62]。Barreto 等致力于比较不同病理的病变在 CT 和 MRI 中的表现，将部分 CT 命名转移到 MRI[63]。

（二）临床肺部磁共振序列

1. 肺部病变的病理表现　与肺结构变化相关的肺病理状况导致肺密度增加 [肺不张，肺泡腔内和（或）肺间质内液体积聚，液体和细胞积聚，肺结节 / 肿块或纤维化] 或肺密度减低（由于空气滞留或肺气肿）[6,7,64,65]。鉴于 MRI 在组织 - 空气界面上的磁化伪影较重的局限性，使肺密度增加继而质子密度的疾病易于检测，但是显示使肺密度降低的疾病具有一定挑战性。然而，肺实质破坏和过度通气的病变（例如肺气肿）多伴随其他肺实质的病变（如肺间质纤维化、小叶间隔增厚、肺实质变形、支气管壁增厚等）。因此，由于过度通气导致缺失信号和伴随肺密度增加的病变，MRI 仍然可以做出正确的诊断[66]。有关空气潴留直接征象的成像技术参阅第11章三（二）1（3）。此外，肺灌注（缺氧性血管收缩，肺栓塞和心衰导致的肺淤血）的改变使 MRI 上肺信号发生变化[33,35]。非增强 MRI 可直接观察血管树以检出大血管病变[3]。

（1）肺信号增加的肺部病变：肺密度增加的病变易于检出。实验研究表明，胸腔积液在 T_2 加权和质子密度加权成像中易于检出[67-70]。可以得出结论，MRI 对胸腔积液的敏感性与胸片和 CT 一致[71,72]。大多数序列基于 T_2 或质子密度加权的 FSE 序列，采用呼吸门控、触发或屏气的采集模式。

另一个关键的临床需求是检出小结节。MRI 对大于 4mm 的肺结节的敏感性为 80%～90%，对于大于 8mm 的肺结节敏感性可达 100%[73]。根据序列技术和病变的信号强度，并且条件是最佳的（即患者可以保持呼吸 20s 或完美的门控/触发），可以假设 MRI 肺结节检测的阈值大小为 4mm[74-76]。与 CT 相比，在 MRI 上肺结节更易显示，因为它们在健康肺组织的深色背景下显示为高信号[76]。由于没有信号，钙化结节无法显示，而对比度增加的血管病变在 T_1 加权图像上易于观察[77]。到目前为止，已经评估了多种 MRI 序列用于肺结节的检出。包括有和没有脂肪饱和的 T_2 加权 FSE 成像[78-81]，反转恢复技术[82]，T_1 加权 SE[80,83] 和 GRE 序列[84,85]。该设计方案要求至少包括一个 T_2 加权或质量密度加权或短时反转恢复（short time inversion recovery, STIR）序列，以检出具有高流体含量的结节病变。这应该与其他序列相结合，以检出 T_1 加权上高信号的结节。尤其对检出高灌注和强化的恶性病变，顺磁性对比剂很有帮助，甚至可以提高检出率。然而，迄今为止没有适当的研究来证实这一点。

（2）肺血管和灌注异常：MR 血管造影和 MR 灌注主要用于研究急性肺栓塞，急性肺栓塞需要较高的诊断准确性。可采用多种成像序列包括直接观察肺动脉内的血栓，针对血流信号的阳性或阴性对比。目前，快速稳态自由进动 GRE 序列（SSFP-GRE）是最有效的技术之一。肺血管呈高信号，与血栓的低信号成为对比。据报道，对急性中央、亚段肺栓塞的敏感性为 90%，特异性为 97%[86-88]。另一种方法使用双反转恢复，凝滞的血凝块呈高信号，但诊断准确性不足[89,90]。

目前，MR 血管造影具有最高的空间分辨率，在屏气时可获得，增强后 T_1 加权 3D GRE 序列[91]。为获得最佳对比度，推荐使用高压注射器和特定的注射方案[92]。一些研究显示 MR 血管造影在疑似肺栓塞患者的检查中取得了良好的结果[93-96]。然而，最近的 PIOPED III 研究涉及 7 个中心和 371 名疑似肺栓塞患者，仅 75% 的患者可获得满意的图像。急性肺栓塞检出的敏感性和特异性分别为 78% 和 99%[97]。图像质量不佳的最常见原因是呼吸困难、咳嗽和对比剂注入的时间不足。

除了肺动脉成像外，采用不同的团注时间，该技术还可用于检测扩张的支气管动脉和肺静脉系统的异常。为了团注时间的问题，其他方法采用快速的 3D GRE 技术多次采集肺容积有利于提高 MR 血管造影的时间分辨率。通过并行成像和数据共享相结合，可以实现 1.5s 或更短的采集时间[98,99]。Ersoy 等通过 4D MR 血管造影或 MRI 动态增强（DCE-MRI），检出肺叶的肺栓塞敏感性为 98%，检出肺段的肺栓塞敏感性为 92%[100]。由于空间分辨率较低，该技术只能检测大血管中的血栓，但无法显示血栓相关的灌注缺损（图 11-1）。

动态增强 MRI 的发展使研究肺栓塞以外的其他疾病中肺实质灌注成为可能。限于一个平面，MRI 灌注 2D 成像，在适宜的空间分辨率下，时间分辨可达 10 幅/秒[101]。由于需要多序列成像和注射对比剂，容积成像难以实现，优先选择 4DMRI。其他技术，如在神经系统成像中应用的基于磁化的固有对比的动脉自旋标记,仍处于研究阶段,但尚未进入临床应用[102,103]。

通过增强前后的图像做减影,使肺实质和肺血管凸显出来,有利于 4D MRI 图像的视觉评估(图 11-1)。应用肺灌注成像可视觉评估和半定量评估 CF 患者由于黏液潴留和缺氧性血管收缩导致的肺灌注缺损,具有一定的临床应用价值(图 11-6 和图 11-7)[99,104-106]。灌注序列可间接评估肺气肿引起的肺实质灌注异常,气胸、浸润或脓肿等。请注意,对 20~30 次采集获得的灌注图无法充分评估灌注延迟区的病变,如动脉供血、容积分流或肺静脉异常。因此,开发了多种后处理软件,但尚未发展到临床应用阶段。

考虑到时间因素,计算的参数包括平均通过时间、达峰时间、峰值增强、PBV 或肺血流量(pulmonary blood flow,PBF),并显示为 3D 颜色编码的参数图,可区分灌注延迟区域[103,107-109]。由于 MR 信号与对比剂浓度成非线性关系,必须谨慎解释诸如 PBV 或 PBF 等定量参数[27]。迄今为止,这些参数已用于评估 COPD 和肺动脉高压[110,111]。

(3)气道和肺部通气障碍:应用 MRI 直接观察气道,要求气道直径大于 3mm 的,除非在 CF 患者中黏液栓导致高信号的病变[112,113]。在年轻的健康受试者中,肺部 MRI 显示气道可达第一亚段水平,但由于心脏搏动,越接近心脏越难以观察气道[114]。高分辨率 CT 对外周小气道的显示优于 MRI。

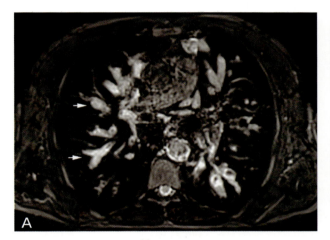
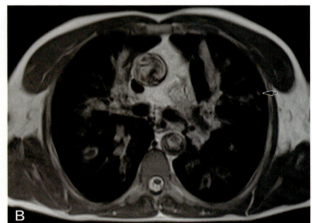
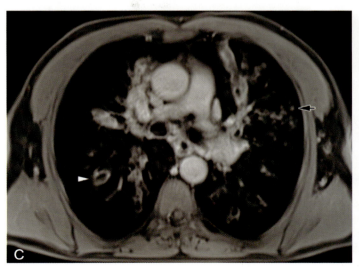
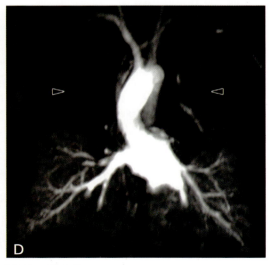

▲ 图 11-6　10 岁肺囊性纤维化晚期的男性患儿

A、B. 在 T_2 加权序列(白箭)上支气管扩张,管壁增厚伴黏液栓呈高信号;C. 在高空间分辨率 T_1 加权序列上,可见树芽征,多反映小气道病变(黑箭)。通过增强检查,可鉴别由炎性反应导致的支气管壁增厚(白色箭头)和黏液;D. 在 5mm 最大强度投影图像上,减影的灌注图显示上叶(黑色箭头)灌注异常和下叶的不均匀灌注

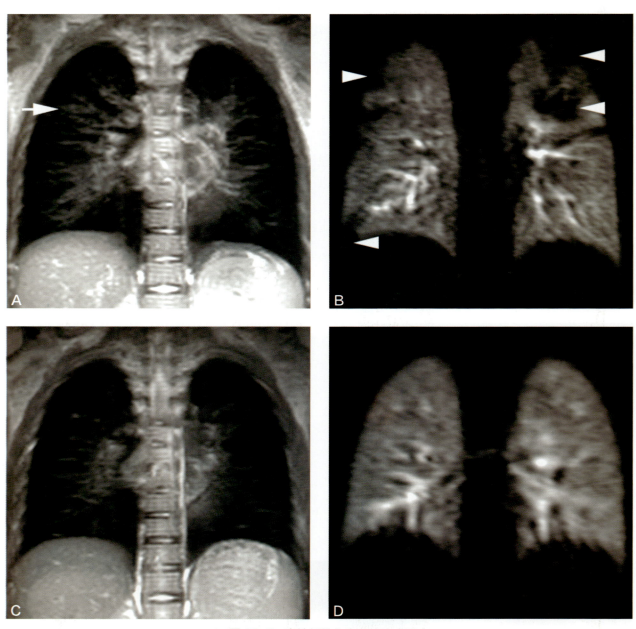

▲ 图 11-7 囊性纤维化患者的治疗反应

在 10 岁女性囊性纤维化患者的自由呼吸模式下获得 T_2 加权导航以及动态增强序列。CF 中的肺部恶化可能与肺黏液含量增加（A，白箭）和广泛的灌注异常（B，白色箭头）有关。抗生素治疗 1 个月后复查 MRI 显示肺黏液（C）和灌注异常减少（D）

然而，MRI 可以用研究肺、中央气道和横膈的呼吸运动。上述 2D + t MRI、3D + t MRI、T_1 加权 GRE 或 bSSFP 序列已应用于此项目[115]，例如，研究儿童的气管支气管软化[116,117] 以及慢性支气管炎，COPD 或 CF 的动态气道塌陷[118]。除气道疾病外，最重要的临床应用是呼吸运动相关的器官放疗[119,120]。

根据局部肺容积变化和动态采集信号变化，或通过肺实质信号较好的吸气、呼气序列评估肺通气[6,121]。由于空气在 MRI 上没有信号，直接评估只能通过吸入超极化惰性气体[122]、对比剂六氟化硫（SF6）[123] 或雾化顺磁对比剂[124] 直观成像，间接评估可以采取氧气增强成像[125]，具体请参阅第 13 章。目前，在单个 2D 平面（2D + t

中使用动态图像采集来研究呼吸运动似乎最接近常规使用。

2. 儿科影像学 无辐射的肺部 MRI 在儿科放射学有很大的应用潜力。由于技术发展和扫描时间缩短，MRI 已成为许多肺部疾病的一线成像技术[126]。可用的序列与成人相同，但是儿科的特征性影响方案的选择。首先，对于 6—8 岁的幼儿，通常不能采取屏气成像。根据患者的大小及其遵守程序和呼吸指令的能力，可使用运动补偿制订个性化扫描序列，优化调整 FOV、扫描层厚、分辨率和信噪比[127]。

两种基本策略是针对运动补偿 bSSFP 或部分傅里叶单次发射序列（例如，HASTE）[128]。即使在低场 MRI 系统上，bSSFP 序列也可在屏气时间小于 10s，快速采集 10 层图像，也可在自由呼吸下完成[129,130]。通常，这些快速序列用于快速浏览，第二步再高分辨率采集。第二种方法，门控或触发采集，增加了采集时间，但可提供良好的空间分辨率和软组织对比度[127,131]。幼儿呼吸频率较高有助于加速采集。非门控采集的差异远小于呼吸频率低的成人受试者。T_2 加权快速自旋回波序列可以施加 2000ms 或更短的重复时间，通常触发在呼气相约 2s，具体取决于个体呼吸频率。该时间帧可完成没有相关的运动伪影的 T_2 加权图像[132]。应用呼吸带或缓冲技术[132]或基于图像（例如，导航器），检测呼吸运动具有良好的效果。K 空间的径向读出方案进一步改善了运动伪影。应用心脏触发在特定情况下可能有所帮助，但会显著增加采集时间[133]。

儿童行 MR 检查多需要在非屏气状态下使用镇静，或在全麻下应用呼吸机控制屏气。低场肺部 MRI 检查仍然存在争议[130,134]。麻醉会导致肺不张，应用异丙酚镇静会导致高达 42% 的背侧肺不张[135]。水合氯醛或苯巴比妥发生肺不张概率较低[136]，但是有可能掩盖其他相似的疾病。因此，需要在俯卧位进行额外扫描。如果需要与 CT 比较相关性，例如，当将随访检查从 CT 切换到 MRI 时，需要抬高手臂进行 MRI 检查，但儿童仅能忍受 15～20min。

（三）肺部序列推荐

1. 基本序列 与 X 线或 CT 相比，MRI 中的图像质量取决于患者长时间的依从性。屏气配合良好、依从性高的青年患者易获得良好的检查图像。相反，依从性差、肥胖、不能屏气配合或无法听从呼吸指令的患者难以达到诊断要求的图像质量。因此，提倡采用快速成像序列，额外的序列可补充任何采集序列的失败[1-3]。快速采集序列和呼吸门控或触发采集方式，部分可以通过自由呼吸获得，但是需要延长采集时间。如果可以使用 T_2 加权 FSE 序列的呼吸触发序列，磁共振室内总时间增加 10min。技术人员应在研究初判断患者的依从性，并相应地调整检查序列。然而，培训患者听从指示是非常重要的，可应用呼吸带在图像采集期间也可监测患者的依从性。

尽管大多数序列是在 1.5T 系统上开发和评估的，但也可在 3T 扫描仪上完成[1,2]。虽然大多数序列，特别是 3D GRE 技术，提高病变与背景对比度有利于病变检出，但是伪影会降低稳态 GRE 序列的图像质量[1,2]。总的来说，应用 3T 磁共振扫描仪，大多数序列获得的图像质量尚可，甚至更好。

调整患者的 FOV 大小，典型的 FOV 在冠状面上为 450～500mm，在横向采集中为约 400mm，矩阵为 256～384 像素（触发的快速自旋回波序列高达 512），像素尺寸小于 1.8mm×1.8mm。2D 采集的层厚为 4～6mm，横向 3D 采集使用 4mm 或更小的层厚，在冠状位肺血管造影成像中层厚可达 2mm 或更小[137]。

基础序列基于 GRE 和 FSE 序列的 T_1 和 T_2 加权图像[2,15]。T_1-GRE 序列可用作 3D 采集，并且可在一次屏气中完成肺部图像采集。T_2 加权 FSE 序列应覆盖至少两个平面，例如，屏气时采用半傅里叶获取冠状位和轴位的图像。有利于浸润性病变和小结节的检出。采用 STIR 或脂肪饱

和 T_2 加权快速自旋回波序列可提高纵隔淋巴结和骨病变（例如转移瘤）的敏感性，肋骨转移易在轴位上检出，脊柱病变易在冠状位检出。应选择在自由呼吸下的冠状位稳态自由进动序列，有助于中央肺栓塞、心脏病或呼吸功能障碍的检出。平扫序列应覆盖大多数常见病变，包括肺炎、肺不张、肺结节或肿块，纵隔肿块（淋巴瘤、甲状腺肿、囊肿和胸腺瘤）和急性中心性肺栓塞。以下推荐的序列涵盖了临床预期特定病变的检出。这只是一个起点，用户可根据自己的需求和经验扩展序列。

2. 扩展 1：肿瘤 根据初始或进一步预期的发现，需要额外使用相同体积的插值 3D GRE 序列完成对比度增强的图像采集，多采用脂肪饱和度以提高对比增强组织和纵隔淋巴结的可见性。尽管 3D 序列覆盖整个胸部，但是在横向或冠状位图像可优化面内分辨率（图 11-8）。在一个屏息时间完成采集，可通过 3D GRE 序列获得轴位和冠状位的图像。特别是对肺癌的分期，采用弥散加权序列有助于检出小淋巴结的转移。两个序列都将总成像时间延长了大约 5min[15]。但是以超过预期扫描时间 15min，可添加运动补偿的 T_2 加权 FSE 序列以提高累及胸壁的病变的检出[2,38]。另一种方法在冠状动脉方向的自由呼吸模式的 bSSFP 序列，聚焦于肿瘤（2D + t 或 MRI 电影），可鉴别肿瘤胸壁侵犯[138]。

3. 扩展 2：肺血管和灌注成像 肺血管系统成像的障碍包括三个部分：首先，多选择自由呼吸 bSSFP 序列，然后是基于 3D GRE 的对比增强 MR 血管造影的两种变化：用于第一次通过灌注成像的时间分辨高，空间分辨率低和用于屏气时采集，空间分辨率高。根据 MR 扫描仪的性能，动态增强序列具有高时间分辨率，优化对比剂团注时间也起着决定作用。这些方案有利于急性和慢性肺栓塞，动静脉畸形（例如，Osler-Weber-Rendu 病），扩张的支气管动脉，肺隔离，肺动脉瘤，肺静脉

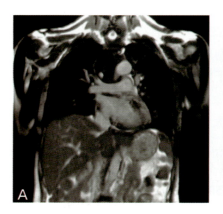
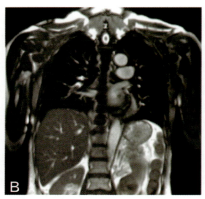
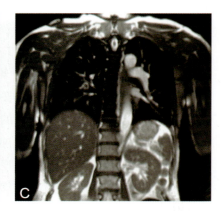
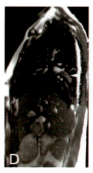
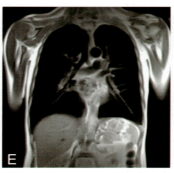
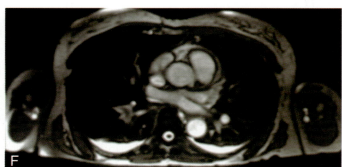

▲ 图 11-8 肺栓塞

59 岁免疫功能低下的女性患者，出现发热和呼吸困难。在自由呼吸的 bSSFP 获得三个平面的图像和在 T_2 加权 HASTE 序列上获得两个平面的图像。A～E. 在 bSSFP 序列检出多个肺段和亚段的肺栓子，两侧胸腔积液。可以排除肺部浸润，并在室内时间（F）10min 内完成该检查

引流异常和肺部血管病变的检出[15]。它也被推荐用于气道疾病（COPD 和 CF）。建议将不同的快速成像序列组合起来，以提高病变检出的灵敏性和特异性[139]。因此，Kluge 等建议联合不同的 MRI 技术检测肺栓塞[88]。肺血管成像可用于血管病理学的研究，例如，在疑似急性肺栓塞或与肿瘤方案组合用于综合评估侵犯血管的中心性肿块。

（四）扩大范围——一站式 MRI？

肺部 MRI 应覆盖可能累及的周围解剖结构，例如，评估相邻的上腹部（肺癌中的肾上腺和肝转移）。广泛的领域是心脏和肺之间的相互作用。最明显的是，应采用全面的心肺序列针对肺动脉高压患者，涵盖肺动脉压升高的一系列潜在病因（例如 COPD、ILD）和右心病变等[140]。在这种情况下，MRI 在测量右心室输出量和右心肥大方面表现出较高的可重复性，后者是死亡率的重要预测因子[141]。相位增强 MRI 可用于确诊大血管中的肺动脉血流。重要的是，慢性血栓栓塞性肺动脉高压可通过的网状物或条带检测，敏感性为 98%，特异性为 94%，通过 MRI 确定中央血栓负荷对手术至关重要[142]。

三、现有技术的临床应用

与其他方式相比，肺部 MRI 具有特定的优点和缺点。在一线检查中，当需要最小化辐射暴露时，MRI 可替换 CT 和 X 射线。典型的适应证是儿童的急性和慢性肺病（肺炎和 CF）、年轻人或孕妇怀疑肺栓塞［参阅第 11 章四（一）］。在某些情况下，肺部 MRI 可以作为有价值的辅助方法（例如，肺癌），用于解决临床问题［参阅第 11 章四（二）］。在肺间质病变中，肺 MRI 是可行的，但与其他检查方法相比不具有优势［参阅第 11 章四（三）］。肺部 MRI 仍然可作为研究或短期随访的选择。随着技术的不断发展，肺部 MRI 的适应证将不断增加。

（一）MRI 一线检查

1. 年轻患者的肺炎 数年前已显示出低场 MRI 和 SSFP 序列取代胸部 X 线的潜力[129,143-146]。肺部 MRI 检出社区获得性肺炎、脓胸、真菌感染和慢性支气管炎等疾病的可行性，已通过体内和体外不同方案的各种研究得到证实[106,132]。通过这些研究证实的序列被整合到推荐的基本方案中。但 3T 磁共振肺部 MRI 应用的经验有限。例如，最近用 HRCT 作为金标准，研究儿童非 CF 慢性肺病，证实和 3T 肺部 MRI 具有极好的相关性[147]，可采用屏气 T_2 和 ECG 触发的 T_1 加权序列。总之，目前肺部 MRI 被认为是检测儿童肺炎的有效工具（图 11-9）。

2. 囊性纤维化 CF 仍然是高加索人中最常见的致死性遗传性疾病，其中肺表型决定死亡率[148]。由于治疗的提高，CF 患者的预期寿命大幅增加，目前的中位生存期约为 40 年[149,150]。影像学检查在疾病管理中起着重要作用，因为临床参数（包括肺功能检测）仅提供整体信息，而观察肺结构和功能的细微变化逐渐被视为 CF 肺活动和病程的重要标志物。患者的年龄（可通过筛查检测到新生儿）和延长的中位生存期，辐射暴露成为主要问题，是肺部 MRI 应用的一个成功案例[151,152]。

据报道，MRI 检测新生儿和成人患者 CF 肺的形态学变化与 CT 相当，MRI 的临床应用正在迅速增长[104,106,112,113,128,153]。此外，当评估肺功能改变时，MRI 优于 CT[99,108]。使用基本的 MRI 序列，可以观察支气管扩张、支气管壁增厚、黏液栓、小气道疾病、气液平、实变和肺破坏[104,106,113]。MRI 检测支气管扩张的准确性取决于许多因素，包括支气管分级水平和直径，壁厚以及支气管壁和管腔内的信号。在 MRI 上可以很好地观察到中央支气管和外周支气管扩张，而在第三级、四级以远正常的外周支气管的难以观察。支气管壁增厚的检出取决于支气管大小和信号[113]。T_2 加权图像上的支气管壁的高信号表示增加的流体，即水肿，可能由炎性反应引起。在注入对比剂后，脂肪抑制

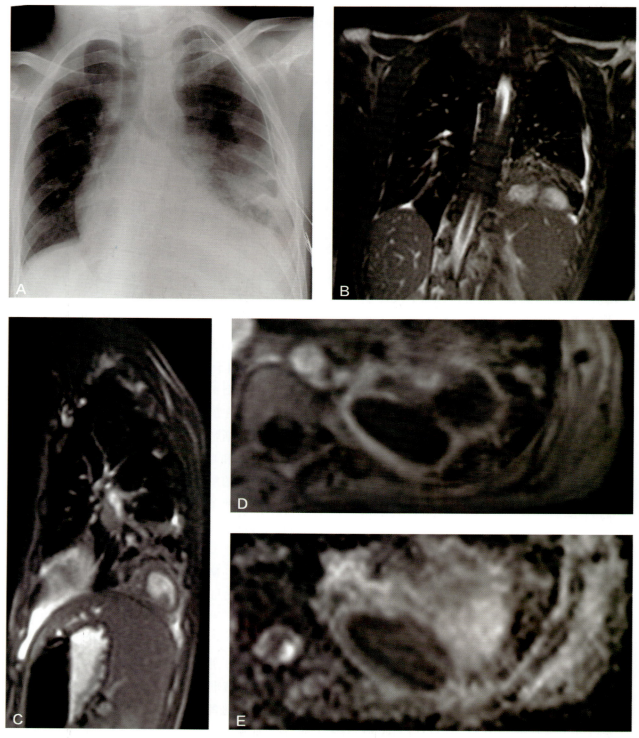

▲ 图 11-9 小儿肺炎并发症的检出

7 岁男性肺炎患儿静脉注射抗生素治疗 1 周后，由于胸腔积液和疑似脓胸插入引流管，但临床症状和发热持续存在。A. 左肺下叶病变没有消退；B、C.bSSFP 显示左肺下叶病变中心呈多个高信号，病变边缘光滑、可见低信号的囊；D. 静脉注射对比剂后囊壁可见强化；E. 扩散加权成像显示某些病变的表观扩散系数降低，最终诊断为肺炎继发肺脓肿

的 T_1 加权图像上支气管壁增强被认为与炎性反应有关。值得注意的是，与 MRI 相比，CT 只能检出支气管壁增厚，但无法说明原因[104,113]。

由于液体在 T_2 上呈信号，MRI 上甚至可以在小气道上显示黏液栓，呈沿支气管分布的 T_2 高信号，可呈分支状、葡萄状或树芽征改变。由于黏液栓无强化，很容易与支气管壁增厚鉴别[104]。支气管内气-液平提示活动性感染，在囊状或静脉曲张型支气管扩张中，呈 T_2 高信号。然而，区分支气管气-液平和严重的支气管管壁增厚伴黏液栓是困难的。在 T_2 和增强的 T_1 加权图像上，气液平易于诊断。

发生在 CF 患者中的肺实变主要是由肺泡充盈引起的炎症因素导致 T_2 加权像的高信号，常伴有肺体积减小。与 CT 相似，MRI 上支气管充气征表现为肺实变内的低信号区域[71,144]。随着疾病的进展，肺段或肺叶的破坏可以在 MRI 和 CT 发生上述类似的改变。

在 CF 患者中，由于缺氧血管收缩反应或组织破坏，区域通气缺陷引起局部肺灌注的变化。使用对比增强 3D MRI，11 例 CF 患儿的灌注缺损与组织破坏程度相关[99,154]。最近研究证实，在 50 名婴儿和学龄前儿童中检测到大约 20% 的灌注异常是由支气管扩张，支气管壁增厚和黏液栓引起的[106]。研究还表明，在 0—6 岁时，肺灌注变化通常比形态学改变更为突出。外周黏液栓可能引起灌注改变，因此灌注成像可能对 CF 中的病理改变更敏感[106]。

MR 信号与应用造影剂浓度之间的非线性关系，使量化肺灌注成为挑战性[27]。Risse 等研究了定性评估对比时间增强的重要性，分析增强的 3D MRI 并将灌注变化分为正常、延迟、减少、减少和延迟以及灌注损失[108]。使用专用的后处理工具，这些数据可以 3D 显示[107,109]。有必要进一步研究灌注数据的临床相关性。临床实践依赖于视觉评估。最近提出的形态功能磁共振成像评分易于临床应用和重复评估，适用于 CF 肺病的大范围光谱的半定量形态学和功能学评估[105]，与常规 CT 评分系统相似[155]。基于目前的状况，形态功能磁共振可应用于几乎所有 CF 患者，评估疾病严重程度以监测治疗效果，并且可能区分可逆和不可逆的病变区域[106]。

3. 年轻人或孕妇的急性肺栓塞 目前用于评估急性肺栓塞的影像学技术是 CT 肺血管造影[156]。与通气和灌注闪烁扫描和 SPECT 相比，它的主要优点是可在较短的时间内完成检查和诊断的准确性。然而，即使最新的研究方案，CT 的辐射暴露仍然是一个问题，特别对于年轻患者和孕妇。与 CT 相比，精简的 MR 检查序列在室内时间 15min 内完成肺血管和肺灌注成像。

虽然 MR 血管造影已被证实是有利于肺栓塞的检出，但大型多中心研究的最新数据表明，这种技术的结果仍然令人不满意[95,97]。联合不同 MRI 技术检测肺栓塞的可能效果更好[88]。该方案进一步修改并扩展为两步法。第一步，应用自由呼吸的稳态 GRE 序列在 5min 内获得两个或三个平面中在检出大的中央栓子，灵敏度为 90%，特异度接近 100%[87,88,157]。检测到的中央肺栓塞可直接转至重症监护病房并给予相应治疗，诊断时间与 CT 肺血管造影一样短。如果第一步检查为阴性或不清楚的结果，则将继续行对比增强检查，包括灌注成像，多相高空间分辨率对比增强 MRA，以及使用容积 3D FLASH 序列轴位采集。尽管它具有多个序列，但两步检查可以在室内时间 15min 内完成，使它可作为日常临床常规的快速检测（图 11-9）。在许多情况下，例如在孕妇中无法使用对比剂，可以采用自由呼吸或屏气的稳态自由进动序列在三个方向上完成第一步检查。此外，由于这些步骤是部分冗余的，因此即使在依从性差的患者中，至少一次采集也是具有诊断性的。最近，Schiebler 及其同事在 190 例疑似肺栓塞患者行 MR 检查发现，诊断准确性达 97.4%[158]。随访 3 个月和 1 年，阴性预测值分别为 97% 和 96%，与多排螺旋 CT 检查结果相似[158]。

（二）MRI 作为补充模态

非小细胞肺癌 当 CT 禁忌时，例如，当不可能使用碘化造影剂时，对胸部恶性肿瘤的检出和分期中，MRI 是一种替代方案。为此，MRI 标准方案可全面评估形态学肿瘤淋巴结转移和分期（TNM）[65]。可在 25min 的室内时间内完成对比增强的检查。直径大于 4~5 mm 的肺内结节或肿块易于检测（图 11-10）。磁共振的软组织对比度高可评估纵隔、肺门和锁骨上淋巴结肿大的程度。其他征象，如暗淋巴结征和对比增强可提高恶性病变检出率（图 11-11）[159]。涉及肝脏、肾上腺和胸部骨骼的转移性疾病可被检出。基于 MRI 的肺癌分期与正电子发射断层扫描（positron emission computed tomography，PET）/CT 比较，证实了其可行性[160-163]。对高风险人群筛查初步结果表明，非增强 MRI 对恶性结节比良性病变更敏感，从而使 MRI 有可能成为肺癌筛查的另一种方式（图 11-10 和图 11-11）[76]。

肺部弥散加权成像（diffusion-weighted imaging，DWI）的作用仍需要进一步评估。DWI 被推荐用于肺癌的全身检出，包括纵隔转移[160,164]。然而，到目前为止，DWI 与胸部其他 MRI 方案相比没有显著优势[165,166]。与 DWI 相比，STIR 序列对肺癌和纵隔转移的检出和分类更敏感[167-169]。DWI 的一个潜在作用是预测临床 I A 期非小细胞肺癌的肿瘤侵袭性，区分肿块与肺不张[170,171]。DWI 序列在鉴别恶性或良性肺病变或鉴别肺癌亚型方面的作用仍存在争议[169,172-174]。根据作者自

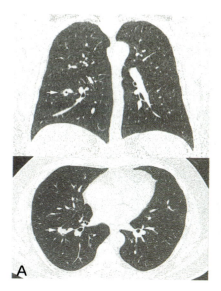
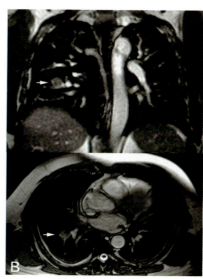
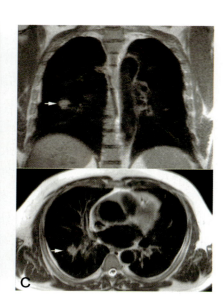

▲ 图 11-10 检测肺结节

A. 冠状位和轴位低剂量 CT（1mm 层厚）检出在 52 岁的重度吸烟者右肺下叶的腺癌，最大直径约为 15mm（白箭）。结节在冠状位和轴位，（B）bSSFP（层厚 4mm，自由呼吸）和（C）T₂（HASTE）序列（层厚 6mm，屏气）中可见

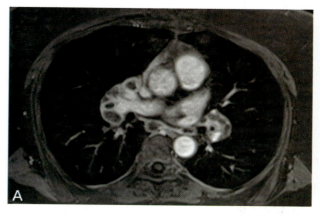
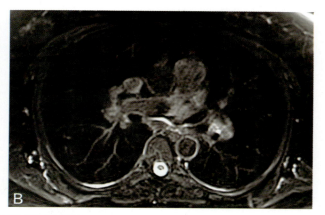

▲ 图 11-11 评估纵隔淋巴结

46 岁女性肺内结节病史。对比增强 T₁ 加权（A）（VIBE）和脂肪抑制 T₂ 加权（B）（BLADE）可见纵隔和肺门淋巴结肿大。在两个序列上淋巴结显示典型的边缘增强、中心为低信号（由 Jonathan H. Chung 教授，丹佛，科罗拉多州提供）

己的经验，DWI 有助于区分胸膜附近的病变，评估纵隔受累情况，并可辅助检出小结节。因此，在肺部 MRI 检查建议包含快速 DWI 采集是有意义的（图 11-12）[64,175]。

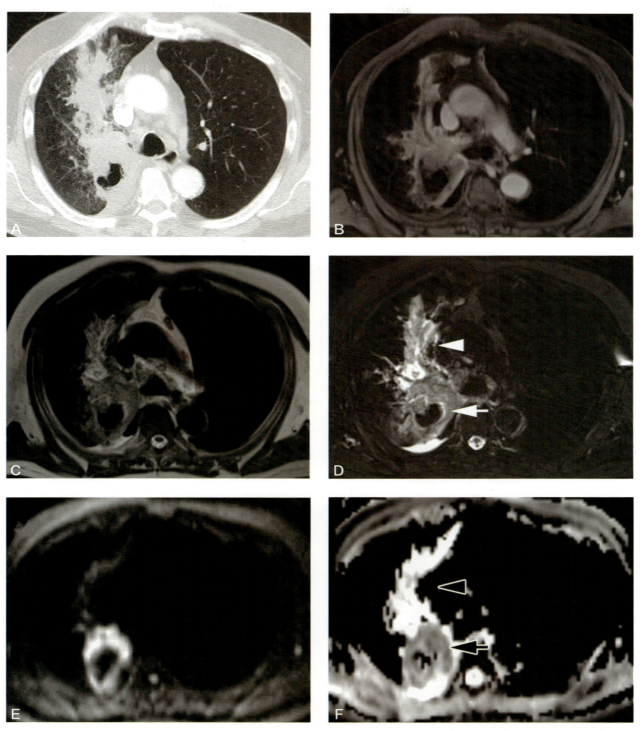

▲ 图 11-12　肿瘤与肺不张的鉴别

A.CT 检测到右肺大肿块伴中央坏死；B. 静脉注射对比剂后 3D GRE（VIBE）序列清楚地显示气管分叉水平纵隔受累的程度；C、D. 特别是 T_2 加权序列（HASTE 和 BLADE）非常适合于区分支气管肺癌（白箭）和相邻的肺不张（白色箭头）。也可以检出胸腔积液；E、F.b = 1000 的 DWI 图像显示肿瘤呈高信号，肺不张呈相对低信号。只有肿瘤表现 ADC 值降低（黑箭），与肺不张（黑色箭头）相反（由德国海德堡大学的胸部 Claus Peter Heussel 教授提供）

在肺部肿块中，MRI 的软组织对比度高，优于 CT，有助于区分肿瘤与肺不张和胸腔积液，可用于图像引导的放射治疗。T_1- 缩短造影剂特异性地检出肿瘤坏死、胸壁或纵隔侵犯、胸膜反应或受累。肺 MRI 可检出肺尖肿瘤（Pancoast 肿瘤）。目前，T_1 椎体水平以上的臂丛神经的受累是手术切除的主要禁忌证。由于其高软组织对比度和多平面能力，MRI 诊断神经根、椎间孔、椎管和臂丛神经受累方面优于 CT[176]。因此，对 Pancoast 肿瘤的患者，应行 MRI 检查（图 11-13）。

此外，MRI 提供全面的呼吸动力学、肿瘤位置[138,177]和肺灌注[178,179]的信息。这些功能成像的研究具有巨大的临床应用潜力。例如，预测术后肺功能，逐渐走向一站式的检查模式[39]。

PET / MRI 在肺癌分期中的作用尚未确定。原则上，PET / MRI 应该将肺部 MRI 的优势即软组织对比度高和功能成像的能力与 PET 的代谢信息相结合。然而，这两个系统的集成在技术上具有挑战性[180]。特别地，混合扫描仪的 3T MR 可能不利于肺 MRI 成像。在 TNM 分期中，PET / MRI 对肺癌局部 T 分期的优势在于鉴别肺不张、实变、局部肿瘤复发或放射治疗后残留瘢痕[181]。在 N 分期中，DWI 和 STIR 序列有助于提高用氟 -2- 脱氧 -d- 葡萄糖 -PET（FDG-PET）分期的灵敏度和特异性[167,182]。然而，对 M 分期，MRI 对于脑、肝和骨转移检出的准确性，PET / MRI 具有极大的临床应用前景[183]。最后，在 PET/MRI 通过 MRI 替换 CT 可减少辐射暴露，有利于年轻患者。此外，非常有前途的方法，如使用 4D MRI 对 PET 行 3D 运动校正，目前还处于研究中（图 11-14）。

（三）肺部 MRI 潜在的未来适应证

1. 肺气肿和 COPD　COPD 是全球发病率和死亡率的主要原因之一。目前，它是成人中第四大常见死亡原因，但其患病率正在增加[184]。COPD 的特征是由于气道阻塞（阻塞性细支气管炎）和实质破坏（肺气肿）的个体间可变组合，不完全可逆的气流阻塞[184]。一个组分的优势通常与不同的临床特征相关，即所谓的表型，对差异疗法具有潜在影响。一些研究表明，COPD 患者的气道阻塞倾向于小于 2mm 的气道[185]。这些

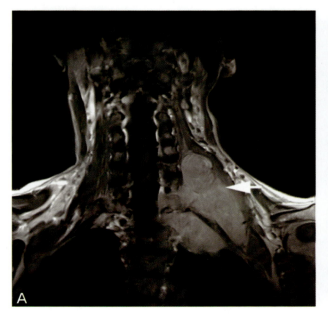
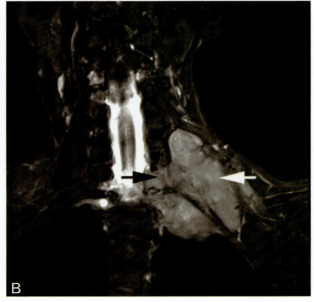

▲ 图 11-13　肺尖肿瘤

肺尖肿瘤中，对比增强的 3D GRE（A）和冠状位脂肪抑制的 T_2 加权快速自旋回波序列（B）是可显示肿瘤边缘。在这种情况下，大肿块（白箭）从左肺尖延伸到颈部软组织，并穿过神经孔进入椎管（黑箭）（由德国海德堡大学胸部 Claus Peter Heussel 教授提供）

Chapter 11 磁共振成像在肺部的临床应用
Clinical Magnetic Resonance Imaging Applications for the Lung

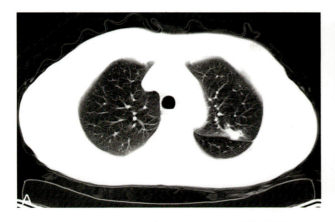
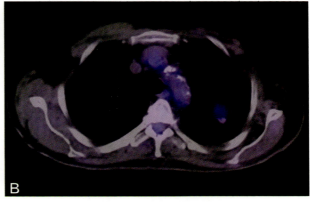
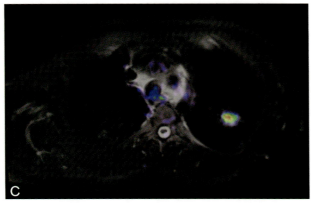

▲ 图 11-14 PET/MRI 成像的潜在价值

71 岁吸烟男性患者行 FDG-PET / CT 检查。A、B. 左肺上叶可见部分实性结节在 6 个月的随访中未见明显改变；B. 因结节对 FDG 摄取不明确，PET / MRI 尚无定论；C. 在 PET / MRI 后直接行运动校正的 PET / CT，与 PET / CT 相比，导致结节的摄取显著增加。组织病理学证实为支气管肺腺癌（由德国海德堡癌症研究中心（DKFZ）H. P. Schlemmer 博士和 O. Sedlaczek 博士提供）

气道位于气管支气管树的第 4 级和第 14 级之间，并且通常不能通过临床成像来观察。

通过肺功能测试和一氧化碳的扩散能力评估 COPD 的严重程度。CT 是 COPD 相关形态学变化成像的参考标准，重点是肺气肿和定量成像。由于缺氧性肺血管收缩导致的肺过度通气、血容量减少以及肺气肿的组织损失（即负性病变）使肺部 ^{1}H-MRI 的进一步减少，导致肺实质信号显著减低（图 11-15）[6]。一项研究表明，MRI 在吸气和呼气相时测量肺实质信号强度的变化与 FEV_1（r = 0.508）作为气流阻塞的预测因子之间存在相关性[7]。

在生理条件下通过 MRI 描绘气道尺寸和气道壁的尺寸仅限于中央支气管树。对于支气管扩张的描述，具有高空间分辨率的序列是必不可少的 [参阅第 11 章四（一）2]。先前描述的 3D 体积内插 GRE 序列具有高空间分辨率，与 CT 相比，对支气管扩张检出的敏感性为 79%、特异性为 98%（图 11-16）[85]。

COPD 的 MRI 成像优势在灌注和呼吸动力学等功能参数的评估[186]。过度通气对膈肌影响严重，降低其机械性能，但对颈部和肋骨肌肉作用降低[187]。COPD 常见的临床参数并未提供关于肺部结构改变、导致呼吸力学功能障碍的信息，尽管对肺量减少、改善肺功能的手术或内窥镜治疗，是通过促进呼吸力学和增加弹性回缩[188,189]。与正常人相比，肺气肿患者经常出现膈肌运动减少、不规则或不同步、膈肌最大振幅显著减低[190,191]。在一些患者中，膈肌运动不协调（例如，半膈膜的腹侧部分向下移动而背侧部分向头部移动）[192]，而反常的膈肌运动与轻度和中度的过度通气相关[193]。严重的外周气流阻塞也会影响亚段支气管到气管的近端。建议在连续呼吸或强迫呼气时采集 MR 电影，以评估气管不稳定性，如气管支气管软化或过度动态气道塌陷，可能模拟小气道阻塞的临床表现[118]。

通过通气和灌注维持肺中的气体交换的最佳状态。在通气减少的地区，发生缺氧性血管收缩[194,195]导致局部 PBF 减少，再分布到更好的通气区[196,197]。肺血管床的减少与实质破坏的严重程度相关；然而，灌注的分布不一定与实质破坏相匹配[198,199]。MR 灌注在检出 COPD 患者肺部异常灌注具有较高的准确性[98,110,200]。此外，MR 灌注比率与放射性核素灌注闪烁显像比率[201,202]相关，可以分析灌注缺损的肺叶和肺段[199]。COPD 的灌注异常不同于血管阻塞引

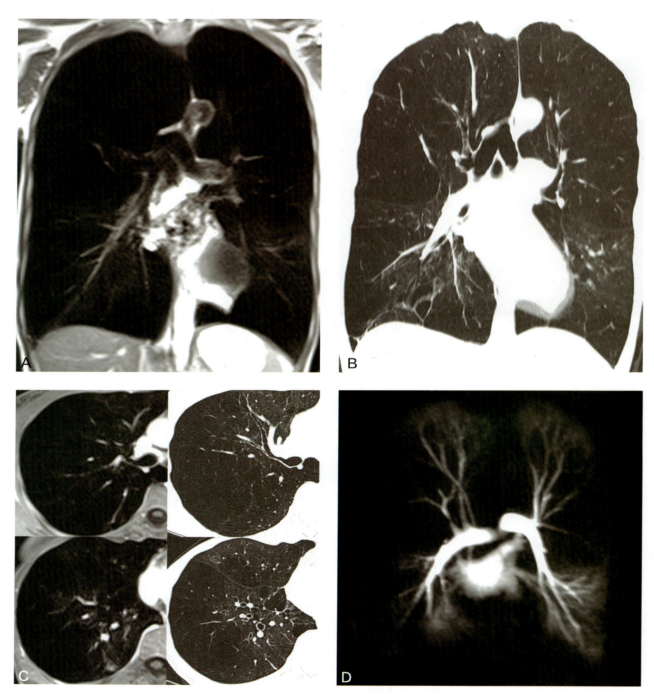

▲ 图 11-15　COPD 的肺气肿表型

A. 冠状位 T_2 加权（HASTE）序列显示重度吸烟者的严重肺气肿，其特征是信号的缺乏；B. 当天行低剂量 CT 的检查。关于组织损失，与伴随的动脉相比，气道显示出宽的腔；C. 由于壁增厚缺失，在对比剂注射后，与相应的 CT（1mm 层厚）相比，在轴向 T_1 加权（VIBE）图像上难以识别支气管；D.MR 灌注成像（TWIST）显示肺气肿肺功能减低与灌注缺损大致匹配（10 mm 冠状位最大强度投影的灌注减影图）

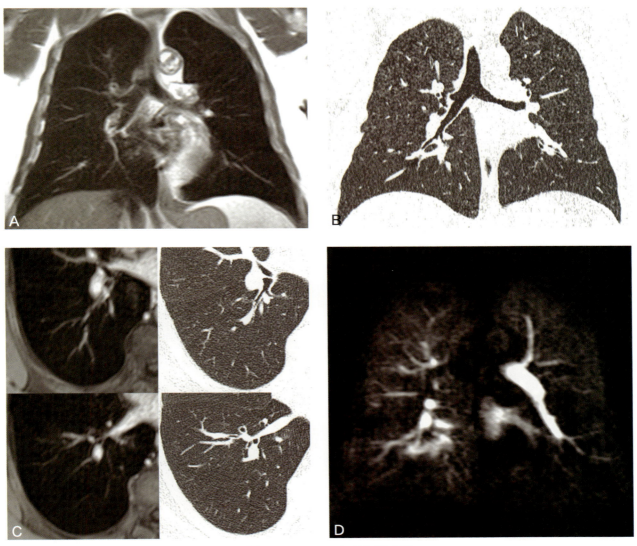

▲ 图 11-16 COPD 的气道表型

A. 重度吸烟者的肺实质在冠状位 T_2 加权（HASTE）序列上显示相对均匀的信号；B. 低剂量 CT 扫描也未显示肺气肿；C. 在造影剂注射后在轴位 T_1 加权（VIBE）图像上可见肺叶和肺段气道壁增厚和狭窄、气道腔重塑。相应的 1mm 层厚上 CT 图像；D.MR 灌注成像（TWIST）显示不均匀分布的斑块状灌注缺损（10mm 冠状位最大强度投影的灌注减影图）

起的灌注异常。栓塞性梗阻中出现楔形灌注缺损，但 COPD 合并肺气肿表现为不均匀强化减低（图 11-15）[65,203]。此外，峰值信号强度降低，这些特征易于区分[204]。在 COPD 患者中，可以使用专用软件量化这些变化：平均 PBF、PBV 和平均通过时间会逐渐减少，并且变化是异质性的[109,110]。

2. 间质性肺病 ILD 包括许多不同病因的病理性疾病，通常表现为肺泡炎性反应，可能向纤维化进展。由于这些疾病的异质性高，因此单独的影像学不足以进行最终诊断，需要将形态学方面与临床和功能数据相结合。CT 阐明了 ILD 浸润性病变的基本改变和形态学特征。随着最近对 IPF 诊断指南的修订，CT 影像学特征起着关键作用[205]。相比 CT，ILD 患者行 MRI 研究的数量非常有限。尽管如此，已公布的数据表明 ILD 中肺 MRI 的至少三种应用可能：形态学变化及病变类型的识别；疾病炎性活动的评估；肺形态学变化影响肺功能参数的研究，如对比增强和灌注。

ILD 的基本形态学变化包括气腔病变和间质病变或两者的结合。因为 MR 信号与质子密度成比例地增加，所以在 T_2 加权图像上出现气腔浸润，表现为对正常肺实质的深色背景的高信号区域。

当肺血管标记未被掩盖时，这些病变与CT的磨玻璃样病变相似（图11-17）[71,206]。更加密集的表现为实变，易于在MRI上评估[72]。与实变相似，可能与不同程度的肺实质扭曲有关，间质病变和纤维化会增加结节和网状影的信号强度[207-209]。在T₂加权图像中通常显示广泛的肺外周和肺门周的纤维化改变，鉴别诊断需要考虑到可疑充血性心力衰竭患者的肺间质水肿。T₁加权VIBE图像提供高空间分辨率，建议采用脂肪抑制序列对比增强后采集，相比胸膜下肌肉、肋骨和正常肺实质，胸膜下肺组织的信号改变增加，使用这种技术[209]可评估蜂窝影。

鉴别活动的炎性反应与纤维化对预测ILD的临床治疗效果具有重要意义。已经研究了炎症和纤维化的MR信号和对比增强的特征。虽然在1.5T的初步研究图像质量欠佳[210-211]，但证实了评估ILD疾病活动性的可行性。最近，Yi等[160]通过与胸壁肌肉信号相比，T₂加权像上的炎症和纤维化病变的MR信号分别是高信号和等信号[209]。动态增强MRI中早期增强和峰值增强的清除可以预测疾病活动[209]。与纤维化相比，较早的增强和快速清除与炎症区域中毛细血管的较高渗透性一致。总之，MRI在ILD研究和临床应用中具有极大的应用前景。

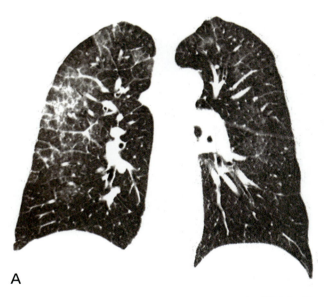
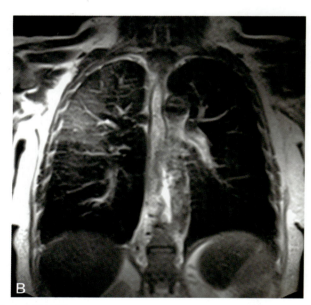

▲ 图11-17 磨玻璃影检测

53岁女性患者因为急性髓系白血病（AML）接受化疗，现因白细胞缺乏而发热。患者同一天接受胸部低剂量CT（A）和平扫MRI（B）检查以检测病变浸润。CT上双肺且以右肺上叶为主的广泛磨玻璃影与MR．T₂加权（HASTE）序列上信号增高相关性很好。请注意：两种检查技术的血管结构均未模糊。患者随后被诊断为病毒性肺炎

参考文献

[1] Wild JM, Marshall H, Bock M, Schad LR, Jakob PM et al. (2012) MRI of the lung (1/3): Methods. *Insights Imaging* 3: 345–353.

[2] Biederer J, Beer M, Hirsch W, Wild J, Fabel M et al. (2012) MRI of the lung (2/3). Why ... when ... how? *Insights Imaging* 3: 355–371.

[3] Biederer J, Mirsadraee S, Beer M, Molinari F, Hintze C et al. (2012) MRI of the lung (3/3)-current applications and future perspectives. *Insights Imaging* 3: 373–386.

[4] Müller CJ, Löffler R, Deimling M, Peller M, Reiser M (2001) MR lung imaging at 0.2 T with T1-weighted true FISP: Native and oxygen-enhanced. *J Magn Reson Imaging* 14: 164–168.

[5] Anjorin A, Schmidt H, Posselt H-G, Smaczny C, Ackermann H et al. (2008) Comparative evaluation of chest radiography, low-field MRI, the Shwachman Kulczycki score and pulmonary function tests in patients with cystic fibrosis. *Eur Radiol* 18: 1153–1161.

[6] Bankier AA, O'Donnell CR, Mai VM, Storey P, De Maertelaer V et al. (2004) Impact of lung volume on MR signal

intensity changes of the lung parenchyma. *J Magn Reson Imaging* 20: 961–966.

[7] Iwasawa T, Takahashi H, Ogura T, Asakura A, Gotoh T et al. (2007) Correlation of lung parenchymal MR signal intensity with pulmonary function tests and quantitative computed tomography (CT) evaluation: A pilot study. *J Magn Reson Imaging* 26: 1530–1536.

[8] Arnold JF, Morchel P, Glaser E, Pracht ED, Jakob PM (2007) Lung MRI using an MR-compatible active breathing control (MR-ABC). *Magn Reson Med* 58: 1092–1098.

[9] Oechsner M, Pracht ED, Staeb D, Arnold JF, Kostler H et al. (2009) Lung imaging under free-breathing conditions. *Magn Reson Med* 61: 723–727.

[10] Lin W, Guo J, Rosen MA, Song HK (2008) Respiratory motion-compensated radial dynamic contrast-enhanced (DCE)-MRI of chest and abdominal lesions. *Magn Reson Med* 60: 1135–1146.

[11] Pruessmann KP, Weiger M, Scheidegger MB, Boesiger P (1999) SENSE: Sensitivity encoding for fast MRI. *Magn Reson Med* 42: 952–962.

[12] Griswold MA, Blaimer M, Breuer F, Heidemann RM, Mueller M et al. (2005) Parallel magnetic resonance imaging using the GRAPPA operator formalism. *Magn Reson Med* 54: 1553–1556.

[13] Heidemann RM, Griswold MA, Kiefer B, Nittka M, Wang J et al. (2003) Resolution enhancement in lung 1H imaging using parallel imaging methods. *Magn Reson Med* 49: 391–394.

[14] Henzler T, Dietrich O, Krissak R, Wichmann T, Lanz T et al. (2009) Half-Fourier-acquisition single-shot turbo spin-echo (HASTE) MRI of the lung at 3 Tesla using parallel imaging with 32-receiver channel technology. *J Magn Reson Imaging* 30: 541–546.

[15] Puderbach M, Hintze C, Ley S, Eichinger M, Kauczor HU et al. (2007) MR imaging of the chest: A practical approach at 1.5T. *Eur J Radiol* 64: 345–355.

[16] Swift AJ, Woodhouse N, Fichele S, Siedel J, Mills GH et al. (2007) Rapid lung volumetry using ultrafast dynamic magnetic resonance imaging during forced vital capacity maneuver: Correlation with spirometry. *Invest Radiol* 42: 37–41.

[17] Biederer J, Hintze C, Fabel M, Dinkel J (2010) Magnetic resonance imaging and computed tomography of respiratory mechanics. *J Magn Reson Imaging* 32: 1388–1397.

[18] Bieri O (2013) Ultra-fast steady state free precession and its application to in vivo H morphological and functional lung imaging at 1.5 tesla. *Magn Reson Med* 70(3): 657–663.

[19] Huang TY, Huang IJ, Chen CY, Scheffler K, Chung HW et al. (2002) Are TrueFISP images T2/T1-weighted? *Magn Reson Med* 48: 684–688.

[20] Hui BK, Noga ML, Gan KD, Wilman AH (2005) Navigator-gated three-dimensional MR angiography of the pulmonary arteries using steady-state free precession. *J Magn Reson Imaging* 21: 831–835.

[21] Miller GW, Mugler JP, Sá RC, Altes TA, Prisk GK et al. (2014) Advances in functional and structural imaging of the human lung using proton MRI. *NMR Biomed* 27(12): 1542–1556.

[22] Hennig J, Nauerth A, Friedburg H (1986) RARE imaging: A fast imaging method for clinical MR. *Magn Reson Med* 3: 823–833.

[23] Bergin CJ, Pauly JM, Macovski A (1991) Lung parenchyma: Projection reconstruction MR imaging. *Radiology* 179: 777–781.

[24] Johnson KM, Fain SB, Schiebler ML, Nagle S (2013) Optimized 3D ultrashort echo time pulmonary MRI. *Magn Reson Med* 70: 1241–1250.

[25] Wilman AH, Riederer SJ (1997) Performance of an elliptical centric view order for signal enhancement and motion artifact suppression in breath-hold three-dimensional gradient echo imaging. *Magn Reson Med* 38: 793–802.

[26] Korosec FR, Frayne R, Grist TM, Mistretta CA (1996) Time-resolved contrast-enhanced 3D MR angiography. *Magn Reson Med* 36: 345–351.

[27] Puderbach M, Risse F, Biederer J, Ley-Zaporozhan J, Ley S et al. (2008) In vivo Gd-DTPA concentration for MR lung perfusion measurements: Assessment with computed tomography in a porcine model. *Eur Radiol* 18: 2102–2107.

[28] Wang T, Schultz G, Hebestreit H, Hebestreit A, Hahn D et al. (2003) Quantitative perfusion mapping of the human lung using 1H spin labeling. *J Magn Reson Imaging* 18: 260–265.

[29] Stadler A, Jakob PM, Griswold M, Barth M, Bankier AA (2005) T1 mapping of the entire lung parenchyma: Influence of the respiratory phase in healthy individuals. *J Magn Reson Imaging* 21: 759–764.

[30] Edelman RR, Hatabu H, Tadamura E, Li W, Prasad PV (1996) Noninvasive assessment of regional ventilation in the human lung using oxygen-enhanced magnetic resonance imaging. *Nat Med* 2: 1236–1239.

[31] Jakob PM, Hillenbrand CM, Wang T, Schultz G, Hahn D et al. (2001) Rapid quantitative lung (1)H T(1) mapping. *J Magn Reson Imaging* 14: 795–799.

[32] Triphan SM, Breuer FA, Gensler D, Kauczor HU, Jakob PM (2015) Oxygen enhanced lung MRI by simultaneous measurement of T1 and T2* during free breathing using ultrashort TE. *J Magn Reson Imaging* 41: 1708–1714.

[33] Bauman G, Puderbach M, Deimling M, Jellus V, Chefd'hotel C et al. (2009) Non-contrast-enhanced perfusion and ventilation assessment of the human lung by means of Fourier decomposition in proton MRI. *Magn Reson Med* 62: 656–664.

[34] Lederlin M, Bauman G, Eichinger M, Dinkel J, Brault M et al. (2013) Functional MRI using Fourier decomposition of lung signal: Reproducibility of ventilation and perfusion-weighted imaging in healthy volunteers. *Eur J Radiol* 82: 1015–1022.

[35] Bauman G, Lutzen U, Ullrich M, Gaass T, Dinkel J et al. (2011) Pulmonary functional imaging: Qualitative comparison of Fourier decomposition MR imaging with SPECT/CT

in porcine lung. *Radiology* 260: 551–559.

[36] Bauman G, Scholz A, Rivoire J, Terekhov M, Friedrich J et al. (2013) Lung ventilation and perfusion-weighted Fourier decomposition magnetic resonance imaging: In vivo validation with hyperpolarized 3He and dynamic contrast-enhanced MRI. *Magn Reson Med* 69: 229–237.

[37] Bauman G, Puderbach M, Heimann T, Kopp-Schneider A, Fritzsching E et al. (2013) Validation of Fourier decomposition MRI with dynamic contrast-enhanced MRI using visual and automated scoring of pulmonary perfusion in young cystic fibrosis patients. *Eur J Radiol* 82: 2371–2377.

[38] Biederer J, Heussel CP, Puderbach M, Wielpuetz MO (2014) Functional magnetic resonance imaging of the lung. *Semin Respir Crit Care Med* 35: 74–82.

[39] Sommer G, Bauman G, Koenigkam-Santos M, Draenkow C, Heussel CP et al. (2013) Non-contrast-enhanced preoperative assessment of lung perfusion in patients with non-small-cell lung cancer using Fourier decomposition magnetic resonance imaging. *Eur J Radiol* 82: e879–e887.

[40] Kjorstad A, Corteville DM, Fischer A, Henzler T, Schmid Bindert G et al. (2014) Quantitative lung perfusion evaluation using Fourier decomposition perfusion MRI. *Magn Reson Med* 72(2): 558–562.

[41] van Beek EJ, Hill C, Woodhouse N, Fichele S, Fleming S et al. (2007) Assessment of lung disease in children with cystic fibrosis using hyperpolarized 3-Helium MRI: Comparison with Shwachman score, Chrispin-Norman score and spirometry. *Eur Radiol* 17: 1018–1024.

[42] Donnelly LF, MacFall JR, McAdams HP, Majure JM, Smith J et al. (1999) Cystic fibrosis: Combined hyperpolarized 3He-enhanced and conventional proton MR imaging in the lung—Preliminary observations. *Radiology* 212: 885–889.

[43] de Lange EE, Altes TA, Patrie JT, Gaare JD, Knake JJ et al. (2006) Evaluation of asthma with hyperpolarized helium-3 MRI: Correlation with clinical severity and spirometry. *Chest* 130: 1055–1062.

[44] Woodhouse N, Wild JM, Paley MN, Fichele S, Said Z et al. (2005) Combined helium-3/proton magnetic resonance imaging measurement of ventilated lung volumes in smokers compared to never-smokers. *J Magn Reson Imaging* 21: 365–369.

[45] Kirby M, Pike D, Coxson HO, McCormack DG, Parraga G (2014) Hyperpolarized He ventilation defects used to predict pulmonary exacerbations in mild to moderate chronic obstructive pulmonary disease. *Radiology*: 140161.

[46] Wild JM, Marshall H, Xu X, Norquay G, Parnell SR et al. (2013) Simultaneous imaging of lung structure and function with triple-nuclear hybrid MR imaging. *Radiology* 267: 251–255.

[47] Marshall H, Kiely DG, Parra-Robles J, Capener D, Deppe MH et al. (2014) Magnetic resonance imaging of ventilation and perfusion changes in response to pulmonary endarterectomy in chronic thromboembolic pulmonary hypertension. *Am J Respir Crit Care Med* 190: e18–e19.

[48] Mentore K, Froh DK, de Lange EE, Brookeman JR, Paget Brown AO et al. (2005) Hyperpolarized HHe 3 MRI of the lung in cystic fibrosis: Assessment at baseline and after bronchodilator and airway clearance treatment. *Acad Radiol* 12: 1423–1429.

[49] Woodhouse N, Wild JM, van Beek EJ, Hoggard N, Barker N et al. (2009) Assessment of hyperpolarized 3He lung MRI for regional evaluation of interventional therapy: A pilot study in pediatric cystic fibrosis. *J Magn Reson Imaging* 30: 981–988.

[50] Thomen RP, Sheshadri A, Quirk JD, Kozlowski J, Ellison HD et al. (2014) Regional ventilation changes in severe asthma after bronchial thermoplasty with He MR imaging and CT. *Radiology*: 140080.

[51] Johansson MW, Kruger SJ, Schiebler ML, Evans MD, Sorkness RL et al. (2013) Markers of vascular perturbation correlate with airway structural change in asthma. *Am J Respir Crit Care Med* 188: 167–178.

[52] Wild JM, Paley MN, Kasuboski L, Swift A, Fichele S et al. (2003) Dynamic radial projection MRI of inhaled hyper polarized 3He gas. *Magn Reson Med* 49: 991–997.

[53] Marshall H, Deppe MH, Parra-Robles J, Hillis S, Billings CG et al. (2012) Direct visualisation of collateral ventilation in COPD with hyperpolarised gas MRI. *Thorax* 67: 613–617.

[54] Swift AJ, Wild JM, Fichele S, Woodhouse N, Fleming S et al. (2005) Emphysematous changes and normal variation in smokers and COPD patients using diffusion 3He MRI. *Eur J Radiol* 54: 352–358.

[55] Altes TA, Mata J, de Lange EE, Brookeman JR, Mugler JP, 3rd (2006) Assessment of lung development using hyperpolarized helium-3 diffusion MR imaging. *J Magn Reson Imaging* 24: 1277–1283.

[56] van Beek EJ, Dahmen AM, Stavngaard T, Gast KK, Heussel CP et al. (2009) Hyperpolarised 3He MRI versus HRCT in COPD and normal volunteers: PHIL trial. *Eur Respir J* 34: 1311–1321.

[57] Kirby M, Svenningsen S, Owrangi A, Wheatley A, Farag A et al. (2012) Hyperpolarized 3He and 129Xe MR imaging in healthy volunteers and patients with chronic obstructive pulmonary disease. *Radiology* 265: 600–610.

[58] Driehuys B, Martinez-Jimenez S, Cleveland ZI, Metz GM, Beaver DM et al. (2012) Chronic obstructive pulmonary disease: Safety and tolerability of hyperpolarized 129Xe MR imaging in healthy volunteers and patients. *Radiology* 262: 279–289.

[59] Cleveland ZI, Cofer GP, Metz G, Beaver D, Nouls J et al. (2010) Hyperpolarized Xe MR imaging of alveolar gas uptake in humans. *PLoS One* 5: e12192.

[60] Mugler JP, 3rd, Altes TA, Ruset IC, Dregely IM, Mata JF et al. (2010) Simultaneous magnetic resonance imaging of ventilation distribution and gas uptake in the human lung using hyperpolarized xenon-129. *Proc Natl Acad Sci USA* 107: 21707–21712.

[61] Stewart NJ, Leung G, Norquay G, Marshall H, Parra Robles J et al. (2014) Experimental validation of the hyperpolarized Xe chemical shift saturation recovery technique in healthy volunteers and subjects with interstitial lung disease. *Magn Reson Med*. doi:10.1002/ mrm.25400.

[62] Hansell DM, Bankier AA, MacMahon H, McLoud TC, Muller NL et al. (2008) Fleischner Society: Glossary of terms for thoracic imaging. *Radiology* 246: 697–722.

[63] Barreto MM, Rafful PP, Rodrigues RS, Zanetti G, Hochhegger B et al. (2013) Correlation between computed tomographic and magnetic resonance imaging findings of parenchymal lung diseases. *Eur J Radiol* 82: e492–e501.

[64] Biederer J, Hintze C, Fabel M (2008) MRI of pulmonary nodules: Technique and diagnostic value. *Cancer Imaging* 8: 125–130.

[65] Wielputz M, Kauczor HU (2012) MRI of the lung: State of the art. *Diagn Interv Radiol* 18: 344–353.

[66] Ley-Zaporozhan J, Ley S, Eberhardt R, Kauczor HU, Heussel CP (2010) Visualization of morphological parenchymal changes in emphysema: Comparison of different MRI sequences to 3D-HRCT. *Eur J Radiol* 73: 43–49.

[67] Biederer J, Busse I, Grimm J, Reuter M, Muhle C et al. (2002) Sensitivity of MRI in detecting alveolar Infiltrates: Experimental studies. *Rofo* 174: 1033–1039.

[68] Kersjes W, Hildebrandt G, Cagil H, Schunk K, von Zitzewitz H et al. (1999) Differentiation of alveolitis and pulmonary fibrosis in rabbits with magnetic resonance imaging after intrabronchial administration of bleomycin. *Invest Radiol* 34: 13–21.

[69] Fink C, Puderbach M, Biederer J, Fabel M, Dietrich O et al. (2007) Lung MRI at 1.5 and 3 Tesla: Observer preference study and lesion contrast using five different pulse sequences. *Invest Radiol* 42: 377–383.

[70] Jacob RE, Amidan BG, Soelberg J, Minard KR (2010) In vivo MRI of altered proton signal intensity and T2 relaxation in a bleomycin model of pulmonary inflammation and fibrosis. *J Magn Reson Imaging* 31: 1091–1099.

[71] Eibel R, Herzog P, Dietrich O, Rieger CT, Ostermann H et al. (2006) Pulmonary abnormalities in immunocompromised patients: Comparative detection with parallel acquisition MR imaging and thin-section helical CT. *Radiology* 241: 880–891.

[72] Rieger C, Herzog P, Eibel R, Fiegl M, Ostermann H (2008) Pulmonary MRI—A new approach for the evaluation of febrile neutropenic patients with malignancies. *Support Care Cancer* 16: 599–606.

[73] Biederer J, Schoene A, Freitag S, Reuter M, Heller M (2003) Simulated pulmonary nodules implanted in a dedicated porcine chest phantom: Sensitivity of MR imaging for detection. *Radiology* 227: 475–483.

[74] Both M, Schultze J, Reuter M, Bewig B, Hubner R et al. (2005) Fast T1 and T2-weighted pulmonary MR-imaging in patients with bronchial carcinoma. *Eur J Radiol* 53: 478–488.

[75] Bruegel M, Gaa J, Woertler K, Ganter C, Waldt S et al. (2007) MRI of the lung: Value of different turbo spin echo, single-shot turbo spin-echo, and 3D gradient-echo pulse sequences for the detection of pulmonary metastases. *J Magn Reson Imaging* 25: 73–81.

[76] Sommer G, Tremper J, Koenigkam-Santos M, Delorme S, Becker N et al. (2014) Lung nodule detection in a high risk population: Comparison of magnetic resonance imaging and low-dose computed tomography. *Eur J Radiol* 83: 600–605.

[77] Gamsu G, de Geer G, Cann C, Muller N, Brito A (1987) A preliminary study of MRI quantification of simulated calcified pulmonary nodules. *Invest Radiol* 22: 853–858.

[78] Kersjes W, Mayer E, Buchenroth M, Schunk K, Fouda N et al. (1997) Diagnosis of pulmonary metastases with turbo-SE MR imaging. *Eur Radiol* 7: 1190–1194.

[79] Chung MH, Lee HG, Kwon SS, Park SH (2000) MR imaging of solitary pulmonary lesion: Emphasis on tuber-culomas and comparison with tumors. *J Magn Reson Imaging* 11: 629–637.

[80] Kirchner J, Kirchner EM (2001) Melanoptysis: Findings on CT and MRI. *Br J Radiol* 74: 1003–1006.

[81] Regier M, Kandel S, Kaul MG, Hoffmann B, Ittrich H et al. (2007) Detection of small pulmonary nodules in high-field MR at 3 T: Evaluation of different pulse sequences using porcine lung explants. *Eur Radiol* 17: 1341–1351.

[82] Baumann T, Ludwig U, Pache G, Gall C, Saueressig U et al. (2008) Detection of pulmonary nodules with move-during-scan magnetic resonance imaging using a free-breathing turbo inversion recovery magnitude sequence. *Invest Radiol* 43: 359–367.

[83] Khalil AM, Carette MF, Cadranel JL, Mayaud CM, Akoun GM et al. (1994) Magnetic resonance imaging findings in pulmonary Kaposi's sarcoma: A series of 10 cases. *Eur Respir J* 7: 1285–1289.

[84] Semelka RC, Cem Balci N, Wilber KP, Fisher LL, Brown MA et al. (2000) Breath-hold 3D gradient-echo MR imaging of the lung parenchyma: Evaluation of reproducibility of image quality in normals and preliminary observations in patients with disease. *J Magn Reson Imaging* 11: 195–200.

[85] Biederer J, Both M, Graessner J, Liess C, Jakob P et al. (2003) Lung morphology: Fast MR imaging assessment with a volumetric interpolated breath-hold technique: Initial experience with patients. *Radiology* 226: 242–249.

[86] Kluge A, Muller C, Hansel J, Gerriets T, Bachmann G (2004) Real-time MR with TrueFISP for the detection of acute pulmonary embolism: Initial clinical experience. *Eur Radiol* 14: 709–718.

[87] Kluge A, Gerriets T, Stolz E, Dill T, Mueller KD et al. (2006) Pulmonary perfusion in acute pulmonary embolism: Agreement of MRI and SPECT for lobar, segmental and subsegmental perfusion defects. *Acta Radiol* 47: 933–940.

[88] Kluge A, Luboldt W, Bachmann G (2006) Acute pulmonary embolism to the subsegmental level: Diagnostic accuracy of three MRI techniques compared with 16-MDCT. *AJR Am J*

Roentgenol 187: W7–W14.

[89] Moody AR, Liddicoat A, Krarup K (1997) Magnetic resonance pulmonary angiography and direct imaging of embolus for the detection of pulmonary emboli. *Invest Radiol* 32: 431–440.

[90] Moody AR (2003) Magnetic resonance direct thrombus imaging. *J Thromb Haemost* 1: 1403–1409.

[91] Biederer J, Liess C, Charalambous N, Heller M (2004) Volumetric interpolated contrast-enhanced MRA for the diagnosis of pulmonary embolism in an ex vivo system. *J Magn Reson Imaging* 19: 428–437.

[92] Matsuoka S, Uchiyama K, Shima H, Terakoshi H, Oishi S et al. (2002) Effect of the rate of gadolinium injection on magnetic resonance pulmonary perfusion imaging. *J Magn Reson Imaging* 15: 108–113.

[93] Meaney JF, Weg JG, Chenevert TL, Stafford-Johnson D, Hamilton BH et al. (1997) Diagnosis of pulmonary embolism with magnetic resonance angiography. *N Engl J Med* 336: 1422–1427.

[94] Gupta A, Frazer CK, Ferguson JM, Kumar AB, Davis SJ et al. (1999) Acute pulmonary embolism: Diagnosis with MR angiography. *Radiology* 210: 353–359.

[95] Oudkerk M, van Beek EJ, Wielopolski P, van Ooijen PM, Brouwers-Kuyper EM et al. (2002) Comparison of contrast-enhanced magnetic resonance angiography and conventional pulmonary angiography for the diagnosis of pulmonary embolism: A prospective study. *Lancet* 359: 1643–1647.

[96] Goyen M, Laub G, Ladd ME, Debatin JF, Barkhausen J et al. (2001) Dynamic 3D MR angiography of the pulmonary arteries in under four seconds. *J Magn Reson Imaging* 13: 372–377.

[97] Stein PD, Chenevert TL, Fowler SE, Goodman LR, Gottschalk A et al. (2010) Gadolinium-enhanced magnetic resonance angiography for pulmonary embolism: A multicenter prospective study (PIOPED III). *Ann Intern Med* 152: 434–443, W142–W433.

[98] Fink C, Puderbach M, Bock M, Lodemann KP, Zuna I et al. (2004) Regional lung perfusion: Assessment with partially parallel three-dimensional MR imaging. *Radiology* 231: 175–184.

[99] Eichinger M, Puderbach M, Fink C, Gahr J, Ley S et al. (2006) Contrast-enhanced 3D MRI of lung perfusion in children with cystic fibrosis—Initial results. *Eur Radiol* 16: 2147–2152.

[100] Ersoy H, Goldhaber SZ, Cai T, Luu T, Rosebrook J et al. (2007) Time-resolved MR angiography: A primary screening examination of patients with suspected pulmonary embolism and contraindications to administration of iodinated contrast material. *AJR Am J Roentgenol* 188: 1246–1254.

[101] Levin DL, Chen Q, Zhang M, Edelman RR, Hatabu H (2001) Evaluation of regional pulmonary perfusion using ultrafast magnetic resonance imaging. *Magn Reson Med* 46: 166–171.

[102] Arai TJ, Henderson AC, Dubowitz DJ, Levin DL, Friedman PJ et al. (2009) Hypoxic pulmonary vasoconstriction does not contribute to pulmonary blood flow heterogeneity in normoxia in normal supine humans. *J Appl Physiol (1985)* 106: 1057–1064.

[103] Hopkins SR, Wielputz MO, Kauczor HU (2012) Imaging lung perfusion. *J Appl Physiol* 113: 328–339.

[104] Wielputz MO, Eichinger M, Puderbach M (2013) Magnetic resonance imaging of cystic fibrosis lung disease. *J Thorac Imaging* 28: 151–159.

[105] Eichinger M, Optazaite DE, Kopp-Schneider A, Hintze C, Biederer J et al. (2012) Morphologic and functional scoring of cystic fibrosis lung disease using MRI. *Eur J Radiol* 81: 1321–1329.

[106] Wielputz MO, Puderbach M, Kopp-Schneider A, Stahl M, Fritzsching E et al. (2014) Magnetic resonance imaging detects changes in structure and perfusion, and response to therapy in early cystic fibrosis lung disease. *Am J Respir Crit Care Med* 189: 956–965.

[107] Kuder TA, Risse F, Eichinger M, Ley S, Puderbach M et al. (2008) New method for 3D parametric visualization of contrast-enhanced pulmonary perfusion MRI data. *Eur Radiol* 18: 291–297.

[108] Risse F, Eichinger M, Kauczor HU, Semmler W, Puderbach M (2011) Improved visualization of delayed perfusion in lung MRI. *Eur J Radiol* 77: 105–110.

[109] Kohlmann P, Strehlow J, Jobst B, Krass S, Kuhnigk J-M et al. (2014) Automatic lung segmentation method for MRI-based lung perfusion studies of patients with chronic obstructive pulmonary disease. *Int J Comput Assist Radiol Surg* 10(4): 403–417.

[110] Ohno Y, Hatabu H, Murase K, Higashino T, Kawamitsu H et al. (2004) Quantitative assessment of regional pulmonary perfusion in the entire lung using three-dimensional ultrafast dynamic contrast-enhanced magnetic resonance imaging: Preliminary experience in 40 subjects. *J Magn Reson Imaging* 20: 353–365.

[111] Ley S, Mereles D, Risse F, Grunig E, Ley-Zaporozhan J et al. (2007) Quantitative 3D pulmonary MR-perfusion in patients with pulmonary arterial hypertension: Correlation with invasive pressure measurements. *Eur J Radiol* 61: 251–255.

[112] Puderbach M, Eichinger M, Haeselbarth J, Ley S, Kopp Schneider A et al. (2007) Assessment of morphological MRI for pulmonary changes in cystic fibrosis (CF) patients: Comparison to thin-section CT and chest x-ray. *Invest Radiol* 42: 715–725.

[113] Puderbach M, Eichinger M, Gahr J, Ley S, Tuengerthal S et al. (2007) Proton MRI appearance of cystic fibrosis: Comparison to CT. *Eur Radiol* 17: 716–724.

[114] Biederer J, Reuter M, Both M, Muhle C, Grimm J et al. (2002) Analysis of artifacts and detail resolution of lung MRI with breath-hold T1-weighted gradient-echo and T2-weighted fast spin-echo sequences with respiratory triggering. *Eur Radiol* 12: 378–384.

[115] Fabel M, Wintersperger BJ, Dietrich O, Eichinger M, Fink C et al. (2009) MRI of respiratory dynamics with 2D steady-state free-precession and 2D gradient echo sequences at 1.5 and 3 Tesla: An observer preference study. *Eur Radiol* 19: 391–399.

[116] Faust RA, Rimell FL, Remley KB (2002) Cine magnetic resonance imaging for evaluation of focal tracheomalacia: Innominate artery compression syndrome. *Int J Pediatr Otorhinolaryngol* 65: 27–33.

[117] Ley S, Loukanov T, Ley-Zaporozhan J, Springer W, Sebening C et al. (2010) Long-term outcome after external tracheal stabilization due to congenital tracheal instability. *Ann Thorac Surg* 89: 918–925.

[118] Heussel CP, Ley S, Biedermann A, Rist A, Gast KK et al. (2004) Respiratory lumenal change of the pharynx and trachea in normal subjects and COPD patients: Assessment by cine-MRI. *Eur Radiol* 14: 2188–2197.

[119] Cai J, Read PW, Altes TA, Molloy JA, Brookeman JR et al. (2007) Evaluation of the reproducibility of lung motion probability distribution function (PDF) using dynamic MRI. *Phys Med Biol* 52: 365–373.

[120] Adamson J, Chang Z, Wang Z, Yin FF, Cai J (2010) Maximum intensity projection (MIP) imaging using slice-stacking MRI. *Med Phys* 37: 5914–5920.

[121] Tetzlaff R, Schwarz T, Kauczor HU, Meinzer HP, Puderbach M et al. (2010) Lung function measurement of single lungs by lung area segmentation on 2D dynamic MRI. *Acad Radiol* 17: 496–503.

[122] Wild JM, Schmiedeskamp J, Paley MN, Filbir F, Fichele S et al. (2002) MR imaging of the lungs with hyperpolar ized helium-3 gas transported by air. *Phys Med Biol* 47: N185–N190.

[123] Scholz AW, Wolf U, Fabel M, Weiler N, Heussel CP et al. (2009) Comparison of magnetic resonance imaging of inhaled SF6 with respiratory gas analysis. *Magn Reson Imaging* 27: 549–556.

[124] Suga K, Ogasawara N, Tsukuda T, Matsunaga N (2002) Assessment of regional lung ventilation in dog lungs with Gd-DTPA aerosol ventilation MR imaging. *Acta Radiol* 43: 282–291.

[125] Molinari F, Puderbach M, Eichinger M, Ley S, Fink C et al. (2008) Oxygen-enhanced magnetic resonance imaging: Influence of different gas delivery methods on the T1-changes of the lungs. *Invest Radiol* 43: 427–432.

[126] Peltola V, Ruuskanen O, Svedstrom E (2008) Magnetic resonance imaging of lung infections in children. *Pediatr Radiol* 38: 1225–1231.

[127] Ley-Zaporozhan J, Ley S, Sommerburg O, Komm N, Muller FM et al. (2009) Clinical application of MRI in children for the assessment of pulmonary diseases. *Rofo* 181: 419–432.

[128] Failo R, Wielopolski PA, Tiddens HA, Hop WC, Mucelli RP et al. (2009) Lung morphology assessment using MRI: A robust ultra-short TR/TE 2D steady state free precession sequence used in cystic fibrosis patients. *Magn Reson Med* 61: 299–306.

[129] Wagner M, Bowing B, Kuth R, Deimling M, Rascher W et al. (2001) Low field thoracic MRI—A fast and radiation free routine imaging modality in children. *Magn Reson Imaging* 19: 975–983.

[130] Rupprecht T, Kuth R, Bowing B, Gerling S, Wagner M et al. (2000) Sedation and monitoring of paediatric patients undergoing open low-field MRI. *Acta Paediatr* 89: 1077–1081.

[131] Serra G, Milito C, Mitrevski M, Granata G, Martini H et al. (2011) Lung MRI as a possible alternative to CT scan for patients with primary immune deficiencies and increased radiosensitivity MRI for lung evaluation in immunodeficiencies. *CHEST J* 140: 1581–1589.

[132] Hirsch W, Sorge I, Krohmer S, Weber D, Meier K et al. (2008) MRI of the lungs in children. *Eur J Radiol* 68: 278–288.

[133] Schaefer JF, Kramer U (2011) Whole-body MRI in chil dren and juveniles. *Rofo* 183: 24–36.

[134] Sanborn PA, Michna E, Zurakowski D, Burrows PE, Fontaine PJ et al. (2005) Adverse cardiovascular and respiratory events during sedation of pediatric patients for imaging examinations. *Radiology* 237: 288–294.

[135] Lutterbey G, Wattjes MP, Doerr D, Fischer NJ, Gieseke J, Jr. et al. (2007) Atelectasis in children undergoing either pro-pofol infusion or positive pressure ventilation anesthesia for magnetic resonance imaging. *Paediatr Anaesth* 17: 121–125.

[136] Blitman NM, Lee HK, Jain VR, Vicencio AG, Girshin M et al. (2007) Pulmonary atelectasis in children anesthetized for cardiothoracic MR: Evaluation of risk factors. *J Comput Assist Tomogr* 31: 789–794.

[137] Biederer J (2009) General requirements of MRI of the lung and suggested standard protocol. In: Kauczor H-U, ed., *MRI of the Lung*. Berlin, Germany: Springer, pp. 3–16.

[138] Seo JS, Kim YJ, Choi BW, Choe KO (2005) Usefulness of magnetic resonance imaging for evaluation of cardio vascular invasion: Evaluation of sliding motion between thoracic mass and adjacent structures on cine MR images. *J Magn Reson Imaging* 22: 234–241.

[139] Stein PD, Gottschalk A, Sostman HD, Chenevert TL, Fowler SE et al. (2008) Methods of Prospective Investigation of Pulmonary Embolism Diagnosis III (PIOPED III). *Semin Nucl Med* 38: 462–470.

[140] Schiebler ML, Bhalla S, Runo J, Jarjour N, Roldan A et al. (2013) Magnetic resonance and computed tomography imaging of the structural and functional changes of pul-monary arterial hypertension. *J Thorac Imaging* 28: 178–193.

[141] Vonk Noordegraaf A, Galie N (2011) The role of the right ventricle in pulmonary arterial hypertension. *Eur Respir Rev* 20: 243–253.

[142] Rajaram S, Swift AJ, Capener D, Telfer A, Davies C et al.

(2012) Diagnostic accuracy of contrast-enhanced MR angiography and unenhanced proton MR imaging compared with CT pulmonary angiography in chronic thromboembolic pulmonary hypertension. *Eur Radiol* 22: 310–317.

[143] Cohen MD, Eigen H, Scott PH, Tepper R, Cory DA et al. (1986) Magnetic resonance imaging of inflammatory lung disorders: Preliminary studies in children. *Pediatr Pulmonol* 2: 211–217.

[144] Rupprecht T, Bowing B, Kuth R, Deimling M, Rascher W et al. (2002) Steady-state free precession projection MRI as a potential alternative to the conventional chest X-ray in pediatric patients with suspected pneumonia. *Eur Radiol* 12: 2752–2756.

[145] Hebestreit A, Schultz G, Trusen A, Hebestreit H (2004) Follow-up of acute pulmonary complications in cystic fibrosis by magnetic resonance imaging: A pilot study. *Acta Paediatr* 93: 414–416.

[146] Abolmaali ND, Schmitt J, Krauss S, Bretz F, Deimling M et al. (2004) MR imaging of lung parenchyma at 0.2 T: Evaluation of imaging techniques, comparative study with chest radiography and interobserver analysis. *Eur Radiol* 14: 703–708.

[147] Montella S, Santamaria F, Salvatore M, Pignata C, Maglione M et al. (2009) Assessment of chest high-field magnetic resonance imaging in children and young adults with noncystic fibrosis chronic lung disease: Comparison to high-resolution computed tomography and correlation with pulmonary function. *Invest Radiol* 44: 532–538.

[148] Gibson RL, Burns JL, Ramsey BW (2003) Pathophysiology and management of pulmonary infections in cystic fibrosis. *Am J Respir Crit Care Med* 168: 918–951.

[149] Dodge JA, Lewis PA, Stanton M, Wilsher J (2007) Cystic fibrosis mortality and survival in the UK: 1947–2003. *Eur Respir J* 29: 522–526.

[150] Stern M, Wiedemann B, Wenzlaff P (2008) From registry to quality management: The German Cystic Fibrosis Quality Assessment project 1995–2006. *Eur Respir J* 31: 29–35.

[151] de Jong PA, Mayo JR, Golmohammadi K, Nakano Y, Lequin MH et al. (2006) Estimation of cancer mortality associated with repetitive computed tomography scanning. *Am J Respir Crit Care Med* 173: 199–203.

[152] O'Connell OJ, McWilliams S, McGarrigle A, O'Connor OJ, Shanahan F et al. (2012) Radiologic imaging in cystic fibrosis: Cumulative effective dose and changing trends over 2 decades. *Chest* 141: 1575–1583.

[153] Sileo C, Corvol H, Boelle PY, Blondiaux E, Clement A et al. (2014) HRCT and MRI of the lung in children with cystic fibrosis: Comparison of different scoring systems. *J Cyst Fibros* 13: 198–204.

[154] Hatabu H, Gaa J, Kim D, Li W, Prasad PV et al. (1996) Pulmonary perfusion: Qualitative assessment with dynamic contrast-enhanced MRI using ultra-short TE and inver-sion recovery turbo FLASH. *Magn Reson Med* 36: 503–508.

[155] de Jong PA, Tiddens HA (2007) Cystic fibrosis specific computed tomography scoring. *Proc Am Thorac Soc* 4: 338–342.

[156] Stein PD, Fowler SE, Goodman LR, Gottschalk A, Hales CA et al. (2006) Multidetector computed tomography for acute pulmonary embolism. *N Engl J Med* 354: 2317–2327.

[157] Kluge A, Gerriets T, Muller C, Ekinci O, Neumann T et al. (2005) Thoracic real-time MRI: Experience from 2200 examinations in acute and ill-defined thoracic diseases. *Rofo* 177: 1513–1521.

[158] Schiebler ML, Nagle SK, Francois CJ, Repplinger MD, Hamedani AG et al. (2013) Effectiveness of MR angiography for the primary diagnosis of acute pulmonary embolism: Clinical outcomes at 3 months and 1 year. *J Magn Reson Imaging* 38: 914–925.

[159] Chung JH, Cox CW, Forssen AV, Biederer J, Puderbach M et al. (2014) The dark lymph node sign on magnetic resonance imaging: A novel finding in patients with sarcoidosis. *J Thorac Imaging* 29: 125–129.

[160] Yi CA, Shin KM, Lee KS, Kim BT, Kim H et al. (2008) Non-small cell lung cancer staging: Efficacy comparison of integrated PET/CT versus 3.0-T whole-body MR imaging. *Radiology* 248: 632–642.

[161] Ohba Y, Nomori H, Mori T, Ikeda K, Shibata H et al. (2009) Is diffusion-weighted magnetic resonance imaging superior to positron emission tomography with fludeoxyglucose F 18 in imaging non-small cell lung cancer? *J Thorac Cardiovasc Surg* 138: 439–445.

[162] Ohno Y, Hatabu H, Takenaka D, Higashino T, Watanabe H et al. (2004) Metastases in mediastinal and hilar lymph nodes in patients with non-small cell lung cancer: Quantitative and qualitative assessment with STIR turbo spin-echo MR imaging. *Radiology* 231: 872–879.

[163] Ohno Y, Koyama H, Nogami M, Takenaka D, Yoshikawa T et al. (2007) Whole-body MR imaging vs. FDG-PET: Comparison of accuracy of M-stage diagnosis for lung cancer patients. *J Magn Reson Imaging* 26: 498–509.

[164] Chen W, Jian W, Li HT, Li C, Zhang YK et al. (2010) Whole-body diffusion-weighted imaging vs. FDG-PET for the detection of non-small-cell lung cancer. How do they measure up? *Magn Reson Imaging* 28: 613–620.

[165] Hasegawa I, Boiselle PM, Kuwabara K, Sawafuji M, Sugiura H (2008) Mediastinal lymph nodes in patients with non-small cell lung cancer: Preliminary experience with diffusion-weighted MR imaging. *J Thorac Imaging* 23: 157–161.

[166] Pauls S, Schmidt SA, Juchems MS, Klass O, Luster M et al. (2012) Diffusion-weighted MR imaging in compari son to integrated [(18)F]-FDG PET/CT for N-staging in patients with lung cancer. *Eur J Radiol* 81(1): 178–182.

[167] Koyama H, Ohno Y, Aoyama N, Onishi Y, Matsumoto K et al. (2010) Comparison of STIR turbo SE imaging and

diffusion-weighted imaging of the lung: Capability for detection and subtype classification of pulmonary adenocarcinomas. *Eur Radiol* 20: 790–800.

[168] Liu H, Liu Y, Yu T, Ye N (2010) Usefulness of diffusion-weighted MR imaging in the evaluation of pulmonary lesions. *Eur Radiol* 20: 807–815.

[169] Tondo F, Saponaro A, Stecco A, Lombardi M, Casadio C et al. (2011) Role of diffusion-weighted imaging in the differential diagnosis of benign and malignant lesions of the chest-mediastinum. *Radiol Med* 116: 720–733.

[170] Kanauchi N, Oizumi H, Honma T, Kato H, Endo M et al. (2009) Role of diffusion-weighted magnetic resonance imaging for predicting of tumor invasiveness for clinical stage IA non-small cell lung cancer. *Eur J Cardiothorac Surg* 35: 706–710; discussion 710–701.

[171] Qi LP, Zhang XP, Tang L, Li J, Sun YS et al. (2009) Using diffusion-weighted MR imaging for tumor detection in the collapsed lung: A preliminary study. *Eur Radiol* 19: 333–341.

[172] Uto T, Takehara Y, Nakamura Y, Naito T, Hashimoto D et al. (2009) Higher sensitivity and specificity for diffusion-weighted imaging of malignant lung lesions without apparent diffusion coefficient quantification. *Radiology* 252: 247–254.

[173] Karabulut N (2009) Accuracy of diffusion-weighted MR imaging for differentiation of pulmonary lesions. *Radiology* 253: 899; author reply 899–900.

[174] Henzler T, Schmid-Bindert G, Schoenberg SO, Fink C (2010) Diffusion and perfusion MRI of the lung and mediastinum. *Eur J Radiol* 76: 329–336.

[175] Regier M, Schwarz D, Henes FO, Groth M, Kooijman H et al. (2011) Diffusion-weighted MR-imaging for the detection of pulmonary nodules at 1.5 Tesla: Intraindividual comparison with multidetector computed tomography. *J Med Imaging Radiat Oncol* 55: 266–274.

[176] Bruzzi JF, Komaki R, Walsh GL, Truong MT, Gladish GW et al. (2008) Imaging of non-small cell lung cancer of the superior sulcus: Part 2: Initial staging and assessment of resectability and therapeutic response. *RadioGraphics* 28: 561–572.

[177] Akata S, Kajiwara N, Park J, Yoshimura M, Kakizaki D et al. (2008) Evaluation of chest wall invasion by lung cancer using respiratory dynamic MRI. *J Med Imaging Radiat Oncol* 52: 36–39.

[178] Ohno Y, Koyama H, Takenaka D, Nogami M, Maniwa Y et al. (2008) Dynamic MRI, dynamic multidetector row computed tomography (MDCT), and coregistered 2-[fluorine-18]-fluoro-2-deoxy-d-glucose-positron emission tomography (FDG-PET)/CT: Comparative study of capability for management of pulmonary nodules. *J Magn Reson Imaging* 27: 1284–1295.

[179] Pauls S, Mottaghy FM, Schmidt SA, Kruger S, Moller P et al. (2008) Evaluation of lung tumor perfusion by dynamic contrast-enhanced MRI. *Magn Reson Imaging* 26: 1334–1341.

[180] Pichler BJ, Kolb A, Nagele T, Schlemmer HP (2010) PET/MRI: Paving the way for the next generation of clinical multimodality imaging applications. *J Nucl Med* 51: 333–336.

[181] Hintze C, Dimitrakopoulou-Strauss A, Strauss LG, Risse F, Thieke C et al. (2007) Fusion of FDG-PET and proton MRI of the lung in patients with lung cancer: Initial results in differentiating tumor from atelectasis. *Fortschr Röntgenstr* 179 – VO_315_3.

[182] Pauls S, Schmidt SA, Juchems MS, Klass O, Luster M et al. (2012) Diffusion-weighted MR imaging in comparison to integrated [(1)(8)F]-FDG PET/CT for N-staging in patients with lung cancer. *Eur J Radiol* 81: 178–182.

[183] Antoch G, Vogt FM, Freudenberg LS, Nazaradeh F, Goehde SC et al. (2003) Whole-body dual-modality PET/ CT and whole-body MRI for tumor staging in oncology. *JAMA* 290: 3199–3206.

[184] Rabe KF, Hurd S, Anzueto A, Barnes PJ, Buist SA et al. (2007) Global strategy for the diagnosis, management, and prevention of chronic obstructive pulmonary disease: GOLD executive summary. *Am J Respir Crit Care Med* 176: 532–555.

[185] Hogg JC, Chu F, Utokaparch S, Woods R, Elliott WM et al. (2004) The nature of small-airway obstruction in chronic obstructive pulmonary disease. *N Engl J Med* 350: 2645–2653.

[186] Ley-Zaporozhan J, Ley S, Kauczor HU (2008) Morphological and functional imaging in COPD with CT and MRI: Present and future. *Eur Radiol* 18: 510–521.

[187] Decramer M, Gosselink R, Troosters T, Verschueren M, Evers G (1997) Muscle weakness is related to utilization of health care resources in COPD patients. *Eur Respir J* 10: 417–423.

[188] Henderson AC, Ingenito EP, Salcedo ES, Moy ML, Reilly JJ et al. (2007) Dynamic lung mechanics in late-stage emphysema before and after lung volume reduction surgery. *Respir Physiol Neurobiol* 155: 234–242.

[189] Sciurba FC, Ernst A, Herth FJ, Strange C, Criner GJ et al. (2010) A randomized study of endobronchial valves for advanced emphysema. *N Engl J Med* 363: 1233–1244.

[190] Suga K, Tsukuda T, Awaya H, Takano K, Koike S et al. (1999) Impaired respiratory mechanics in pulmonary emphysema: Evaluation with dynamic breathing MRI. *J Magn Reson Imaging* 10: 510–520.

[191] Wielputz MO, Eberhardt R, Puderbach M, Weinheimer O, Kauczor HU et al. (2014) Simultaneous assessment of airway instability and respiratory dynamics with low dose 4D-CT in chronic obstructive pulmonary disease: A technical note. *Respiration* 87: 294–300.

[192] Iwasawa T, Yoshiike Y, Saito K, Kagei S, Gotoh T et al. (2000) Paradoxical motion of the hemidiaphragm in patients with emphysema. *J Thorac Imaging* 15: 191–195.

[193] Iwasawa T, Kagei S, Gotoh T, Yoshiike Y, Matsushita K

et al. (2002) Magnetic resonance analysis of abnormal diaphragmatic motion in patients with emphysema. *Eur Respir J* 19: 225–231.

[194] Euler U, Liljestrand G (1946) Observations on the pulmonary arterial blood pressure in the cat. *Acta Physiol Scand* 12: 301–320.

[195] Theissen IL, Meissner A (1996) Hypoxic pulmonary vasoconstriction. *Anaesthesist* 45: 643–652.

[196] Morrison NJ, Abboud RT, Muller NL, Miller RR, Gibson NN et al. (1990) Pulmonary capillary blood volume in emphysema. *Am Rev Respir Dis* 141: 53–61.

[197] Cederlund K, Hogberg S, Jorfeldt L, Larsen F, Norman M et al. (2003) Lung perfusion scintigraphy prior to lung volume reduction surgery. *Acta Radiol* 44: 246–251.

[198] Sandek K, Bratel T, Lagerstrand L, Rosell H (2002) Relationship between lung function, ventilation-perfusion inequality and extent of emphysema as assessed by high-resolution computed tomography. *Respir Med* 96: 934–943.

[199] Ley-Zaporozhan J, Ley S, Eberhardt R, Weinheimer O, Fink C et al. (2007) Assessment of the relationship between lung parenchymal destruction and impaired pulmonary perfusion on a lobar level in patients with emphysema. *Eur J Radiol* 63: 76–83.

[200] Sergiacomi G, Sodani G, Fabiano S, Manenti G, Spinelli A et al. (2003) MRI lung perfusion 2D dynamic breath hold technique in patients with severe emphysema. *In Vivo* 17: 319–324.

[201] Ohno Y, Koyama H, Nogami M, Takenaka D, Matsumoto S et al. (2007) Postoperative lung function in lung cancer patients: Comparative analysis of predictive capability of MRI, CT, and SPECT. *AJR Am J Roentgenol* 189: 400–408.

[202] Molinari F, Fink C, Risse F, Tuengerthal S, Bonomo L et al. (2006) Assessment of differential pulmonary blood flow using perfusion magnetic resonance imaging: Comparison with radionuclide perfusion scintigraphy. *Invest Radiol* 41: 624–630.

[203] Amundsen T, Torheim G, Kvistad KA, Waage A, Bjermer L et al. (2002) Perfusion abnormalities in pulmonary embolism studied with perfusion MRI and ventilation-perfusion scintigraphy: An intra-modality and inter-modality agreement study. *J Magn Reson Imaging* 15: 386–394.

[204] Alford SK, van Beek EJ, McLennan G, Hoffman EA (2010) Heterogeneity of pulmonary perfusion as a mechanistic image-based phenotype in emphysema susceptible smokers. *Proc Natl Acad Sci USA* 107: 7485–7490.

[205] Raghu G, Collard HR, Egan JJ, Martinez FJ, Behr J et al. (2011) An official ATS/ERS/JRS/ALAT statement: Idiopathic pulmonary fibrosis: Evidence-based guidelines for diagnosis and management. *Am J Respir Crit Care Med* 183: 788–824.

[206] Muller NL, Mayo JR, Zwirewich CV (1992) Value of MR imaging in the evaluation of chronic infiltrative lung diseases: Comparison with CT. *AJR Am J Roentgenol* 158: 1205–1209.

[207] Lutterbey G, Grohe C, Gieseke J, von Falkenhausen M, Morakkabati N et al. (2007) Initial experience with lung MRI at 3.0T: Comparison with CT and clinical data in the evaluation of interstitial lung disease activity. *Eur J Radiol* 61: 256–261.

[208] Yi CA, Lee KS, Han J, Chung MP, Chung MJ et al. (2008) 3-T MRI for differentiating inflammation and fibrosis predominant lesions of usual and nonspecific interstitial pneumonia: Comparison study with pathologic correlation. *AJR Am J Roentgenol* 190: 878–885.

[209] McFadden RG, Carr TJ, Wood TE (1987) Proton magnetic resonance imaging to stage activity of interstitial lung disease. *Chest* 92: 31–39.

[210] Berthezene Y, Vexler V, Kuwatsuru R, Rosenau W, Muhler A et al. (1992) Differentiation of alveolitis and pulmonary fibrosis with a macromolecular MR imaging contrast agent. *Radiology* 185: 97–103.

[211] Gaeta M, Blandino A, Scribano E, Minutoli F, Barone M et al. (2000) Chronic infiltrative lung diseases: Value of gadolinium-enhanced MRI in the evaluation of disease activity—Early report. *Chest* 117: 1173–1178.

Chapter 12
胸膜和膈

Pleura and Diaphragm

Francesco Molinari 著

宋 兰 译

宋 伟 校

目录　CONTENTS

一、胸膜 / 242

二、胸膜肿瘤 / 245

磁共振（MRI）过去不作为胸膜和膈的首选影像学检查。然而，现在研究表明 MRI 也是评估胸部病变安全有效的方法，尤其是 MRI 相关序列对胸部一些特定病变的诊断效果得到提高。此外，对于临床医师而言，当他们的患者是短期内需要多次影像学检查的年轻人时，MRI 无电离辐射的特性受到广大年轻人的欢迎。因此，胸部 MRI 的临床适应证越来越广泛，并已成为评估胸膜和横膈病变的较好的影像学检查方法。

一、胸膜

（一）解剖与功能

胸膜指的是覆盖在胸壁、横膈、纵隔内侧表面（如壁胸膜）和肺叶表面（如脏胸膜）的两层间皮细胞。正常情况下胸膜腔不可见，是由于肺-胸壁间壁胸膜与脏胸膜紧密相连及叶间裂层面两层脏胸膜紧密贴合。壁胸膜通过胸膜外脂肪和胸内筋膜的作用向外附着于胸部肋骨边缘。肋骨间隙则填充着肋间肌肉、血管和脂肪。胸膜和胸膜腔参与肺和胸壁淋巴管引流。

（二）胸膜疾病

胸膜病变多种多样，通常需要进行特定的胸部影像学评估。接下来，我们将论述 MRI 在胸膜病变中的诊断作用。

1. 胸腔积液　正常情况下胸膜腔含有 5ml 的液体。当胸膜腔内液体过多时则会出现胸腔积液。根据形成机制、部位、形态学和成分，胸膜渗出分为不同种类。

胸腔积液若由毛细血管压力不均衡（静水压增大或渗透压减小）导致则称为漏出液。左心衰竭、缩窄性心包炎、低白蛋白血症、肝硬化及肾病综合征等都是产生漏出液的主要原因。漏出液通常是可移动的，且主要积聚在胸膜腔最低点。站立位时，少量胸腔积液可积聚在下肺区域，即肺下叶下面和膈肌之间。仰卧位时，漏出液主要位于后肋膈角区。因此，漏出液多流动至围绕肺表面的空腔。

胸腔积液若是由胸膜和毛细血管渗透性改变导致的则被称为渗出液。典型的渗出液包括无菌性肺炎旁胸腔积液、积脓和恶性肿瘤导致的胸腔积液。胸腔渗出液可伴随胸膜增厚和胸膜粘连。因此，这些渗出液进一步可局限于某处形成包裹性积液（图 12-1）。血胸、脓胸、气胸或感染性胸膜炎最易形成分隔。多发分隔也常常取决于粘连的位置和数量（图 12-2），胸膜-肺表面或叶间裂内的分叶状胸腔积液可表现为肿块样病变（图 12-3）。

常规胸片、CT 和超声是诊断和定性胸腔积液的首选影像学检查。MRI 在特定临床状态下也可作为一种检查手段，尤其在判断不明来源的胸腔积液的性质（如漏出液或渗出液）或评估胸腔积液伴随组织损伤的存在具有重要意义。

与漏出液相比，渗出液在注射钆对比剂后表现为更高程度的强化（Frolaetal，1997），弥散加权图像根据表观扩散系数值有利于区分渗出液和漏出液（Baysal 等，2004）。此外，MRI 可直接定性胸腔积液中的血性和脂肪成分。T_1 和 T_2 加权像上的信号特点可帮助区分胸腔积液中血红蛋白的种类，并根据其成分（氧合血红蛋白、脱氧血红蛋白、高铁血红蛋白和含铁血黄素）区分

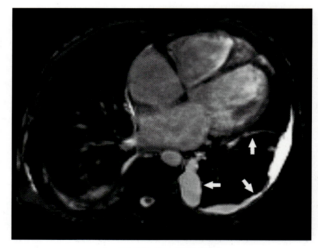

▲ 图 12-1　胸腔积液
患者自由呼吸梯度回波序列。MRI 影像显示左侧胸腔积液呈分叶状和左侧叶间裂积液（白箭），右侧也有少量胸腔积液（未标明）

Chapter 12　胸膜和膈
Pleura and Diaphragm

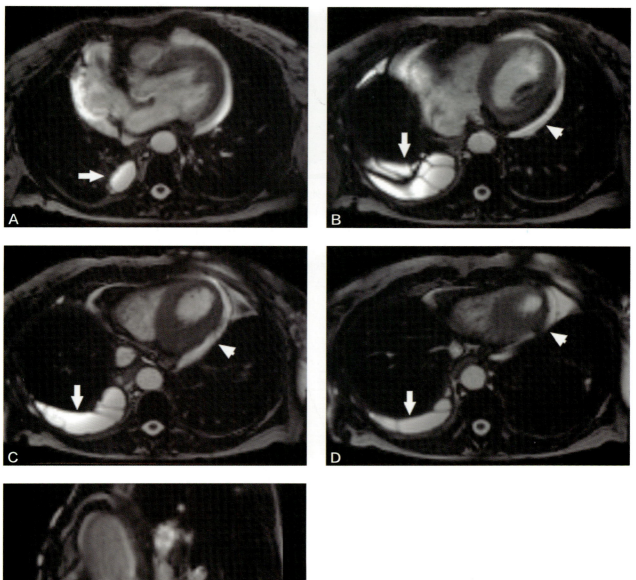

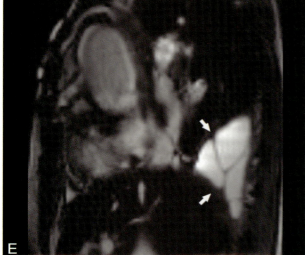

▲ 图 12-2　胸腔积液

轴位（A～D）和矢状位（E）平面自由呼吸平衡梯度回波 MR 图像。该患者右侧胸膜腔包裹性积液（白箭），伴有心包积液（白色箭头）。胸腔积液与邻近肺组织分界清晰。胸膜层和内隔中度增厚。邻近肺组织移位伴中度受压。MRI 平衡梯度回波序列为胸膜腔内高信号液体及低信号分隔提供了较好的对比

亚急性和慢性胸腔积血（Mitchell，2003）。这有利于临床做出正确诊治（例如创伤、肿瘤转移、抗凝治疗等），尤其是对于高危患者可避免有创治疗（图 12-3）。非分叶状胸腔积液 T_1 加权序列高信号提示较多脂肪成分，其很有可能为纵隔肿瘤导致的乳糜胸所致（McLoud 和 Flower，1991）。MRI 发现脓胸中存在气液平面则提示支气管 - 胸膜瘘。MRI 上发现不规则或结节状胸膜增厚则提示为恶性胸腔积液（见下文）。

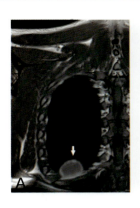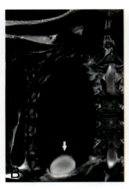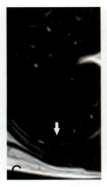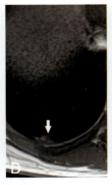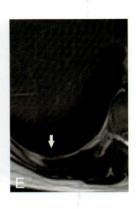

▲ 图 12-3　外伤后胸膜血肿

A、B. 梯度回波序列 MR 图像显示右肋后胸膜呈椭圆形病变（白箭），与邻近组织分界清晰。该患者最近有严重创伤史。MRI 检查是因为可疑脊柱损伤。病变在 T_1 和 T_2 加权图像上表现为外周边缘厚层环形高信号，其内部成分在 T_1 加权图像上（A）为稍高信号，T_2 加权图像上（B）与肌肉组织相比表现为中度高信号，与急性血肿类似；C～E. 首次 MRI 检查后 6 个月随访，病变大小明显吸收缩小，表现为轻微分叶状胸膜结节（白箭），在 T_1 加权快速梯度回波序列图像上（D）为中度高信号，在平衡梯度回波序列和 T_2 加权快速自旋回波序列图像（C、E）上为低信号。患者没有做后续 MRI 随访

2. 组织病变

胸膜增厚和斑块

（1）弥漫性胸膜增厚常由严重和（或）慢性胸膜炎导致。炎症常由胸膜感染导致（如脓胸和结核感染），但也可见于非感染性病变（如胸膜出血、创伤、射线损伤、肺栓塞、药物治疗、胶原血管疾病、肿瘤及职业暴露史）。无论感染与非感染因素，胸膜增厚常伴有胸膜钙化。胸膜增厚伴钙化最常见于陈旧性肺结核、细菌性脓胸、血胸或石棉肺。由于胸膜增厚的弥漫性，胸膜纤维化可导致纤维胸，使同侧胸廓扩张进行性受限。因此当患者伴有弥漫胸膜增厚时应通过查体、胸部影像学检查和肺功能检查进行评估。

（2）胸膜斑是透明胶原蛋白沉积在壁胸膜形成，推测可能是石棉纤维导致胸膜炎症，并沿淋巴管转移至胸膜表面造成的。双侧散发胸膜钙化斑块与长期接触石棉有关（Peacock 等，2000）。在 60%～70% 的接触石棉工人中观察到了这种现象（Falaschi 等，1995），在吸入石棉纤维后，非钙化斑块平均潜伏期约为15 年，钙化斑块的潜伏期至少为 20 年（Muller，1993）。尽管胸膜斑块不是恶变征象，也不提示潜在疾病风险，但其仍提示着石棉暴露史。由于石棉暴露史是间皮瘤（大约 3 倍危险）、肺癌等一些恶性肿瘤的高危因素（Mossman 和 Gee，1989；Schwartz，1991），因此影像学发现石棉斑有重要意义。

CT 是诊断和定性弥漫性胸膜增厚和胸膜斑块的金标准（Lynch 等，1989）。MRI 很少用于诊断良性胸膜改变。但发现胸膜病变对正确评估患者病情依然重要。因此不能忽视 MRI 中偶然发现的良性胸膜病变。

弥散性胸膜增厚形态学诊断标准定义如下：厚度 >3mm，头尾方向长度 >8cm，沿一侧胸壁长度 >5cm。通常为双侧。在 T_1 和 T_2 加权图像上，表现为肋下弥漫性线样低信号。壁层胸膜外脂肪组织沉积可能是由于胸膜下脂肪收缩牵拉胸膜的结果。胸膜下脂肪在 MRI 上表现为 T_1 和 T_2 上线样高信号，压脂相上为低信号。

胸膜斑常出现于胸膜增厚的中心区域，多位于靠近肋骨的壁胸膜处，尤其是第 6～9 肋骨及膈胸膜处（图 12-4）。胸膜斑在肋间隙和脏层胸膜少见，也不会出现在肋膈角及肺尖处。胸膜斑块可表现为线状、带状或结节状，部分可侵犯邻近肺实质。当侵犯肺间质时表现为胸膜下线影，提示局灶肺纤维化。非钙化胸膜斑块在 MRI 上表现为 T_1 和 T_2 中至低信号。在 T_1 和 T_2 加权图像上，钙化的胸膜斑表现为局灶点状或带状极低信号、

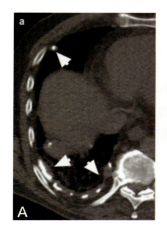 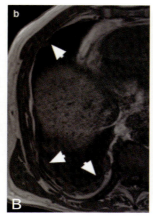 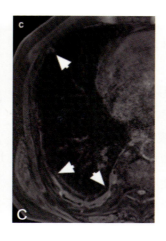 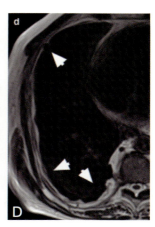

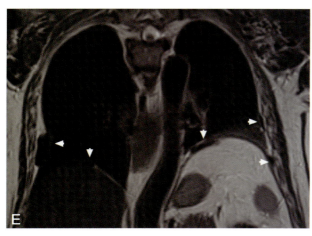

▲ 图12-4　胸膜斑和钙化

A.CT图像为石棉接触史患者，胸壁中部后外侧肋胸膜和膈胸膜多个钙化（白色箭头）和斑块；在长TE和长TR在单向快速自旋回波序列中的应用，胸膜斑块中的非钙化成分在T_1梯度回波加权序列（B）和压脂T_1梯度回波加权序列（C）中与肌肉相比表现为略高信号，而在T_2单向快速自旋回波序列（D）则表现为显著的信号缺失，这是由于单次快速自旋回波测量所使用的长TE和TR。钙化的斑块成分由于其信号的快速衰减，其在T_1和T_2加权图像上均表现为明显低信号；E.冠状位T_2加权单向快速自旋回波序列上显示清晰胸膜斑块的形态及分布。增厚的显著低信号病变同时位于肋胸膜和膈胸膜（白色箭头）

易被发现，这是由于在标准快速自旋回波序列上，钙质信号快速衰减所致。T_2^*加权图像上（梯度回波序列）钙化点周围也可见环状伪影。使用高分辨率超短TE序列伴辐射状K空间采样的先进MRI技术也被用于胸膜斑评估的研究（Weber等，2004），这对胸膜斑钙化成分的评估具有一定意义。

二、胸膜肿瘤

根据2006年WHO组织学分型，胸膜肿瘤分为间皮瘤（包括弥漫性恶性间皮瘤和局限性恶性间皮瘤）和间叶细胞来源肿瘤（包括孤立性纤维瘤和淋巴增殖性病变）。然而大部分胸膜肿瘤为转移性疾病，而原发性胸膜恶性肿瘤罕见。

当怀疑存在胸膜肿瘤时，首先要根据其影像学特征判断良恶性，其次是缩小恶性胸膜病变的鉴别诊断范围。影像学评估胸膜肿瘤最重要的检查方法是碘对比剂增强多排螺旋CT，钆对比剂增强MRI对胸膜恶性肿瘤的评估有较高的敏感性和特异性。但是因其不易获得，常规胸部检查中较少用到（Downer等，2013）。

无论选择哪种断层影像学检查（CT或MRI）对可疑胸膜肿瘤患者进行评估，提示恶性病变的特征总是一定的：结节状和不规则增厚；侵犯纵隔胸膜；环周增厚；增厚厚度超过1cm。恶性胸膜病变倾向于侵犯整个胸膜表面，而反应性胸膜炎通常不会累及纵隔胸膜，但结核性脓胸除外（Hierholzer等，2000）。

（一）转移

胸膜转移是最常见的累及胸膜的恶性肿瘤。最常见的转移至胸膜的恶性肿瘤依次为肺癌（40%）、乳腺癌（20%）以及淋巴瘤（10%）。其他可能转移至胸膜的肿瘤包括结肠癌、胰腺癌、肾癌或卵巢癌（30%）。远处的原发恶性肿瘤可通过血行转移至胸膜，邻近恶性肿瘤或胸膜下肿瘤可通过直接侵犯（如淋巴瘤）或种植（如胸腺瘤或支气管来源癌）转移至胸膜。

对怀疑存在胸膜转移的患者，CT通常是首选的影像学检查方法。胸部MRI也能发现胸膜转移的影像学征象。胸膜转移的表现多种多样，既可表现为仅出现伴胸腔积液的正常胸膜，也可表现为均匀增厚、局限性肿块或者广泛性结节样增厚。广泛性环状胸膜增厚可能与叶间裂结节状增厚及患侧肺容积缩小有关。如同前文所示，这些表现提示存在胸膜转移，但并不是胸膜转移的特异性表现。尤其是广泛性环周结节状胸膜增厚伴患侧肺体积缩小时，应考虑胸膜转移或间皮瘤可能。

（二）原发肿瘤

原发性胸膜病变直接起源于胸膜层。下述段落将主要论述最常见的原发性胸膜肿瘤。

恶性胸膜间皮瘤

恶性胸膜间皮瘤（malignant pleural mesothelioma，MPM）是一种罕见的、隐匿性的、高度侵袭性的肿瘤，预后很差。可来源于体内任何间皮细胞，如胸膜、心包、腹膜或鞘膜。80%来源于胸膜。

恶性胸膜间皮瘤可分为不同的组织学亚型，其中肉瘤是预后最差的组织学亚型。长期石棉接触史的患者最易罹患MPM，其发病率是非石棉接触史患者的1000倍（80%的MPM患者有石棉接触史）。因此MPM在职业病医院更常见。从首次接触石棉，到出现间皮瘤的临床表现，其潜伏期20～40年（Kishimoto等，2003）。石棉接触史患者发生间皮瘤的高发年龄是50—70岁。在发达国家，预计2010—2030年该病的发病率将达到峰值。

大多数MPM患者在检出肿瘤之前的数月中，患者肺部临床表现不具有特异性。当确诊时，肿瘤已是晚期。MPM的发病率和死亡率主要与其局部侵袭有关。随着肿瘤的扩散，其逐渐闭塞胸膜腔，包绕侵袭肺部、心脏或心包等胸部的重要结构，并通过膈肌向腹腔延伸。肿瘤远处转移也可发生在对侧肺、脑部和其他肺外部位。患者主要死于肿瘤局部浸润和呼吸衰竭。

胸部影像学作为常规评估非特异性患者肺部症状的手段，有时可最终发现间皮瘤。在这些患者中，常规胸片往往表现为单侧胸腔积液，引流后可复发，最终通过轴位图像进行进一步评估。在CT或MRI上，最常见的肿瘤影像学表现包括：胸膜呈结节状同心圆样增厚，厚度大于1cm，并侵犯叶间胸膜；同侧胸腔积液；肿瘤厚壁包裹肺，可导致同侧纵隔移位；单侧肺体积缩小；胸壁浸润和肋骨破坏；肺内、心脏、心包转移（图12-5至图12-7）。

胸部CT轴位图像是目前评估MPM及对其分期主要的影像学检查手段（Layer等，1999；Marom等，2002；Wang等，2004）。由于CT对钙化的显示优于MRI，因此CT能提示弥漫性或多灶性胸膜增厚钙化的良性表现。然而，MPM并不以钙化样肿瘤的形式出现，也不由钙化斑块恶性转化而来。MPM主要为软组织成分，而MRI对软组织分辨率高，因此MRI对肿瘤的形态学评估，尤其是局限性侵犯有明显的优势。MPM在T_1加权上表现为不均匀低至中等信号，在T_2加权图像上表现为高信号，增强扫描有强化（图12-5至图12-7）（Bonomo等，2000）。与肋间肌相比，在T_2加权图像和MRI T_1增强扫描上表现为高信号提示为恶性疾病。MRI诊断胸膜恶性肿瘤的敏感性与特异性分别为100%和93%（Hierholzer等，2000）。

最近的研究表明，MRI有助于显示肿瘤局部浸润，尤其适用于MPM患者外科切除（Patz等，1992；Wang等，2004）。MRI特别适用于评估肿瘤胸腔内筋膜、胸壁和横膈的侵犯，以及肿瘤经横膈的生长。最近动态MRI也是评估MPM的一种方法。在之前的研究中，MRI可在静态时测量肺容积（Qanadli等，1999；Ley等，2004），并能在呼吸周期的不同阶段（Whitelaw 1987；Plathow等，2004；Haage等，2005）通过相关参数评估疗效（Plathow 等，2006）。动态 MRI 技术应用快速低角度成像（FLASH）序列和真实稳态进动快速成像（true fast imaging with steady state precession, true FISP）序列可定性和定量评估胸廓体积在 MPM 治疗中的改变并通过吸气呼气相评估治疗效果。动态增强（dynamic susceptibility contrast, DCE）MRI 也可以作为一种有效手段无创评价对比剂通过肿瘤微循环和邻近组织的到达及廓清。结果表明，钆对比剂的强化方式可用于治疗监测时定性肿瘤微血管的特点并显示肿瘤的异质性（Giesel 等，2006，2008）。

尽管 CT 和 MRI 表现可高度提示胸膜恶性病变，但是诊断 MPM 不具有特异性，因为与转移性胸膜病变非常相似。MPM 的诊断需要组织病理学检查，不能仅仅依靠临床或影像学检查，即使患者有石棉暴露史也应如此。当患者伴有胸

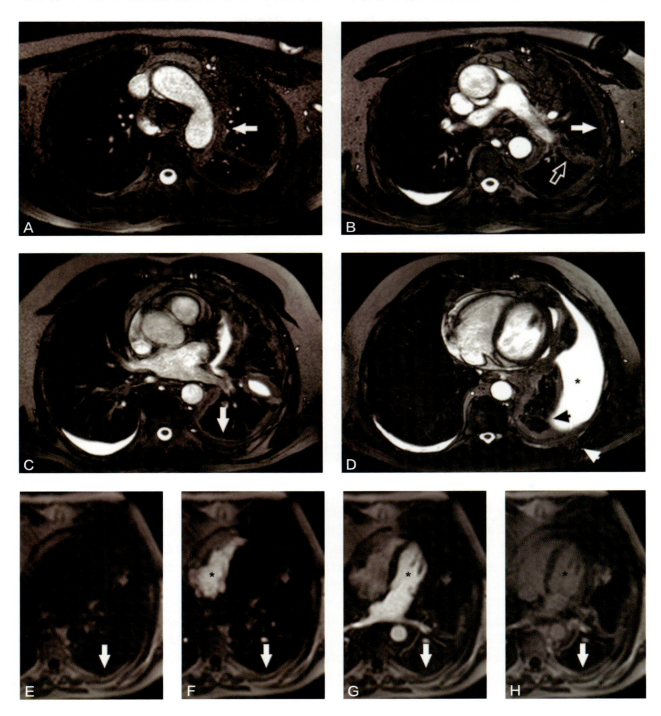

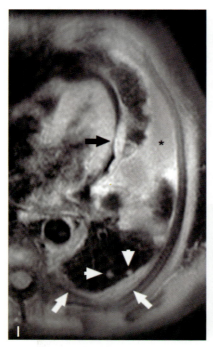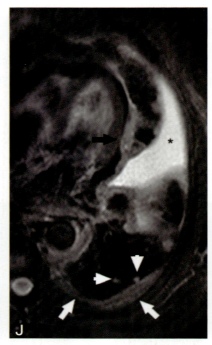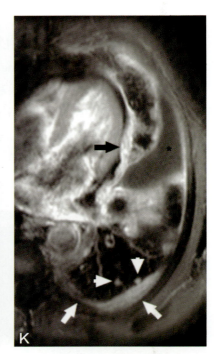

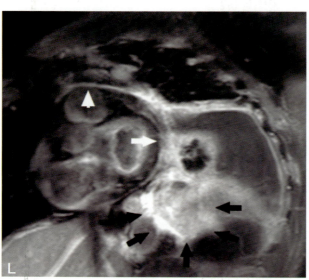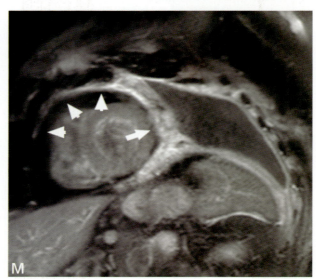

▲ 图 12-5　胸膜间皮瘤

A～D. 梯度回波序列 MR 图像示多分叶的融合胸膜肿块，表现为左侧胸膜表面弥漫不规则增厚（白箭），增厚的胸膜延伸至肋间、纵隔、横膈（白箭）以及叶间裂（黑箭），并引起左侧肺环周增厚，患侧胸腔缩小，轻微的同侧纵隔移位。胸膜渗出浸润下方的肺实质主要延伸至小叶间隔（黑色箭头）。还需要注意的是渗出也会通过肋间隙浸润后胸壁（白色箭头）。左侧胸腔积液伴随浸润性胸膜增厚（黑色星号），由于肿瘤组织的胸膜固定，对侧纵隔无移位（冰冻胸）；E～H. 四张灌注图像是从 60 张动态增强图像中选取的，动态增强应用快速梯度回波 MR 序列并使用静脉注射单一钆对比剂（0.1mmol/kg）。平扫 T_1 加权图像（E）显示胸膜增厚，表现为与肌肉类似的高信号（白箭）。动态增强早期（F，注意对比剂在右心腔，黑色星号），胸膜病变无明显强化（F，白箭）。当对比剂通过左心腔时（G，黑色星号）和增强后期（H，黑色星号），胸膜增厚呈渐进性强化；I～K. 显示 T_1 加权、T_2 加权和增强后 T_1 加权成像的特征。在 T_1 加权压脂快速自旋回波序列（I，白箭）及 T_2-STIR 快速自旋回波序列（J，白箭）上，以胸膜增厚为基础的融合占位与肌肉相比呈略高信号。增强后 T_1 加权压脂快速自旋回波图像（K）显示胸膜肿瘤明显强化（白箭）。纵隔和心包胸膜浸润（黑箭）。注意左肺下叶两个结节（白色箭头）提示肿瘤肺内血行转移。胸腔积液（黑色星号）由于含有血性成分，因此在平扫 T_1 加权（I）、T_2 加权（J）图像上均表现为高信号；L、M. 显示增强后 T_1 加权压脂快速自旋回波图像对肿瘤横膈和心包播散的评估。胸膜肿瘤浸润胸膜下部表面，并沿着上腹部膈面转移（L，黑箭），心包（白色箭头）及心外膜脂肪（白箭）亦受侵

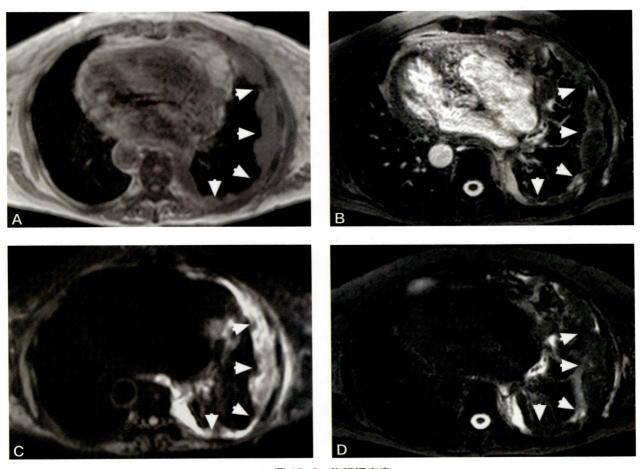

▲ 图 12-6　胸膜间皮瘤

MRI 图像示多分叶融合的胸膜间皮瘤（白色箭头），表现为右侧胸膜弥漫不规则增厚（白色箭头）。胸膜增厚在 T_1 加权快速梯度回波图像上（B）表现为中高信号，在 T_2 加权压脂快速自旋回波图像上（C 和 A）为稍高信号，DWI 图像上（D）为高信号

腔积液，胸腔穿刺细胞学检查和闭式胸膜活检通常是初步的诊断过程。然而，这种方法可能不能提供足够的组织学样本做出恶性诊断，也不能区分间皮瘤和其他肿瘤。胸腔穿刺和（或）胸膜活检阴性也不能排除间皮瘤的诊断。如果初步的胸腔穿刺和胸膜活检无法诊断，外科干预（通过胸腔镜活检或开放式胸腔手术切除）有更高的诊断率。

（三）其他原发胸膜肿瘤

其他相对常见的原发的胸膜肿瘤包括脂肪瘤和纤维瘤。

1. 胸膜脂肪瘤　脂肪瘤是罕见的良性肿瘤，典型者含有均一的脂肪成分。好发于上胸部沿第 2 或第 3 肋骨。也可见于胸部其他部位。脂肪成分在 CT（脂肪的 CT 值为 $-100 \sim -50 HU$）和 MRI（T_1 加权和 T_2 加权序列上均为高信号，压脂相上为低信号）上都很容易显示，故诊断较容易。

2. 胸膜孤立性纤维瘤　胸膜孤立性纤维瘤（solitary fibrous tumor of the pleura，SFTP，也叫局限性纤维瘤）来源于间充质细胞（Travis 等，2004；Cardillo 等，2012）。SFTP 占原发性胸膜肿瘤的比例不到 5%，与间皮瘤和石棉沉着无明显关系。组织学上相同的肿瘤也可发现在其他部位（Wignall 等，2010）。尽管大多数 SFTP 为良性，但也有一些恶性肿瘤的组织学特征，如有丝分裂的数目、坏死的存在、细胞增多或核异质性。恶性 SFTP 较良性 SFTP 生长更快，完整的外科手术切除是 SFPT 的标准治疗方法（Lahon 等，2012）。

SFTP 的平均发病年龄为 55—65 岁（Magdeleinat，2002）。大多数 SFTP 患者起病时无症状，或由于是胸腔内肿块而表现为非特异性肺部症状（Lahon 等，2012；Lococoet 等，2012）。无症状患者可经胸片偶然发现肺内肿块。20% 的患者中伴有肥厚性肺骨关节病（Pierre Marie–Bamberger 综合征），5% 的患者伴有难治性低血糖症（Doege–Potter 综合征）。SFTP 的诊断依靠病理检查，经胸部穿刺活检通常不足以诊断。大多数情况下，SFTP 的诊断是在病灶完全切除后作出的。

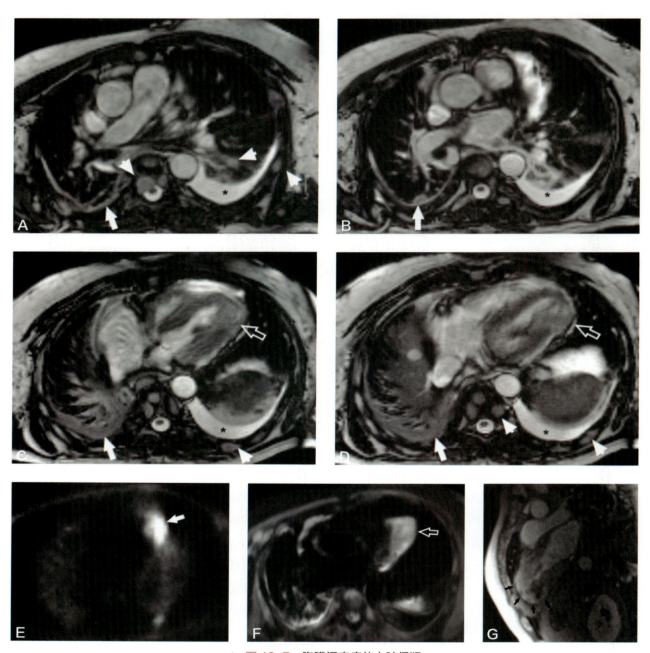

▲ 图 12-7　胸膜间皮瘤伴心脏侵犯

A～D. 梯度回波图像显示双侧多分叶状胸膜肿块和胸膜增厚（白箭），患者为晚期间皮瘤，并通过血行转移至肺、肋骨和脊柱（白色箭头）。可见左肺胸腔积液（黑色星号）。心尖和左心室顶外侧段边缘不规则、信号不均匀（黑箭）；E. 在 FDG-PET 扫描上，心脏损伤表现为高代谢肿块（白箭）；F. DWI 图像上表现为心脏相同区域高信号（黑箭）；G. 增强后快速梯度回波图像显示左心室不均匀强化，并伴有不规则浸润（黑箭）

在常规胸片和横断面图像（CT 或 MRI）上，SFTP 通常表现为边界清楚的 5～30cm 的胸廓肿块，偶尔呈分叶状（图 12-8 和图 12-9）。病变常位于椎旁区域，也可位于其他部位，肿瘤也可发生于叶间裂，类似于肺内肿块。若不经外科手术，原发部位常不明确（如胸膜）。40% 的肿块带有蒂，因此病变可移动，在影像学检查中若改变体位常可发现病变活动性。该征象有利于缩窄鉴别诊断的范围（Desser 和 Stark，1998）。SFTP 典型的特征为结构复杂。黏液样变中囊性和坏死成分在 T_2 加权 MR 图像上可表现为高信号。肿块内钙化少见（约 7%），由于肿块内有丰富的血管，因此强化后肿块内部或边缘可见到膈动脉血管及其分支（图 12-9）。胸膜孤立性纤维瘤一般不伴有为胸腔积液（De Perrot 等，2002）。虽然 MRI 在此类胸膜病变中诊断价值有限，但与 CT 相比，MRI 对大病变与邻近纵隔及主要血管结构的关系及形态学的显示优于 CT。

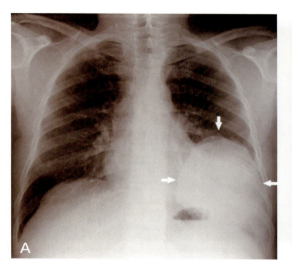
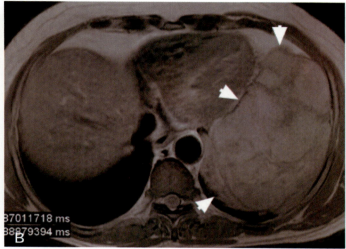
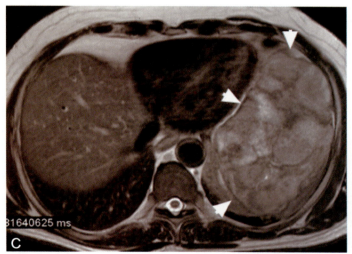

▲ 图 12-8 胸膜孤立性纤维瘤
A. 胸片示胸膜孤立性纤维瘤（SFTP）。左肺底可见直径超过 10cm 的类圆形轻度分叶状肿块（白箭）。MRI T_1 加权快速自旋回波（B）和 T_2 加权（C）图像显示明显不均匀信号的占位，没有胸膜来源的表现（白色箭头）

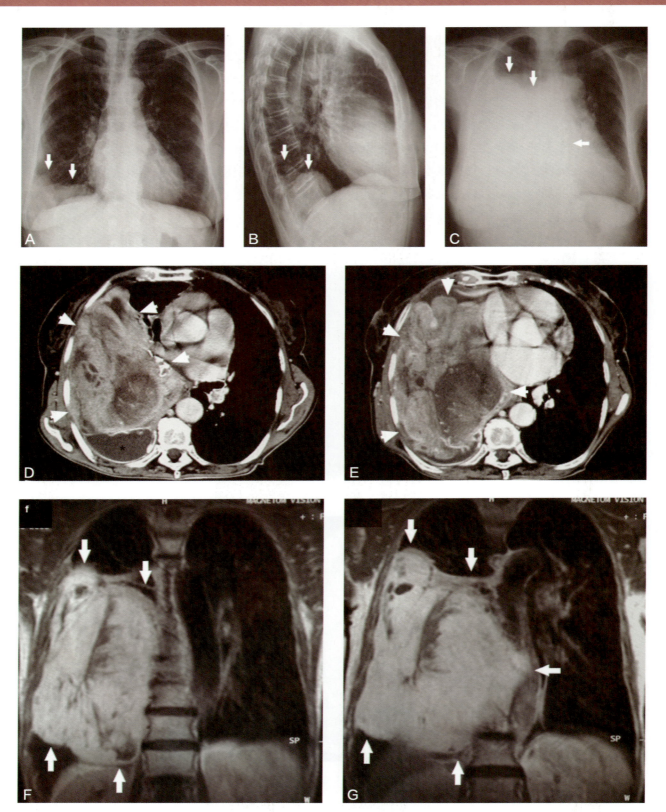

▲ 图 12-9 胸膜孤立性纤维瘤

A 胸片显示胸膜孤立性纤维肿瘤（SFTP）。无症状患者拒绝接受外科治疗，右侧后肋膈角可见分叶状肿块（白箭）。基线胸片检查检出病变 9 个月后胸片随访。右侧胸腔几乎完全被肿块填充，纵隔轻度向左移位（白箭）。肿瘤快速进展提示其为恶性。在胸部 CT 上，肿块呈明显不均匀强化，其内可见囊性低密度坏死区（白箭）。肿块边缘增粗的血管可能来源于膈动脉。在胸部 MRI 中，T_1 加权自旋回波图像（白箭）较好地显示了肿块平扫及增强信号不均匀

参考文献

[1] Baysal T, Bulut T, Gokirmak M, Kalkan S, Dusak A, Dogan M. Diffusion-weighted MR imaging of pleural fluid: Differentiation of transudative vs exudative pleural effusions. *Eur Radiol* 2004;14(5):890–896.

[2] Bonomo L, Feragalli B, Sacco R, Merlino B, Storto ML. Malignant pleural disease. *Eur J Radiol* 2000;34(2): 98–118.

[3] Cardillo G, Lococo F, Carleo F, Martelli M. Solitary fibrous tumors of the pleura. *Curr Opin Pulm Med* 2012;18:339.

[4] De Perrot M, Fischer S, Brundler MA, Sekine Y, Keshavjee S. Solitary fibrous tumors of the pleura. *Ann Thorac Surg* 2002;74(1):285–293.

[5] Desser TS, Stark P. Pictorial essay: Solitary fibrous tumor of the pleura. *J Thorac Imaging* 1998;13(1):27

[6] Downer NJ, Ali NJ, Au-Yong IT. Investigating pleural thickening. *BMJ* 2013;346:e8376. doi: 10.1136/bmj.e8376.

[7] Falaschi F, Battolla L, Paolicchi A et al. High-resolution com-puted tomography compared with the thoracic radio-gram and respiratory function tests in assessing workers exposed to silica. *Radiol Med* 1995;89(4):424–429.

[8] Frola C, Cantoni S, Turtulici I et al. Transudative vs exudative pleural effusions: Differentiation using Gd-DTPA enhanced MRI. *Eur Radiol* 1997;7(6):860–864.

[9] Giesel FL, Bischoff H, von Tengg-Kobligk H et al. Dynamic contrast-enhanced MRI of malignant pleural mesothelioma: A feasibility study of noninvasive assessment, therapeutic follow-up, and possible predictor of improved outcome. *Chest* 2006;129(6):1570–1576.

[10] Giesel FL, Choyke PL, Mehndiratta A et al. Pharmacokinetic analysis of malignant pleural mesothelioma-initial results of tumor microcirculation and its correlation to microvessel density (CD-34). *Acad Radiol* 2008;15(5): 563–570.

[11] Haage P, Karaagac S, Spuntrup E et al. Feasibility of pulmonary ventilation visualization with aerosolized magnet resonacne contrast media. *Invest Radiol* 2005;40:85–88.

[12] Hierholzer J, Luo L, Bittner RC et al. MRI and CT in the differential diagnosis of pleural disease. *Chest* 2000;118:604–609.

[13] Kishimoto T, Ohnishi K, Saito Y. Clinical study of asbestos related lung cancer. *Ind Health* 2003;41(2):94–100.

[14] Lahon B, Mercier O, Fadel E et al. Solitary fibrous tumor of the pleura: Outcomes of 157 complete resections in a single center. *Ann Thorac Surg* 2012;94(2):394–400.

[15] Layer G, Schmitteckert H, Steudel A et al. MRT, CT, and sonography in the preoperative assessment of the primary tumor spread in malignant pleural mesothelioma. *Rofo* 1999;170(4):365–370.

[16] Ley S, Zaporozhan J, Morbach A et al. Functional evaluation of emphysema using diffusion-weighted 3Helium-magnetic resonance imaging, high-resolution computed tomography, and lung function tests. *Invest Radiol* 2004;39:427–434.

[17] Lococo F, Cesario A, Cardillo G et al. Malignant solitary fibrous tumors of the pleura: Retrospective review of a multicenter series. *J Thorac Oncol* 2012;7:1698.

[18] Lynch DA, Gamsu G, Aberle DR. Conventional and high resolution computed tomography in the diagnosis of asbestos-related diseases. *RadioGraphics* 1989;9(3): 523–551.

[19] Magdeleinat P, Alifano M, Petino A et al. Solitary fibrous tumors of the pleura: Clinical characteristics, surgical treatment and outcome. *Eur J Cardiothorac Surg* 2002;21(6): 1087–1093.

[20] Marom EM, Erasmus JJ, Pass HI, Patz EF, Jr. The role of imag ing in malignant pleural mesothelioma. *Semin Oncol* 2002;29(1):26–35.

[21] McLoud TC, Flower CD. Imaging the pleura: Sonography, CT, and MR imaging. *AJR Am J Roentgenol* 1991;156(6):1145–1153.

[22] Mitchell JD. Solitary fibrous tumor of the pleura. *Semin Thorac Cardiovasc Surg* 2003;15(3):305–309.

[23] Mossman BT, Gee JB. Asbestos-related diseases. *N Engl J Med* 1989;320(26):1721–1730.

[24] Muller NL. Imaging of the pleura. *Radiology* 1993;186(2): 297–309.

[25] Patz EF Jr, Shaffer K, Piwnica-Worms DR et al. Malignant pleural mesothelioma: Value of CT and MR imaging in predicting resectability. *AJR* 1992;159(5):961–966.

[26] Peacock C, Copley SJ, Hansell DM. Asbestos-related benign pleural disease. *Clin Radiol* 2000;55(6):422–432.

[27] Plathow C, Klopp M, Schoebinger M et al. Monitoring of lung motion in patients with malignant pleural mesothelioma using two-dimensional and three-dimensional dynamic magnetic resonance imaging: Comparison with spirometry. *Invest Radiol* 2006;41(5):443–448.

[28] Plathow C, Ley S, Fink C et al. Evaluation of chest motion and volumetry during the breathing cycle by dynamic MRI in healthy subjects—comparison with pulmonary function tests. *Invest Radiol* 2004;39:202–209.

[29] Qanadli SD, Orvoen-Frija E, Lacombe P, Di Paola R, Bittoun J, Frija G. Estimation of gas and tissue lung volumes by MRI: Functional approach of lung imaging. *J Comput Assist Tomogr* 1999;23(5):743–748.

[30] Schwartz DA. New developments in asbestos-induced pleural disease. *Chest* 1991;99(1):191–198.

[31] Travis WD, Churg A, Aubry MC et al. Mesenchymal tumours. In: *Tumours of the Lung, Pleura, Thus and Heart*, Travis WD, Brambilla E, Muller-Hermelink HK, and Harris CC. (Eds), IARC Press, Lyon, France, 2004, p.142.

[32] Wang ZJ, Reddy GP, Gotway MB et al. Malignant pleural mesothelioma: Evaluation with CT, MR imaging, and PET. *RadioGraphics* 2004;24(1):105–119.

[33] Weber MA, Bock M, Plathow C et al. Asbestos-related pleural disease: Value of dedicated magnetic resonance imaging techniques. *Invest Radiol* 2004;39(9):554–564.

[34] Whitelaw WA. Shape and size of the human diaphragm in vivo. *J Appl Physiol (1985)* 1987;62(1):180–186.

[35] Wignall OJ, Moskovic EC, Thway K, Thomas JM. Solitary fibrous tumors of the soft tissues: Review of the imaging and clinical features with histopathologic correlation. AJR Am J Roentgenol 2010;195:W55.

Chapter 13 肺及肺血管的功能性磁共振成像

Functional Magnetic Resonance Imaging of the Lung and Pulmonary Vasculature

Saeed Mirsadraee, Andrew J. Swift,
Jim M. Wild, Edwin J.R. van Beek 著

宋 兰 译

宋 伟 校

目录 CONTENTS

一、MR 技术 / 256

二、临床应用 / 260

肺部标准成像技术，如高分辨率CT，具有很多局限性，不是总在早期做出诊断，不能提供生理学信息。尽管已经开发了其他方法，但它们需要增加辐射剂量、吸气和呼气容积CT以及一些先进的软件工具，而这些工具通常在报告工作流程中无法立即获得。

肺功能成像已经逐渐成为传统形态学评估的重要补充，日益被人们所认识。功能成像可通过CT（利用吸气、呼气以及对比剂增强的方法），但是由于辐射剂量的限制，一个总体的评估是很困难的。因此，磁共振成像（MRI）拥有使肺功能成像蓬勃发展的有利条件：在无辐射下它速度很快，而且可对肺的各个子系统进行多重评估并对心脏进行综合评估。

MRI采用增强和平扫的方法通过评估肺灌注和通气、肺动脉血流动力学及运动来研究肺和气道功能。在这一章，讨论了新的成像技术在肺功能评估中的应用。最后，将讨论MRI在肺动脉高压评估中的作用。

一、MR 技术

由于质子浓度低，MR信号的加速衰减，以及运动（呼吸）的影响，肺部成像具有挑战性（Wielpütz 和 Kauczor，2012；Wildand 等，2012）。最近，磁共振技术的发展使得肺部成像成为可能，其在一次或多次屏气中，或者在呼吸门控的自由呼吸期间，具有足够的时间和空间分辨率。本章将讲述适用于功能性肺成像的多种MR技术的使用。

（一）灌注成像

MR灌注成像可以对组织中微血管水平的血流量进行描述和量化（Harris等，2009）。这项技术已经被用于研究各种良性和恶性的肺部疾病，如肺栓塞（Sebastian 和 Julia，2012）和肺癌（Ohno等，2014）。成像技术需要高时间分辨率（如1.5s）和足够的空间分辨率进行全部或部分肺成像。灌注成像可在有或无静脉造影的情况下进行。

1. 对比剂增强肺灌注成像 最常见的定量灌注成像方法是时间分辨率（重复）成像，同时使用顺磁性造影剂[钆 - 二乙烯三胺五乙酸（gadotinmm-diethylenetriamine pentaacetic acid, DPTA）]。重T_1加权三维扰相梯度回波序列（短TR和高旋转角来抑制不增强的组织）是血管造影和灌注成像中最常用的脉冲序列（Wild等，2012）。最常见的替代成像序列是运用K空间填充时间分辨动态MR血管造影（表13-1）。并行成像可以应用于屏气时间受限时。灌注成像技术的目的是实现时间分辨率和对比-噪声比的最佳结合。据报道，对于反褶积算法的正确应用，需要约2s的时间分辨率。图像噪声高将导致对肺血流量（pulmonary blood flow，PBF）的评估有很大的低估。采用较低的加速因子（如2）和增加体素尺寸来提高信噪比（Ingrisch等，2010）。

钆-DTPA缩短了T_1，从而在重T_1加权成像上增强结构的信号增高。造影剂的注射通常是在屏气和成像开始时进行，或在短暂延迟（3～5s）之后开始。时间分辨信号数据将定义动脉输入函数的时间 - 信号曲线（arterial input functions, AIF；肺动脉），它将被用于灌注量化的数学处理（图13-1）。单次屏气（20～30s）通常足以从正常的肺实质中获得时间 - 信号曲线（部分或完全），但在有或没有呼吸门控的情况下，可能需要更长的图像采集时间来充分评估伴有延迟对比转化时

表13-1 用于对比剂增强灌注成像的MRI序列缩略语

序列类型	飞利浦	西门子	GE	日立	东芝
扰相梯度回波序列	T_1-FFE	FLASH	SPGR MPSPGR	RSSG	RF-spoiled FE
运用K空间的动态MR血管成像	Keyhole（4D-TRAK）	TWIST	TRICKS	—	—

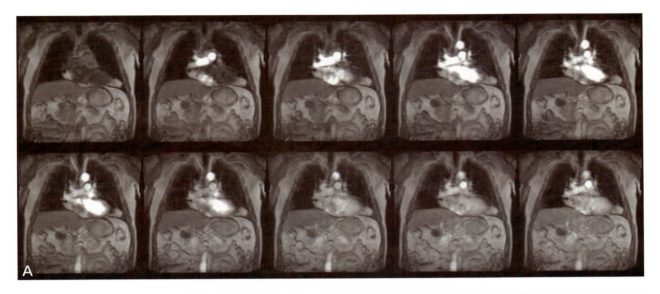

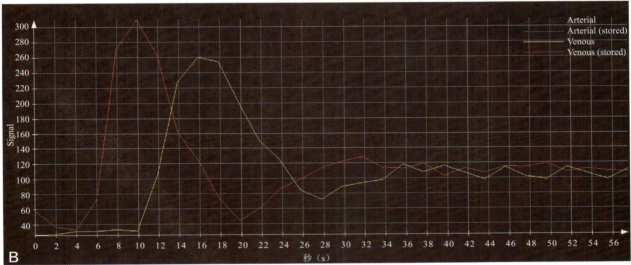

▲ 图 13-1 动态增强磁共振灌注成像

A. 冠状位图像显示从右心到左心的通过密度对比，以及随后的稀释后再循环的对比（时间分辨率：1.5s）；B. 显示肺动脉（红色）和左心房（黄色）感兴趣区的时间 - 信号强度曲线

间的区域（如肿瘤）的增强和洗脱模式。超过 20～30s 的成像通常是在浅腹式呼吸时进行，需要应用后处理（如非刚性配准）来减少运动的影响。

最优注射方案的目的是团注一个密集的对比剂团，然后以生理盐水冲洗，以达到短暂的首过峰值增强，在肺动脉和肺实质中快速冲洗。为了达到这个目的，在中等口径的静脉（如前肘静脉）使用大口径静脉器快速（4～5ml/s）注射造影剂。通过预加热到体温，对比剂的黏度可以降低 50%。双侧静脉路线可以用来改善造影剂的

输送。与碘造影剂相比，在造影剂量和 CT 值之间存在线性关系时，MR 信号与钆之间的关系是非线性的，导致在较高的血药浓度下信号饱和。信号饱和使灌注量化更加复杂，为了避免对 MRI 的影响，必须保持最低的对比浓度（Puderbach 等，2008）。在更高磁场强度（如 3T 和 1.5T）和较低浓度的钆 -DTPA（0.05 mmol/kg）时效果较好。在肺灌注成像技术中应用了双团注法来克服这个问题（Risse 等，2006）。在这种方法中，给予低剂量对比剂（如在 1.5T 时 0.05mmol/kg）是为了在 AIF 中实现线性信号 - 时间曲线，接着是

标准剂量注射（如，在1.5T时为0.1mmol/kg）（Hueper等，2013）以观察肺组织的增强情况。虽然该技术避免了输入函数的信号饱和，但由于AIF的低估，导致灌注值的低估。之前的研究已经报道了纠正这种影响的技术。

肺灌注定义为肺实质的毛细血管供血（PBF），以ml/（100g/min）为单位测量。为了对灌注进行量化，必须在主肺动脉（Sebastian和Julia，2012）或右心室（Hueper等，2013）中放置一个感兴趣区，以获得AIF。肺组织的功能性反应由肺实质的感兴趣区决定（Sebastian和Julia，2012）。数据分析由有效的软件进行。该软件利用逐像素分析提供参数彩色图谱。根据时间-信号强度曲线，采用多种模型对灌注量进行量化。假设信号与造影剂浓度之间存在线性关系，信号-时间曲线可以转换为浓度-时间曲线（Risse等，2006），并计算了各种灌注值。肺血容量（pulmonary blood volume，PBV；ml/100ml肺组织）是通过将组织浓度-时间曲线下的面积正常化为AIF积分来计算的（Ley，2012）。

通过绘制感兴趣区的信号强度变化，在输入函数（如肺动脉）和肺实质中构造时间-信号强度曲线。根据时间-信号强度曲线计算灌注参数。达到峰值的时间定义为从注射造影剂开始到最大组织增强的时间，以秒为单位。肺组织血流量（PBV）是一种衡量成像体素（组织和血管；ml/100 g）内总血容量的指标，它是由组织时间-信号曲线下面积的数学积分决定的，如前一段所述（Aksoy和Lev，2000；Allmendinger等，2012）。PBF被定义为单位时间内某一特定区域的血流容积[ml/（100mg·min）]，代表肺组织中的毛细血管流动。平均通过时间是所有对比剂分子通过组织体积的平均通过时间，以秒为单位，并根据中心体积原理大概估算：平均通过时间＝PBV/PBF（Allmendinger等，2012）。各种模型被用来计算时间-密度曲线的灌注值，包括反渗透技术。灌注量的绝对值取决于测量时的心脏输出量。为了比较患者的灌注值，建议将这些数值统一为心输出量（Miles，2001）。

为了避免灌注分析中包含肺动脉分支而导致灌注值过高，相关分析技术可用于抑制肺灌注MRI中的肺血管。在该技术中，与肺动脉和左心房具有高相关系数的像素被认为是动脉或静脉，被排除在进一步分析之外。据报道，这种校正可导致与包含所有血管结构相比PBF与PBV值分别下降15%和25%（Risse等，2009）。

2. MR平扫肺灌注技术 动脉自旋标记已被用作对比剂增强灌注成像的替代序列。在这项技术中，供应动脉中的血液质子被磁性标记（标记物），通常带有反转恢复脉冲，并用作内源性对比剂（Rizi等，2003）。组织磁化随灌注状态而改变。由于没有使用其他的对比剂，该技术可以重复。该技术比对比剂增强的灌注MRI速度慢，更容易出现运动伪影，但最近，它已经可近似于对比剂增强灌注成像（Martrorosin等，2010）。其他平扫灌注技术使用单层时间分辨平衡稳态自由进动序列，然后应用傅里叶分解获得来自实质内的时间信号灌注数据（参阅第11章）（Kj-rstad等，2014）。

（二）通气显像

通气显像可以通过不同的对比机制实现。通气显像包括以质子为基础的方法，注射顺磁造影剂（氧和雾化钆溶液）和非质子的方法（超极性化惰性气体）（Ohno等，2008；Mugler等，2010；Wild等，2012；Mirsadraee和van Beek，2015）。

显然，通过在肺部成像方法中增加通气功能，它完成了评估肺部主要功能的整体能力：通过匹配的通气和灌注来交换氧气和二氧化碳。

超极化气体MR成像技术已经开发了20多年，进展缓慢，受到了一些限制和压力，包括需要先进的硬件（包括专用调谐射频发射/接收线圈、用于生产超极化气体的偏振片，以及与一些其他需求 ^{3}He的竞争）（Van Beek等，2004；

Chapter 13　肺及肺血管的功能性磁共振成像
Functional Magnetic Resonance Imaging of the Lung and Pulmonary Vasculature

Mugler 等，2010）。尽管如此，这项技术现在可以在专门的临床研究中应用，而且多中心研究是可行的（Van Beek 等，2009；Kirby 等，2014）。

与 ³He 平行，偏光镜领域的硬件开发已经提高极性化水平和体积生产（Becker 等，1994），允许重新引入 ¹²⁹Xe 作为潜在的对比剂（Hersman 等，2008）。其他新型气体正在试验中，如 ¹⁹F，未来这也可能是有用的（Couch 等，2013）。

所有上述气体都需要经过能量输入（超极化），这使得它们可以在镜面调谐的射频系统中被探测到。随着射频脉冲的使用，偏振被破坏，因此，为了避免去极化，需要对 IP 角减小的成像序列采取不同的方法。

引入的高信号超极性气体使这项技术相对较少地依赖于场强，大多数研究是在 1.5T 系统上进行的，在大多数医院中可行。非标准成像序列已被开发，允许最大限度地利用超极化。超极化惰性气体的作用使人们对病理生理学关系及其在各种临床条件下作为疾病和治疗反应的定量生物标记物的潜力有了认识（Kirby 等，1985；Samee 等，2003；Woodhouse 等，2009；Ireland 等，2010；Kirby 等，2011；Couch 等，2013）。

正常受试者会有相对均匀的通气分布，并伴有轻微的依赖肺过度通气（实际上与灌注相匹配）（De Lange 等，1999）。患有一系列肺和肺部血管疾病的患者会出现通气障碍（De Lange 等，1999；Marshall 等，2014），这往往与疾病的程度有关，并提供了通气分布的研究。特别令人感兴趣的是，这项技术无辐射，可以应用于短期和长期随访。这样就可以直接评估 5—6 岁儿童的通气挑战（如过敏挑战）和对治疗的反应（如支气管扩张器或物理疗法）。此外，MRI 通气技术可研究小气道（下至肺泡水平）的大小，以及通气功能的分布（Saam 等，2000；Salerno 等，2002；Fichele 等，2004）。气体进入肺部的动力学（Salerno 等，2001；Wild 等，2003），以及从肺部到血液的氧摄取（Wild 等，2005；Hamedani 等，2015）。最近，¹²⁹Xe 被证明能够应用于研究肺泡 - 血屏障（间质）厚度和有效气体交换膜的总面积（Mugler 等，2010；Patz 等，2007；Muradyan 等，2013）。

这项技术已经应用于各种肺部疾病的评估，包括哮喘、囊性纤维化、慢性阻塞性肺病（chronic obstructive pulmonary disease, COPD）、肺癌和肺移植排斥反应的评估。

（三）氧增强 ¹H MRI

氧增强磁共振成像技术通过应用氧的顺磁性特性获得肺通气的图像。该原理是呼吸门控中心重排反转 - 恢复单点快速自旋回波超声脉冲序列，在呼气时得到肺的蒙片图像，然后在受试者被允许呼吸 100% 的氧气 5min 后，再进行相同的成像序列（Ohno 等，2014）。这些图像随后被减影去除，由于质子 MR 图像通过氧气的顺磁效应去相位从而产生信号差异。

这种方法已经在一些中心进行了试点，但到目前为止还没有完全进入临床应用。尽管如此，这项技术是相对直接的，不需要额外的硬件（通常在任何 MRI 序列中都可以使用氧气），将其转化为临床实践应该是可行的。最近的研究表明，采用基于多回声 2D 超短 TE（ultrashort TE, UTE）的分段的反转 - 恢复 Look- Locker 多次回声序列，对难以处理的 T_1 和 T_2^* 的定量分析方法是可行的，分别与肺泡气体中溶解性分子氧浓度有关（Triphan 等，2015）。这些发展使得这种方法有可能在不久的将来进入临床常规。

（四）运动的动态成像

MRI 可用于评估胸腔内结构的移动性（如膈肌、气道和周围肿瘤）。利用时间分辨成像技术，如扰相梯度回波（如 FLASH）或平衡稳态自由进动脉冲序列，用来评估吸气和呼气期间的移动性（图 13-2）。因此，追踪膈肌的运动并显示膈肌病变，与肺活量测量也有很好的相关性（Cluzel 等，2000；Voorhees 等，2005；Swift 等，2007）。

二、临床应用

（一）肺灌注成像的临床应用

通过动态增强磁共振成像评估肺灌注。灌注改变的区域会显示缓慢且强度较低的增强，或者没有灌注（梗死组织）。

肺灌注显像已被应用于肺血栓栓塞的评估（图13-3）。一些研究报道表明，动态磁共振灌注成像在预测急性肺血栓栓塞后疾病严重程度和预后方面优于MR和CT血管造影术（Ohno等，2010）。对肺叶和节段性肺栓塞的敏感性分别为98%和92%（Ersoy等，2007）。MR在慢性血栓栓塞性疾病患者的评估中使用的最广泛，这一问题将在本章稍后讨论（Tsai等，2011；Pena等，2012）。

最近，据报道无造影剂的傅里叶分解MRI可用于区域肺通气和灌注的定性评估，可与传统的单光子发射计算机断层扫描/CT（Bauman等，2011）相媲美。第11章讨论了这一技术。

人们对慢性阻塞性肺疾病（COPD）患者的灌注成像颇有兴趣（图13-4和图13-5）。这是基于对在本病发病机制中起关键作用的内皮功能障碍和异常肺血管反应的认识（Kanazawa等，2003；Barr等，2007）。肺气肿形成时，肺泡表面积减少伴随毛细血管体积减小（Morrison等，1990；Barberà等，1994），因此，灌注量进一步减少（Pansini等，2009）。肺气肿肺部MRI的挑战是由于额外的空气容积和质子密度的进一步降低导致的T_2^*效应。多重定量和半定量MR灌注研究表明，与正常肺相比，肺气肿患者的肺灌注减少了（Amundsen等，2002a；Sergiacomi等，2003；Ohno等，2004b；Hueper等，2013）。

一项小规模的研究使用动态增强MRI和通气-灌注（V-Q）闪烁显像在各种肺疾病（PE 20例，急性肺炎11例，COPD加重13例）的增强模式（Amundsen等，2002）。灌注MRI在自由呼吸和无心脏门控的情况下进行。定性评价了对比增强模式。在测量中，运动的潜在影响尚未被研究。在评估灌注异常时方法间的一

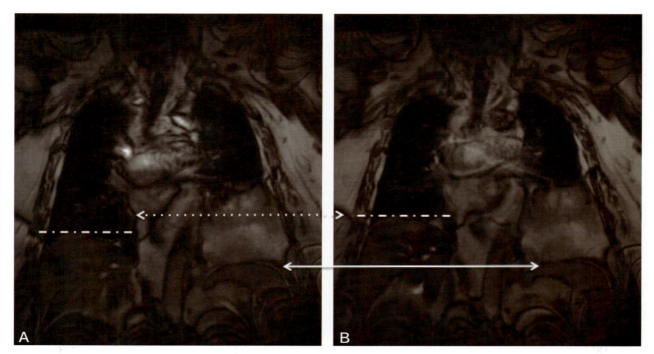

▲ 图13-2　肺动态MRI

62岁男性，CT上显示有分叶状肿块。实时稳态自由进动成像显示右半膈肌运动正常，但是左半膈肌麻痹，提示有膈神经麻痹的可能。这就排除了肿瘤手术切除的适宜性。A. 吸气相；B. 呼气相。注意右膈（虚线）水平的变化而左膈水平没变化

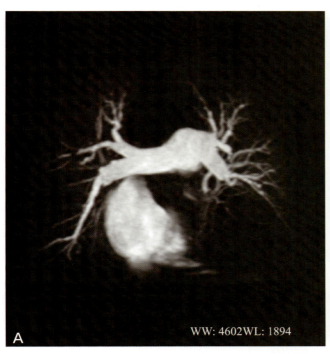 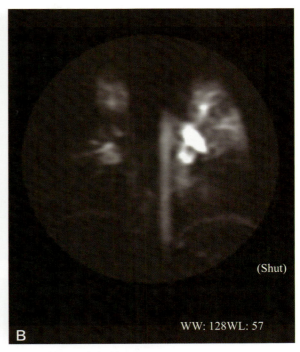

▲ 图 13-3　1 例既往有肺栓塞病史和进行性呼吸急促的患者

磁共振血管成像（MRA）（A）显示广泛的慢性血栓栓塞性疾病和 MR 灌注图像（B）中相匹配的节段性肺灌注缺损。这个患者患有慢性血栓栓塞性肺动脉高压（注意近端肺动脉分支的大小）

致性（kappa 值）范围从 0.52～0.57。在肺炎中，实变与周围正常肺组织相比，在增强前、后呈明显高信号强度。与正常的肺组织相比，COPD 合并肺气肿的增强程度一般较低。在急性肺栓塞中，可观察到无明显强化的肺区域（灌注缺损）。时间 - 信号强度曲线在早期没有达到信号峰值，仅是信号的微弱延迟增加。MR 灌注成像与 V-Q 显像相比，能更高比例地观察到有灌注缺损的肺。

对 30 例重度肺气肿患者进行另一种半定量肺灌注评估与 V-Q 显像法检测灌注异常相比，MR 检测灌注异常有较高的敏感性（86.7%）和良好的特异性（80.0%）。同样地，肺气肿区观察到的峰值信号强度也较低（Sergiacomi 等，2003）。一项针对 143 例患者（80 例 COPD 患者）的更大规模的研究应用了双团注 MR 灌注。该研究结果表明定量和半定量 MRI 参数间有密切的相关性（r=0.86）。该研究报道称，MRI 衍生的灌注测量与全肺灌注（心输出量除以总肺容积）和肺弥散量（Hueper 等，2013）相关。

与肺气肿相似，微血管异常如微血管血栓形成和损伤在肺纤维化的发病机制中起着重要作用（Magro 等，2003），因此，成像技术已经被用来绘制这些患者的灌注图。一项研究报道了肺纤维化合并肺气肿患者的平均通过时间和达到峰值强化时间都延长了（Sergiacomi 等，2010）。与标准的 MR 技术相比，它不能区分炎症和纤维化（Jacob 等，2010），3-T 动态增强 MRI 在静脉注射造影剂前和注射后 1、3、5 和 10min 后 T_1 加权序列分别显示不同的增强模式，其在区分炎症和纤维为主的变化方面敏感性、特异性和准确性分别是 82%、92% 和 88%。在大多数炎症为主的病变中可发现早期增强，在纤维化为主的病变中可见晚期 / 持续性增强（Yi 等，2008）。图 13-6 显示了纤维化区域的灌注改变。图 13-7 显示了 1 例继发于肺纤维化的肺动脉高压患者。

据报道，动态 MR 灌注可研究肺结节的特征。多项研究报道其敏感性 52%～100%，特异性 17%～100%，准确性 58%～96%（Hittmair 等，1995；Gückel 等，1996；Ohno 等，2002，2008b；Kim 等，2004；Schaefer 等，2004；Kono 等，

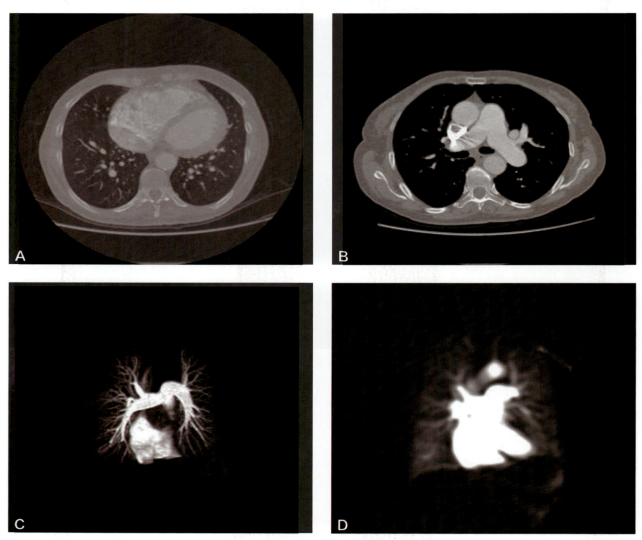

▲ 图 13-4　55 岁男性慢性支气管炎患者

A. 心室中段水平轴位 CT 图像。右心室（RV）是肥大的，这在 COPD 患者中是常见的；B. 主肺动脉水平的轴位 CT 图像。肺动脉扩张，直径 3.5cm（正常上限范围 3.3cm）；C、D. 3D MR 血管造影冠状位图像和冠状位灌注图像显示正常的肺动脉分支和灌注

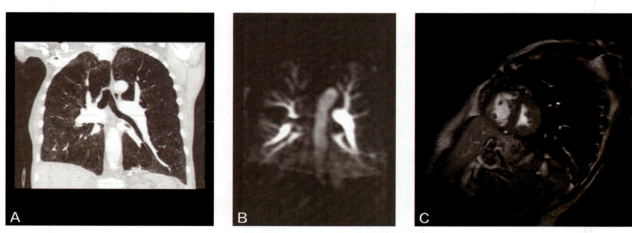

▲ 图 13-5　肺气肿患者的 MR 灌注

A. 典型上叶优势型小叶中心性肺气肿患者的冠状位 CT；B. 显示匹配的冠状位 MR 灌注图像，显示肺破坏区域灌注不良；C. 显示该患者肺气肿对肺血管系统的作用，导致 RV 后负荷增高伴 RV 扩张和室间隔肥厚及反常偏离

2007；Zou 等，2008）。

用病理变化来解释灌注模式的差异。先前的研究显示，肿瘤的异常血管结构和间质腔隙会最终影响肿瘤的增强特性（Less 等，1991）。恶性结节与良性结节比较时，在灌注、细胞外间隙体积和毛细血管通透性方面存在差异，可通过灌注成像进行

研究（Ohno 等，2014b）。

与正常肺大部分灌注都来自肺动脉相比，肺结节多来源于支气管动脉供血（Wright，1967；Milne，1976，1987），导致了肺动脉成像阶段洗入减少和阻碍流动（Ohno 等，2004b）。类似地，与正常肺相比，血管内对比剂的洗脱主要是通过支

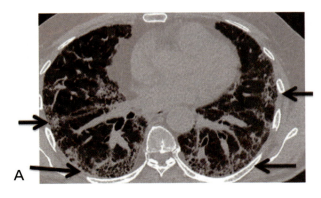

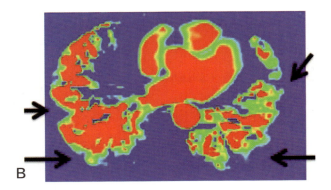

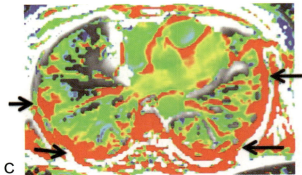

▲ 图 13-6　1 例 67 岁患有特发性肺纤维化的患者的 MR 灌注成像

A. 肺高分辨率计算机断层扫描（CT）显示胸膜下间质改变（箭），提示肺纤维化。参数灌注图显示在与纤维性变化相对应的胸膜下区域肺血流量（PBF）减少（B）和平均通过时间延长（C）。参数图中根据灌注程度像素被颜色编码（PBF 值从高到低：红、黄、绿、蓝，平均通过时间值从高到低：红、黄、绿）

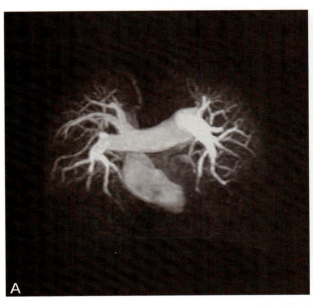

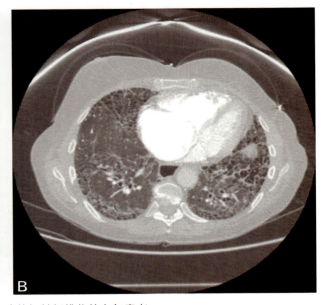

▲ 图 13-7　1 例结缔组织病伴相关纤维化的老年患者

A. 磁共振血管成像（MRA）显示肺动脉显著扩张及血管结构扭曲；B. 显示肺基底段的纤维化改变及其所继发的心脏右心室和心房扩张及右心室肥厚

气管静脉而不是肺静脉分支。此外，间质腔隙也没有正常的淋巴洗脱。所有这些都会导致肺结节的延迟洗脱和对比剂保留（Littleton 等，1990）。

炎症结节主要是由增多、增大的支气管动脉供血。在大多数情况下，由于小动脉水平弥漫血栓形成，肺动脉供应减少。这导致血供的消失和延迟。相比之下，通过对流和扩张淋巴管的弥散增加使间质腔隙对比剂的冲洗增强（Ohno 等，2014b）。亦有报道称薄的外周强化与良性结节的相关性强，其被认为是炎性反应（Schaefer 等，2004）。

（二）肺部疾病的通气成像

肺部通气 MRI 在真正的常规临床机构中的应用仍处于起步阶段（图 13-8 和图 13-9）。尽管进行了许多（主要是小的）研究，但目前还没有使用该方法的临床适应证。然而，有一些进展需要被视为临床应用的前体（无论是常规还是临床试验的一部分）。

氧增强成像开始在临床中使用。显然，这种方法最容易引入，因为不需要特定的硬件或软件，通常可在 1.5T 扫描仪上进行（Renne 等，2015b）。上述段落中描述的技术能够预测肺癌进行肺切除术患者的预后，在一项研究中，30 名接受氧增强 MRI 检查的患者与术前和术后肺功能检查相比较（Ohno 等，2005）。两种方法之间存在极好的相关性，提示该方法可以预测术后肺功能，也可提供肺功能检查无法获得的功能和区域信息。

在另一项研究中，30 例哮喘患者，动态氧增强 MRI 与定量 CT 测量和肺功能测试进行了比较（Ohno 等，2014a）。与定量 CT 测量相比，哮喘患者的洗入时间与肺功能检查的相关性更好。

一项针对 9 例哮喘患者和 4 例健康个体的

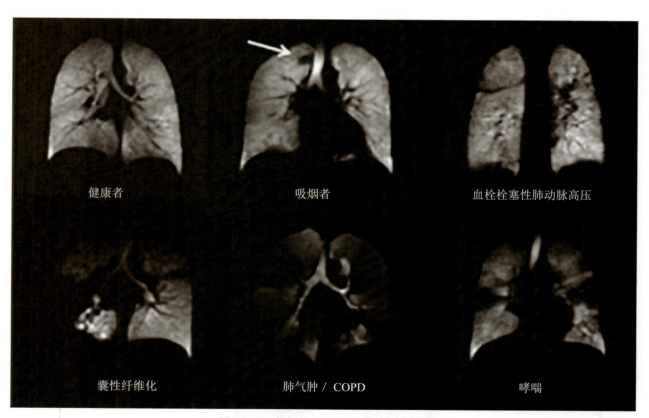

▲ 图 13-8　超极化 3-Helium MRI 通气成像

正常志愿者的图像显示均匀信号（正常通气）。在吸烟者中，右上叶（箭）发现了一个小的通气缺损。在患有慢性血栓栓塞性肺动脉高压的患者中显示为略微不均匀的通气。在囊性纤维化的患者中，主要在右肺中显示出大的通气缺损和通气量减少。肺气肿 / COPD 患者的图像显示大的节段性通气缺损。在哮喘患者中，通气缺损特别易在外周（亚段）中出现

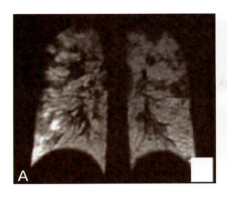 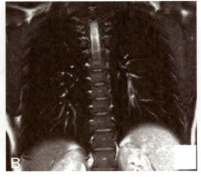 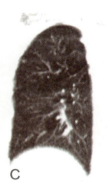 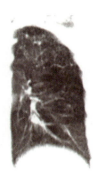

▲ 图 13-9 超极化 3-Helium

图像显示上部区域通气缺损显著（A）而质子 MRI（B）正常。CT 扫描（C）显示低密度相应区域与空气滞留相一致以及由于黏液堵塞导致的一些小叶中心结节

小型研究比较了过敏源激发前后的氧增强 MRI，并证明了其显示和量化区域过敏反应效应的可行性（Renne 等，2015a）。

超极化惰性气体成像目前仅用于小规模的临床试验。它的使用主要限于具有适当硬件和知识基础的中心。另外，气体相对昂贵且不易获得（如，^{3}He）或在常规临床机构中不易使用（如，^{129}Xe）。虽然这种方法被用于证明干预措施有效，如通过支气管高反应性刺激 / 缓解试验，并且已经证明其倾向于对小气道形态学和复杂的通气 / 灌注相互作用进行详细的生理分析，但不太可能将它用于常规的临床实践。

（三）肺动脉高压 MRI

肺动脉高压是一种以肺血管内血压升高为特征的疾病（Kiely 等，2013）（图 13-7，图 13-10 至图 13-13）。这导致进行性右心室（right ventricle，RV）衰竭并最终死亡。如果不治疗，肺动脉高压预后不良，诊断后中位生存时间仅为 2.8 年（D'Alonzo 等，1991）。然而，最近的治疗进展提高了该疾病预后，成为开发生物标志物的动力，这些生物标志物可以跟踪治疗的反应并对患者风险进行分层。

心脏 MRI 被认为是评估和管理肺动脉高压的

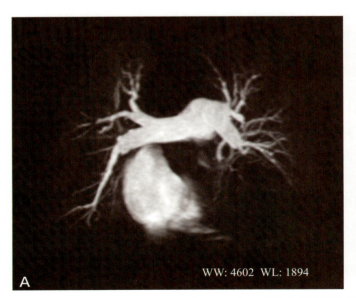 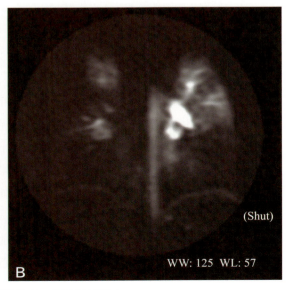

▲ 图 13-10 1 例气短进行性加重的患者，既往肺栓塞史

A.MRA 图像显示广泛慢性血栓栓塞性疾病 ;B. 与 MR 灌注图像中节段性灌注缺损模式相符合。该患者有慢性血栓栓塞性肺动脉高压（注意近端肺动脉分支的大小）

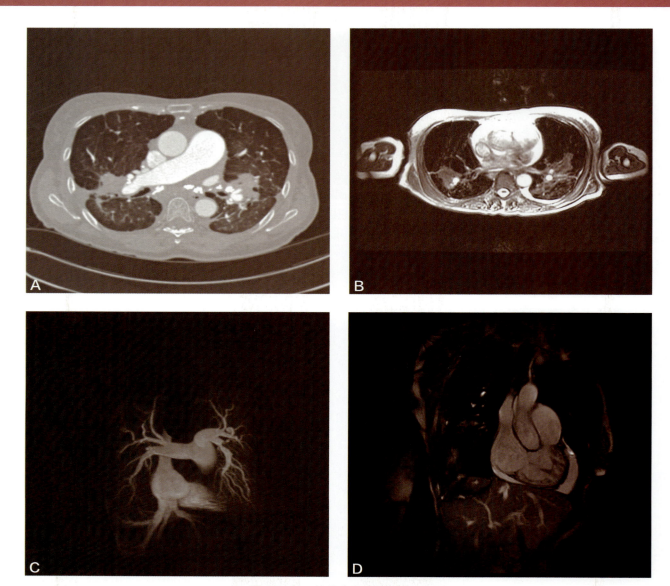

▲ 图 13-11 结节病患者的肺动脉高压

CT（A）和 MRI（B）显示肺结节病患者的间质增厚、聚集结节和淋巴结增大。血管造影（C）显示由于肺动脉高压导致的肺动脉扩张和肺动脉分支扭曲。冠状稳态自由进动成像（D）显示右心房扩张和右心室肥厚伴有心包积液

一种越来越重要的成像方式（Swift 等，2014b）。MRI 具有以下优点：无创、无辐射，提供优异的对比分辨率、时间分辨率，并且可在任意平面成像。此外，MRI 对血流的敏感性，允许测量血流速度和流量，增强后成像允许评估心肌、肺血管和灌注（Bradlow 等，2012）。

1. 心脏成像 MRI 通常用于评估心血管疾病的心脏形态、室腔容积、心肌质量和心脏功能（图 13-11 至图 13-13）。晚期钆成像的出现彻底改变了心脏成像，可显示病理为各种缺血性和炎症性心肌组织改变的特征。

心脏和呼吸运动、幽闭恐惧症、相对较长的扫描采集时间以及对体内金属植入物的特定禁忌限制了 MRI 的应用。加快扫描时间的方法包括开发并行成像技术（Wieben 等，2008）。此外，诸如 k-t blast（Kozerke 等，2004）和压缩感知（Gamper 等，2008）之类的新序列可缩短采集时间，同时保持高信噪比。心脏运动的解决方案是通过心电（electrocardiogram，ECG）门控，在多次心跳下经常在获取成像数据同时采集 ECG，在某些情况下实时成像是有利的。进一步的挑战与植入金属装置患者的安全性以及对图像

质量的影响相关；然而，现在大多数植入的金属装置都是用 MRI 兼容的材料制造的。

（1）右心室：心脏 MRI 是一种可用于量化心室容积、质量和功能的高度可重复的方法（Grothues 等，2002；Grothues 等，2004）（图 13-11 和图 13-12）。平衡稳态自由进动 MRI 被认为是测定心室容积的金标准方法，通过采集心脏多层图像实现。每个心腔的典型测量值包括舒张末期容积，即心电图 R 波收缩时相前最大心室腔容积，以及每个短轴切片上的收缩末期容积或最小室腔容积。

多个 MRI 参数在疑似肺动脉高压患者的检查中具有潜在的优势。MR 心室质量指数，定义为右心室质量除以左心室质量，与肺动脉压密切相关（Saba 等，2002；Hagger 等，2009），是一种诊断标志物。此外，在黑血图像上观察到心室间转折点钆剂延迟强化和肺动脉流动伪影的出现，有助于预测未经选择的疑似肺血管疾病患者的肺动脉高压的存在。

室间隔位置可以通过其角度或通过其曲率的测量来评估（Roeleveld 等，2005；Dellegrottaglie 等，2007）；隔膜角度易于快速测量，并且作为诊断标记物非常准确。此外，显示了隔膜角度与心室质量指数相结合的附加值。隔膜角度和心室质量指数的综合指数提高了诊断的准确性和与 mPAP 的相关性。

此外，可以通过 MRI 无创地评估肺血管阻力，分别通过额外的肺毛细血管楔压的替代标志物、心脏输出左心房容积和相位对比 MRI，所有主要的血流动力学测量值均可通过 MRI 无创评估。

基线时 RV 测量评估相对于 RV 后负荷增加的代偿性扩张水平。对 RV 后负荷增加 RV 适应性失败所致的进行性扩张导致右心室衰竭和死亡（van Wolferen 等，2007）。64 例特发性肺动脉高压患者的单中心预后研究发现右心室舒张末期容积（right ventricular end-diastolic volume，RVEDV）指数 > 84 ml/m^2 与生存率低有关（$P = 0.011$）。此外，在 1 年随访中，RVEDV 指数的变化与预后独立相关（van Wolferen 等，2007）。在一组 110 例肺动脉高压患者的队列中，基线时，RV 射血分数独立地指向预后不良，随访时 RV 射血分数的变化与生存风险比 0.93 独立相关（95% CI 0.88 ～ 0.99）。RV 舒张末期和收缩末期容积是基线和随访时肺动脉高压患者不良预后的预测因素。在两个体积状态中，RV 收缩末期容积已被证明具有相应更大的预后价值，可能是它代表了室腔的扩张和低收缩功能（Swift 等，2014a）。

（2）左心室：肺动脉高压时每搏输出量是比心脏输出量更重要的预后因素，因为当每搏输出量不再增加时，患者可以通过增加心率来维持心输出量（van Wolferen 等，2007）。Holverda 等（2006）研究了一个非常小的队列，包括 10 例功能Ⅲ级特发性肺动脉高压的患者。将这些患者与 10 例年龄和性别匹配的对照组进行比较。患有肺动脉高压的患者体力活动时不能增加每搏输出量以产生足够的心输出量。在几项研究中，左心室（每搏输出量）已被证明是预后不良的一致指标（van Wolferen 等，2007；Swift 等，2014a）。

低 LV 舒张末期容积与肺动脉高压预后较差有关；这被假设是由于 RV 容积超过负荷、LV 压缩及 LV 充盈不良造成的。LV 充盈不足导致 LV 每搏输出量少，这也是肺动脉高压患者不良预后

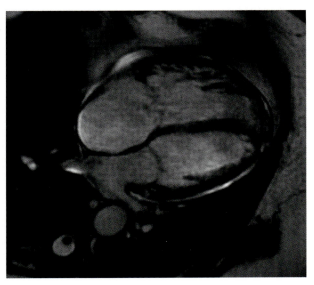

▲ 图 13-12 肺动脉高压患者四腔 CINE 心脏 MR 图像
该图像显示不良的预后特征，RV 扩张和少量心包积液

的有力指标。此外，已发现 LV 舒张末期容积的变化是肺动脉高压治疗反应的标志。

2. 肺血管成像 以前的影像学研究主要集中在可疑肺动脉高压患者的肺动脉大小的临床应用上（Devaraj 和 Hansell，2009；Devaraj 等，2010）（图 13-13）。肺动脉大小在肺动脉高压筛查中具有价值，但在疾病严重程度的评估中作用有限。这是因为肺动脉扩张的程度与病情的持续时间有关，而不是与平均肺动脉压（mPAP）直接相关（Boerrigter 等，2010）。

肺动脉相对面积变化（relative area change，RAC）的缺失是轻度肺血管疾病的标志，可用与肺血管阻力成反比关系来解释，肺血管阻力的小幅增加导致 RAC 更大比例的减少。这证实了先前的一项研究（Sanz 等，2009），该研究提出 RAC 作为一种敏感的标志物，通过识别运动性肺动脉高压患者显著降低的 RAC 来检测临床前疾病。在患有轻度肺血管疾病的患者中，RAC 减少，而 RV 体积和功能没有显著改变，这与肺动脉在 RV 功能丧失之前变得僵硬的理论一致。

慢性血栓栓塞性肺动脉高压（chronic thromboembolic pulmonary hypertension，CTEPH）是肺血栓栓塞性疾病的严重并发症，并且具有相当高的发病率和死亡率（Riedel 等，1982）。据估计，高达 3.8% 的患有急性肺栓塞症状的患者将在 2 年内发生 CTEPH（Pengo 等，2004），甚至在急性期间接受适当治疗的患者中，血栓可能无法完全消退，导致 CTEPH（Remy-Jardin 等，1997；Ribeiro 等，1999；Wartski 和 Collignon，2000）。

CTEPH 的诊断主要通过成像来进行。传统上，肺血管造影被认为是对慢性血栓栓塞诊断的确诊性研究，特别是在外科手术计划的背景下（Daily 等，1980；Jamieson 等，1993）。随着多排 CT 扫描仪的出现，CTPA 取代了肺血管造影（Kauczor 等，1994；Remy-Jardin 等，1992；Wittram 等，2006）。

高空间分辨率 MR 血管造影能够显示肺血管的中心部分。高空间分辨率肺动脉成像的屏气持续时间可长达 25s，对于肺动脉高压有明显呼吸困难的患者而言，屏气时间过长。并行成像技术可以提高空间分辨率，并且可以通过更短的憋气时间来实现全肺容积覆盖。

通过时间分辨 MRA 技术，区分特发性肺动脉高压患者和 CTEPH 患者，显示肺动脉至节段水平。此外，额外的 3D MR 灌注成像可以帮助观察灌注缺损的特征模式。对于疑似 CTEPH 的患者，非电离 3D MR 肺部灌注成像在可疑的 CTEPH 患者具有较高的诊断准确性，与灌注闪烁扫描相当，正常的 MR 肺灌注研究排除了可动手术的 CTEPH（Rajaram 等，2013）。

3. 肺血流特点成像 相位对比是用 MRI 估计血流的有效方法（Lotz 等，2002；Gatehouse 等，2005）。基础相位对比 MRI 的基本原理是在磁场梯度方向上移动的质子自旋经历与速度成正比的相位移动。血流动力学测量可以确定如前向流动、逆行流动、平均速度和峰值速度。

几项研究已将心输出量确定为 PAH 患者

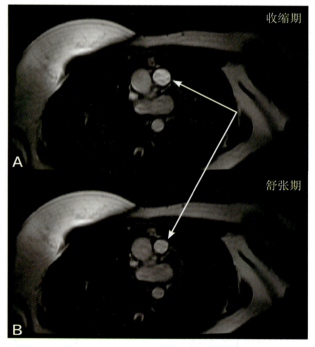

▲ 图 13-13 心脏收缩期（A）和心脏舒张期（B）

与主肺动脉正交的 CINEMRI 显示肺动脉具有良好的搏动性，随着心动周期血管直径变化，收缩期管径增宽。肺动脉搏动是肺血管系统顺应性的替代标记物，且是长期存活的良好预后标记物

不良预后的关键独立标志物（D'Alonzo等，1991；Sandoval等，1994；McLaughlin等，2002；Sitbon等，2002；Humbert等，2010）。有几种无创性MRI方法非常适合评估心输出量和每搏输出量。MR容积可以准确且可重复地评估健康和患病状态下RV和LV腔室的容积变化（Heusch等，1999；Benza等，2008；Mooij等，2008；Bradlow等，2010；Marrone等，2010），相位对比成像是一种评估肺动脉和主动脉血流的稳健方法（Kondo等，1991；Gatehouse等，2005；Ley等，2007；Sanz等，2007；Mauritz等，2008）。相位对比MRI衍生的测量结果也被证明与压力和阻力的创伤性测量结果相关。如，Sanz等已证实肺动脉压力与肺动脉主干血流的平均速度呈负相关（Sanz等，2007），肺血管阻力通过射血期间快速容积计算流率最大变化率来评估（Mousseaux等，1999）。此外，最近的一项研究表明，早期逆向分流是肺动脉高压患者的一个特征（Helderman等，2011）。

参考文献

[1] Aksoy FG, Lev MH. Dynamic contrast-enhanced brain perfusion imaging: Technique and clinical applications. *Semin Ultrasound CT MR*. 2000 Dec;21(6):462–477.

[2] Allmendinger AM, Tang ER, Lui YW et al. Imaging of stroke: Part 1, Perfusion CT—Overview of imaging technique, interpretation pearls, and common pitfalls. *AJR Am J Roentgenol*. 2012;198:1, 52–62.

[3] Amundsen T, Torheim G, Kvistad KA, Waage A, Bjermer L, Nordlid KK, Johnsen H, Asberg A, Haraldseth O. Perfusion abnormalities in pulmonary embolism studied with perfusion MRI and ventilation-perfusion scintigraphy: An intra-modality and inter-modality agreement study. *J Magn Reson Imaging*. Apr 2002;15(4):386–394.

[4] Barberà JA, Riverola A, Roca J et al. Pulmonary vascular abnormalities and ventilation-perfusion relationships in mild chronic obstructive pulmonary disease. *Am J Respir Crit Care Med*. 1994;149(2 Pt 1):423–429.

[5] Barr RG, Mesia-Vela S, Austin JH et al. Impaired flow-mediated dilation is associated with low pulmonary function and emphysema in ex-smokers: The Emphysema and Cancer Action Project (EMCAP) Study. *Am J Respir Crit Care Med* 2007;176:1200–1207.

[6] Bauman G, Lützen U, Ullrich M et al. Pulmonary functional imaging: Qualitative comparison of Fourier decomposition MR imaging with SPECT/CT in porcine lung. *Radiology*. 2011;260(2):551–559.

[7] Becker J, Heil W, Krug B et al. Study of mechanical compression of spin-polarized 3He gas. *Nucl Instrum Meth A* 1994;346:45–51.

[8] Benza R, Biederman R, Murali S, Gupta H. Role of cardiac magnetic resonance imaging in the management of patients with pulmonary arterial hypertension. *J Am Coll Cardiol*. 2008;52:1683–1692.

[9] Boerrigter B, Mauritz GJ, Marcus JT, Helderman F, Postmus PE, Westerhof N, Vonk-Noordegraaf A. Progressive dilatation of the main pulmonary artery is a characteristic of pulmonary arterial hypertension and is not related to changes in pressure. *Chest*. 2010;138(6):1395–1401.

[10] Bradlow WM, Gibbs JS, Mohiaddin RH. Cardiovascular magnetic resonance in pulmonary hypertension. *J Cardiovasc Magn Reson*. 2012;14:6.

[11] Bradlow WM, Hughes ML, Keenan NG, Bucciarelli-Ducci C, Assomull R, Gibbs JS, Mohiaddin RH. Measuring the heart in pulmonary arterial hypertension (pah): Implications for trial study size. *J Magn Reson Imaging*. 2010;31:117–124.

[12] Cluzel P, Similowski T, Chartrand-Lefebvre C et al. Diaphragm and chest wall: Assessment of the inspiratory pump with MR imaging preliminary observations. *Radiology*. 2000;215: 574–583.

[13] Couch MJ, Ball IK, Li T et al. Pulmonary ultrashort echo time 19F MR imaging with inhaled fluorinated gas mixtures in healthy volunteers: Feasibility. *Radiology*. 2013;269:903–909. D'Alonzo GE, Barst RJ, Ayres SM et al. Survival in patients with primary pulmonary hypertension. Results from a national prospective registry. *Ann Inter Med*. 1991;115:343–349.

[14] Daily PO, Johnston GG, Simmons CJ, Moser KM. Surgical management of chronic pulmonary embolism: Surgical treatment and late results. *J Thorac Cardiovasc Surg*. 1980;79:523–531.

[15] De Lange EE, Mugler III JP, Brookeman JR et al. Lung air spaces: MR imaging evaluation with hyperpolarized 3He gas. *Radiology*. 1999;210:851–857.

[16] Dellegrottaglie S, Sanz J, Poon M, Viles-Gonzalez JF, Sulica R, Goyenechea M, Macaluso F, Fuster V, Rajagopalan S. Pulmonary hypertension: Accuracy of detection with left ventricular septal-to-free wall curvature ratio measured at cardiac MR. *Radiology*. 2007;243:63–69.

[17] Devaraj A, Hansell DM. Computed tomography signs of pul-monary hypertension: Old and new observations. *Clin Radiol*. 2009;64:751–760.

[18] Devaraj A, Wells AU, Meister MG, Corte TJ, Wort SJ, Hansell DM. Detection of pulmonary hypertension with multi detector ct and echocardiography alone and in combination. *Radiology*. 2010;254:609–616.

[19] Ersoy H, Goldhaber SZ, Cai T et al. Time-resolved MR angiography: A primary screening examination of patients with suspected pulmonary embolism and contraindications to administration of iodinated contrast material. *AJR Am J Roentgenol.* 2007;188:1246–1254.

[20] Fichele S, Woodhouse N, Swift AJ et al. MRI of Helium-3 gas in healthy lungs: Posture related variation of alveolar size. *J MRI.* 2004;20:331–335.

[21] Gamper U, Boesiger P, Kozerke S. Compressed sensing in dynamic MRI. *Magn Reson Med.* 2008;59:365–373.

[22] Gatehouse PD, Keegan J, Crowe LA, Masood S, Mohiaddin RH, Kreitner KF, Firmin DN. Applications of phase-contrast flow and velocity imaging in cardiovascular MRI. *Eur Radiol.* 2005;15:2172–2184.

[23] Grothues F, Moon JC, Bellenger NG, Smith GS, Klein HU, Pennell DJ. Interstudy reproducibility of right ventricular volumes, function, and mass with cardiovascular magnetic resonance. *Am Heart J.* 2004;147:218–223.

[24] Grothues F, Smith GC, Moon JC, Bellenger NG, Collins P, Klein HU, Pennell DJ. Comparison of interstudy reproduc-ibility of cardiovascular magnetic resonance with two dimensional echocardiography in normal subjects and in patients with heart failure or left ventricular hypertrophy. *Am J Cardiol.* 2002;90:29–34.

[25] Gückel C, Schnabel K, Deimling M, Steinbrich W. Solitary pulmonary nodules: MR evaluation of enhancement pat-terns with contrast-enhanced dynamic snapshot gradient-echo imaging. *Radiology.* 1996;200:681–686.

[26] Hagger D, Condliffe R, Woodhouse N, Elliot CA, Armstrong IJ, Davies C, Hill C, Akil M, Wild JM, Kiely DG. Ventricular mass index correlates with pulmonary artery pressure and predicts survival in suspected systemic sclerosis-associated pulmonary arterial hypertension. *Rheumatology.* 2009;48:1137–1142.

[27] Hamedani H, Kadlecek SJ, Ishii M et al. Alterations of regional alveolar oxygen tension in asymptomatic current smokers: Assessment with hyperpolarized 3He MR imaging. *Radiology.* 2015;274:585–596.

[28] Harris AD, Coutts SB, Frayne R. Diffusion and perfusion MR imaging of acute ischemic stroke. *Magn Reson Imaging Clin N Am.* 2009;17(2):291–313.

[29] Helderman F, Mauritz GJ, Andringa KE, Vonk-Noordegraaf A, Marcus JT. Early onset of retrograde flow in the main pulmonary artery is a characteristic of pulmonary arterial hypertension. *J Magn Reson Imaging.* 2011;33:1362–1368.

[30] Hersman FW, Ruset IC, Ketel S et al. Large production system for hyperpolarized 129Xe for human lung imaging studies. *Acad Radiol.* 2008;15:683–692.

[31] Heusch A, Koch JA, Krogmann ON, Korbmacher B, Bourgeois M. Volumetric analysis of the right and left ventricle in a porcine heart model: Comparison of three-dimensional echocardiography, magnetic resonance imaging and angiocardiography. *Eur J Ultrasound.* 1999;9:245–255.

[32] Hittmair K, Eckersberger F, Klepetko W, Helbich T, Herold CJ. Evaluation of solitary pulmonary nodules with dynamic contrast-enhanced MR imaging: A promising technique. *Magn Reson Imaging.* 1995;13:923–933.

[33] Hueper K, Parikh MA, Prince MR et al. Quantitative and semi-quantitative measures of regional pulmonary microvascular perfusion by magnetic resonance imaging and their relationships to global lung perfusion and lung diffusing capacity: The multiethnic study of atherosclerosis chronic obstructive pulmonary disease study. *Invest Radiol.* 2013 Apr;48(4):223–230.

[34] Humbert M, Sitbon O, Chaouat A et al. Survival in patients with idiopathic, familial, and anorexigen-associated pulmonary arterial hypertension in the modern management era. *Circulation.* 2010;122:156–163.

[35] Ingrisch M, Dietrich O, Attenberger UI, Nikolaou K, Sourbron S, Reiser MF, Fink C (2010) Quantitative pulmonary perfusion magnetic resonance imaging: Influence of temporal resolution and signal-to-noise ratio. *Invest Radiol.* 45:7–14.

[36] Ireland RH, Din O, Swinscoe JA et al. Detection of radiation-induced lung injury in non-small cell lung cancer patients using hyperpolarized helium-3 magnetic resonance imaging. *Radiother Oncol* 2010;97: 244–248.

[37] Jacob RE, Amidan BG, Soelberg J, Minard KR. In vivo MRI of altered proton signal intensity and T2 relaxation in a bleomycin model of pulmonary inflammation and fibrosis. *J Magn Reson Imaging.* 2010;31(5):1091–1099.

[38] Jamieson SW, Auger WR, Fedullo PF, Channick RN, Kriett JM, Tarazi RY, Moser KM. Experience and results with 150 pulmonary thromboendarterectomy operations over a 29-month period. *J Thorac Cardiovasc Surg.* 1993;106:116–126; discussion 126–117.

[39] Kanazawa H, Asai K, Hirata K et al. Possible effects of vascular endothelial growth factor in the pathogenesis of chronic obstructive pulmonary disease. *Am J Med.* 2003;114: 354–358.

[40] Kauczor HU, Schwickert HC, Mayer E, Schweden F, Schild HH, Thelen M. Spiral ct of bronchial arteries in chronic thromboembolism. *J Comput Assist Tomogr.* 1994;18:855–861.

[41] Kiely DG, Elliot CA, Sabroe I, Condliffe R. Pulmonary hypertension: Diagnosis and management. *BMJ.* 2013;346:f2028.

[42] Kim JH, Kim HJ, Lee KH, Kim KH, Lee HL. Solitary pulmonary nodules: A comparative study evaluated with contrast-enhanced dynamic MR imaging and CT. *J Comput Assist Tomogr.* 2004;28:766–775.

[43] Kirby M, Heydarian M, Wheatley A et al. Evaluating bronchodilator effects in chronic obstructive pulmonary disease using diffusion-weighted hyperpolarized helium-3 magnetic resonance imaging. *J Appl Physiol (1985).* 2012;112:651–657.

[44] Kirby M, Mathew L, Heydarian M et al. Chronic obstructive pulmonary disease: Quantification of bronchodilator

effects using hyperpolarized 3He MR imaging. *Radiology*. 2011;261:283–292.

[45] Kirby M, Pike D, Coxson HO et al. Hyperpolarized 3He ventilation defects used to predict pulmonary exacerbations in mild to moderate chronic obstructive pulmonary disease. *Radiology*. 2014;273:887–896.

[46] Kjørstad Å, Corteville DM, Fischer A, Henzler T, Schmid-Bindert G, Zöllner FG, Schad LR. Quantitative lung perfusion evaluation using Fourier decomposition perfusion MRI. *Magn Reson Med*. 2014 Aug;72(2):558–562.

[47] Kondo C, Caputo GR, Semelka R, Foster E, Shimakawa A, Higgins CB. Right and left ventricular stroke volume measurements with velocity-encoded cine MR imaging: In vitro and in vivo validation. *AJR*. 1991;157:9–16.

[48] Kono R, Fujimoto K, Terasaki H et al. Dynamic MRI of solitary pulmonary nodules: Comparison of enhancement patterns of malignant and benign small peripheral lung lesions. *AJR*. 2007;188:26–36.

[49] Kozerke S, Tsao J, Razavi R, Boesiger P. Accelerating cardiac cine 3d imaging using k-t blast. *Magn Reson Med*. 2004;52:19–26.

[50] Less JR, Skalak TC, Sevick EM, Jain RK. Microvascular architecture in a mammary carcinoma: Branching patterns and vessel dimensions. *Cancer Res*. 1991;51:265–273.

[51] Ley S, Mereles D, Puderbach M, Gruenig E, Schock H, Eichinger M, Ley-Zaporozhan J, Fink C, Kauczor HU. Value of MR phase-contrast flow measurements for functional assessment of pulmonary arterial hypertension. *Eur Radiol*. 2007;17:1892–1897.

[52] Ley S, Ley-Zaporozhan J. Pulmonary perfusion imaging using MRI: Clinical application. *Insights Imaging*. 2012;3(1):61–71.

[53] Littleton JT, Durizch ML, Moeller G, Herbert DE. Pulmonary masses: Contrast enhancement. *Radiology*. 1990;177:861–871

[54] Lotz J, Meier C, Leppert A, Galanski M. Cardiovascular flow measurement with phase-contrast MR imaging: Basic facts and implementation. *RadioGraphics*. 2002;22:651–671.

[55] Magro CM, Allen J, Pope-Harman A et al. The role of microvascular injury in the evolution of idiopathic pulmonary fibrosis. *Am J Clin Pathol*. Apr 2003;119(4):556–567.

[56] Marrone G, Mamone G, Luca A, Vitulo P, Bertani A, Pilato M, Gridelli B. The role of 1.5t cardiac MRI in the diagnosis, prognosis and management of pulmonary arterial hypertension. *Int J Cardiovasc Imaging*. 2010;26:665–681.

[57] Marshall H, Kiely DG, Parra-Robles J et al. Magnetic resonance imaging of ventilation and perfusion changes in response to pulmonary endarterectomy in chronic thromboembolic pulmonary hypertension. *Am J Resp Crit Care Med*. 2014;190:e18–e19.

[58] Martirosian P1, Boss A, Schraml C, Schwenzer NF, Graf H, Claussen CD, Schick F. Magnetic resonance perfusion imaging without contrast media. *Eur J Nucl Med Mol Imaging*. 2010 Aug;37(Suppl 1):S52–S64.

[59] Mauritz GJ, Marcus JT, Boonstra A, Postmus PE, Westerhof N, Vonk-Noordegraaf A. Non-invasive stroke volume assessment in patients with pulmonary arterial hypertension: Leftsided data mandatory. *J Cardiovasc Magn Reson*. 2008;10:51.

[60] McLaughlin VV, Shillington A, Rich S. Survival in primary pulmonary hypertension: The impact of epoprostenol therapy. *Circulation*. 2002;106:1477–1482.

[61] Miles KA, Griffiths MR, Fuentes MA. Standardized perfusion value: Universal CT contrast enhancement scale that correlates with FDG PET in lung nodules. *Radiology*. 2001;220:548–53.

[62] Milne EN. Circulation of primary and metastatic pulmonary neoplasms: a postmortem micro-arteriographic study. *AJR*. 1967;100:603–619.

[63] Milne EN. Pulmonary metastases: vascular supply and diagnosis. *Int J Radiat Oncol Biol Phys*. 1976;1:739–742.

[64] Milne EN, Zerhouni EA. Blood supply of pulmonary metastases. *J Thorac Imaging*. 1987;2:15–23.

[65] Mirsadraee S, van Beek EJR. Functional imaging: CT and MRI. *Clin Chest Med*. 2015;36(2):349–363.

[66] Mooij CF, de Wit CJ, Graham DA, Powell AJ, Geva T. Reproducibility of MRI measurements of right ventricular size and function in patients with normal and dilated ventricles. *J Magn Reson Imaging*. 2008;28:67–73.

[67] Morrison NJ, Abboud RT, Müller NL et al. Pulmonary capillary blood volume in emphysema. *Am Rev Respir Dis*. 1990;141(1):53–61.

[68] Mousseaux E, Tasu JP, Jolivet O, Simonneau G, Bittoun J, Gaux JC. Pulmonary arterial resistance: Noninvasive measurement with indexes of pulmonary flow estimated at velocity-encoded MR imaging—preliminary experience. *Radiology*. 1999;212:896–902.

[69] Mugler JP 3rd, Altes TA, Ruset IC et al. Simultaneous magnetic resonance imaging of ventilation distribution and gas uptake in the human lung using hyperpolarized xenon 129. *Proc Natl Acad Sci USA*. 2010;107:21707–21712.

[70] Muradyan I, Butler JP, Dabaghyan M et al. Single-breath xenon polarization transfer contrast (SB-XTC): Implementation and initial results in healthy humans. *J MRI*. 2013;37:457–470.

[71] Ohno Y, Hatabu H, Higashino T et al. Oxygen-enhanced MR imaging: Correlation with postsurgical lung function in patients with lung cancer. *Radiology*. 2005;236:704–711.

[72] Ohno Y, Hatabu H, Murase K et al. Quantitative assessment of regional pulmonary perfusion in the entire lung using three-dimensional ultrafast dynamic contrast enhanced magnetic resonance imaging: Preliminary experience in 40 subjects. *J Magn Reson Imaging*. 2004a;20:353–365.

[73] Ohno Y, Hatabu H, Takenaka D et al. Dynamic MR imaging: Value of differentiating subtypes of peripheral small adenocarcinoma of the lung. *Eur J Radiol*. 2004b;52:144–150.

[74] Ohno Y, Hatabu H, Takenaka D, Adachi S, Kono M,

Sugimura K. Solitary pulmonary nodules: Potential role of dynamic MR imaging in management—Initial experience. *Radiology*. 2002;224:503–511.

[75] Ohno Y, Iwasawa T, Seo JB et al. Oxygen-enhanced magnetic resonance imaging versus computed tomography: Multicentre study for clinical stage classification of smoking-related chronic obstructive pulmonary disease. *Am J Respir Crit Care Med*. 2008a;177:1095–1102.

[76] Ohno Y, Koyama H, Matsumoto K et al. Dynamic MR perfusion imaging: Capability for quantitative assessment of disease extent and prediction of outcome for patients with acute pulmonary thromboembolism. *J Magn Reson Imaging*. May 2010;31(5):1081–1090.

[77] Ohno Y, Koyama H, Takenaka D et al. Dynamic MRI, dynamic multidetector-row computed tomography (MDCT), and coregistered 2-[fluorine-18]-fluoro-2-deoxy-d-glucose-positron emission tomography (FDG-PET)/CT: Comparative study of capability for management of pulmonary nodules. *J Magn Reson Imaging* 2008b;27:1284–1295.

[78] Ohno Y, Nishio M, Koyama H et al. Asthma: Comparison of dynamic oxygen-enhanced MR imaging and quantitative thin-section CT for evaluation of clinical treatment. *Radiology*. 2014a;273:907–916.

[79] Ohno Y, Nishio M, Koyama H, Miura S, Yoshikawa T, Matsumoto S, Sugimura K. Dynamic contrast-enhanced CT and MRI for pulmonary nodule assessment. *AJR Am J Roentgenol*. Mar 2014b;202(3):515–529.

[80] Pansini V, Remy-Jardin M, Faivre JB et al. Assessment of lobar perfusion in smokers according to the presence and severity of emphysema: Preliminary experience with dualenergy CT angiography. *Eur Radiol*. Dec 2009;19(12):2834–2843.

[81] Patz S, Hersman PW, Muradyan I et al. Hyperpolarized (129) Xe MRI: A viable functional lung imaging modality? *Eur J Radiol* 2007;64:335–344.

[82] Pena E, Dennie C, Veinot J et al. Pulmonary hypertension: How the radiologist can help. *RadioGraphics*. 2012;32:9–32.

[83] Pengo V, Lensing AW, Prins MH et al. Incidence of chronic thromboembolic pulmonary hypertension after pulmonary embolism. *N Engl J Med*. 2004;350:2257–2264.

[84] Puderbach M, Risse F, Biederer J, Ley-Zaporozhan J, Ley S, Szabo G, Semmler W, Kauczor HU. In vivo Gd-DTPA concentration for MR lung perfusion measurements: Assessment with computed tomography in a porcine model. *Eur Radiol*. 2008 Oct;18(10):2102–2107.

[85] Rajaram S, Swift AJ, Telfer A et al. 3d contrast-enhanced lung perfusion MRI is an effective screening tool for chronic thromboembolic pulmonary hypertension: Results from the aspire registry. *Thorax*. 2013;68(7):677–678.

[86] Remy-Jardin M, Louvegny S, Remy J, Artaud D, Deschildre F, Bauchart JJ, Thery C, Duhamel A. Acute central thromboembolic disease: Posttherapeutic follow-up with spiral ct angiography. *Radiology*. 1997;203:173–180.

[87] Remy-Jardin M, Remy J, Wattinne L, Giraud F. Central pulmonary thromboembolism: Diagnosis with spiral volumetric CT with the single-breath-hold technique–comparison with pulmonary angiography. *Radiology*. 1992;185:381–387.

[88] Renne J, Hinrichs J, Schonfeld C et al. Noninvasive quantification of airway inflammation following segmental allergen challenge with functional MR imaging: A proof of concept study. *Radiology*. 2015a;274:267–275.

[89] Renne J, Lauermann P, Hinrichs J et al. Clinical use of oxygen enhanced T1 mapping MRI of the lung: Reproducibility and impact of closed versus loose fit oxygen delivery system. *J MRI*. 2015b;41:60–66.

[90] Ribeiro A, Lindmarker P, Johnsson H, Juhlin-Dannfelt A, Jorfeldt L. Pulmonary embolism: One-year follow-up with echocardiography Doppler and five-year survival analysis. *Circulation*. 1999;99:1325–1330.

[91] Riedel M, Stanek V, Widimsky J, Prerovsky I. Longterm follow up of patients with pulmonary thromboembolism. Late prognosis and evolution of hemodynamic and respiratory data. *Chest*. 1982;81:151–158.

[92] Risse F, Kuder TA, Kauczor HU, Semmler W, Fink C. Suppression of pulmonary vasculature in lung perfusion MRI using correlation analysis. *Eur Radiol*. 2009;19:2569–2575.

[93] Risse F, Semmler W, Kauczor HU, Fink C. Dual-bolus approach to quantitative measurement of pulmonary perfusion by contrast-enhanced MRI. *J Magn Reson Imaging*. 2006 Dec;24(6):1284–1290.

[94] Rizi RR, Lipson DA, Dimitrov IE, Ishii M, Roberts DA. Operating characteristics of hyperpolarized 3He and arterial spin tagging in MR imaging of ventilation and perfusion in healthy subjects. *Acad Radiol*. 2003 May;10(5):502–508.

[95] Roeleveld RJ, Marcus JT, Faes TJ, Gan TJ, Boonstra A, Postmus PE, Vonk-Noordegraaf A. Interventricular septal configuration at MR imaging and pulmonary arterial pressure in pulmonary hypertension. *Radiology*. 2005;234:710–717.

[96] Saam BT, Yablonskiy DA, Kodibagkar VD et al. MR imaging of diffusion of 3He gas in healthy and diseased lungs. *Magn Reson Med*. 2000;44:174–179.

[97] Saba TS, Foster J, Cockburn M, Cowan M, Peacock AJ. Ventricular mass index using magnetic resonance imaging accurately estimates pulmonary artery pressure. *Eur Respir J*. 2002;20:1519–1524.

[98] Salerno M, Altes TA., Brookeman JR, de Lange EE, Mugler JP 3rd. Dynamic spiral MR imaging of pulmonary gas flow using hyperpolarized 3He: Preliminary studies in healthy and diseased lungs. *Magn Reson Med*. 2001;46:667–677.

[99] Salerno M, de Lange EE, Altes TA, Truwit JD, Brookeman JR, Mugler III JP. Emphysema: Hyperpolarized helium 3 diffusion MR imaging of the lungs compared with spirometric indexes-initial experience. *Radiology*. 2002;222:252–260.

[100] Samee S, Altes T, Powers P et al. Imaging the lungs in asthmatic patients by using hyperpolarized helium-3 magnetic resonance: Assessment of response to methocholine and exercise challenge. *J Allergy Clin Immunol*.

[101] Sandoval J, Bauerle O, Palomar A, Gomez A, Martinez-Guerra ML, Beltran M, Guerrero ML. Survival in primary pulmonary hypertension. Validation of a prognostic equation. *Circulation*. 1994;89:1733–1744.

[102] Sanz J, Kariisa M, Dellegrottaglie S, Prat-Gonzalez S, Garcia MJ, Fuster V, Rajagopalan S. Evaluation of pulmonary artery stiffness in pulmonary hypertension with cardiac magnetic resonance. *JACC Cardiovasc Imaging*. 2009;2:286–295.

[103] Sanz J, Kuschnir P, Rius T, Salguero R, Sulica R, Einstein AJ, Dellegrottaglie S, Fuster V, Rajagopalan S, Poon M. Pulmonary arterial hypertension: Noninvasive detection with phase-contrast MR imaging. *Radiology*. 2007;243:70–79.

[104] Schaefer JF, Vollmar J, Schick F et al. Solitary pulmonary nodules: Dynamic contrast-enhanced MR imaging– perfusion differences in malignant and benign lesions. *Radiology*. 2004;232:544–553.

[105] Sebastian L, Julia L-Z. Pulmonary perfusion imaging using MRI: Clinical application. *Insights Imaging*. Feb 2012;3(1):61–71.

[106] Sergiacomi G, Bolacchi F, Cadioli M et al. Combined pulmonary fibrosis and emphysema: 3D time-resolved MR angiographic evaluation of pulmonary arterial mean transit time and time to peak enhancement. *Radiology*. Feb 2010;254(2):601–608.

[107] Sergiacomi G, Sodani G, Fabiano S, Manenti G, Spinelli A, Konda D, Di Roma M, Schillaci O, Simonetti G. MRI lung perfusion 2D dynamic breath-hold technique in patients with severe emphysema. *In Vivo*. Jul–Aug 2003;17(4):319–324.

[108] Sitbon O, Humbert M, Nunes H, Parent F, Garcia G, Herve P, Rainisio M, Simonneau G. Long-term intravenous epoprostenol infusion in primary pulmonary hypertension: Prognostic factors and survival. *J Am Coll Cardiol*. 2002;40:780–788.

[109] Swift AJ, Rajaram S, Campbell MJ, Hurdman J, Thomas S, Capener D, Elliot C, Condliffe R, Wild JM, Kiely DG. Prognostic value of cardiovascular magnetic resonance imaging measurements corrected for age and sex in idiopathic pulmonary arterial hypertension. *Circ Cardiovas Imaging*. 2014a;7:100–106.

[110] Swift AJ, Wild JM, Nagle SK et al. Quantitative magnetic resonance imaging of pulmonary hypertension: A practical approach to the current state of the art. *J Thorac Imaging*. 2014b;29:68–79.

[111] Swift AJ, Woodhouse N, Fichele S, Siedel J, Mills GH, van Beek EJR, Wild JM. Rapid lung volumetry using ultrafast dynamic magnetic resonance imaging during forced vital capacity maneuver. Correlation with spirometry. *Invest Radiol*. 2007;42:37–41.

[112] Triphan SMF, Breuer FA, Gensler D, Kauczor HU, Jakob PM. Oxygen enhanced lung MRI by simultaneous measurement of $T1$ and $T2^*$ during free breathing using ultrashort TE. *J MRI*. Jul 7 2015;41(6):1708–1714.

[113] Tsai IC, Tsai WL, Wang KY et al. Comprehensive MDCT evaluation of patients with pulmonary hypertension: Diagnosing underlying causes with the updated Dana Point 2008 classification. *Amer J Roentgenol*. 2011;197:W471–W481.

[114] Van Beek EJR, Dahmen AM, Stavngaard T et al. Comparison of hyperpolarised 3-He MRI and HRCT in normal volunteers, patients with COPD and patients with alpha-1-antitrypsin deficiency—PHIL trial. *Eur Resp J*. 2009;34:1–11.

[115] Van Beek EJR, Wild JM, Kauczor HU, Schreiber W, Mugler JP 3rd, De Lange EE. Functional MRI of the lung using hyperpolarized 3-Helium gas. *J MRI*. 2004;20:540–554.

[116] van Wolferen SA, Marcus JT, Boonstra A, Marques KM, Bronzwaer JG, Spreeuwenberg MD, Postmus PE, Vonk-Noordegraaf A. Prognostic value of right ventricular mass, volume, and function in idiopathic pulmonary arterial hypertension. *Eur Heart J*. 2007;28:1250–1257.

[117] Voorhees A, An J, Berger KI et al. Magnetic resonance imaging-based spirometry for regional assessment of pulmonary function. *Magn Reson Med*. 2005;54:1146–1154.

[118] Wartski M, Collignon MA. Incomplete recovery of lung perfusion after 3 months in patients with acute pulmonary embolism treated with antithrombotic agents. Thesee study group. Tinzaparin ou heparin standard: Evaluation dans l'embolie pulmonaire study. *J Nucl Med*. 2000;41:1043–1048.

[119] Wieben O, Francois C, Reeder SB. Cardiac MRI of ischemic heart disease at 3 t: Potential and challenges. *Eur J Radiol*. 2008;65:15–28.

[120] Wielpütz M, Kauczor HU. MRI of the lung: State of the art. *Diagn Interv Radiol*. 2012 Jul–Aug;18(4):344–353.

[121] Wild JM, Fichele S, Woodhouse N, Paley MNJ, Kasuboski L, van Beek EJR. 3D Volume-localized pO2 measurement in the human lung with 3He MRI. *Magn Reson Med*. 2005;53:1055–1064.

[122] Wild JM, Marshall H, Bock M, Schad LR, Jakob PM, Puderbach M, Molinari F, Van Beek EJ, Biederer J. MRI of the lung (1/3): Methods. *Insights Imaging*. 2012 Aug;3(4):345–353.

[123] Wild JM, Paley MNJ, Kasuboski L et al. Dynamic radial projection MRI of inhaled hyperpolarized 3He. *Magn Reson Med*. 2003;49:991–997.

[124] Wittram C, Kalra MK, Maher MM, Greenfield A, McLoud TC, Shepard JA. Acute and chronic pulmonary emboli: Angiography-CT correlation. *AJR Am J Roentgenol*. 2006;186:S421–S429.

[125] Woodhouse N, Wild JM, van Beek EJR et al. Hyperpolarized 3He-MRI for the evaluation of CF therapies. *J MRI* 2009;30:981–988.

[126] Wright RD. The blood supply of abnormal tissues in the

lungs. *J Pathol Bacteriol*. 1938;47:489–499.

[127] Yi CA, Lee KS, Han J, Chung MP, Chung MJ, Shin KM. 3-T MRI for differentiating inflammation and fibrosis predominant lesions of usual and nonspecific interstitial pneumonia: Comparison study with pathologic correla tion. *AJR Am J Roentgenol*. 2008;190(4):878–885.

[128] Zou Y, Zhang M, Wang Q, Shang D, Wang L, Yu G. Quantitative investigation of solitary pulmonary nodules: Dynamic contrast-enhanced MRI and histopathologic analysis. *AJR*. 2008;191:252–259.

Chapter 14
乳腺 MRI

Breast MRI

Diana L. Lam，Habib Rahbar 著

王 磊 郑福玲 译

隋 昕 校

目录　CONTENTS

一、乳腺 MRI 的检查适应证 / 276

二、技术研究 / 282

三、常见伪影 / 286

四、正常乳腺的 MRI 解剖 / 286

五、乳腺 MR 报告及释义 / 287

六、乳腺 MRI 良性发现 / 306

七、乳腺 MRI 恶性征象 / 312

八、乳腺 MRI 上的高危病变 / 317

九、硅胶乳房植入假体的评价 / 317

十、MRI 上可疑病变的组织病理学取样 / 320

十一、总结 / 322

在20世纪70年代早期，MRI首次被提出作为一种用来检测癌症的影像方法[1]。随后，人们发现在体外纵向弛豫时间（T_1）和横向弛豫时间（T_2）可以分辨正常乳腺组织和异常乳腺组织的组织差异[2]。80年代早期，用MRI成功地在切除的乳腺标本中辨别出了乳腺癌，随后第一篇研究人体正常乳腺组织和异常乳腺组织鉴别特征的报道出现了[3,4]。直到证明单独应用钆造影剂增强扫描MRI就能可靠地发现乳腺癌后，乳腺MRI才成为一种检测乳腺恶性肿瘤可靠的临床工具[5]。确定乳腺MRI的最佳临床适应证后，人们创建了一个标准化的报告系统（即美国放射学会乳腺成像报告和数据系统，BI-RADS），建立了更加统一的跨领域技术方法。乳腺MRI被广泛认为是检测乳腺癌最敏感的影像检查，也是评估病变范围最精准的成像方式[6]。

一、乳腺MRI的检查适应证

乳腺MRI检查主要有六种适应证，总结如下。

（一）筛查

近些年，美国癌症协会建议那些终身罹患乳腺癌概率>20%的妇女，进行过年度乳腺X线检查后要使用MRI进行补充筛查，其中包括有明确乳腺或卵巢癌家族史、10—30岁间有胸部放射治疗史、BRCA基因突变携带者（或未做过检测的一级亲属）、患有遗传综合征（或未做过检测的一级亲属）的这些会有较高的患乳腺癌的风险的妇女（表14-1）[7]。虽然乳腺MRI对乳腺癌检测的敏感性比当前其他任何成像方式都高（图14-1），但它的特异性还是稍低。假阳性的存在以及患者对乳腺MRI检查相对于乳腺X线的高昂费用的担心影响了乳腺MRI在一般人群筛查中的应用。然而，越来越多的证据支持MRI在中度风险人群中的应用（终身罹患乳腺癌概率为15%～20%），这其中包括了曾患乳腺癌的病史或诊断有高危病变的患者，如小叶瘤样病变，这些都与增加患乳腺癌风险是相关的[8-11]。

（二）新发乳腺癌患者的评估

目前，美国国家综合癌症网络（National Comprehensive Cancer Network，NCN）实践指南建议新发乳腺癌患者用乳腺MRI来评估患侧乳腺的病变范围以及筛查对侧乳腺[12]。在临床应用中，乳腺MRI还有多种潜在的应用价值。首先，MRI提供了最精确的病变范围的影像学评估，这使得临床医师能够更自信地评价单侧乳房中有无多灶性病变（发于乳腺单个象限内的多个病变）或多中心（多象限）病变（图14-2和图14-3）[6]。在一份已发表的综述中，10%～34%的患者在术前的乳腺MRI检查中会发现在临床及乳腺X线中漏诊的同侧乳腺内的病变（图14-4）[13]。此外，乳腺MRI还可以帮助评估病变对周围组织的累及程度，包括胸肌、胸壁（包括肋骨和肋间肌肉）以及邻近的皮肤（图14-5和图14-6）。乳腺MRI也可评估腋窝和乳房内的可疑淋巴结转移，这

表14-1 根据2007年美国癌症协会指南需每年进行乳房MRI检查的适应证

每年必须进行乳腺MRI筛查的适应证	非每年必须进行乳腺MRI筛查情形
• BRCA基因突变携带者未做过基因检测的一级亲属* • BRCA基因突变（BRCA1或BRCA2）* • 家族史阳性者依据BRCAPRO或其他易感基因模型检测患病风险>20%* • 10—30岁有过胸部放射治疗史 • Li-Fraumeni综合征及其一级亲属 • Cowden综合征和Bannayan–Riley–Ruvalcaba综合征及其一级亲属	• 家族史阳性者依据BRCAPRO或其他易感基因模型检测患病风险<15%～20% • 小叶原位癌（lobular carcinoma in-situ，LCIS）或非典型小叶增生（atypical lobular hyperplasia，ALH） • 非典型导管增生（atypical ductal hyperplasia，ADH） • 乳腺钼靶X线检查可见，乳腺异质致密或密度极高 • 有乳腺癌史的妇女，包括导管内原位癌（ductal carcinoma in situ，DCIS）

*. 基于非随机临床试验和观察性研究的结果

Chapter 14 乳腺 MRI
Breast MRI

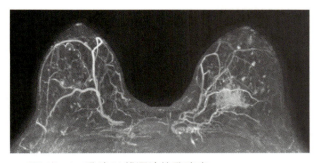

▲ 图 14-1 乳腺 X 线漏诊的乳腺癌

48 岁女性，有 20% 的终身患乳腺癌风险，右乳部分切除活检显示原位小叶癌。增强扫描横轴位最大密度投影显示在左侧乳房内上象限有边缘带毛刺的不规则肿块，病理示浸润性小叶癌

有助于术前在超声引导下的对可疑淋巴结穿刺活检（图 14-7）[14]。最后，乳腺 MRI 常常发现被临床及乳腺 X 线漏诊的新发乳腺癌患者对侧乳腺内的乳腺癌。一个大型多中心试验表明，被 MRI 发现的被临床和乳腺 X 线漏诊的同侧或对侧乳腺的乳腺癌占新诊断为乳腺癌妇女的 3%（图 14-8）[12]。虽然还没有大型试验来评估乳腺 MRI 对实施了保乳手术的患者的长期影响，例如切缘阳性、复发率和死亡率[13]，但已有证据表明接受过保乳手术的早期乳腺癌患者，如果术前做过乳

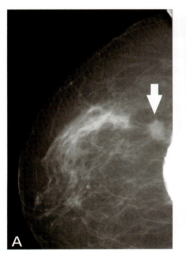 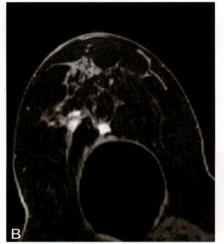 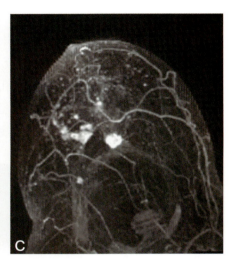

▲ 图 14-2 多灶病变

患浸润性导管癌的 61 岁女性。MRI 用来观察病变范围。乳腺 X 线在乳腺后部见一边缘有毛刺的不规则肿块（A，箭）。增强扫描横轴位 T_1 脂肪抑制序列（B）及最大密度投影（C）显示在一个象限有多个相似表现的不规则肿块。病理显示为多发浸润性导管癌

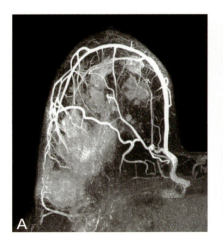 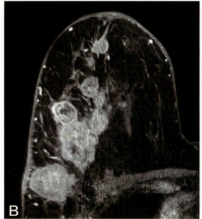 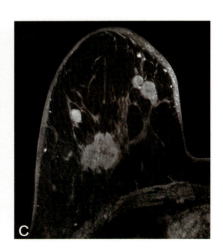

▲ 图 14-3 多中心病变

61 岁女性患者，新近诊断为浸润性导管癌。用 MRI 来确定在已知肿瘤区域（未显示）内非肿块样强化的范围。横轴位最大密度投影（A）及增强横轴 W 位 T_1 加权图像（B、C）显示不同层面在不同象限有多个病灶，与多中心病变相一致

腺 MRI 检查，那么其比未做过检查的患者的再切除率要降低[15]。

（三）解决临床或影像检查中的可疑发现

使用 MRI 来进一步对临床或影像学上的可疑发现进行评估至今仍存在争议。乳腺 MRI 的应用有时被称为"解决问题"，但目前还没有得到很好的文献支持[13]。乳腺 MRI 检查有较高的准确性及安全性[16]，可以减少乳腺 X 线检查导致的不必要的活检，包括相对价格较低的图像引导下的穿刺活检。另外乳腺 MRI 检查还对减少 Bi-RADS 提示的可疑病变的活检有高阴性预测值（约98%）[13]，只是高昂的价格是其广泛应用的障碍。最近的研究表明，在有任何可疑的乳腺 X 线或临床发现的情况下，MRI 对该临床指征的阴性预测值范围为 76%[17]，对评估乳腺 X 线上有可疑乳

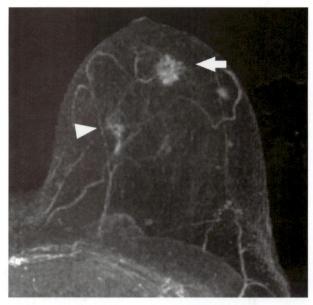

▲ 图 14-4 乳腺 X 线漏诊的同侧乳腺内病变

52 岁女性患者，触诊发现左乳浸润性导管癌，乳腺 X 线未能发现。横轴位最大密度投影显示活检证实的浸润性导管癌在 12 点钟位置（白箭）。在肿瘤后内侧的非肿块样强化区为低级别导管原位癌（箭头）

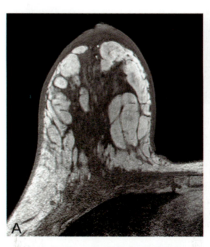
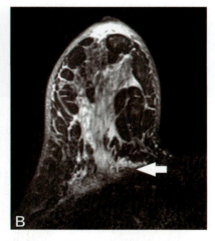
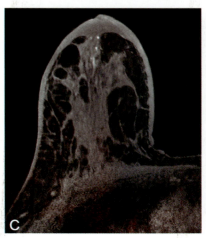
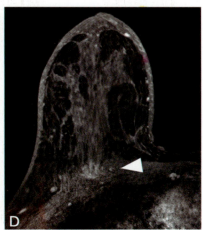

◀ 图 14-5 胸肌受侵

64 岁女性患者，右侧乳腺癌治疗后，右侧乳癌复发侵犯右侧胸肌。平扫轴位 T_1 加权（A），T_2 加权 SPAIR（B），T_1 加权压脂像（C），增强 T_1 加权压脂像（D）显示胸肌强化（箭），其与胸肌受累相符。需注意的是弥漫增厚的皮肤与之前有过放射治疗相关

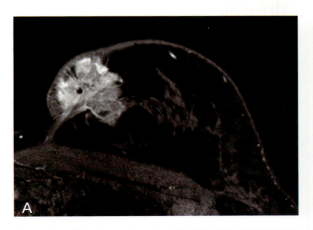
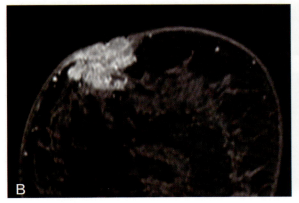
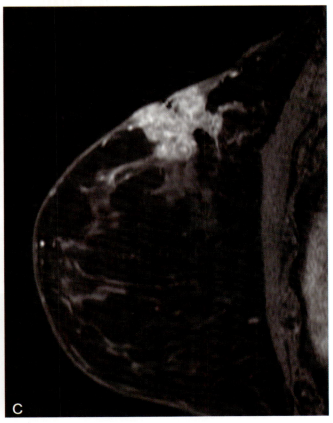

▲ 图 14-6 皮肤受累

31 岁女性患者，新诊断复发性左乳腺浸润性导管癌。MRI 行病情评估，增强轴位（A），冠状位（B），矢状位（C）T_1 加权脂肪抑制序列图像示在先前肿块切除术区前 11 点钟方向一不规则肿块，其边缘有毛刺并累及相邻皮肤

腺钙化的病灶阴性预测值可达 85%[18]。笔者的研究发现，乳腺 MRI 对这种临床表现具有高度的敏感性和高阴性预测价值，但能比其他的检查多发现的乳腺癌数量还是太少，所以还无法常规推荐乳腺 MRI[19]。有趣的是，在这一组病例中有 2/3 的乳腺癌都是存在可疑乳头溢液并且乳腺 X 线检查和超声检查结果为阴性（图 14-9），因而在这种特殊的临床表现中，乳腺 MRI 的作用也正在被积极研究[20]。

（四）原发灶不明的转移性腋窝腺癌患者的评估

虽然临床上发生没有明确的原发灶的腋窝淋巴结转移性腺癌是非常少见的，但是这些转移经常发生在同侧乳腺患有乳腺癌的女性身上（图 14-10）。对所有可利用的研究做完 Meta 分析后表明，乳腺 MRI 可以识别大约 61% 临床和乳腺 X 线检查没有异常发现而仅表现为腋窝转移性淋巴结肿大的隐匿癌患者[13]。

（五）乳腺癌新辅助化疗疗效评价

在美国乳腺癌大肠癌外科辅助治疗计划组织 B-18 项目中（NSABP B-18），进行了在可手术的乳腺癌患者中进行术前（新辅助）和术后（辅助）化疗的比较研究。在两组患者中总的生存率和无病生存率均无统计学意义。然而，在新辅助化疗组中更多的患者能够成功地进行保乳手术，而不是乳房切除术。此外，原发肿瘤对化疗的反应在术前进行了临床评估，以及新辅助化疗对患者预后的影响（取决于手术切除范围的大小）。这让我们有兴趣研究使用 MRI 以改善对治疗早期反应的评估和手术前对疾病范围的

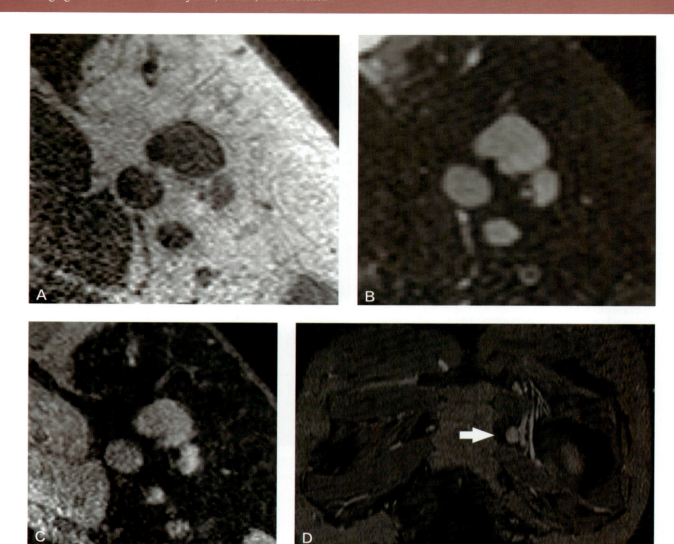

▲ 图 14-7 异常淋巴结的鉴别

27 岁女性，诊断为浸润性导管癌。平扫横轴位 T_1 加权像（A），T_2 加权像 SPAIR（B），增强 T_1 加权压脂像（C）图像示 I 级腋窝淋巴结，其外观呈圆形，伴脂肪门消失。增强冠状位 T_1 加权压脂像（D）示异常增大的内乳淋巴结（白箭），怀疑转移可能

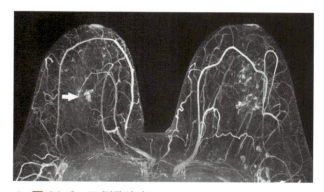

▲ 图 14-8 双侧乳腺癌

67 岁女性，被诊断为右侧乳腺癌。横轴位最大密度投影示右乳一边缘伴有毛刺的不规则肿块（白箭）。左侧乳房见不对称点状非肿块样强化，活检证实为导管内原位癌

治疗评估[21,22]。初步研究发现用 MRI 观察早期治疗反应，MRI 检测到的病灶大小或体积以及增强动力曲线的变化与治疗反应是相关的[23,24]，这也证明对于那些对肿瘤治疗反应较差的女性，MRI 可以帮助调整新辅助化疗方案（图 14-11 和图 14-12）。其他单中心研究还表明，在新辅助化疗治疗后，在对残存病变的评估中，MRI 检查是优于乳腺触诊、乳腺 X 线及超声检查的[25,26]，但是不能依此而证明残存病灶消失了[25]。由美国放射影像网络协会（ACRIN 6657）发起的多地点试验的最新结果证实，MRI 影像发现比临床

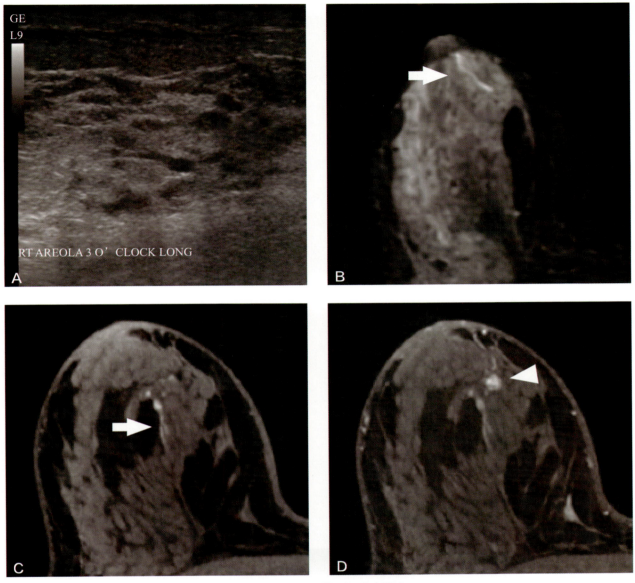

▲ 图 14-9 评估可疑乳头溢液

46 岁女性患者，乳头自发性溢出血性分泌物。乳腺 X 线（未显示）及超声检查均未见异常（A），遂行双侧乳腺 MRI 检查。横轴位 T_2 加权 SPAIR（B）和 T_1 加权压脂像（C）平扫图像显示导管扩张呈高信号（白箭），这与扩张的导管内含有液体及组织残骸是相符的。增强 T_1 加权压脂像（D）图像显示一圆形的导管内肿块，边缘清晰，强化不均匀（箭头）。病理显示导管内乳头状瘤伴导管增生

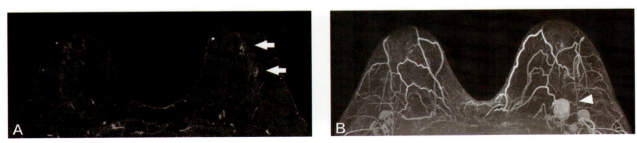

▲ 图 14-10 原发灶不明的腋窝淋巴结转移癌

63 岁女性患者，腋窝淋巴结转移癌合并不明的乳腺原发恶性肿瘤。A.MRI 横轴位增强减影图示左乳外上象限内不连续的非肿块样强化病灶（白箭）；B. 横轴位最大密度投影图像显示左腋窝多个肿大淋巴结（箭头）。病理为浸润性小叶癌

评估更能预测病灶对新辅助化疗的病理反应[27]。其他 ACRIN 赞助的研究正在进行中，研究如弥散加权成像（diffusion weighted image，DWI）和波谱（magnetic resonance spectrum，MRS）等先进的 MRI 技术，以进一步提高 MRI 在评估对新辅助治疗早期反应中的能力。

（六）硅胶植入物完整性评价

自 2006 年以来，隆胸术是美国每年最多的整形外科手术。植入物可由单腔或双腔组成，其内包含生理盐水、硅胶或者两者兼而有之。植入术后的并发症是非常常见的，超过一半的患者在植入的 12 年内发生硅胶植入物破裂[28]。因为通常生理盐水可以在 5～14d 内被身体重新吸收，这造成了乳房体积明显缩小，所以盐水植入物出现并发症在临床检查中很容易确诊[29]。因此，通常不会对盐水植入物的完整性进行影像学检查。然而，对含有硅胶的植入物完整性的评估在临床检查中很困难。尽管当在纤维囊外和乳腺实质内见到高密度的有机硅材料时，乳腺 X 线可以显示硅胶植入物破裂的征象，但乳腺 X 线对检测硅胶植入物破裂的灵敏度还是较低（11%～69%），尤其是当出现囊内破裂的情况[13]。MRI 已经被证明是检测硅胶植入物并发症最敏感（6%～98%）的影像学检查，而且还具有良好的特异性（55%～92%）[30-34]。另外，当出现临床特征不明显的硅胶植入物破裂时，乳腺 MRI 是检查的首选方法。

二、技术研究

虽然在各个医院之间乳腺 MRI 检查序列有所不同，但是高质量的 MRI 都有一些共同的基本技术原则。这些包括包覆足够范围的乳房和腋窝，有足够的空间和时间分辨率以及防止和最小化伪影的方法，这样才能充分显示出病变的特征。

（一）检查体位及注意事项

乳腺 MRI 采集时患者应该俯卧位，这样会使得患者的乳房位于乳腺线圈合适的位置中[35]，另外这样的体位还可以减少心脏和呼吸的运动干扰，同时这样也有助于延展乳房以便乳房组织尽量覆盖于线圈内。要尽量缩短扫描时间以及在动态增强扫描（dynamic contrast enhanced，DCE）开始之前给予患者清晰的指令也是同样重要的，这样才可以限制患者在扫描时的呼吸运动。

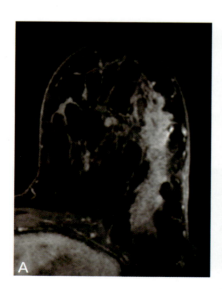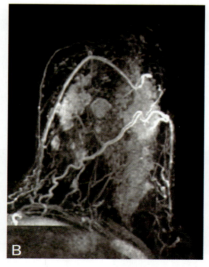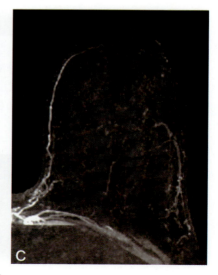

▲ 图 14-11　肿瘤对新辅助化疗的反应

39 岁女性患者，多点活检证实浸润性导管癌。A. 增强横轴位 T_1 加权压脂像显示非肿块样强化（NME）沿乳房外侧分布；B. 横轴位最大密度投影显示病变为多中心病变；C. 患者接受了新辅助化疗后，在横轴位最大密度投影图像上显示多个肿块和 NME 完全消失，这与病变对新辅助化疗反应良好是相符的

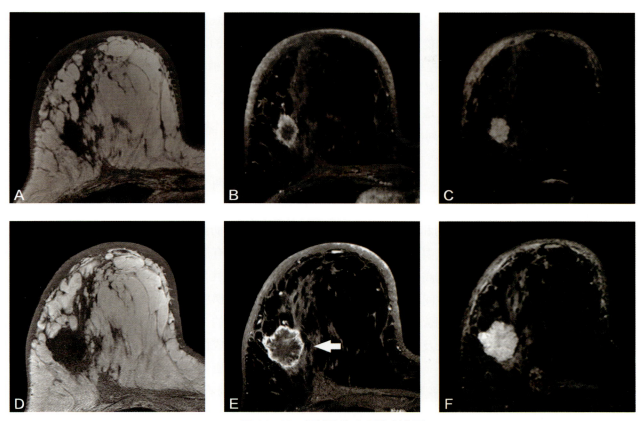

▲ 图 14-12 新辅助化疗后肿瘤进展

51 岁女性患者，患有浸润性导管癌和炎性乳腺癌接受新辅助化疗。在新辅助化疗前、后分别行乳腺 MRI 检查以评估治疗反应。横轴位（A、D），增强加权压脂像（B、E），T_2 加权 SPAIR 像（C、F）图像显示边缘不规则的不规则形肿块增大，边缘强化（白箭）伴中央坏死，坏死区在 T_2 加权图像上呈高信号。弥漫性皮肤增厚和强化与炎性乳腺癌的临床表现相一致

（二）采集双侧乳腺影像

因为乳腺 MRI 采集双侧乳腺影像在技术上和临床上都有明显的优点，所以几乎所有的临床适应证都推荐使用这种检查。首先，采集双乳影像可以在相位编码梯度平面尽量避免卷褶伪影，并且在左右方向上还能尽量减小心脏运动对图像的影响[36]。其次，采集双侧乳腺影像可以对乳腺和腋窝同时评估，这就对于乳癌高危的妇女筛查或新诊断乳腺癌患者的病情评估显得尤为重要[37]。此外，同传统乳腺 X 线一样，对双乳影像进行对称性观察能够提高诊断的准确性[38]。例如，可以利用对称性建立背景实质强化（background parenchymal enhancement，BPE；下文会详述这种正常生理学现象）的形式和程度，并可以识别与 BPE 不同的特殊可疑强化区域。最后，采集双侧乳腺影像可以帮助诊断双侧、多发性的良性肿瘤，如乳腺内淋巴结和纤维腺瘤。

（三）线圈

乳腺 MRI 必须使用专门的乳腺表面线圈，因为体线圈提供的信号不够强，无法对乳房进行最优的成像。最理想的方法是使用带大量线圈元件的乳腺线圈（目前有 7～32 个同步射频通道），以便使用并行成像。并行成像对于乳腺显像来说是非常有效的[39]，并有助于减少扫描时间或提高空间分辨率。

（四）造影剂

虽然如 DWI 和 MR 波谱等一些非对比技术正在被研究用于乳腺癌检测，但是目前临床上乳腺 MRI 仍需要用钆造影剂来检测或评估乳腺癌。通常，钆对比剂是按 0.1mg/kg 的剂量加

20ml 的盐水用高压注射器以大约 2ml/s 的速度进行注射，这样就确保了对比剂能迅速到达体内的血管内，并且在整个检查过程中保持强化的一致。然而，需要注意的是注射钆对比剂会导致 T_2 和 T_2^* 弛豫时间减少，所以在造影剂注射前应该首先采集对液体敏感的成像序列，比如 T_2 加权序列[40]。

（五）空间和时间分辨率

在乳腺 MRI 扫描中，高空间和时间分辨率对病变的识别和描述来说是至关重要的。然而，两者在技术上是需要平衡的，实现高空间分辨率就需要较长的成像时间，从而在时间分辨率上就需要权衡了。因此，一个最好的乳腺 MRI 检查就需要了解这些错综复杂的技术要求及其对临床工作的意义。

在作者的观点中，对于大多数的临床目的来说，乳腺 MRI 应该强调空间分辨率而不是时间分辨率。这是由于高空间分辨率能最大化地展现解剖细节，使得放射科医师能够更好评估病变的形态特征以及病变可能累及的乳头-乳晕复合体、皮肤和胸壁。一般来说，形态学特征比对时间分辨率要求高的动态增强特性具有更大的诊断价值[18]。为了观察一些最特殊的 MRI 形态细节，比如毛刺征（通常是恶性的）或病灶内部低信号隔膜影（通常是良性的），要求在平面像素尺寸空间分辨率不大于 1mm。

时间分辨率，或动态增强扫描的速度，决定了动态增强信息的成像采样点。通常情况下，浸润性乳腺癌表现为增强早期的快速强化和延时后强化消退。先前的研究已经证明，这种最初的快速强化发生在注射造影剂之后的 60~120s 内[41]。尽管乳腺癌表现出早期快速强化和延时强化消退的现象可能比良性的乳房病变更常见，但是乳腺的良恶性病变的增强动力曲线还是存在大量重叠[42]。高时间分辨率技术已经展现出可以提供高质量药物动力学信息，这可能被证明对了解疾病特征及监测治疗反应具有很高的价值[43,44]，但是这种技术常规应用在临床实践中的话还是需要进行额外研究的。近来出现的耦合技术是一种采用新的 K 空间抽样的方法，它可以在获得高时间分辨率图像之后立刻得到高空间分辨率的图像。

（六）关键脉冲序列与重建的图像

乳腺 MRI 检查的基本序列包括含有平扫、增强早期及至少两个延时期的 T_1 加权动态增强扫描序列，以及平扫的液体敏感序列。如果动态增强扫描用主动脂肪抑制技术的话，应该在平扫的时候先做一个没有脂肪抑制 T_1 加权序列，这样能有效地确认脂肪性坏死和内乳淋巴结等良性病变中的脂肪含量。梯度回波（gradient echo，GRE）序列应用于检查的 T_1 加权部分，以便以可接受的速度实现高质量成像。为了避免任何类 T_2 加权效应或条纹伪影，应该尽量不使用 GRE 脉冲序列[45]。由于 GRE 序列不能提供真正的 T_2 加权图像[45]，平扫液体敏感序列需要使用自旋回波、快速自旋回波或短时反转恢复（short time inversion recovery，STIR）技术。

有用的重建图像包括轴位减影序列（增强动态强化图像减掉增强前的平扫图像），重建后的最大密度投影（MIP）图像，以及用原来增强序列图像重建的垂直平面图像（矢状面和冠状面）。

（七）脂肪抑制：饱和与减影

因为乳腺内的强化病变可以被与脂肪相关的高信号所掩盖，因此使用脂肪抑制技术是非常重要的，这样可以避免脂肪对诊断乳腺内病变的干扰。脂肪抑制可以通过脂肪饱和技术在图像采集过程中实现，也可以通过减影技术在后处理时来消除脂肪（与其他的平扫的 T_1 加权信号）[36]。

脂肪饱和，也称为主动脂肪抑制，通常是通过施加额外的射频脉冲来消除脂肪或通过选择性激发水信号来实现的[46]。与减影技术相比，脂肪饱和技术的主要缺点是图像数据采集时间较长，因此，一般应用在空间分辨率比时间分辨率更重要的技术中。此外，要获得成功的脂肪抑

Chapter 14 乳腺 MRI
Breast MRI

制图像，需要在整个视野范围内有均匀的磁场（B_0）（图 14-13）[46]。因为在较高场强下脂肪和水的谱峰有更大的分布，在 3T 等高 B_0 场强下，脂肪抑制技术才可能更有效 [47]。

减影技术从增强 T_1 加权序列采集的数据中减去平扫 T_1 加权序列采集的数据，这样就消除了 T_1 加权像中没有强化的呈高信号的脂肪和其他结构。然而，仅仅依赖这种方法来抑制脂肪的话会有明显的缺点，因为患者在扫描过程中如果有轻微的移动就可以产生运动伪影甚至出现可疑强化。特别是，在强调空间分辨率的扫描序列中，这个问题就显得更严重了，因此，推荐在优先考虑时间分辨率的扫描序列中采用这个技术。

作者倾向于脂肪饱和和减影技术结合使用，这样通过叠加平扫 T_1 高信号与增强图像来消除令人混淆组织结构，以便让放射科阅片医师能快速评估减影图像的强化区域，同时也允许医师对照脂肪饱和动态增强图像来分辨出减影扫描序列中患者运动产生的需要注意的"伪增强"伪影（图 14-14）。

（八）磁场强度（B_0）与均匀性

乳腺磁共振的信噪比（signal-to-noise ratio，SNR）需要最大化才能满足其对时空分辨率的要求。理论上，SNR 与 B_0 强度成正比，因此，不推荐较低磁场强度（小于 1～1.5T）的核磁机用于乳腺成像 [46]。更高的场强也改善了两乳区域的 B_0 均匀性，这样可以使脂肪饱和度更稳定 [35,36]。磁场不均匀也会导致信号丢失，比如在空气 - 软组织界面（图 14-15）。乳腺磁共振检查越来越多地应用于 3T 场强，其能提供更高的 SNR，并可以转化为更高的空间分辨率改善脂肪抑制。然而，值得注意的是，迄今为止很少有公开的数据支持在大于 1.5T 场强的 3T 场强下进行乳腺 MRI 检查有明确的临床效益，只有一项已发表的研究表明，与 1.5T 场强相比，在 3T 场强下检查提高了诊断准确率 [48]。

（九）相位编码梯度

由于乳腺与心脏和肺相对较近，运动伪影可能对乳腺的成像产生影响。因此，应该选择应用相位编码梯度方向，以使运动伪影产生的影响达到最小。对于双乳轴位成像，相位梯度应该在左 - 右方向上，以防止心脏和呼吸运动伪影传导到乳腺。同样，当进行冠状或矢状位图像采集时，相位编码梯度应该在上下方向。

（十）评估硅胶假体的技术要求

很多平扫序列可用在对于硅胶假体完整性的评估上。在作者的经验中，最有用的序列是使用 silicone-only 技术，其采集的图像中脂肪和水的信号都是低信号，这样评估假体囊内和囊外破裂就有很高的敏感度。和其他乳腺磁共振成像序列

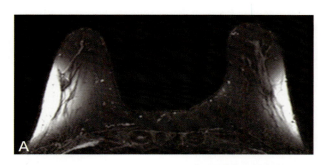
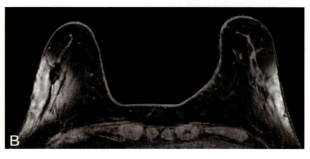
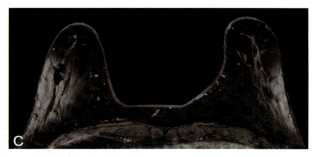

▲ 图 14-13　压脂不完全
35 岁女性，行 MRI 高危筛查。横轴位 T_2 SPAIR 序列（A）、平扫（B）、增强 T_1（C）压脂像示由于磁场（B_0）的不均匀，乳房两侧的脂肪饱和度较低

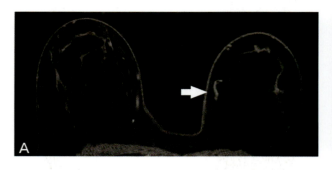
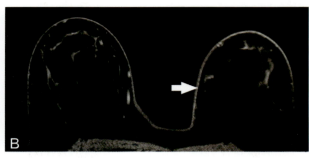
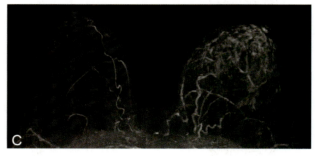

▲ 图 14-14 在减影技术中，扫描中患者的运动产生的伪增强

58 岁女性，行 MRI 高危筛查。在平扫（A）和增强（B）轴位 T_1 加权的脂肪饱和图像中，相同的层面（白箭）图像比较下，从纤维腺体组织的差异可以看出，左乳有明显的运动。这造成了在减影的最大密度投影图像（C）上看到的右侧乳房和左侧乳房背景实质强化不对称的错觉

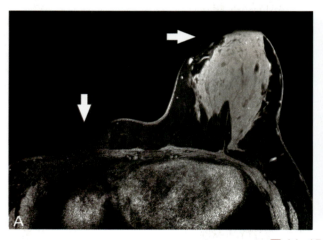
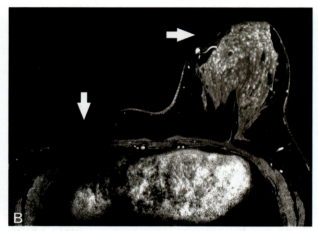

▲ 图 14-15 磁场不均匀

33 岁女性，右乳导管内原位癌乳腺切除术后。行 MRI 高危筛查。平扫（A）及增强（B）轴位 T_1 加权脂肪抑制图像显示右前胸壁及左前部乳（白箭）附件信号缺失，这是由于磁场（B_0）不均匀产生的伪影

一样，这项研究采用患者俯卧位。因为硅胶破裂在 MRI 图像上可能只有微小的表现，所以这项检查最好在高场强（至少 1T）的机器上进行。

三、常见伪影

在磁检查中有许多常见的伪影，其中一些可能与病理学改变相仿，所以在阅片时要注意这种情况。对于伪影的详细讨论超出了本章的范围，然而，正如上面提到的，要认识这些伪影

是非常重要的，特别是运动伪影、不均匀脂肪抑制、磁化率伪影和幻影伪影（图 14-15 至图 14-20）。

四、正常乳腺的 MRI 解剖

成年女性乳房由三个主要部分组成：皮肤、皮下组织和乳腺组织[49]。乳房的外上象限包含了乳腺组织中最大的部分，它是由包括腺泡和导管的功能结构（实质）以及由脂肪、结缔组织、血管、神经和淋巴管构成的支撑结构（间质）组成的。网状

结构的 Cooper 韧带连接着浅筋膜来支撑着乳房。乳房的皮肤很薄（在 MRI 图像上不到 3mm），含有毛囊、皮脂腺和汗腺。乳头通常有 5～9 个导管开口，周围乳晕内有蒙氏结节，它代表了蒙哥马利腺导管开口。淋巴管分布在皮下组织和乳腺间质内，大部分淋巴液回流到腋窝淋巴结（97%），余下的淋巴液流向内乳淋巴链。乳房内淋巴结的数目分布不均，其中大部分位于乳房的外上象限。腋窝淋巴结解剖分区以胸小肌为基础划分：Ⅰ区淋巴结位于胸小肌外侧缘外侧，Ⅱ区淋巴结是位于胸小肌体部后方间隙，Ⅲ区淋巴结位于胸小肌内侧缘内侧（图 14-21 和图 14-22）。乳房的大部分血液供应来自内乳动脉和发自腋动脉的胸外侧动脉。这些血管在增强图像上显示得很明显，尤其是在 MIP 图像上。

乳腺 MRI 正常具有代表性的图像及相关的解剖展示在图 14-23 上。在无脂肪饱和的平扫 T_1 加权图像上，乳腺（纤维腺体）组织、淋巴结、肌肉和皮肤显示为中等信号强度，这样可以很容易地与含有较高信号强度的脂肪组织区分开来。在乳房实质内的导管导致了乳头 - 乳晕复合体内可能含有包括脂肪和蛋白质在内的液体，因此，其在 T_1 和（或）T_2 加权图像上可能表现为高信号。在平扫 T_2 加权图像中，纤维腺体组织（fibrograndular tissue，FGT）通常具有比肌肉组织更高的信号强度，但比邻近的皮下血管的信号强度要低。在增强的图像中，正常乳腺组织强化程度是可变的，这被称为背景实质强化（BPE）。乳头 - 乳晕复合体由于有丰富的血管，通常在增强图像上强化明显（图 14-24 和图 14-25）其他强化的正常结构还包括血管和乳头 - 乳晕复合体。正常皮肤和脂肪不强化。

动态增强曲线（下文将详细描述）与动态增强技术也可以帮助区分乳腺 MRI 中的正常组织和异常组织。一般来说，纤维腺体组织（FGT）在增强早期有轻度缓慢强化，而肌肉组织则在早期具有轻度快速强化。乳腺恶性肿瘤一般比周围正常的乳腺实质具有更明显的强化，通常表现为独特的动力学增强曲线，下面将更详细地描述。

五、乳腺 MR 报告及释义

美国放射学会（American College of Radiology, ACR）乳腺影像报告和数据系统（BI-RADS）[50]中有关 MRI 的进展，有助于规范报告和解释，提高放射科医师和不同机构间建议的一致性。如乳腺 X 线和超声，结合 BI-RADS 标准用一致的方法来解释 MRI 发现是必不可少的，从而提供给临床医师准确、有针对性的与临床相关的乳腺 MRI 报告和建议[51]。框 14-1 概述了作者建议的逐一解释乳腺 MRI 的方法。

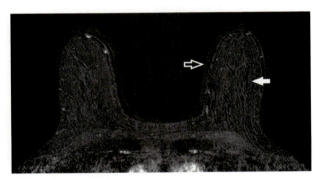

▲ 图 14-16 层间运动伪影

60 岁女性，行高危乳腺筛查 MRI。轴位增强压脂序列显示信号多个线样信号缺失区域（白箭），在乳房外也可以看到信号（黑箭）。这表示在平扫和增强 T_1 加权图像之间由于运动导致了减法图像上发生了重叠错误。这有可能会掩盖病变或模拟线样导管增强。除了可以最大限度地提高患者的舒适性和得到清晰的图像，检查时对乳房施以的较小压力可以避免检查时乳房的运动（例如浅呼吸）

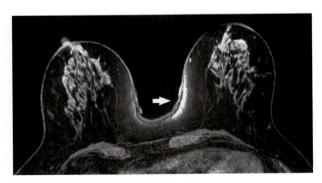

▲ 图 14-17 脂肪饱和不完全

71 岁女性，行高危乳腺筛查 MRI。平扫脂肪饱和 T_1 加权图像示在乳房内侧出现脂肪饱和不完全（白箭）。这种现象在乳腺边缘特别常见，不应该被错误地认为是皮肤增厚或皮肤的强化

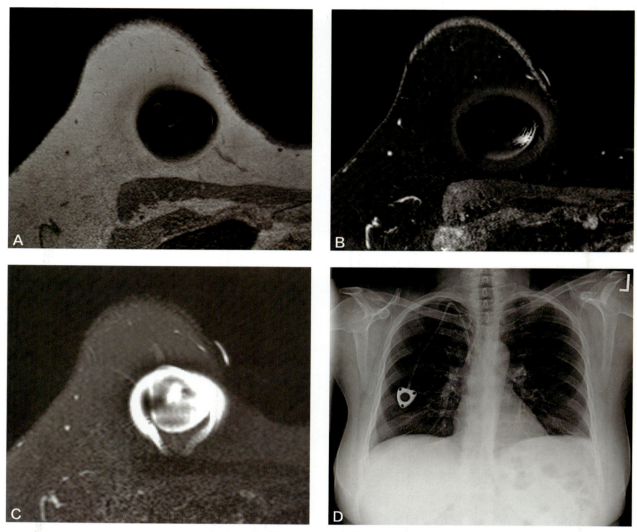

▲ 图 14-18 磁化率伪影

66 岁女性，左侧乳腺浸润性导管癌。平扫 T_1 加权像（A）及增强脂肪饱和 T_1 加权像（B）示右上内乳见一个大圆形信号缺失区。在 T_2 加权像显示为主要以高信号为主的圆形混杂信号区（C）。在胸片上可见此信号为中心静脉导管口（D），伪影有可能会掩盖 MRI 的一些发现

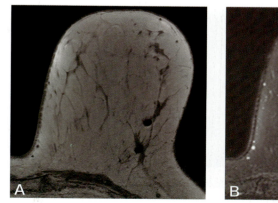 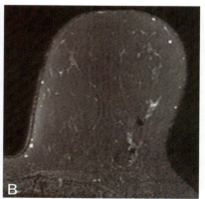 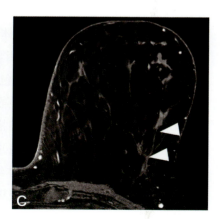

▲ 图 14-19 磁化率伪影

66 岁女性，左乳浸润性导管癌。平扫 T_1 加权（A）及 T_2 加权 SPAIR（B）序列显示在左乳外上象限有两个点状信号缺失影。这些缺失影对应为 MRI 活检标记物。需要注意的是，这些伪影在增强 T_1 脂肪饱和图像中（箭头）（C）显示比较模糊。因此非脂肪饱和序列是评估活检夹和手术钉的最佳序列

Chapter 14 乳腺 MRI
Breast MRI

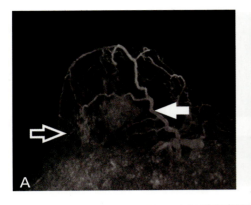
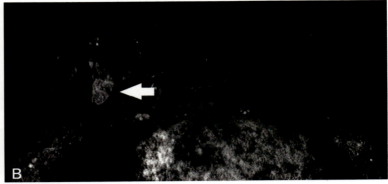
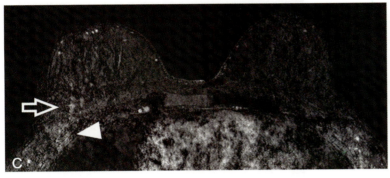
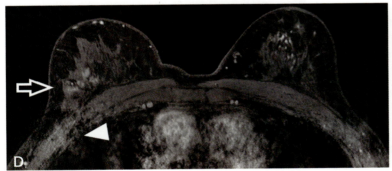
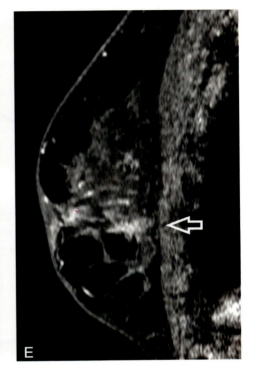

▲ 图 14-20 幻影伪影

61 岁女性，活检证实右乳浸润性导管癌（白箭），另外在增强的最大密度投影像（A）及轴位减影像（B）上的 7 点方位可见非肿块样强化（NME）（黑箭）。幻影伪影是指在相位编码方向上出现的界面的折叠或者明亮区域的重叠显示，在本例中，增强轴向减影（C）和 T_1 加权脂肪抑制图像（D）上伪影的出现造成了胸肌受侵的假象（箭头）。当乳腺 MRI 轴向采集信号时，应选择左右方向相位编码梯度，这样就避免了乳腺实质内出现伪影。增强 T_1 加权像矢状位重建图像（E）证实了 NME（黑箭）没有真正侵犯胸肌

框 14-1 乳腺 MRI 检查法的说明	框 14-1 乳腺 MRI 检查法的说明

• 评估患者病史和临床症状
• 回顾之前的影像学研究（乳腺摄影、超声和 MRI）
• 对比前后的研究以评估运动伪影
• 查看 MIP 图像以评估背景实质增强，评估对称性并识别明显的病变
• 查看减影图像，并进一步评估及确认可疑焦点增强
• 回顾 T_1 初期对比后研究
   - 确认背景实质增强
   - 进一步评估在 MIP 和减影上发现的任何病变的形态
	• 查看 T_2 加权图像
	   - 评估双侧囊肿和扩张导管
	   - 进一步表征良性肿块（例如囊肿发炎，乳内淋巴结肿大和纤维腺瘤）
	• 回顾 T_1 加权对比前研究
	   - 评估 FGT
	   - 评估出血性或蛋白质性囊肿或导管液
	• 查看计算机辅助检测软件的信息，以了解增强质量的动力学曲线

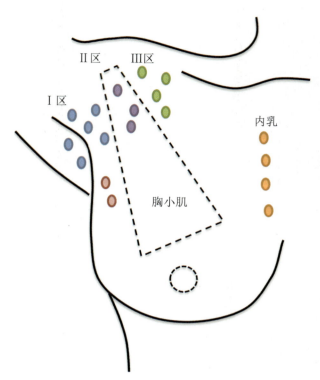

▲ 图 14-21　腋窝淋巴结分区

腋窝淋巴结的三分区是由淋巴结相对于胸小肌的位置确定的Ⅰ区淋巴结（蓝色）位于胸小肌外缘的外侧，Ⅱ区淋巴结（紫色）位于胸小肌后方间隙，Ⅲ区淋巴结（绿色）位于胸小肌内缘的内侧。内乳淋巴结（橙色）和乳房内淋巴结（红色）也可见到。胸肌间淋巴结（或 Rotter 节点，未标识）位于胸大肌和胸小肌之间

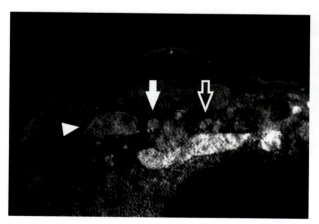

▲ 图 14-22　腋窝淋巴结肿大

61 岁女性，筛查发现浸润性导管癌和导管原位癌，活检证实右腋窝转移性淋巴结肿大。轴位增强 T_1 加权像示异常显示的Ⅰ区（箭头）、Ⅲ区（黑箭）及胸肌间淋巴结（白箭）

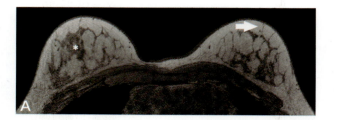
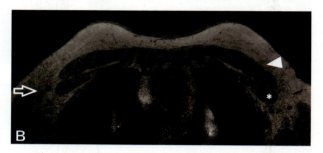
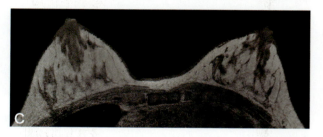
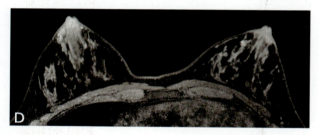
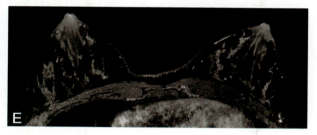

▲ 图 14-23　正常乳腺 MRI

有乳腺癌家族史的 28 岁女性。行乳腺 MRI 高危筛查。轴位平扫 T_1 加权像示（A）在乳头水平由间质和实质组成的纤维腺体组织为等信号（星号），Cooper 韧带（箭）呈线样，线样等信号从纤维腺体组织延伸至皮肤，这些组织以网状方式连接在一起。轴位平扫 T_1 加权图像（B）更好地显示出等信号的正常腋窝淋巴结（黑箭）、皮肤、胸大肌（箭头）和胸小肌（*）肌肉组织。轴位平扫 T_1 加权（C）、T_2 加权 SPAIR（D）和增强脂肪饱和 T_1 加权图像（E）在同一水平显示出正常乳头 - 乳晕复合体。需要注意的是 T_2 加权像上的纤维腺体组织的正常高信号

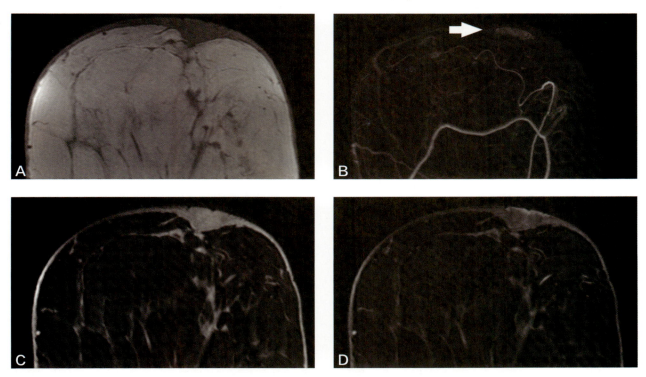

▲ 图 14-24 乳头－乳晕复合体

52 岁女性，行高危筛查乳腺 MRI 检查。平扫轴位 T_1 加权像（A），最大密度投影（B），脂肪饱和 T_1 加权像（C），和增强脂肪饱和 T_1 加权像（D）显示乳头 - 乳晕复合体的正常强化（白箭）

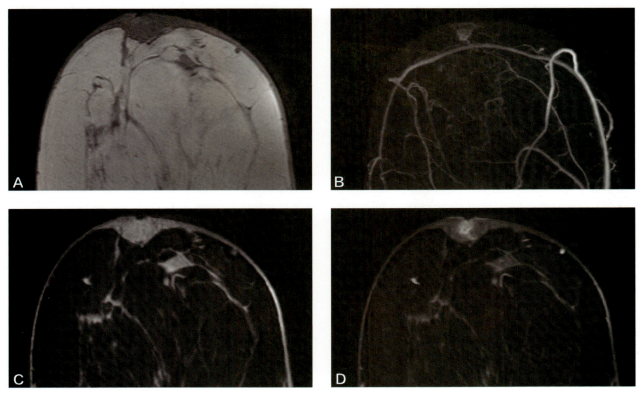

▲ 图 14-25 乳头内陷

52 岁女性，行高危筛查乳腺 MRI 检查。平扫轴位 T_1 加权像（A），最大密度投影（B），脂肪饱和 T_1 加权像（C），和增强脂肪饱和 T_1 加权像（D）显示出在强化的乳晕下似一个强化了的肿块样的内陷乳头影

(一)乳腺纤维腺体组织(fibrograndular tissue, FGT)数量

与乳腺X线影像上的乳房密度相似，乳腺纤维腺体数量也可以在MRI上进行表征。平扫T_1加权像是最好的评估方式，根据ACR BI-RADS词汇定性评价分为四组：几乎全部脂肪、散在纤维腺体组织、混杂纤维腺体组织和致密纤维腺体组织（框14-2，图14-26）。

> **框14-2　乳腺组成**（按体积计算的致密腺体组织的量）
> - 几乎全部脂肪（0%～25%纤维腺体组织）
> - 散在纤维腺体组织（25%～50%纤维腺体组织）
> - 混杂纤维腺体组织（50%～75%纤维腺体组织）
> - 致密纤维腺体组织（>75%纤维腺体组织）

(二)乳腺背景实质强化

背景实质增强（background parenchymal enha

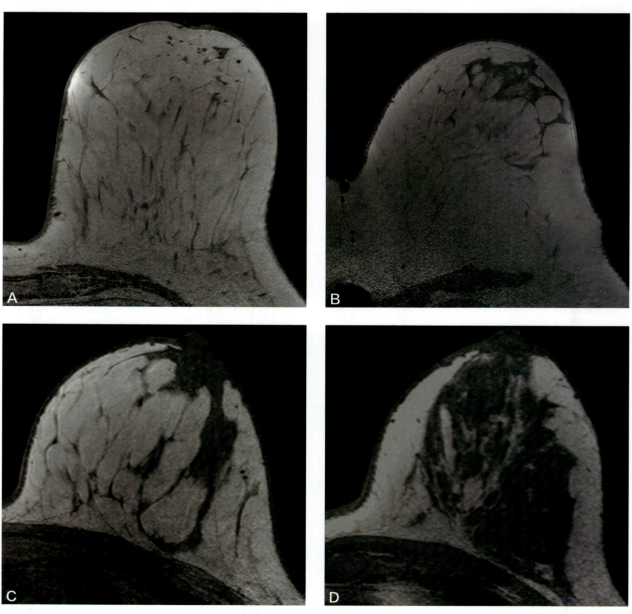

▲ 图14-26　乳腺组成

轴位T_1加权图像上纤维腺体组织数量的示例：几乎全部脂肪（A），散在纤维腺体组织（B），混杂纤维腺体组织（C），致密纤维腺体组织（D）

ncement, BPE）是指正常乳腺组织的良性、激素相关性增强。背景实质强化的量在患者自身和患者之间各不相同，取决于绝经前状态或绝经状态、绝经前患者的月经周期阶段和外源激素或激素治疗方法。背景实质强化评估基于增强后的第一幅图像，其中心 K 空间填充时间约为 90s。一般来说，随着时间的推移，背景实质强化显示逐渐增强的强化，并且在延迟期更为明显。根据第 5 版 ACR BI-RADS 标准（第 2 版 MRI），背景实质强化应根据纤维腺体数量分为 4 类：极少、轻度、中度或显著（框 14-3，图 14-27 和图 14-28）。

乳腺 MRI 上未知的背景实质强化数量可以掩盖或被误认为是乳腺癌的强化，从而对乳腺 MR 评判产生不利的影响。然而，背景实质强化的增

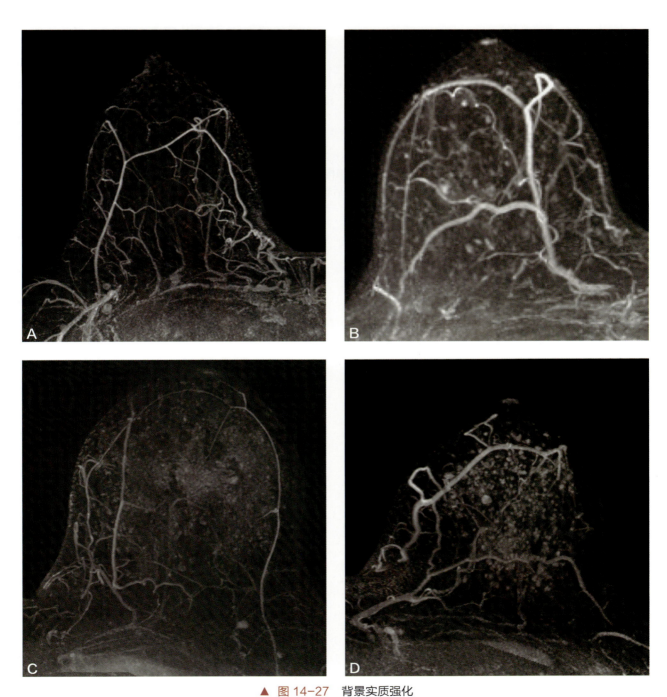

▲ 图 14-27　背景实质强化

最大强度投影图像上背景实质强化的典型示例：极少（A），轻度（B），中度（C），显著（D）

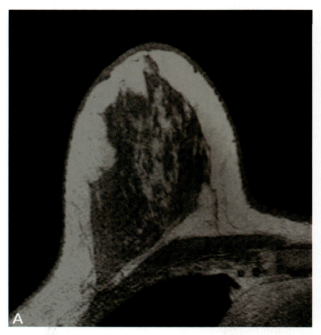 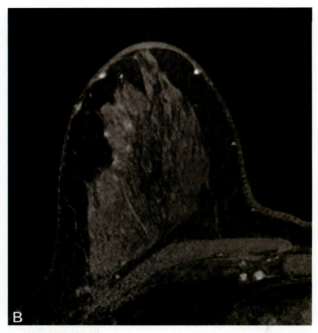

▲ 图 14-28 乳腺构成与背景实质强化

48岁女性，轴位 T_1 加权像上有大量纤维腺体组织（A）。增强后轴位脂肪饱和 T_1 加权像（B）显示极少的背景实质强化。注意：纤维腺体组织的数量与背景实质强化的数量不直接相关

框 14-3　乳腺背景实质强化
• 极少（1%～25%）
• 轻度（25%～50%）
• 中度（50%～75%）
• 显著（>75%）

加与活检阳性率、MRI 的肿瘤发现率、敏感性或特异性无显著差异等无关[52]。增加的背景实质强化的增加与较高的异常判读率相关，这可能导致额外的成像[52,53]。因此，对绝经前患者进行更多的选择性检查，如高危筛查，最好是在月经周期开始后 7～10d（背景实质强化处于最低点）进行成像（图 14-29）。然而，对新近诊断乳腺癌的患者应用 MRI 成像评估病变范围是不宜推迟检查时间的。

虽然通常乳腺背景实质强化是对称性的，偶尔也会是非对称性的。这通常见于既往接受过乳腺癌治疗的妇女（图 14-30）。典型地，如放射治疗后最初受影响的乳腺组织中背景实质强化相对于未受影响的乳腺增加，之后随着时间的推移而减少。良性的不对称性背景实质强化也可发生在实质上乳腺组织不对称和哺乳期仅单侧哺乳的女性。无解剖或生理原因的不对称背景实质强化应疑诊乳腺炎或恶性肿瘤，需要密切的临床相关性证据。

（三）病变评估

病变在 MRI 上被定义为增强后 T_1 加权像上发现的独有的背景实质强化。每个增强病灶可以进一步由 ACR BI-RADS 标准描述其特定形态和动力学曲线增强特征。此外，根据病变类型，平扫 T_1 加权和 T_2 加权（或其他液体敏感序列）上的附加特征可以有助于病变定性。

1. 形态学　美国放射学会 BI-RADS 标准描述了三种常见病变类型：局灶性病变、肿块和非肿块增强（non-mass enhancement, NME）。除了局灶性病变，每种病变类型都可以用形态学描述来进一步表述，用以评估恶性肿瘤的疑似程度。一般来说，形态学是 MRI 鉴别良恶性病变的最重要的因素[18]。

（1）局灶性病变：在增强图像上，局灶性病变被用来描述典型小于 5mm 的强化病变，无形

Chapter 14 乳腺 MRI
Breast MRI

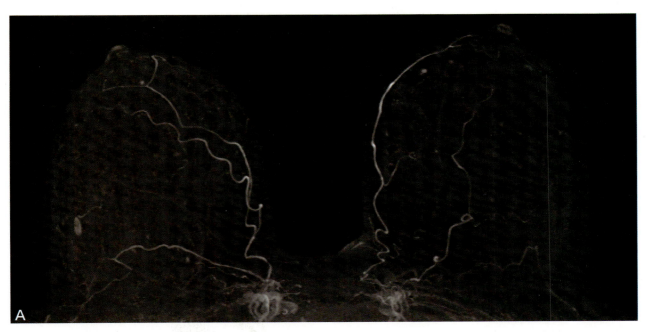

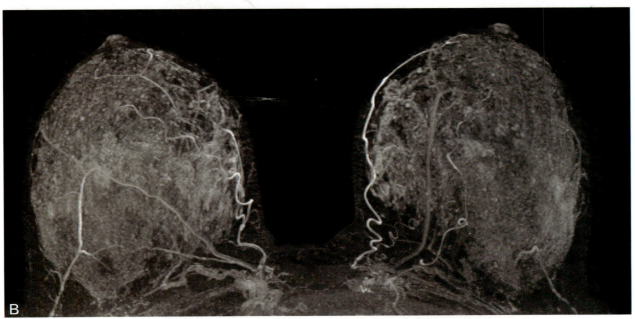

▲ 图 14-29 月经周期内不同阶段背景实质强化的差异

31 岁女性，乳腺癌高危筛查的 MRI 表现。在最近的检查中，患者背景实质强化极少（A）；然而她一年前的检查呈显著的背景实质强化（B）。这源于月经周期不同阶段激素水平的变化

态学特征，并且在平扫 T_1 加权图像上没有相应的发现（图 14-31）。这些病变本质上是非特异性的，通常是最不可疑的乳腺 MRI 病变。虽然局灶性病变可以代表小的恶性肿瘤，但大多数是背景实质强化（尤其是双侧时）、乳房内淋巴结或良性病变。如果局灶性病变被认为是唯一的（即与背景实质强化相比突出，或与乳腺内其他病灶相比更大和

更显著），遵循检查清单确定恶性肿瘤疑似度和处理方法是有用的。表 14-2 总结了在评估唯一病灶时要考虑的特征。一般来说，在 T_2 加权像上显示高信号的病灶和在动态增强序列上具有稳定或持久延迟增强动力学特征、与其先前的检查相比稳定或在基线检查中确定是良性的，可以被安全地忽略或影像学随诊。代表乳内小淋巴结的病

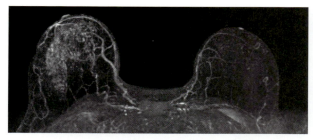

▲ 图 14-30 放射治疗引起的不对称性背景实质强化

48 岁女性，左侧乳腺癌治疗史。MRI 用于高危筛查。增强后轴位最大强度投影显示不对称的背景实质强化，左侧呈极少背景实质强化、右侧中度背景实质强化；这归因于左侧乳腺放射治疗史

灶常在 T_2 加权像上呈高信号，而在非脂肪饱和的 T_1 加权像上呈少量的脂肪内陷（或"脂肪缺口"）。然而，如果唯一的病灶与先前的研究相比是新发的，并且没有表现出这些典型的良性特征，则应考虑活检。最后，应该注意的是，并非所有小于 5mm 的唯一病变都被强制分类为局灶性病变。随着 MRI 技术的改进，尤其是磁场强度的提高和对高空间分辨率成像的重视，预计越来越多的小病灶将满足被描述为肿块的标准。

（2）肿块：乳腺 MRI 上肿块是一种占位的三

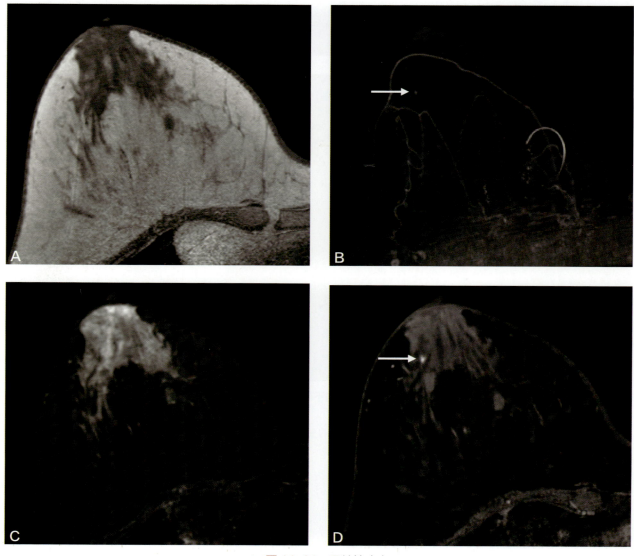

▲ 图 14-31 局灶性病变

54 岁女性，MRI 用于高危筛查。平扫轴位 T_1 加权像（A），最大强度投影（B），脂肪抑制 T_2 加权像（C）及增强后压脂 T_1 加权像（D）显示在 9 点钟位置一个 3mm 病灶（箭）。注意：在 T_1 加权图像上没有相关性，并且这在 T_2 加权图像上不表现出高信号

维病灶，具有不同的形状、边缘和内部增强特征。虽然基于美国放射学会 BI-RADS 标准定义是相当具体的，但在局灶性病变和肿块之间存在重叠，有时可能难以区分。一个有用的经验法则来区分小肿块和病灶是评估病变是否可以描述可疑形状和边缘：如果小强化病灶具有不规则形状、和（或）不确定边缘，则应称为肿块。

与病灶相比，肿块应以更高的怀疑指数和较低的阈值来推荐活检。由于相关的新生血管而迅速增强，因此在第一期增强后 T_1 加权图像上评估肿块的形状和边缘是最有用的。根据第 5 版 BI-RADS 标准，形容肿块的形状可以用 3 个术语来描述：卵圆形（包括分叶状，意味着 2~3 个轻微的起伏）、圆形或不规则形。肿块的边缘可被界定（与周围的乳房组织分界清晰）或不可界定（不规则或毛刺状边缘）（如图 14-32 和图 14-33）。与乳腺 X 线一样，界限清晰的肿块比有毛刺或不规则边缘的肿块更可能是良性的；然而，重要的是要认识到，根据扫描的空间分辨率、平均容积等因素可导致边缘有毛刺的肿块在 MRI 图像上表现为局限性的。

内部结构和动态强化特征也有助于区分良性和恶性病变。表现为均质（融合和均一）增强的肿块常提示良性，而异质性增强则提示恶性病变。还有两种特殊的增强模式：病变内无强化分隔和边缘环形增强。据报道，与其他良性形态学和动力学特征相结合，病变内无强化低信号分隔对纤维腺瘤诊断有特异性。然而，当使用这种增强特性来确定疑似病变时应谨慎，因为先前的研究发现单独的无强化分隔不能预示良性[54]。第二种边

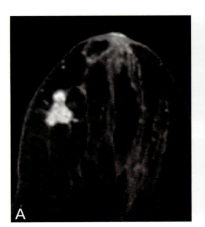 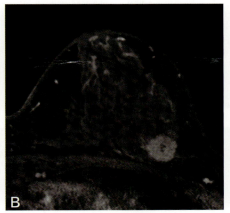 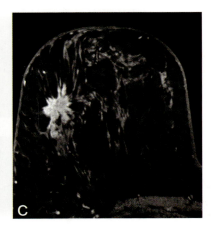

▲ 图 14-32 疑似恶性的形状及边缘

3 例不同女性患者的增强后轴位压脂 T_1 加权图像：A.49 岁女性浸润性导管癌患者表现为一分叶状边界清晰的肿块；B.55 岁女性浸润性导管癌患者表现为边缘不规则的不规则肿块，内部呈不均匀强化；C.40 岁女性浸润性小叶癌患者表现为不规则肿块伴边缘毛刺和内部不均匀强化

表 14-2 有助于确定病理取样需要的病灶特征

良性可能	可疑恶性
不是唯一的背景实质强化	显著的背景实质强化
液体敏感序列呈高信号	液体敏感序列呈低信号
初始中等强化伴延迟渐进型或平台型强化曲线	初始快速强化伴延迟流出型强化曲线
边界清晰的圆形或卵圆形病变	边界不清不规则形（注意：如果这些特征出现，应描述为肿块）
形态学提示为乳内淋巴结（表现为"脂肪缺口"）	
基线研究稳定或确定	与先前检查比较为新发病变

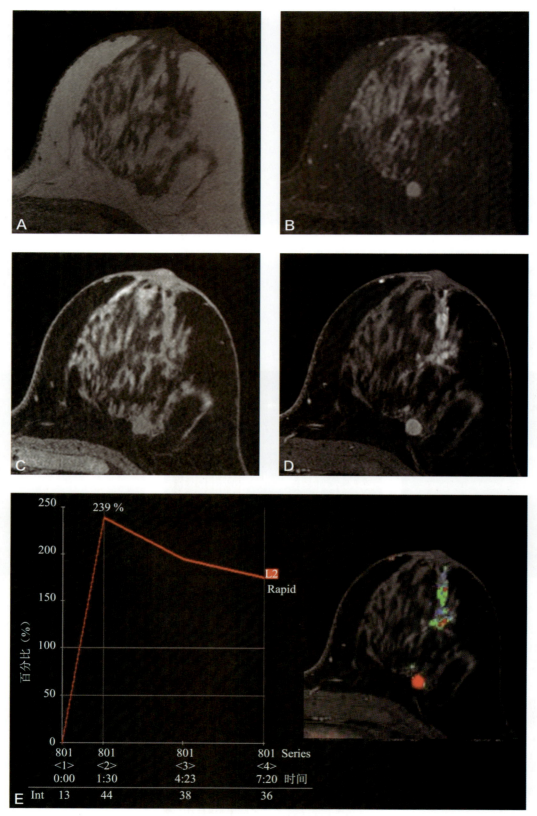

▲ 图 14-33 圆形边界清晰肿块

57 岁女性，初诊浸润性导管癌和导管内原位癌。MRI 评估病变范围。平扫轴位 T_1 加权像（A）、脂肪抑制 T_2 加权像（B），脂肪饱和 T_1 加权像（C），增强后脂肪饱和 T_1 加权像（D）显示乳腺中心深部一界限清晰的圆形肿块，呈边缘强化。动力学增强曲线（E）呈快速初始增强、延迟后期流出。活检为纤维囊性改变，常见于导管增生和硬化性腺病缘增强方式，除炎性囊肿或脂肪坏死（图14-34）等明显相关的病例外，被认为高度怀疑恶性（图14-35）。通常，基于病变平扫内部信号特性，良性囊肿和脂肪坏死可以很容易和恶性肿瘤坏死或黏液性恶性肿瘤的边缘强化区别开。边缘强化肿块样炎症囊肿，典型地表现是 T_2 和（或）T_1 加权图像上的高信号，这取决于囊肿内容物。在脂肪坏死的情况下，其内部信号特征应遵循 T_1 加权图像上的脂肪信号特点（不压脂为高信号、脂肪抑制序列呈黑色）。

（3）非肿块强化：非肿块样强化（NME）描述了与正常乳腺组织背景实质强化（background parenchymal enhancement, BPE）不同的增强模式，但不适于局灶性病变或肿块的定义。非肿块样强化的范围可以很小抑或很大，可以根据它们的分布进行分类（表14-3）。

非肿块样强化的线性和节段性分布与恶性肿瘤相关（图14-36至图14-38），特别是乳腺导管内原位癌，而区域性或弥漫性分布提示良性。多中心癌也可能有这些表现，血流动力学强化曲线可以帮助区分良恶性病变。非肿块样强化的内部增强特性也可以用 BI-RADS 标准来描述，即均匀、不均匀、聚集和聚集环状强化。

2. 动态增强 MRI 的血流动力学强化特征
乳腺癌的异常动力学增强特征是基于肿瘤血管生成与异常、增多的导管周围或基质血管增多所致

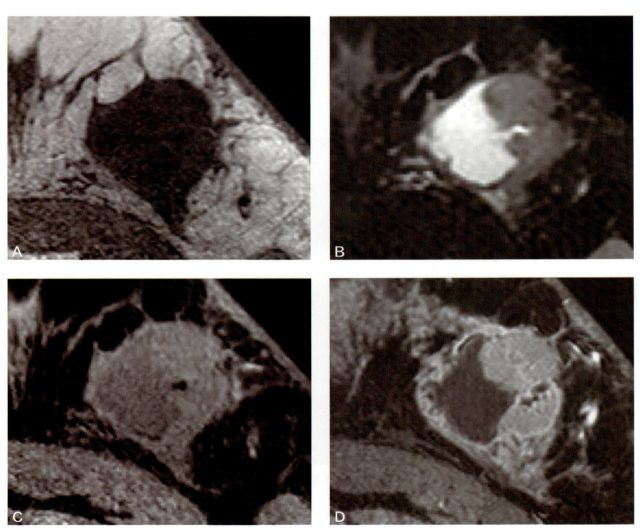

▲ 图 14-34　边缘强化

27 岁浸润性导管癌患者。平扫轴位 T_1 加权像（A）、脂肪抑制 T_2 加权像（B），脂肪饱和 T_1 加权像（C），增强后脂肪饱和 T_1 加权像（D）显示一不规则肿块、边缘不规则，增强后边缘强化。T_2 加权像肿块内部见高信号，可能表示坏死

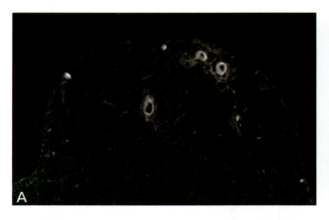
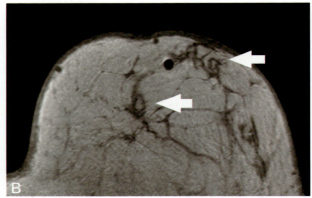
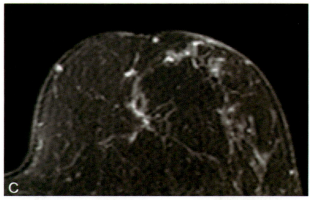

▲ 图 14-35 脂肪坏死的边缘强化

69 岁女性乳房缩小成形术后。增强后轴位减影图像（A）、平扫 T_1 加权像（B）、脂肪抑制 T_2 加权像（C）显示多个分散的边缘增强肿块，其中心呈脂肪信号（箭），T_2 加权像与脂肪坏死一致肿块内并没有信号增高

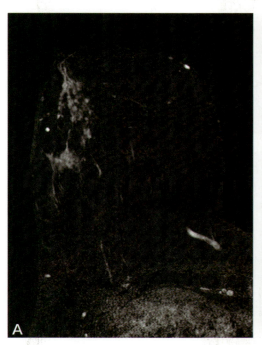

▲ 图 14-36 节段性非肿块样强化

50 岁女性，新近诊断乳腺导管内原位癌。增强后减影图像（A）显示节段性非肿块样强化延伸至乳头，经活检证实是乳腺导管内原位癌。从患者乳腺 X 线影像中对应的点压放大相（B）显示节段性分布的细小多形性钙化

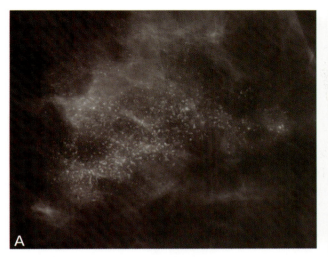
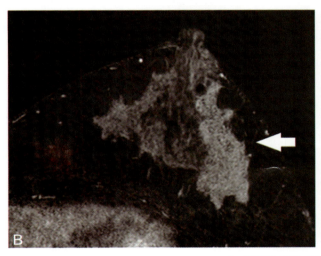
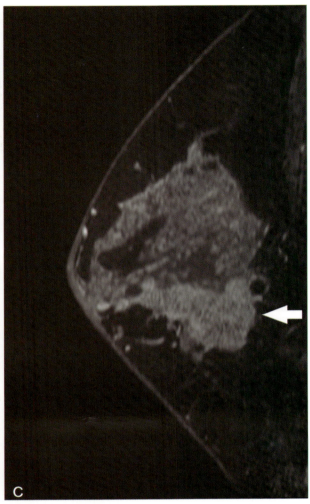

▲ 图 14-37　节段性非肿块样强化

36 岁诊乳腺导管内原位癌患者，乳腺 X 线示乳腺内节段分布细小多形性钙化（A）。脂肪饱和平扫 T_1 加权像轴位（B）及矢状位（C）图像显示节段性非肿块样增强（箭），从乳房实质后缘延伸至乳头，具有均匀的内部增强

表 14-3　非肿块样强化分布

强化分布	强化范围
局部	小于乳腺的 1 个象限即在单一的乳导管系统内
线性	单一乳导管内
节段性	三角形或锥形的，顶端朝向乳头
区域性	跨越至少 1 个象限，其面积大于单一乳导管系统。缺少一个凸出向外的轮廓，因此不定义为肿块
多区域性	强化范围至少 2 个由正常腺体组织或脂肪分离的区域
弥漫性	均匀分布，广泛的增强区域，类似于整个乳房组织

灌注和渗漏血管增加。对于准确地确定动态增强特征所需的扫描时间没有共识，但是大多数协议包括至少 3 个增强后时相点，通常以 K 空间为中心，大约在注射造影剂后 90s、270s 及 450s 时扫描。获得的动态增强信息可以评估增强的两个主要阶段：初始增强与后期增强（图 14-39）。初始阶段增强特征在到达到峰值增强为止（通常发生在注射造影剂后的 2min 内）。延迟后期增强阶段，在峰值增强后发生。延迟后期强化可以用 3 种主要的曲线类型来描述：缓慢上升型、平台型和流出型。

在增强的初始阶段，依照信号强度增强率分类为"慢""中""快"，对应信号强化增强率 < 50%、

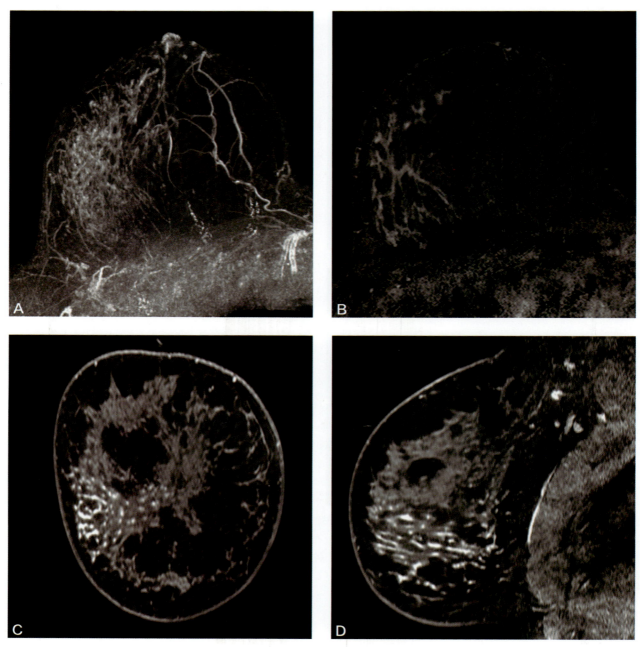

▲ 图 14-38 节段性非肿块样强化

31 岁女性，新近诊断左乳复发性浸润性癌，MRI 评估病变范围。轴位最大强度投影（A），轴位增强后减影图像（B），增强后脂肪饱和 T_1 加权像轴位（C）和矢状位（D）图像显示外下象限节段性线状、分支状非肿块强化伴树突状内部强化。经活检证实为导管内原位癌

50%～100% 和＞100%，其中信号强度增强率运用公式计算：

$$SI_{\%increase} = [(SI_{post} - SI_{pre})/SI_{pre}] \times 100\%$$

式中 SI_{pre} 是感兴趣区域的基线信号强度，而 SI_{post} 是注射对比剂后相同感兴趣区域的信号强度。在延迟阶段，主要有三种强化曲线类型：渐进型、平台型和流出型。渐进型延迟增强被定义为持续增强的强化超过 10% 的初始增强，被认为是最良性的延迟强化曲线。平台型延迟增强指的是达到峰值后信号强度恒定（±10% 初始增强），中等程度疑似恶性。流出型延迟增强指峰值增强后信号强度降低超过 10% 的初始增强，此为高度

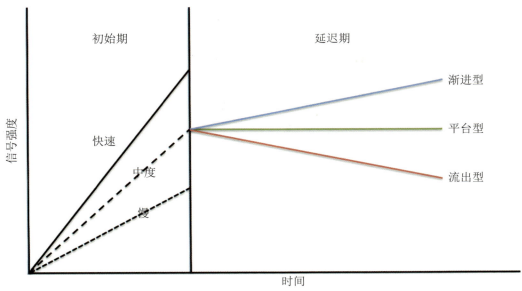

▲ 图 14-39　动态增强血流动力学强化曲线

动态增强 MRI 中表现出不同的初始和延迟期相动力学增强曲线的代表性图像。可见有缓慢、中等或快速的初始阶段增强，以及渐进型、平台型或流出型延迟增强

提示恶性病变的强化曲线类型。

虽然恶性乳腺病变最典型的强化曲线类型是快速的初始强化，然后是早期的流出（图 14-40），但在良性病变和恶性病变中，半定量血流动力学强化曲线类型有明显的重叠。因此，应在其他重要的临床和影像学特征（如患者病史、病变形态学和对比研究）的背景下解释动力学强化特征。在我们的经验中，不具备良性形态学特征的病变，结合动力学增强曲线评估最有助于证实病变的良性。可疑恶性形态特征的病灶应活检，而不考虑其增强特性。计算机辅助分析工具被用来评估病变血流动力学强化，通过设置不同的增强阈值来显示强化超过一定范围的组织（例如信号强度增加 50%～100%）。

除了标准的半定量血流动力学参数外，开发先进的 MRI 技术是非常有意义的，这些技术可以采用药物动力学模型来获得高度定量的信息，这些信息可以作为恶性肿瘤的生物标志物（例如，容量转移常数，Ktrans）。这些参数虽然是有前途的，但对技术要求苛刻，并且在有限的时间内具有重复性，因此不推荐作为常规临床应用。

3. T_2 加权像（T_2-Weighted Imaging）

一般而言，T_2 加权图像上相对于正常乳腺组织的均匀高信号，而没有强化的病变代表良性（框 14-4）。这些病变包括囊肿（也可能表现为周边强化）和充满液体的扩张乳导管。T_2 加权图像也有助于确认小的边界清晰的均匀强化肿块为良性（通常小于 10mm）：T_2 加权像高信号者最有可能是纤维腺瘤或乳内淋巴结，因此可以在短时间内安全地忽略或随访。T_2 加权图像上的高信号表现不应用于排除任何具有可疑恶性形态学发现的肿块或其他可疑发现的活检。事实上，已知一些恶性肿瘤亚型在 T_2 加权上常常表现出高信号，如乳腺黏液癌和化生性癌。

4. 乳腺磁共振成像的新进展

虽然动态增强 MRI 技术对乳腺癌的检测提供了非常高的灵敏度（90%），但其特异性中等（约 72%）[55] 需要对比剂，且相对高的价格限制它的应用。最近，多项研究表明，弥散加权成像（DWI）作为一种非对比增强技术，它测量水在组织内自由扩散的

框 14-4　在 T_2 加权像上呈高信号的肿块

- 囊肿
- 扩张乳导管
- 乳内淋巴结
- 纤维腺瘤
- 黏液癌或化生癌

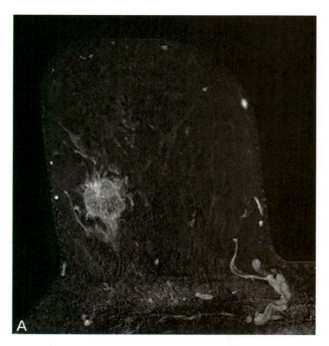
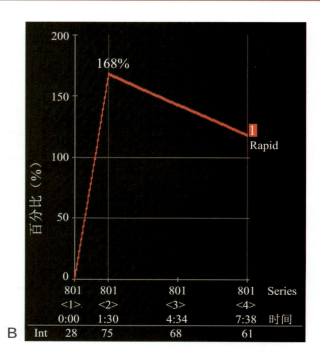
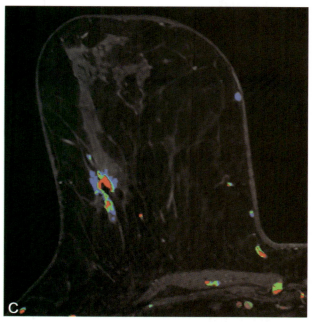

▲ 图 14-40 流出型动力学增强曲线

50 岁女性，新近诊断浸润性导管癌行乳腺 MRI 评估病变范围。增强后轴位 T_1 加权像（A）显示一不规则肿块伴不规则边缘及内部不均匀强化。动力学增强曲线（B）在活检被证实的恶性肿瘤部分显示快速的初始增强和延迟期流出（红色覆盖）（C）

能力，有助于提高动态增强 MRI 的特异性和阳性预测值，从而减少假阳性 MRI 发现和不必要的活检[56]。此外，最近的研究表明 DWI 有作为一种独立的非对比筛选技术的潜力[57]，这可以降低检查成本、同时增加对肾功能不全或对比剂过敏患者的 MRI 检查的可行性。MR 波谱（magnetic resonance spectroscopy，MRS）是一种能够测量体内化学信息并广泛应用于脑和前列腺的成像技术，它也显示了鉴别乳腺良恶性病变的可能[58]。然而，尽管这些技术潜能有助于提高乳腺 MRI 性能和（或）增加乳腺 MRI 的使用率，但仍存在显著未解决的技术和标准化问题，因此，不能作为常规临床使用。由美国放射影像学网络（ACRIN 试验 6698、6657 和 6702）赞助的几项关于乳腺癌的 DWI 和 MRS 应用的多中心研究正在进行，这将提高这些技术临床应用可能性。

(四)病变位置

以一致的方式描述病灶的位置非常重要,清楚地表述该病变的位置,以便在其他相关成像、随访 MRI 及手术规划、穿刺引导定位中容易被识别。与乳腺 X 线一样,乳房在患者面对医师时被视为钟面,除了钟面之外,象限的使用也避免混乱(图 14-41)。在报告描述中,首先给出病灶是哪一侧,其次是位置、然后是深度。通过将乳房组织分为三部分(前、中、后)来报告病灶深度(图 14-42)。与乳头的距离,即从病变前缘至乳头画线,也可以用来帮助确定深度和位置。如果病变仅位于乳头深处,也可以使用乳晕下区来描述。当中心、乳晕下区和腋窝尾部描述更为合适时也可以代替象限使用。

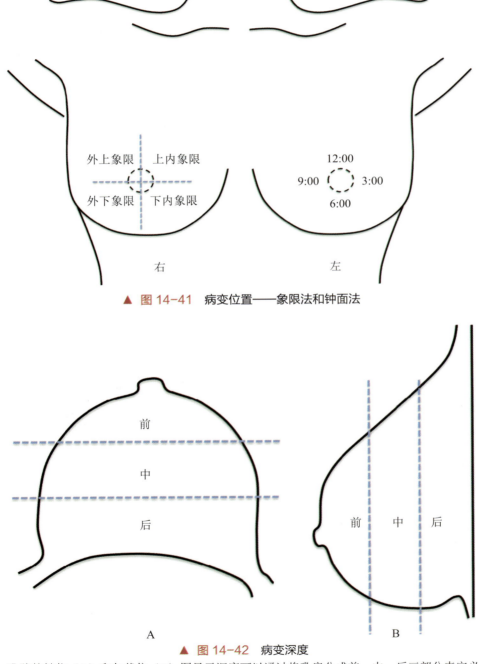

▲ 图 14-41 病变位置——象限法和钟面法

▲ 图 14-42 病变深度
乳腺的轴位(A)和矢状位(B)图显示深度可以通过将乳房分成前、中、后三部分来定义

六、乳腺 MRI 良性发现

与恶性肿瘤相比，MRI 能鉴别出一系列的良性发现，对放射科医师来讲熟悉它们的表现是很重要的。

（一）液性囊肿

囊肿是常见的良性病变，MRI 具有鉴别特征。像身体其他部位囊肿一样，单纯囊肿呈边界清晰的圆形或椭圆形。一般而言，单纯囊肿在液体敏感序列上具有高信号、无强化（图 14-43），并且可能有薄的分隔。含有高蛋白成分或可能含有血液产物的囊肿，在液体敏感成像序列上呈较低的信号，并且在平扫 T_1 加权图像上呈高信号（图 14-44）。囊肿内部从不强化。然而，有时囊肿壁在发炎时增强 T_1 加权像可见强化（图 14-45）。只要强化是均匀的、薄的，无结节性或相关的内部增强，那这就是一个良性的病灶。

（二）乳导管扩张

乳导管扩张或扩张充满液体的导管倾向于从乳头向外辐射，表现为类似于囊肿的信号强度，呈分支状。这些管状结构在充满蛋白质成分时可在平扫 T_1 加权图像上呈现出高信号（图 14-46）。这是一个正常表现，也与增加乳腺癌风险没有相关性。然而，还需认真观察乳导管有无增强或导管内肿块存在，这样才能诊断乳导管扩张症，特别是对于孤立性乳导管扩张者。如果出现乳导管周围聚集环状强化或乳导管内出现强化时，则应怀疑为恶性肿瘤。

（三）纤维囊性改变

纤维囊性改变指的是一组良性、非增生性乳腺病变，与乳腺癌的风险增加无关。这些病变包括如单纯乳房囊肿、乳头状瘤改变、上皮相关性钙化和常见型轻度增生[49]。很少有研究评估乳腺纤维囊性改变的 MRI 特征，因为病变通常是根据临床发现诊断的。纤维囊性改变可表现为与对侧乳腺不对称的节段性非肿块样强化（图 14-47），并且通常在 T_2 加权图像上呈相应的高信号。

（四）淋巴结

发现乳内淋巴结是常见的，特别是在乳腺的外上象限，这些良性结节必须与可疑恶性结节相鉴别。乳内淋巴结通常较小，为直径小于 5mm 边界清晰的椭圆形结节（通常有轻微的小叶），皮层呈均匀高 T_2 信号。良性淋巴结的第二个表现是中央脂肪门的存在，这可以在非脂肪抑制的 T_1 加权图像上看到，并与血管密切相关。

动态增强动力学特征通常无法帮助区分正

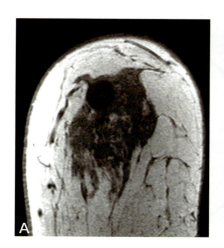 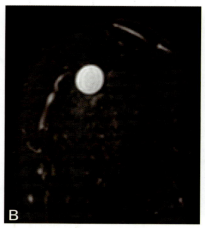 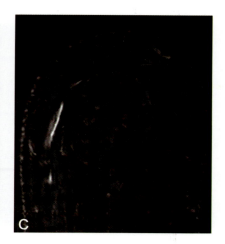

▲ 图 14-43 单纯囊肿

54 岁右侧乳腺癌患者术前 MRI 评估病变范围。平扫轴位 T_1 加权像（A），脂肪抑制 T_2 加权像（B）及增强 T_1 减影图像（C）显示一边界光整的圆形肿块，T_2 呈均匀高信号、T_1 减影图像无内部强化，符合单纯囊肿

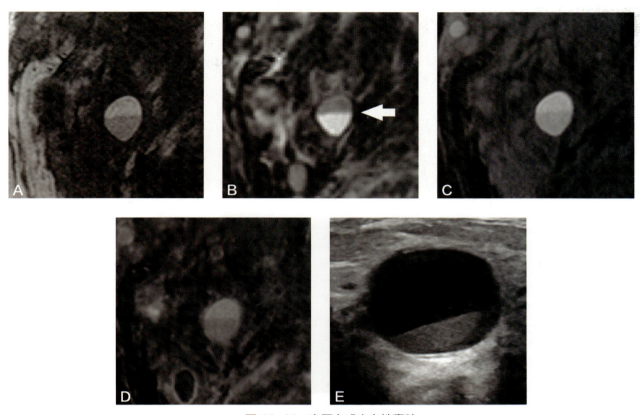

▲ 图 14-44 高蛋白或出血性囊肿

63 岁女性，既往双侧乳腺囊肿病史做乳腺 MRI 高危筛查。平扫轴位 T_1 加权像（A），脂肪抑制 T_2 加权像（B），脂肪饱和 T_1 加权像（C），以及增强脂肪饱和 T_1 加权像（D）显示一个边界清晰的椭圆形肿块，其内可见液 - 液平面（箭），没有与出血性或蛋白质性成分并存的异常强化。注意，患者趴在核磁机上，确定图像方向，使得"前方"处于图像的上方。T_1 加权像上的高信号强度和 T_2 加权像上的低信号强度表现为出血或蛋白质成分，而 T_1 加权像上的低信号和 T_2 加权图像上的高信号是简单的液体成分。仰卧位（E）的靶向超声表现为边界清晰的椭圆形肿块，液 - 液平面与出血或蛋白质成分呈分层状态有关

常淋巴结和恶性病变，因为它们均可表现出快速的初始阶段增强与平台型或流出型晚期延迟增强。因此，人们必须严重依赖 T_2 加权图像上的形态和信号特征（图 14-48）。偶尔，疑似乳内淋巴结的小肿块在乳腺 MRI 上呈现出不明确的形态和信号。在这种情况下，靶向超声有助于明确它们是否为乳房内淋巴结。如果用这样的方式，超声也无异常发现或不明确的情况下，则建议基于 MRI 特征给出明确的 BI-RADS 评估（例如，BI-RADS 类别 3 或 4）。

异常淋巴结，包括乳腺原发性病变或其他全身性恶性疾病如淋巴瘤等，都表现为脂肪门缺失、圆形肿大（与肾豆状相反）或局灶性偏心性皮质增厚（图 14-49）。不幸的是，形态学和动力学特征都没有足够的能力区分出恶性淋巴结与良性 / 反应性增生淋巴结，对于初诊乳腺癌患者还无法取代传统手术分期[37]。

（五）纤维腺瘤

纤维腺瘤是良性纤维上皮肿瘤，在所有年龄段妇女中最常见的实体瘤，最常见于 30 岁。根据其成熟阶段，纤维腺瘤在乳腺 MRI 上表现多样。其最常见的乳腺 MRI 表现为椭圆形或小叶状界限清晰的强化肿块，T_2 加权像上呈高信号。然而，随着一些纤维腺瘤逐渐纤维化，由于其成分硬化它们在 T_2 加权图像上往往变暗（图 14-50）。大约 20% 的纤维腺瘤可见无强化的内分隔（图 14-51）。因为乳腺叶状肿瘤通常具有纤维腺瘤的

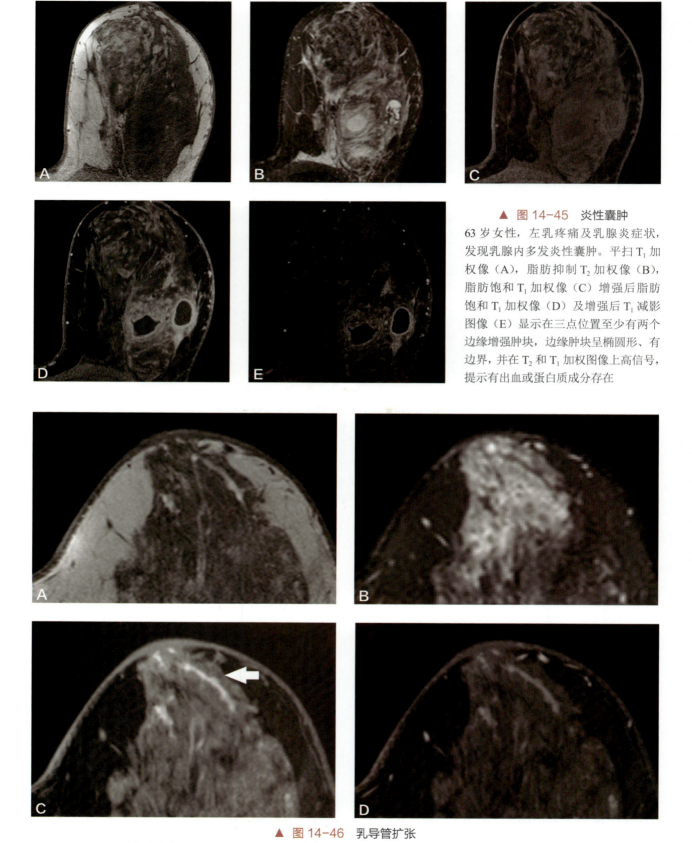

▲ 图 14-45 炎性囊肿

63 岁女性，左乳疼痛及乳腺炎症状，发现乳腺内多发炎性囊肿。平扫 T_1 加权像（A），脂肪抑制 T_2 加权像（B），脂肪饱和 T_1 加权像（C）增强后脂肪饱和 T_1 加权像（D）及增强后 T_1 减影图像（E）显示在三点位置至少有两个边缘增强肿块，边缘肿块呈椭圆形、有边界，并在 T_2 和 T_1 加权图像上高信号，提示有出血或蛋白质成分存在

▲ 图 14-46 乳导管扩张

55 岁初诊浸润性乳腺癌患者，乳腺 MRI 评估病变范围。平扫轴位 T_1 加权像（A），脂肪抑制 T_2 加权像（B），脂肪饱和 T_1 加权像（C）及增强脂肪饱和 T_1 加权像（D）示含蛋白质成分填充的正常扩张乳导管（箭）。无导管内强化

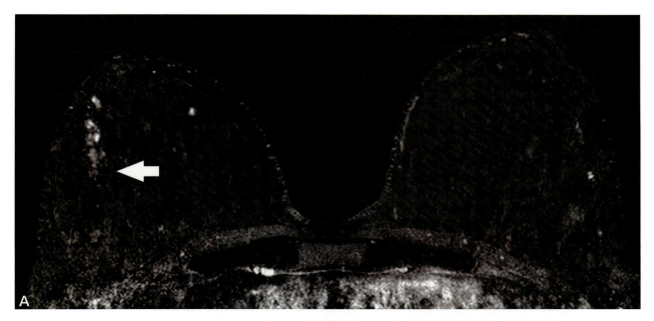

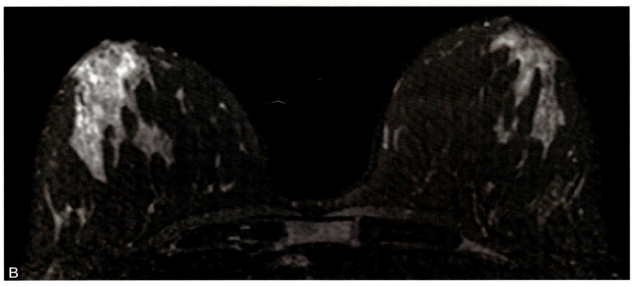

▲ 图 14-47 纤维囊性改变和普通型乳导管增生

37 岁女性，明确乳腺癌家族史。增强减影图像（A）显示右乳内与对侧乳腺不对称的节段性非肿块样强化及团状内部强化（箭）。非肿块样强化在 T_2 加权像上呈高信号，然而，对于在形态学上可疑恶性病变者 MRI 上的液性信号不能作为其良性病理的指征

形态学特征，故两者难以区分[59]，因此，任何具有纤维腺瘤影像学特征的肿块（不能被生理激素状态所解释的，如妊娠）应予活检和（或）切除。

乳腺纤维腺瘤血流动力学强化一般呈缓慢至中度的初始期增强，渐进型的延迟强化。然而，并非所有纤维腺瘤都表现出良性的增强动力学曲线，黏液样纤维腺瘤表现特殊为初始阶段快速增强[60]。最后，硬化性纤维腺瘤通常内部无任何强化，并可能表现出与乳腺 X 线上显示的"爆米花"样钙化相对应的不规则内部信号空洞。

（六）导管内乳头状瘤

乳腺导管内乳头状瘤是一种由增殖的导管上皮和肌上皮细胞构成的肿瘤，可能有纤维血管蒂。最常见在乳晕下区出现乳导管内小肿块（直径＜5mm），临床上有血性乳头溢液。关于导管内乳

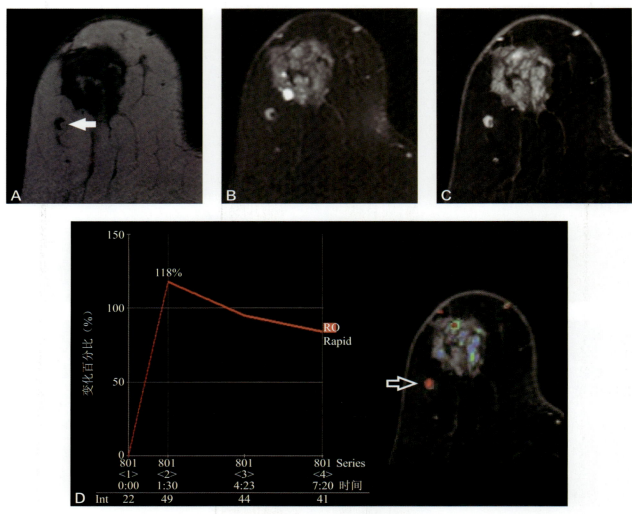

▲ 图 14-48 正常乳内淋巴结

平扫 T_1 加权像（A），脂肪抑制 T_2 加权像（B），增强脂肪饱和 T_1 加权像（C）显示一正常的乳内淋巴结，脂肪门（箭）、T_2 加权图像上呈高信号。注意该良性淋巴结（黑箭）的动态对比增强动力学曲线（D）显示了快速初始增强和流出型延迟强化，这对于区分正常乳腺内淋巴结和恶性病变没有帮助，因此，这种情况下最重要的是形态学评估

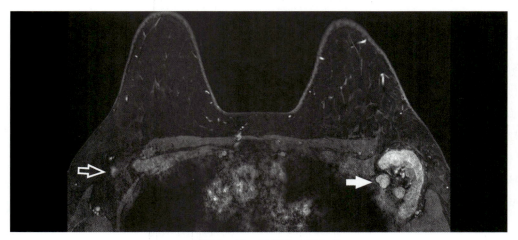

▲ 图 14-49 异常乳内淋巴结

66 岁乳腺浸润性导管癌患者。增强轴位脂肪饱和 T_1 加权像显示左腋窝多发肿大和形态异常的淋巴结，呈皮质增厚和无脂肪门的圆形结构（白箭）。右侧可见正常腋窝淋巴结显示（黑箭）

Chapter 14 乳腺 MRI
Breast MRI

头状瘤或相关的高危病变在手术切除时升级为恶性肿瘤的比率，各种报道的数据不同。因此，是否手术切除常常是依赖于医疗机构[61-63]。在 MRI 上，导管内乳头状瘤可被视为一个充满液体的乳导管远端有明显强化的肿块。平扫 T_1 或 T_2 加权序列上的高信号的乳导管中可识别出导管内的低信号肿块，类似于乳导管造影的充盈缺损（图 14-52）。时间 - 强度曲线通常呈快速的初始强化及流出型延迟强化[64]。

（七）术后改变

术后瘢痕组织的强化可持续性存在于手术后 2 年以上。一般来说，在大约 6 个月内恢复，但会根据伤口愈合能力而变化。最常见的术后瘢痕可通过增强程度与复发或残留恶性肿瘤区别开。通常，瘢痕组织呈沿切口部位均匀的轻度强化，而复发或残留肿瘤常表现为多结节状的快

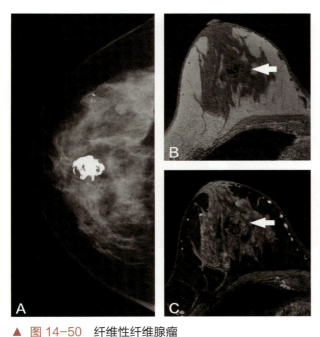

▲ 图 14-50 纤维性纤维腺瘤

61 岁新近诊断浸润性乳腺癌患者，行 MRI 评估病变治疗范围。头足位乳腺 X 线（A）显示乳腺中央粗大钙化，符合纤维性纤维腺瘤。平扫 T_1 加权像呈低信号（B），增强脂肪饱和 T_1 加权像（C）无强化（箭）

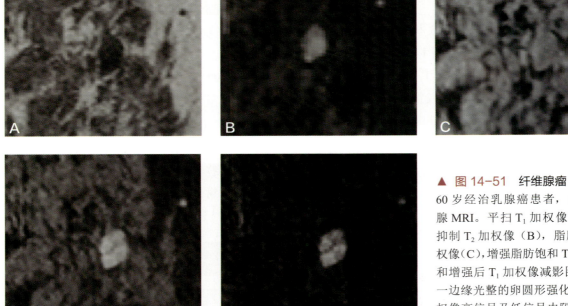

▲ 图 14-51 纤维腺瘤

60 岁经治乳腺癌患者，高危筛查乳腺 MRI。平扫 T_1 加权像（A），脂肪抑制 T_2 加权像（B），脂肪饱和 T_1 加权像（C），增强脂肪饱和 T_1 加权像（D）和增强后 T_1 加权像减影图（E）显示一边缘光整的卵圆形强化肿块，T_2 加权像高信号及低信号内隔膜，符合纤维腺瘤

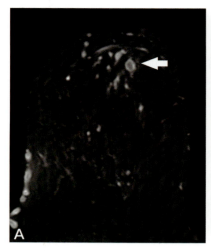 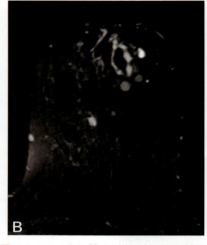 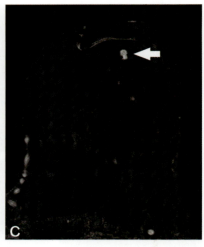

▲ 图 14-52　乳导管内肿块引起的导管扩张症

54 岁女性，新近诊断右乳浸润性乳腺癌，MRI 评估病变范围。在乳腺中，乳晕下区域是导管内卵圆形肿块（箭），其在轴位脂肪抑制 T_2 加权像（A）上扩张导管内的液体。其他层面脂肪抑制 T_2 加权像显示多个扩张积液的乳导管（B）。增强 T_1 加权减影图像（C）显示是此卵圆形、边界清晰的肿块呈明显不均匀增强。活检显示为硬化性乳头状瘤伴局灶性非典型小叶增生

速强化并可引起肿块效应。在术后乳腺中脂肪坏死也很常见，表现为形态不规则且在边缘呈明显环状强化的肿块。脂肪坏死的特征是在肿块中心存在与脂肪相一致的信号。在平扫 T_1 加权序列上呈同脂肪一样的高信号，而脂肪饱和图像上信号被抑制（图 14-53）。

术后或活检后的皮下积液和血肿中充满液体，其内部信号强度多变（图 14-54）。血肿由于其内血液成分的存在，通常在 T_1 加权像上表现出高信号，而皮下积液在 T_2 加权像上更为明亮。皮下积液和血肿均表现为均匀菲薄的环状强化。若有更多的结节性强化区域时应该怀疑有残留或复发的恶性肿瘤。

七、乳腺 MRI 恶性征象

恶性肿瘤有些特殊的影像特征已被证明是有高度特异性的，这将在下面更详细地描述。除了评估原发病灶外，可评估乳腺癌的其他相关或继发征象，如乳头退缩或浸润同样主要（图 14-55 和图 14-56）。相关征象列述于框 14-5。仔细观察 MRI 视野中的乳腺癌常见转移的常见部位同样重要，特别是对于确诊晚期乳腺癌的患者，这些部位包括胸骨和肋骨（图 14-57）、胸膜间隙（恶性胸腔积液）和肝脏。

（一）浸润性乳腺癌

浸润性乳腺癌（无论任何组织病理学亚型）最常见的 MRI 表现为肿块。先前的多个研究已经证实，边缘毛刺状的特殊形态（阳性预测值 76%～88%）和边缘强化（阳性预测值 79%～92%）对浸润性乳腺癌的诊断具有高度的预测作用[65]。研究还表明，大小在 10mm 以上的形态不规则或者边缘有毛刺状改变伴有内部不均匀强化的肿块病变[66,67]，而那些显示边缘光滑且有均匀增强的肿瘤恶性概率非常低[67]。如果有初始快速增强[66]和延迟流出[68]这样的动力学强化特征则预测存

框 14-5　乳腺癌的相关特征和继发征象

- 皮肤增厚、内陷或受侵（通过直接浸润或炎性乳腺癌）
- 乳头内陷或受侵
- 侵犯肌肉
- 侵犯乳房悬韧带（Cooper 韧带）
- 结构变形
- 圆形或无"脂肪门"的腋窝淋巴结

Chapter 14 乳腺 MRI
Breast MRI

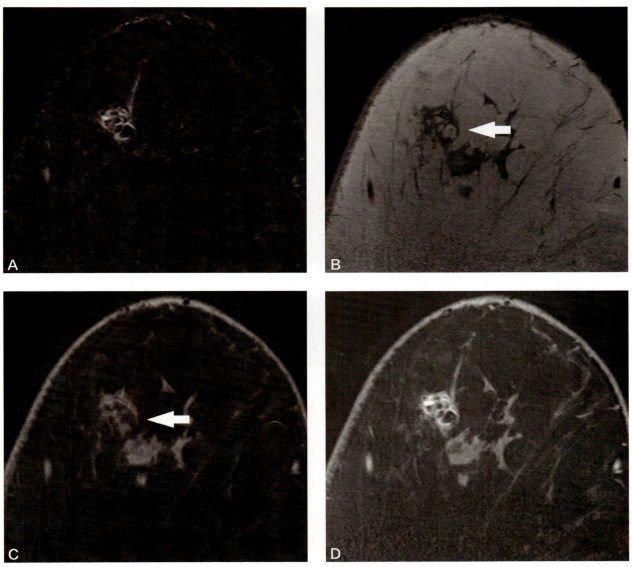

▲ 图 14-53 脂肪坏死

52 岁女性，近期左乳固定术后。轴位增强后 T_1 加权减影图（A），平扫 T_1 加权像（B），脂肪抑制 T_2 加权像（C）及增强脂肪饱和 T_1 加权像（D）显示左乳上内象限一分叶状肿块伴有边缘强化，其中心 T_1 高信号（箭）和 T_2 低信号（箭）经脂肪饱和序列证实为脂肪信号。这些发现符合脂肪坏死表现

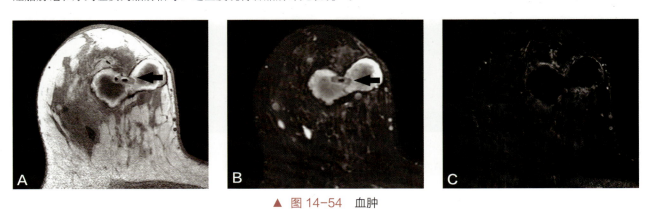

▲ 图 14-54 血肿

54 岁女性，近期经皮穿刺活检术后。平扫 T_1 加权像（A），脂肪抑制 T_2 加权像（B）及增强减影图像（C）显示一"双瓣状"不均质信号团，轻微的薄环状边缘强化，符合血肿表现。其中心可见活检标记（箭）

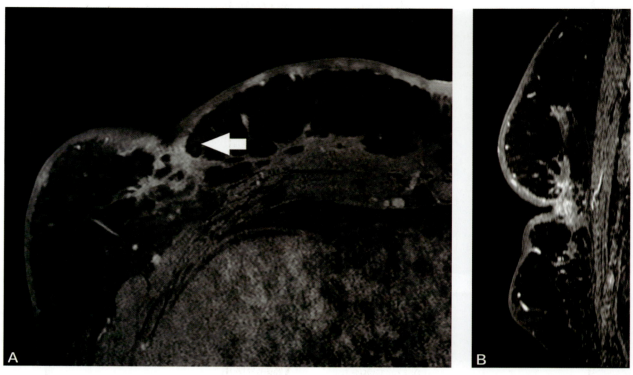

▲ 图 14-55 乳头内陷

71 岁浸润性导管癌女性患者。在轴位（A）和矢状位（B）增强脂肪饱和 T_1 加权像可见继发于已知恶性肿瘤的乳头内陷征象

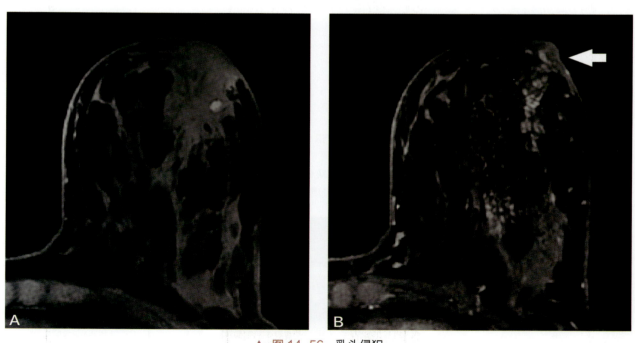

▲ 图 14-56 乳头侵犯

39 岁女性高危筛查乳腺 MRI。平扫（A）、增强后（B）轴位脂肪饱和 T_1 加权像示外侧乳腺非肿块样强化且强化范围延伸至乳头，表明乳头受侵（箭）。活检证实为浸润性导管癌

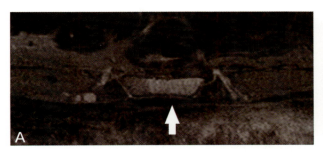 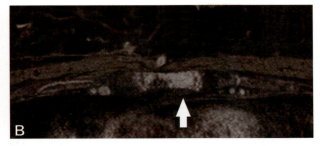

▲ 图 14-57 胸骨转移

70 岁右侧乳腺癌 IV 期患者。乳腺 MRI 对治疗反应进行评估。增强后轴位 T_1 加权像显示胸骨内两个不同层面的转移病变（箭）强化

在恶性肿瘤，但总体上预测值比形态学的特征预测值要低[54]。

浸润性导管癌占浸润性乳腺癌的绝大多数（70%～90%），通常表现为上述 MRI 特征（图 14-58）。浸润性小叶癌是浸润性乳腺癌的第二大常见亚型，由于其浸润性生长方式而被公认在乳腺 X 线上有高度隐匿性。然而，MRI 对浸润性小叶癌的检测灵敏度约为 93%，并不明显低于浸润性导管癌[69]。此外，虽然大多数的浸润性小叶癌在磁共振成像中表现为肿块，但那些显示为非肿块样强化的患者更有可能是乳腺 X 线成像中隐匿的小叶癌，其表现为弥漫性浸润性生长方式（图 14-59）。

浸润性乳腺癌的几个特殊亚型，包括浸润性乳头状癌、黏液性癌、化生癌和髓质癌，更常在 MRI 上表现为相对良性的影像学特征，如圆形或椭圆形的肿块和边界分明的边缘[70]。浸润性乳头状癌预后良好，多见于绝经后妇女，表现为均匀的内部强化。黏液性和化生性癌在老年妇女中也较为常见，并且由于黏液（对于黏液性癌）或囊性变性（对于化生性癌）的存在，两者在 T_2 加权图像上都表现出高信号区。黏性癌通常也表现出不同的 T_1 加权信号，这取决于病变中蛋白质的含量（图 14-60）。在化生性和黏液性肿瘤中，病变周围的存活的肿瘤细胞通常会导致在 MRI 上表现为不规则的边缘增强及多变的动力学强化特征。髓样癌多见于较年轻的患者，约 60% 的患者年龄小于 50 岁。除了卵圆形或圆形的形态外，这些癌症也常常表现出边缘强化或无强化的内部隔膜[71]，有时难以和纤维腺瘤区分。

恶性叶状肿瘤最常见于 50 岁以上女性。这些肿瘤比其他原发性乳腺癌更接近于组织病理学上的肉瘤样病变，而且它们通常表现为圆形或卵圆形，在 MRI 上界限清晰，这使得它们很难单纯依靠 MRI 特征与纤维腺瘤区分开。虽然 MRI 对早期诊断不太有用，但当已知的恶性叶状瘤难以仅通过临床评估和（或）标准影像学来确定时，MRI 可能对确定外科规划切除病变的全部范围有用[49]。

炎性乳腺癌是局部进展期乳腺癌的一种形式，它可以与任何乳腺浸润性腺癌的病理亚型相关，最常见的是浸润性导管癌。炎性乳腺癌的临床诊断依据表皮红斑、水肿（皮肤橘皮样改变）和乳腺肿胀如果皮肤淋巴管受累则可以确定诊断，但由于只有 75% 的皮肤活组织检查存在，故不作为诊断的必要条件。与乳腺 X 线相似，MRI 提示炎性乳腺癌的征象包括单侧乳房增大、皮肤增强和弥漫性乳腺水肿（图 14-61）[72]。MRI 对于鉴别原发性癌症（敏感性为 98% 到 68%）特别有用，可以表现为肿块或非肿块强化；并且与乳腺 X 线检查相比，MRI 可确定胸壁肌肉和区域淋巴结链是否受侵[73]。此外，MRI 在确定新辅助化疗反应方面优于其他所有方式，新辅助化疗因其能够降低转移扩散率和优化局部控制而成为炎性乳腺癌治疗的主要手段。

（二）乳腺导管内原位癌

乳腺导管内原位癌（ductal carcinoma in situ, DCIS）是侵袭性乳腺癌的前驱病变，由于筛查更为普遍，其被诊断出的频率更高。乳腺 MRI 最初

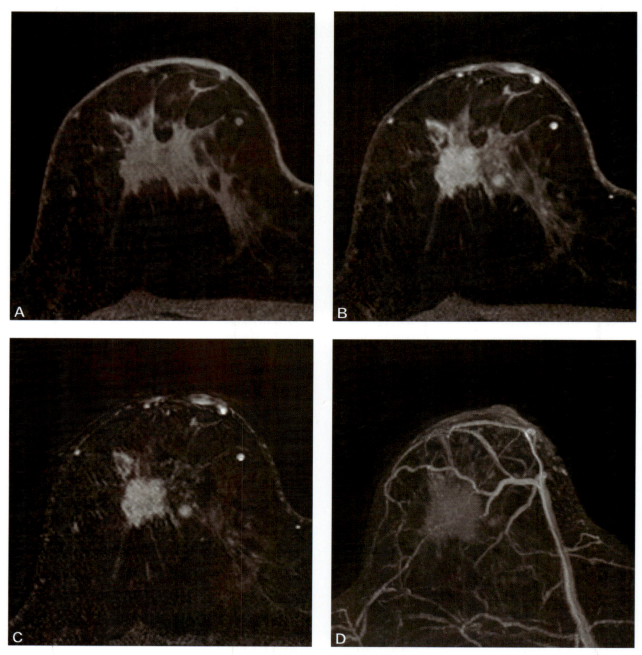

▲ 图 14-58 浸润性导管癌

42 岁新近诊断乳腺癌患者，乳腺 MRI 评估病变范围。平扫（A）和增强（B）轴位脂肪饱和 T_1 加权像，增强 T_1 加权减影图像（C），最大强度投影图像（D）显示一不规则肿块伴边缘毛刺，不均匀强化；活检证实为浸润性导管癌

被认为是对导管内原位癌评价能力相对较差，假阴性率高[74]。随着磁共振成像技术从强调高时间分辨率转向高空间分辨率，常代表导管内原位癌的形态学特征（如非肿块强化等）逐渐被识别。此后多项研究显示，与乳腺 X 线成像相比，MRI 在诊断导管内原位癌的灵敏度（92%～56%）[12] 和评价最近诊断的导管内原位癌疾病程度的准确性上都具有优势[75]。有趣的是，与乳腺 X 线检查相比，MRI 也能鉴别出更多的高级别病变[38]。因为据估计，如果不进行治疗，多达一半的诊断导管内原位癌病变不会对女性的生命产生不利影响，因此 MRI 可能优先识别导管内原位癌的生

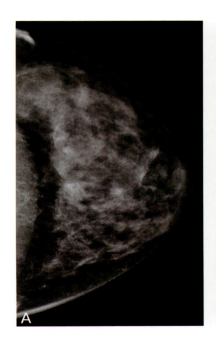
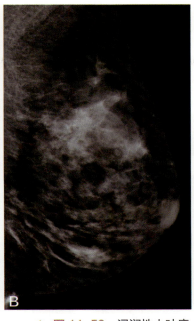
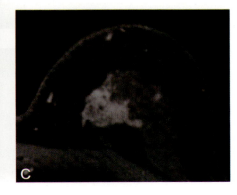

▲ 图 14-59 浸润性小叶癌

48 岁女性，小叶原位癌病史。左乳乳腺 X 线头足位及内外侧斜位（A、B）均未见异常。高危筛查的 MRI 中发现不规则肿块伴边缘毛刺。活检证实为浸润性小叶癌

物侵袭形式，这引起了导管内原位癌风险的潜在 MRI 生物标志物的研究[76]。

导管内原位癌在乳腺 MRI 上最常表现为节段性或导管性非肿块强化，具有成簇状的内部增强形态学特征，占 MRI 上可见导管内原位癌病变的 60%～80%。导管内原位癌在 MRI 上少见的表现包括增强肿块（14%～34%）和增强灶（1%～12%）[77-79]。导管内原位癌具有可变的动力学强化特征，从快速的初始增强伴流出到 5%～10% 的病例没有增强（图 14-62）[80]。

八、乳腺 MRI 上的高危病变

高危病变包括各种各样的乳腺病理，当通过空心针穿刺活检诊断时，由于对病变的采样不足或核心样本病理解释的差异，很有可能在手术切除后升级为恶性肿瘤。因此，最初由 MRI 检查发现为高风险病变升级为恶性病变的比率从 13%～57% 不等[81]。

这些病变包括不典型导管增生、小叶肿瘤［包括原位小叶癌（lobular carcinoma in situ，LCIS）和不典型小叶增生］、放射状瘢痕/复杂硬化病变、乳头瘤和扁平上皮非典型增生。对其中一些病变的治疗（手术切除与观察）仍有争议，而且各机构也各不相同，特别是对于放射状瘢痕/复杂硬化病变和非异型性乳头状瘤。不幸的是，目前没有特定的形态学或动力学强化特征用以鉴别 MRI 上的高危病灶，或确定适合于随访的时间而不是手术切除[82]。无论如何，与良性病变一样，任何在 MRI 上被认为是高度可疑的恶性肿瘤发现（例如，不规则形状的肿块边缘呈毛刺状，呈异质性或边缘强化，初始阶段快速延迟期流出的动力学强化曲线）与穿刺活检诊断病理不一致，应追加病理取样。

九、硅胶乳房植入假体的评价

MRI 是评价硅胶乳房植入假体并发症的最灵敏和最特异的影像学方式[30,32,83]。单腔型硅胶植入物由填充液体硅树脂的弹性体壳组成。在 silicone-only 序列图像上，硅凝胶应该是明亮的，弹性体壳本身不应该有信号，表现为一条细黑线。植入物自身并不能考虑到乳房的自然弯曲度，因此，在成像中，植入物可能有正常的波

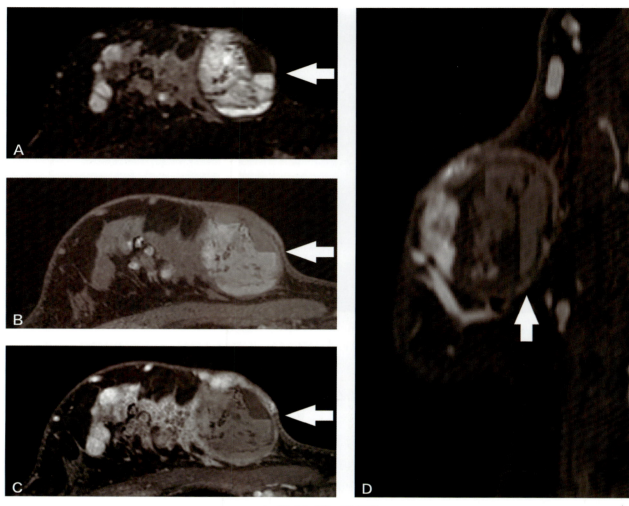

▲ 图 14-60 黏液癌

44 岁女性，新近诊断黏液癌。平扫轴位脂肪抑制 T_2 加权像（A），轴位平扫脂肪饱和 T_1 加权像（B），增强轴位（C）和矢状位（D）脂肪饱和 T_1 加权像显示一边界局限的卵圆形肿块，伴结节状强化，T_2 加权像上呈不均匀高信号伴液 - 液平面（箭）。注意前平扫 T_1 加权像的固有高信号。这与病理证实的黏液型肿瘤一致

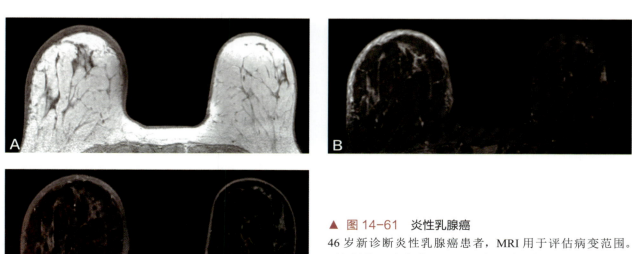

▲ 图 14-61 炎性乳腺癌

46 岁新诊断炎性乳腺癌患者，MRI 用于评估病变范围。平扫轴位 T_1 加权像（A），脂肪抑制 T_2 加权像（B），增强脂肪饱和 T_1 加权减影图像（C）显示皮肤增厚、水肿和强化，与左乳对比右乳轻度增大，符合炎性乳腺癌表现

Chapter 14 乳腺 MRI
Breast MRI

动或被称为"径向皱褶"的褶皱，这可能会在评估破裂时引起混淆（图 14-63）。随着时间的推移，身体在植入物周围形成了一个纤维囊，它也应该表现为一条细黑线，并且由于它的位置靠近外壳，通常不能从一个正常的植入物的弹性体外壳中分辨出独特的结构。

植入假体是根据成分和位置来描述的。如前所述，MRI 可用于怀疑有硅胶植入物并发症的患者，而生理盐水植入物破裂有典型的临床表现。植入假体可能位于两个部位之一：胸肌前（也称为腺下、腺后或乳房后）或胸肌下。胸肌前植入物位于胸肌前，但位于纤维腺体组织后，而胸肌下植入物位于胸大肌后（但通常位于胸小肌前）。

硅胶植入假体并发症

植入物植入年限已被证明是导致植入物破裂的最重要因素，研究表明，植入物完好无损的患者人数随着植入物植入年限的增加而减少[31]。一项研究预测植入物的完好曲线从 8 年后的 89% 下降到 14 年后的 29%，再到 20 年后的 5%[28]。

硅胶植入物破裂主要有两种类型：囊内破裂和囊外破裂。在囊内破裂中，植入物外壳破裂，然而，外部纤维囊仍然完好无损，因此，硅凝胶在外壳外面，但仍然被纤维囊所包裹。在囊外破裂中，弹性外体壳和纤维囊都被破坏，这使得硅凝胶扩散到正常的乳腺组织中。在这些情况下，可能会有硅胶通过淋巴引流到腋窝和乳房内的淋巴结（图 14-64）。随着时间的推移，将会发生肉芽肿炎，并且与囊外硅凝胶相关的组织信号可能降低。

外伤是硅胶植入物破裂的最常见原因，它可以从植入时开始，这时可以产生一个小裂缝，允许硅胶泄漏到外壳外。硅油可以从凝胶中分离出来，通过弹性体壳扩散，随着时间的推移，会导致弹性体壳与纤维囊的粘连。由于硅胶无法在植入体外壳和纤维囊之间自由移动，这才造成更多的局灶性囊内破裂。随着时间的推移，硅胶会引起植入物外壳的局部塌陷，并以"反相环"或"锁孔"的形式出现，显示出未塌陷的囊内破裂（图

14-65A）。随着渗漏的进展，硅胶可能在外壳和纤维囊之间交叉，导致"包膜下线征"（图 14-65B）。随着渗漏的继续，植入物外壳可以折叠在其自身上，从而产生一堆低信号线。泄漏的硅凝

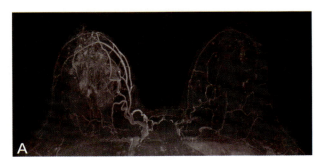
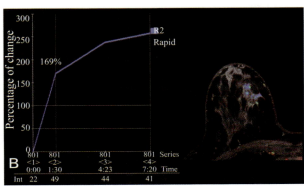

▲ 图 14-62 导管内原位癌

53 岁右乳导管内原位癌患者，MRI 评估病变范围。轴位最大强度投影（A）右乳内不对称的节段性非肿块强化，非均匀的内部强化从乳头 - 乳晕复合体延伸至距胸壁 10mm 处。计算机辅助的增强动力学评估（B）显示初始快速增强（强化率 >100%）。然而，有持续的后期强化特征，这在良性病变中更典型，但在导管内原位癌中比较常见。这说明良性和恶性病变之间的动力学强化特征存在重叠，而动力学曲线的评估只能在形态学特征的背景下进行

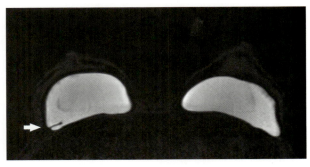

▲ 图 14-63 径向褶皱

50 岁女性，双侧胸肌前硅胶假体植入，高危筛查。轴位 silicone-only 序列显示一细线状低信号，其可以追溯到周围的种植入体壳，与径向褶皱一致，这是一个正常的发现

胶会慢慢地包围植入物囊，它将表现为暗的或波浪状的"浮动"线，有时称为囊内破裂的"舌征"。这是植入体破裂的特异性征象（图 14-66）。

长的径向皱襞可与囊内破裂的扁面条征混淆，然而，这可以通过追溯回完整的弹性体壳来解决。放射状褶皱应始终追溯到植入物外壳，而由于囊内破裂塌陷所致的黑线影则不会。尽管如此，有时很难诊断，复杂的径向折叠可能被错误地解释为囊内破裂。

十、MRI 上可疑病变的组织病理学取样

当乳腺 MRI 发现可疑病变时，需要组织病理学评估以明确诊断。为了实现这一点，通常有两种方法：靶向超声评估超声发现的可疑病灶，然后在超声或 MRI 引导下进行空心针穿刺活检。对 MRI 可疑的发现进行靶向超声有以下几个优点，第一，它允许对 MRI 的发现进行进一步的特性描述，有时部分发现可定义为良性（例如，乳内淋巴结）。第二，超声引导活检比 MRI 引导活检费用低，对患者而言更舒适。第三，超声允许更大程度地显露后部和腋窝组织，并可检出与胸前植入物密切相关的病变。

常规进行靶向超声来进一步评估 MRI 可疑病变也有很大的风险。有时，确定超声与 MRI 可疑发现之间的相关性是很有挑战性的，尤其是在非肿块强化、小于 5～10mm 的小病变以及在超声上有非均质乳腺组织的患者。此外，常规进行靶向超声检查以评估 MRI 表现，可能会导致患者在检查和最终诊断病变时出现不必要的延误。最后，由于 MRI 检测到的 43%～53% 恶性肿瘤超声无相关发现，因此，阴性的超声结果不能排除对 MRI 检测到的可疑发现进行组织病理学取样的必要性[84,85]。由于这些因素，作者提倡只在乳腺磁共振检查后进行有针对性的超声检查，这时在超声引导下极有可能发现病变。一般来说，这是用于较大肿块（通常至少为 10mm），在一个非常有利于超声识别的位置，或位于腋窝，或靠近胸前的植入物。由于超声识别的可能性较低，我们不建议常规通过超声评估可疑非肿块强化或病灶[85]。当建议靶向超声时，放射科医师提供明确的说明是非常必要的，如果可能的话，在超声不能识别病灶的情况下，应在 MRI 指导下进行病变取样。

无论用什么方式及设备或系统，在 MRI 引导下进行乳腺活检的基本要求和步骤是相似的。对于每个系统如何进行 MRI 引导下活检的详细指导已超出了本章的范围。为了总结基本步骤，首先使用专用乳腺线圈患者呈俯卧位，将包含感兴趣

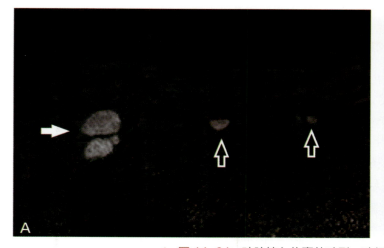
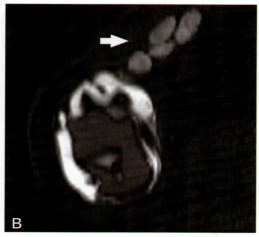

▲ 图 14-64　硅胶植入体囊外破裂，硅凝胶沉积于腋窝淋巴结

轴位（A）和矢状位（B）只显示硅胶序列患者双侧双腔假体植入后，内侧腔内为盐水，外侧腔内为硅胶。囊外破裂，伴腋窝（白箭）及乳内淋巴结（黑箭）硅胶沉积

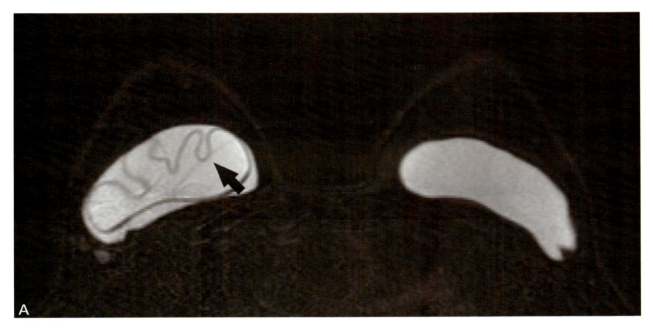
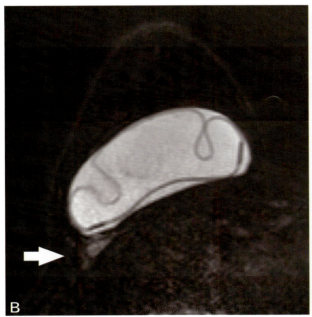
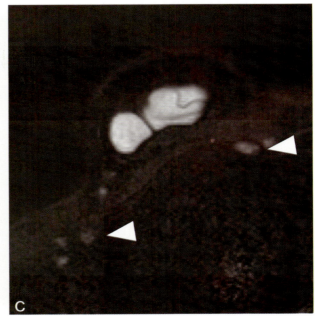

▲ 图 14-65 非塌陷性囊内破裂

60 岁双侧胸前区硅胶假体植入，MRI 评估破裂情况。轴位 silicone-only 成像序列双乳（A）及右乳不同层面图像（B、C）除了在右侧硅胶植入物的后外侧高信号（白箭）外，还显示了囊内破裂的"匙孔征"（黑箭）。此外，在 1 级腋窝淋巴结和单个内乳腺淋巴结中存在高硅信号，这与硅胶沉积一致，从而进一步证明了囊外破裂（箭头）

病灶的乳腺压缩在包含基准标记的网格中，该基准标记在 T_1 加权序列上可见。获得平扫和增强图像（通常在矢状位方向上，因为大多数技术只允许内侧或外侧入路），然后确定病变的位置（使用手动方法或借助软件辅助），允许网格上适当的方框进入皮肤，并确定正确的进针深度。完成皮肤灭菌消毒后，进行局部麻醉，并经过皮肤将 MRI 活检同轴系统的外部组件（可选择使用手术刀，作者认为很少需要）引入至乳房内的适当深度。同轴护套通过塑料针导向器（通常有 9 个隧道的方形塑料盒）放置在合适的格栅空间内，并用塑料闭孔器将内管芯取出并更换。然后，进

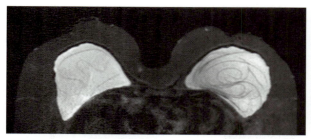

▲ 图 14-66　硅胶植入体囊内破裂的"发丝征"

76 岁女性，保留皮肤双侧乳腺切除术后胸大肌后硅胶假体重建术后。轴位有机硅成像序列显示双侧植入体囊内破裂的"发丝征"，有多个无法延续到外壳的薄的低信号线影

行乳房扫描以确认鞘的位置，并用 MRI 兼容的真空辅助乳腺活检装置代替闭孔器。通常会得到 8～12 个样本，并在鞘内放置活检标志夹。最后，进行 MRI 扫描和双视图常规乳腺 X 线检查，以确定夹子的留置和位置。夹子的留置是必要的，因为它有利于在必要时进行乳腺 X 线定位，这比 MRI 引导定位更容易执行，也更便宜。

十一、总结

乳腺 MRI 是一种强大的成像工具，为乳腺癌和硅胶植入物并发症的检测提供了最高的灵敏度，并提供了无与伦比的影像上的病变特征，有助于评估乳腺癌患者对新辅助化疗的病情程度和治疗反应。与超声和常规乳腺 X 线相比，它的成本相对较高，并且其特异性还不完善，乳腺 MRI 必须慎重使用，应评估适应证，以使其临床价值可以最大化。此外，有必要全面了解高质量 MRI 采集的基本技术要求，以避免次佳的图像和伪影。最后，如美国放射学会 BI-RADS 词汇所概述的，使用标准化报告是必要的，以便提供具有一致性并与临床密切相关的报告和诊断。

关注焦点

● 乳腺 MRI 适应证包括高危患者（超过 20% 一生中罹患癌症的风险）筛查，评估新诊断乳腺癌患者疾病的程度，评价新辅助化疗，原发灶不明的腋窝转移性的诊断隐匿性乳腺癌，以及评价硅胶植入物的完整性。

● 乳腺 MRI 应用高场强磁体和专用乳腺线圈进行，以获得高空间分辨率和时间分辨率的动态对比增强图像。

● 全面了解 BI-RADS 的标准化报告对提供重点和临床相关的 MRI 评估及诊断至关重要。

● MRI 最可疑的发现应该用来指导 BI-RADS 评估，可疑的形态学特征优于看似优越的动态增强曲线。

● 由于乳腺 MRI 的特异性还不完美，所以乳腺 MRI 上的可疑发现在影响临床决策之前需进行活检，这些病例需在 MRI 或超声引导下进行。

参考文献

[1] Damadian R. Tumor detection by nuclear magnetic resonance. *Science (New York)*. 1971;171(3976):1151–1153.

[2] Bovee WM, Getreuer KW, Smidt J, Lindeman J. Nuclear magnetic resonance and detection of human breast tumor. *Journal of the National Cancer Institute*. 1978;61(1):53–55.

[3] Mansfield P, Morris PG, Ordidge RJ, Pykett IL, Bangert V, Coupland RE. Human whole body imaging and detection of breast tumours by n.m.r. *Philosophical Transactions of the Royal Society of London Series B, Biological Sciences*. 1980;289(1037):503–510.

[4] Ross RJ, Thompson JS, Kim K, Bailey RA. Nuclear magnetic resonance imaging and evaluation of human breast tissue: Preliminary clinical trials. *Radiology*. 1982;143(1):195–205.

[5] Kaiser WA, Zeitler E. MR imaging of the breast: Fast imaging sequences with and without Gd-DTPA. Preliminary observations. *Radiology*. 1989;170(3 Pt 1):681–686.

[6] Orel SG, Schnall MD. MR imaging of the breast for the detection, diagnosis, and staging of breast cancer. *Radiology*. 2001;220(1):13–30.

[7] Saslow D, Boetes C, Burke W et al. American Cancer Society guidelines for breast screening with MRI as an adjunct to mammography. *CA: A Cancer Journal for Clinicians*. 2007;57(2):75–89.

[8] Mainiero MB, Lourenco A, Mahoney MC et al. ACR appropriateness criteria breast cancer screening. *Journal of the American College of Radiology: JACR*. 2013;10(1):11–14.

[9] Brennan S, Liberman L, Dershaw DD, Morris E. Breast MRI screening of women with a personal history of breast cancer. *AJR American Journal of Roentgenology*. 2010;195(2):510–516.

[10] Sung JS, Malak SF, Bajaj P, Alis R, Dershaw DD, Morris EA. Screening breast MR imaging in women with a history of lobular carcinoma in situ. *Radiology*. 2011;261(2):414–420.

[11] Schacht DV, Yamaguchi K, Lai J, Kulkarni K, Sennett CA, Abe H. Importance of a personal history of breast cancer as a risk factor for the development of subsequent breast cancer: Results from screening breast MRI. *AJR American Journal of Roentgenology*. 2014;202(2):289–292.

[12] Lehman CD, Gatsonis C, Kuhl CK et al. MRI evaluation of the contralateral breast in women with recently diagnosed breast cancer. *The New England Journal of Medicine*. 2007;356(13):1295–1303.

[13] DeMartini W, Lehman C. A review of current evidence-based clinical applications for breast magnetic resonance imaging. *Topics in Magnetic Resonance Imaging: TMRI*. 2008;19(3):143–150.

[14] Liberman L. Breast MR imaging in assessing extent of disease. *Magnetic Resonance Imaging Clinics of North America*. 2006;14(3):339–349, vi.

[15] Sung JS, Li J, Costa GD et al. Preoperative breast MRI for early-stage breast cancer: Effect on surgical and long-term outcomes. *AJR American Journal of Roentgenology*. 2014;202(6):1376–1382.

[16] Lee CI, Bensink ME, Berry K et al. Performance goals for an adjunct diagnostic test to reduce unnecessary biopsies after screening mammography: Analysis of costs, benefits, and consequences. *Journal of the American College of Radiology: JACR*. 2013;10(12):924–930.

[17] Cilotti A, Iacconi C, Marini C et al. Contrast-enhanced MR imaging in patients with BI-RADS 3–5 microcalcifications. *La Radiologia Medica*. 2007;112(2):272–286.

[18] Bluemke DA, Gatsonis CA, Chen MH et al. Magnetic resonance imaging of the breast prior to biopsy. *JAMA*. 2004;292(22):2735–2742.

[19] Yau EJ, Gutierrez RL, DeMartini WB, Eby PR, Peacock S, Lehman CD. The utility of breast MRI as a problem solving tool. *The Breast Journal*. 2011;17(3):273–280.

[20] Lorenzon M, Zuiani C, Linda A, Londero V, Girometti R, Bazzocchi M. Magnetic resonance imaging in patients with nipple discharge: Should we recommend it? *European Radiology*. 2011;21(5):899–907.

[21] Fisher B, Bryant J, Wolmark N et al. Effect of preoperative chemotherapy on the outcome of women with operable breast cancer. *Journal of Clinical Oncology: Official Journal of the American Society of Clinical Oncology*. 1998;16(8):2672–2685.

[22] Wolmark N, Wang J, Mamounas E, Bryant J, Fisher B. Preoperative chemotherapy in patients with operable breast cancer: Nine-year results from National Surgical Adjuvant Breast and Bowel Project B-18. *Journal of the National Cancer Institute Monographs*. 2001(30):96–102.

[23] Martincich L, Montemurro F, De Rosa G et al. Monitoring response to primary chemotherapy in breast cancer using dynamic contrast-enhanced magnetic resonance imaging. *Breast Cancer Research and Treatment*. 2004;83(1):67–76.

[24] Pickles MD, Lowry M, Manton DJ, Gibbs P, Turnbull LW. Role of dynamic contrast enhanced MRI in monitoring early response of locally advanced breast cancer to neoadjuvant chemotherapy. *Breast Cancer Research and Treatment*. 2005;91(1):1–10.

[25] Rosen EL, Blackwell KL, Baker JA et al. Accuracy of MRI in the detection of residual breast cancer after neoadjuvant chemotherapy. *AJR American Journal of Roentgenology*. 2003;181(5):1275–1282.

[26] Weatherall PT, Evans GF, Metzger GJ, Saborrian MH, Leitch AM. MRI vs. histologic measurement of breast cancer following chemotherapy: Comparison with x-ray mammography and palpation. *Journal of Magnetic Resonance Imaging*. 2001;13(6):868–875.

[27] Hylton NM, Blume JD, Bernreuter WK et al. Locally advanced breast cancer: MR imaging for prediction of response to neoadjuvant chemotherapy— results from ACRIN 6657/I-SPY TRIAL. *Radiology*. 2012;263(3):663–672.

[28] Robinson OG, Jr., Bradley EL, Wilson DS. Analysis of explanted silicone implants: A report of 300 patients. *Annals of Plastic Surgery*. 1995;34(1):1–6; discussion 7.

[29] Brenner RJ. Evaluation of breast silicone implants. *Magnetic Resonance Imaging Clinics of North America*. 2013;21(3):547–560.

[30] Ahn CY, DeBruhl ND, Gorczyca DP, Shaw WW, Bassett LW. Comparative silicone breast implant evaluation using mammography, sonography, and magnetic resonance imaging: Experience with 59 implants. *Plastic and Reconstructive Surgery*. 1994;94(5):620–627.

[31] Berg WA, Caskey CI, Hamper UM et al. Diagnosing breast implant rupture with MR imaging, US, and mammography. *Radio Graphics: A Review Publication of the Radiological Society of North America, Inc*. 1993;13(6):1323–1336.

[32] Everson LI, Parantainen H, Detlie T et al. Diagnosis of breast implant rupture: Imaging findings and relative efficacies of imaging techniques. *AJR American Journal of Roentgenology*. 1994;163(1):57–60.

[33] Reynolds HE, Buckwalter KA, Jackson VP, Siwy BK, Alexander SG. Comparison of mammography, sonography, and magnetic resonance imaging in the detection of silicone-gel breast implant rupture. *Annals of Plastic Surgery*. 1994;33(3):247–255; discussion 56–57.

[34] Weizer G, Malone RS, Netscher DT, Walker LE, Thornby J. Utility of magnetic resonance imaging and ultrasonography in diagnosing breast implant rupture. *Annals of Plastic Surgery*. 1995;34(4):352–361.

[35] Hendrick RE. High-quality breast MRI. *Radiologic Clinics of North America*. 2014;52(3):547–562.

[36] Rausch DR, Hendrick RE. How to optimize clinical breast MR imaging practices and techniques on Your 1.5-T system. *RadioGraphics: A Review Publication of the Radiological Society of North America, Inc.* 2006;26(5): 1469–1484.

[37] Rahbar H, Partridge SC, Javid SH, Lehman CD. Imaging axillary lymph nodes in patients with newly diagnosed breast cancer. *Current Problems in Diagnostic Radiology.* 2012;41(5):149–158.

[38] Kuhl CK, Schrading S, Bieling HB et al. MRI for diagnosis of pure ductal carcinoma in situ: A prospective observational study. *Lancet.* 2007;370(9586):485–492.

[39] Nnewihe AN, Grafendorfer T, Daniel BL et al. Custom fitted 16-channel bilateral breast coil for bidirectional parallel imaging. *Magnetic Resonance in Medicine.* 2011;66(1):281–289.

[40] Hendrick RE, Haacke EM. Basic physics of MR contrast agents and maximization of image contrast. *Journal of Magnetic Resonance Imaging.* 1993;3(1):137–148.

[41] Kuhl CK. Breast MR imaging at 3T. *Magnetic Resonance Imaging Clinics of North America.* 2007;15(3):315–320, vi.

[42] Wang LC, DeMartini WB, Partridge SC, Peacock S, Lehman CD. MRI-detected suspicious breast lesions: Predictive values of kinetic features measured by computer-aided evaluation. *AJR American Journal of Roentgenology.* 2009;193(3):826–831.

[43] Huang W, Tudorica LA, Li X et al. Discrimination of benign and malignant breast lesions by using shutter-speed dynamic contrast-enhanced MR imaging. *Radiology.* 2011;261(2):394–403.

[44] Li X, Huang W, Yankeelov TE, Tudorica A, Rooney WD, Springer CS, Jr. Shutter-speed analysis of contrast reagent bolus-tracking data: Preliminary observations in benign and malignant breast disease. *Magnetic Resonance in Medicine.* 2005;53(3):724–729.

[45] Bitar R, Leung G, Perng R et al. MR pulse sequences: What every radiologist wants to know but is afraid to ask. *RadioGraphics.* 2006;26(2):513–537.

[46] Kuhl CK. Current status of breast MR imaging. Part 2. Clinical applications. *Radiology.* 2007;244(3):672–691.

[47] Rahbar H, Partridge SC, DeMartini WB, Thursten B, Lehman CD. Clinical and technical considerations for high quality breast MRI at 3 Tesla. *Journal of Magnetic Resonance Imaging: JMRI.* 2013;37(4):778–790.

[48] Kuhl CK, Jost P, Morakkabati N, Zivanovic O, Schild HH, Gieseke J. Contrast-enhanced MR imaging of the breast at 3.0 and 1.5 T in the same patients: Initial experience. *Radiology.* 2006;239(3):666–676.

[49] Calhoun KE, Allison KA, Kim JN, Rahbar H, Anderson BO. Phyllodes tumors. In *Diseases of the Breast*, 5th edn, Harris JR, Lippman ME, Morrow M, Osborne CK (eds), 2014. Wolters Kluwer Health, Philadelphia, PA.

[50] Morris EA, Comstock CE, Lee CH et al. *ACR BI-RADS Atlas, Breast Imaging Reporting and Data System.* Reston, VA, American College of Radiology; 2013.

[51] Burnside ES, Sickles EA, Bassett LW et al. The ACR BI-RADS experience: Learning from history. *Journal of the American College of Radiology: JACR.* 2009;6(12):851–860.

[52] DeMartini WB, Liu F, Peacock S, Eby PR, Gutierrez RL, Lehman CD. Background parenchymal enhancement on breast MRI: Impact on diagnostic performance. *AJR American Journal of Roentgenology.* 2012;198(4):W373–W380.

[53] Hambly NM, Liberman L, Dershaw DD, Brennan S, Morris EA. Background parenchymal enhancement on baseline screening breast MRI: Impact on biopsy rate and short-interval follow-up. *AJR American Journal of Roentgenology.* 2011;196(1):218–224.

[54] Schnall MD, Blume J, Bluemke DA et al. Diagnostic architectural and dynamic features at breast MR imaging: Multicenter study. *Radiology.* 2006;238(1):42–53.

[55] Peters NH, Borel Rinkes IH, Zuithoff NP, Mali WP, Moons KG, Peeters PH. Meta-analysis of MR imaging in the diagnosis of breast lesions. *Radiology.* 2008;246(1):116–124.

[56] Partridge SC, McDonald ES. Diffusion weighted magnetic resonance imaging of the breast: Protocol optimization, interpretation, and clinical applications. *Magnetic Resonance Imaging Clinics of North America.* 2013;21(3):601–624.

[57] Kuroki-Suzuki S, Kuroki Y, Nasu K, Nawano S, Moriyama N, Okazaki M. Detecting breast cancer with non-contrast MR imaging: Combining diffusion-weighted and STIR imaging. *Magnetic Resonance in Medical Sciences: MRMS: An Official Journal of Japan Society of Magnetic Resonance in Medicine.* 2007;6(1):21–27.

[58] Bolan PJ. Magnetic resonance spectroscopy of the breast: Current status. *Magnetic Resonance Imaging Clinics of North America.* 2013;21(3):625–639.

[59] Wurdinger S, Herzog AB, Fischer DR et al. Differentiation of phyllodes breast tumors from fibroadenomas on MRI. *AJR American Journal of Roentgenology.* 2005;185(5):1317–1321.

[60] Brinck U, Fischer U, Korabiowska M, Jutrowski M, Schauer A, Grabbe E. The variability of fibroadenoma in contrast-enhanced dynamic MR mammography. *AJR American Journal of Roentgenology.* 1997;168(5):1331–1334.

[61] Lewis JT, Hartmann LC, Vierkant RA et al. An analysis of breast cancer risk in women with single, multiple, and atypical papilloma. *The American Journal of Surgical Pathology.* 2006;30(6):665–672.

[62] Liberman L, Tornos C, Huzjan R, Bartella L, Morris EA, Dershaw DD. Is surgical excision warranted after benign, concordant diagnosis of papilloma at percutaneous breast biopsy? *AJR American Journal of Roentgenology.* 2006;186(5):1328–1334.

[63] Jaffer S, Bleiweiss IJ, Nagi C. Incidental intraductal papillomas (<2 mm) of the breast diagnosed on needle core biopsy do not need to be excised. *The Breast Journal.* 2013;19(2):130–133.

[64] Daniel BL, Gardner RW, Birdwell RL, Nowels KW, Johnson D. Magnetic resonance imaging of intraductal papilloma of

the breast. *Magnetic Resonance Imaging*. 2003;21(8):887–892.

[65] Heller SL, Hernandez O, Moy L. Radiologic-pathologic correlation at breast MR imaging: What is the appropriate management for high-risk lesions? *Magnetic Resonance Imaging Clinics of North America*. 2013;21(3):583–599.

[66] Mahoney MC, Gatsonis C, Hanna L, DeMartini WB, Lehman C. Positive predictive value of BI-RADS MR imaging. *Radiology*. 2012;264(1):51–58.

[67] Gutierrez RL, DeMartini WB, Eby PR, Kurland BF, Peacock S, Lehman CD. BI-RADS lesion characteristics predict likelihood of malignancy in breast MRI for masses but not for nonmasslike enhancement. *AJR American Journal of Roentgenology*. 2009;193(4):994–1000.

[68] Kuhl CK, Mielcareck P, Klaschik S et al. Dynamic breast MR imaging: Are signal intensity time course data useful for differential diagnosis of enhancing lesions? *Radiology*. 1999;211(1):101–110.

[69] Mann RM, Hoogeveen YL, Blickman JG, Boetes C. MRI compared to conventional diagnostic work-up in the detection and evaluation of invasive lobular carcinoma of the breast: A review of existing literature. *Breast Cancer Research and Treatment*. 2008;107(1):1–14.

[70] Yoo JL, Woo OH, Kim YK et al. Can MR Imaging contribute in characterizing well-circumscribed breast carcinomas? *RadioGraphics*. 2010;30(6):1689–1702.

[71] Jeong SJ, Lim HS, Lee JS et al. Medullary carcinoma of the breast: MRI findings. *AJR American Journal of Roentgenology*. 2012;198(5):W482–W487.

[72] Chow CK. Imaging in inflammatory breast carcinoma. *Breast Disease*. 2005;22:45–54.

[73] Le-Petross HT, Cristofanilli M, Carkaci S et al. MRI features of inflammatory breast cancer. *AJR American Journal of Roentgenology*. 2011;197(4):W769–W776.

[74] Boetes C, Strijk SP, Holland R, Barentsz JO, Van Der Sluis RF, Ruijs JH. False-negative MR imaging of malignant breast tumors. *European Radiology*. 1997;7(8):1231–1234.

[75] Berg WA, Gutierrez L, NessAiver MS et al. Diagnostic accuracy of mammography, clinical examination, US, and MR imaging in preoperative assessment of breast cancer. *Radiology*. 2004;233(3):830–849.

[76] Rahbar H, Partridge SC, Demartini WB et al. In vivo assessment of ductal carcinoma in situ grade: A model incorporating dynamic contrast-enhanced and diffusion-weighted breast MR imaging parameters. *Radiology*. 2012;263(2):374–382.

[77] Jansen SA, Newstead GM, Abe H, Shimauchi A, Schmidt RA, Karczmar GS. Pure ductal carcinoma in situ: Kinetic and morphologic MR characteristics compared with mammographic appearance and nuclear grade. *Radiology*. 2007;245(3):684–691.

[78] Rosen EL, Smith-Foley SA, DeMartini WB, Eby PR, Peacock S, Lehman CD. BI-RADS MRI enhancement characteristics of ductal carcinoma in situ. *The Breast Journal*. 2007;13(6):545–550.

[79] Menell JH, Morris EA, Dershaw DD, Abramson AF, Brogi E, Liberman L. Determination of the presence and extent of pure ductal carcinoma in situ by mammography and magnetic resonance imaging. *The Breast Journal*. 2005;11(6):382–390.

[80] Kuhl CK. Concepts for differential diagnosis in breast MR imaging. *Magnetic Resonance Imaging Clinics of North America*. 2006;14(3):305–328, v.

[81] Heller SL, Moy L. Imaging features and management of high-risk lesions on contrast-enhanced dynamic breast MRI. *AJR American Journal of Roentgenology*. 2012;198(2):249–255.

[82] Strigel RM, Eby PR, Demartini WB et al. Frequency, upgrade rates, and characteristics of high-risk lesions initially identified with breast MRI. *AJR American Journal of Roentgenology*. 2010;195(2):792–798.

[83] Gorczyca DP, DeBruhl ND, Ahn CY et al. Silicone breast implant ruptures in an animal model: Comparison of mammography, MR imaging, US, and CT. *Radiology*. 1994;190(1):227–232.

[84] LaTrenta LR, Menell JH, Morris EA, Abramson AF, Dershaw DD, Liberman L. Breast lesions detected with MR imaging: Utility and histopathologic importance of identification with US. *Radiology*. 2003;227(3):856–861.

[85] Demartini WB, Eby PR, Peacock S, Lehman CD. Utility of targeted sonography for breast lesions that were suspicious on MRI. *AJR American Journal of Roentgenology*. 2009;192(4):1128–1134.

Chapter 15
肝脏扫描技术与肝脏弥漫性疾病

Liver: Technique and Diffuse Pathology

Michele Di Martino，Carlo Catalano 著

冯 冰 译

马霄虹 校

目录 CONTENTS

一、MR 扫描技术 / 328

二、肝的解剖 / 340

三、血管解剖与变异 / 340

四、肝脏弥漫性病变 / 341

在过去几十年里，随着能够获取快速成像序列的新型软件和硬件的发展，磁共振（magnetic resonance，MR）成像技术克服了肝脏研究中运动伪影的主要问题。另外，与计算机断层扫描技术（computed tomography，CT）相比，MR 具备更好的对比分辨率，能够区分同一实质内的不同成分（例如，脂肪、水和血液）。然而大多数情况下，上述功能并不足以正确发现并反映肝脏疾病的特征[1]。选择合适的技术设备以获得质量良好的图像至关重要。肝脏 MR 检查应在具备快速梯度的高场强设备（≥1.5T）中进行，采用相控阵体表线圈提高图像信噪比（signal-to-noise，SNR）及空间分辨率，同时使用并行采集技术减少扫描时间[2-4]。引入以钆为基础对比剂也提高了 MR 诊断的准确度，与对比增强 CT 具有相似的价值。此外在临床实践过程中，肝脏特异性对比剂的引入除了提供形态学特征还可以提供功能学信息。MR 新技术的开发，如扩散、灌注、波谱及弹性成像，在临床实践中扮演着越来越重要的角色。

一、MR 扫描技术

目前，体部 MR 检查常用磁场强度是 1.5T。在当前的发展状况下，该场强可以提供信噪比与扫描速度的最佳组合，使快速采集技术的最优化得以实现，同时又将作用于人体的能量沉积率保持在政府机构限定的范围内。该磁共振系统在依赖于磁场强度的 T_1 值与可获得组织对比效果之间提供了良好的平衡。此外，随场强增加而增加的磁场失真和顺磁性效应可能导致不良的图像伪影，而这是在 1.5T 场强设备允许范围内的。开发体部 MR 更高场强的设备理论上是支持的，并正在努力将应用于 1.5T 磁共振设备的技术迁移至 3.0T 磁共振设备上。然而，显而易见的是，先前用于将较低场强技术转移到较高场强（1.5T）的方法未成功应用于 1.5T 场强技术转移到 3.0T 场强。用于研究肝脏疾病的 MR 扫描方案包括 T_1 加权序列、T_2 加权序列、脂肪抑制 T_2 加权序列及静脉注射对比剂后增强 T_1 加权序列。

（一）T_2 加权序列

目前，快速自旋回波（turbo spin echo，TSE 或 fast spin echo，FSE）T_2 加权序列用于肝实质的研究（图 15-1）。半傅里叶采集单次激发快速自旋回波序列（the half-Fourier single-shot turbo spin echo，HASTE），又名单次激发快速自旋回波序列（single-shot FSE，SS-FSE）对不配合的、病情不稳定的以及幽闭恐惧症患者是有帮助的[5]。HASTE 序列仅采集略多于 1/2 K 空间的数据（比 1/2 空间多数行，以进行必要的边缘相位修正），然后利用软件进行重建。尽管该序列有效地缩短了扫描时间，但是降低了图像的信噪比[6]。磁敏感性高的序列，比如 T_2^* 加权序列，可用于血色素沉着病或注射超顺磁氧

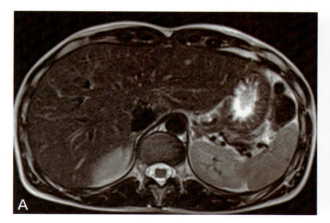
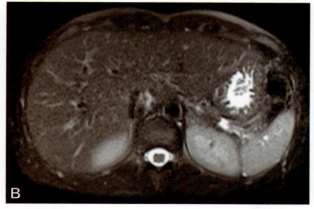

▲ 图 15-1 肝脏 T_2 加权图像
A. 快速自旋回波 T_2 加权磁共振图像；B. 脂肪抑制快速自旋回波 T_2 加权磁共振图像

化铁（superparamagnetic iron oxide，SPIO）对比剂后局灶性肝脏疾病的研究。与 T_2 加权序列相比，梯度回波（gradient-recalled-echo，GRE）T_2^* 加权序列对 SPIO 的作用更加敏感，因为缺少 180°重聚脉冲，因此对局部磁场不均匀所致的磁敏感效应增加[7]。T_2 加权序列对鉴别液性和实性成分非常有帮助：与周围肝实质信号相比，液性成分在 T_2 上表现为高信号，而实性成分表现为等信号或稍高信号（图 15-2）。

（二）T_1 加权序列

T_1 加权序列和 T_2 加权序列常规应用于评价肝脏疾病。平扫 T_1 加权序列有助于显示纤维成分和液性成分，这些成分在平扫 T_1 加权上通常表现为低信号；相比之下，比如脂肪、蛋白质和血液成分（出血/出血性囊肿）等成分在平扫 T_1 加权

上表现为高信号。抑制脂肪信号有助于显示含脂肪的病变。在注射对比剂之后，建议应用脂肪抑制序列增加病变与邻近结构之间的对比度。扰相梯度回波（spoiled gradient echo，SGE）T_1 加权序列是研究上腹部脏器的最佳序列，其相对较长的射频脉冲重复时间（TR）和较短的回波时间（TE），联合并行成像技术能够在单次屏气约 20s 的时间内完成感兴趣区（region of interest，ROI）的扫描。在 MR 脂肪抑制技术中，同相位/反相位（in-phase/out-of-phase）成像，又称双回波成像（dual-echo imaging）可用于反映同一体素内同时存在脂肪和水的病变，另一用途则是反映与铁沉积相关的顺磁性效应[8]。在第二个较长的回波时间内（1.5T 设备的回波时间为 4.4ms），由于 T_2^* 效应，铁质会导致组织信号丢失[9,10]。增强扫描前脂肪抑制图像主要用于发现蛋白质（黏蛋白和黑色素）和

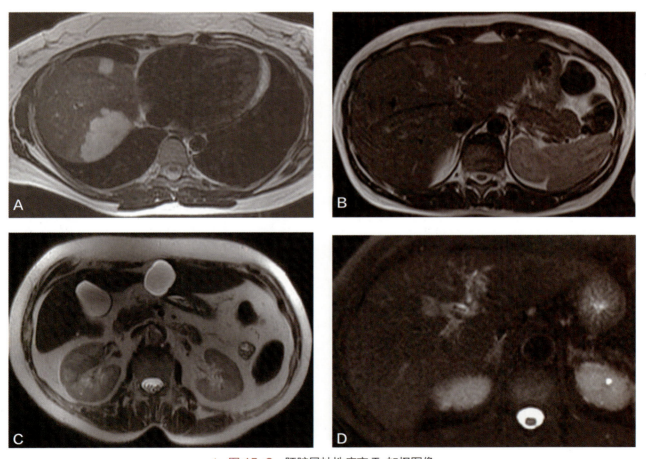

▲ 图 15-2 肝脏局灶性病变 T_2 加权图像
A. 血管瘤；B. 局灶性结节性增生；C. 肝囊肿；D. 肝转移瘤，肝囊肿的信号强度与胆囊信号强度相近

血液成分[11]。脂肪抑制技术是在获取序列前通过调节射频脉冲选择性激励脂肪质子得以实现的，图像所使用的参数和标准 SGE 序列相近。

在目前 MRI 设备中，脂肪抑制 SGE 序列可以在一次 20s 屏气时间内得到 22 层脂肪抑制较均匀的图像（图 15-3）。除了用于平扫 T_1 加权图像，SGE 序列还用于静脉注射对比剂后的多期增强扫描，该序列扫描时间短，可以根据血供情况（动脉期、静脉期及平衡期）研究肝实质。

（三）对比剂

肝脏成像中使用对比剂主要用于显示血管和肝实质，并用于发现局灶性或弥漫性疾病。目前，关于肝脏 MR 检查中必须使用对比剂的方面已达成共识。现已研发出不同种类的对比剂，并依据其在体内的分布不同和作用靶点不同，分为细胞外对比剂、肝细胞特异性对比剂、网状内皮细胞对比剂和血管内对比剂。细胞外对比剂是亲水性的小分子钆螯合物，静脉注射该对比剂后，药物迅速从血管内进入到细胞外间质，不会进入完整的细胞内，并经泌尿系统从体内排出。最常用于肝脏 MR 检查的钆对比剂包括：钆喷酸葡胺（gadopentetate dimeglumine, Gd-DTPA，马根维显，拜耳）、钆特酸葡甲胺（gadoterate meglumine, Gd-DOTA，多它灵，加柏）、钆双胺（gadodiamide, Gd-DTPA-BMA，欧乃影，安盛药业）、钆特醇（gadoteridol, Gd-HP-DO3A，普朗斯，博莱科）。作为一种顺磁性物质，其原理是通过缩短 T_1 弛豫时间来增加组织信号强度，这种作用在 T_1 加权图像上显示得最好[11-14]。由于钆螯合物能够迅速地从血管内再分布到细胞外间隙，因此对比剂必须以静脉团注的方式迅速给药，通常以 2ml/s 的速度静脉注射对比剂，然后以同样的速度静脉团注 20ml 生理盐水（0.9% 氯化钠）冲管，随后在一次屏气下对整个肝脏行多期动态增强扫描。肝脏具有双血供特点，肝脏

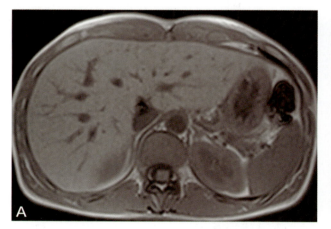
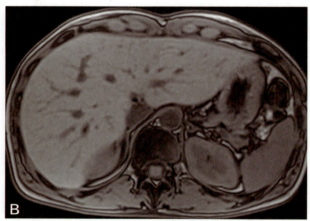
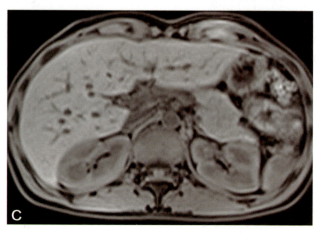

▲ 图 15-3 T_1 加权图像

肝脏梯度回波 T_1 加权图像：A. 同相位；B. 反相位；C. 选择性脂肪抑制序列

血供的 25% 来自肝动脉，75% 来自门静脉，使用快速扫描序列如 2D/3D 扰相 GRE T_1 加权序列，可以依据肝脏双血供特点研究不同增强时相的肝实质。静脉团注对比剂后 15s 首先出现肝动脉强化，并在 30s 时肝动脉强化达峰，30s 后对比剂通过门静脉系统从腹腔内器官返回肝实质，肝实质强化达峰时间在 60～70s，约 3min 后对比剂在肝脏细胞内外达到平衡，肝实质强化进入平衡期。

肝脏动脉期是最重要的增强扫描时相[15]。动脉期能突出显示富血供病变，而此时肝实质呈相对未强化状态（图 15-4）。实现这一目的的关键是在合适的时间进行 K 空间填充。动脉期扫描最佳的标志是肝动脉和门静脉强化而肝静脉未强化，肾皮质明显强化，并且脾脏呈花斑样强化（图 15-5）。应使用不同技术以获得最佳动脉期：固定扫描延迟时间，在注射对比剂后约 25s 开始扫描[16,17]；小剂量测试团注技术，在正式注射对比剂之前，先团注 1～2ml 对比剂以评估对比剂通过时间；对比剂团注自动监测与触发技术（CARE-bolus, SmartPrep）；最佳动脉期是在第 9 胸椎水平达到峰值后 8s 获得（图 15-6）[16,18,19]。

静脉期的标志是肝实质明显强化，大约是在注射对比剂后 60s。在静脉期，门静脉和肝静脉明显强化，因此可以明确地显示血管腔内的血栓（图 15-7）。乏血供转移和静脉内血栓在该期能够更好地显示（图 15-8）。

延迟期时间跨度较大，为 90s～5min，该阶段对比剂在血管内和肝脏间质内分布达到平衡（图 15-9），通常在注射对比剂后 180s 开始扫描。该期对于评价乏血供病变的强化（胆管细胞癌和血管瘤）、富血供病变强化均匀减低（局灶性结节性增生和腺瘤）以及肝细胞癌的"包膜样"强化和"廓清"征象十分重要（图 15-10）[20-24]。

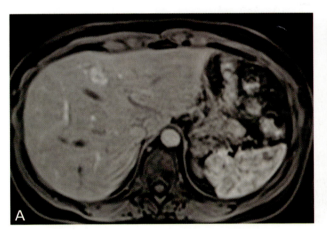
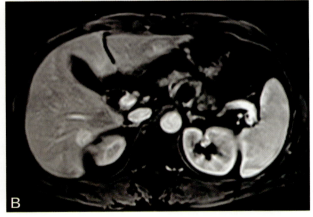
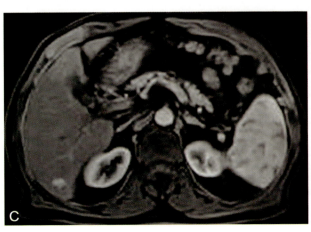

▲ 图 15-4　肝脏动脉期

肝脏富血供病例：A. 局灶性结节性增生；B. 血管瘤；C. 肝转移瘤

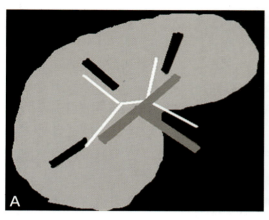 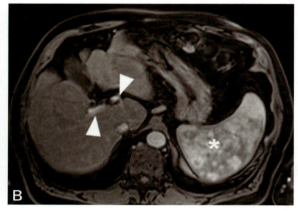

▲ 图 15-5　肝脏动脉期

A. 肝脏动脉期绘图；B. 肝脏动脉期 MR 图像：主要特征包括脾脏"花斑样"外观（星号）门静脉轻度强化（箭头）以及肾皮质明显强化。肝静脉一定不强化

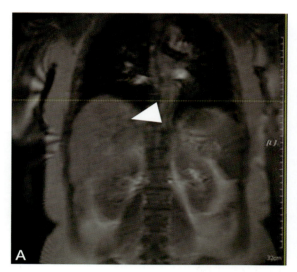 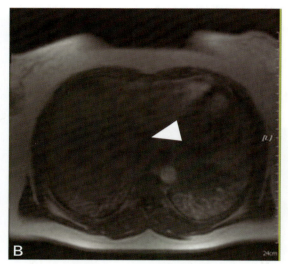

▲ 图 15-6　动脉期 CARE 技术

轴位触发器位于第 9 胸椎：序列从对比剂到达后 8s 开始进行扫描

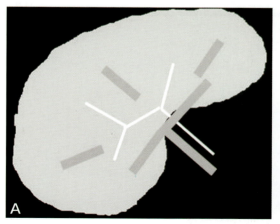 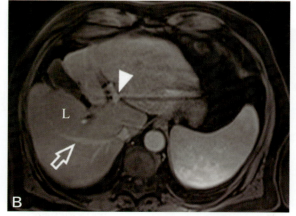

▲ 图 15-7　肝脏静脉期

A. 静脉期绘图；B. 静脉期 MR 图像表明了该期主要影像特征：肝实质（L）、门静脉（箭头）以及肝静脉（空心箭）明显强化

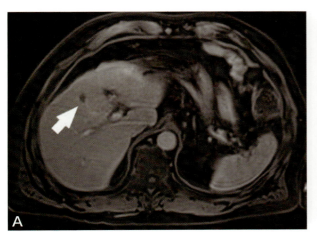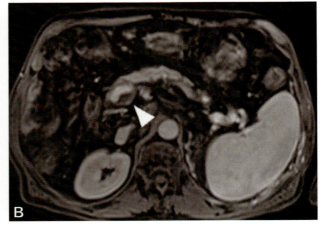

▲ 图 15-8 静脉期

A. 在静脉期，肝实质与乏血供转移灶之间对比 - 噪声比更高（白箭）；B. 静脉期也有助于发现血管内血栓（箭头）

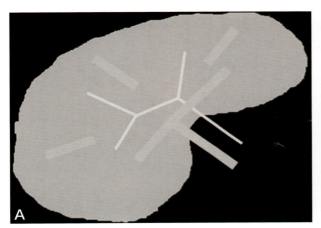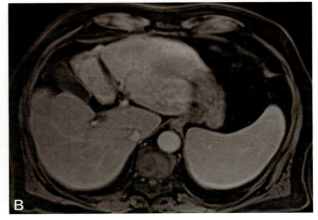

▲ 图 15-9 肝脏延迟期

A. 延迟期绘图；B. 延迟期 MR 图像表明了对比剂在血管内对比剂和肝实质内分布达到平衡

（四）肝脏特异性对比剂

1. 网状内皮系统特异性对比剂 网状内皮系统特异性对比剂是一种氧化铁颗粒，能够被存在于肝脏、脾脏和骨髓中的网状内皮系统（reticuloendothelial system，RES）细胞选择性摄取，并由于其磁敏感效应导致 T_2 信号减低[25]。SPIO 氧化铁颗粒平均直径为 50nm，而超微型 SPIO 颗粒直径小于 50nm。网状内皮系统特异性对比剂的超顺磁性能够缩短 T_2 和 T_1 弛豫时间，采用梯度回波 T_1 和 T_2^* 加权序列以及自旋回波 T_2 加权序列进行扫描。菲立磁通过静脉注射的方式给药[26,27]。首先在注射前使用梯度回波 T_1 及 T_2 加权序列对肝脏进行扫描，在注射药物后约 30min 使用相同的成像序列再次进行肝脏 MRI 扫描。此类对比剂通过肝脏（80%）及脾脏（12%）中的网状内皮系统从血浆中清除，只有极少量被淋巴结及骨髓组织摄取。铁羧葡胺可直接以小剂量（< 2ml）团注的方式给药，使用梯度回波 T_1 加权序列进行肝脏动态增强扫描。在延迟期（注射后 20min），库普弗细胞（Kupffer 细胞）中铁颗粒摄取明显增加，肝实质信号明显减低，尤其是在 T_2 加权图像上[28]。

2. 肝细胞特异性对比剂 肝胆特异性对比剂是一种顺磁性化合物，能够被有功能的肝细胞摄取，并通过胆汁排出。由于其具有顺磁性，该对比剂在 T_1 加权图像上可以使肝脏胆道及一些含

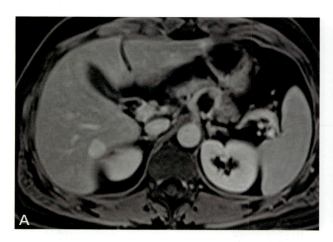
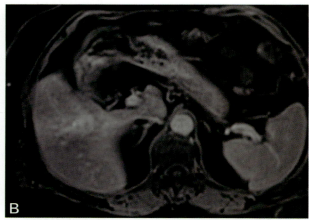
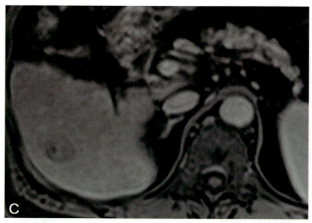

▲ 图 15-10 肝脏延迟期
延迟期是显示晚期强化的重要时相，例如典型的血管瘤（A）或胆管癌（B）或肝细胞癌"廓清"征象（C）

肝细胞病变的信号强度增加。这类对比剂既可以仅由肝细胞摄取，也可同时分布在肝细胞内外。这两种对比剂都是 T_1 阳性对比剂，缩短 T_1 弛豫时间，致 T_1 加权图像上信号强度增加，但是后一种对比剂应用更加广泛。在临床实践中，有两种结合血管和肝细胞特异性对比剂特性的化合物：钆贝葡胺（gadobenate dimeglumine, Gd-BOPTA, 博莱科, 意大利米兰）及钆塞酸（gadoxetic acid, Gd-EOB-DTPA, 拜耳, 德国柏林）。Gd-BOPTA 具有更高的弛豫率，但肝细胞摄取率仅为 5%；相比之下，Gd-EOB-DTPA 的肝细胞摄取率约 50%，决定了肝脏与病灶之间有更高的对比度[29-31]。Gd-EOB-DTPA 的肝细胞摄取率较高，在给药后 20min 达到肝胆期，而 Gd-BOPTA 在给药后 45min 后才可达到肝胆期；也有作者认为 Gd-EOB-DTPA 在给药后 10min 后即可获得肝胆期[32,33]。肝胆特异性对比剂在确定病变中是否含有功能性肝细胞具有独特优势（含有功能性肝细胞的病变，如局灶性结节性增生；不含功能性肝细胞的病变，如囊肿、血管瘤、腺瘤、转移瘤）（图 15-11）。在肝硬化时，使用肝胆特异性对比剂诊断肝硬化相关结节（再生结节、不典型增生结节及肝细胞癌）仍然存在一些挑战，主要原因在于这些结节在组织学和影像学表现存在重叠以及由于纤维化及血流动力学的改变造成的肝硬化使肝脏呈现不均质的外观。由于 Gd-EOB-DTPA 的高胆管排泄率，应将其用于研究胆管树，为 MR 胆管成像提供更多有效信息。在显示对比增强胆管系统方面，冠状位 / 斜位 3D GRE T_1 加权序列具有最佳的空间分辨率（图 15-12）。

（五）扩散加权成像

扩散加权成像（diffusion-weighted imaging, DWI）的主要应用领域是神经放射学：DWI 在发现超急性期（0～6h）脑缺血起着至关重要的作用；有助于鉴别实性及囊性病变（如脓肿

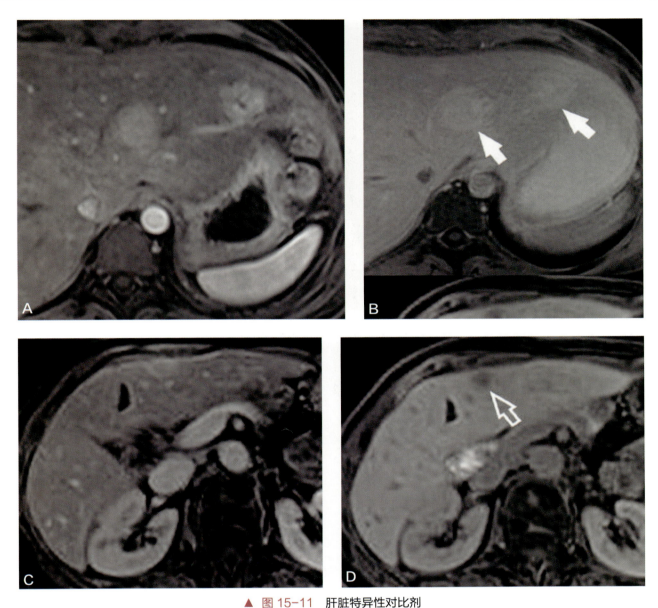

▲ 图 15-11 肝脏特异性对比剂

A、B. 肝脏局灶性病变例如局灶性结节性增生含有功能性肝细胞，能够摄取保留肝胆特异性对比剂（白箭）；C、D. 非肝细胞起源的局灶性病变不摄取对比剂（例如转移瘤，空心箭）

和肿瘤），近期还用于评价脱髓鞘病变。尽管如此，DWI 易产生运动伪影和磁敏感伪影，使其在腹部研究中仍然存在问题，这主要是由于心跳、肠蠕动以及各种实质 - 气体界面的存在所引起的伪影。超高速成像技术（平面回波成像，echoplanar sequences，EPI）的发展减少了运动伪影，并将其对空间分辨率的影响降至最低[34]。该序列应使用高场强超导设备（1.5T 或更高），配备梯度场强应在 23～30mT/m，梯度切换率为 150mT/m，并使用相控阵表面线圈[35]。

DWI 是使用自旋回波单次激发平面回波序列（spin echo sequence performed with the single-shot echoplanar technique，SE-EPI-SSh）获得，具体扫描参数如下：TR=2883，TE=61，反转角（flip angle，FA）=90°，扫描视野（field of view，FOV）根据具体情况而定，矩阵 =128×256，b 值 0 和 500s/mm²（最近，多 b 值序列通常使用以下 b 值：0、50、400、800s/mm²）。另外，并行采集技术的使用具有潜在优势，这种技术可以减少采集时间或增加矩阵，从而在不改变采集时间的情况下提高空间

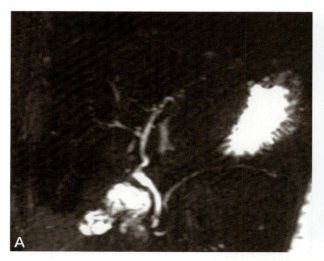 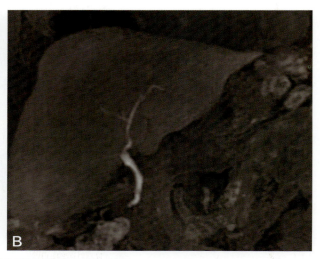

▲ 图15-12 肝胆特异性对比剂MR胆管成像

A. 厚层块T_2加权序列胆管成像；B. 肝胆期冠状位T_1加权成像。两者显示胆管轮廓相近

分辨率，并且不会明显降低图像质量（敏感度，SENSE）[35,36]。对原始DWI图像进行后处理可以得到相应的ADC图，在ADC图上对感兴趣区进行勾画，可以对相应部位的信号进行定量分析。如上所述，由于b值选择的不同，而因此产生扩散加权程度不同的问题亟待解决。一个病灶如果在低b值DWI图像上与周围肝实质相比表现为轻至中等程度高信号，在高b值DWI图像上仍表现如上（扩散受限），则通常认为该病灶是恶性的，另外该病灶在ADC图上与周围肝实质相比应呈低信号（图15-13）。

（六）灌注成像

MR灌注成像是反映组织血流动力学（如组织的微循环）的一种成像技术，超出了直接肉眼观察MR图像所能达到的分辨率，该技术可以定量分析肝脏实质和肿瘤微循环的改变[37]。目前，肝脏局灶性病变的灌注特征主要基于肝脏三期增强扫描的强化速率及强化模式。MR灌注成像可以通过定量指标反映肝脏局灶性病变的血流动力学特点，为目前用于肝脏局灶性病变鉴别诊断的定性评估提供了新思路。MR灌注成像通常采用3D T_1加权序列并行采集技术来获取图像，以减少扫描时间并提高时间分辨率。MR扫描参数如下：TR 2.7mms，TE 1ms，层厚8mm，矩阵256×159，FA=14°，带宽90Hz，温度分辨率1.98[38]。

（七）磁共振波谱

在扩散成像中，磁共振波谱（MR spectroscopy，MRS）已被应用于显示不同神经系统疾病的特征。在过去几十年里，MRS也被尝试用于弥漫性和局灶性肝脏疾病的评估。MRS反映了组织中化学物质或代谢物的信号变化，这些信号主要通过其频率来识别，并以其相对于标准频率的变化表示出来[39]。在质子MRS（^{1}H-MRS）中，代谢物或化学物质的频率位置取决于化合物中质子构型。组织中含水量丰富，通常以其频率位置作为体内^{1}H-MRS的常规标准频率，这意味着所有其他化学物质都是通过比较它们的频率位置（频移）与水的频率位置来识别的。为了获得足够的信噪比，需要使用高场强设备（1.5T或更高），并用体部相控阵线圈接收信号。肝脏单体素MRS需选取10～20mm³的体素、避开肝内大血管，并距离肝脏边缘至少10mm。使用化学位移选择性饱和技术（chemical shift saturation pulse，CHESS）抑制水的信号，并采用点解析波谱序列（pointresolved spectroscopy，PRESS）获得波谱图像（在TR 2000～3000ms和TE 20～30ms内进行128次采集）[40,41]。肝

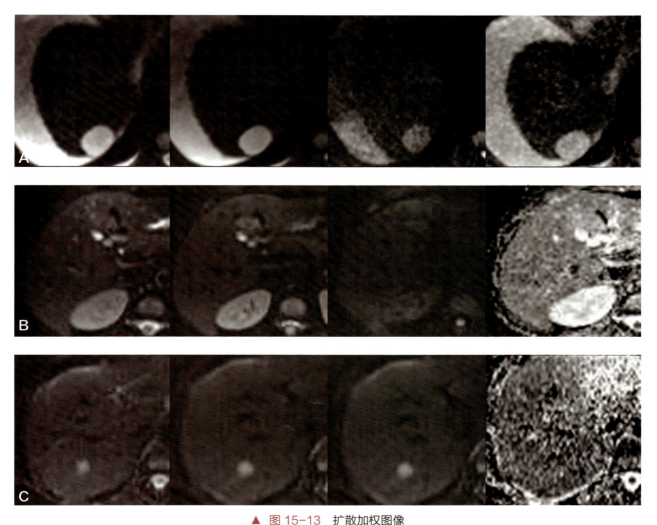

▲ 图 15-13　扩散加权图像

分子扩散受限的肝脏局灶性病变在 ADC 图像可进行评估：A. 肝囊肿；B. 局灶性结节性增生；C. 转移瘤

脏 MRS 采用自由呼吸的方式进行扫描以获得更高的信噪比。应用具有多种算法的软件对磁共振波谱数据进行后处理。后处理包括运动校正（频率和相移校正）、自动水抑制、残余水信号的低频滤波、傅里叶转换以及洛伦兹 - 高斯转换，后处理过程可以全部或部分自动化。MRS 是非侵入性定量评价脂肪肝的金标准，因为 MRS 能够量化体素内的甘油三酯（图 15-14）。目前，MRS 在发现肝脏局灶性病变中仍存在一定的局限性，主要是在评价小病灶时，运动伪影及体素大小的限制是最显著的缺陷。胆碱是一种代谢产物，通常用于评价恶性肿瘤，比如肝细胞癌，因为它反映了细胞更新周期活跃[42]。然而，尚不能可靠地鉴别良恶性肿瘤和正常的肝实质[43-45]。

（八）MR 弹力成像

肝实质弹性与肝脏纤维化程度密切相关，并与血管阻力增加有关，如门静脉高压[46]。在首次提出的基于超声的弹性成像技术中，我们使用多普勒超声观察外部压缩脉冲，表现为瞬时剪切波在肝实质内传播，其直接依赖于肝实质本身的弹性[47]。当能观察全器官的 MR 代替仅能观察有限部分器官的多普勒超声时，这一相对较新的技术可以定量评估肝脏弹性，特别适用于评估肝脏纤维化[48]。MR 弹性成像将作用于肝实质的外部正弦振动波与 2D 梯度回波 MR 弹性成像序列相结合，该序列需在选层方向上施加运动敏感梯度回波以探测该方向上的正弦波运动，同时外部

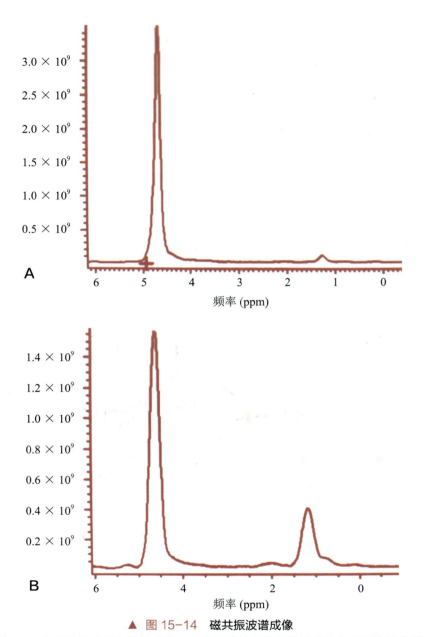

▲ 图 15-14 磁共振波谱成像

A. 健康志愿者的肝脏 MRS 未显示相对于水的脂质峰；B. 非酒精性脂肪肝男性患者由于肝脏轻度脂肪变性，肝脏 MRS 显示出相对于水的小脂质峰

的机械波驱动器和运动敏感梯度必须在频率和相位上保持一致[49]。

（九）高场强 MR（3T）

3.0TMR 设备可以提供比 1.5TMR 设备更好的图像信噪比和对比噪声比（Contrast-to-noise ratio，CNR），能够提高图像质量并缩短扫描时间。在肝脏 MR 成像中，3.0T 设备的 T_2 加权图像具有更好的信噪比和更高的分辨率，可以更好地发现肝脏恶性病变。2D GRE T_1 加权序列在 3.0T 系统上仍然难以优化；然而，使用 3D GRE T_1 加权序列可以提供相似的病灶对比度和更好的图像信噪比（图 15-15）。在较高场强下提高的图像对比度很大程度上是外源性对比剂如钆的结果，钆是一种破坏局部磁场导致 T_1 弛豫时间缩短的顺磁性物质[50]。即使使用了顺磁性物质，如钆，T_1 弛

Chapter 15 肝脏扫描技术与肝脏弥漫性疾病
Liver: Technique and Diffuse Pathology

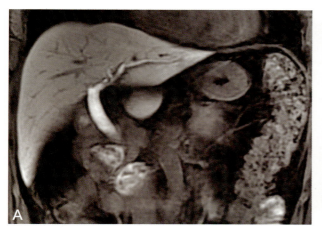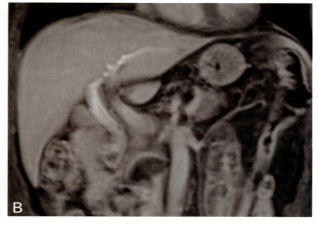

▲ 图 15-15 高场强 MR

A.3.0T 设备获取的肝胆期冠状位 T_1 加权图像；B. 同一患者 1.5T 设备获取的肝胆期冠状位 T_1 加权图像；在高场强设备上图像信噪比明显提高

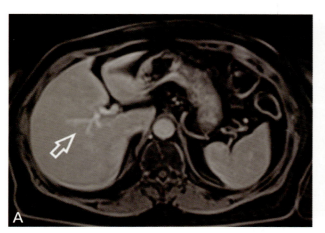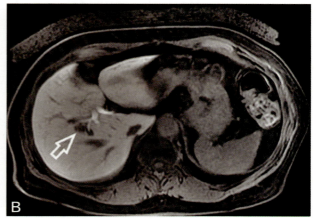

▲ 图 15-16 高场强 MR

A.1.5T 设备上显示的肝转移瘤；B. 同一患者 3.0T 设备上显示的肝转移瘤；病变在高场强设备上显示更突出（空心箭）

豫时间在 3.0TMR 成像设备上也会延长。然而，正是由于钆的 T_1 弛豫时间比软组织 T_1 弛豫时间短，被钆强化的组织就会在背景中显著突出。通过增加的对比度提高了诊断敏感性（图 15-16），而这种改善反过来为减少钆使用剂量提供了机会。通过优化成像参数和序列设计以及硬件系统的持续开发对检查方案进行了实质性修改，这将会提高了 3.0T 设备在腹部 MR 检查中的地位。DWI 从 3.0T 设备提高的信噪比中获益颇多，对扩散受限部位的敏感性提高。然而，由于磁化率增加引起的图像失真极大地导致了 3.0T 图像质量的下降。磁化率伪影可用并行采集技术加以限制。然而，使用 1.5T 所致的差异在临床上并不重要。3.0T 设备化学位移效应的增加可以提高波谱分辨率[51]，使得代谢物峰分离得到改善，这可以使 MRS 能更精确地量化单个代谢物[52]。信噪比的增加还缩短了整体成像时间。与其他应用程序一样，使用更小的体素，信噪比的增加可以转换成更高的空间分辨率。随着信噪比和对比噪声比的增加，关于能量沉积、射频脉冲场强的不均匀性、磁化率和化学位移伪影以及 MR 设备兼容性的问题也随之增加。目前，3.0T MRI 技术并不能提供足够的图像质量提升以证明其在腹部和肝脏评价中的应用价值。此外，关于临床上使用 3.0T MRI 设备的成本和设计问题在临床决策中占很大比重。

二、肝的解剖

根据 Couinaud 提出的肝脏分段法，后由 Bismuth 修订，肝实质在影像学上被分为 8 段，每一段均有独立的血管和胆管系统[53,54]，为外科手术提供了具有可重复性及必要的临床所需的细节描述。除了尾状叶和左叶内侧段，肝实质其他部分由三支主肝静脉所形成的纵向切面和左右门静脉分支所形成的横截面进行分段。肝脏 Ⅰ 段是尾状叶，Ⅱ - Ⅲ - Ⅳ 段位于肝左叶，Ⅴ - Ⅵ - Ⅶ - Ⅷ 段位于肝右叶（图 15-17）。每一部分有独立的血供（动脉和静脉）和胆汁引流。Bismuth 分类法又将Ⅳ段分为Ⅳa 和Ⅳb 亚段。最常见的解剖变异是 Riedel 叶，是肝右叶向下的一个舌状突起。Riedel 叶不是病理性改变，是一种正常的解剖变异，可以延伸至骨盆，经常会被误认为胆囊扩张或肝脏肿瘤。

其他肝脏解剖变异包括肝叶发育不全。复杂的先天性心脏病可以合并对称肝。完全或部分内脏器官转位畸形可以伴发左位肝。

三、血管解剖与变异

肝动脉供血量仅占肝脏血供的 25%～30%。肝总动脉通常起源于腹腔干。肝总动脉在胃幽门部发出胃十二指肠动脉后，形成肝固有动脉；肝固有动脉行于肝十二指肠韧带内，在门

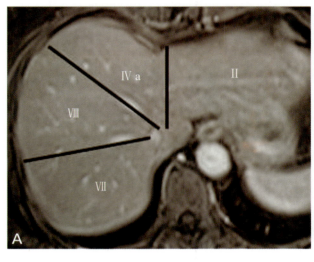
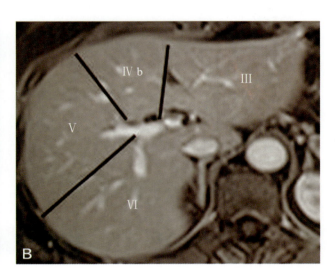
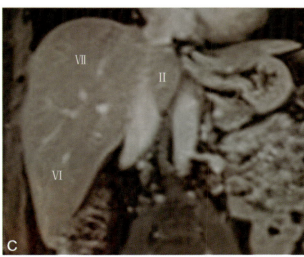
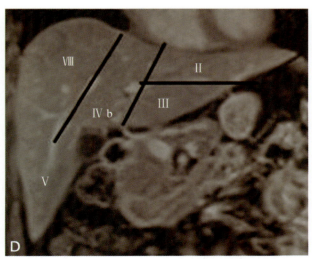

▲ 图 15-17 肝脏解剖

A、B. 肝脏 Couinaud 分段轴位 T_1 加权图像；C、D. 肝脏 Couinaud 分段冠状位 T_1 加权图像

静脉前内侧及胆管前方上行至肝门，于肝门处分为左、右支。为肝脏Ⅳ段供血的肝中动脉起源于肝左动脉或肝右动脉。典型的肝动脉供血分布仅略多于50%，45%会出现一种及以上的变异。最常见的变异包括肝左动脉起源于胃左动脉（10%～25%）以及肝右动脉起源于肠系膜上动脉（11%～17%）（图15-18）[55]。门静脉分为左、右两支，与肝左、右动脉以及胆管伴行。在肝右叶内，门静脉右支分为前、后两支，进入相应肝段。门静脉系统可能会受解剖变异的影响，例如门静脉主干分出三支血管（8%～10%）；其他解剖变异包括门静脉发育不全或萎缩，合并相应肝实质萎缩。在经典解剖中，三支主要的肝静脉最终汇入下腔静脉；肝左静脉收集肝脏Ⅱ段和Ⅲ段的血液；肝中静脉回收肝脏Ⅳ段、Ⅴ段及Ⅷ段的血液；肝右静脉接收肝脏Ⅴ段、Ⅵ段及Ⅶ段的血液。在大约60%的人群中，肝中静脉与肝左静脉形成共干后汇入下腔静脉。最常见的解剖变异是副肝右静脉收集肝脏Ⅵ段血液后直接汇入下腔静脉（图15-19）[56]。

四、肝脏弥漫性病变

肝脏弥漫性病变，包括慢性肝脏疾病的所有病因，影响着全世界数百万人。随着获取治疗手段愈加便利，对于诊断评估的需求日益增长。MRI在无创性评估肝脏特征方面展现了其独特的诊断能力，超过了肝脏活检的诊断效能。在评价肝脏弥漫性病变，包括评价肝实质及血供情况的研究中，注射对比剂前后获取标准MRI序列的使用得到了逐步改善。最近MRI技术的发展已经产生了可以量化肝脏重要代谢产物（包括脂肪和铁）以及肝脏纤维化的方法，肝脏纤维化是慢性肝脏疾病的标志。肝脏弥漫性病变通常分为沉积性疾病、血管系统疾病以及炎性疾病。

（一）沉积性疾病

1. 脂肪沉积　肝脏脂肪变性是肝细胞内甘油三酯沉积，可以是局灶性或弥漫性。脂肪肝的严重程度涵盖了从显性非炎症性脂肪肝到脂肪性肝炎、肝脏纤维化和肝硬化。肝脏脂肪变性的主要原因与酗酒有关；非酒精性脂肪肝（non-alcoholic fatty liver disease, NAFLD）与肥胖、2型糖尿病以及血脂异常有关，这些疾病均是代谢综合征的表现[57,58]。最近，基因和环境因素与NAFLD发病的相互作用也得到了证实，尤其是证实了PNAPLA3基因的rs738409多态性与NAFLD具有很强的相关性[59]。肝脏脂肪变性分为局灶性和弥漫性。基于病变的典型发病部位如韧带和肝门周围，以及病变内有正常血管穿行的

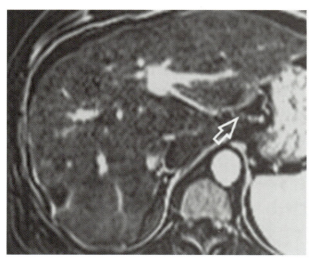

▲ 图15-18　肝动脉解剖变异
动脉期剪影图像显示肝左动脉起源于胃左动脉（黑箭）

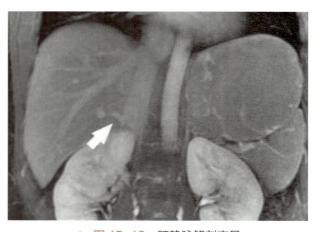

▲ 图15-19　肝静脉解剖变异
MR延迟期增强图像最大强度投影（Maximum intensity projection, MIP）显示副肝右下静脉收集肝Ⅳ段血液直接汇入下腔静脉

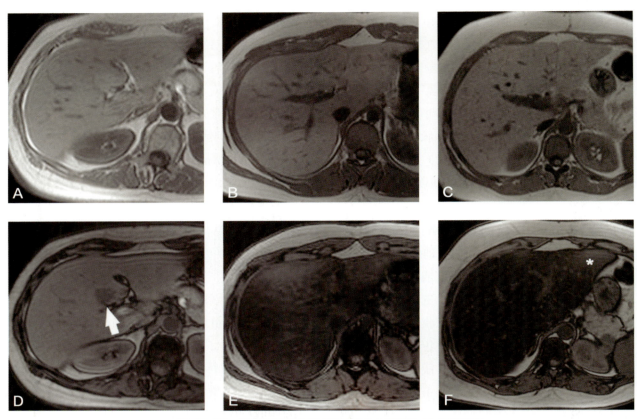

▲ 图 15-20 脂肪沉积双回波梯度回波（GRE）T_1 加权图像

A 和 D. 局灶脂肪变性在同相位 T_1 加权图像上呈高信号，在反相位 T_1 加权图像上呈低信号；B 和 E. 肝实质斑片样脂肪变性；C 和 F. 肝实质弥漫均匀脂肪变性；星号所示区域表示肝脏Ⅱ段乏脂肪区域

特点，局灶性脂肪肝通常较易确诊。多灶性或斑片状局灶性脂肪肝也较常见，可能会被误诊为浸润性肿瘤（图 15-20）[60]。MRI 是无创检测肝脏脂肪变性的最佳诊断方法。MRI 化学位移成像无疑是诊断肝脏脂肪变性最简单的方法：在反相位 T_1 加权序列上，图像信号下降是诊断脂肪肝非常准确的征象。使用 MRS 进行肝脏脂肪定量分析被认为是检测和量化肝脏中生化脂肪含量的唯一无创性参考标准，它能够定量分析体素内的甘油三酯（图 15-21）[61]。MRS 已被用于多项研究中，但它的临床适用性或实用性有限，因为 MRS 需要复杂的后处理方法，并不是每台 MRI 设备都常规配备 MRS 的能力。同时，在过去几年里也开发了一些 MR 序列作为可替代的和更快的量化分析肝脏脂肪变性的方法：两点法 Dixon 水脂分离技术、非对称回波三点法 IDEAL 水脂分离技术及三回波及六回波 GRE 化学位移序列[62-65]。关于量化分析肝脏脂肪变性的最佳 FAST-MR 方法，在文献中仍存在争论。

2. 铁过度沉积 肝脏内铁超负荷是指在肝细胞、库普弗细胞（Kupffer cell）或两者中铁的异常沉积。肝脏铁沉积源自肠道的异常吸收和红细胞受损（遗传性血色素沉着症、铁粒幼红细胞性贫血以及镰状细胞疾病）。输血所致铁超负荷主要是由于经肠道外注射红细胞引起，导致铁储存在肝脏、脾脏、胰腺和骨髓中红细胞中[66]。肝细胞内铁超负荷会产生氧化应激，导致终末期肝硬化，肝衰竭甚至发展成肝细胞癌[67]。MRI 不直接对铁进行成像，而是检测铁对感兴趣区中水质子的影响。MRI 检测铁元素的基础是铁作为超顺磁性元素可以加快 T_2 弛豫时间和 T_2^* 信号衰减，从而导致自旋回波/快速自旋回波 T_2 加权图像和梯度回波 T_2^* 加权图像上信号减低；后者对铁的检测灵敏度更高，对铁的分布范围显示更清楚（图

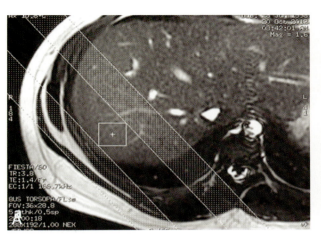
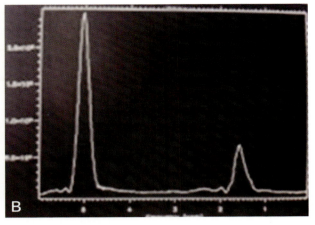

▲ 图 15-21　脂肪沉积磁共振波谱（MRS）图像
A. 轴位 T_2 加权图像显示了 MRS 体素在肝脏Ⅶ段中的正确位置；B. 儿童肝脏波谱显示了相对于水的小脂质峰

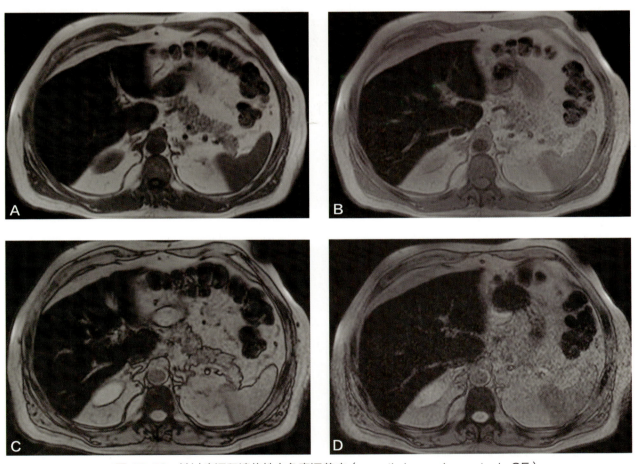

▲ 图 15-22　铁过度沉积遗传性血色素沉着症（genetic hemochromatosis, GE）
不同的 T_2^* 加权序列对铁沉积进行量化分析

15-22 和图 15-23）[68]。骨骼肌信号强度作为信号强度参考标准，以比较其他器官信号强度的变化并进行定量分析[69]。铁和脂肪可能会同时出现，定量分析可能会更加复杂。

3. 肝豆状核变性（Wilson's Disease, Wilson 病） 肝豆状核变性，通常被称为 Wilson 病，是一种常染色体隐性遗传病，其特征是肠道铜吸收增加所致铜异常沉积，主要好发部位是肝脏、大脑和角膜。虽然 Wilson 病恶化成肝细胞癌的可能性很小，但可表现为急性甚至急性重型肝炎，并迅速发展为大结节型肝硬化。临床上，患者的血浆铜蓝蛋白水平极低。目前，据我们所知，Wilson 病的 MR 图像没有表现出可以区别于其他慢性肝病的特征（图 15-24）。在

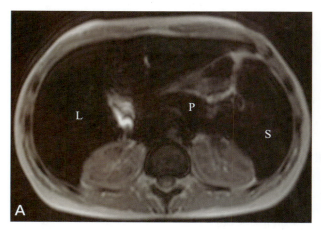
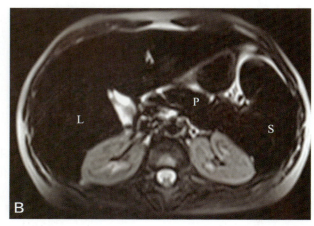

▲ 图 15-23 铁沉积

输血所致铁沉积 GRE T_2^* 加权图像显示肝脏（L）、脾脏（S）和胰腺（P）呈低信号；胰腺的异常低信号说明输注的铁含量已经超过了红细胞的铁储存能力

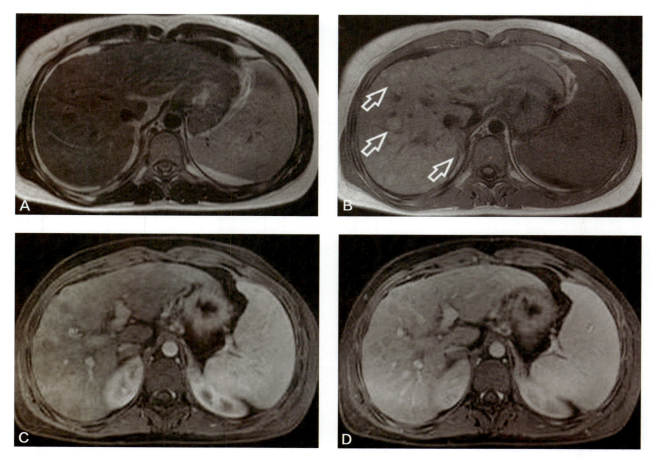

▲ 图 15-24 Wilson 病

A、B. 轴位 T_1 和 T_2 加权图像显示肝脏边缘不规则，伴多发肝实质结节（空心箭）；C、D. 轴位增强延迟期 T_1 加权图像这些结节未显示；MR 图像表现不具有特异性，并且与肝硬化表现相似

Wilson病引起的肝炎或肝功能衰竭临床病例中,可以观察到早期非特异性斑片状强化,伴肝实质钆摄取的明显延迟的特点[70]。有些笔者描述了Wilson病不常见的影像表现,如肝周脂肪层、多发性富血供结节以及无肝尾状叶肥大[71]。

4. 肝糖原贮积病 糖原贮积病患者的特征在于不能将6-磷酸-葡萄糖转化为葡萄糖;然而,它们可以内源性地产生葡萄糖。与骨髓信号相比,肝细胞内糖原贮积导致T_1加权图像上信号强度增加。患有该疾病的患者也可能患肝细胞腺瘤[72]。

(二) 血液系统疾病

1. 遗传性出血性毛细血管扩张症 (Osler-Weber-Rendu综合征) 遗传性出血性毛细血管扩张症又称Osler–Weber–Rendu综合征,是一种常染色体显性遗传性血管发育异常型疾病,其发病率为1~2/100 000,肝脏受累率达8%~31%[73]。遗传性毛细血管扩张症的特征性表现在于皮肤黏膜或内脏器官血管异常增生性病变,后者常见于肝脏、肺、大脑以及胃肠道。肝脏受累的特征在于存在肝脏血管畸形,包括肝动脉扩张、肝内毛细血管扩张、肝动脉-肝静脉瘘、肝动脉-门静脉瘘、异常汇聚的血管团及肝动脉瘤[74,75]。17例(74%)患者出现结节性再生性增生,9例(39%)患者出现缺血性胆管炎[76]。动静脉畸形通常在肝内弥漫性分布,这可能与肝动脉扩张、肝门区及肝小叶中央区血管增粗、迂曲有关。在Osler病中,肝实质动脉灌注增加常导致继发性再生结节,可能被误诊为肝脏恶性肿瘤。这些假性肿瘤,例如局灶性结节增生,代表了肝细胞局部过度增殖,而不是真正的肿瘤。肝脏受累的患者可能无症状,但已有报道患者出现心力衰竭、门体分流性脑病、胆管炎、门静脉高压以及肝硬化[75]。在MRI上,毛细血管扩张在平扫T_1加权图像上表现为低或等信号小病灶,在T_2加权图像上表现为高或等信号病灶;动态增强MRI上表现为动脉期明显强化,门静脉期及

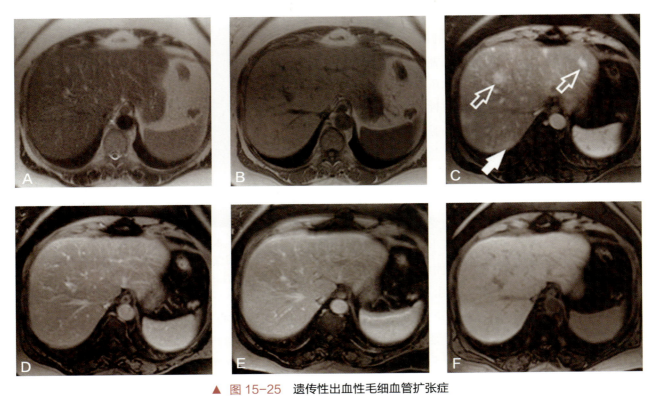

▲ 图15-25 遗传性出血性毛细血管扩张症

A,B.肝脏局灶性病变在T_2加权图像及T_1加权图像未显示;C.动脉晚期T_1加权图像显示肝实质内(空心箭)及肝被膜下(白箭)血管增生性病变,包括动静脉畸形和血管扩张;D,F.动脉期之后获取的图像显示肝实质均匀强化

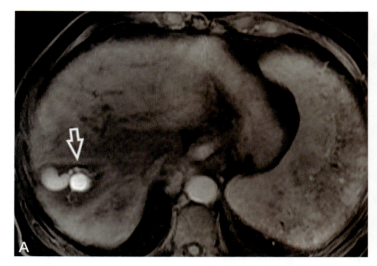
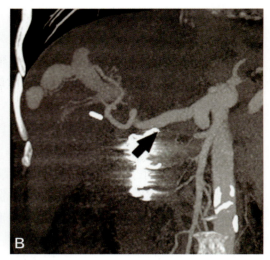

▲ 图 15-26 遗传性出血性毛细血管扩张症

A. 增强后轴位 T_1 加权图像显示异常扩张的血管进入肝实质；B. 在动脉期获得的冠状位 MIP 图像显示动脉 - 门静脉分流，扩张的肝动脉（黑色箭）与门静脉相通

平衡期与周围肝实质相比呈等信号；通过使用肝胆对比剂，可以发现在肝胆期病灶正常强化（图 15-25）。而在平扫 T_1 加权图像及 T_2 加权图像上难以发现动静脉分流，但是在动静脉分流附近通常可以看到迂曲、扩张的血管（图 15-26）。

2. 肝淤血 肝淤血是由于肝静脉回流障碍导致肝实质内血液淤滞引起。肝淤血是充血性心力衰竭和缩窄性心包炎的常见并发症，由于其解剖关系密切，升高的中心静脉压直接从右心房传至肝静脉。即使是短暂的缺血性创伤，肝细胞也会非常敏感，可能会被各种心脏引起的循环系统紊乱所损伤，包括动脉缺氧、急性左心衰竭致使心输出量下降以及中心静脉高压[77]。在急性右心衰竭时，血液淤滞会导致肝静脉扩张和且血窦淤血。肝小叶中央区的肝细胞受压、萎缩、坏死程度不一，并可能发生轻度肝小叶中央区脂肪浸润。在慢性肝淤血时，持续性低氧阻止了肝细胞再生，导致纤维组织增生由小叶中央区向周边发展，与邻近小叶中央区延伸的纤维组织联结，并以门静脉为中心形成纤维化，最终发展成为心源性肝硬化（槟榔肝）。下腔静脉和肝静脉扩张是肝淤血的主要特征：肝右静脉主干直径超过 8mm 被认为是病理性扩张[78]。另外，当静脉团注对比剂进入衰竭的右心房时，对比剂可能

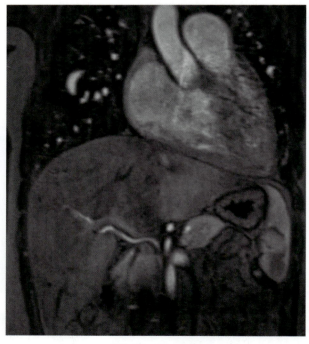

▲ 图 15-27 肝淤血

增强后 T_1 加权图像显示肝实质肿大以及肝静脉扩张，并伴有肝静脉逆行性浑浊

不正常进入右心室，而是直接进入下腔静脉和肝静脉，出现逆行性浑浊（retrograde opacification）（图 15-27）。在 T_2 加权图像上，由于血管周围淋巴水肿，沿着门静脉周围间隙可能会出现稍高信号影；注射对比剂后，会出现由线样低信号影所形成的网格样改变，也称"马赛克征"：注射对比

剂1～2min后，肝实质强化变得更均匀。

3. 布-加综合征（Budd-Chiari syndrome） Budd-Chiari综合征是由各种原因引起的肝静脉流出道阻塞，由此产生的一种临床综合征，阻塞部位可发生在从肝小静脉到下腔静脉与右心房交界处的任何水平[79]。Budd-Chiari综合征根据病因分为原发性和继发性，原发性主要是由于内源性静脉腔内隔膜或血栓形成所致，继发性主要由外源性压迫或肿瘤侵犯引起[80-82]。肝静脉及其开口以上的下腔静脉膜性阻塞，也称为原发性Budd-Chiari综合征，是由于纤维肌性隔膜或后天获得性病变所致。隔膜起源于血管壁，可部分或完全闭塞静脉管腔[83]。这种类型的病变被认为是长期血栓形成的后遗症[84]。显然静脉血栓形成的病因是所需要考虑的重要因素。血液系统疾病如骨髓增殖性疾病；阵发性睡眠性血红蛋白尿；抗磷脂抗体综合征；遗传性蛋白C、蛋白S及抗凝血酶Ⅲ缺乏；凝血因子V Leiden突变；凝血酶原基因突变以及亚甲基四氢叶酸还原酶突变是导致Budd-Chiari综合征的主要原因[83,85]。其他促使Budd-Chiari综合征发展的因素包括妊娠、产后即刻以及使用口服避孕药。继发性Budd-Chiari综合征是由腔外占位性病变的外源性压迫或者恶性肿瘤腔内侵犯（肾细胞癌、肝细胞肝癌、肾上腺皮质腺癌、肝转移瘤以及原发性下腔静脉平滑肌瘤）所致[82-85]。肝脏形态的改变主要包括肝外周区域萎缩、肝尾状叶和中央区肥大以及肝实质结节样改变（图15-28）[86,87]。急性期时肝实质中央区强化程度高于外周区（flip-flop sign），慢性期肝实质强化更均匀[87]。

文献中已描述了与慢性Budd-Chiari综合征相关的再生结节[86,88-90]。Budd-Chiari综合征的良性再生结节发病机制尚不清楚。肝细胞生长因子和肝脏微循环障碍可能是影响其进展的重要因素[90,92]。Budd-Chiari综合征的再生结节通常为多发（>10个）、小的（<4cm）的富血供结节。在MRI上，良性再生结节常在T_1加权图像上表现为高信号，在T_2加权图像上表现为等/低信号[90-93]。结节的动脉供血量增加对应在动态增强图像上表现为致密强化影，在MR血管成像连续多时相扫描过程中，许多这样的肝结节逐渐强化，并且强化持续到静脉晚期。慢性终末期肝病患者发生肝细胞癌的风险会增加。因此，区分良性再生结节和肝细胞癌很重要（图15-29）。通常增强前的信号特征以及强化模式可以区分这两种病变，但是某些情况下基于MR信号特征也难以区分两者。

4. 肝梗死 肝梗死是指局部缺血引起肝细胞凝固性坏死的区域，主要是由于血栓或栓子阻塞了受累区域的循环。由于肝脏有肝动脉和门静

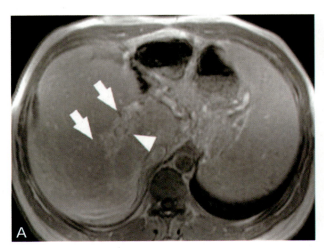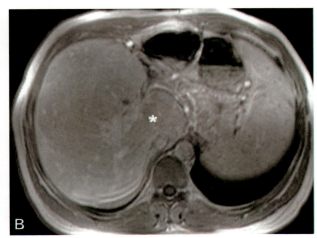

▲ 图15-28 布-加综合征
A、B. 在静脉期获得的增强后T_1加权图像显示肝实质肿大，尾状叶肥大为主（星号）；肝静脉不能误认为门静脉（箭头），肝静脉表现为扩张的侧支血管（白箭）

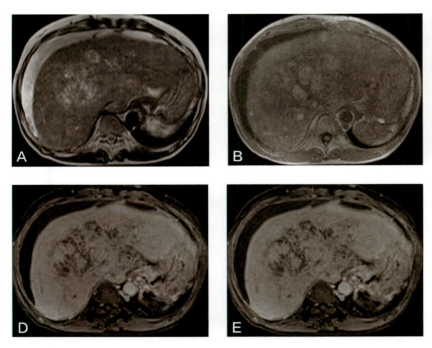

▲ 图 15-29 Budd-Chiari 综合征

A、B. T_1 和 T_2 加权图像显示肝实质信号不均，伴有坏死区域及多发结节样表现；注射对比剂后，在动脉期（C）结节轻度强化，而静脉期（D）和延迟期（E）未见廓清征象；这些结节有时难以和肝细胞肝癌区分

脉双重血供，因此肝梗死发生相对罕见。肝梗死可能是医源性（经动脉化疗栓塞）或创伤性（肝动脉或门静脉撕裂）；可以是肝移植术后并发症，也可能继发于血管炎或感染[33]。在被报道的近 3% 的成人肝移植受试者中，肝动脉血栓形成所致的肝梗死最常见。在 T_1 加权图像上，肝梗死表现为边界清楚的低信号区；在 T_2 加权图像上，肝实质表现为不均匀高信号；注射对比剂后，肝梗死表现为灌注缺损区，与周围肝实质相比呈低信号（图 15-30）。尽管大多数情况下肝梗死诊断比较明确，但是仍然可能与局灶性脂肪浸润、脓肿甚至肿瘤相混淆[37]。

（三）炎性疾病

1. 肝硬化　肝硬化是由于肝内纤维间隔形成及肝细胞结节样再生所致的肝脏组织结构不可逆性重构的一类肝脏疾病[94]。肝硬化最常见的病因是乙型和丙型肝炎病毒感染或慢性酒精中毒；其他尚有胆系疾病，隐源性和代谢性疾病所致肝硬化。常见的临床表现主要由于门静脉高压、门体分流以及肝功能不全引起。常见的并发症主要有腹水、上消化道出血、肝性脑病以及凝血功能障碍。肝硬化早期，肝脏大小、形态正常；在疾病晚期，影像学检查可能会出现一些典型征象，如肝脏结节状轮廓，肝右叶萎缩，尾状叶及左叶外侧段代偿性肥大，肝右后缘切迹征（the notch sign），门静脉周围间隙增宽（图 15-31）[95-99]。尾状叶横径与肝右叶横径之比≥ 0.65 是诊断肝硬化的阳性指标，具有很高的准确性（图 15-32）。有研究提出了一种改良的测量尾状叶宽度与右叶宽度比值的方法，这种方法使用门静脉右支代替门静脉主干作为两者的边界[100]。在慢性肝脏疾病进展过程中，肝脏组织结构改变以及纤维间隔形成导致肝血窦的血管阻力增加，增加的压力梯度被称为门静脉高压，并引起一系列并发症，如腹水、脾大、侧支循环开放，最终可能会形成食管胃底静脉曲张（图 15-33）[101]。附脐静脉和胃左静脉回流入门静脉，也会重新开放形成门 - 体侧支循环。其他门 - 体侧支循环还包括脾肾静脉交通支、肛管直肠下段交通支、腹壁静脉以及腹膜后交通支。如上所述，肝硬化的主要特征之一是肝脏纤维化：它的典型表现是斑片状纤维化，呈花边样改变（lacelike pattern）或融合成肿块。花边样纤维化表现为围绕再生结节的薄或厚的带状结构。在终末期肝硬化可见局灶融合性纤维化，通常表现为位于肝脏Ⅳ、Ⅴ或Ⅷ段被膜下楔形

Chapter 15 肝脏扫描技术与肝脏弥漫性疾病
Liver: Technique and Diffuse Pathology

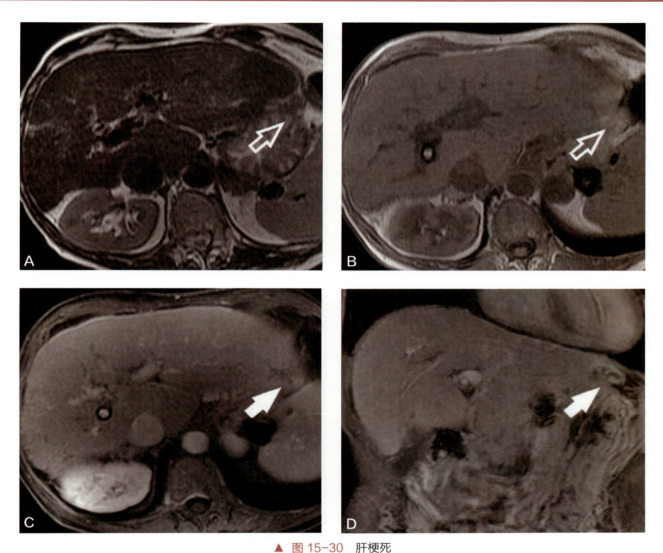

▲ 图 15-30 肝梗死
A、B. T_2 和 T_1 加权图像显示肝脏外周楔形、信号不均匀区域，伴肝脏表面皱缩（空心箭）；C、D. 静脉期轴位和冠状位增强图像上，该区域与周围肝实质相比呈低信号（白箭）

病灶，伴相应被膜皱缩（图 15-34）[102]。有时局灶融合性纤维化动脉期有强化，可能会被误诊为肝细胞肝癌；延迟期持续强化，楔形皱缩和被膜皱缩，这些是肝纤维化的典型表现，可能有助于鉴别两者。肝硬化第二个最重要的特征是肝细胞结节：大多数肝细胞结节是良性的（再生结节）；但是，再生结节可能会沿着已知的癌变途径进展为不典型增生结节（低级别和高级别）或肝细胞肝癌[103]。再生结节是最常见的与肝硬化相关的肝细胞结节；根据大小可分为小结节型（< 3mm）和大结节型（≥ 3mm）。在 MRI 图像上，再生结节边界清楚。在平扫 T_2 加权及 T_2^* 加权图像上，结节通常表现为低信号，在 T_1 加权图像上信号多变[104]。与同相位图像相比，含脂再生结节在反相位 GRE 图像及平扫非对称自旋回波图像上信号减低。增强图像的影像学特征较平扫图像在诊断上更具有特异性。注射细胞外对比剂后，大多数再生结节强化与邻近肝实质强化相同，或在动脉期和门静脉期强化略高于周围肝实质。这些结节摄取和排泄肝脏特异性对比剂的能力保留。因此，在肝细胞期获得的图像中，所有的再生结节与周围肝实质的信号强度相近（图 15-35）。少数情况下，再生结节可能具有足够的肝细胞功能中摄取肝细胞对比剂的能力，但不能

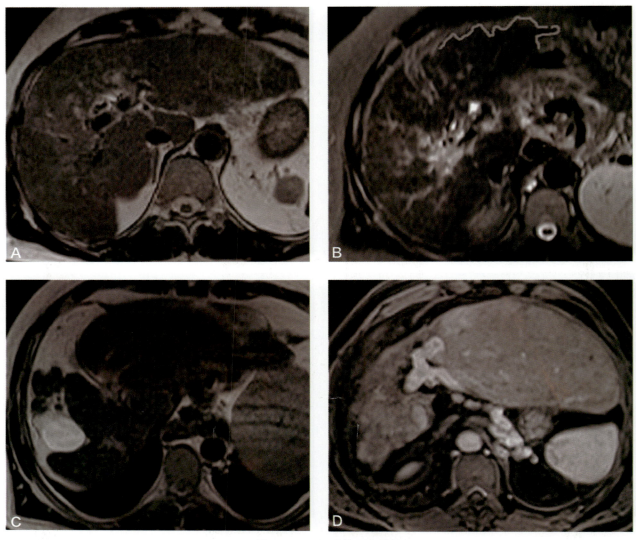

▲ 图 15-31　肝硬化形态特征

A～C. T_2 加权图像上显示肝右后缘切迹：这一特征在酒精性肝硬化更常见；B. 肝脏不规则边缘；C. 胆囊窝扩大；D. 增强后 T_1 加权图像显示肝右叶萎缩及肝左叶代偿性肥大

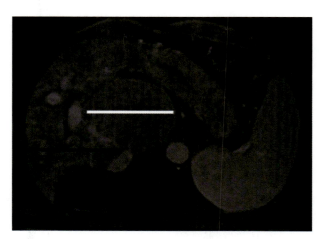

▲ 图 15-32　肝硬化尾状叶之比

增强后 T_1 加权图像显示肝尾状叶明显增大与萎缩的肝右叶之比，为 1.15

排泄肝细胞对比剂，因此这些结节在肝细胞期呈高信号[105]。最后，因为大多数再生结节保留了吞噬功能，这些结节能摄取 SPIO，因此在 SPIO 增强 T_2 及 T_2^* 加权图像上呈低信号。

铁质沉着结节是再生性或不典型增生结节，含有高水平内源性铁。尽管"铁质沉着结节"一词没有纳入国际词典内，但是放射科医师创造了该词，描述了含铁量高的肝硬化相关结节。铁质沉着结节在平扫 T_1 加权图像及 T_2^* 加权图像上呈低信号[106]。

不典型增生结节在 MR 图像上表现各异，它们的信号强度与再生结节及分化好的肝细胞肝癌

Chapter 15 肝脏扫描技术与肝脏弥漫性疾病
Liver: Technique and Diffuse Pathology

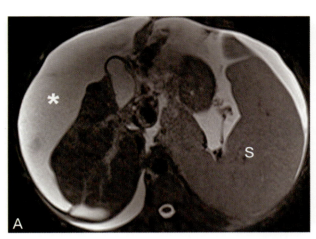
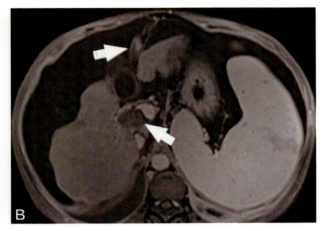

▲ 图 15-33　肝硬化肝周特征

A.T₂ 加权图像显示由于门静脉高压引起的巨脾（S）和大量腹水（星号）；B. 增强后 T₁ 加权图像显示血液流入附脐静脉和门静脉血栓形成（白箭）

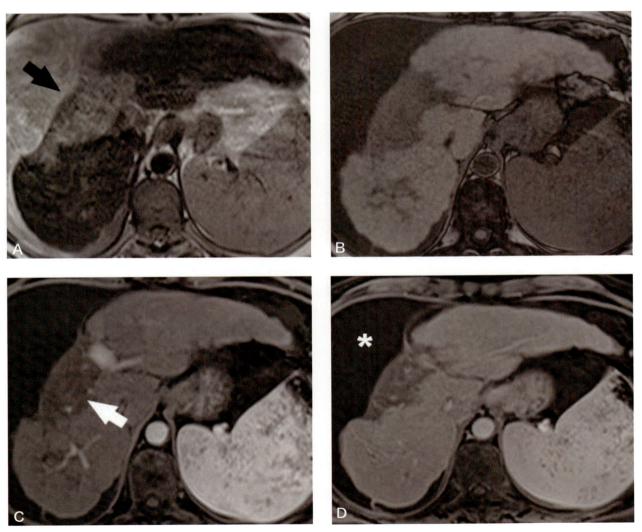

▲ 图 15-34　肝硬化融合性肝纤维化

A，B.T₂ 加权图像和 T₁ 加权图像分别显示肝脏中央区高信号和低信号区，伴不规则边缘及肝被膜皱缩（黑色箭）；C、D. 动脉期和延迟期增强 MR 图像显示肝右叶前段楔形病灶（白箭），信号低于邻近肝实质；星号所示是腹腔大量积液

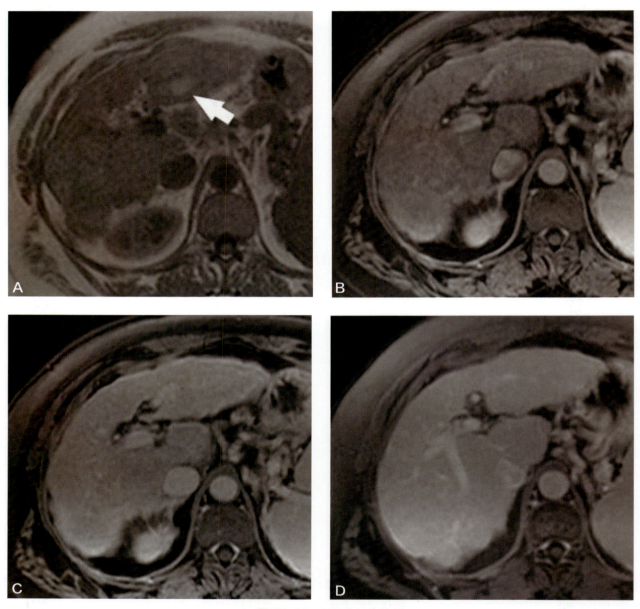

▲ 图 15-35 肝硬化再生结节

A.T$_1$ 加权图像显示肝脏Ⅲ段稍高信号局灶性病变；B～D. 注射对比剂后动脉期、延迟期及肝胆期，肝实质内未发现病变；该结节在肝移植中得以证实

有重叠。在 T$_2$ 加权图像上，不典型增生结节相对周围肝实质呈低信号[107]。T$_1$ 加权图像没有帮助，因为它们在 T$_1$ 加权图像上信号多变（低、中及高信号）。在钆对比剂和 SPIO 增强图像上，低级别不典型增生结节通常在动脉期不强化；此外，一些不典型增生结节在延迟期呈现"廓清"（图 15-36）[108]。动脉期强化提示高级别不典型增生结节内出现肝细胞癌灶，即 MRI 上的结节中结节[109]。MR 比 CT 能够更好地发现和鉴别不典型增生结节，但是只有 15% 的病例可以准确诊断。

2. 硬化性胆管炎 原发性硬化性胆管炎（primary sclerosing cholangitis, PSC）是一种以炎性纤维化和肝内外胆管破坏为特征的慢性胆汁淤积性疾病。PSC 好发于中年男性，平均年龄为 40 岁。大约 75% 的患者与炎症性肠病有关，例如溃疡性结肠炎和克罗恩病[110,111]。PSC 被认为是胆管癌的危险因素，10%～15%PSC 可伴发恶变[112,113]。尽管涉及多种危险因素，但是单一的发病机制尚不清楚。PSC 被认为与自身免疫有关，因为该病与体液和细胞介导的免疫过程异常以及 HLA Ⅱ类抗原在胆管上皮细胞表达异常有关。PSC 与腹膜后纤维化、纵隔纤维化以及干燥综合征等免疫类疾病之间的关联也提示该病可能为自身免疫性疾病[114,115]。PSC 的典型表现与胆管的进行性炎症和纤维化有关，导致胆管的节段性扩张与狭窄或闭塞[116]。MR 胆管造影（MR cholangiography, MRC）能够清楚地显示 PSC 胆管造影的特征。最常见的表现就是肝内外胆管弥漫性或多发性的胆管环状狭窄，交替出现正常或轻度扩张胆管，呈现"串珠状"改变。其他胆管造影表现包括环状狭窄征、憩室征以及结石。环状狭窄征是指胆管壁局灶性厚 1~2mm 的不完全环形狭窄区域。传统胆管造影术中，胆管内压力增高可能会导致胆管局灶性扩张，致使环状狭窄区转变为憩室。另外，肝实质也会发生形态学改变，包括尾状叶肥大和外侧段及后段萎缩。

注射对比剂后，病灶动脉期轻度强化[117,118]（图15-37）。

3. 肝炎 肝炎是肝脏对多种致病因素的一种非特异性炎性反应。最常见的病因是病毒感染（HBV、HCV、EBV、HAV），主要通过临床或血清学检查诊断；其他病因有细菌或真菌感染、自身免疫反应、药物诱导损伤以及放射治疗所致。

横断位成像并不作为肝炎主要诊断方法的一部分。急性病毒性肝炎的典型 MR 表现是肝大合并肝被膜水肿。暴发型急性病毒性肝炎中，MR 图像可以发现弥漫性或局灶性坏死区（图15-38）。在慢性肝炎的患者中，进行横断位成像，尤其是MRI，用以确定是否存在肝硬化及腹水及筛查是否存在肝细胞肝癌。在急性或慢性活动性肝炎患者的 T_2 加权图像上，经常会发现围绕门静脉分支的高信号区；但被认为是非特异征象。另外，在 T_2 加权图像上可以发现弥漫性或局限性高信号区[119]。患有病毒性肝炎的患者通常在肝门区

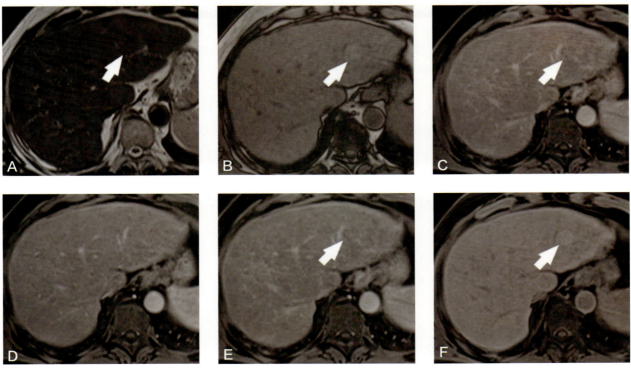

▲ 图 15-36 肝硬化不典型增生结节

A. T_2 加权图像上显示肝脏Ⅱ段稍低信号结节；B. T_1 加权图像上，该结节呈高信号，可能是由于脂肪或糖蛋白沉积；注射对比剂后，该结节呈乏血供，在延迟期显示"廓清征象"（C～E）；F. 在肝胆期 T_1 加权图像上，该结节与周围肝实质相比呈高信号

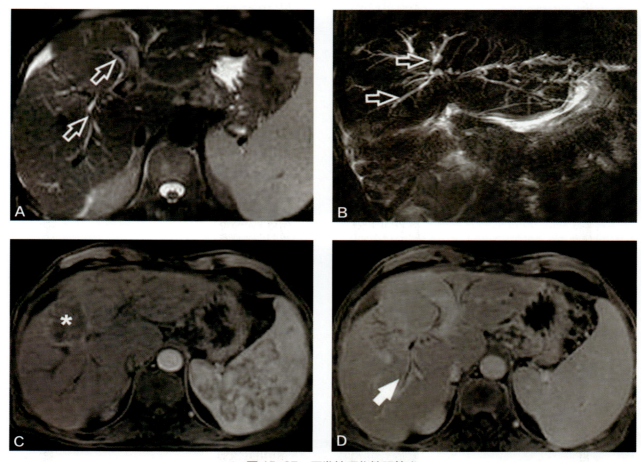

▲ 图 15-37 原发性硬化性胆管炎

A、B. 轴位 T_2 加权图像和 MIP 图像显示肝周区域边缘不规则的扩张胆管（空心箭）；C、D. 注射对比剂后，由于炎症和纤维化部分胆管出现强化（箭）；星号标注为肝脏Ⅷ段融合性纤维化区

出现孤立性或融合状肿大淋巴结。但是，与转移淋巴结不同的是，门静脉和其他结构不会呈受压改变，保持正常管径。

由于肝脏大小及在腹部的解剖位置，肝脏经常受到肝外恶性肿瘤放射治疗的影响。在放射性损伤 6 个月内，可以看到肝脏弥漫水肿，在 T_2 加权图像上信号增高，在 T_1 加权图像上信号减低[119]。在放射性损伤的区域门静脉血流量会减少，与伴随脂肪浸润的患者相似，这些区域的脂肪沉积通常会减少（图 15-39）[120]。

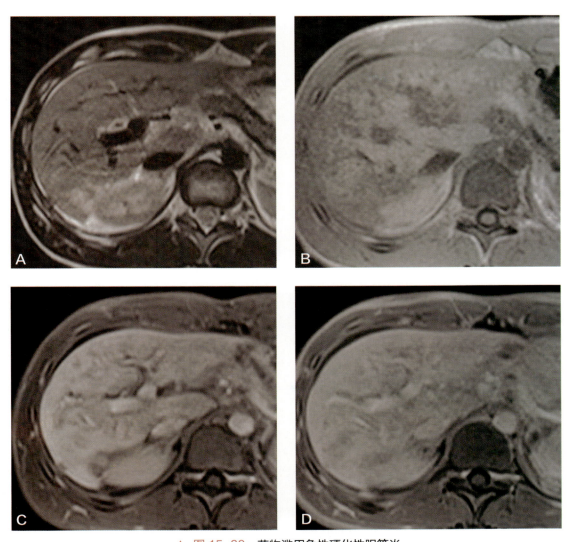

▲ 图 15-38　药物滥用急性硬化性胆管炎

A、B.T_2 加权图像及 T_1 加权图像显示肝周信号不均；C、D. 注射对比剂后，肝实质动脉不均匀强化，延迟期强化变均匀

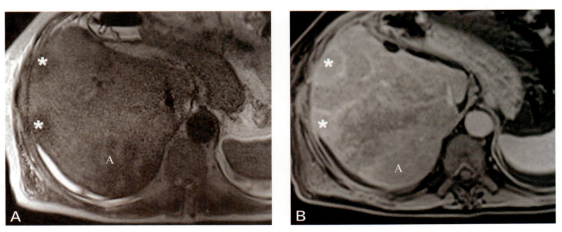

▲ 图 15-39　放射性栓塞期间辐射照射引起的慢性肝炎

A.T_2 加权图像显示由于组织水肿导致的肝实质弥漫高信号；B. 增强后 T_1 加权图像显示肝实质弥漫低信号，在肝Ⅵ段为正常肝实质区域；星号标记处为 2 个转移灶

参考文献

[1] Bartolozzi C, Cioni D, Donati F et al. (2001) Focal liver lesions: MR imaging-pathologic correlation. *Eur Radiol* 11:1374–1388.

[2] Keogan MT, Edelman RR (2001) Technologic advances in abdominal MR imaging. *Radiology* 220:310–320.

[3] Morrin MM, Rofsky NM (2001) Techniques for liver MR imaging. *Magn Reson Imaging Clin N Am* 9:675–696.

[4] Schwartz LH, Panicek DM, Thomson E et al. (1997) Comparison of phased-array and body coils for MR imaging of liver. *Clin Radiol* 52:745–749.

[5] Helmberger TK, Schroder J, Holzknecht N et al. (1999) T_2-weighted breathhold imaging of the liver: A quantitative and qualitative comparison of fast spin echo and half Fourier single shot fast spin echo imaging. *MAGMA* 9:42–51.

[6] Kim TK, Lee HJ, Jang HJ et al. (1998) T_2-weighted breath hold MRI of the liver at 1.0 T: Comparison of turbo spin-echo and HASTE sequences with and without fat suppression. *J Magn Reson Imaging* 8:1213–1218.

[7] Ward J, Robinson PJ, Guthrie JA et al. (2005) Liver metastases in candidates for hepatic resection: Comparison of helical CT and gadolinium and SPIO-enhanced MR imaging. *Radiology* 237:170–180.

[8] Siegelman ES (1997) MR imaging of diffuse liver disease: Hepatic fat and iron. *Magn Reson Imaging Clin N Am* 5:347–365.

[9] Engelhardt R, Langkowski JH, Fischer R et al. (1994) Liver iron quantification: Studies in aqueous iron solutions, iron overloaded rats, and patients with hereditary hemochromatosis. *Magn Reson Imaging* 12:999–1007.

[10] Ernst O, Sergent G, Bonvarlet P et al. (1997) Hepatic iron overload: Diagnosis and quantification with MR imaging. *AJR Am J Roentgenol* 168:1205–1208.

[11] Ferrucci JT (1998) Advances in abdominal MR imaging. *RadioGraphics* 18:1569–1586.

[12] Schneider G, GrazioliL, Saini S (2006) *MR Imaging of the Liver*, 2nd edition. Springer, New York.

[13] Larson RE, Semelka RC, Bagley AS, Molina PL, Brown ED, Lee JK (1994) Hypervascular malignant liver lesions: Comparison of various MR imaging pulse sequences and dynamic CT. *Radiology* 192:393–399.

[14] Low RN, Francis IR, Sigeti JS, Foo TK (1993) Abdominal MR imaging: Comparison of T_2-weighted fast conventional spin-echo, and contrast-enhanced fast multiplanar spoiled gradient-recalled imaging. *Radiology* 186:803–811.

[15] Yamashita Y, Mitsuzaki K, Yi T et al. (1996) Small hepatocellular carcinoma in patients with chronic liver damage: Prospective comparison of detection with dynamic MR imaging and helical CT of the whole liver. *Radiology* 200:79–84.

[16] Hussain HK, Londy FJ, Francis IR et al. (2003) Hepatic arterial phase MR imaging with automated bolus detection three-dimensional fast gradient-recalled echo sequence: Comparison with test-bolus method. *Radiology* 226:558–566.

[17] Kanematsu M, Semelka RC, Matsuo M et al. (2002) Gadolinium-enhanced MR imaging of the liver: Optimizing imaging delay for hepatic arterial and portal venous phases-A prospective randomized study in patients with chronic liver damage. *Radiology* 225:407–415.

[18] Mori K, Yoshioka H, Takahashi N et al. (2005) Triple arterial phase dynamic MRI with sensitivity encoding for hypervascular hepatocellular carcinoma: Comparison of the diagnostic accuracy among the early, middle, late, and whole triple arterial phase imaging. *AJR Am J Roentgenol* 184:63–69.

[19] Goshima S, Kanematsu M, Kondo H et al. (2009) Optimal acquisition delay for dynamic contrast-enhanced MRI of hypervascular hepatocellular carcinoma. *AJR Am J Roentgenol* 192:686–692.

[20] Hussain HK, Londy FJ, Francis IR et al. (2003) Hepatic arterial phase MR imaging with automated bolus detection three-dimensional fast gradient-recalled echo sequence: Comparison with test-bolus method. *Radiology* 226:558–566.

[21] Whitney WS, Herfkens RJ, Jeffrey RB et al. (1993) Dynamic breath-hold multiplanar spoiled gradient recalled MR imaging with gadolinium enhancement for differentiating hepatic hemangiomas from malignancies at 1.5 T. *Radiology* 189:863–870.

[22] Mathie D, Rahmouni A, Anglade MC et al. (1991) Focal nodular hyperplasia of the liver: Assessment with contrast-enhanced Turbo-FLASH MR imaging. *Radiology* 180:25–30.

[23] Mahfouz AE, Hamm B, Wolf KJ (1994) Peripheral wash out: A sign of malignancy on dynamic gadolinium enhanced MR images of focal liver lesions. *Radiology* 190:49–52.

[24] Low RN, Sigeti JS, Francis IR et al. (1994) Evaluation of malignant biliary obstruction: Efficacy of fast multiplanar spoiled gradient-recalled MR imaging vs. spin echo MR imaging, CT and cholangiography *AJR Am J Roentgenol* 162:315–323.

[25] Ros PR, Freeny PC, Harms SE et al. (1995) Hepatic MR imaging with ferumoxides: A multicenter clinical trial of the safety and efficacy in the detection of focal hepatic lesions. *Radiology* 196:481–488.

[26] Balci NC, Semelka RC (2005) Contrast agents for MR imaging of the liver. *Radiol Clin North Am* 43:887–898.

[27] Semelka RC, Helmberger T.K.G (2001) Contrast agent for MR imaging of the liver. *Radiology* 218:27–38.

[28] Bellin MF, Zaim S, Auberton E et al. (1994) Liver metastases: Safety and efficacy of detection with superparamagnetic iron oxide in MR imaging. *Radiology* 193:657–663.

[29] Winter III TC, Freeny PC, Nghiem HV et al. (1993) MR imaging with i.v. superparamagnetic iron oxide: Efficacy in the detection of focal hepatic lesions. *AJR Am J Roentgenol* 161:1191–1198.

[30] Kirchin MA, Pirovano GP, Spinazzi A (1998) Gadobenate dimeglumine (Gd-BOPTA). An overview. *Invest Radiol* 33:798–809.

[31] Huppertz A, Haraida S, Kraus A et al. (2005) Enhancement of focal liver lesions at gadoxetic acid-enhanced MR imaging: Correlation with histopathologic findings and spiral CT—Initial observations. *Radiology* 234:468–478.

[32] Bashir MR, Breault SR, Braun R, Do RK, Nelson RC, Reeder SB (2014) Optimal timing and diagnostic ade quacy of hepatocyte phase imaging with gadoxetate enhanced liver MRI. *Acad Radiol* 21:726–732.

[33] Van Kessel CS, Veldhuis WB, van den Bosch MA, van Leeuwen MS (2012) MR liver imaging with Gd-EOB DTPA: A delay time of 10 minutes is sufficient for lesion characterisation. *Eur Radiol* 22:2153–2160.

[34] Colagrande S1, Carbone SF, Carusi LM, Cova M, Villari N (2006) Magnetic resonance diffusion-weighted imaging: Extraneurological applications. *Radiol Med* 111:392–419.

[35] Taouli B, Martin AJ, Qayyum A et al (2004) Parallel imaging and diffusion tensor imaging for diffusion-weighted MRI of the liver: Preliminary experience in healthy vol unteers. *AJR Am J Roentgenol* 183:677–680.

[36] Yoshikawa T, Kawamitsu H, Mitchell DG et al. (2006) ADC measurement of abdominal organs and lesions using parallel imaging technique. *AJR Am J Roentgenol* 187:1521–1530.

[37] Thng CH, Koh TS, Collins DJ, Koh DM. Perfusion magnetic resonance imaging of the liver. *World J Gastroenterol* 16:1598–1609.

[38] Jackson A, Haroon H, Zhu XP et al. (2002) Breath-hold perfusion and permeability mapping of hepatic malig nancies using magnetic resonance imaging and a first pass leakage profile model. *NMR Biomed* 15:164–173.

[39] Qayyum A (2009) MR Spectroscopy of the liver: Principles and clinical applications *RadioGraphics* 29:1653–1664.

[40] Noworolski SM, Tien PC, Merriman R, Vigneron DB, Qayyum A (2009) Respiratory motion-corrected proton magnetic resonance spectroscopy of the liver. *Magn Reson Imaging* 27:570–576.

[41] Cowin GJ, Jonsson JR, Bauer JD et al. (2008) Magnetic resonance imaging and spectroscopy for monitoring liver steatosis. *J Magn Reson Imaging* 28:937–945.

[42] Soper R, Himmelreich U, Painter D et al. (2002) Pathology of hepatocellular carcinoma and its precursors using proton magnetic resonance spectroscopy and a statistical classification strategy. *Pathology* 34:417–422.

[43] Li CW, Kuo YC, Chen CY et al. (2005) Quantification of choline compounds in human hepatic tumors by proton MR spectroscopy at 3 T. *Magn Reson Med* 53:770–776.

[44] Wu B, Peng WJ, Wang PJ et al. (2006) In vivo 1H magnetic resonance spectroscopy in evaluation of hepatocellular carcinoma and its early response to transcatheter arterial chemoembolization. *Chin Med Sci J* 21:258–264.

[45] Kuo YT, Li CW, Chen CY, Jao J, Wu D, Liu GC (2004) In vivo proton magnetic resonance spectroscopy of large focal hepatic lesions and metabolite change of hepatocellular carcinoma before and after transcatheter arterial chemoembolization using a 3.0 T MR scanner. *J Magn Reson Imaging* 19:598–604.

[46] Hernandez-Guerra M, Garcia-Pagan JC, Bosch J (2005) Increased hepatic resistance: A new target in the pharmacologic therapy of portal hypertension. *J Clin Gastroenterol* 39:S131–S137.

[47] Ganne-Carrié N, Ziol M, de Ledinghen V et al. (2006) Accuracy of liver stiffness measurement for the diagnosis of cirrhosis in patients with chronic liver diseases. *Hepatology* 44:1511–1517.

[48] Talwalkar JA, Yin M, Fidler JL, Sanderson SO, Kamath PS, Ehman RL (2008) Magnetic resonance imaging of hepatic fibrosis: Emerging clinical applications. *Hepatology* 47:332–342.

[49] Yin M, Talwalkar JA, Glaser KJ et al. (2007) Assessment of hepatic fibrosis with magnetic resonance elastography. *Clin Gastroenterol Hepatol* 5:1207–1213.

[50] Elster AD (1997) How much contrast is enough? Dependence of enhancement on field strength and MR pulse sequence. *Eur Radiol* 7(suppl 5):276–280.

[51] Chang KJ, Kamel IR, Macura KJ, Bluemke DA (2008) 3.0-T MR imaging of the abdomen: Comparison with 1.5 T. *RadioGraphics* 28:1983–1998.

[52] Barth MM, Smith MP, Pedrosa I, Lenkinski RE, Rofsky NM (2007) Body MR imaging at 3.0 T: Understanding the opportunities and challenges. *Radio Graphics* 27:1445–1462.

[53] Couinaud C (1957) *Le foie: Études anatomiques et chirurgi cales*. Masson, Paris, France, pp. 9–12.

[54] Bismuth H (1982) Surgical anatomy and anatomical surgery of the liver. *World J Surg* 6:3–8.

[55] Catalano OA, Singh AH, Uppot RN et al. (2008) Vascular and biliary variants in the liver: Implications for liver surgery *RadioGraphics* 28:359–378.

[56] Makuuchi M, Hasegawa H, Yamazaki S et al. (1983) The inferior right hepatic vein ultrasonic demonstration. *Radiology* 148:213–217.

[57] Charlton M (2004) Non-Alcoholic fatty liver disease: A review of current understanding and future impact. *Clin Gastroenterol Hepatol* 2:1048–1058.

[58] Fabbrini E, Sullivan S, Klein S (2010) Obesity and no alcoholic fatty liver disease: Biochemical, metabolic, and clinical implications. *Hepatology* 51:679–689.

[59] Romeo S, Kozlitina J, Xing C, Pertsemlidis A, Cox D, Pennacchio LA, Boerwinkle E, Cohen JC, Hobbs HH (2008) Genetic variation in PNPLA3 confers susceptibility to nonalcoholic fatty liver disease. *Nat Genet* 40:1461–1465.

[60] Prasad SR, Wang H, Rosas H et al. (2005) Fat-containing lesions of the liver: Radiologic-pathologic correlation. *RadioGraphics* 25:321–331.

[61] Qayyum A (2009) MR spectroscopy of the liver: Principles and clinical applications. *RadioGraphics* 29:1653–1664.

[62] Kim H, Taksali SE, Dufour S et al. (2008) Comparative MR

study of hepatic fat quantification using single-voxel proton spectroscopy, two-point dixon and three-point IDEAL. *Magn Reson Med* 59:521–527.

[63] Hussain HK, Chenevert TL, Londy FJ et al. (2005) Hepatic fat fraction: MR imaging for quantitative measurement and display—Early experience. *Radiology* 237:1048–1055.

[64] Guiu B, Petit JM, Loffroy R et al. (2009) Quantification of liver fat: Comparison of triple-echo chemical shift gradient-echo imaging and in vivo proton MR Spectroscopy. *Radiology* 1:95–102.

[65] Shwartz LH, Panicek DM, Koutcher JA et al. (1995) Adrenal masses in patients with malignancy: Prospective comparison of echo-planar, fast spin echo, and chemical shift MR Imaging. *Radiology* 197:421–425.

[66] Siegelman ES, Mitchell DG, Semelka RC (1996) Abdominal iron deposition: Metabolism, MR findings, and clinical importance. *Radiology* 199:13–22.

[67] Sirlin CB, Reeder SB (2010) Magnetic resonance imaging quantification of liver iron. *Magn Reson Imaging Clin N Am* 18:359–381.

[68] Alústiza JM, Artetxe J, Castiella A et al. (2004) MR quantification of hepatic iron concentration. *Radiology* 230:479–484.

[69] Li TQ, Aisen AM, Hindmarsh T (2004) Assessment of hepatic iron content using magnetic resonance imaging. *Acta Radiol* 45:119–129.

[70] Vogl TJ, Steiner S, Hammerstingl R et al. (1994) MRT of the liver in Wilson's disease. *Rofo* 160:40–45.

[71] Akhan O, Akpinar E, Karcaanticaba M et al. (2009) Imaging findings of liver involvement of Wilson's disease. *Eur Radiol* 69:147–155.

[72] Tani I, Kurihara Y, Kawaguchi A et al. (2000) MR imaging of diffuse liver disease. *AJR Am J Roentgenol* 174:965–971.

[73] Buscarini E, Buscarini L, Civardi G, Arruzzoli S, Bossalini G, Piantanida M (1994) Hepatic vascular malformations in hereditary hemorrhagic telangiectasia: Imaging findings. *AJR Am J Roentgenol* 163:1105–1110.

[74] Dakeishi M, Shioya T, Wada Y et al. (2002) Genetic epidemiology of hereditary hemorrhagic teleangiectasia in a local community in the northern part of Japan. *Hum Mutat* 19:140–148.

[75] Milot L, Kamaoui I, Gautier G, Pilleul F (2008) Hereditary hemorrhagic telangiectasia: One-step magnetic resonance examination in evaluation of liver involvement. *Gastroenterol Clin Biol* 32:677–685.

[76] Memeo M, Stabile Ianora AA, Scardapane A et al. (2004) Hepatic involvement in hereditary hemorrhagic telean giectasia: CT findings. *Abdom Imaging* 29:211–220.

[77] Hennksson L, Hedman A, Johansson A, Lindstrom K (1982) Ultrasound assessment of liver veins in congestive heart failure. *Acta Radiol* 23:361–363.

[78] Moulton JS, Miller BL, Dodd GD, Vu DN (1988) Passive hepatic congestion in heart failure: CT abnormalities. *AJR* 51:939–942.

[79] Janssen HL, Garcia-Pagan JC, Elias E et al. (2003) Budd Chiari syndrome: A review by an expert panel. *J Hepatol* 38:364–71.

[80] Dilawari JB, Bambery P, Chawla Y et al. (1994) Hepatic outflow obstruction (Budd-Chiari syndrome). Experience with 177 patients and a review of the literature. *Medicine* 73:21–36.

[81] Ludwig J, Hashimoto E, McGill DB, van Heerden JA (1990) Classification of hepatic venous outflow obstruction: Ambiguous terminology of the Budd-Chiari syndrome. *Mayo Clin Proc* 65:51–55.

[82] Noone TC, Semelka RC, Siegelman ES et al. (2000) Budd Chiari syndrome: Spectrum of appearances of acute, subacute, and chronic disease with magnetic resonance imaging. *J Magn Reson Imaging* 11:44–50.

[83] Bogin V, Marcos A, Shaw-Stiffel T (2005) Budd-Chiari syn drome: In evolution. *Eur J Gastroenterol Hepatol* 17:33–35.

[84] Lim JH, Park JH, Auh YH (1992) Membranous obstruction of the inferior vena cava: Comparison of findings at sonography, CT, and venography. *AJR Am J Roentgenol* 159:515–520.

[85] Kimura C, Matsuda S, Koie H, Hirooka M (1972) Membranous obstruction of the hepatic portion of the inferior vena cava: Clinical study of nine cases. *Surgery* 72:551–559.

[86] MenonKV, ShahV, Kamath PS (2004) The Budd-Chiari syndrome. *N Engl J Med* 350:578–585.

[87] Stark DD, Hahn PF, Trey C, Clouse ME, Ferrucci Jr JT (1986) MRI of the Budd-Chiari syndrome. *AJR Am J Roentgenol* 146:1141–1148.

[88] Soyer P, Lacheheb D, Caudron C, Levesque M (1993) MRI of adenomatous hyperplastic nodules of the liver in Budd-Chiari syndrome. *J Comput Assist Tomogr* 17:86–89.

[89] Federle MP (2004) *Diagnostic Imaging. Abdomen*. Amirsys, Salt Lake City, Utah.

[90] Vilgrain V, Lewin M, Vons C et al. (1999) Hepatic nodules in Budd-Chiari syndrome: Imaging features. *Radiology* 210:443–450.

[91] Brancatelli G, Federle MP, Grazioli L, Golfieri R, Lencioni R (2002) Large regenerative nodules in Budd-Chiari syn drome and other vascular disorders of the liver: CT and MR imaging findings with clinicopathologic correlation. *AJR Am J Roentgenol* 178:877–883.

[92] Maetani Y, Itoh K, Egawa H et al. (2002) Benign hepatic nodules in Budd-Chiari syndrome: Radiologic–patho-logic correlation with emphasis on the central scar. *AJR Am J Roentgenol* 178:869–875.

[93] Boll DT, Merkle EM (2009) Diffuse liver disease: Strategies for hepatic CT and MR imaging. *RadioGraphics* 29:1591–1614.

[94] Hanna RF, Aguirre DA, Kased N et al. (2008) Cirrhosis associated hepatocellular nodules: Correlation of histopathologic and MR Imaging Features. *RadioGraphics* 28:747–769.

[95] Giorgio A, Amoroso P, Lettieri G et al. (1986) Cirrhosis:

Value of caudate to right lobe ratio in diagnosis with US. *Radiology* 161:443–445.

[96] Stark DD, Goldberg HI, Moss AA, Bass NM (1984) Chronic liver disease: Evaluation by magnetic resonance. *Radiology* 150:149–151.

[97] Okazaki H, Ito K, Fujita T, Koike S, Takano K, Matsunaga N (2000) Discrimination of alcoholic from virus-induced cirrhosis on MR imaging. *AJR Am J Roentgenol* 175:1677–1681.

[98] Ito K, Mitchell DG, Kim MJ, Awaya H, Koike S, Matsunaga N (2003) Right posterior hepatic notch sign: A simple diagnostic MR sign of cirrhosis. *J Magn Reson Imag* 18:561–6.

[99] Ito K, Mitchell DG, Gabata T, Hussain SM (1999) Expanded gallbladder fossa: Simple MR imaging sign of cirrhosis. *Radiology* 211:723–6.

[100] Brancatelli G, Federle MP, Ambrosini R et al. (2007) Cirrhosis: CT and MR imaging evaluation. *Eur J Radiol* 61:57–69.

[101] Vilgrain V (2001) Ultrasound of diffuse liver disease and portal hypertension. *Eur Radiol* 11:1563–77.

[102] Ohtomo K, Baron RL, Dodd III GD et al. (1993) Confluent hepatic fibrosis in advanced cirrhosis: Evaluation with MR imaging. *Radiology* 189:871–874.

[103] Coleman WB (2003) Mechanisms of human hepatocarcinogenesis. *Curr Mol Med* 3:573–588.

[104] Hussain SM, Zondervan PE, IJzermans JN, Schalm SW, de Man RA, Krestin GP (2002) Benign versus malignant hepatic nodules: MR imaging findings with patho-logic correlation. *RadioGraphics* 22:1023–1036; discussion 1037–1039.

[105] Manfredi R, Maresca G, Baron RL et al. (1998) Gadobenate dimeglumine (BOPTA) enhanced MR imaging: Patterns of enhancement in normal liver and cirrhosis. *J Magn Reson Imaging* 8:862–867.

[106] Krinsky GA, Lee VS, Nguyen MT et al. (2000) Siderotic nodules at MR imaging: Regenerative or dysplastic? *J Comput Assist Tomogr* 24:773–776.

[107] Krinsky GA, Lee VS, Theise ND et al. (2001) Hepatocellular carcinoma and dysplastic nodules in patients with cirrhosis: Prospective diagnosis with MR imaging and explanation correlation. *Radiology* 219:445–454.

[108] Di Martino M, Anzidei, M, Zaccagna F, Saba L, Catalano C (2014) Gadoxetic Acid MR Imaging in the characterization of the "grey zone" of the hepatocarcinogenesis. In: *Scientific Assembly and Annual Meeting*, Chicago, IL, Radiological Society of North America.

[109] Mitchell DG, Rubin R, Siegelman ES, Burk Jr DL, Rifkin MD (1991) Hepatocellular carcinoma within siderotic regenerative nodules: Appearance as a nodule within a nodule on MR images. *Radiology* 78:101–103.

[110] Cohen SA, Siegel JH, Kasmin FE (1996) Complication of diagnostic and therapeutic ERCP. *Abdom Imaging* 21:385–394.

[111] Silverman WB, Kaw M, Rabinovitz M et al. (1994) Complication rate of endoscopic retrograde cholangiopancreatography (ERCP) in patients with primary sclerosing cholangitis: Is it safe? *Gastroenterology* 106:359.

[112] Lee YM, Kaplan MM (1995) Primary sclerosing cholangitis. *N England J Med* 332:924–933.

[113] Boberg KM, Schrumpf E (2004) Diagnosis and treatment of cholangiocarcinoma. *Curr Gastroenterol Rep* 6:52–59.

[114] Chapman RW, Jewell DP (1985) Primary sclerosing cholangitis: An immunologically mediated disease? *West J Med* 143:193–195.

[115] Crippin JS, Lindor KD (1992) Primary sclerosing cholangitis: Etiology and immunology. *Eur J Gastroenterol Hepato* 4:261–265.

[116] McCarty RC, LaRusso NF, Wiesner RH et al. (1983) Primary sclerosing cholangitis: Findings on cholangiography and pancreatography. *Radiology* 149:39–44.

[117] Bader TR, Beavers KL, Semelka RC (2003) MR imaging features of primary sclerosing cholangitis: Patterns of cirrhosis in relationship to clinical severity of disease. *Radiology* 226:675–685.

[118] Ito K, Mitchell DG, Outwater EK et al. (1999) Primary sclerosing cholangitis: MR imaging features. *AJR* 172:1527–1533.

[119] Matsui O, Kadoya M, Takashima T, Kameyama T, Yoshikawa J, Tamura S (1989) Intrahepatic periportal abnormal intensity on MR images: An indication of various hepatobiliary diseases. *Radiology* 171:335–338.

[120] Unger EC, Lee JK, Weyman PJ (1987) CT and MR imaging of radiation hepatitis. *J Comput Assist Tomogr* 11:264–268.

Chapter 16
肝脏局灶性病变

Liver: Focal Pathology

Michele Di Martino，Carlo Catalano 著

冯 冰 译

马霄虹 校

目录 CONTENTS

一、囊性局灶性病变 / 362

二、肝脏良性局灶性疾病 / 365

三、其他肝脏良性病变 / 376

四、肝恶性局灶性病变 / 377

五、其他肝脏恶性病变 / 386

六、治疗后评估 / 388

肝脏局灶性病变十分常见，普通人群的患病率超过 20%。在过去的几十年里，随着技术革新发展，磁共振（MR）的灵敏度和特异性已经超越了计算机断层扫描（CT），在评估肝脏局灶性病变方面发挥着主导作用。

一、囊性局灶性病变

肝脏的囊性局灶性病变是一类复杂的异质性疾病的集合，这些疾病在发病机制、临床表现、影像表现和治疗管理方面各有不同，可分为先天性、炎症性和肿瘤性肝囊肿[1]。先天性肝囊肿包括多种不同疾病［肝囊肿、胆道错构瘤、多囊肝和先天性肝内胆管扩张（Caroli 病）］，也可被称为"纤维多囊性肝病"，这一术语是指由于不同阶段胚胎胆管板发育紊乱所引发的一类疾病[2]。炎症性肝囊肿可能是肝内包虫囊肿形成的脓肿，而肿瘤性肝囊肿可能是囊腺瘤或囊腺癌、未分化肉瘤、囊性转移瘤等。

（一）肝囊肿

肝囊肿是常见的肝脏疾病，在普通人群中的发生率高达 2.5%[3]。它们可以是单发或多发，大小不等（从几毫米到 5cm 及以上），不与胆管树相通，内容物为浆液性成分，有时可合并出血或感染则称为复杂性肝囊肿。在 MR 成像中，肝囊肿在 T_1 加权图像上呈均匀低信号，在 T_2 加权图像上呈均匀高信号。增强扫描无强化，囊壁一般不能显示（图 16-1）。

（二）胆管错构瘤

胆管错构瘤，也称为 von Meyenburg 复合体，由一个或多个内衬胆管上皮的扩张胆管及纤维性基质组成。它们通常为多发、散在分布，大小一般不超过 1.5cm，不与胆管树相通。根据错构瘤的均一性和胆管扩张情况，胆管错构瘤分类如下：第 1 类为实性病变合并胆管狭窄，第 2 类为胆管轻度或局限性扩张，第 3 类为胆管明显扩张[4]。在 MR 成像中，胆管错构瘤 T_1 加权图像呈低信号，T_2 加权图像呈显著高信号（图 16-2）。研究人员观察到在增强扫描后这些病灶可以出现均匀强化或环状强化[5-8]。在肿瘤患者中，胆管错构瘤可能被误诊为肝转移瘤[9]。

（三）多囊肝

常染色体显性多囊肝的特点是多发囊性病灶，有时多到难以计数，通常合并多囊肾[3]。它被认为是由胆管错构瘤中的异常胆管逐渐扩张

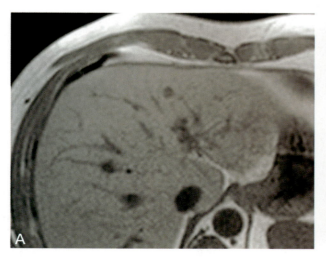 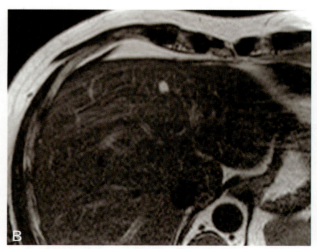

▲ 图 16-1　肝囊肿

A. 轴位 T_1 加权图像示肝内一均匀、圆形、边界清晰的低信号病灶；B. 在 T_2 加权图像上，病变显示出明显的高信号

形成，属于肝内小胆管水平的胆管板发育异常的一部分。与胆管错构瘤类似，它们不与胆管树相通。患者通常无症状，也可出现腹胀、腹部不适和呼吸困难等症状。在影像学检查中，肝实质增大，取而代之的是直径从几毫米到 12cm 或更大的弥漫分布的肝囊肿（图 16-3）[10]。囊肿的特征与单纯囊肿的特征相同：T_1 加权图像上呈均匀低信号，T_2 加权图像呈均匀高信号；其中一些可能合并出血和（或）感染而出现信号不均的表现。

囊壁可能出现钙化，恶变极为罕见，对于有症状的患者应进行肝移植。

（四）Caroli 病

Caroli 病是大的肝内胆管板发育畸形的结果。在文献中，Caroli 病有两种类型：一种是 Caroli 病，主要累及肝内较大胆管；另一种是 Caroli 综合征，主要累及周围性胆管及胆总管。在 MR 成像中，Caroli 病表现为胆管多发囊状扩张，T_1 加权图像呈

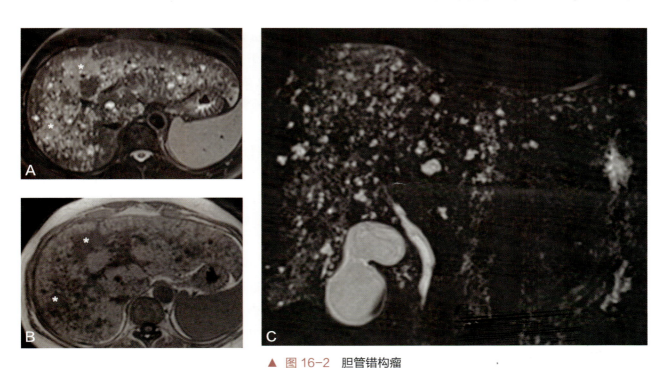

▲ 图 16-2 胆管错构瘤

A、B. T_1 加权图像和 T_2 加权图像示多个小的（直径 1.5cm）结节，与胆管错构瘤表现一致；C. 冠状位 MR 胆管造影示所有病灶直径均小于 1.5cm 且不与胆管树相通。注意广泛的肝脏纤维化（星号）

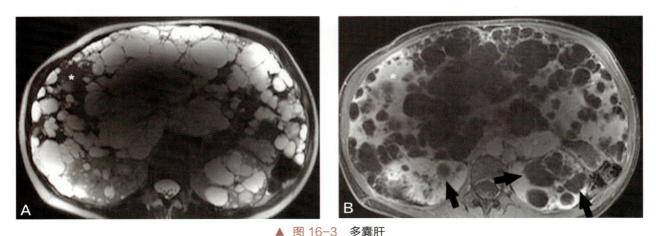

▲ 图 16-3 多囊肝

T_1 加权图像和 T_2 加权图像示多发肝囊肿典型 MR 表现，还要注意肾脏受累（黑色箭）

低信号，T_2 加权图像呈高信号，增强扫描在囊状扩张的胆管腔内可见强化的门静脉小分支，称为"中心点征"（图 16-4）[11]。磁共振胰胆管造影（magnetic resonance cholangiopancreatography，MRCP）非常适用于显示囊状或梭形扩张的胆管与胆管树相通的情况，有时可见充盈缺损代表合并肝内胆管结石（图 16-4）[12]。Caroli 病的主要并发症是胆管炎、结石和脓肿；在 Caroli 综合征中，除了上述并发症外，还可能出现继发性胆汁性肝硬化和门静脉高压。Caroli 病患者胆管癌的患病率高于一般人群[13]。

（五）肝脓肿

肝脓肿可分为化脓性、阿米巴性或真菌性肝脓肿。化脓性肝脓肿最常见的致病菌是梭菌属和革兰阴性菌，如大肠埃希菌、克雷伯菌、肠球菌，它们通过门静脉系统或胆管树等途径到达肝脏[14]。

在早期阶段，化脓性脓肿表现为簇状分布多发小病灶，之后可融合成一个较大的脓腔。它也可表现为大的多房肿物，内见分隔，增强后环状强化；边缘强化是由肉芽组织引起的。在 MR 成像中，这些脓肿的特征包括钆增强早期边缘和分隔明显强化，钆增强晚期持续强化，边缘及分隔的强化厚度及强化程度的变化可忽略不计（图 16-5）[15]。

阿米巴性肝脓肿是阿米巴病最常见的肠外并发症，发生率为 3%～9%。其特征是大的厚壁单房囊腔，周围可见水肿。中央囊性区域由出血、颗粒状坏死物质和称为"鲲鱼酱"的细胞碎片组成[16]。在 MR 成像中，T_1 加权图像和 T_2 加权图像信号强度多变，主要取决于囊内容物的成分；钆增强后，通常可以看到脓肿壁的快速强化（图 16-6）。

（六）肝包虫囊肿

肝包虫囊肿是一种严重的常见寄生虫病。它通常是由于感染棘球属带绦虫（绦虫）的幼虫所致。MR 成像可以清楚地显示外囊、囊内容物和子囊。外囊在 T_1 加权图像和 T_2 加权图像均呈环状低信号，是由于外囊主要是纤维性成分，常出现钙化。囊内容物（囊"沙"）在 T_1 加权图像上呈低信号，在 T_2 加权图像上呈明显高信号，如果存在子囊时，子囊 T_2 加权图像信号比囊内容物信号低，增强后病灶无明显强化[17]（图 16-7）。

（七）胆管囊腺瘤/囊腺癌

胆管囊腺瘤是一种罕见的、生长缓慢的多房性囊性肿瘤，在肝内胆管源性囊性病变中所占比例不到 5%。主要好发于中年妇女（平均年龄 38 岁），并被认为是癌前病变，因为它可以

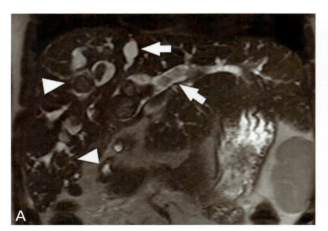 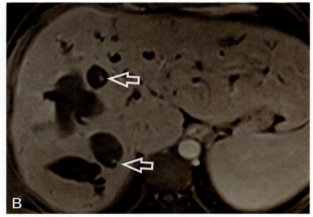

▲ 图 16-4 Caroli 病
A. 冠状位 T_2 加权图像显示多发高信号囊状扩张（白箭）和结石（箭头）；B. 注射对比剂之后，可见中央纤维血管束（中心点征）（空心箭）

进展为囊腺癌，手术切除是首选的治疗方式。胆管囊腺瘤通常位于肝内（85%），但是也有报道一些病变发生在肝外。胆囊腺瘤的直径范围为 1.5～35cm。肿瘤内部有蛋白质性、黏液性液体，偶尔是胶状、化脓性或血性液体[18]。MR 成像上典型表现是多房囊性肿块，在 T_1 加权图像上通常表现为均匀低信号，在 T_2 加权图像上表现为均匀高信号[19]。T_1 加权图像和 T_2 加权图像上信号强度的变化取决于实性成分、出血和蛋白质的含量[20]（图 16-8）。如果病变出现囊壁不规则增厚、实性壁结节、粗大钙化和乳头状突起提示囊腺癌。最近研究表明肿瘤标志物肿瘤相关糖蛋白（TAG）72 在鉴别单纯性囊肿和囊腺瘤方面优于癌胚抗原（carcino-embryonic antigen，CEA）、糖类抗原（carbohydrate antigen，CA）19-9[21]。

（八）囊性转移瘤

囊性转移瘤不如实性转移瘤（富血供和乏血供）常见。它们被定义为瘤内有大片液性区域，增强后边缘有微弱强化。对于囊性转移瘤的起源目前有两种解释：富血供转移瘤生长速度过快而血供不足而使瘤内发生坏死（神经内分泌肿瘤、胃肠间质瘤）和黏液腺癌（结肠和卵巢）的转移瘤产生黏蛋白[22]。卵巢黏液腺癌通常通过腹膜种植转移，因此，转移瘤表现为种植在肝脏表面浆膜的囊性病灶，而不是在肝实质内的病灶。囊性转移瘤表现为单房或多房囊肿，囊壁不规则增厚，其内缘可以不光整，可散在多个壁结节。增强后表现为环状强化或其内结节成分强化[15]（图 16-9）。

二、肝脏良性局灶性疾病

随着影像检查的广泛使用，在 MR 检查中经常会检出良性肝脏病变，其中最常见的肝脏良性肿瘤包括血管瘤（4%），局灶性结节性增生（focal nodular hyperplasia，FNH；0.4%）和肝腺瘤（0.004%）。

（一）血管瘤

肝血管瘤是最常见的良性肝脏肿瘤，在一

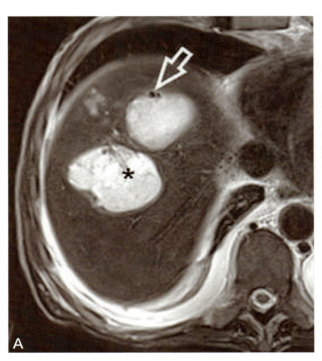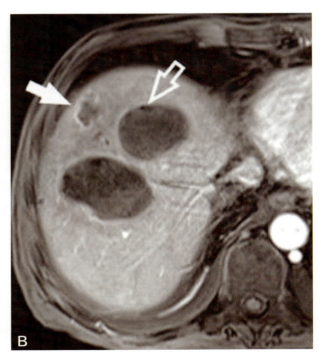

▲ 图 16-5 化脓性脓肿

A. 轴位 T_2 加权图像显示一个多房肿物被另一个较小的病变包围。病灶内可见气泡（空心箭）；B. 轴位静脉期 T_1 加权图像显示较小病变边缘强化（白箭）。注意引流管（星号）的存在

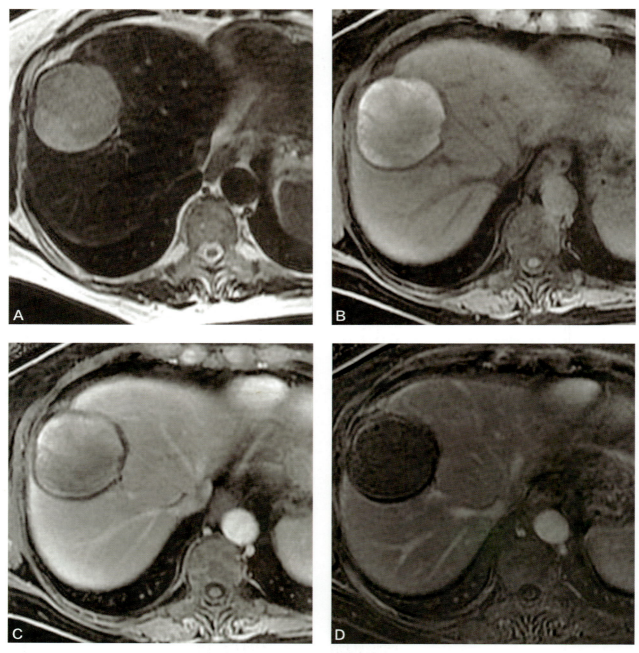

▲ 图 16-6 阿米巴脓肿

A、B.T_1 加权图像和 T_2 加权图像显示肝右叶一大的、圆形、边界清晰的囊性肿块，其内信号不均并可见出血；C、D. 静脉期 T_1 加权图像和相应减影图像上病变内未见强化

般人群中患病率为 2%～20%。临床上通常无症状，肿块较大时可出现并发症，例如压迫邻近结构和（或）肿瘤破裂后出血[23,24]。血管瘤在高达 50% 的病例中可以是多发的，并且可合并其他局灶性病变，如局灶性结节性增生（FNH）[25]。在组织学上，肿瘤由多发内衬单层血管内皮细胞的血管窦及薄层纤维基质组成。大的血管瘤组成成分比较复杂，可以出现纤维化、坏死、囊变和钙化。

在 MR 成像中，肝血管瘤表现为边界清晰的类圆形肿块，T_1 加权图像呈低信号，T_2 加权图像呈均匀的高亮信号，T_2 加权图像序列在鉴别诊断中起着非常重要的作用。注射钆对比剂后，血管瘤可以有两种不同的强化方式：小血管瘤（< 1.5

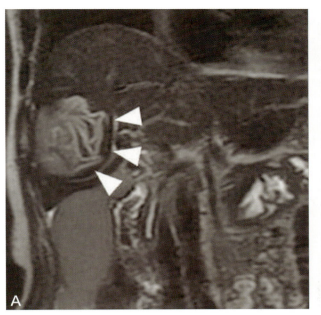
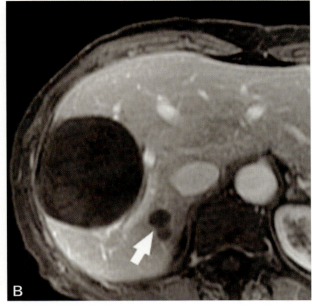

▲ 图 16-7　肝包虫囊肿

A. 冠状位 T_2 加权图像显示大的信号不均的肿块伴有低信号假包膜（箭头）；B. 轴位静脉期 T_1 加权图像显示主要病变与子囊（白箭）

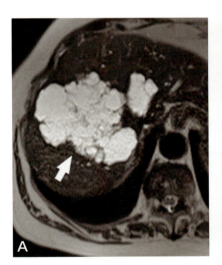
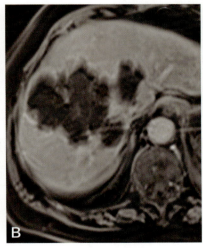
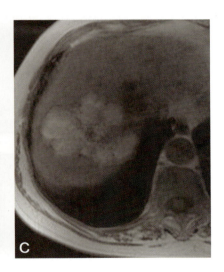

▲ 图 16-8　胆管囊腺瘤

A. 轴位 T_2 加权图像显示肝右叶的多房、内有分隔的肿物（白箭）；B. 相应的静脉期 T_1 加权 MR 图像示包膜和分隔的强化；C. 在后续的成像中，增强前 T_1 加权图像证明了病变内内容物含黏蛋白成分

cm）通常在动脉期均匀强化，门静脉期及延迟期仍持续强化。这些特征也可以在其他富血供肿瘤中观察到，如 FNH、肝细胞癌（hepatocellular carcinoma，HCC）和富血供转移瘤（图 16-10）。典型的血管瘤和大血管瘤动脉期表现为边缘结节状强化，门静脉期和延迟期向心性渐进性强化（图 16-11 和图 16-12）。应用 T_2 加权自旋回波和动态钆增强 T_1 加权梯度回波序列诊断血管瘤的灵敏度和特异性为 98%，准确度为 99%[26]。肝血管瘤很少出现钙化[27,28]。

（二）局灶性结节性增生

局灶性结节性增生（FNH）是第二常见的肝脏良性肿瘤，其患病率为 3%～8%。多见于 30 或 50 岁左右中青年女性（男女比例约为 8∶1）[29]。FNH 是由有功能的肝细胞组成的结节，周围是正常或近似正常的肝实质[30]。其发病机制尚不清楚，可能与血管畸形和血管损伤有关[31]。FNH 分为两种类型：经典型和非经典型。非经典型 FNH 包含三种亚型：毛细血管扩张型 FNH，具有细胞异型性的 FNH 和混合性增生性和腺瘤性 FNH[29]。约 20% 的患者中 FNH 为多发，既可以是有多个不同类型的 FNH 病灶，也可以合并以下一种或多种病变——肝血管瘤、中枢神经系统血管畸形、脑膜瘤、星形细胞瘤——被称为多发 FNH 综合征[32,33]。经典型 FNH 的大体病理表现为分叶状外形，实质部分被发自中央瘢痕的纤维间隔分隔呈多个结节。FNH 无肿瘤包膜，但在一些 FNH 病灶周围可见明显的假包膜结构。组织学分析显示，经典型 FNH 为结节增生的肝实质，这些结节可以被环状或短纤维间隔完全或部分完全包绕，肝板是由中度增厚的肝细胞组成。中央

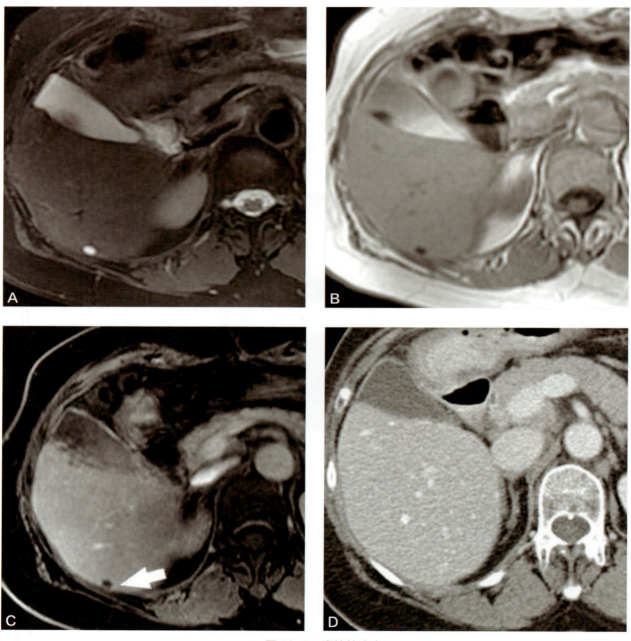

▲ 图 16-9　囊性转移瘤

A、B. T_2 加权图像和 T_1 加权图像显示肝脏被膜下 Ⅵ 段的囊样病变；C. 轴位 T_1 加权静脉期图像显示周围微弱的环形强化；D.3 个月前的 CT 图像未显示任何病灶

瘢痕含有纤维结缔组织、被炎性细胞浸润包绕的增殖的胆管和不同大小的畸形血管。

与超声和CT相比，MR对诊断FNH具有更高的灵敏度（70%）和特异性（98%）[34]。在MR成像中，典型的FNH在T_1加权图像上呈等信号或稍低信号，在T_2加权图像上呈稍高或等信号[35]。注射对比剂后，FNH在动脉期均匀明显强化，在门静脉和平衡期呈等信号。中央瘢痕在T_2加权图像上呈稍高信号，在T_1加权图像上呈低信号，并且注射对比剂后呈延迟强化（图16-13和图16-14）。

随着在临床实践中MR肝脏特异性对比剂（肝胆管和网状内皮细胞）的应用，FNH的诊断情况显著改善。注射顺磁性肝胆特异性对

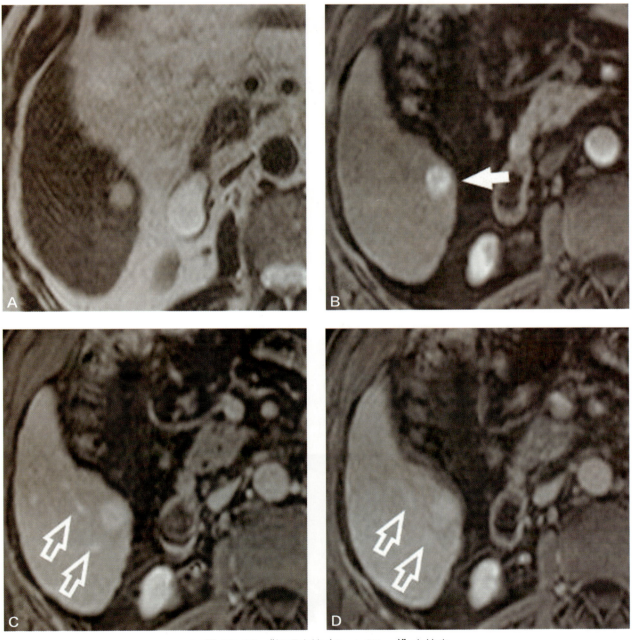

▲ 图 16-10 "闪现充填（flash filling）"血管瘤

A. T_2加权图像显示肝Ⅴ段一高亮信号的圆形病变，信号均匀；B. 动脉期T_1加权 MR 图像示小病灶（白箭）立即均匀强化；C、D. 静脉期和延迟期T_1加权 MR 图像示病变持续强化，强化程度类似于肝血管（空心箭）

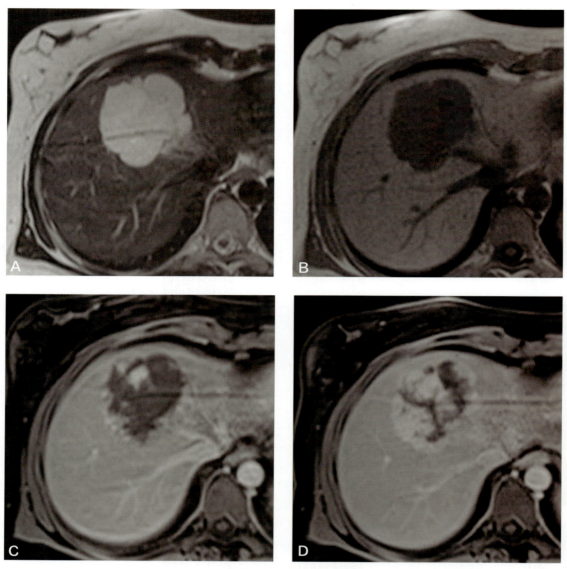

▲ 图 16-11 海绵状血管瘤

A、B. T_1 加权图像和 T_2 加权图像显示肝Ⅳ、Ⅷ段之间一信号均匀、圆形、边界清晰的病变。动脉期（C）和延迟期（D）对比增强的 MR 序列示边缘结节状渐进性强化，高度提示血管瘤

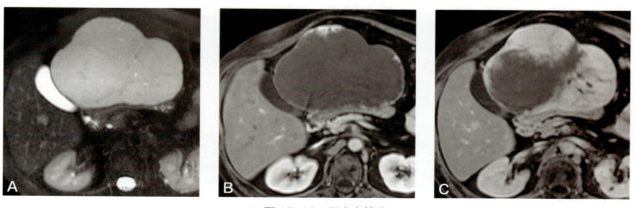

▲ 图 16-12 巨大血管瘤

A～C. T_2 加权图像和动脉期和延迟期对比增强的 T_1 加权图像示整个肝左叶内一局灶性病变，具有典型血管瘤影像表现

比剂后，与周围肝实质相比，FNH 呈高信号或等信号，这是因为对比剂往往留在未分化良好的胆管系统内[36,37]。这个影像表现的灵敏度为 92%～96.9%（图 16-15）。肝胆期中不典型的 FNH 可以出现低信号，其可能解释是病灶存在大的中央瘢痕、病变内富含脂肪成分或是毛细血管扩张型 FNH（图 16-16）[38]。应用含有超顺磁性氧化铁（SPIO）对比剂时，FNH 结节在 T_2 加权图像和 T_2^* 加权图像图像上信号减低，这与病灶内 Kupffer 细胞摄取氧化铁颗粒有关。因此，当使用这种对比剂时,中央瘢痕显示得更加明显（图 16-15）[39]。肝脏特异性造影剂是鉴别诊断 FNH 与其他富血供肿瘤（如肝细胞腺瘤，HCC 和富血供转移瘤）及"快速充盈"血管瘤非常有用的工具。由于肝细胞腺瘤中缺乏胆管系统，HCC 和富血供转移瘤缺乏有功能的肝细胞，因此这些病变不会摄取肝脏特异性对比剂。

（三）肝细胞腺瘤

肝细胞腺瘤（hepatocellular adenoma，HA）是一种少见的良性肿瘤，通常好发于中青年女性。通常是单发的（70%～80%），遇到两三个腺瘤的情况并不罕见；多发腺瘤（>10个）则称为"肝细胞腺瘤病"[40]。肿瘤的发病机制尚不清楚，但很可能是由多种因素引起的。肝细胞腺瘤最常见的两种并发症是破裂出血和进展为 HCC。

肝细胞腺瘤目前分为 3 种不同的组织病理学亚型：炎症型肝细胞腺瘤，肝细胞核因子 1α（HNF-1α）- 突变型肝细胞腺瘤和 β- 连锁蛋白突变型肝细胞腺瘤[41]。

炎症型肝细胞腺瘤是最常见的亚型，占所有肝细胞腺瘤的 40%～50%。常见于口服避孕药的

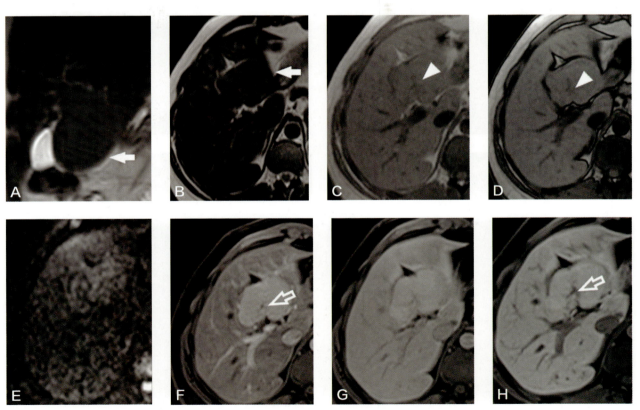

▲ 图 16-13　局灶性结节性增生伴瘢痕

A、B. 在冠状位和轴位 T_2 加权图像上，FNH 信号与周围肝实质比呈等信号，但由于占位效应仍然可被观察到；C、D. 在轴位同相位和反相位 T_1 加权图像上，FNH 与周围肝实质比呈等信号，中央瘢痕呈稍低信号（箭头）；E. 在 b-400 EPI DW 图像上，病变的信号强度与肝实质相似；F.轴位动脉期图像：FNH 表现为非常明显且均匀的强化而中央瘢痕无强化（空心箭）；G、H. 静脉期和延迟期 FNH 强化程度与周围肝实质相仿

女性及肥胖患者[42]。大体病理学上，炎症型肝细胞腺瘤因充血和明显的出血区表现为不均质。组织病理学上，炎症型肝细胞腺瘤可见明显的多形性细胞浸润、明显的血窦扩张或淤血以及动脉壁增厚[43]。在 T_2 加权图像上通常是高信号；在 T_1 加权图像上通常是等信号或高信号，反相位上信号不减低。增强后，炎症型 HA 显示均匀强化，门静脉期和延迟期持续强化[44,45]。

在 MR 成像中，HNF-1α 突变型肝细胞腺瘤在 T_1 加权图像图像上主要为高信号或等信号，反相位上可见弥漫性信号减低；相比之下，在 T_2 加权图像上则表现为等至稍高信号。增强后，HNF-1α 突变型肝细胞腺瘤在动脉期略有强化，不伴有门静脉期及延迟期持续强化。β-连锁蛋白突变型肝细胞腺瘤尚无相应的特征性 MRI 表现，在 T_1 加权图像和 T_2 加权图像上，这些肿瘤可表现为均匀或不均匀高信号，这取决于是否存在出血和（或）坏死。β-连锁蛋白突变型肝细胞腺

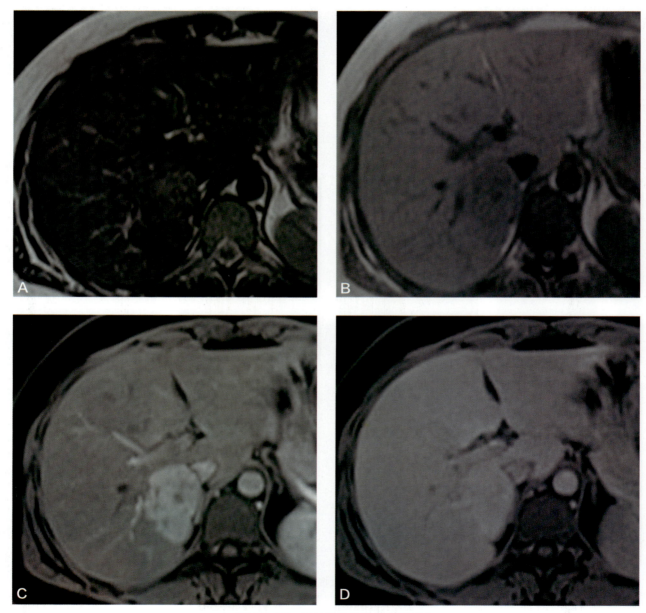

▲ 图 16-14　局灶性结节性增生无瘢痕
A，B. 平扫序列示肝脏Ⅶ段病变在 T_2 加权图像上呈稍高信号、T_1 加权图像上稍低信号；C，D. 增强后，病变在动脉期可见强化，延迟期信号均匀

瘤通常动脉期明显强化，门静脉期和延迟期可持续性强化，也可无持续性强化。这类肿瘤的影像表现可能和肝细胞癌类似。

由于 HA 缺乏胆管，因此与正常肝细胞相比，HA 内肝细胞在物质转运方面有所改变。虽然 HA 可能含有功能性肝细胞，这类细胞可以摄取顺磁性肝脏特异性对比剂，但由于缺乏跨肝窦膜的主动转运，不能形成细胞内转运梯度，因此在肝胆期与周围正常肝实质相比 HA 病灶表现为低信号。这是用来鉴别 HA 与 FNH 非常准确的方式（图 16-17 和图 16-18）[35,36]。

腺瘤通常不摄取 SPIO 颗粒，因此在 T_2 加权图像上表现为信号减低。在注射肝细胞特异性对比剂后，通常没有明显的对比剂摄取。在肝胆期，约 4% 的肝腺瘤可表现出摄取肝脏特异性对比剂。但是不幸的是，这种现象的解释是未知的（图 16-19）[36]。

在肝腺瘤病中，同一患者中会存在多个腺瘤，病变可小可大，可复杂或不复杂。此外，部分结节可能出现脂肪变性，而其他结节可能信号均匀。由于这些原因，肿瘤的强化的特点会因不同的病灶而不同（图 16-20）。

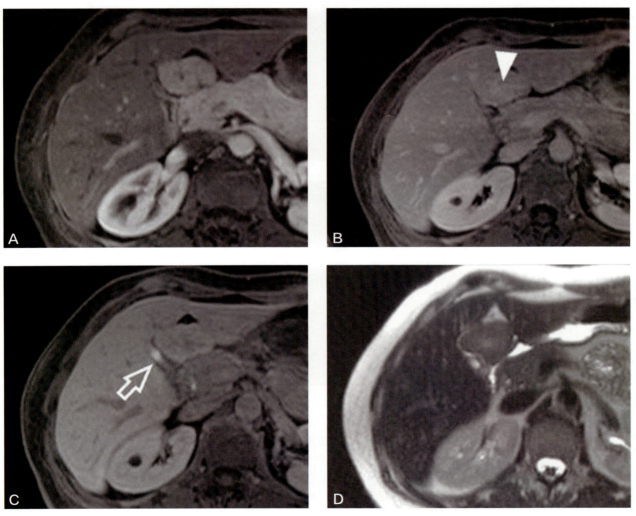

▲ 图 16-15 局灶性结节性增生：肝脏特异性对比剂强化模式

A，B. 轴位动脉期和延迟期示肝Ⅳ段局灶性的富血供病变，延迟期与肝实质相比呈等信号。注意延迟期中央瘢痕的强化（箭头）；C. 在注射顺磁性对比剂后的 T_1 加权肝胆期图像上，病灶为等至高信号，证明了病灶内功能性肝细胞的存在。注意对比剂通过胆管树排泄（空心箭）；D. 注射超顺磁性对比剂 T_2 加权肝胆期图像上，同一病灶与周围肝实质相比呈等信号

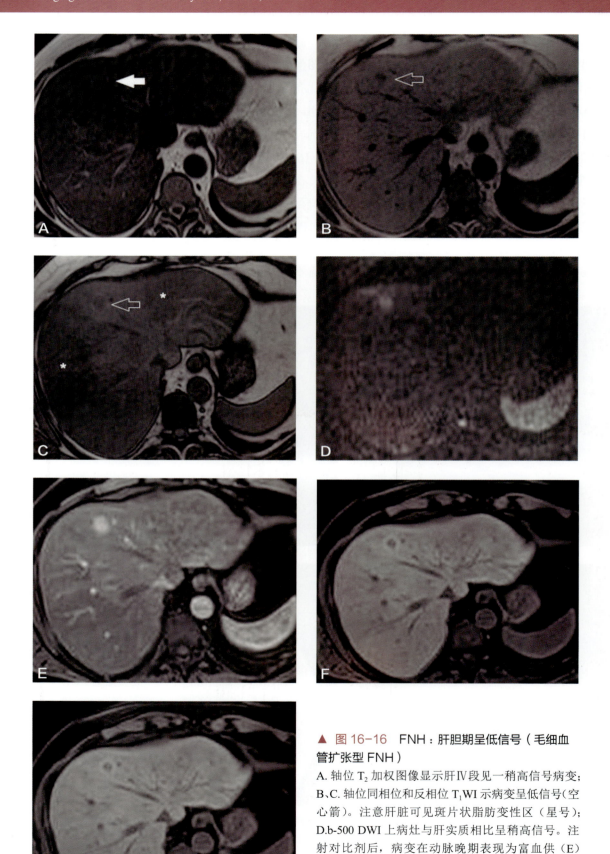

▲ 图 16-16 FNH：肝胆期呈低信号（毛细血管扩张型 FNH）

A. 轴位 T_2 加权图像显示肝Ⅳ段见一稍高信号病变；B、C. 轴位同相位和反相位 T_1WI 示病变呈低信号（空心箭）。注意肝脏可见斑片状脂肪变性区（星号）；D.b-500 DWI 上病灶与肝实质相比呈稍高信号。注射对比剂后，病变在动脉晚期表现为富血供（E）并且在延迟期（F）呈等信号，并可见薄层边缘；G. 在 T_1 加权肝胆期图像上，病变与周围的肝实质相比呈低信号

Chapter 16 肝脏局灶性病变
Liver: Focal Pathology

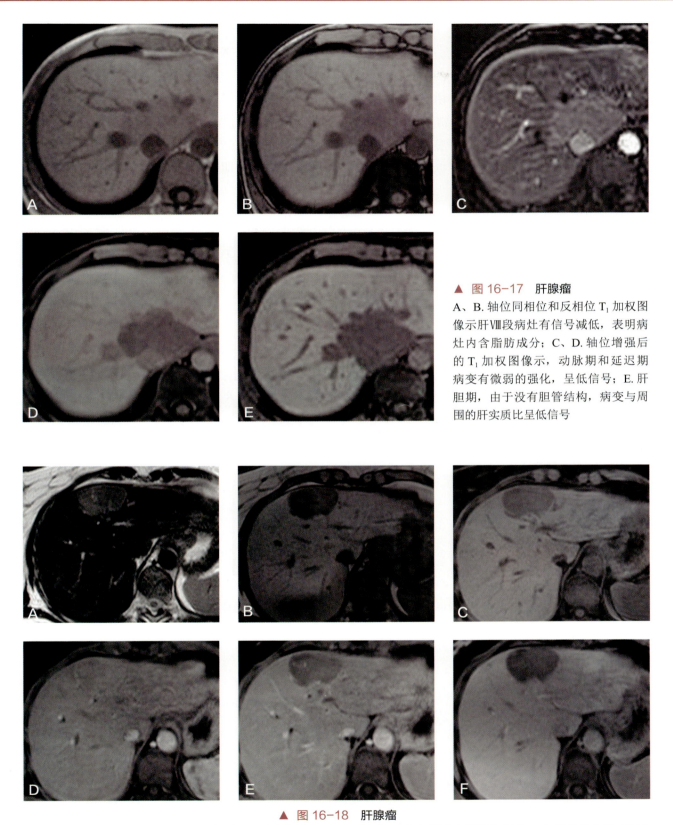

▲ 图 16-17 肝腺瘤

A、B. 轴位同相位和反相位 T_1 加权图像示肝Ⅷ段病灶有信号减低，表明病灶内含脂肪成分；C、D. 轴位增强后的 T_1 加权图像示，动脉期和延迟期病变有微弱的强化，呈低信号；E. 肝胆期，由于没有胆管结构，病变与周围的肝实质比呈低信号

▲ 图 16-18 肝腺瘤

A. 在 T_2 加权图像上，病变与周围肝实质比呈略高信号；B、C. 反相位 T_1 加权图像和脂肪抑制的 T_1 加权图像上显示存在脂质成分；D、E. 注射对比剂后，动脉期病变与肝实质呈等信号，延迟期呈低信号；F. 肝胆期由于病变内没有胆管结构而呈低信号

三、其他肝脏良性病变

（一）平滑肌瘤

平滑肌瘤是一种良性肿瘤，由交织的平滑肌纤维束组成[46]。尽管这类病变常发生于泌尿生殖系和胃肠道，但是目前已有肝脏原发性平滑肌瘤的少数病例报道。临床表现可以是偶然发现的小病灶、无明显症状，也可以是可触及的上腹部大肿块（最大直径达 15cm）、常伴有腹痛。虽然肝脏的原发性平滑肌瘤很少恶变，但通常需要进行肝脏切除以明确诊断。在 MR 成像中，小的肝平滑肌瘤在 T_1 加权图像上呈低信号，在 T_2 加权图像上呈等至高信号。增强扫描后，动脉期明显强化，门静脉期和延迟期持续强化且无对比剂退

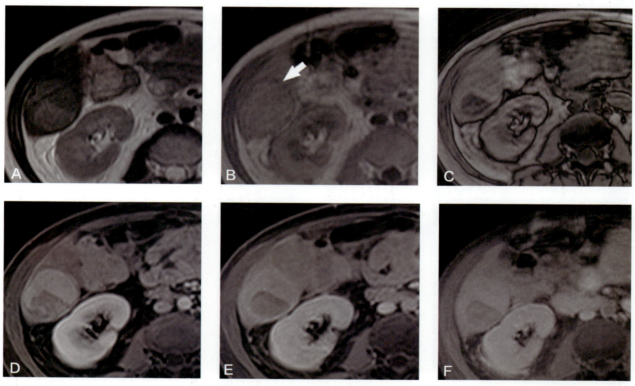

▲ 图 16-19　肝腺瘤

A. 轴位 T_2 加权图像显示肝Ⅵ段中的圆形、边界清晰的稍高信号病变；B、C. 轴位同相位和反相位 T_1 加权图像可见信号减低，这表明存在脂肪成分，还可以见到病变周围有一层薄的包膜（白箭）；D. 动脉晚期的轴位 T_1 加权图像示不均匀强化；E、F. 延迟期和肝胆期，病变与周围肝实质比呈等信号

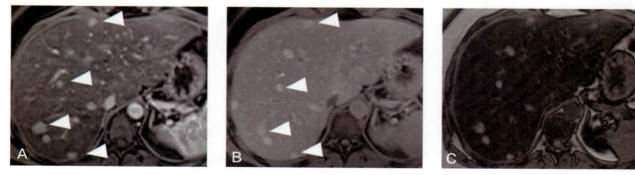

▲ 图 16-20　肝腺瘤病

A、B. 增强后的 T_1 加权图像中动脉期和延迟期可见多发圆形、边界清晰的腺瘤（箭头）；C. 由于肝脏脂肪变性背景，病变呈相对高信号

出表现[47]。在肝胆期，由于缺乏功能性肝细胞，与周围的肝实质相比肿瘤表现为低信号[48]（图16-21）。

（二）血管平滑肌脂肪瘤

肝血管平滑肌脂肪瘤（hepatic angiomyolipoma，HAML）是一种罕见的良性间质性肿瘤，由不同数量的平滑肌细胞、脂肪和血管成分组成[49]。

由于存在不同的成分，HAML 的诊断有时非常困难。它通常表现包膜不完整和无包膜的结节，内含脂肪成分和明显的中央血管。T_1 加权图像和 T_2 加权图像脂肪抑制序列可检测肿瘤内脂肪成分[50]。增强后，HAML 在动脉期明显不均匀强化。延迟期总体上仍是持续性强化，但强化程度可能会有所降低[51]（图 16-22）。在肝胆期中，由于病变内缺乏功能性肝细胞，因此与周围肝实质相比表现为低信号。HAML 的鉴别诊断包括 HCC、腺瘤、FNH、脂肪瘤和局灶性脂肪肝，这也说明了 MR 影像诊断 HAML 十分困难，有时需要活检。

四、肝恶性局灶性病变

恶性肿瘤可发生在正常肝脏或有慢性肝病背景的肝脏中。在正常肝脏中最常见的恶性病变是肝外原发肿瘤的血行播散转移。肝细胞癌（HCC）和一小部分肝内胆管细胞癌（intrahepatic cholangiocarcinomas，IHC）主要发生在有慢性肝病背景的肝脏中，是最常见的原发性肝脏恶性肿瘤。

（一）肝细胞癌

HCC 是肝脏最常见的原发性肿瘤，在男性常见恶性肿瘤中排名第五，女性常见恶性肿瘤中排名第七。这种疾病预后很差，是全球肿瘤相关死亡率的第三大原因，2008 年估计有 694 000 人死亡[52]。HCC 主要发生在患有慢性肝病或肝硬化的患者中，是这类患者主要死亡原因。HCC 发病率逐渐增加，好发于男性。在高发病率国家中，男女比例可能高达 7∶1 或 8∶1[53-57]。HCC 的发生可以是新生（de novo）肝癌形成的结果或是由肝内再生结节多步演变而成，即肝内再生结节经过低级和高级别不典型增生结节最终演变为 HCC[58,59]。HCC 可有不同的生长方式。最常见的是单发小结节或大肿块，可有包膜或无包膜。第二常见的生长方式是多灶性 HCC，其特征表现是多个独立的结节。弥漫型 / 浸润型 HCC 表现为

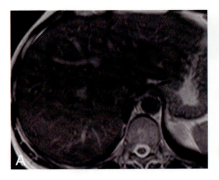
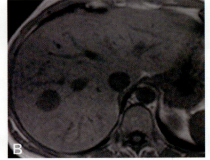
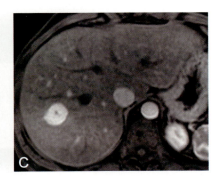
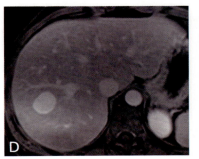
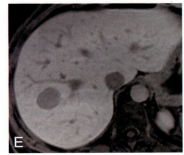

▲ 图 16-21 平滑肌瘤
A. 脂肪抑制轴位 T_2 加权图像上肝Ⅷ段见稍高信号病灶；B. 轴位增强前 T_1 加权图像可见边界清晰的低信号病变，边缘光滑；C、D. 轴位 T_1 加权图像动脉晚期表现为明显的富血供病变，延迟期持续强化；E. 增强后 T_1 加权图像肝胆期病变呈低信号，证明病灶内没有功能性肝细胞

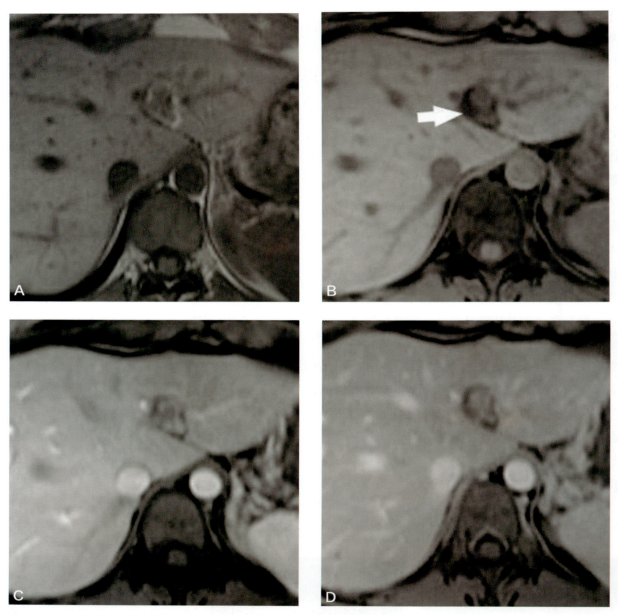

▲ 图 16-22　血管平滑肌脂肪瘤

A、B. 轴位同相位和反相位 T_1 加权图像示肝 Ⅱ 段同相位高信号病变，在反相位图像上可见信号减低（白箭）。注射对比剂后，动脉晚期（C），病变呈不均匀强化，延迟期持续强化（D）

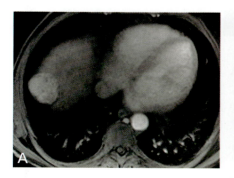
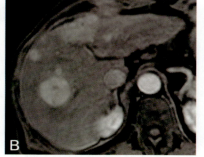
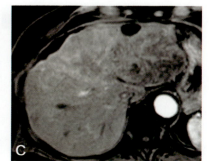

▲ 图 16-23　肝细胞癌：形态学模式

A. 孤立结节；B. 多发结节；C. 浸润性病变

肝内弥漫分布的多个小肿瘤病灶，与肝硬化结节类似[60]（图 16-23）。

最近发布的指南指出，每 6 个月应用超声联合甲胎蛋白（alpha-fetal protein，AFP）是最具成本效益的监测手段[61]。虽然在肝硬化患者中 AFP 是筛查最常用的血清化验指标，但是有研究显示其假阴性也相对常见，特别是对于小病变[62-64]。虽然应用超声检测 HCC 的敏感性较好，但该技术在特异性不高，主要是有较多的假阳性病例[61,65,66]。在 MR 成像中，小 HCC 病灶在 T_1WI 信号变化较大，通常是呈低信号，但是已经报道有 34% 和 61% 小 HCC 病灶在 T_1WI 上呈高信号[67,68]。在 T_2WI 上，与周围肝实质相比，HCC 表现为等至高信号[69]。一般来说，T_1 加权图像呈高信号、T_2 加权图像上呈等信号的病灶分化程度较好，这是由于脂肪和（或）糖蛋白的存在（图 16-24）。相比之下，T_1 加权图像上低信号、T_2 加权图像上的高信号的病灶一般是中/低分化的 HCC[70,71]。肿瘤动脉血供增多是鉴别癌前病变和 HCC 最重要的特征，因此，增强后动脉期强化是 HCC 的主要影像特征。

小 HCC 均匀强化，而大 HCC 则表现为不均匀强化，一些病灶可能出现日冕状强化（corona enhancement），约 7% 为乏血供病灶[72]（图 16-25）。

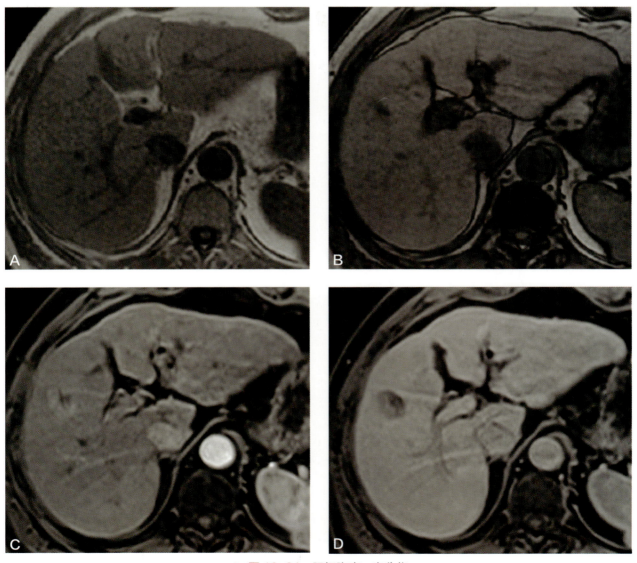

▲ 图 16-24　肝细胞癌：高分化
轴位及同相位（A、B）T_1 加权示典型 HCC 结节（C、D）内含脂质成分，这与分化好的肿瘤相关

然而，在肝硬化患者中并非所有动脉期强化病灶都是HCC，其他局灶性病变，如"闪现充填"的血管瘤、动脉-门静脉分流、一过性肝脏血供异常以及肝再生结节，这些都有可能是导致误诊的原因[73,74]。延迟期信号减低，也就是"快出"征，是HCC第二大重要影像特征，这个影像特征显著提高了HCC检出的灵敏度和特异性，可能是HCC最强的独立预测因子[74-76]（图16-24和图16-26）。肿瘤包膜是另一个提示恶性的重要征象：T_1加权图像上为稍低信号环，在T_2加权图像为稍高信号。在延迟期，肿瘤包膜强化程度高于周围肝实质，这是由于肿瘤包膜存在纤维基质成分（图16-26）。在临床实践中应用肝特异性对比剂，超顺磁性和顺磁性对比剂，显著提高了HCC的检出和诊断，特别是对于1～2cm的病变。使用顺磁对比剂时，恶性肿瘤缺乏功能性肝细胞，因此病变在肝胆期呈低信号（图16-27）。然而，不到20%的高分化和中分化HCC在肝胆

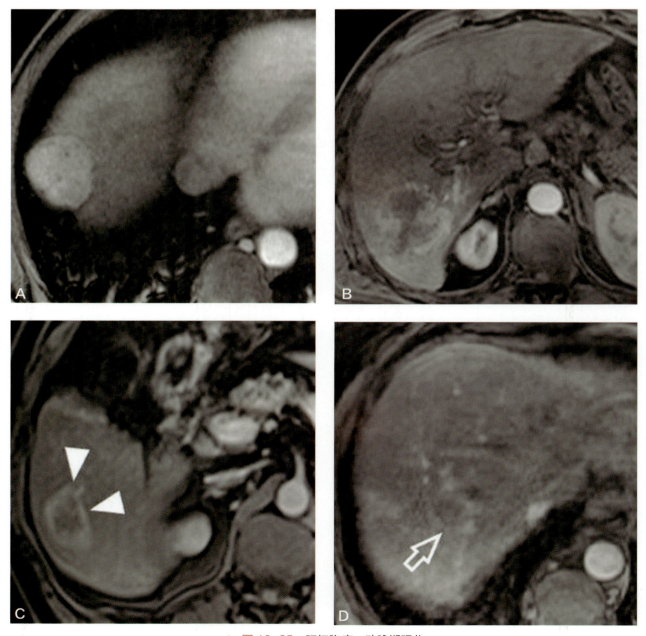

▲ 图16-25 肝细胞癌：动脉期强化
A. 均匀；B. 不均匀；C. 日冕状强化（箭头）；D. 乏血供（空心箭）

期呈等或高信号[77-79]。含有 SPIO 对比剂有助于检出肝硬化背景中的小 HCC。最近有文献[80]研究了 HCC 和 DN 中 Kupffer 细胞数量与 SPIO 摄取程度之间的关系。该研究表明，肿瘤组织与非肿瘤组织中 Kupffer 细胞数量的比例随着细胞分化程度的降低而降低。肝脏磁共振扩散加权成像（diffusion weighted imaging, DWI）最近引起了人们的兴趣，这一成像方法可以显著改善肝脏病变的检出，并可使用表观扩散系数（apparent diffusion coefficient, ADC）对病变进行诊断[81]。

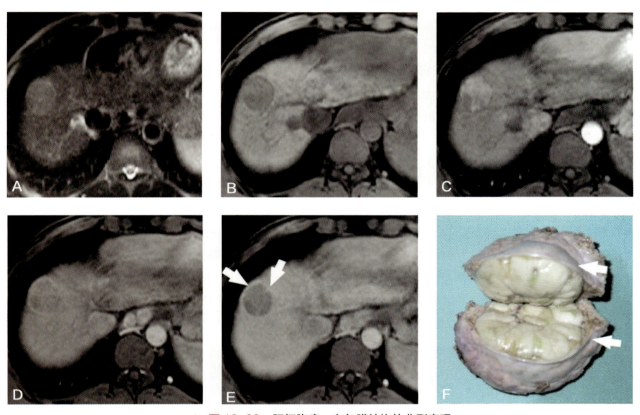

▲ 图 16-26　肝细胞癌：有包膜结构的典型表现

A. 轴位 T_2 加权图像显示肝Ⅷ段高信号病变；B. T_1 加权图像上呈低信号；C. 注射钆对比剂后，动脉期病灶可见强化；D、E. 静脉期和延迟期强化程度减低（wash-out 征）。肿瘤包膜在延迟期更明显（白箭）；F. 大体标本照片可见一有包膜的病变（白箭）

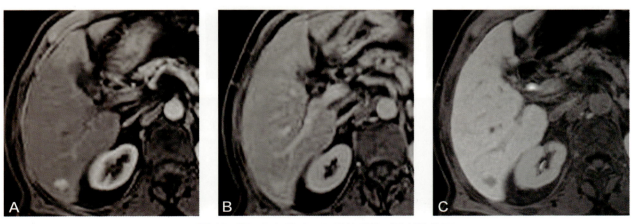

▲ 图 16-27　肝细胞癌：肝脏特异性对比剂的作用

A~C. 小的富血供 HCC 在延迟期没有强化减低；C. 胆期病灶呈低信号，这表明病灶内缺乏功能性肝细胞，这被认为是恶性肿瘤的标志。文献报道肝脏特异性对比剂显著改善了 MR 对小 HCC（1~2cm）诊断的准确性

对于 HCC，一些研究表明 DW-MR 图像能够改善 HCC 的检出，并且可能有助于对动态增强表现不典型的小 HCC 进行诊断[82,83]。然而，关于 DWI 定量和定性分析在 HCC 评估中的作用仍然存在争论，一些作者认为它仅能略微提高诊断的灵敏度[84-86]（图 16-28）。HCC 可以发生在没有肝硬化背景的肝脏上，甚至是没有目前已知的相关危险因素。这种情况通常表现为中年男性的肝脏上发现有症状的肿块。这个肝脏病变可能是一个瘤体较大的孤立性肿块，呈分叶状，边缘可能会有包膜结构。其 MR 影像表现与肝硬化患者 HCC 影像表现类似[87-89]（图 16-29）。

纤维板层肝细胞癌是 HCC 的少见亚型，具有相当独特的特征[90]。常见于青年患者，无肝硬化病史。出血或坏死不常见。在大体病理上，与 FNH 类似。在 MR 成像上，T_1WI 为低信号，T_2WI 为高信号。病变内有中心瘢痕，在 T_1WI 和 T_2WI 上均为低信号，这一信号特点与 FNH 中的中央瘢痕不同，FNH 中央瘢痕在 T_2 加权图像上为高亮信号[91]。在钆动态增强图像上，纤维板层肝细胞癌早期为弥漫性不均匀强化，之后强化趋向均匀、呈等信号[92]。

（二）肝内胆管细胞癌

肝内胆管细胞癌（intrahepatic cholangiocarcinoma, ICC）是起源于胆管上皮的腺癌，是第二常见的肝脏原发性肿瘤。根据起源部位，可将其分为周围型和肝门部（Klatskin 肿瘤）胆管细胞癌[93]。前者被认为起自肝内胆管二级分支，而后者起自于肝内胆管一级分支、肝左管、肝右管及两者汇合处。这两类肿瘤的影像表现和治疗方式明显不同。

周围型胆管细胞癌约占胆管癌的 10%，它与肝内胆管结石、原发性硬化性胆管炎、Caroli 病、华支睾吸虫感染和暴露于氧化钍悬浮液（Thorotrast）有关[94]。最常见的症状是腹痛、疲劳和体重下降。依据大体表现及生长方式，周围型胆管细胞癌分为 3 种类型：肿块型、导管内生长型和导管周围浸润型[95]。在 MR 成像中，与周围肝实质相比，胆管癌在 T_1 加权图像上为均

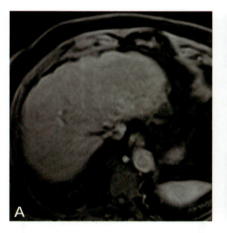
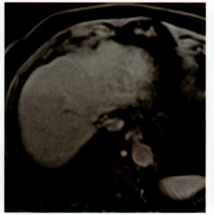
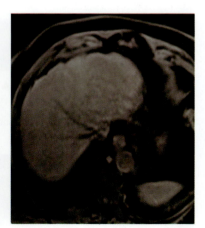
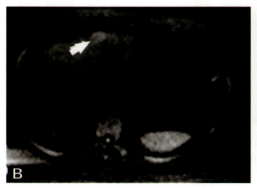
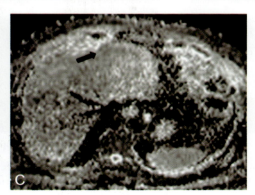

▲ 图 16-28　肝细胞癌：DWI

A～C. 增强后 T_1 加权图像动脉期、静脉期和延迟期肝 Ⅱ 段未见任何局灶性病变。b 值 400 的 DWI 上肝被膜下可见局灶性扩散受限区域，在 ADC 图上可以确证

匀低信号，但在 T_2 加权图像上可以从明显高信号到轻度高信号之间变化。肿瘤信号的变化取决于肿瘤内黏液性物质、纤维组织、出血和坏死成分的多少[96]。虽然中央瘢痕不是 ICC 的特异性表现，但是它所反映的严重纤维化是 ICC 的一个特征。动态钆增强 MR 表现为动脉期边缘轻度或中度强化，在 3min 和 5min 后的延迟期可见渐进性向心性强化[97,98]。这种强化特点与肿瘤内部纤维性成分有关，并且是周围型 ICC 典型表现（图 16-30）。在 DWI 上，在高肿瘤细胞密度区域水扩散受限，因此在高 b 值 DWI 上表现为高信号；一些学者提出 DWI 上的靶征可以鉴别小 ICC 和小 HCC[99]。

在注射肝脏特异性对比剂或非特异性钆对比剂的多期动态增强阶段，肝内胆管细胞癌的 MR 影像表现类似。然而，在使用顺磁性对比剂在肝胆期延迟扫描时病灶中的纤维成分会出现强化（图 16-31）。但是由于 ICC 内没有 Kupffer 细胞，因此在注射 SPIO 后病灶未观察到对比剂的摄取[100]。ICC 的主要鉴别诊断包括肝转移瘤、HCC、淋巴瘤和类癌。特别需要注意的是，混合型 CCC/HCC 肿瘤是一种血供十分丰富的肿瘤，

在动脉期表现为明显、均匀强化，延迟期仍持续强化。

肝门部胆管癌（通常表现为黄疸）大体病理类型通常分为三类：浸润型、外生型和乳头型。在磁共振胆管造影（MR cholangiography，MRC）图像上，肝门部胆管癌表现为胆管壁中度不规则增厚，其上游肝内胆管不对称扩张。浸润型表现为管腔狭窄，外生型常表现为胆管的完全梗阻，而乳头型表现为腔内结节状突起。

在 MR 图像上，与周围肝实质相比，T_1 加权图像上呈低信号，T_2 加权图像上呈中高信号。肝门部胆管癌是一种乏血供肿瘤，增强后表现为不均匀、渐进性强化（图 16-32）。肝门部胆管癌中很少出现卫星结节和中央瘢痕[101,102]。MRC 与 MR 联合使用可以有效评估肿瘤侵犯范围和血管受累情况。特别是放射科医师在评估肝内二级胆管根部、肝叶动脉和门静脉左右分支的受累情况时要十分谨慎。通常，如果肿瘤累及双侧上述一个或更多结构时，则肿瘤不可切除[103]。肝门部胆管癌的主要鉴别诊断有原发性硬化性胆管炎、炎症、假性肿瘤、Mirizzi 综合征、复发性化脓性胆管炎和黄色肉芽肿性胆管炎[104]。

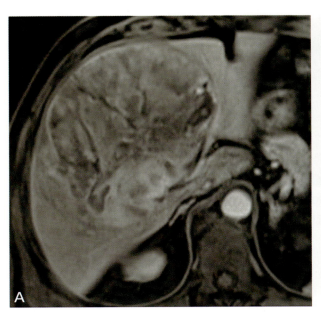 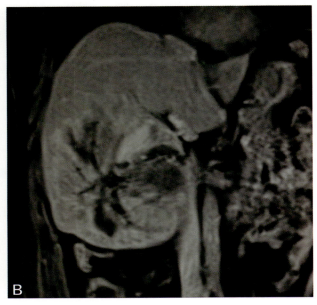

▲ 图 16-29　无危险因素的患者的肝细胞癌

A，B. 轴位增强后 T_1 加权图像动脉期和冠状位延迟期可见一大的、孤立的、有包膜的、信号不均的富血供肿块，延迟期可见对比剂流出

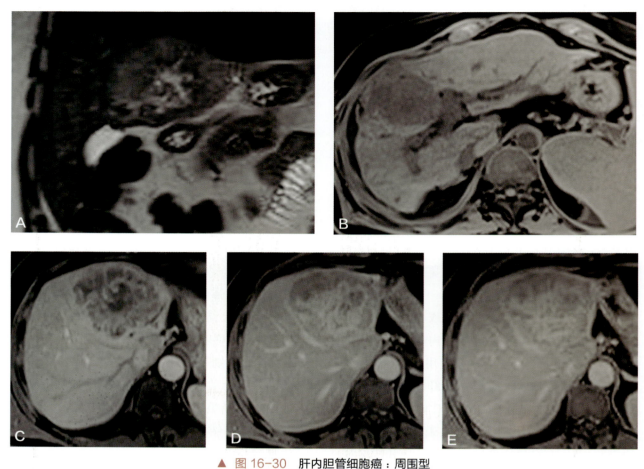

▲ 图 16-30 肝内胆管细胞癌：周围型

A、B. T_2 加权图像和 T_1 加权图像显示肝Ⅳ段肿物、信号不均匀；C～E. 注射对比剂后，病变不均匀边缘强化（C）、静脉期（D）和延迟期（E）渐进性强化

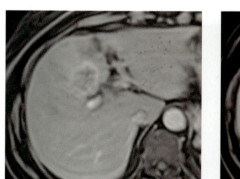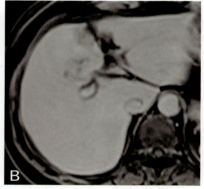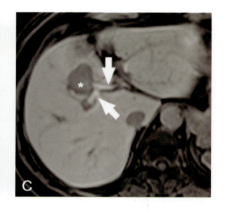

▲ 图 16-31 胆管癌：肝门部

A，B. 增强后图像显示为典型的胆管细胞癌强化方式；C. 肝胆期主要病变（星号）和肝内一级胆管（白箭）清晰可见

（三）转移瘤

转移瘤是最常见的肝脏恶性肿瘤，也是肝脏影像检查的最常见指征。肝脏是主要的肿瘤转移器官，仅次于区域淋巴结[105]。肝转移瘤的检出对肿瘤正确分期和确定最佳治疗方法非常重要。

肝转移瘤有几种形态学特征：在 T_1 加权图像上转移瘤通常是低信号，可有类似"甜甜圈"的表现（内部低信号、边缘高信号）或少许情况下因存在黑色素或蛋白质而表现为高信号。在 T_2 加权图像上呈稍高信号并具有不同的特征，如晕环征、靶征、

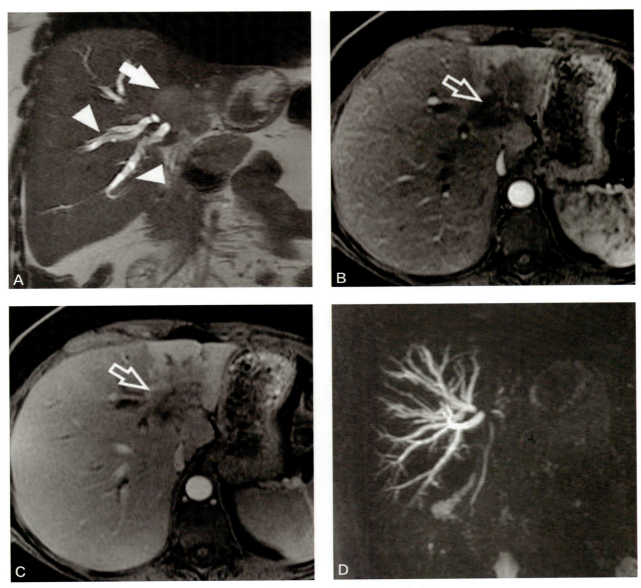

▲ 图 16-32　肝内胆管细胞癌：肝门部

A. 冠状位 T_2 加权图像病变信号略高于周围肝实质（白箭）和胆管扩张（箭头）；B. 动脉期轴位 T_1 加权图像肝门部病灶呈低信号（空心箭）伴有延迟强化（C）；D. MRCP 显示肝右管梗阻伴肝内胆管扩张

灯泡征或无定形征[106]（图 16-33）。在注射对比剂后，与周围肝实质相比，转移瘤可分为乏血供和富血供两类。乏血供转移瘤通常来自原发性胃肠道肿瘤（胰腺、结肠、胃）、肺癌和一些乳腺癌亚型；由于在静脉期病变与肝实质之间的对比噪声比（CNR）最高，因此病变在静脉期显示得最清晰（图 16-34）。乏血供转移瘤最常见的鉴别诊断是周围型胆管癌、脓肿和纤维性肿瘤。富血供转移瘤来自于血供丰富的肿瘤，如肾透明细胞癌、黑色素瘤、类癌、胰岛细胞肿瘤、甲状腺癌、嗜

肝转移瘤形态学特征

T_2		
- 无定型征	45%	●
- 靶征	19%	●
- 晕环征	26%	●
- 灯泡征	10%	●

T_1		
- 低信号伴有晕环，类似"甜甜圈"	80%	●
- 高信号蛋白质、黑色素、高铁血红蛋白	10%	●

▲ 图 16-33　MR 平扫序列肝转移瘤的形态学特征

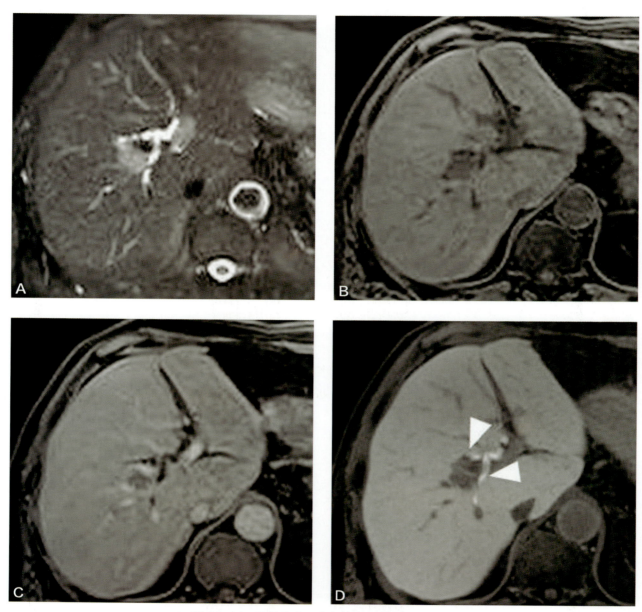

▲ 图 16-34　肝转移瘤：来自结直肠癌的乏血供转移瘤
A. 轴位 T_2 加权图像显示肝门部的高信号病变；B. T_1 加权图像上呈低信号；C. 增强后病变与周围肝实质相比呈低信号；D. 肝胆期病灶不摄取对比剂。注意肝胆期与主要的胆管（箭头）相邻

铬细胞瘤和乳腺癌，富血供转移瘤在动脉期的检出率更高[107]（图 16-35 和图 16-36）。在 10% 的富血供转移瘤中，可以观察到对比剂流出（washout）的征象[108]。对于富血供转移瘤，最常见的鉴别诊断是局灶性结节增生（FNH），"闪现充填（flash filling）"的血管瘤和局灶性脂肪沉积区。在注射顺磁性肝脏特异性对比剂后延迟扫描的肝胆期图像中，与周围强化的正常肝实质相比，所有转移瘤都显示为显著的低信号[109]（图 16-37）。但是，偶尔会观察到一些对比剂的滞留[110,111]。

五、其他肝脏恶性病变

（一）肝上皮样血管内皮瘤

肝上皮样血管内皮瘤（hepatic epithelioid hemangioendothelioma, HEHE）是由上皮样细胞、内皮细胞或树突细胞组成的罕见交界性肿瘤[112]。HEHE 不仅发生于软组织，也可发生在其他

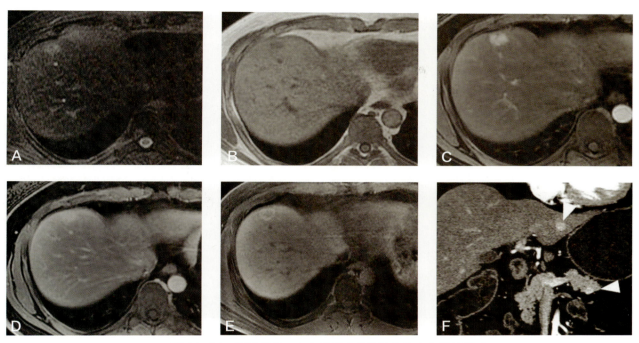

▲ 图 16-35　肝转移瘤：来自神经内分泌肿瘤的富血供转移瘤

A. 轴位 T_2 加权图像上肝Ⅷ段可见一稍高信号病灶；B. T_1 加权图像上呈低信号。增强后 T_1 加权图像动脉期，病变呈富血供表现；C、D. 延迟期呈等信号。肝胆期病变呈低信号，周围有薄层边缘；E. 冠状位 CT 动脉期胰腺尾部可见一微小的富血供病变，肝Ⅱ段也有一个富血供病变（箭头）

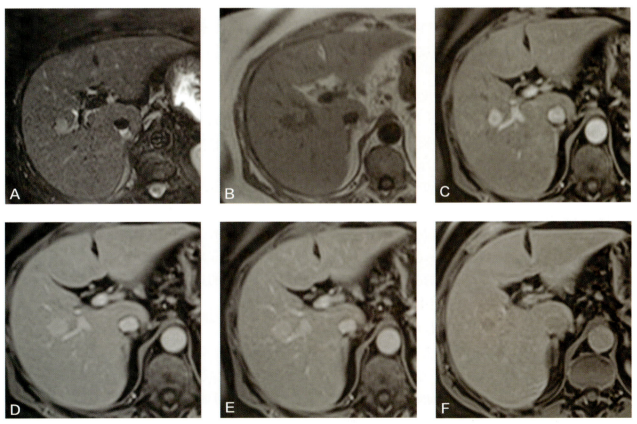

▲ 图 16-36　肝转移瘤：来自黑色素瘤的富血供转移瘤

黑色素的肝转移瘤与神经内分泌的肝转移瘤具有相同的 MR 影像特征

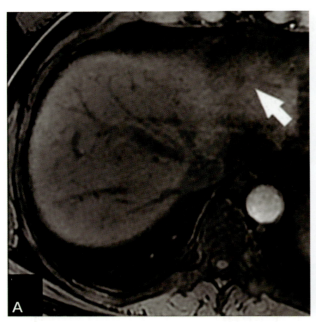 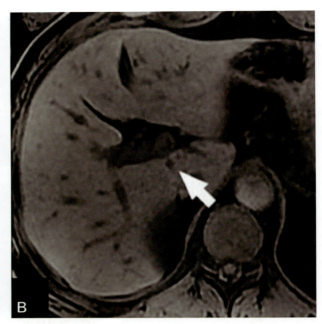

▲ 图 16-37　肝转移：肝胆期的作用
2 例来自结肠直肠癌的微小富血供转移瘤，仅在肝胆期可见

器官，如肺、骨、脑、心脏、唾液腺、静脉和胸膜[113,114]。该病好发于女性（60%），发病年龄高峰在 30—50 岁。尽管大多数患者病灶表现为多灶性生长，但在初次诊断时，1/3 的患者就已经出现转移灶，肝上皮样血管内皮瘤的预后被认为比其他肝脏恶性肿瘤的预后好[115,116]。

文献中对于肝上皮样血管内皮瘤的 MRI 特征有很详尽的描述。有两大主要的影像特征：靶征，其特征是中心区域呈低信号和外周呈高信号或等信号；晕环征，表现为中心及边缘呈低信号，两者之间有一层高信号环。病变附近可出现"被膜皱缩"[117,118]。

在 MR 肝胆期中，病变不摄取对比剂，表示其内部没有功能性肝细胞（图 16-38）。HEHE 的无创诊断是困难的，可能被误诊为肝脏转移性疾病、胆管癌（周围型），局灶性融合性纤维化、血管瘤。因此，组织病理学的确诊是必要的。

（二）原发性肝淋巴瘤

原发性肝淋巴瘤（primary hepatic lymphoma，PHL）是一种非常罕见的恶性肿瘤，通常没有特异性症状，导致延误诊断。在所有原发性结外 NHL 中，肝脏原发性淋巴瘤仅占 0.4%。PHL 主要有三种表现形式：孤立性的肝脏肿块、多灶性的肝脏病变和弥漫浸润性肝脏病变。PHL 最常见的表现是单发、边界清晰的肝脏病变[119]。在 MR 成像上，与周围肝实质相比，肝脏淋巴瘤典型表现为 T_1 加权图像上呈低信号和 T_2 加权图像上呈高信号。注射对比剂后，PHL 表现为低信号病灶，边缘出现薄层环形强化，这可能与肿瘤诱发邻近肝实质出现血管炎有关（图 16-39）[120,121]。

六、治疗后评估

有几种治疗策略可用于治疗肝脏的原发性和继发性肿瘤。了解治疗后肝脏的正常表现和病理表现对于患者的正确管理和随访至关重要。

（一）射频消融

射频消融（radio frequency，RF）是治疗肝脏原发性和继发性肿瘤最有前景的非手术治疗方式[122,123]。目前的临床经验表明，与手术相比，RF 有效、安全、相对简单、并发症发生率低、治疗时间较短和住院费用较低[124,125]。RF 的主要限

Chapter 16　肝脏局灶性病变
Liver: Focal Pathology

制因素与以下几种情况有关：超声上病灶的可显示性（有些病变在超声上不显示）；病变应小于 4cm，可以显著降低复发风险；肿瘤靠近大血管可能会使"加热"不够（由于血流引起的散热）；肿瘤靠近中央胆管，患者易出现胆道并发症。消融的过程是在肝实质内产生坏死区域。射频消融产生的肝脏缺损区域的形状是可变的，通常是圆形或卵圆形，有时因针道或接近大血管而呈现出更复杂的几何形状。在 T_2 加权图像上，治疗后的肿瘤呈低信号，而有活性的肿瘤组织呈高信号[126]。

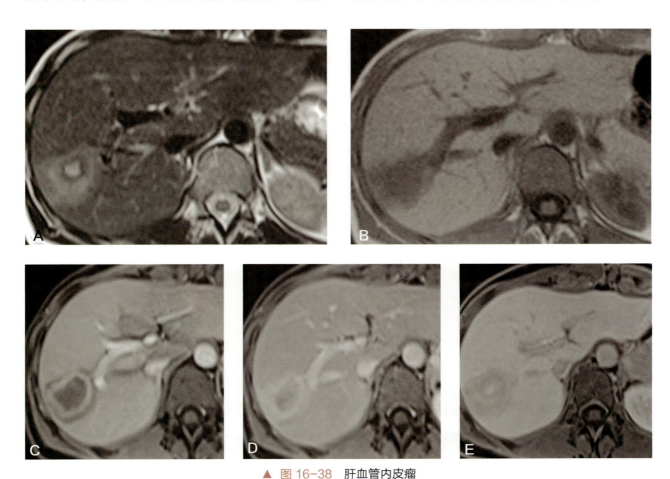

▲ 图 16-38　肝血管内皮瘤

A. T_2 加权图像显示肝Ⅷ段肿块，信号不均；B. 在 T_1 加权图像上呈低信号；C、D. 增强后动脉期和延迟期病变呈"靶征"，是血管内皮瘤的特征性表现；E. 肝胆期病变未摄取肝脏特异性对比剂

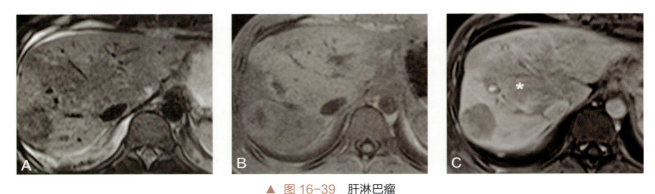

▲ 图 16-39　肝淋巴瘤

A、B. 增强前 T_1 加权图像和 T_2 加权图像上肝Ⅶ段可见一类圆形、边界清晰的病变；C. 增强后 MR 图像可见一大的低信号肿物。注意肝中叶可见一弥漫性、混杂信号区域，这是因为该患者患有肝炎（星号）

在早期随访中，缺损区域的坏死碎片通常在 T_2WI 上表现为不均匀高信号伴边缘低信号。在注射对比剂后，完全消融的病灶内的坏死区域无强化，但是在缺损区域周围可以出现强化，给诊断带来困难[127]（图 16-40）。完全消融的另一个重要标准是缺损区域的大小随时间的演变。虽然大小的演变是不可预测的，但如果消融是完全的，缺损区域的大小可以保持稳定或减小。任何缺损区域的增大都代表肿瘤生长[128]。不完全消融和疾病复发被定义为随访过程中在距离治疗的病变 2cm 内的区域出现新病变，其在治疗后的病变中发生率在 2%～10% 的范围内。疾病复发的主要原因是病变组织病理学分级高、微血管侵犯和邻近血管结构（图 16-41）。RF 术后并发症的发生率为 9% 和死亡率为 0.5%，包括早期并发症和晚期并发症。一些重要的早期并发症包括血栓形成（肝静脉和门静脉）、血肿、梗死、动静脉瘘、胆道梗阻、胸腔积液和气胸（图 16-42）。晚期并发症包括感染和肿瘤种植[129,130]。

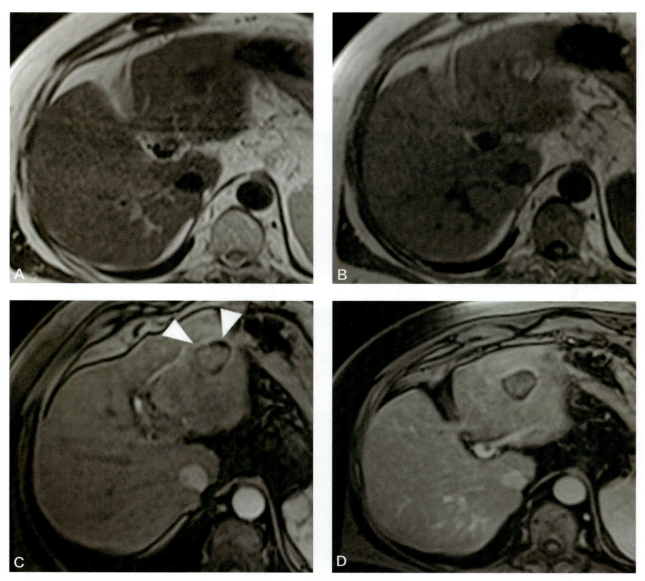

▲ 图 16-40　HCC 的射频消融治疗

A、B. 由于治疗后病灶内出血坏死，在增强前 T_2 加权图像上呈低信号，T_1 加权图像上呈高信号；C、D. 增强后病灶内及周围既无富血供表现，也无对比剂流出征象。病灶边缘可能出现薄层强化，这是由于治疗后充血所致（箭头）

Chapter 16　肝脏局灶性病变
Liver: Focal Pathology

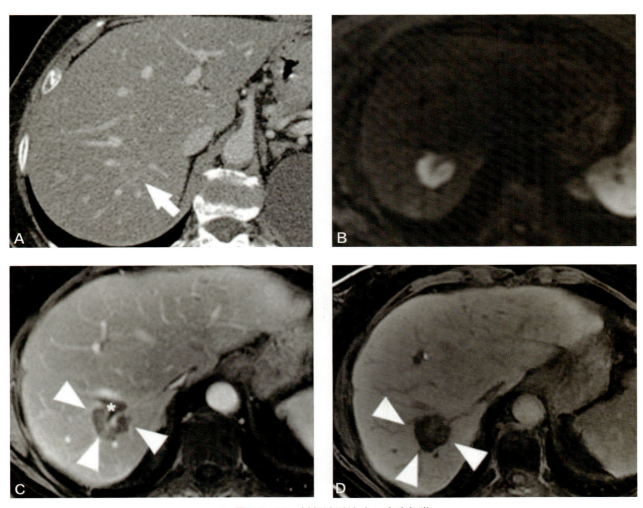

▲ 图 16-41　射频消融治疗：疾病复发

A.CT 扫描显示肝Ⅶ段乏血供转移瘤；B. 随访过程中，DWI 上治疗后的病灶周围的可见扩散限制区域，这是恶性肿瘤的标志；C、D. 增强后静脉期和肝胆期证实了在治疗后病灶（箭头）坏死区域（星号）周围存在病理组织

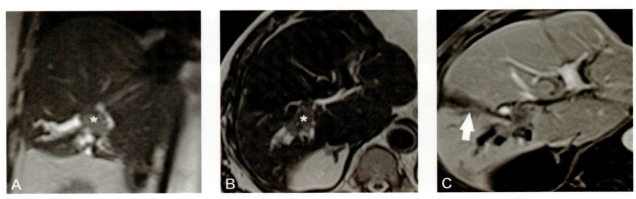

▲ 图 16-42　射频消融并发症：胆管扩张

A，B. 轴位和冠状位 T_2 加权图像显示"肝门部"肝脏坏死区域（星号）伴胆管扩张；C. 增强后，治疗后的病变没有强化。针道也清晰可见（白箭）

（二）肝动脉化疗栓塞术

肝动脉化疗栓塞术（transarterial chemoembolization, TACE）是将化疗药物注入肝动脉治疗肿瘤的一种姑息性方法，适用于肝脏原发性和继发性富血供肿瘤[131]。它是中期 HCC 患者和不能手术、肝移植或射频消融的患者的首选治疗方法，还可应用于超过米兰标准或 USCF（University Of California, San Francisco）标准的患者降期治疗，或作为肝移植等待间隔时间较长的患者的桥接治疗。TACE 是一种经导管介入技术，结合局部化疗和栓塞，增加细胞毒性药物的停留时间并诱导肿瘤内部缺血。新型 TACE 术中应用药物洗脱微球，可以提高药物投放的精确度。近期另外一项新进展是近距离放射治疗技术，经肝动脉注射钇-90（90Y）微球，其优先沉积在富血供肿瘤内并发射 β 射线（放射性栓塞）。TACE 技术的主要限制因素与肝功能（不适合 Child-Pugh 评分 > 8 或胆红素值高的患者）和门静脉血栓形成有关。

确定肿瘤治疗反应的标准参数是肿瘤大小，可根据修改后的实体瘤疗效评价标准（mRECIST）对治疗反应程度进行分类[132]。TACE 术后 6 个月后复发率为 37%，1 年后复发率为 67%，主要影响因素包括病变大小（> 3cm）、多结节型肿瘤和肝外血管供血（内乳动脉、心包膈动脉和肾上腺膈动脉）[133]（图 16-43）。TACE 的主要并发症是肝梗死、动脉破裂、脓肿、出血和动脉-门静脉短路，轻微的并发症可能是发热和疼痛[134,135]。

（三）手术治疗

在肝脏原发性和继发性肿瘤患者中有多种不同治疗策略，在其中一部分患者中，手术切除可为患者提供长期生存的最佳机会，甚至可能治愈[136]。

对无肝病背景和早期肝病背景（Child-Pugh A）的孤立性结节 HCC 患者，手术切除是最有效的治疗方法。更准确的肝功能评估、借助更精准的影像检查提高对肝脏分段解剖的理解以及手术技术进步是降低死亡率的最重要因素，预

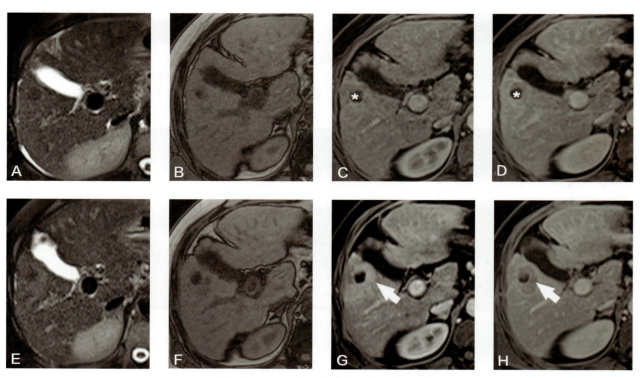

▲ 图 16-43 肝动脉化疗栓塞术：疾病复发

A～D. TACE 术后 3 个月的随访图像上在坏死区域内或周围未见任何强化或病理组织（星号）；E～H. 6 个月的随访图像上胆囊窝附近可见富血供组织，并在延迟期可见对比剂流出，这是典型的 HCC

期 5 年生存率为 70%。手术切除也可用于治疗原发性结直肠癌的肝转移，这类患者 5 年生存率为 24%～58%[137]。然而，除结肠直肠癌以外的其他原发性肿瘤的肝转移进行手术治疗效果并不明显，并且高度依赖于原发性肿瘤的类型。主要手术方式包括解剖性（节段性）和非解剖性（楔形）切除术：第一种是根据 Couinaud 分类切除肝段；第二种方法是完全切除肿瘤而不考虑肝段解剖（即肝段Ⅷ肿物的切除）。肝大部切除是指切除 3 个及以上肝段。术前 MR 检查的作用包括肝脏疾病分期、肿瘤定位、确定病变与肝脏主要血管（肝动脉、门静脉和肝静脉分支）和胆管的关系，最后需要评估术后残肝是否足以满足肝功能需要[138]。术后行 MR 检查有助于检出术后并发症，如血肿/出血、脓肿、胆漏或胆汁瘤[139]（图 16-44 和图 16-45）。胆汁瘤或脓肿在 T_1 加权图像上呈低到高信号，通常在 T_2 加权图像上呈高信号。胆汁瘤和脓肿增强后中央无强化；但如果可以看到明显的边缘强化，则表明是脓肿壁，患者可能需要介入引流或外科修补术治疗[140]。在胆漏的情况下，通常可以使用肝胆特异性 MR 对比剂确定胆漏的准确位置。在这种情况下，可以通过胆管损伤部位的对比剂外渗来显示漏口的位置（图 16-45）。不幸的是，疾病复发比较常见，可以沿着切除边缘累及残余实质或出现肝外转移[141]。

（四）肝移植

肝移植（liver transplantation，LT）是慢性肝病和急性肝衰竭导致肝功能不全患者的首选治疗方法[142]。在过去的几十年中，手术技术、器官保存、免疫抑制治疗和早期发现术后并发症等方面的进展提高了 LT 后的生存率，因为它的 1 年生存率约为 85%[143]。早期发现术后并发症对于移植物和患者的生存至关重要。由于外科手术的复杂性和可用于移植的肝源短缺，移植物失功是一个严重的问题。排异是移植失败的最常见原因。在这种情况下，影像检查起次要作用，因为临床症状和实验室检查提出可疑诊断，并且只能通过肝脏活检的组织病理学分析来确诊。可能会有一些非特异性的影像表现，例如门静脉-胆管周围间隙水肿、肝边缘形态不规则和增强后不均匀强化[144]。LT 的主要并发症累及手术吻合部位：肝动脉、门静脉、下腔静脉、肝静脉及胆管。肝动脉并发症包括血栓形成、狭窄和假性动脉瘤（图 16-46 和图 16-47）。2%～11% 的肝移植受者发生肝动脉血栓形成和狭窄。它们可导致胆管缺血，因为肝动脉是胆管血供的唯一来源。门静脉并发症相对

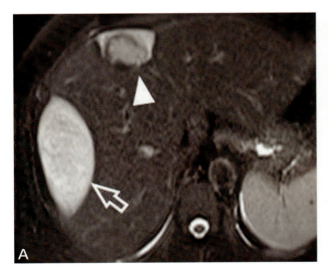 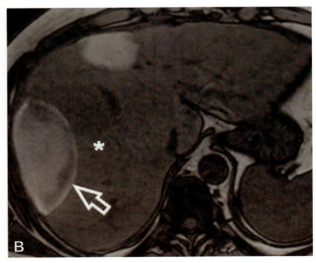

▲ 图 16-44　手术并发症：血肿

A. T_2 加权图像显示肝Ⅳ段楔形切除术后，肝被膜下可见液体积聚，在 T_1 加权图像上呈高信号；B. 典型的出血。注意 T_1 加权图像反相位肝实质呈低信号是由于肝脏脂肪变性（星号）

罕见，包括血栓形成和狭窄。门静脉血栓形成发生在 1%～2% 的病例中[145,146]。IVC 和肝静脉的并发症发生率较低（＜1%）。技术性因素，如供体和受体血管之间的大小差异或肝上下腔静脉从器官旋转扭结，可能导致急性 IVC 狭窄[147,148]。胆道疾病是仅次于排异之后移植物功能障碍的最常见原因，发生率约 25%，通常在前 3 个月内出现[149]。这些并发症包括胆管梗阻、吻合口和

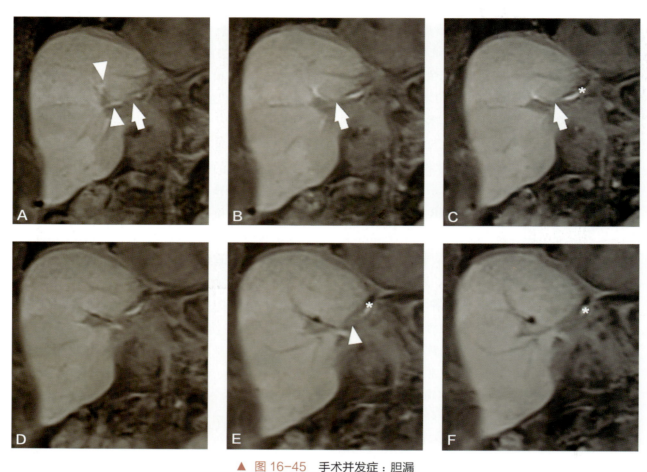

▲ 图 16-45　手术并发症：胆漏
A～F. 使用肝胆特异性对比剂后连续冠状图像上可见胆汁树（白箭）之间的轨迹（箭头）和液体积聚（星号）

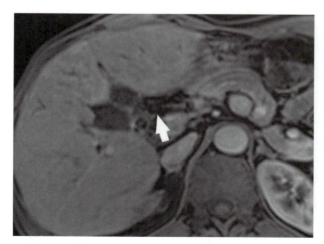

▲ 图 16-46　肝移植并发症
动脉期 T_1 加权图像示肝动脉支架内血栓

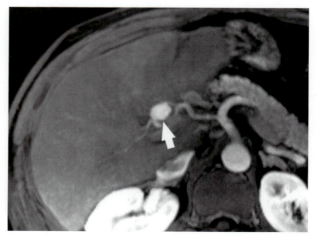

▲ 图 16-47　肝移植并发症
动脉期 T_1 加权图像示肝动脉的假性动脉瘤

非吻合口胆管狭窄、结石形成、胆漏和胆汁瘤（图 16-48 至图 16-51）。胆管狭窄是最常见的胆道并发症：吻合口部位的狭窄通常继发于瘢痕形成，而非吻合处的胆管狭窄继发于缺血（通常是肝动脉血栓形成或狭窄）、感染性胆管炎或移植前硬化性胆管炎[150]。在这种情况下，MR 胆管造影在胆道狭窄的无创诊断中起重要作用。LT 后的肿瘤相关并发症包括卡波西肉瘤、黑色素瘤或非霍奇金淋巴瘤。移植后也可出现肝细胞癌复发，肝脏是继肺部后第二常见的部位[151]。

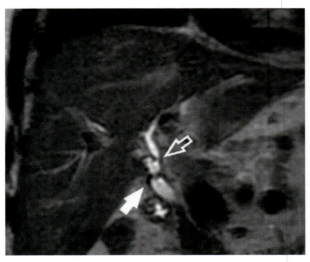

▲ 图 16-48 肝移植并发症

冠状为 T_2 加权图像显示吻合口狭窄（白箭）。同样值得注意的是非吻合口的狭窄，狭窄部位在肝左管的汇入处狭窄（黑箭）

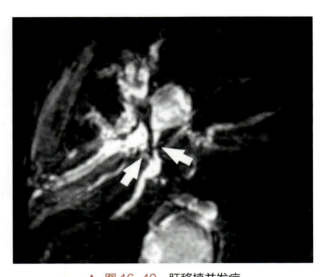

▲ 图 16-49 肝移植并发症

厚层状磁共振胆道成像显示出一种非吻合口处狭窄（白箭），在肝右管和肝左管汇合处

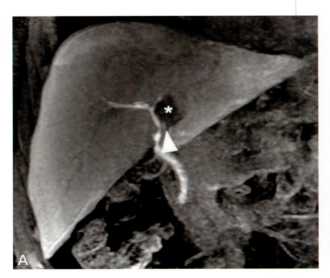

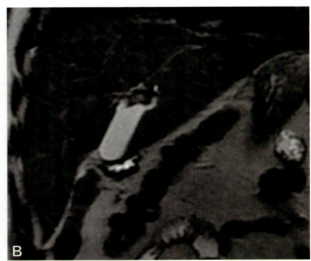

▲ 图 16-50 肝移植并发症

A. 在肝胆期冠状位 T_1 加权图像显示液体积聚（星号）不与胆管树（箭头）相同；B. 相应的 T_2 加权图像显示"肝门部的胆汁瘤"

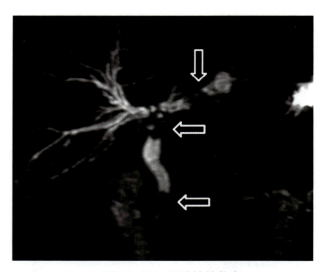

▲ 图 16-51　肝移植并发症

厚层块磁共振胆道成像示左肝内胆管、吻合口处和壶腹周围区域多发胆管结石

参考文献

［1］Brancatelli G1, Federle MP, Vilgrain V et al. Fibropolycystic liver disease: CT and MR Imaging Findings. *RadioGraphics*. 2005;25: 659–670.

［2］Desmet VJ. What is congenital hepatic fibrosis? *Histopathology*. 1992;20:465–477.

［3］Mortelé KJ, Ros PR. Cystic focal liver lesions in the adult: Differential CT and MR Imaging Features. *RadioGraphics*. 2001;21:895–910.

［4］Lev-Toaff AS, Bach AM, Wechsler RJ, Hilpert PL, Gatalica Z, Rubin R. The radiologic and pathologic spectrum of biliary hamartomas. *AJR Am J Roentgenol*. 1995;165:309–313.

［5］Mortele B et al: Hepatic bile duct hamartomas (von Meyenburg Complexes): MR and MR cholangiography findings. *J Comput Assist Tomogr*. 2002;126:438–443.

［6］Semelka RC, Hussain SM, Marcos HB, Woosley JT. Biliary hamartomas: Solitary and multiple lesions shown on current MR techniques including gadolinium enhancement. *J Magn Reson Imaging*. 1999;10:196–201.

［7］Wohlgemuth WA, Böttger J, Bohndorf K. MRI, CT, US and ERCP in the evaluation of bile duct hamartomas (von Meyenburg complex): A case report. *Eur Radiol*. 1998;8:1623–1626.

［8］Song JS, Noh SJ, Cho BH, Moon WS. Multicystic biliary hamartoma of the liver. *Korean J Pathol*. 2013;47:275–278.

［9］Iha H, Nakashima Y, Fukukura Y et al. Biliary hamartomas simulating multiple hepatic metastasis on imaging findings. *Kurume Med J*. 1996;43:231–235.

［10］van Sonnenberg E, Wroblicka JT, D'Agostino HB et al. Symptomatic hepatic cysts: Percutaneous drainage and sclerosis. *Radiology*. 1994;190:387–392.

［11］Zangger P, Grossholz M, Mentha G, Lemoine R, Graf JD, Terrier F. MRI findings in Caroli's disease and intrahepatic pigmented calculi. *Abdom Imaging*. 1995;20:361–364.

［12］Pavone P, Laghi A, Catalano C, Materia A, Basso N, Passariello R. Caroli's disease: Evaluation with MR cholangiopancreatography (MRCP). *Abdom Imaging*. 1996;21:117–119.

［13］Baghbanian M, Salmanroghani H, Baghbanian A. Cholangiocarcinoma or Caroli disease: A case presentation. *Gastroenterol Hepatol Bed Bench*. 2013;6:214–216.

［14］Rahimian J, Wilson T, Oram V, Holzman RS. Pyogenic liver abscess: Recent trends in etiology and mortality. *Clin Infect Dis*. 2004;39:1654–1659.

［15］Qian LJ, Zhu J, Zhuang ZG, Xia Q, Liu Q, Xu JR. Spectrum of multilocular cystic hepatic lesions: CT and MR imaging findings with pathologic correlation. *RadioGraphics*. 2013;33:1419–1433.

［16］Van Sonnenberg E, Mueller PR, Schiffman HR et al. Intrahepatic amebic abscesses: Indications for and results of percutaneous catheter drainage. *Radiology*. 1985;156:631–635.

［17］Marani SA, Canossi GC, Nicoli FA et al. Hydatid disease: MR imaging study. *Radiology*. 1990;175:701–706.

［18］Buetow PC, Midkiff RB. MR imaging of the liver. Primary malignant neoplasms in the adult. *Magn Reson Imaging Clin N Am*. 1997;5:289–318.

［19］Kim HG. Biliary cystic neoplasm: Biliary cystadenoma and biliary cystadenocarcinoma. *Korean J Gastroenterol*. 2006;47:5–14.

［20］Kele PG, van der Jagt EJ. Diffusion weighted imaging in the liver. *World J Gastroenterol*. 2010;16:1567–1576.

［21］Fuks D, Voitot H, Paradis V, Belghiti J, Vilgrain V, Farges O. Intracystic concentrations of tumour markers for the diagnosis of cystic liver lesions. *Br J Surg*. 2014;101:408–416.

［22］Lewis KH, Chezmar JL. Hepatic metastases. *Magn Reson Imaging Clin N Am*. 1997;5:241–253.

［23］Semelka RC, Sofka CM. Hepatic hemangiomas. *Magn Reson Imaging Clin N Am*. 1997;5:241–253.

［24］Vilgrain V, Boulos L, Vullierme MP, Denys A, Terris B, Menu Y. Imaging of atypical hemangiomas of the liver with pathologic correlation. *RadioGraphics*. 2000;20:379–397.

［25］Brancatelli G, Federle MP, Blachar A et al. Hemangioma in the cirrhotic liver: Diagnosis and natural history. *Radiology*. 2001;219:69–74.

［26］Soyer P, Gueye C, Somveille E et al. MR diagnosisf hepatic metastases from neuroendocrine tumors versus hemangiomas: Relative merits of dynamic gado linium chelate-enhanced gradient-recalled echo and unenhanced spin-echo images. *AJR Am J Roentgenol*. 1995;165:1407–1413.

［27］Darlak JJ, Moshowitz M, Kattan KR. Calcifications in the liver. *Radiol Clin North Am*. 1990;18:209–219.

［28］Scatarige JC, Fishman EK, Saksouk FA, Siegelman S. Computed tomography of calcified liver masses. *J Comput Assist Tomogr*. 1983;7:83–89.

［29］Nguyen BN, Flejou JF, Terris B et al. Focal nodular hyperplasia of the liver: A comprehensive pathologic study of 305 lesions and recognition of new histologic forms. *Am J Surg Pathol*. 1999;23:1441–1454.

[30] International Working Party. Terminology of nodular hepatocellular lesions. *Hepatology*. 1995;22:983–993.

[31] Wanless IR, Mawdsley C, Adams R. On the pathogenesis of focal nodular hyperplasia of the liver. *Hepatology*. 1985;5:1194–1200.

[32] Marin D, Brancatelli G, Federle MP et al. Focal nodular hyperplasia: Typical and atypical MRI findings with emphasis on the use of contrast media. *Clin Radiol*. 2008;63:577–585.

[33] Morteleˊ KJ, Praet M, Van Vlierberghe H, Kunnen M, Ros PR. CT and MR imaging findings in focal nodular hyperplasia of the liver: Radiologic-pathologic correla tion. *AJR Am J Roentgenol*. 2000;175:687–692.

[34] Hussain SM, Terkivatan T, Zondervan PE et al. Focal nodular hyperplasia: Findings at state-of-the-art MR imaging, US, CT, and pathologic analysis. *RadioGraphics*. 2004;24:3–17.

[35] Vilgrain V. Focal nodular hyperplasia. *Eur J Radiol*. 200;58:236–245.

[36] Grazioli L, Bondioni MP, Haradome H et al. Hepatocellular adenoma and focal nodular hyperplasia: Value of gadoxetic acid-enhanced MR imaging in differ ential diagnosis. *Radiology*. 2012; 262:520–529.

[37] Grazioli L, Morana G, Kirchin MA, Schneider G. Accurate differentiation of focal nodular hyperplasia from hepatic adenoma at gadobenate dimeglumine enhanced MR imaging: Prospective study. *Radiology*. 2005;236:166–177.

[38] Ba-Ssalamah A, Schima W, Schmook MT et al. Atypical focal nodular hyperplasia of the liver: Imaging features of nonspecific and liver-specific MR contrast agents. *AJR Am J Roentgenol*. 2002;179:1447–1456.

[39] Terkivatan T, van den Bos IC, Hussain SM et al. Focal nodular hyperplasia: Lesion characteristics on state of-the-art MRI including dynamic gadolinium enhanced and superparamagnetic iron-oxide-uptake sequences in a prospective study. *J Magn Reson Imaging*. 2006;24:464–472.

[40] Grazioli L, Federle MP, Brancatelli G et al. Hepatic adenomas: Imaging and pathologic findings. *RadioGraphics*. 2001;21:877–892.

[41] Katabathina VS, Menias CO, Shanbhogue AKP et al. Genetics and imaging of hepatocellular adenomas: 2011 update. *RadioGraphics*. 2011;31:1529–1543.

[42] Bioulac-Sage P, Rebouissou S, Thomas C et al. Hepatocellular adenoma subtype classification using molecular markers and immunohistochemistry. *Hepatology*. 2007;46:740–748.

[43] Bioulac-Sage P, Laumonier H, Laurent C, Zucman-Rossi J, Balabaud C. Hepatocellular adenoma: What is new in 2008. *Hepatol Int*. 2008;2:316–321.

[44] Lewin M, Handra-Luca A, Arrivé L et al. Liver ade nomatosis: Classification of MR imaging features and comparison with pathologic findings. *Radiology*. 2006;241:433–440.

[45] Laumonier H, Bioulac-Sage P, Laurent C, Zucman Rossi J, Balabaud C, Trillaud H. Hepatocellular adenomas: Magnetic resonance imaging features as a function of molecular pathological classification. *Hepatology*. 2008;48:808–818.

[46] Wachsberg RH, Cho KC, Adekosan A. Two leiomyomas of the liver in an adult with AIDS: CT and MR appearance. *J Comput Assist Tomogr*. 1994;18:156–157.

[47] Santos I, Valls C, Leiva D, Serrano T, Martinez L, Ruiz S. Primary hepatic leiomyoma: Case report. *Abdom Imaging*. 2011;36:315–317.

[48] Marin D, Catalano C, Rossi M et al. Gadobenate dimeglumine-enhanced magnetic resonance imaging of primary leiomyoma of the liver. *J Magn Reson Imaging*. 2008;28:755–758.

[49] Ahmadi T, Itai Y, Takahashi M et al. Angiomyolipoma of the liver: Significance of CT and MR dynamic study. *Abdom Imaging*. 1998;23:520–526.

[50] Balci NC, Akinci A, Akun E et al. Hepatic angiomyolipoma: Demonstration by out of phase MRI. *Clin Imaging*. 2002;26:418–420.

[51] Hussain S. *Liver MR*. Springer, Berlin, Germany, 2007.

[52] International Agency for Research on Cancer, World Health Organization (WHO). GLOBOCAN 2008: Cancer incidence, mortality and prevalence worldwide in 2008. Available at: http://globo can.iarc.fr. Accessed April 19, 2012.

[53] Stroffolini T, Andreone P, Andriulli A et al. Characteristics of hepatocellular carcinoma in Italy. *J Hepatol*. 1998;29:944–952.

[54] El-Serag HB, Mason AC. Rising incidence of hepatocellular carcinoma in the United States. *N Engl J Med*. 1999;340:745–750.

[55] Deuffic S, Poynard T, Buffat L, Valleron AJ. Trends in pri mary liver cancer. *Lancet*. 1998;351:214–215.

[56] Taylor-Robinson SD, Foster GR, Arora S, Hargreaves S, Thomas HC. Increase in primary liver cancer in the UK, 1979–1994. *Lancet*. 1997;350:1142–1143.

[57] International Agency for Cancer Reseach. GLOBOCAN 2002. Available at: http://www-dep.iarc.fr. Accessed January 20, 2010.

[58] Coleman WB. Mechanisms of human hepatocarcinogen esis. *Curr Mol Med*. 2003;3: 573–588.

[59] Efremidis SC, Hytiroglou P. The multistep process of hepatocarcinogenesis in cirrhosis with imaging correlation. *Eur Radiol*. 2002;12:753–764.

[60] Okuda K, Noguchi T, Kubo Y, Shimokawa Y, Kojiro M, Nakashima T. A clinical and pathological study of diffuse type hepatocellular carcinoma. *Liver*. 1981;1:280–289.

[61] Bruix J, Scherman M. Management of hepatocellular carcinoma: An update. *Hepatology*. 2011;53:1020–1022.

[62] Peterson MS, Baron RL, Marsh JW, Oliver III JH, Confer SR, Hunt LE. Pretransplantation surveillance for pos sible hepatocellular carcinoma in patients with cirrhosis: Epidemiology and CT-based tumor detection rate in 430 cases with surgical pathologic correlation. *Radiology*. 2000;217:743–749.

[63] Trojan J, Raedle J, Zeuzem S. Serum tests for diagnosis and follow-up of hepatocellular carcinoma after treat ment. *Di-*

gestion. 1998;59(Suppl. 2):72–74.
[64] Lok AS, Sterling RK, Everhart JE et al. Des-gamma Carboxy Prothrombin and alpha-fetoprotein as biomarkers for the early detection of hepatocellular carcinoma. *Gastroenterology.* 2010;138:493–502.
[65] Reinhold C, Hammers L, Taylor CR et al. Characterization of focal hepatic lesions with Duplex sonogrphy: Findings in 198 patients. *AJR Am J Roentgenol.* 1995;164:1131–1135.
[66] Di Martino M, De Filippis G, De Santis A et al. Hepatocellular carcinoma in cirrhotic patients: Prospective comparison of US, CT and MR imaging. *Eur Radiol.* 2013;23:887–896.
[67] Kadoya M, Matsui O, Takashima T, Nonomura A. Hepatocellular carcinoma: Correlation of MR imaging and histopathologic findings. *Radiology.* 1992;183:819–825.
[68] Ebara M, Fukuda H, Kojima Y et al. Small hepatocellular carcinoma: Relationship of signal intensity to histopath ologic findings and metal content of the tumor and surrounding hepatic parenchyma. *Radiology.* 1999;210:81–88.
[69] Takayama Y1, Nishie A, Nakayama T et al. Hypovascular hepatic nodule showing hypointensity in the hepatobiliary phase of gadoxetic acid-enhanced MRI in patients with chronic liver disease: Prediction of malignant transformation. *Eur J Radiol.* 2012;81:3072–3078.
[70] Lencioni R, Cioni D, Crocetti L et al. Magnetic resonance imaging of liver tumors. *J Hepatol.* 2004;40:162–171.
[71] Shinmura R, Matsui O, Kobayashi S et al: Cirrhotic nod - ules: Association between MR imaging signal intensity and intranodular blood supply. *Radiology.* 2005;237:512–519.
[72] Kim CK, Lim JH, Park CK et al. Neoangiogenesis and sinusoidal capillarization in hepatocellular carcinoma: Correlation between dynamic CT and density of tumor microvessels. *Radiology.* 2005;237:529–534.
[73] Brancatelli G, Baron RL, Peterson MS, Marsh W. Helical CT screening for hepatocellular carcinoma in patients with cirrhosis: Frequency and causes of false-positive interpretation. *AJR Am J Roentgenol.* 2003;180:1007–1014.
[74] Marrero JA, Hussain HK, Nghiem HV et al. Improving the prediction of hepatocellular carcinoma in cirrhotic patients with an arterially-enhancing liver mass. *Liver Transpl.* 2005;11:281–289.
[75] Lim JH, Chooi D Kim SH et al. Detection of hepatocellular carcinoma:Value of adding delayed phase imaging to dual - phase helical CT. *AJR Am J Roentgenol.* 2002;179:67–73.
[76] Iannaccone R, Laghi A, Catalano C et al. Hepatocellular carcinoma of unenhanced and delayed phase multi detector row helical CT in patients with cirrhosis. *Radiology.* 2005;234:460–467.
[77] Di Martino M, Marin D, Guerrisi G et al. Intraindividual comparison of gadoxetate disodium-enhanced MR imaging and 64-section multidetector CT in the detec tion of hepatocellular carcinoma in patients with cirrhosis. *Radiology.* 2010;256:806–816.
[78] Vogl TJ, Stupavsky A, Pegios W et al. Hepatocellular carcinoma: Evaluation of dynamic and static gadobenate dimeglumine-enhanced MR imaging and histopato logic correlation. *Radiology.* 1997;205:721–728.
[79] Grazioli L, Morana G, Caudana R et al. Hepatocellular carcinoma: Correlation between gadobenate dimeglumine-enhanced MRI and pathologic findings. *Invest Radiol.* 2000;35:25–34.
[80] Imai Y, Murakami T, Yoshida S et al. Superparamagnetic iron oxide-enhanced magnetic resonance images of hepatocellular carcinoma: Correlation with histological grading. *Hepatology.* 2000;32:205–212.
[81] Mannelli L, Bhargava P, Osman SF et al. Diffusion weighted imaging of the liver: A comprehensive review. *Curr Probl Diagn Radiol.* 2013;42:77–83.
[82] Kim DJ, Ju JS, Kim JH, Chung JJ, Kim KW. Small hypervascular hepatocellular carcinomas: Value of diffusion weighted imaging compared with "washout" appearance on dynamic MRI. *Br J Med.* 2012;9:1–8.
[83] Mannelli L, Kim S, Hajdu CH et al. Assessment of tumor necrosis of hepatocellular carcinoma after chemoem bolization: Diffusion-weighted and contrast-enhanced MRI with histopathologic correlation of the explanted liver. *AJR Am J Roentgenol.* 2009;193:1044–1052.
[84] LeMoigne F, DurieuxM, Baincel B et al. Impact of diffusion weighted MRimaging on the characterization of small hepatocellular carcinoma in the cirrhotic liver. *Magn Reson Imaging.* 2012;30:656–665.
[85] Di Martino M, Di Miscio R, De Filippis G, Lombardo CV, Saba L, Geiger D, Catalano C. Detection of small (≤2 cm) HCC in cirrhotic patients: Added value of diffusion MR-imaging. *Abdom Imaging.* 2013;38:1254–1262.
[86] Park MS, Kim S, Patel J et al. Hepatocellular carcinoma: Detection with diffusion-weighted versus contrast enhanced magnetic resonance imaging in pretransplant patients. *Hepatology.* 2012;56:140–148.
[87] Di Martino M, Saba L, Bosco S et al. Hepatocellular carcinoma (HCC) in non-cirrhotic liver: Clinical, radiological and pathological findings. *Eur Radiol.* 2014;24:1446–1454.
[88] Iannaccone R, Piacentini F, Murakanmi T et al. Hepatocellular carcinoma in patients with nonalco holic fatty liver disease: Helical CT and MR Imaging with clinical-pathologic correlation findings. *Radiology.* 2007;243:422–430.
[89] Brancatelli G, Federle MP, Grazioli L, Carr BI. Hepatocellular carcinoma in non-cirrhotic liver: CT, clinical and pathological findings in 39 U.S. residents. *Radiology.* 2002;222:89–94.
[90] Berman MA, Burnham JA, Sheahan DG. Fibrolamellar carcinoma of the liver: An immunohistochemical study of 19 cases and a review of the literature. *Hum Pathol.* 1988;19:784–794.
[91] Ichikawa T, Federle MP, Grazioli L, Madariaga J, Nalesnik M, Marsh W. Fibrolamellar hepatocellular carcinoma: Imaging and pathologic findings in 31 recent cases. *Radiology.* 1999;213:352–361.
[92] McLarney JK, Rucker PT, Bender GN, Goodman ZD,

Kashitani N, Ros PR. Fibrolamellar carcinoma of the liver: Radiologic-pathologic correlation. *RadioGraphics*. 1999;19:453–471.

[93] Won JL, Lim HK, Jang KM et al. Radiologic spectrum of cholangiocarcinoma: Emphasis on unusual manifestations and differential diagnoses. *RadioGraphics*. 2001;21:S97–S116.

[94] Soyer P, Bluemke DA, Reichle R et al Imaging of intra hepatic cholangiocarcinoma:1. Peripheral cholangiocar cinomo. *AJR Am J Roentgenol*. 1995;165:1427–1431.

[95] Liver Cancer Study Group of Japan. *Classification of Primary Liver Cancer*. Kanehara, Tokyo, Japan, 1997; pp. 6–8.

[96] Worawattanakul S, Semelka RC, Noone TC et al. Cholangiocarcinoma: Spectrum of appearances on MR images using current techniques. *Magn Reson Imaging*. 1998;16:993–1003.

[97] Maetani Y, Itoh K, Watanabe C et al. MR imaging of intrahepatic cholangiocarcinoma with pathologic correlation. *AJR Am J Roentgenol*. 2001;176:1499–1507.

[98] Vilgrain V, Van Beers BE, Flejou JF et al. Intrahepatic cholangiocarcinoma: MRI and pathologic correlation in 14 patients. *J Comput Assist Tomogr*. 1997;21:59–65.

[99] Park HJ, Kim YK, Park MJ, Lee WJ. Small intrahepatic mass-forming cholangiocarcinoma: Target sign on diffusion-weighted imaging for differentiation from hepa tocellular carcinoma. *Abdom Imaging*. 2013;38:793–801.

[100] Schneider G, Grazioli L, Saini S. *MR Imaging of the Live*, 2nd ed. Springer, Berlin, Germany, 2006.

[101] Manfredi R, Masselli G, Maresca G, Brizi MG, Vecchioli A, Marano P. MR imaging and MRCP of hilar cholangiocarcinoma. *Abdom Imaging*. 2003;28:319–325.

[102] Guthrie JA, Ward J, Robinson PJ. Hilar cholangiocarcinomas: T_2-weighted spin-echo and gadolinium-enhanced FLASH MR imaging. *Radiology*. 1996;201:347–351.

[103] Chryssou E, Guthrie JA, Ward J, Robinson PJ. Hilar cholangiocarcinoma: MR correlation with surgical and histological findings. *Clin Radiol*. 2010;65:781–788.

[104] Menias CO, Surabhi VR, Prasad SR, Wang HL, Narra VR, Chintapalli KN. Mimics of cholangiocarcinoma: Spectrum of disease. *RadioGraphics*. 2008;28:1115–1129.

[105] Pedro MS, Semelka RC, Braga L. MR imaging of hepatic metastases. *Magn Reson Imaging Clin N Am*. 2002;10:15–29.

[106] Semelka RC, Braga L, Armao D et al. Liver. In: Semelka RC, ed. *Abdominal-Pelvic MRI*, 1st ed. Wiley-Liss, New York, 2002; pp. 101–134.

[107] Danet IM, Semelka RC, Leonardou P, Spectrum of MRI appearances of untreated metastases of the liver. *AJR Am J Roentgenol*. 2003;181:809–817.

[108] Nino-Murcia M, Olcott EW, Jeffrey RB Jr, Lamm RL, Beaulieu CF, Jain KA. Focal liver lesions: Pattern-based classification scheme for enhancement at arterial phase CT. *Radiology*. 2000;215:746–751.

[109] Caudana R, Morana G, Pirovano GP et al. Focal malignant hepatic lesions: MR imaging enhanced with gadolinium benzyloxypropionictetra-acetate (BOPTA) preliminary results of phase II clinical application. *Radiology*. 1996;199:513–520.

[110] Ha S, Lee CH, Kim BH et al. Paradoxical uptake of Gd-EOB-DTPA on the hepatobiliary phase in the evaluation of hepatic metastasis from breast cancer: Is the "target sign" a common finding? *Magn Reson Imaging*. 2012;30:1083–1090.

[111] Kim A, Lee CH, Kim BH et al. Gadoxetic acid-enhanced 3.0T MRI for the evaluation of hepatic metastasis from colorectal cancer: Metastasis is not always seen as a "defect" on the hepatobiliary phase. *Eur J Radiol*. 2012;81:3998–4004.

[112] Ishak KG, Sesterhenn IA, Goodman ZD, Rabin L, Stromeyer FW: Epithelioid hemangioendothelioma of the liver: A clinicopathologic and follow-up study of 32 cases. *Hum Pathol*. 1984;15:839–852.

[113] Kopniczky Z, Tsimpas A, Lawson DD et al. Epithelioid hemangioendothelioma of the spine: Report of two cases and review of the literature. *Br J Neurosurg*. 2008;22:793–797.

[114] Lee YJ, Chung MJ, Jeong KC et al. Pleuralepithelioid hemangioendothelioma. *Yonsei Med J*. 2008;49:1036–1040.

[115] Mehrabi A, Kashfi A, Fonouni H et al. Primary malignant hepatic epithelioid hemangioendothelioma: A comprehensive review of the literature with emphasis on the surgical therapy. *Cancer*. 2006;107:2108–2121.

[116] Weitz J, Klimstra DS, Cymes K et al. Management of primary liver sarcomas. *Cancer*. 2007;109:1391–1396.

[117] Van Beers B, Roche A, Mathieu D et al. Epithelioid hemangioendothelioma of the liver: MR and CT find ings. *J Comput Assist Tomogr*. 1992;16:420–424.

[118] Lin J, Ji Y. CT and MRI diagnosis of hepatic epithelioid hemangioendothelioma. *Hepatobiliary Pancreat Dis Int*. 2010;9:154–158.

[119] Maher MM, McDermott SR, Fenlon HM et al. Imaging of primary non-Hodgkin's lymphoma of the liver. *Clin Radiol*. 2001;56:295–301.

[120] Gazelle GS, Lee MJ, Hahn PF, Goldberg MA, Rafaat N, Mueller PR. US, CT and MRI of primary and secondary liver lymphoma. *J Comput Assist Tomogr*. 1994;18:412–415.

[121] Weissleder R, Stark DD, Elizondo G. MRI of hepatic lymphoma. *Magn Reson Imaging*. 1988;6:675–681.

[122] Garra BS, Shawker TH, Chang R, Kaplan K, White RD. The ultrasound appearance of radiation-induced hepatic injury. Correlation with computed tomography and magnetic resonance imaging. *J Ultrasound Med*. 1988 Nov;7(11):605–609.

[123] McGahan JP, Dodd GD 3rd. Radiofrequency ablation of the liver. *AJR Am J Roentgenol*. 2001;176:3–16.

[124] Gazelle GS, Goldberg SN, Solbiati L, Livraghi T. Tumor ablation with radio-frequency energy. *Radiology*. 2000;217:633–646.

[125] Wood TF, Rose DM, Chung M, Allegra DP, Foshag LJ, Bilchik AJ. Radiofrequency ablation of 231unresectable hepatic tumors: Indications, limitations, and complications. *Ann Surg Oncol.* 2000;7:593–600.

[126] Livraghi T, Meloni F, Di Stasi M et al. Sustained complete response and complications rates after radiofrequency ablation of very early hepatocellular carcinoma in cirrhosis: Is resection still the treatment of choice? *Hepatology.* 2008;47:82–89.

[127] Sironi S, Livraghi T, Meloni F, De Cobelli F, Ferrero CG, Del Maschio A. Small hepatocellular carcinoma treated with percutaneous RF ablation: MR imaging follow-up. *AJR Am J Roentgenol.* 1999;173:1225–1229.

[128] Choi H, Loyer EM, DuBrow RA et al. Radio-frequency ablation of liver tumors: Assessment of therapeutic response and complications. *RadioGraphics.* 2001;21:S41–S54.

[129] Kuszyk BS, Boitnott JK, Choti MA et al. Local tumor recurrence following hepatic cryoablation: Radiologic histopathologic correlation in a rabbit model. *Radiology.* 2000;217:477–486.

[130] Rhim H, Dodd GD 3rd, Chintapalli KN et al. Radiofrequency thermal ablation of abdominal tumors: Lessons learned from complications. *RadioGraphics.* 2004;24:41–52.

[131] Kalva SP, Thabet A, Wicky S. Recent advances in transarterial therapy of primary and secondary liver malignancies. *RadioGraphics.* 2008;28:101–117.

[132] Lencioni R, Llovet JM. Modified RECIST (mRECIST) assessment for hepatocellular carcinoma. *Semin Liver Dis.* 2010;30:52–60.

[133] Kim HC, Chung JW, Lee W, Jae HJ, Park JH. Recognizing extrahepatic collateral vessels that supply hepato cellular carcinoma to avoid complications of trans catheter arterial chemoembolization. *RadioGraphics.* 2005;25:S25–S39.

[134] Gates J, Hartnell GG, Stuart KE, Clouse ME. Chemoembolization of hepatic neoplasms: Safety, complications, and when to worry. *RadioGraphics.* 1999;19:399–414.

[135] Ramsey DE, Kernagis LY, Soulen MC, Geschwind JF. Chemoembolization of hepatocellular carcinoma. *J Vasc Interv Radiol.* 2002;13:S211–S221.

[136] Shin DS, Ingraham CR, Dighe MK et al. Surgical resection of a malignant liver lesion: What the surgeon wants the radiologist to know. *AJR Am J Roentgenol.* 2014;203:W21–W33.

[137] Donadon M, Ribero D, Morris-Stiff G, Abdalla EK, Vauthey JN. New paradigm in the management of liver-only metastases from colorectal cancer. *Gastrointest Cancer Res.* 2007;1:20–27.

[138] Morris-Stiff G, Gomez D, Prasad R. Quantitative assessment of hepatic function and its relevance to the liver surgeon. *J Gastrointest Surg.* 2009;13:374–385.

[139] Huynh-Charlier I, Taboury J, Charlier P, Vaillant J, Grenier P, Lucidarme O. Imaging of the postsurgical liver. *J Radiol.* 200;90:888–904.

[140] Sadamori H, Yagi T, Shinoura S et al. Risk factors for major morbidity after liver resection for hepatocellular carcinoma. *Br J Surg.* 2013;100:122–129.

[141] Arii S, Teramoto K, Kawamura T et al. Characteristics of recurrent hepatocellular carcinoma in Japan and our surgical experience. *J Hepatobiliary Pancreat Surg.* 2001;8:397–403.

[142] Mazariegos GV, Molmenti EP, Kramer DJ. Early complications after orthotopic liver transplantation. *Surg Clin North Am.* 1999;791:109–129.

[143] Caiado AH, Blasbalg R, Marcelino AS et al. Complications of liver transplantation: Multimodality imaging approach. *RadioGraphics.* 2007;27:1401–1417.

[144] Nghiem HV. Imaging of hepatic transplantation. *Radiol Clin North Am.* 1998;36:429–443.

[145] Singh AK, Nachiappan AC, Verma HA et al. Postoperative imaging in liver transplantation: What radiologists should know. *RadioGraphics.* 2010;30:339–351.

[146] Wozney P, Zajko AB, Bron KM, Point S, Starzl TE. Vascular complications after liver transplantation: A 5-year experience. *AJR Am J Roentgenol.* 1986;147:657–663.

[147] Glockner JF, Forauer AR, Solomon H et al. Vascular complications after orthotopic liver transplantation. *Am J Surg.* 1991;161:76–82.

[148] Varma CR, Perman WH. Three-dimensional gadolinium enhanced MR angiography of vascular complications after liver transplantation. *AJR Am J Roentgenol.* 2000;174:1447–1453.

[149] Haberal M. Liver transplantation: Experience at our center. *Transplant Proc.* 2006;38:2111–2116.

[150] Fulcher AS, Turner MA. Orthotopic liver transplantation: Evaluation with MR cholangiography. *Radiology.* 1999;211:715–722.

[151] Aseni P, Vertemati M, De Carlis L et al. De novo cancers and post-transplant lymphoproliferative disorder in adult liver transplantation. *Pathol Int.* 2006;56:712–715.

Chapter 17
胆囊

Gallbladder

Ganeshan Dhakshinamoorthy, Nicolaus Wagner-Bartak, Rafael Andres Vicens, Shelby Kent, Neeraj Lalwani, Priya Bhosale 著

马霄虹 译

赵心明 校

目录 CONTENTS

一、正常解剖 / 402

二、成像技术 / 404

胆囊（gallbadder，GB）是梨形的囊状中空性器官，有助于储存肝脏产生的胆汁。虽然胆结石是胆囊最常见的疾病之一，但是许多其他疾病也可以累及胆囊。在许多胆囊疾病中可有右上腹疼痛和（或）黄疸的表现，但通常情况下患者没有特异性的临床表现，因此影像学检查在诊断和指导治疗方面起着关键作用。超声检查（ultrasound，US）是评估 GB 疾病最常见的主要影像检查方式，但是计算机断层扫描（CT）和磁共振成像（MRI）正越来越多地应用于临床以提高诊断的准确性。

在本章中，我们要讨论胆囊的胚胎学和正常解剖，并回顾胆囊的各种先天性、炎症性、传染性、肿瘤性、医源性及其他各种疾病，重点在于 MRI 在各类疾病的诊断和治疗中的作用。

一、正常解剖

（一）胚胎学

胆囊、胆道、腹侧胰腺和肝脏均起源于肝憩室，肝憩室在胚胎发育第 4 周出现在原始前肠尾端的腹侧壁。肝脏、肝总管（common hepatic duct，CHD）和肝内胆管来自于憩室的头侧部分（肝原基），而胆囊和胆囊管来自憩室的尾侧部分（胆囊憩室）[1]。胚胎发育第 5 周初，肝胆管的所有组成部分，包括胆囊、胆囊管、肝管、胆总管（common bile duct，CBD）和腹侧胰腺就都可以辨认识别了。胚胎发育第 5 周期间，肝外胆管快速延长，伴随上皮细胞增生，管腔内被细胞实性成分充填。胚胎发育第 6 周，胆总管的管腔从远端开始再通，然后向近端延伸。胆囊管再通出现在胚胎发育第 8 周。

解剖

胆囊是位于肝右叶下表面梨形囊状结构（图 17-1）。它大小可变，大小可达到 10cm×4cm，并容纳约 50ml 的胆汁。胆囊分为胆囊底、胆囊体、漏斗部和颈部四部分。Hartmann 囊是指漏斗部的下表面的凸起，胆囊结石常常在此处存留。胆囊管长约 4cm，起自胆囊颈部，与肝总管汇合形成胆总管。胆总管进入胰腺头部并与主胰管汇合，并在十二指肠大乳头处形成 Vater 壶腹。Oddi 括约肌，即环形的平滑肌束，包绕胆总管的远端和 Vater 壶腹水平的主胰管。Luschka 管是胆管的一种正常的解剖变异，是指走行在胆囊床的小胆管，人群中发生率约 50%。这个解剖变异对手术很有意义，在胆囊切除术中可能会损伤 Luschka 管，如果没有妥善结扎会导致医源性胆瘘。

胆囊是由胆囊动脉供血（肝右动脉或肝总动脉的一个分支）和胆囊静脉（门静脉的一个属支）回流。胆囊受迷走神经和腹腔神经丛支配。胆囊的淋巴引流非常重要，这解释了根治性手术切除通常很困难的原因，因为胆囊具有广泛的淋巴引流途径。大量研究显示胆囊有 3 条主要的淋巴引流途径[2]。

（1）胆囊 - 胰后区引流途径，是主要的引流途径，沿着胆总管的前后表面引流至胰头后方的门静脉后淋巴结。

（2）胆囊 - 腹腔引流途径，沿着肝十二指肠韧带引流至腹腔淋巴结。

（3）胆囊 - 肠系膜引流途径，沿着门静脉前表面引流至肠系膜上动脉根部淋巴结。

这些引流途径进一步汇入左肾静脉附近的腹

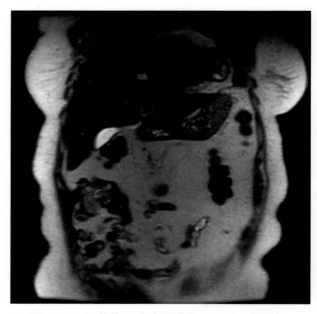

▲ 图 17-1　冠状位 T_2 加权图像显示梨形正常胆囊

膜后淋巴结并进入腹主动脉下腔静脉间淋巴结。

（二）解剖变异与先天发育异常

胆囊的先天畸形比较罕见，据报道发生率约为 0.15%[3]。虽然不常见，但是却非常重要，因为它们经常与胆管和血管的变异和发育异常相关，这对避免胆囊切除手术并发症至关重要。此外，胆囊先天畸形也可能与其他器官的先天畸形有关，这也是容易出现并发症的因素之一。

胆囊发育不全罕见，发生率为 0.02%～0.15%，是由于原始肝憩室的尾支未正常发育所致[4]。约 65% 的胆囊发育不全患者也有合并其他脏器异常，包括先天性心脏病、多脾、肛门闭锁和直肠阴道瘘[5]。完全肝内胆囊偶尔可能会被误认为是胆囊发育不全，但横断面成像，尤其是 CT 或 MRI，可以清楚地识别 GB 的位置，并有助于做出正确的诊断。实际上，通过影像进行术前诊断，可以使症状性胆囊发育不全患者避免不必要的手术[6,7]。胆囊发育不良比发育不全更常见。发育不良的小胆囊可以直接贴附于肝总管或通过非常短的胆囊管与肝总管相连，这可能会被误认为是胆总管。

大约每 4000 人中就有 1 人是双胆囊（图 17-2），是由于原始胆囊的不完全再空泡化而导致的。双叶胆囊、折叠胆囊及胆囊憩室与双胆囊有相似之处（图 17-3），CT 或 MRI 的横断面成像可确定 2 个独立的 GB 腔的存在，每个腔都有独立的胆囊管，有助于做出正确的诊断。双胆囊可导致胆结石、继发性胆汁性肝硬化及胆囊癌等并发症。

胆囊形状的异常包括 Phrygian 帽（因其与古希腊奴隶获得自由后所戴的帽子相似而命名）、胆囊分隔及胆囊憩室。Phrygian 帽（图 17-4）是一种较常见的变异，发病率 1%～6%，但并无临床意义，而胆囊分隔及胆囊憩室可导致胆石症。

胆囊先天性变异导致的解剖位置异常并不常见，包括"游走胆囊"和"异位胆囊"，可导致胆汁淤积。游走胆囊指胆囊系膜很长，使胆囊"游走"到异常位置，包括骨盆、椎间隙和小网膜囊，这可能导致胆囊扭转，因而有重要的临床意义。胆囊也可发生异位（图 17-5），可完全位于肝内，诊断比较困难，也可位于肝上、肝后，甚至可能位于腹膜后。左侧胆囊（图 17-6）是罕见的先天性异常，可是内脏转位的一部分，也可是孤立的异常[8,9]。这可能由于胆囊向肝脏左侧迁移，或者由于原始胆囊萎缩而继发第二胆囊，这可能与门静脉系统和胰胆管树的异常有关。

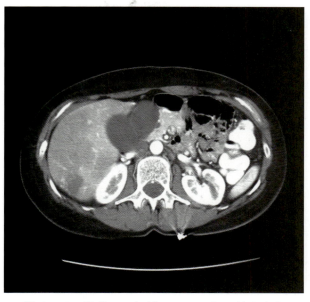

▲ 图 17-2　轴位 CT 扫描显示 52 岁男性患者折叠胆囊

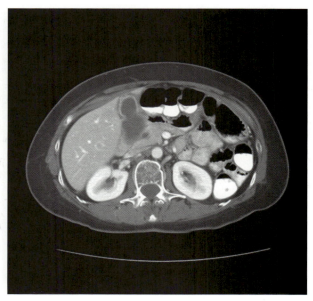

▲ 图 17-3　轴位 CT 扫描显示 61 岁男性患者的胆囊憩室

(三) 胆囊管

胆囊管的走向、长度以及其位置均可以变化。例如，胆囊管可以平行于肝总管并且进入其内侧位置。观察影像图像时，发现并报道这种变异解剖结构很重要，因为如果在胆囊切除术中没有发现，术中夹紧和牵拉切除胆囊时会增加肝总管损伤的风险。

胆囊管汇入胆总管的位置可较低，位于十二指肠乳头（8%～14%）水平，也可较高，位于肝门水平。此外，胆囊管可汇入右肝管、左肝管或胆管汇合处。

二、成像技术

腹部X线在评估GB疾病或诊断右上腹疼痛病例中的价值不大，发现胆结石的灵敏度低（15%～20%）。此外，即使X线提示胆结石，也不能确定是否存在胆囊炎。根据目前美国放射学会（American College of Radiology，ACR）指南，超声是评估右上腹疼痛患者的首选影像学方法[11]。它应用广泛、费用较低，而且可以在床边快速操作，非常适合评估有无胆囊结石、胆囊壁厚度、胆囊息肉、肿块、胆囊周围积液及胆管扩张（图17-7至图17-9）。超声也有助于评估是否存在墨菲征（Murphy征），是诊断急性胆囊炎非常有意义的征象。

有研究表明，胆管闪烁显像在诊断急性胆囊炎中有很高的敏感性和特异性（图17-10）。最近一项META分析显示，胆管闪烁显像检查的敏感性为96%、特异性为90%，而超声的敏感性为81%、特异性为83%[10]。然而尽管其诊断急性胆囊炎的效能较高，但由于多种原因，如超声检查便捷、可更广泛应用、提供有关胆管状态的

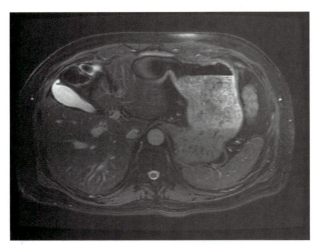

▲ 图17-4 轴位T₂加权MRI显示胆囊Phrygian帽，是一种正常的变异

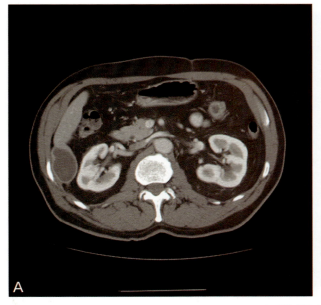
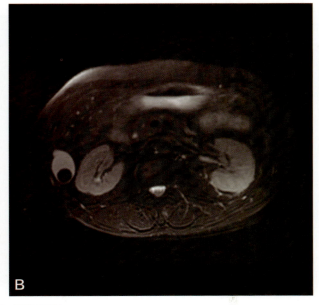

▲ 图17-5 异位胆囊

轴位CT扫描（A）和轴位T₂加权MRI（B）显示位于肝脏后方的胆囊。MRI显示胆结石，在CT扫描中无法清晰显示

信息并且没有辐射,因此首选检查为超声。使用 ^{99m}Tc-IDA（亚氨基二乙酸）的胆管闪烁显像也可用于诊断非结石性胆囊炎,鉴别急慢性胆囊炎,以及评估胆汁漏。

增强 CT 在评估 GB 疾病方面非常有意义,包括急性炎症和胆囊恶性肿瘤。CT 特别适用于评估胆囊炎的并发症,如坏疽性胆囊炎,气肿性胆囊炎,出血性胆囊炎和胆囊穿孔[12-16]（图 17-11 至图 17-20）。研究表明 CT 还有助于临床制订术前计划,胆囊壁不强化和（或）胆囊颈部存在结石增加了从腹腔镜转为开腹胆囊切除术的必要性[17]。因此,这些影像结果有助于指导临床选择合适的手术方法。另外,CT 对于排除由其他原因引起的右上腹疼痛也非常有价值。

MRI 目前尚未被提倡作为评估急性右上腹疼痛或其他胆囊疾病的主要影像学检查手段,但一些研究表明 MRI 对于难以用超声评估或结果不确

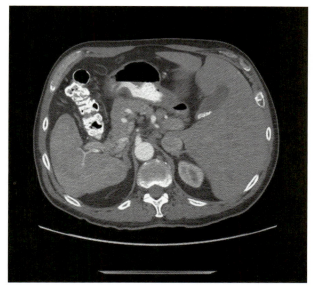

▲ 图 17-6　47 岁的男性患者,左侧胆囊,患者内脏转位

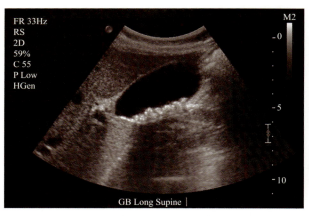

▲ 图 17-7　纵向超声声像图示多发胆囊结石

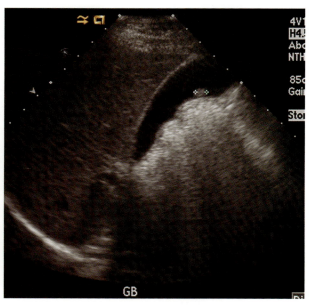

▲ 图 17-9　纵向超声声像图示胆囊息肉

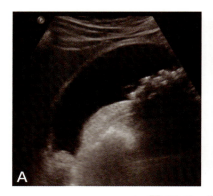
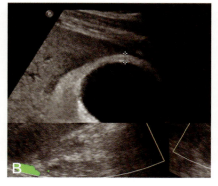
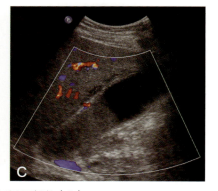

▲ 图 17-8　纵向和横向超声声像图示胆囊结石（A、B）和胆囊炎（C）

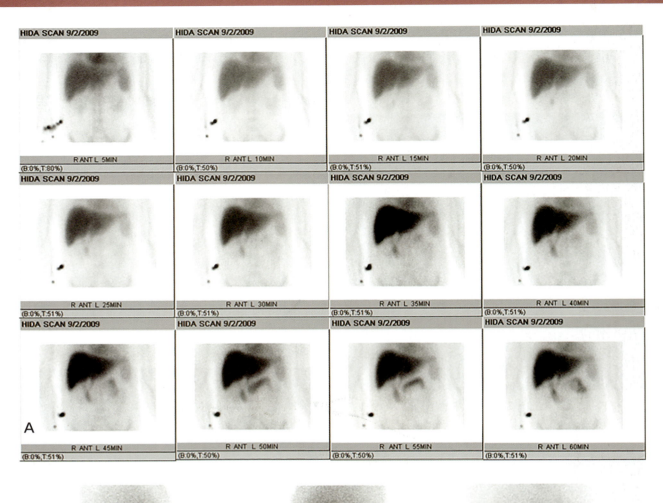

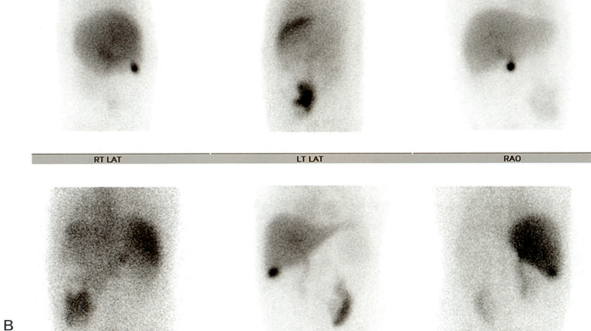

▲ 图 17-10 胆管闪烁显像用于诊断急性胆囊炎

HIDA 扫描（A）显示最初 60min 胆囊未显像。在注射 4mg 硫酸吗啡（B）后 30min，上腹部的连续静态图像显示胆囊显像。既往超声检查显示胆囊壁增厚。结果符合慢性胆囊炎

Chapter 17 胆囊
Gallbladder

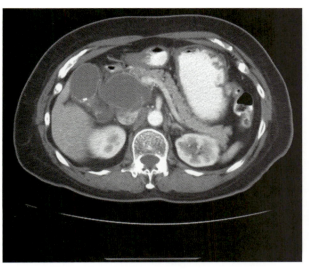

▲ 图 17-11 轴位 CT 扫描显示胆囊穿孔伴脓肿形成

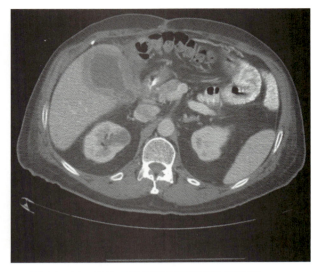

▲ 图 17-14 轴位 CT 扫描显示坏疽性胆囊炎

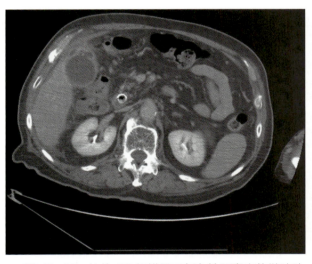

▲ 图 17-12 轴位 CT 扫描显示复杂性胆囊炎伴微脓肿

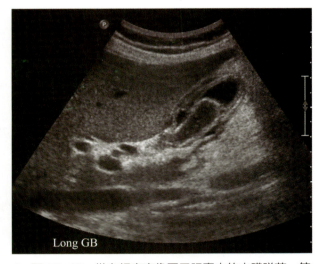

▲ 图 17-15 纵向超声声像图示胆囊中的内膜脱落，符合坏疽性胆囊炎

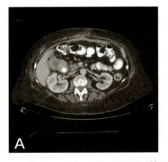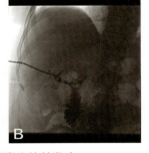

▲ 图 17-13 CT 用于评估胆囊炎的并发症
轴位 CT（A）显示重症胆囊炎，十二指肠壁明显增厚。胆囊造口术随访（B）显示胆囊十二指肠瘘，胆囊直接与十二指肠降段相通

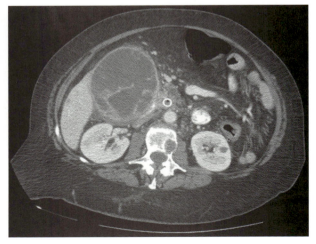

▲ 图 17-16 轴位 CT 扫描显示胆囊中内膜脱落，符合坏疽性胆囊炎

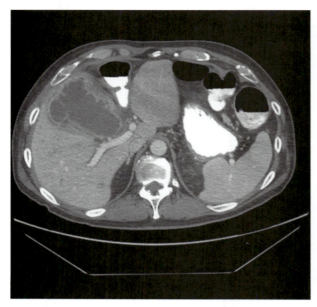

▲ 图 17-17　轴位 CT 扫描显示坏疽性胆囊炎伴穿孔

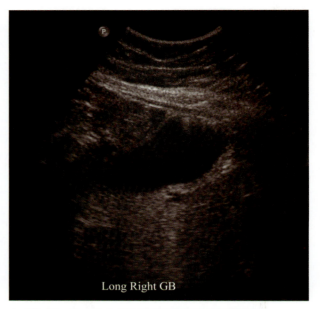

▲ 图 17-19　纵向超声声像图示气肿性胆囊炎

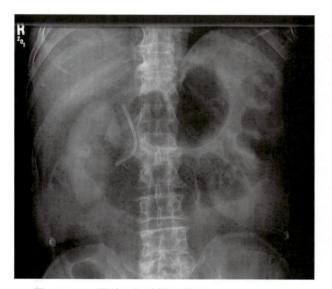

▲ 图 17-18　平片示气肿性胆囊炎

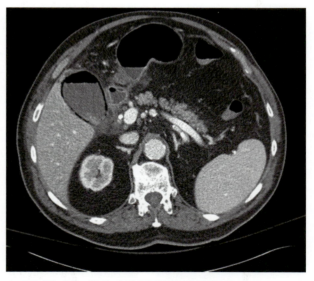

▲ 图 17-20　轴位 CT 显示气肿性胆囊炎

定的患者是可靠的替代检查。在 META 分析中，MRI 对急性胆囊炎的敏感性为 85%，特异性为 81%[10]。此外，MRI 尤其适用于妊娠不能受放射线照射的患者，MRI 也可用于确定是否存在并发症以及评估肝内、外胆管系统。此外，MRI 有利于鉴别良、恶性胆囊疾病以及胆囊恶性肿瘤的诊断和分期。

MRI 和 MR 胰胆管造影（MRCP）是用于评估 GB 和胆道病变的无创性成像技术（图 17-21）。MRCP 的重 T_2 加权序列可形成高的胆汁 - 背景对比度，从而提高胆管和胆囊的显影。脂肪饱和序列也有助于更好地显示胆囊和胆管系统。静脉注射钆对比剂后增强图像可用于评估胆囊壁增厚，胆囊肿块以及胆囊恶性肿瘤的分期（图 17-22）。初步研究报道，扩散加权成像可能有助于鉴别良性和恶性 GB 息肉样病变[18,19]。用于评估 GB 疾病的 MRI 序列的选择可能因机构不同而异，但标准方案[20,21]包括冠状位 T_2 加权单次快速自旋回波序列，轴位呼吸门控 T_2 加权快速自旋回波序列（用于评估涉及胆囊壁

Chapter 17 胆囊
Gallbladder

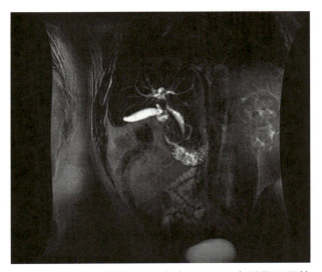

▲ 图 17-21 冠状位重 T_2 加权 MRCP 序列显示胆管和胆囊

的软组织异常），以及重 T_2 加权流体敏感采集技术，如单次激发快速涡流自旋回波半傅里叶采集（HASTE），轴位屏气梯度 T_1 加权同相位和反相位（屏气扰相梯度回波技术优于自旋回波序列，因为它们减少了呼吸伪影），MRCP 序列用于胆道成像，如斜冠状位屏气厚层块重 T_2 加权 2D 快速自旋回波序列或重 T_2 加权快速恢复快速自旋回波 3D 序列，以及增强前与动态增强后的轴位脂肪饱和的屏气三维梯度回波序列[20,21]。轴位多 b 值（例如 0、500、1000 s/mm²）呼吸触发脂肪抑制单次回波平面成像的扩散加权成像和表观扩散系数（ADC）图越来越多地用于评估胆囊疾病。

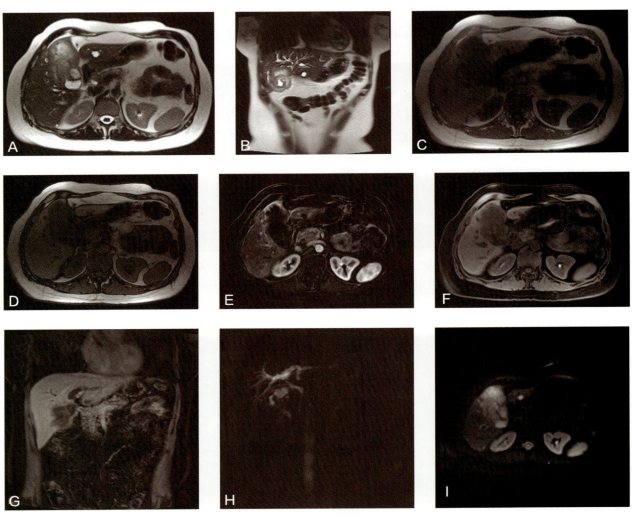

▲ 图 17-22　1 例患有胆囊癌的 56 岁患者

A. 轴位 T_2 HASTE；B. 冠状位 HASTE；C. 轴位同相位；D. 反相位 T_1 加权图像；早期（E）和延迟期（F）增强后 VIBE 图像；G. 冠状位增强图像；MRCP 序列（H）和 b 值 500（I）的轴位扩散加权图像示晚期胆囊癌胆囊壁弥漫性增厚

(一) GB 的正常 MR 表现

胆囊壁在 T_1 加权图像上呈等信号，在 T_2 加权图像上呈低信号，并且在钆对比增强图像上表现为光滑且均匀的强化特点（图 17-23）。胆囊壁的正常厚度可达到 3mm。在 T_2 加权图像和 MRCP 中，GB 呈高信号，因为它由静态液体胆汁组成（图 17-24）。在 T_1 加权图像上，胆汁的信号强度可能从低信号到高信号变化（图 17-25），这取决于胆汁浓度和内部成分，长时间禁食导致胆汁中水的再吸收，从而增加胆固醇、胆汁盐和磷脂的浓度，这种浓缩的胆汁在 T_1 加权图像上显示为高信号[22,23]。

(二) 胆石症

胆石症在世界范围内的总患病率为 10%～20%。胆囊排泄功能受损和胆汁过饱和的人患胆石症的风险增加。胆结石的危险因素包括妊娠、肥胖、快速体重减轻、糖尿病及饮酒。大多数胆结石患者无症状，临床症状出现时，最常见的是胆绞痛，即由胆结石引起的胆囊管间歇性梗阻导致的短暂性腹痛。超声是评估胆石症的首选检查，但 MRI 可能有助于诊断胆石症及其相关并发症，并有助于区分胆结石和胆囊息肉。

在 MRI 上，在 T_2 加权图像和 MRCP 上，所有成分的胆结石相对于胆汁呈低信号（图 17-26）。若胆汁充满了裂隙可能表现为 T_2 中心高信号。如前所述，胆结石在 T_1 加权图像上信号强度可变，这取决于结石的成分。胆固醇结石呈低信号，而胆色素结石相对于胆汁呈高信号[24]（图 17-27 和图 17-28）。除非受到影响，否则它们通常存在于

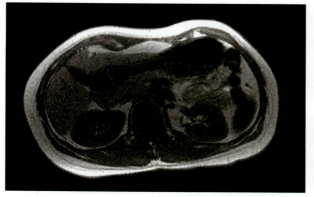

▲ 图 17-23 胆囊壁
轴位 T_1 加权 MRI 显示正常胆囊壁的中等信号强度

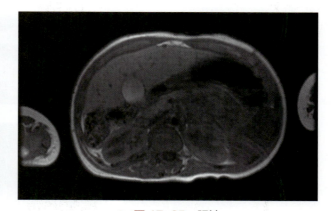

▲ 图 17-25 胆汁
轴位 T_1 加权 MRI 显示胆汁的高信号强度。胆汁的信号强度可以在 T_1 加权图像上变化

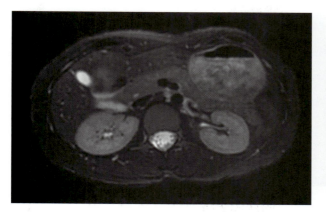

▲ 图 17-24 胆囊腔
轴位 T_2 加权 MRI 显示胆囊腔内的高信号

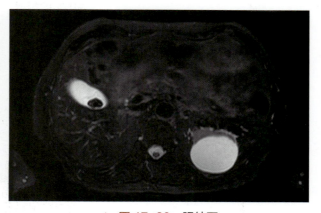

▲ 图 17-26 胆结石
轴位 T_2 加权 MRI 显示胆结石低信号

胆囊中的重力方向位置。由于胆结石在 T_1 加权对比增强图像中无强化，可以与胆囊息肉进行鉴别。

（三）胆囊炎

1. 急性结石性胆囊炎 急性结石性胆囊炎是指由胆结石阻塞胆囊颈或胆囊管引起的急性胆囊炎。由于胆囊压力增加，阻碍胆囊的静脉和淋巴回流。如果不及时治疗，可能会进一步发展为缺血、穿孔。患者通常出现恶心、呕吐及右上腹部疼痛，大多数患者既往有胆绞痛发作的病史。超声通常是用于诊断急性胆囊炎的首选检查。MRI 可在超声不能确定的病例中使用[25]。

急性胆囊炎时 MRI 可显示胆囊壁增厚（图 17-29）。当胆囊壁的厚度超过 3mm 时，通常认为增厚。在 T_2 加权图像中，胆囊壁显示高信号（图 17-30），胆囊周围可能存在积液，可以在 T_2 加权图像或 MRCP 图像上看到胆结石。钆增强图像显示胆囊壁的高强化及相邻肝实质的一过性强化。这些结果被认为更适用于急性胆囊炎的诊断，因为它们反映了导致血流量增加的炎症过程。增强早期图像可显示胆囊内壁的首先强化，但延迟图像通常表现出更弥漫的强化。胆囊壁强化百分比可用于区分急性和慢性胆囊炎[26]。在最近的一项研究中，Altun 等报道，MRI 检测急性胆囊炎的敏感性为 95%，特异性为 69%[27]。

在增强扫描图像上，胆囊壁强化程度增加，

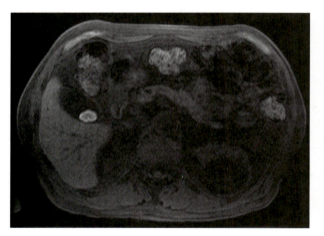

▲ 图 17-27 胆色素结石
同一患者的轴位 T_1 加权 MRI 显示胆结石呈高至中等信号强度

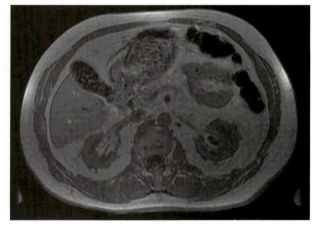

▲ 图 17-28 胆固醇结石
轴位 T_1 加权 MRI 显示多个呈低信号强度的胆结石。根据其组成，胆结石的信号强度可以在 T_1 加权图像变化

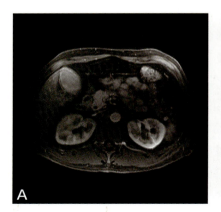

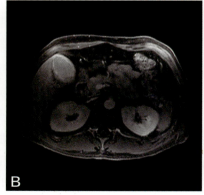

▲ 图 17-29 胆囊炎
对比增强轴位 T_1 加权 MRI 显示胆囊壁轻度增厚，符合胆囊炎

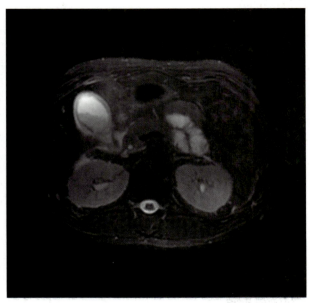

▲ 图 17-30 胆囊炎患者的胆囊壁
轴位 T_2 加权图像示胆囊炎患者增厚的胆囊壁

壁厚度增加，以及胆囊周围肝脏的一过性异常强化提示急性胆囊炎。在 T_2 加权图像上，除了显示胆结石、壁增厚以及胆囊周围水肿之外，T_2 加权图像还可以显示壁内脓肿，其表现为胆囊壁高信号。据报道，胆囊壁强化程度增加和邻近肝脏一过性强化是两个最有意义的表现，可以帮助区分急性和慢性胆囊炎。肝细胞特异性对比剂的延迟图像上，胆囊管内对比剂截断和胆囊内充盈缺损有助于诊断急性结石性胆囊炎[28,29]。

胆囊壁增厚并不是诊断胆囊炎的特异性指标。实际上，与胆囊无关的几种情况都可导致胆囊壁增厚，包括慢性肝病、低白蛋白和慢性肾衰竭。然而，与急性胆囊炎不同，在这些情况下，增强图像并不会表现出胆囊壁强化程度增加和邻近肝实质一过性强化。

对比增强图像也有助于发现胆囊炎的并发症，如穿孔、脓肿形成及坏疽性胆囊炎。可以通过观察胆囊壁强化不连续来确定胆囊穿孔。这与胆囊窝局部积液的边缘强化有关。当胆囊壁表现为弥漫性或斑片状无强化时，可诊断坏疽性胆囊炎，无强化部分对应于坏死区域[30]。在气肿性胆囊炎和胆肠瘘中胆囊内可见气体，在胆囊内液体的衬托下表现为低信号，胆囊壁和周围组织中的气体对于诊断气肿性胆囊炎非常重要。由气体引起的磁场不均匀性导致信号损失而呈低信号[31]。通过 T_1 和 T_2 加权图像上胆囊壁和腔内的出血信号，可以更容易地在 MRI 上诊断出血性胆囊炎。根据出血的时间，血液分解产物在 T_1 和 T_2 加权序列上显示不同的信号强度。

2. 胆结石的其他并发症 除急性胆囊炎外，胆结石还会引起其他几种急性并发症，包括胰腺炎、胆道瘘、胆总管结石、胆石性肠梗阻及 Mirizzi 综合征（图 17-31）。Mirizzi 综合征是胆囊管或胆囊颈部结石导致肝总管狭窄及胆道梗阻。有两种类型：第一种是胆总管的单纯阻塞，而第二种伴有胆总管壁的侵蚀，可能导致形成瘘。MRI 对于术前诊断非常有价值，对预防医源性胆管损伤非常重要，因为它不同于超声和 CT，它可以显示阻塞的原因和程度，并有助于区分 1 型和 2 型。MRI 还有助于术前识别胆囊管解剖变异，这也是手术前的重要信息。

（四）非结石性胆囊炎

非结石性胆囊炎并不常见，仅占急性胆囊炎的 5%～15%，但预后较差。通常发生在 ICU 的重症患者中，可能由于蠕动降低、胆囊动脉血流减少或细菌感染而发生，患者出现不明原因的败血症。诊断通常很困难，这是由于存在多种并发症和非特异性体征和症状。如果不及时发现，非结石性胆囊炎可能并发穿孔和坏疽性胆囊炎。在没有胆囊结石的情况下，MRI 证实胆囊扩张伴壁增厚，增厚的壁在 T_2 加权图像上呈高信号，可能有胆囊周围积液[15]。这些重症患者通常通过经皮胆囊造口术治疗。

缺血/化学性胆囊炎

由于化疗药物进入胆囊动脉，缺血性/化学性胆囊炎是肝脏化疗栓塞的潜在并发症。由于胆囊动脉起源于肝右动脉，大多数患者更可能在右肝病变的化疗栓塞后出现。这些患者数周内可能没有任何症状或仅非特异性腹痛。疾病过程通常是自限性的，因此很少需要治疗。MRI 显示胆囊

Chapter 17 胆囊
Gallbladder

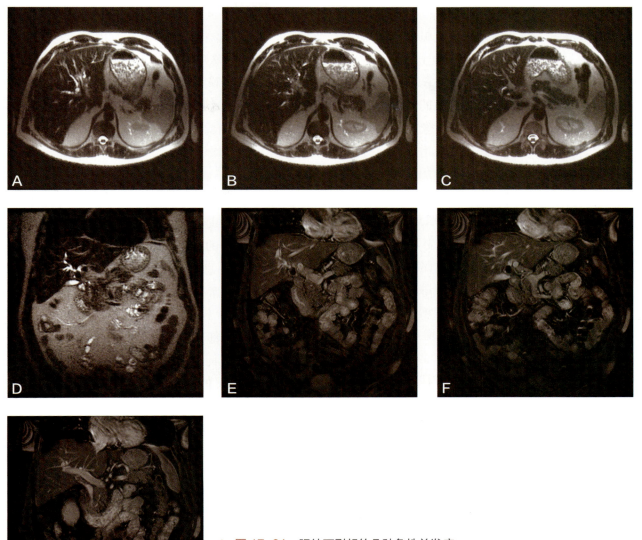

▲ 图 17-31 胆结石引起的几种急性并发症
轴向（A～C）和冠状位（D）SSFSE 图像和冠状位 FIESTA（E～G）显示出明显的肝内胆管扩张。肝总管也扩张，但胆总管没有扩张。胆道梗阻起源于胆囊内的结石，累及肝总管，符合 Mirizzi 综合征。这些结果在手术中得到了证实

扩张，在对比增强的图像上，可见明显的壁水肿、强化程度增加和一过性胆囊周围强化。由于该过程与化学治疗剂的反流有关，因此不涉及胆结石。

（五）慢性胆囊炎

慢性胆囊炎通常与胆石症相关，患者可能无症状或复发性胆绞痛发作。MRI 显示胆囊壁增厚和胆结石。由于纤维化，一些患者的胆囊可能会收缩，并且可能表现出延迟强化。慢性胆囊炎中未见邻近肝实质的短暂强化，这一特征可用于与急性胆囊炎鉴别[15]。此外，胆囊壁上可形成钙化（瓷样胆囊），尽管在 CT 和超声上更容易识别钙化，但 MRI 也可在钙化区域显示信号缺失。此外，瓷样胆囊患者具有较高的胆囊癌风险，特别是增强后图像出现不规则的结节样强化有助于发现肿瘤病变。

黄色肉芽肿性胆囊炎是一种罕见的胆囊炎性疾病，占胆囊疾病的 1%～13%，主要发生在 60—70 岁的老年女性中[32-35]。发病机制尚不清楚，但罗阿窦的闭塞被认为是一种影响因素，导致胆汁外渗入胆囊壁，随后形成壁内黄色肉芽肿。正确诊断非常重要，因为它在临床和影像上胆囊癌

类似。MRI 显示 T_2 加权图像上的局灶性或弥漫性 GB 壁增厚，以及增强图像上胆囊壁强化程度增加（图 17-32）。在 T_2 加权图像上呈等或略高信号的区域，在动态增强研究中显示早期轻度强化和延迟的明显强化，这可能反映的是大量黄色肉芽肿区域[36]。坏死在 T_2 加权图像上表现为明显高信号，而增强后无强化。与壁增厚型胆囊癌很难鉴别，但最近的研究表明扩散加权成像可能有帮助[37]。

胆囊腺肌增生症 胆囊腺肌增生症的特征是良性非炎症性胆囊壁黏膜增生，并侵入肥大的肌层，导致罗阿窦的形成，这是肌层内的黏膜种植。虽然局灶性病变常见，但腺肌增生症也可能导致弥漫性壁增厚或节段性壁增厚。最常见于胆囊底部，导致胆囊底新月形增厚。由于肌层增厚，节段型可能导致胆囊呈"沙漏"样外观。在大多数（＞ 90%）病例中，腺肌增生症和胆结石之间存在关联。因此，腺肌增生症不被认为是一种癌前病变[38]。然而，腺肌增生症可能同时合并腺癌，可能是由于同时存在慢性炎症和胆结石，特别是在节段型腺肌增生症中常见。

罗阿窦经常含有胆固醇晶体沉积物，超声检查表现为从增厚的胆囊壁延伸出来的呈彗尾征。在 MRI 上，胆囊壁表现为局部或弥漫性增厚，罗阿窦在 T_2 加权图像中表现为胆囊壁中的高信号，T_1 加权图像上呈低信号，增强后无强化。这些窦在 T_2 加权图像（图 17-33）和 MRCP 上的环状排列被称为"珍珠项链征"或"串珠征"，据报道这一征象在诊断腺肌增生病（＞ 90%）中具有很高的特异性[38]。增强图像可能显示早期黏膜强化（图 17-34）和晚期均匀增强，但在大多数患者中，腺肌增生症的对比增强模式可类似胆囊癌。

（六）胆囊息肉

胆囊息肉是指起源于胆囊壁并突向胆囊腔的病变。胆囊的息肉样病变包括多种病理改变，从良性胆固醇息肉到癌前病变腺瘤及明显恶性的癌。它们通常在影像上偶然发现或是胆囊切除术后在病理学上被诊断出来。其中大多数是良性的；而一小部分是癌前病变或恶性，需要及早发现和治疗，而良恶性的鉴别存在困难[39]。在 T_2 加权和 MRCP 图像上，GB 息肉表现为低信号的充盈缺损并突向胆囊腔（图 17-35）。与结石不同，它们可能位于与胆囊壁相邻的非重力位置。在钆增强图像上，息肉可见强化。影像上若表现为大于 1cm，无蒂，孤立性息肉，逐渐增长及合并胆结石时，应当警惕恶性可能[39]。如果息肉大于 10mm，则患者应进行胆囊切除术。6～10mm 的息肉通常在 6 个月内进行超声复查。如果期间息肉增大、患者有症状、年龄超过 50 岁、或有原发

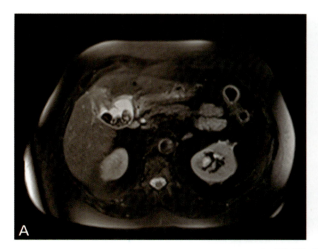
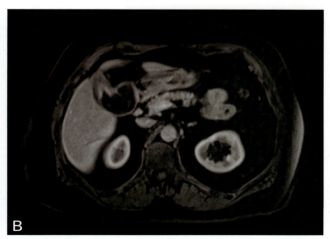

▲ 图 17-32 胆囊壁增厚

轴位脂肪抑制 T_2 加权图像（A）和对比增强 T_1 加权图像（B）显示胆囊底部壁增厚和胆结石。患者接受了胆囊切除术和手术证实黄色肉芽肿性胆囊炎

Chapter 17 胆囊
Gallbladder

性硬化性胆管炎病史，则应将 6~10mm 的息肉行胆囊切除术。

1. 胆囊癌 GB 癌是美国第五位常见的胃肠道恶性肿瘤，通常与慢性炎症和胆结石相关。它是胆道最常见的癌。大多数胆囊癌是腺癌（高达 90%），但也可能发生鳞状细胞癌和小细胞癌。每年每 100 000 人中约 2.5 例发病。由于发现病变时大多已经是进展期，中位生存时间仅 3 个月。5 年总生存率为 5%。GB 癌在女性中的发病率高于男性，可能是由于女性胆结石的发病率高。

患者可能完全无症状或出现非特异性症状，特别是在早期阶段。进展期患者常出现右上腹疼痛，厌食，体重减轻和（或）发热。由于胆管阻塞，黄疸也可能是晚期症状。患者通常是老年人，发病平均年龄为 65 岁。尽管不到 1% 的胆结石患者可发展为胆囊癌，但 90% 的胆囊癌患者与胆结石有关。高危因素包括慢性炎症（通常与胆结石有关）、瓷样胆囊（图 17-36）、胰胆管过长、慢性胆道感染、肥胖和慢性伤寒携带状态。

胆囊癌可以是弥漫性或局灶性胆囊壁增厚（图 17-22 和图 17-37），或局灶性息肉样腔内生长的肿块。弥漫型比局灶型更常见，常生长到胆囊壁外，并侵犯相邻的肝脏。壁增厚型占胆囊癌的 15%~30%，息肉型是最少见的。

分期采用美国肿瘤联合委员会（American Joint Committeeon Cancer，AJCC）的 TNM 分期[40]。T_1 期肿瘤侵入肌层固有层（1a）或肌层（1b）；T_2 期肿瘤侵入肌层周围结缔组织，但没有侵及浆

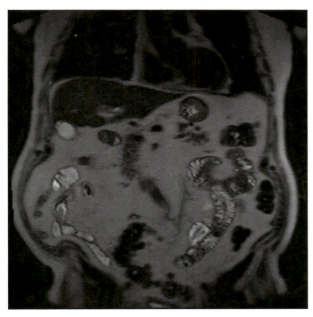

▲ 图 17-33 腺肌增生症
冠状位 T_2 加权 MRI 显示胆囊底部局灶性腺肌增生症

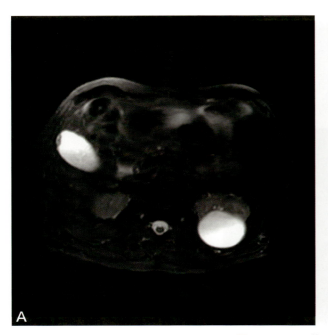 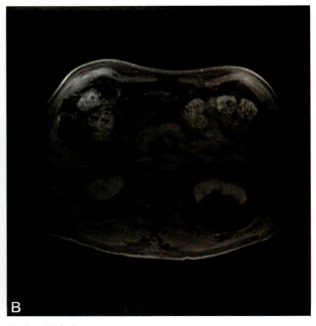

▲ 图 17-34 早期强化腺肌增生症
轴位 T_2 加权图像（A）和对比增强后 T_1 加权图像（B）显示早期强化腺肌增生症

膜外或肝脏；T_3 期肿瘤侵透浆膜并直接侵及肝脏和（或）邻近结构；T_4 期肿瘤侵入门静脉主干或肝动脉或侵入至少两个肝外器官。

N_1 是沿胆囊管、胆总管、肝动脉、门静脉的淋巴道转移；N_2 是淋巴结转移至主动脉周围，肠系膜上动脉和（或）腹腔动脉淋巴结。M_1 是远处转移（《AJCC 癌症分期手册》2010 版可从 www.cancer.gov 获取）。

Ⅰ期（$T_1N_0M_0$）被认为是局限性疾病，恶性肿瘤局限于胆囊壁，可以完全切除区域淋巴管，淋巴结也可切除。如果疾病局限于黏膜层，则 5 年生存率接近 100%，但如果浸润或超出肌层，则降至不到 15%。Ⅱ～Ⅳ期可涉及 T_2～T_4、N_1～N_2 和（或）M_1 疾病，大多数病例是Ⅱ～Ⅳ期，通常无法切除，主要采取姑息治疗。

影像

MRI 有多种表现，可以表现为局灶性息肉样肿块、胆囊壁增厚，或胆囊完全被肿块取代。

肿块型 胆囊窝肿块样病变的鉴别诊断包括原发性恶性肿瘤、转移瘤和周围脓肿。胆囊恶性肿瘤最常见的形式是肿块型，MRI 表现为 T_2 不均匀高信号，T_1 中等强度等信号，增强扫描呈早期及延迟强化（图 17-38），在肿块中可见胆结石。同时可能会发现淋巴结、邻近脂肪和肝实质的侵犯。增强扫描图像有助于确定侵及邻近器官的程度和胆管的受累程度，这些信息对于术前制订治疗计划至关重要。

壁增厚型 胆囊壁增厚的鉴别诊断较多，包括胆囊炎、恶性肿瘤、腺肌增生病和非胆囊病症，如低蛋白血症和肾衰竭。胆囊壁局灶性或弥散性增厚、大于 1cm 是恶性肿瘤的特征。与肝脏相比，肿瘤在 T_2 加权图像上的呈不均匀高信号，T_1 加权图像上呈低信号或等信号，增强表现为不规则的不均匀强化，这有助于与慢性胆囊炎鉴别。

息肉型 腔内息肉样肿块的鉴别诊断包括恶性肿瘤、息肉、局灶性腺肌增生症、血凝块和肿瘤块样污泥（tumefactive sludge）。恶性息肉样肿块大多数大于 1cm。可通过缺乏活动性将息肉样恶性肿瘤、腺肌增生症和息肉与真菌灶鉴别。息肉样肿块表现为 T_1 加权图像中等信号、T_2 加权图像高信号、增强早期和延迟期中度强化。在对比

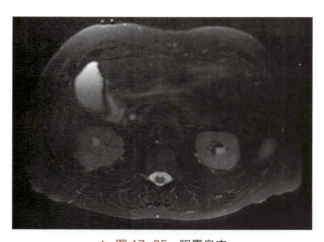

▲ 图 17-35 胆囊息肉

轴位 T_2 加权图像显示胆囊壁中的许多微小的低信号影，符合微小的息肉。小于 6mm 的胆囊息肉没有临床意义

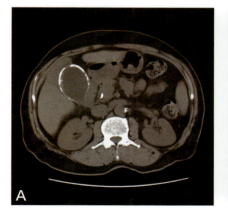
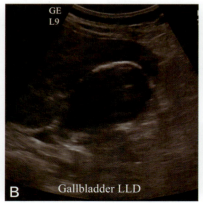
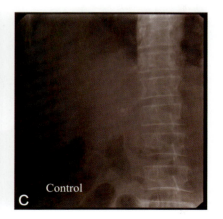

▲ 图 17-36 瓷样胆囊

轴位 CT（A）、纵向超声声像图（B）和 X 线片（C）示瓷样胆囊

增强图像上，胆囊癌表现为早期不规则强化，延迟持续强化。良性病变表现为早期强化，延迟期不持续强化。最近，扩散加权成像在鉴别胆囊恶性肿瘤与良性疾病中的应用受到了极大的关注，早期的研究结果令人鼓舞[41,42]。

2. 其他胆囊恶性肿瘤 包括转移性病变和淋巴瘤。已经有报道来自黑色素瘤、乳腺癌和肾细胞癌的胆囊转移。在 T_1 加权图像上，黑素瘤转移可能出现高信号。类似地，来自肾细胞癌和乳腺癌的转移可以表现为息肉样病变强化。淋巴瘤累及胆囊很少见，通常胆囊淋巴瘤倾向于继发性非霍奇金淋巴瘤，原发性淋巴瘤极少见。它表现为胆囊壁增厚或胆囊区域的肿块样病变，通常与肝门区淋巴结肿大相关，影像上很难鉴别淋巴瘤和胆囊癌。

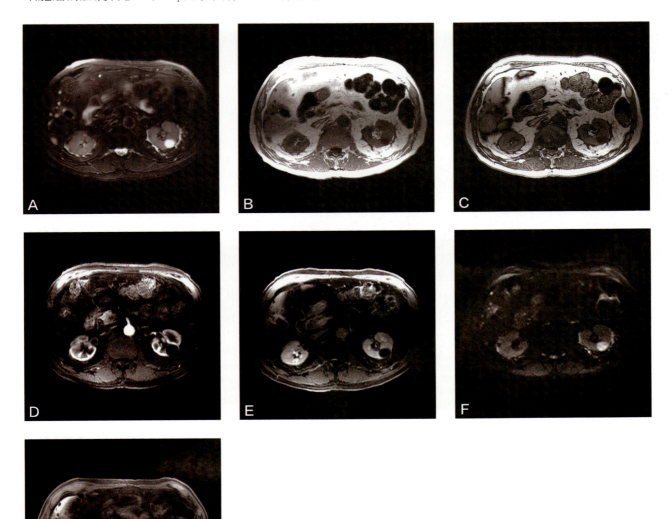

▲ 图 17-37 胆囊癌
轴位 T_2（A）、同相位（B）、反相位（C）、早期（D）和延迟期（E）增强后图像，b 值为 500 的 DWI 显示局灶性不规则胆囊壁增厚。EOVIST 随访研究 20min 延迟扫描序列（G）证实了肿瘤范围。手术证实是胆囊癌

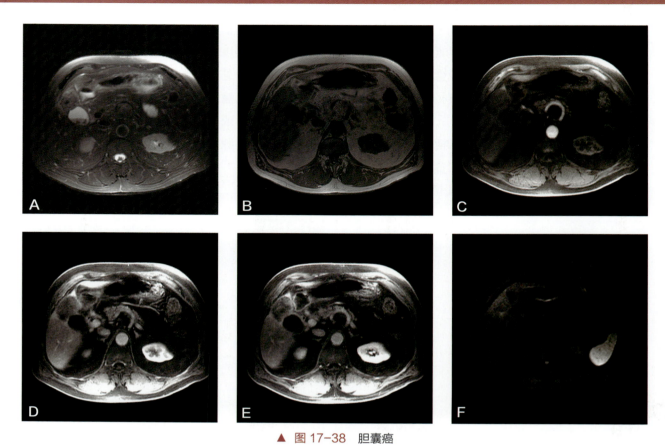

▲ 图 17-38 胆囊癌

轴位 T_2（A）、T_1 加权图像（B）、增强扫描动脉期（C）、门静脉期（D）和延迟期（E）图像，b 值为 500（F）的 DWI 显示胆囊底不规则增厚。手术证实是胆囊癌

参考文献

[1] Ando H. Embryology of the biliary tract. *Dig Surg* 2010; 27:87–89.

[2] Sato T, Ito M, Sakamoto H. Pictorial dissection review of the lymphatic pathways from the gallbladder to the abdominal para-aortic lymph nodes and their relation- ships to the surrounding structures. *Surg Radiol Anat* 2013; 35:615–621.

[3] Bronshtein M, Weiner Z, Abramovici H, Filmar S, Erlik Y, Blumenfeld Z. Prenatal diagnosis of gall bladder anomalies—Report of 17 cases. *Prenat Diagn* 1993; 13:851–861.

[4] Bani-Hani KE. Agenesis of the gallbladder: Difficulties in management. *J Gastroenterol Hepatol* 2005; 20:671–675.

[5] Senecail B, Nonent M, Kergastel I, Patin-Philippe L, Larroche P, Le Borgne A. Ultrasonic features of con genital anomalies of the gallbladder. *J Radiol* 2000; 81:1591–1594.

[6] Balakrishnan S, Singhal T, Grandy-Smith S, El-Hasani S. Agenesis of the gallbladder: Lessons to learn. *JSLS* 2006; 10:517–519.

[7] Piccolo G, Di Vita M, Zanghi A, Cavallaro A, Cardi F, Capellani A. Symptomatic gallbladder agenesis: Never again unnecessary cholecystectomy. *Am Surg* 2014; 80:E12–E13.

[8] Idu M, Jakimowicz J, Iuppa A, Cuschieri A. Hepatobiliary anatomy in patients with transposition of the gallblad der: Implications for safe laparoscopic cholecystectomy. *Br J Surg* 1996; 83:1442–1443.

[9] Carbajo MA, Martin del Omo JC, Blanco JI et al. Congenital malformations of the gallbladder and cystic duct diagnosed by laparoscopy: High surgical risk. *JSLS* 1999; 3:319–321.

[10] Kiewiet JJ, Leeuwenburgh MM, Bipat S, Bossuyt PM, Stoker J, Boermeester MA. A systematic review and meta-analysis of diagnostic performance of imaging in acute cholecystitis. *Radiology* 2012; 264:708–720.

[11] Yarmish GM, Smith MP, Rosen MP et al. ACR appropriateness criteria right upper quadrant pain. *J Am Coll Radiol* 2014; 11(3):316–322.

[12] Bennett GL, Balthazar EJ. Ultrasound and CT evaluation of emergent gallbladder pathology. *Radiol Clin North Am* 2003; 41:1203–1216.

[13] Bennett GL, Rusinek H, Lisi V et al. CT findings in acute gangrenous cholecystitis. *AJR Am J Roentgenol* 2002; 178:275–281.

[14] Shakespear JS, Shaaban AM, Rezvani M. CT findings of acute cholecystitis and its complications. *AJR Am J Roentgenol* 2010; 194:1523–1529.

[15] Smith EA, Dillman JR, Elsayes KM, Menias CO, Bude RO. Cross-sectional imaging of acute and chronic gall- bladder inflammatory disease. *AJR Am J Roentgenol* 2009; 192:188–

196.

[16] Tsai MJ, Chen JD, Tiu CM, Chou YH, Hu SC, Chang CY. Can acute cholecystitis with gallbladder perforation be detected preoperatively by computed tomography in ED? Correlation with clinical data and computed tomography features. *Am J Emerg Med* 2009; 27:574–581.

[17] Fuks D, Mouly C, Robert B, Hajji H, Yzet T, Regimbeau JM. Acute cholecystitis: Preoperative CT can help the surgeon consider conversion from laparoscopic to open cholecystectomy. *Radiology* 2012; 263:128–138.

[18] Irie H, Kamochi N, Nojiri J, Egashira Y, Sasaguri K, Kudo S. High b-value diffusion-weighted MRI in differentia tion between benign and malignant polypoid gallbladder lesions. *Acta Radiol* 2011; 52:236–240.

[19] Ogawa T, Horaguchi J, Fujita N et al. High b-value diffusion-weighted magnetic resonance imaging for gall- bladder lesions: Differentiation between benignity and malignancy. *J Gastroenterol* 2012; 47:1352–1360.

[20] Elsayes KM, Oliveira EP, Narra VR, El-Merhi FM, Brown JJ. Magnetic resonance imaging of the gallbladder: Spectrum of abnormalities. *Acta Radiol* 2007; 48:476–482.

[21] Tan CH, Lim KS. MRI of gallbladder cancer. *Diagn Interv Radiol* 2013; 19:312–319.

[22] Demas BE, Hricak H, Moseley M et al. Gallbladder bile: An experimental study in dogs using MR imaging and proton MR spectroscopy. *Radiology* 1985; 157:453–455.

[23] Bilgin M, Shaikh F, Semelka RC, Bilgin SS, Balci NC, Erdogan A. Magnetic resonance imaging of gallbladder and biliary system. *Top Magn Reson Imaging* 2009; 20:31–42.

[24] Tsai HM, Lin XZ, Chen CY, Lin PW, Lin JC. MRI of gallstones with different compositions. *AJR Am J Roentgenol* 2004; 182:1513–1519.

[25] Yusoff IF, Barkun JS, Barkun AN. Diagnosis and management of cholecystitis and cholangitis. *Gastroenterol Clin North Am* 2003; 32:1145–1168.

[26] Loud PA, Semelka RC, Kettritz U, Brown JJ, Reinhold C. MRI of acute cholecystitis: Comparison with the normal gallbladder and other entities. *Magn Reson Imaging* 1996; 14:349–355.

[27] Altun E, Semelka RC, Elias J, Jr. et al. Acute cholecystitis: MR findings and differentiation from chronic cholecys-titis. *Radiology* 2007; 244:174–183.

[28] Catalano OA, Sahani DV, Kalva SP et al. MR imaging of the gallbladder: A pictorial essay. *RadioGraphics* 2008; 28:135–155; quiz 324.

[29] Choi IY, Cha SH, Yeom SK et al. Diagnosis of acute cho- le-cystitis: Value of contrast agent in the gallbladder and cystic duct on Gd-EOB-DTPA enhanced MR cholangiog-raphy. *Clin Imaging* 2014; 38(2):174–178.

[30] Pedrosa I, Guarise A, Goldsmith J, Procacci C, Rofsky NM. The interrupted rim sign in acute cholecystitis: A method to identify the gangrenous form with MRI. *J Magn Reson Imaging* 2003; 18:360–363.

[31] Koenig T, Tamm EP, Kawashima A. Magnetic resonance imaging findings in emphysematous cholecystitis. *Clin Radiol* 2004; 59:455–458.

[32] Casas D, Perez-Andres R, Jimenez JA et al. Xanthogranulomatous cholecystitis: A radiological study of 12 cases and a review of the literature. *Abdom Imaging* 1996; 21:456–460.

[33] Duber C, Storkel S, Wagner PK, Muller J. Xanthogranulomatous cholecystitis mimicking carci noma of the gallbladder: CT findings. *J Comput Assist Tomogr* 1984; 8:1195–1198.

[34] Ros PR, Goodman ZD. Xanthogranulomatous cholecysti tis versus gallbladder carcinoma. *Radiology* 1997; 203:10–12.

[35] Shetty GS, Abbey P, Prabhu SM, Narula MK, Anand R. Xanthogranulomatous cholecystitis: Sonographic and CT features and differentiation from gallbladder carci noma: A pictorial essay. *Jpn J Radiol* 2012; 30:480–485.

[36] Shuto R, Kiyosue H, Komatsu E et al. CT and MR imag ing findings of xanthogranulomatous cholecystitis: Correlation with pathologic findings. *Eur Radiol* 2004; 14:440–446.

[37] Kang TW, Kim SH, Park HJ et al. Differentiating xanthogranulomatous cholecystitis from wall-thickening type of gallbladder cancer: Added value of diffusion- weighted MRI. *Clin Radiol* 2013; 68:992–1001.

[38] Boscak AR, Al-Hawary M, Ramsburgh SR. Best cases from the AFIP: Adenomyomatosis of the gallbladder. *RadioGraphics* 2006; 26:941–946.

[39] Andren-Sandberg A. Diagnosis and management of gallbladder polyps. *N Am J Med Sci* 2012; 4:203–211.

[40] Edge SB, Byrd DR, Compton CC, Fritz AG, Greene FL, Trotti A eds. *AJCC Cancer Staging Manual*, 7th edn., 2010. New York, NY: Springer.

[41] Kim SJ, Lee JM, Kim H, Yoon JH, Han JK, Choi BI. Role of diffusion-weighted magnetic resonance imaging in the diagnosis of gallbladder cancer. *J Magn Reson Imaging* 2013; 38:127–137.

[42] Lee NK, Kim S, Kim TU, Kim DU, Seo HI, Jeon TY. Diffusion-weighted MRI for differentiation of benign from malignant lesions in the gallbladder. *Clin Radiol* 2014; 69:e78–e85.

Chapter 18 胆道系统磁共振成像

Magnetic Resonance Imaging of Biliary Tract

Sachin Kumbhar, Manjiri K.Dighe, Ganeshan Dhakshinamoorthy, Neeraj Lalwani 著

李登峰 马霄虹 译

赵心明 校

目录 CONTENTS

一、胆道系统 MRI 序列与技术 / 422

二、胆道的正常解剖表现 / 423

三、胆道梗阻 / 425

四、胆道肿瘤 / 428

五、胆囊的 MRI 表现 / 429

胆道由胆囊和胆管系统（包括肝内和肝外胆管）组成，其主要作用是贮存胆汁并将胆汁从肝脏运输到其活性作用部位十二指肠。胆道系统可发生包括良性及恶性疾病在内的多种疾病。影像学检查在胆道疾病的诊断以及病变部位的准确定位中具有重要作用。

磁共振成像（MRI）在胆道疾病的诊断中得到了广泛应用，因为它不受胆管梗阻部位和严重程度的影响，可以对整个胆管树系统进行完整的评估。标准 MRI 技术可用于评估胆管壁和胆管外病变。磁共振胆胰管成像（MR cholangiopancreatography，MRCP）可显示腔内充满液体的胆囊和胆管，更适合于评估胆道系统管腔内的病变。肝细胞特异性 MRI 对比剂在动态评估胆管病变的应用中显示出了良好的应用前景。

一、胆道系统 MRI 序列与技术

磁共振胆胰管成像（MRCP）与 T_1 加权成像、T_2 加权成像和 T_1 增强扫描序列一起用于评估胆管病变。MRCP 技术多种多样，然而所有这些技术都有一个共同点：基于重 T_2 加权成像。在这些重 T_2 加权成像序列中，来自胆管壁和胆管外组织结构的背景信号会被抑制，与此同时胆道内静止态胆汁的高信号得以突出显示。胃肠道内的液体在 MRCP 上往往也表现为高信号。因此，口服阴性对比剂可以用来抑制胃肠道产生的信号[1]。患者应在检查前禁食至少 4h，有助于胆囊充盈。MRCP 图像可以使用具有呼吸触发功能的非屏气扫描序列通过 2D 或 3D 采集方式来获得。或者是使用屏气扫描序列，如单次激发快速自旋回波序列（single shot fast spin echo，SSFSE）和半傅里叶采集单次激发快速自旋回波序列（half-Fourier acquisition single-shot turbo spin-echo，HASTE）。这些可以通过薄层准直或厚层采集来完成[2]。

（一）屏气扫描序列

MRCP 的屏气采集序列扫描时间更短。这种采集方式可以在单次屏气过程中或自由呼吸期间完成，因此在一些无法配合呼吸指令的患者中也可以使用。这些采集方式避免了由于呼吸运动和校正不准引起的伪影。SSFSE 序列采用无限重复时间（repetition time，TR）和非常长的回波链来减少扫描时间和采集时间，通常在 30s 内完成。长回波时间（echo time，TE）超过 600ms 可以抑制包括脂肪在内的胆管外实性组织的信号。因此，这种采集方式中不需要脂肪抑制。改良的快速自旋回波序列如弛豫增强快速采集（rapid acquisition with relaxation enhancement，RARE）和 HASTE 采集已经在屏气 MRCP 扫描中广泛应用。由于受运动伪影干扰较少，以上所有这些采集序列都具有较高信噪比（signal-to-noise ratio，SNR）[3]。

这些屏气扫描序列可以以一次单层厚层扫描或多层薄层扫描获得。在厚层图像采集中，获取代表整个成像容积的平均值作为单个图像。采集一幅图像仅需不到 2s 的时间。通常，这种采集在不同的方向和不同的平面上重复，以提供胆管树的多个投影图像。然而，采用这种平均显示方式的图像可能会导致小病灶或隐匿性病灶显示模糊。因此，厚层采集图像的敏感度较低，并且必须通过获取多个薄层图像来作为补充。这些是使用 3～4mm 的图像层厚并且通常在斜冠状位中获得的。这些图像尤其适合显示胆管内小的腔内充盈缺损病变[3]。

（二）非屏气扫描序列

非屏气扫描序列可以使用膈肌导航技术实现，这种扫描序列可以评估膈肌的位置。导航器位于冠状位图像上右侧膈肌和肺部的交界面处。MRI 扫描器监测该界面的位置，并当其位置在预设窗口内时触发 MRCP 采集。非屏气序列可以是 3D 或 2D 采集。利用这些图像可以生成最大密度投影（maximal intensity projection，MIP）图像。MIP 图像是由沿着垂直于投影平面的方向投影的整个成像体内最高信号强度的像素组成。这些图像与传统的胆管造影图像类似[1]。

（三）促胰液素刺激状态下的 MRCP

促胰液素是由十二指肠释放的激素，其作用于胰腺外分泌细胞并刺激它们释放富含碳酸氢盐成分的液体。当静脉注射体外合成的促胰液素时，它通过增加其管径来改善胰管的显示效果[4]，并且可以用于早期慢性胰腺炎的诊断。促胰液素的作用效果在注射后 2~5min 达到峰值并在注射后约 10min 消退。

（四）对比剂增强 MRCP

有些含钆的对比剂一部分经过肝脏排泄到胆汁中，另一部分经由肾脏排泄。这类对比剂被称为肝细胞特异性对比剂，包括钆塞酸和钆贝酸。在静脉内注射后，这些对比剂在一定时间后出现在胆汁中，这取决于肝脏对钆剂排泄的相对比例。此外，如果肝功能降低，它们在胆汁中的出现会延迟。通常在 20min 后使用 T_1 加权脂肪抑制序列进行延迟成像。对比增强 MRCP 特别有助于证明囊状结构与胆管的沟通关系以及证明胆漏的存在[5]。

二、胆道的正常解剖表现

根据 Couinaud 分类，根据门静脉和肝静脉的走行关系将肝脏分为 8 段。每个肝段都有其独立的一套门静脉供血，以及独立的肝静脉和胆管引流。右肝管引流 5~8 肝段。它是由引流 5 段和 8 段的右前胆管与引流 6 段和 7 段的右后胆管的汇合而成。左肝管引流 2~4 肝段。左右肝管汇合形成肝总管（common hepatic duct，CHD）（图 18-1）。引流 1 段的胆管既可以汇入右肝管，也可以汇入左肝管。肝总管与从胆囊发出的胆囊管汇合成胆总管（common bile duct，CBD）（图 18-1）。胰管与胆总管在壶腹附近汇合。然而，胆道解剖结构变异情况并不少见。

除非在胆管扩张情况下，MRCP 通常不会显示外周的肝内胆管。正常胆总管的直径最大为 6mm。虽然正常情况下，胆总管的直径可能超过 6mm，但这种情况应结合患者的临床表现和肝功能检查考虑。此外，胆总管的直径也会随着年龄的增长而增加。在 50 岁以上的患者中，其直径可以达到 8mm。对于摘除胆囊的患者，胆总管的最大直径达到 10mm 也应该被考虑为正常情况[6]。

（一）胆道的解剖学变异

胆道引流路径的解剖学变异并不少见。识别这些解剖学变异有时很重要，因为它们可能易患疾病。此外，在进行肝胆手术之前识别任何形式的解剖学变异至关重要，这样可以避免发生潜在的严重并发症。

左、右肝管以及肝总管汇合处最常发生解剖学变异。正常情况下，右后胆管和右前胆管汇合形成右肝管，接着再与左肝管汇合形成肝总管（图 18-2）。然而，在有些个体中，右后胆管引流汇入左肝管，然后再与右前胆管汇合形成肝总管。这是一种最常被报道的胆道解剖变异[7]。另一种常见变异情况是右前胆管、右后胆管和左肝管同时汇合形成肝总管，此时右肝管不存在。还有一种不常见的情况，右后胆管引流汇入肝总管（图 18-3）。在潜在的活肝供体上检测到这些解剖学变

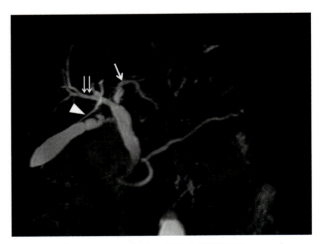

▲ 图 18-1 MRCP 上的正常胆道解剖结构
从 MRCP 序列处理得到的 MIP 图像显示了胆管的类似 ERCP 的投影图像。右后肝管（箭头）与右前肝管（双箭）汇合形成右肝管，其与左肝管（白箭）汇合而成肝总管

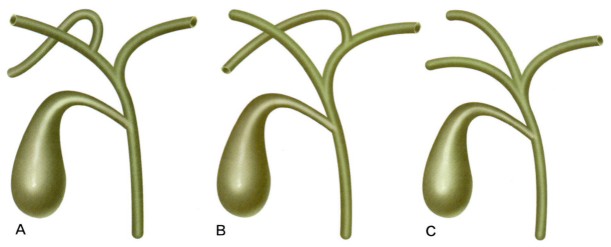

▲ 图 18-2　胆道的常见解剖变异

A. 右后胆管与右前胆管汇合形成右肝管。然后右肝管再与左肝管汇合形成肝总管。这是最常见的胆道解剖结构；B. 右后胆管汇入左肝管，然后左肝管再与右前胆管汇合形成肝总管。右肝管缺如；C. 右前胆管，右后胆管以及左肝管同时汇合形成肝总管

异是至关重要的，因为存在此种变异时，（肝移植）需要多次胆道吻合术，从而增加并发症发生的机会[8]。此外，精确确定胆道解剖结构有助于移植外科医师规划制订手术方案[9]。

胆囊管的解剖变异通常不会产生临床后果。然而，由于胆囊切除术经常通过腹腔镜进行，因此重要的是要确定这些变异以避免在腹腔镜操作期间对胆总管和右肝管的潜在损伤。胆囊管可以在胆总管的远端 1/3 处汇入，也可能与胆总管紧邻并行走行。胆囊管很少会汇入右肝管。如果在手术前未发现这些变异，则存在无意中结扎和切断右肝管或胆总管的风险[10,11]。这可能导致术后出现病态改变和可能危及生命的并发症。MRCP 可以较为容易地识别这些解剖变异并避免这种不良事件。

胆总管和胰管通常在开口进入十二指肠之前有 4～5mm 长的共同通道汇合在一起。该汇合处被 Oddi 括约肌所包围。有的情况下，胰管和胆总管可能分别具有进入十二指肠的独立开口。异常胰胆管汇合（anomalous pancreaticobiliary junction，APBJ）是一种很罕见的情况，此时胆总管和胰管在十二指肠外部汇合并且汇合处位于 Oddi 括约肌近端。共同通道长度通常超过 15mm。由于汇合处在 Oddi 括约肌近端，胆汁可能会反流进入胰管，同时胰腺分泌液可能会反流进入胆

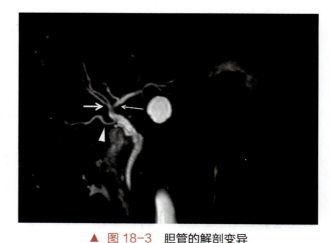

▲ 图 18-3　胆管的解剖变异
右前胆管（粗白箭）与左肝管（细白箭）汇合形成肝总管。右后胆管（箭头）直接汇入肝总管

总管。有推测认为这是 APBJ 与胆总管囊肿、胆管癌和反复发作性胰腺炎高度相关的原因[12,13]。

（二）先天性胆道异常

胆管囊肿（Choledochal 囊肿）

胆管囊肿是以肝外和（或）肝内胆管的囊性或囊状扩张为特征的先天性疾病。女性发病率较高，大部分病例在儿童期被诊断。典型的三联症状包括右上腹疼痛、腹部肿块以及黄疸。然而，这些征象并不见于所有患者。胆管囊肿通常会导致并发症，如胆管炎、胰腺炎、胆总管结石、

胆汁性肝硬化以及胆管癌。因此，治疗需要用 Roux-en-Y 肝脏空肠吻合术将囊肿完全切除。如果病变累及肝内胆管，则可能需要通过部分肝切除或肝移植来治疗[14,15]。

根据 Todani 所提出的分类学说，胆管囊肿被分为以下五类（图18-4）[16]。Ⅰ型是最常见的类型，表现为胆总管的梭形扩张（图18-5），而Ⅱ型主要表现为胆总管憩室。MRCP 图像上可以观察到胆总管的扩张或者与胆总管相通的囊状结构。Ⅲ型胆总管囊肿通常表现为十二指肠腔内的局限性囊性扩张（图18-5）。与输尿管囊肿类似，其鉴别诊断包括十二指肠重复囊肿和胰腺囊性病变。Ⅳ型胆管囊肿表现为累及肝内胆管或同时累及肝内及肝外胆管的多发囊状扩张。Ⅴ型胆管囊肿也被称为 Caroli 病，仅累及肝内胆管，造成肝内胆管多发扩张。影像学在疾病的诊断、评估病变范围以及并发症的检出中发挥重要作用[17]。

三、胆道梗阻

内镜逆行胰胆管造影（endoscopic retrograde cholangiopancreatography, ERCP）被认为是诊断可疑胆道梗阻的金标准。MRI 在评估胆道梗阻性病变方面非常有用。MRI 一次检查可以显示从肝内胆管末梢到胆胰壶腹的整个胆管树结构，也可以同时显示胆管内和胆管外的病变。与 ERCP 不同，MRCP 可以同时显示胆道阻塞部位的近端和远端胆管，并生成与类似 ERCP 的图像。同时，它还避免了射线暴露所带来的损害，以及与 ERCP 有关的操作和麻醉相关并发症。MRCP 在诊断胆道梗阻方面的敏感性与 ERCP 接近，敏感性接近 100%[18]。MRI 能够证实胆道梗阻并且还能够确定梗阻的准确部位。在 T_2 加权图像上，胆管内病变比如结石表现为高信号胆汁中的充盈缺损。此外，压迫胆管的胆管外病变诸如肿大淋

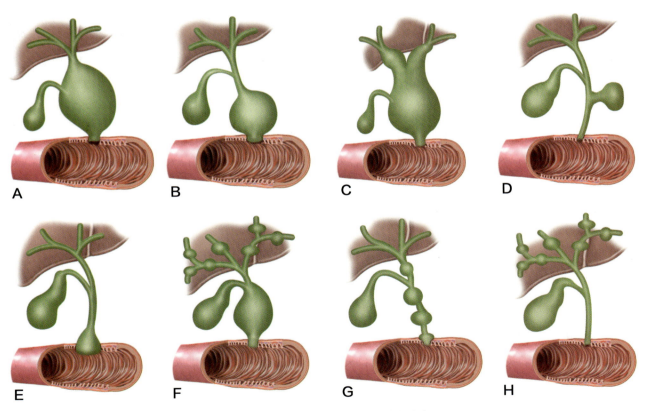

▲ 图 18-4　Todani 对胆管囊肿的分类

A. Ⅰa 型胆管囊肿，胆管的囊性扩张；B. Ⅰb 型胆管囊肿，局灶性胆总管扩张；C. Ⅰc 型，累及整个肝外胆管树梭形扩张；D. Ⅱ型胆管囊肿，胆总管憩室；E. Ⅲ型胆管囊肿（胆总管囊肿），十二指肠壁内段胆总管扩张；F. Ⅳa 型胆管囊肿，多发肝内和肝外管扩张；G. Ⅳb 型胆管囊肿，肝外胆管多发扩张；H. Ⅴ型胆管囊肿（Caroli 病），肝内胆管多发扩张

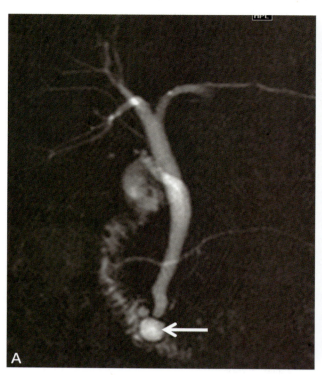
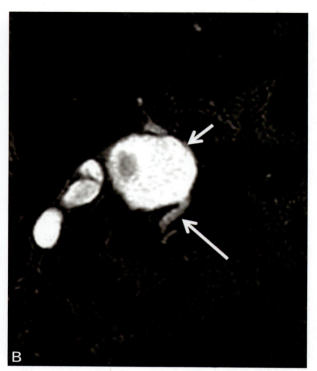

▲ 图 18-5 胆管囊肿

A. Ⅲ型胆管囊肿，胆总管十二指肠壁内段局限性扩张；B. Ⅰ型胆管囊肿

巴结和胰头部肿块，也可以在 MRCP 上得到显示。

（一）胆管结石

胆管中存在的结石被称为胆管结石。胆管结石是胆道梗阻最常见的原因。MRI 检出胆管结石的准确性主要取决于结石本身的大小。MRCP 检测胆管结石的敏感性、特异性和准确性分别为 90%、88% 和 89%。对于 6mm 或更大的结石，灵敏度、特异性和准确性分别增加到了 100%、99% 和 99%[19]。MRCP 在诊断胆总管结石方面与 ERCP 相当，在诊断肝内胆管结石方面优于 ERCP。

在 T_2 加权图像和 MRCP 图像上，胆管结石相对于邻近高信号的胆汁表现为低信号管腔内充盈缺损（图 18-6）。在 T_1 加权图像上，胆色素结石可能相对于胆汁呈现高信号。小结石通常难以发现，例如位于肝内胆管内的小结石或者挤压进入壶腹部的小结石。薄层 MRCP 图像和轴位图像有助于检出小结石。其他会导致胆管内充盈缺损的病变可能为气泡、血凝块和肿瘤[20]。结石与气泡可以通过轴位图像区分开来，石头由于重力作用存在于靠近下部的位置，而气泡通常上升到胆管的上部[21]。血凝块通常具有不规则的形状，这一点与胆道结石的圆形或椭圆形不同。血液凝块也可能在 T_1 图像上显示高信号，这取决于出血的时间长短。肿瘤则通常表现为在注射含钆造影剂后在 T_1 加权图像上有强化。

一些 MRI 伪影可能表现为胆管中的充盈缺损，可能被误诊为结石。由手术后金属夹和邻近的肠管内肠气以及流动伪影所导致的磁敏感伪影可以造成类似于胆管结石的表现。在流动伪影的案例中，MR 血管成像可以显示胆管中的流动伪影。相邻血管的动脉搏动可能导致胆管的外压性变窄，这可能被错误地解读为胆管的病理性狭窄。同样，MR 血管成像可以显示导致胆管外压性狭窄的动脉[21]。

Mirizzi 综合征有必要特别提及，其原因是由于邻近胆囊管中的结石压迫（肝总管）而导致的肝总管梗阻。术前诊断有助于避免手术过程中发生的并发症，因为该区域的炎症粘连可能使解剖结构显示不清，以及胆总管可能被误认为是胆囊管[22]。

（二）胆管炎

1. 原发性硬化性胆管炎 原发性硬化性胆管炎（primary sclerosing cholangitis,PSC）是胆管的慢性炎性疾病，其特点是肝内和肝外胆管特发性的、进行性炎症和纤维化（图18-7A）。虽然目前确切的病因尚不清楚，但它被认为是一种自身免疫性疾病，因为本病与炎症性肠病的发病具有很高的相关性。PSC最终发展为肝硬化和肝衰竭。也可合并出现门静脉高压症或胆管癌（图18-7B）。肝移植是唯一的治疗方法[23]。

ERCP一直是诊断PSC的金标准。然而，在最近的研究中，与ERCP相比MRCP可以更好地观察肝外和肝内胆管。MRI还可评估肝脏情况并检查出相关发症[24]。在MRI上最常见的病变是肝内胆管的狭窄和扩张。在疾病发展的早期，胆管狭窄段较短并且与扩张的胆管交替分布，形成胆管的串珠状外观。相较于胆管狭窄的严重程度，胆管扩张通常低于预期。随着疾病的进展，周围胆管的闭塞，逐渐形成修剪的树木样外观。在MRI的其他序列上可以观察到胆管壁的增厚和强化[25]。

肝脏的形态学改变与疾病的进展阶段有关。在疾病早期，肝实质表现正常。随着疾病的进展，可以观察到门静脉周围肝实质内的T_2高信号区域，这代表炎性水肿的存在。由于炎症和纤维化的发展导致肝脏的灌注模式改变，可能会出现外周高信号和动脉期强化。在疾病晚期，肝右叶和左叶发生萎缩，同时伴有尾状叶肥大。在这些患者中，门淋巴结肿大的情况并不少见[25]。

2. 感染性胆管炎 感染性胆管炎或上行感染性胆管炎是由于在胆道梗阻的情况下，由来源于肠道的革兰阴性菌感染胆管。感染性胆管炎可

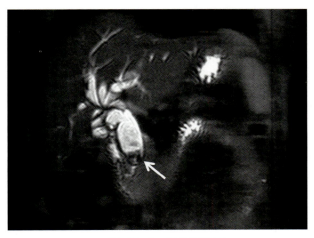

▲ 图 18-6 胆总管结石

冠状位T_2加权HASTE图像显示胆总管下段狭窄合并结石（白箭），近端胆总管和肝内胆管普遍扩张

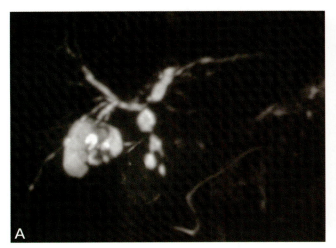 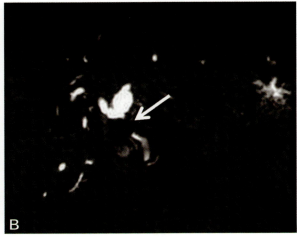

▲ 图 18-7 原发性硬化性胆管炎

A.MRCP图像显示受累胆管多发狭窄和扩张形成胆管成串珠状改变；B.MRCP图像显示由于出现胆管癌导致胆管不成比例扩张，右肝管较左肝管明显扩张（白箭）

能危及生命，通常表现为发热、黄疸和腹痛，同时可能会并发脓毒血症。治疗包括支持治疗、抗生素治疗以及减轻胆道梗阻。MRCP 显示胆管扩张，无串珠状或外周修剪树枝状表现。本病可能会合并胆管结石[26]。可表现为胆总管壁弥漫性增厚以及肝内胆管壁强化。炎症扩展到肝实质后可表现为肝脏实质外周楔形或门静脉周边片状区域在 T_2 加权图像上呈高信号，对应区域在注射含钆对比剂后明显强化。感染性胆管炎可能会进展并形成肝脓肿，表现为肝实质内有外周强化的局灶性病变[27]。

3. 复发性化脓性胆管炎 复发性化脓性胆管炎或东方型胆管炎以及反复发作性胆管炎，肝内胆色素性结石以及胆管扩张为特征。其发病与寄生虫感染有关，例如蛔虫或华支睾吸虫感染（图 18-8）。通常认为胆管存在这些寄生虫所引发的慢性感染导致了炎症，胆管狭窄以及结石形成。患者通常会出现反复发作性胆管炎[28]。MRCP 显示肝内胆管狭窄以及末端陡然变细，肝内中央胆管和肝外胆管多发扩张。约 80％ 的患者可以见到肝内胆管结石，由于结石内含有胆红素成分，这些结石往往在 T_1 加权图像上显示高信号（图 18-9）。同时可能会见到胆道积气和肝脓肿。在慢性病例中可发生肝脏萎缩[27]。

4. 艾滋病（AIDS）相关胆道疾病 艾滋病相关胆道疾病包括一系列发生在 HIV 感染者中的可影响胆道的疾病。这些疾病包括隐孢子虫和巨细胞病毒在内的病原体所造成的胆管机会性感染，会导致非结石性胆囊炎或淋巴瘤。艾滋病胆道病变的 MRI 表现通常为胆管扩张或狭窄，局灶性胆管壁增厚以及壶腹部狭窄[29]。

四、胆道肿瘤

（一）胆管细胞癌

胆管细胞癌是起源于胆管上皮的恶性肿瘤。多发生于 60—70 岁的人群。某些胆道慢性疾病会增加发生胆管细胞癌的风险。这些包括原发性硬化性胆管炎（PSC）、胆管囊肿、慢性胆总管结石、胆管乳头状瘤以及肝吸虫感染等。然而，在大多数情况下，人们无法确定发病的危险因素。患者通常表现出厌食、体重减轻、腹痛、黄疸及瘙痒[30]。

根据发生位置不同，胆管细胞癌分为 3 种不同的形式。肝内胆管细胞癌起源于肝内外周胆管，是仅次于肝细胞癌的第二常见的肝脏原发性恶性肿瘤。肝门部胆管癌起源于右肝管、左肝管或它们的汇合处。这些是最常见的胆管癌类型，也被

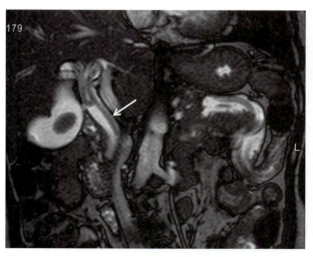

▲ 图 18-8 胆道蛔虫病
T_2 加权冠状 MRI 部分显示胆管中的蛔虫为长管状充盈缺损（白箭），其上端盘绕。胆管的寄生虫感染与复发性胆管炎有关

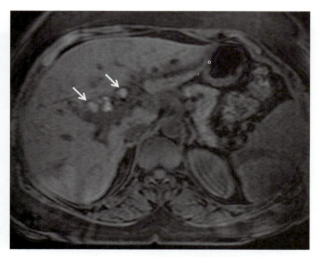

▲ 图 18-9 复发性化脓性胆管炎
轴位 T_1 加权 MRI 图像显示肝内胆管多发胆色素性结石，T_1 加权图像上呈高信号（白箭），这种情况通常在复发性化脓性胆管炎中比较常见

称为 Klatskin 肿瘤。胆管癌的第三种解剖学亚型是肝外胆管癌，起源于肝总管或胆总管。在组织学上，大多数胆管细胞癌属于硬化型腺癌[30]。

肝内胆管细胞癌在 MRI 上通常表现为无包膜的局灶性实性肿块。肿块通常在 T_1 加权图像上呈低信号，在 T_2 加权图像上呈高信号。在一些患者中，由于中心纤维瘢痕的存在，在 T_2 加权图像上可能出现相对应的中心低信号表现。当这种征象存在时，肿块中心低信号可用于区分肝内胆管细胞癌与肝转移瘤。在注射含钆对比剂后的动态增强图像上，动脉期病灶边缘强化，在随后的门静脉期内肿块渐进性向心强化（图 18-10）。延迟扫描很重要，因为某些肿瘤可能仅仅在延迟扫描时可见。MRI 上的其他可见征象包括局限性肝被膜皱缩以及肿瘤周围肝内胆管局限性轻度扩张[31]。

肝门部及肝外胆管癌通常是环周浸润状生长。这些征象通常难以在常规 T_1 或 T_2 加权图像上被观察到。MRCP 序列通过显示由于局灶性狭窄所引起的近端胆管扩张以及胆管突然变细的征象，间接地显示肿瘤的存在和位置。胆管壁的局灶性增厚有可能会在 MRCP 上显示，有时则不会显示。不常见的是，它们可以表现为小肿块。在这种情况下，它们的信号强度特征和增强模式与肝内胆管细胞癌相似。比较罕见的是，肝门部胆管癌和肝外胆管癌可以主要表现为管腔内息肉样生长，并且在 MRCP 上表现为充盈缺损。这种生长类型具有相对较好的预后[31]。

MRI 有助于术前对胆管细胞癌进行分期，并确定这些病变是否具有可切除性以及具体的手术方法。门静脉淋巴结肿大并不是转移的特异性表现，因为其他原因如原发性硬化性胆管炎（PSC），感染或支架置入都可以导致肝门部淋巴结肿大。确定是否存在腹膜和肝转移病灶至关重要。原发病灶的可切除性主要通过对胆管、血管和肝段的受累程度和范围进行评估来确定。对于肝内胆管细胞癌，受累肝段相对于剩余肝脏的体积的评估有助于外科手术切除方案的制订[31]。对于肝门部和肝外胆管癌，可切除性和手术程序的类型取决于肿瘤与胆道汇合处的接近程度以及肝门部、左右肝管及其二级分支汇合处的受累情况。基于这些因素，肝门部和肝外胆管癌可以根据 Bismuth 分类进行分型（图 18-11）[32]。

（二）壶腹部病变

肝胰（Vater）壶腹或十二指肠大乳头是十二指肠降段内侧壁上的突起，内部含有胆总管和胰管的共同开口。正常的壶腹结构在 MRI 有时无法显示。有时在 MRI 图像上可显示，直径通常小于 10mm，强化方式通常与邻近十二指肠黏膜强化模式类似[33]。在壶腹部位发生梗阻时，MRCP 可显示胆总管扩张至壶腹水平，而此时引起胆道梗阻的壶腹病变本身可能无法被观察到。壶腹部位梗阻的原因可能是由于壶腹部痉挛、炎症性狭窄、结石以及各种良性或恶性肿瘤等原因所致[34]。这些疾病的影像学特征经常互有重叠。

在壶腹部痉挛和壶腹部狭窄的情况下，除了壶腹部的胆道梗阻外，通常观察不到其他异常表现。乳头发生急性炎症可表现为远端胆总管管壁轻度增厚，管壁仍显示光滑，同时伴有乳头明显强化。壶腹癌是起源于覆盖在壶腹表面的十二指肠上皮的腺癌。MRI 有时无法显示出较小的壶腹癌，在这种情况下，可能无法与其他原因引起的壶腹部梗阻相鉴别。然而，当壶腹癌增大到一定程度时表现为低强化的壶腹部肿块，同时伴有乳头形态不规则[33]。

五、胆囊的 MRI 表现

（一）技术

推荐患者在进行胆囊磁共振成像检查前至少禁食 4h，以使胆囊充分扩张。用于腹部 MRI 检查的常规序列如 T_1 和 T_2 加权序列均可用于对胆囊进行成像。MRCP 序列也会被使用，尤其是对于胆囊管和小结石的显示具有优势。如果有需要，还可以对胆囊进行含钆对比剂增强 T_1 加权扫描。

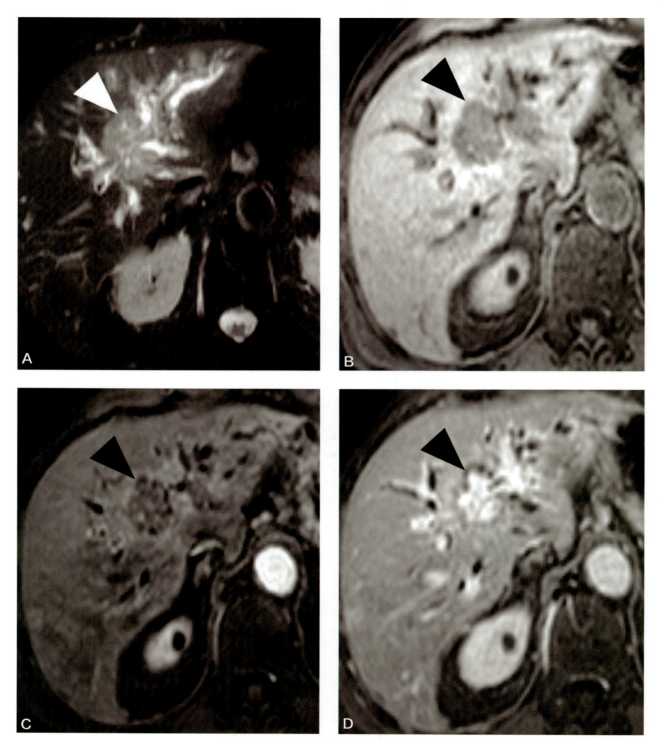

▲ 图 18-10 肝门部胆管癌（箭头）

A. T_2 加权轴位 MRI 图像显示肝门部胆管癌呈高信号；B. 肿瘤在 T_1 加权图像上呈低信号；C. 含钆对比剂增强 T_1 加权动脉期图像显示胆管癌外周强化；D. 含钆对比剂增强 T_1 加权延迟期图像显示肿瘤延迟强化

（二）胆囊的正常表现

胆囊腔在 T_2 加权图像和 MRCP 上显示为高信号，因为腔内充满静止的液态胆汁。在 T_1 加权图像上，由于胆汁的浓度和成分不同，其信号强度表现多种多样，可能会表现为从低信号到高信号之间的各种信号。延长禁食时间会导致胆汁中的水分重吸收，从而会增加胆固醇、胆盐和磷脂的浓度。这种浓缩的胆汁在 T_1 加权图像中显示为中高信号[2]。胆囊壁在 T_2 加权图像上呈低信号，在 T_1 加权图像上呈中等信号，在注射含钆对比剂增强后图像上表现光滑和均匀一致的强化。胆囊壁的正常厚度最大为 3mm[35]。胆囊管连接胆囊并于肝总管汇合形成。正常胆囊管的长度是可以变化的，其直径可达 5mm。

（三）胆结石症

胆结石症在世界范围内的总发病率为 10%～20%。胆囊运动性受损以及胆汁过饱和会增加个体患胆石病的风险。胆囊结石的危险因素包括妊娠、肥胖、快速体重下降、糖尿病和酗酒。大多数胆囊结石患者无症状。当临床症状出现时，最常出现症状是胆绞痛，是由于胆囊结石导致胆囊管间歇性梗阻引发的阵发性腹痛[36]。超声是评估胆囊结石疾病的首选检查方法。

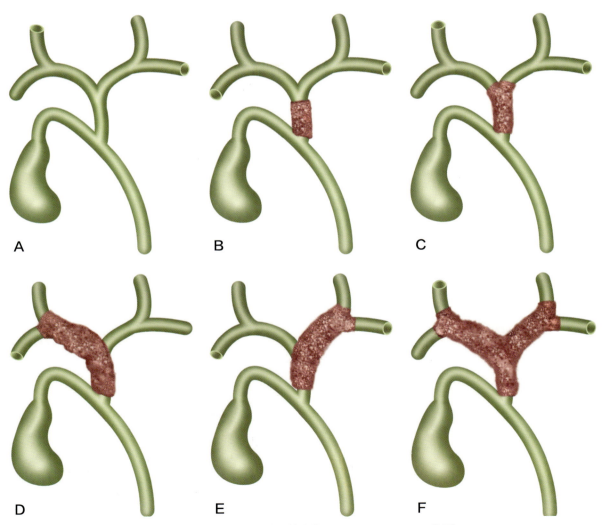

▲ 图 18-11　肝门部胆管癌的 Bismuth-Corlette 分型

A. 胆道正常解剖结构；B. Ⅰ型，胆管癌局限于左右肝管汇合处远端的肝总管；C. Ⅱ型，胆管癌累及肝左右管汇合处；D. Ⅲa 型，胆管癌延伸至右肝管的分叉处；E. Ⅲb 型，胆管癌延伸至左肝管的分叉处；F. Ⅳ型，胆管癌同时延伸至右肝管和左肝管的分叉处

在MRI图像上，各种成分的胆囊结石在T_2加权图像和MRCP上均表现为高信号胆汁内的低信号影（图18-12）。由于结石中心裂缝由液体充填，可能会在T_2加权图像上表现为中心高信号。如前所述，胆囊结石在T_1加权图像上信号强度变化较大，这取决于其组成成分不同。胆固醇结石呈低信号，而胆色素结石相对于胆汁呈现高信号[37]。胆囊结石通常存在于胆囊中的重力依赖性位置，除非其受到外界影响。

（四）胆囊炎

1. 急性结石性胆囊炎 急性结石性胆囊炎是指由胆结石阻塞胆囊颈或胆囊管而引起的胆囊急性炎症。梗阻会导致胆囊中的压力逐渐增加，进一步导致胆囊的静脉和淋巴引流受阻。如果治疗不及时，可能会进展为胆囊缺血坏死或穿孔。患者通常出现恶心、呕吐和右上腹部疼痛。回顾性分析大多数患者既往有胆绞痛发作病史。超声通常是诊断急性胆囊炎的首选成像方法。MRI可以用于疑难病例[38]。

急性胆囊炎时，MRI可显示胆囊壁增厚（图18-13）。当图像上显示壁的厚度超过3mm时，可认为胆囊壁增厚。急性炎症时的胆囊壁在T_2加权图像上呈高信号。胆囊周围可见积液，以上所有这些特征都是非特异性的，同时也可以在如慢性肝病等其他疾病中观察到。胆囊结石可以在T_2加权或MRCP图像上被观察到。注射含钆对比剂增强后图像显示胆囊壁明显强化以及相邻肝实质的一过性强化，这些征象被认为是诊断急性胆囊炎的更具有特异性的征象。肝细胞特异性对比剂可以在延迟期图像上显示胆囊管的突然截断以及胆囊内的充盈缺损，有助于诊断急性结石性胆囊炎[35,39]。

对比增强扫描也有助于检出胆囊炎的并发症，如穿孔、脓肿形成和坏疽性胆囊炎。强化的胆囊壁连续性中断对于胆囊穿孔具有提示性意义。它可能与胆囊窝中的边缘强化的局部液体积聚有关。当胆囊壁出现弥漫性或斑片状无强化区域时，可以诊断为坏疽性胆囊炎。无强化区域对应相应的坏死区[40]。在气肿性胆囊炎和胆囊-肠瘘中可以观察到胆囊积气。它以胆囊腔内出现游离的低信号区域以及液平面形成。胆囊壁和胆囊周围组织积气应高度怀疑气肿性胆囊炎。空气呈现为低信号区域，这是由于空气介导的磁场不均匀性导致的信号缺失所引起[41]。出血性胆囊炎可以在T_1和T_2加权图像上检测到胆囊壁和胆囊腔内高信号出血，以此来进行诊断。

2. 慢性胆囊炎 慢性胆囊炎是指胆囊发生

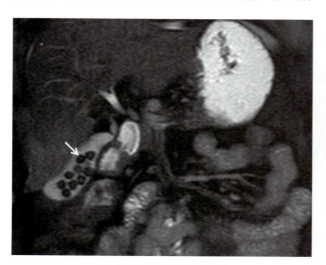

▲ 图18-12 胆囊结石
胆囊内多发低信号结石影（白箭）。注意这些结石内部的高信号裂隙

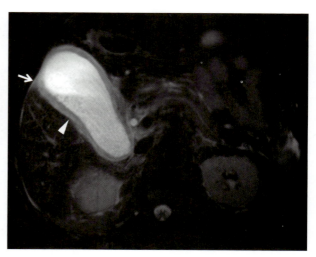

▲ 图18-13 急性胆囊炎
轴位脂肪抑制T_2加权图像显示胆囊明显扩张，胆囊壁增厚呈弥漫性中高信号（箭头）以及胆囊周围积液（白箭）。这些征象在特定的临床情况中对急性胆囊炎具有指示性意义

的慢性炎症，通常与胆石症发作有关。患者可能无症状或者出现反复发作性胆绞痛。MRI可以显示胆囊壁增厚和胆囊结石。在某些患者中由于胆囊纤维化可以出现收缩，表现为延迟强化。慢性胆囊炎中不会见到邻近肝实质的一过性强化，这一特征可用来鉴别急慢性胆囊炎[42]。

3. 非结石性胆囊炎 非结石性胆囊炎通常发生在ICU的重症患者中。患者出现不明原因的败血症。由于存在多种合并症和非特异性体征和症状，通常不能直接做出诊断。如果不及时发现，非结石性胆囊炎可能会并发穿孔和坏疽性胆囊炎。MRI显示胆囊内无结石，胆囊扩张，胆囊壁增厚并在T_2加权图像呈高信号。同时可能出现胆囊周围积液[42]。这些重症患者通常通过经皮胆囊造瘘进行治疗。

4. 胆囊腺肌增生症 胆囊腺肌增生症是黏膜层的增生、肌层肥大、同时增生的黏膜憩室突入肌层内所形成。这些胆囊壁内黏膜憩室被称为Rokitansky-Aschoff窦。本病与胆结石症有关，不被认为是一种癌前病变[43]。然而，本病可能与胆囊腺癌共存。

在MRI上显示胆囊腺肌增生症并不罕见。胆囊壁表现为局灶或弥漫性增厚。Rokitansky-Aschoff窦表现为T_2加权图像上胆囊壁中高信号囊状结构。这些结构在T_1加权图像上呈低信号，含钆对比剂增强扫描无强化。这些Rokitansky-Aschoff窦在T_2加权图像和MRCP上呈花环状排列，此征象被称为"珍珠项链征"（图18-14）[43]。

（五）息肉

胆囊息肉是起源于胆囊壁并突入胆囊腔内的病变。有不同种类包括良性病变如胆固醇性息肉和良性肿瘤以及恶性肿瘤如胆囊腺癌和转移瘤。它们通常在影像学检查中偶然发现并诊断，或者是在胆囊切除术后通过病理偶然诊断。在影像学检查发现病变时，将良性息肉与恶性息肉区分开至关重要。然而有时并不完全能够将它们鉴别开来[44]。

在T_2加权图像和MRCP图像上，胆囊息肉表现为突入胆囊腔内的低信号充盈缺损。与结石不同，它们可以位于与胆囊壁相邻的非重力依赖性位置。在含钆对比剂增强后的图像上，息肉可见强化。应该予以重视的可能恶变的征象有息肉直径超过1cm、无蒂性息肉、孤立性息肉、进行性长大的息肉以及息肉与胆囊结石共存[44]。

（六）胆囊癌

胆囊癌是世界范围内最常见的胆道恶性肿瘤。女性发病更常见，其发病率随年龄增长而增加。不幸的是，由于本病早期症状不具有特异性，大多数患者被诊断时已经进入了疾病进展期。症状包括腹部隐痛、体重减轻及黄疸。有些胆囊癌是在胆囊切除术后病理检查时被诊断出来。胆囊癌的危险因素包括胆石症、慢性胆道感染、肥胖和瓷化胆囊[45]。

早期癌表现为胆囊壁的局限性或不对称性增厚。胆囊壁增厚超过10mm时应警惕为恶性。胆囊癌相对于邻近肝实质在T_2加权图像上呈高信号，在T_1加权图像上呈等信号或低信号。在增强扫描图像上，胆囊癌表现出早期不均匀

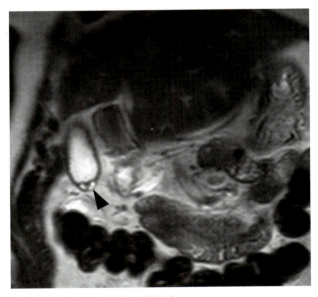

▲ 图18-14 胆囊腺肌增生症
冠状位T_2加权MRI图像显示胆囊底壁的局灶性增厚。注意增厚的胆囊壁内的T_2高信号囊肿（箭头）。胆囊腺肌增生中的胆囊壁内部黏膜憩室被称为Rokitansky-Aschoff窦

强化。这种强化在延迟期仍持续存在。良性病变往往表现出早期强化而在强化不会持续到延迟期。然而，在胆囊良恶性疾病之间图像特征存在显著重叠[45]。

进展期癌表现为胆囊区域实性肿块。胆囊可能已无法辨认。肿块通常与胆囊结石有关，胆囊结石可显示为被肿块所吞没包绕。肿块可以通过直接侵犯蔓延至肝脏Ⅴ段和Ⅳa段。病变也可能沿胆囊管浸润至胆总管。病变表现为T_1低信号和T_2不均匀高信号。MRI还有助于检出有无邻近器官、血管和胆管的受侵，有无淋巴结转移、腹膜和远处转移等[35]。

（七）胆囊其他恶性肿瘤

胆囊其他恶性肿瘤包括转移瘤及淋巴瘤。目前已有报道黑色素瘤、乳腺癌和肾细胞癌转移到胆囊。在T_1加权图像上，黑色素瘤转移灶往往呈现高信号。淋巴瘤胆囊受累的情况很少见，主要表现为胆囊壁增厚或胆囊区域实性肿块。然而，仅仅从图像特点上无法准确区分胆囊淋巴瘤与胆囊癌。

参考文献

[1] Griffin N, Charles-Edwards G, Grant LA. Magnetic resonance cholangiopancreatography: The ABC of MRCP. *Insights Imaging*. Feb 2012;3(1):11–21.

[2] Bilgin M, Shaikh F, Semelka RC, Bilgin SS, Balci NC, Erdogan A. Magnetic resonance imaging of gallbladder and biliary system. *Top Magn Reson Imaging*. Feb 2009;20(1):31–42.

[3] Vitelas KM, Keogan MT, Spritzer CE, Nelson RC. MR cholangio-pancreatography of bile and pancreatic duct abnormalities with emphasis on the single-shot fast spin echo technique. *RadioGraphics*. 2000;20:939–957.

[4] Sanyal R, Stevens T, Novak E, Veniero JC. Secretin-enhanced MRCP: Review of technique and application with proposal for quantification of exocrine function. *AJR Am J Roentgenol*. Jan 2012;198(1):124–132.

[5] Gupta RT, Brady CM, Lotz J, Boll DT, Merkle EM. Dynamic MR imaging of the biliary system using hepa-tocyte-specific contrast agents. *AJR Am J Roentgenol*. Aug 2010;195(2):405–413.

[6] Senturk S, Miroglu TC, Bilici A, Gumus H, Tekin RC, Ekici F et al. Diameters of the common bile duct in adults and postcholecystectomy patients: A study with 64-slice CT. *Eur J Radiol*. Jan 2012;81(1):39–42.

[7] Mortelé KJ, Ros PR. Anatomic variants of the biliary tree: MR cholangiographic findings and clinical applica tions. *AJR Am J Roentgenol*. Aug 2001;177(2):389–394.

[8] Lim JS, Kim M-J, Kim JH, Kim S IL, Choi J-S, Park M-S et al. Preoperative MRI of potential living-donor-related liver transplantation using a single dose of gadobenate dimeglumine. *AJR Am J Roentgenol*. Aug 2005;185(2):424–431.

[9] Bassignani MJ, Fulcher AS, Szucs RA, Chong WK, Prasad UR, Marcos A. Use of imaging for living donor liver transplantation. *RadioGraphics*. 2001;21(1):39–52.

[10] Yu J, Turner MA, Fulcher AS, Halvorsen RA. Congenital anomalies and normal variants of the pancreaticobiliary tract and the pancreas in adults: Part 1, Biliary tract. *AJR Am J Roentgenol*. Dec 2006;187(6):1536–1543.

[11] Wu Y-H, Liu Z-S, Mrikhi R, Ai Z-L, Sun Q, Bangoura G et al. Anatomical variations of the cystic duct: Two case reports. *World J Gastroenterol*. Jan 7, 2008;14(1):155–157.

[12] Itoh S, Fukushima H, Takada A, Suzuki K, Satake H, Ishigaki T. Assessment of anomalous pancreaticobiliary ductal junction with high-resolution multiplanar reformatted images in MDCT. *AJR Am J Roentgenol*. Sep 2006;187(3):668–675.

[13] Rizzo RJ, Szucs RA, Turner MA. Congenital abnormalities of the pancreas and biliary tree in adults. *RadioGraphics*. Jan 1995;15(1):49–68.

[14] Bhavsar MS, Vora HB, Giriyappa VH. Choledochal cysts: A review of literature. *Saudi J Gastroenterol*. 2005;18(4):230–236.

[15] Baek S-J, Park J-Y, Kim D-Y, Kim J-H, Kim Y-M, Kim Y-T et al. Stage IIIC epithelial ovarian cancer classified solely by lymph node metastasis has a more favorable prognosis than other types of stage IIIC epithelial ovarian cancer. *J Gynecol Oncol*. Dec 2008;19(4):223–228.

[16] Todani T, Watanabe Y, Narusue M, Tabuchi K, Okajima K.Congenital bile duct cysts: Classification, operative procedures, and review of thirty-seven cases including cancer arising from choledochal cyst. *Am J Surg*. Aug 1977;134(2):263–269.

[17] Singham J, Yoshida EM, Scudamore CH. Choledochal cysts: Part 1 of 3: classification and pathogenesis. *Can J Surg*. Oct 2009;52(5):434–440.

[18] Adamek HE, Albert J, Weitz M, Breer H, Schilling D, Riemann JF. A prospective evaluation of magnetic resonance cholangiopancreatography in patients with sus pected bile duct obstruction. *Gut*. Nov 1998;43(5):680–683.

[19] Guarise A, Baltieri S, Mainardi P, Faccioli N. Diagnostic accuracy of MRCP in choledocholithiasis. *Radiol Med*. Mar 2005;109(3):239–251.

[20] Eason JB, Taylor AJ, Yu J. MRI in the workup of biliary tract filling defects. *J Magn Reson Imaging*. May

[21] Irie H, Honda H, Kuroiwa T, Yoshimitsu K, Aibe H, Shinozaki K, Masuda K. Pitfalls in MR cholangiopancreatographic interpretation. *RadioGraphics*. Jan-Feb 2001; 21(1):23–37.

[22] Becker CD, Hassler H, Terrier F. Preoperative diagnosis of the Mirizzi syndrome: Limitations of sonography and computed tomography. *AJR Am J Roentgenol*. Sep 1984; 143(3):591–596.

[23] Enns RA, Spritzer CE, Baillie JM, Nelson RC. Radiologic manifestations of sclerosing cholangitis with emphasis on MR cholangiopancreatography. *RadioGraphics*. 2000;20(4):959–975.

[24] Variability CI, Vaswani KK, Bennett WF, Tzalonikou M, Mabee C, Kirkpatrick R et al. MR cholangiopan- creatography in patients with primary sclerosing. Aug 2002;179:399–407.

[25] Ito K, Mitchell D, Outwater EK, Blasbalg R. Primary sclerosing MR imaging features. Jun 1999;172:1527–1533.

[26] Bader TR, Braga L, Beavers KL, Semelka RC. MR imaging findings of infectious cholangitis. *Magn Reson Imaging*. Jul 2001;19(6):781–788.

[27] Catalano OA, Sahani DV, Forcione DG, Czermak B, Liu C-H, Soricelli A et al. Biliary infections: Spectrum of imaging findings and management. *RadioGraphics*. Nov 2009;29(7):2059–2080.

[28] Heffernan EJ, Geoghegan T, Munk PL, Ho SG, Harris AC. Recurrent pyogenic cholangitis: From imaging to inter vention. *AJR Am J Roentgenol*. Jan 2009;192(1):W28–W35.

[29] Bilgin M, Balci NC, Erdogan A, Momtahen AJ, Alkaade S, Rau WS. Hepatobiliary and pancreatic MRI and MRCP findings in patients with HIV infection. *AJR Am J Roentgenol*. Jul 2008;191(1):228–232.

[30] Vanderveen KA, Hussain HK. Magnetic resonance imaging of cholangiocarcinoma. *Cancer Imaging*. Jan 2004;4(2):104–115.

[31] Choi BI, Lee JM, Han JK. Imaging of intrahepatic and hilar cholangiocarcinoma. *Abdom Imaging*. 2004;29(5):548–557.

[32] Sainani NI, Catalano OA, Holalkere NS, Zhu AX, Hahn PF, Sahani DV. Cholangiocarcinoma: Current and novel imaging techniques. *RadioGraphics* 2008;28:1263–1287.

[33] Kim TU, Kim S, Lee JW, Woo SK, Lee TH, Choo KS et al. Ampulla of Vater: Comprehensive anatomy, MR imaging of pathologic conditions, and correlation with endoscopy. *Eur J Radiol*. Apr 2008;66(1):48–64.

[34] Chung YE, Kim M-J, Kim HM, Park M-S, Choi J-Y, Hong H-S et al. Differentiation of benign and malignant ampullary obstructions on MR imaging. *Eur J Radiol*. Nov 2011;80(2):198–203.

[35] Catalano OA, Sahani DV, Kalva SP, Cushing MS, Hahn PF, Brown JJ, Edelman RR. MR imaging of the gallbladder: A pictorial essay. *RadioGraphics* 2008;28:135–155.

[36] Reshetnyak VI. Concept of the pathogenesis and treatment of cholelithiasis. *World J Hepatol*. Mar 27, 2012;4(2):18–34.

[37] Tsai H, Lin X, Chen C, Lin P, Lin J. MRI of gallstones with different compositions. *AJR Am J Roentgenol* 2004;182:1513–1519.

[38] Yusoff IF, Barkun JS, Barkun AN. Diagnosis and management of cholecystitis and cholangitis. *Gastroenterol Clin North Am*. Dec 2003;32(4):1145–1168.

[39] Choi IY, Cha SH, Yeom SK, Lee SW, Chung HH, Je BK et al. Diagnosis of acute cholecystitis: Value of contrast agent in the gallbladder and cystic duct on Gd-EOB- DTPA enhanced MR cholangiography. *Clin Imaging*. Oct 30, 2013;38:1–5.

[40] Pedrosa I, Guarise A, Goldsmith J, Procacci C, Rofsky NM. The interrupted rim sign in acute cholecystitis: A method to identify the gangrenous form with MRI. *J Magn Reson Imaging*. Oct 2003;18(3):360–363.

[41] Koenig T, Tamm EP, Kawashima A. Magnetic resonance imaging findings in emphysematous cholecystitis. *Clin Radiol*. May 2004;59(5):455–458.

[42] Smith EA, Dillman JR, Elsayes KM, Menias CO, Bude RO. Cross-sectional imaging of acute and chronic gallbladder inflammatory disease. *AJR Am J Roentgenol*. Jan 2009;192(1):188–196.

[43] Boscak AR, Al-Hawary M, Ramsburgh SR. Best cases from the AFIP: Adenomyomatosis of the gallbladder. *RadioGraphics*. 2006;26(3):941–946.

[44] Andrén-Sandberg A. 3Diagnosis and management of gallbladder polyps. *N Am J Med Sci*. May 2012;4(5):203–211.

[45] Tan CH, Lim KS. MRI of gallbladder cancer. *Diagn Interv Radiol*. 2013;19(4):312–319.

Chapter 19 脾脏磁共振成像新进展

Update in Magnetic Resonance Imaging of the Spleen

Luis Luna Alcalá, Antonio Luna, Christine Menias 著

徐 飞 译

冯 冰 校

目录 CONTENTS

- 一、解剖 / 440
- 二、MRI 技术 / 440
- 三、正常 MRI 表现 / 442
- 四、正常变异 / 442
- 五、多脾综合征 / 443
- 六、脾大 / 443
- 七、血色沉着病（含铁血黄素沉着症和镰状细胞病）/ 444
- 八、外伤 / 444
- 九、感染性病变（感染）/ 444
- 十、囊肿 / 446
- 十一、血管源性病变 / 449
- 十二、非血管源性肿瘤 / 459
- 十三、其他脾脏病变 / 466
- 十四、总结 / 469

脾脏可能是放射学文献中研究最少的腹部器官。虽然它是原发疾病的罕见部位，但脾脏在创伤、血管、炎症、血液、肿瘤或贮积类疾病中的受累并不罕见。然而，脾脏出现异常的频率很低，大多数为偶然，无明显临床症状。从这个角度来看，脾脏疾病的发现和特征描述对于放射科医师来说是具有挑战性的。

超声（US）和计算机断层扫描（CT）已成为脾脏评估的主要无创性方式，在检出和描述脾脏局灶性和弥漫性病变中呈现出不同的结果[1]。磁共振成像（MRI）的最新进展已经能够开发更精确的序列来评估脾脏。即时和延迟采集的增强动态成像的使用可以更好地检出脾脏局灶性病变。对于偶发的脾脏局灶性病变，增强 MRI 检查可区分囊性和实性病变，在绝大多数病例中可区分良恶性[2]。

在本章中，我们描述了 MRI 扫描方案，并回顾了脾脏不同类型的疾病（表 19-1），包括其常见和不常见的 MR 特征。

表 19-1 脾脏病变的 MRI 特征

	范围	T₁WI	T₂WI	动态增强序列
继发性含铁血黄素沉着症和镰状细胞病	弥漫	低	低	增强早期呈弥漫性低血供
脓肿	局灶	低至等	高	轻度边缘强化
念珠菌病	局灶（多发微脓肿）	低至等	高	急性期无强化；慢性期轻度强化
包虫囊肿	局灶	多样	高	无强化
囊肿	局灶	低	高	无强化
假性囊肿	局灶	低至高 取决于蛋白质性或出血性成分	高/混合性	无强化
血管瘤	局灶	低至等	典型：高 硬化性：低 大：高，伴中央瘢痕	不同模式的渐进性强化 ①边缘渐进性强化至延迟期的均匀强化 ②早期均匀强化，持续强化 ③向心性填充
窦岸细胞血管瘤	局灶/弥漫	低	多样	动脉期轻度不均匀强化，延迟期均匀强化
血管内皮瘤	局灶/弥漫	低	低	低血供 实性部分不均匀强化
硬化性血管瘤样结节性转化	局灶	低	磁敏感区域的低信号（铁质沉着）	增强早期边缘强化伴轮辐状结构，延迟期持续强化
血管肉瘤	局灶/弥漫	多样	多样	明显强化，不均匀
血管外皮细胞瘤	局灶/弥漫	低	高	实性成分明显强化
脾梗死	局灶/弥漫	低（出血性梗死为高信号）	高，不均匀（慢性期梗死为低信号）	无强化

Chapter 19　脾脏磁共振成像新进展
Update in Magnetic Resonance Imaging of the Spleen

（续 表）

	范　围	T$_1$WI	T$_2$WI	动态增强序列
血肿	局灶	急性期：高 亚急性期：高 慢性期：低	急性期：低 亚急性期：高 慢性期：低	无强化或轻度边缘强化
动静脉畸形	局灶	多发流空信号	多发流空信号	早期迂曲强化
血管瘤病	弥漫	多样	多样	明显强化，不均匀
淋巴管瘤	局灶/弥漫	低；如果含蛋白质或出血成分为高信号	高	无强化
紫癜	局灶/弥漫	多样	高	边缘及分隔强化
错构瘤	局灶	等	高，不均匀	动脉期不均匀强化，延迟期均匀强化
脂肪瘤	局灶	高（脂肪抑制序列信号减低）	高（脂肪抑制序列信号减低）	无强化
淋巴瘤	局灶/弥漫	局灶：等	局灶：等至低	弥漫性：不规则高低信号区域混杂 局灶性：增强早期为低强化，第1分钟为等信号，延迟期渐进性强化
白血病（绿色瘤）	弥漫/局灶	等至低	高	增强早期为低强化，延迟期渐进性强化
转移瘤	局灶	等（急性出血或黑色素成分为高信号）	等至高	增强早期为低强化，延迟期为等信号
脾脏多形性未分化肉瘤	局灶	多样	多样	渐进性不均匀强化
脾脏囊腺癌	局灶	低	高	边缘、分隔及实性成分强化
Gaucher 病	局灶	等	白结节：低 红结节：高	无文献报道
Niemann-Pick 病	局灶		多样	延迟强化
淀粉样变	弥漫	低	低	低血供
结节病	弥漫	低	低	轻度、延迟强化
Gamna-Gandy 小体	局灶	信号缺失（GRE 同相位可见晕状伪影）	信号缺失	无强化
炎性假瘤	局灶	等至低	低	延迟期不均匀强化
髓外造血	弥漫/局灶	急性：中 慢性：低	急性：高 慢性：低	急性：轻度 慢性：无强化

一、解剖

脾脏是由被膜包裹的腹部器官，富含血管和淋巴组织，位于胃底和膈肌之间，在左上腹深处。成人脾脏的正常大小是 12cm×7cm×4cm，最大头尾径 10～12cm[3]。该器官具有膈面和脏面，呈月牙形，外侧凸面与腹壁和左半膈相接，内侧凹面与胃和左肾相接。脾门在前内侧，有脾血管和神经进出。

脾脏由脾肾韧带和胃脾韧带固定[4]。脾肾韧带来源于腹膜，它在脾脏和左肾之间延伸并连接脾门和左肾，内含胰尾和脾动静脉。胃脾韧带是小网膜囊和大网膜囊联合形成，连接脾门和胃，内含脾动脉的胃短支和胃网膜左支。最后，膈结肠韧带连接脾下极和结肠脾曲及膈肌。

脾是一个血液过滤器官，在功能可上分为三个部分：红髓、边缘区和白髓（图 19-1）。在显微镜下，红髓由许多薄壁的有孔血窦形成，细胞容易通过，被由巨噬细胞、网状细胞和网状纤维组成的脾索分隔。该结构为全身循环血液提供物理性和功能性的过滤。脾索内有淋巴细胞和造血细胞，在脾索之间的区域内，有不同类型的血细胞[5]。白髓由淋巴滤泡组成，主要是 B 细胞，其内含有中央小动脉，并被以 T 细胞为主动脉周围淋巴鞘（periarteriolar lymphoid sheaths, PALS）所包绕。包含边缘区的白髓与动脉树和红髓相联系，并与引流的静脉系统相联系。

在新生儿中，脾脏主要由红髓组成，随着年龄增长和进行性的抗原刺激，白髓逐渐增加，在成人脾实质中白髓所占比例高达 20%[6]。

二、MRI 技术

在许多情况下，脾脏病变是在 MRI 上偶

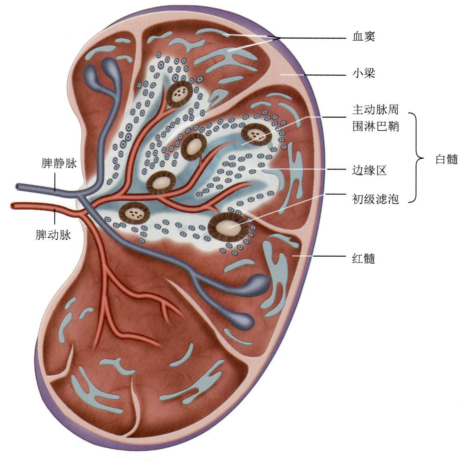

▲ 图 19-1　脾脏结构示意图

然发现的。大多数情况下，常规腹部 MRI 方案足以评估脾脏，但在可能的情况下，我们更倾向于使用特定的方案（表 19-2），其中包括：①冠状 T_2 加权半傅立叶变换单次激发快速自旋回波（HASTE）采集；②轴位屏气梯度回波（gradient echo，GE）T_1 加权化学位移同反相位序列；③轴位屏气快速自旋回波（turbo spin echo，TSE）T_2 加权序列（包含或不包含脂肪抑制）；④轴位 3D 脂肪抑制 GRE 动态系列采集，含增强前和增强后早期（对比剂注射后 10～12s）、增强后 1min 和 5min 采集。更常见的是，我们采用增强 T_1 加权高分辨率各向同性体素激发（e-THRIVE）作为动态增强序列。

评估脾脏实质的另一种方法是使用超顺磁氧化铁（superparamagnetic iron oxide，SPIO）颗粒。这种静脉内对比剂被脾脏和肝脏中的网状内皮系统（reticular endothelial system，RES）摄取。在 T_2 加权序列中，正常脾脏实质表现为低信号，脾脏局灶性病变显示为较高信号，相比于脾脏背景而言病灶会显示得更加明显[7]。超微 SPIO（ultrasmall superparamagnetic iron oxide，USPIO）颗粒的使用还可以增加脾脏病变的检出率，其血池半衰期更长，因而具有进一步描述血管瘤特征[8]并有更长的可采集时间窗[9]的优势。钆动态增强序列的结果与应用 SPIO 或 USPIO 对比剂的结果是相似的[8]。虽然这种方法很有前景，但它从未在临床领域广泛使用，可能是因为其管理复杂。

表 19-2 MRI 序列

	HASTE	T_2 TSE	Dual/FFE	Diffusion	DCE-MRI
（a）1.5T					
方向	冠状位	轴位	轴位	轴位	轴位
像素大小（mm）	1.5/1.5/7	1.2/1.2/5	1.5/1.9/6	3/3/7	2/2.2/2.2
SENSE	1.5	1.5	1.5	2	1.7
TE（ms）	80	120	2.3/4.6	70	2.2
TR（ms）	540	2500	136	1636	4.4
呼吸补偿	屏气	屏气	屏气	无	屏气
b 值（s/mm²）				4（b0;b250;b500;b1000）	
总扫描时间（s）	0:14.9	2:20	0:29.9	3:13	1:12.5
（b）3T					
像素大小（mm）	1/1.5/7	1/1.5/7	2/1/5	3/3/7	1.6/1.6/1.6
SENSE	2	1.3	2	2	2
TE（ms）	103	80	1.15/2.3	54	1.4
TR（ms）	924	778	150	1150	3
呼吸补偿	触发	屏气	屏气	触发	屏气
b 值（s/mm²）				4（b0;b250;b500;b1000）	
总扫描时间（s）	1:21	47	41	2:50	1:30

注：DCE-MRI. 动态造影增强 MRI；FFE. 快速场回波；HASTE. 半傅立叶采集单脉冲涡轮自旋回波；SENSE. 敏感度编码；TE. 回波时间；TR. 重复时间；TSE. 涡轮自旋回波

三、正常 MRI 表现

与肝实质相比，正常脾脏实质 T_1 加权图像上呈低信号，T_2 加权图像上呈高信号（图 19-2）。

增强早期序列能更好地鉴别正常和异常的脾脏区域[10]，因为此时它们之间的血供差异达到最大值。正常脾脏在增强早期通常表现为高低信号区域混杂的弓形模式。在稍延迟的采集序列中（1min 或更晚），脾脏实质信号变得均匀。目前据报道脾脏还有其他的早期增强模式（图 19-3）[11]。在炎症、肿瘤性病变或脂肪肝的情况下，脾脏的均匀强化通常表现为均匀的高信号。增强早期整个脾脏信号强度的下降与输血性铁负荷过载有关。识别增强早期的脾脏强化模式对于提高脾脏病变的检出率很重要。

在扩散加权图像（diffusion weighted imaging, DWI）上，由于该器官的细胞丰富，正常脾脏表现为高 b 值扩散受限。扩散加权成像在脾脏中的应用尚未被文献验证。根据我们自己的经验，正常脾脏扩散受限。初步研究数据表明，表观扩散系数（apparent diffusion coefficient, ADC）随着年龄增加而降低，而在存在肝硬化和门静脉高压时脾脏 ADC 值增加[12,13]。在这一点上，DWI 在评估脾脏方面是否有任何作用，仍需要进一步验证。

四、正常变异

由于存在切迹或裂缝，脾脏可能呈现出结节状轮廓或断裂的外观[1]。这些胚胎小叶的残余在平扫 CT 或 MRI 上可能被误认为是脾结节。MRI 的多平面成像和在所有序列中均表现为与脾脏等信号可以区分这些假性病灶。

副脾是一种常见的胚胎变异，在多达 40% 的人群中可见[14]（图 19-4）。它们是小的球形病灶，其信号及增强模式与脾脏相同。通常它们的直径小于 4cm，可能是单发或多发[15]。虽然它们可

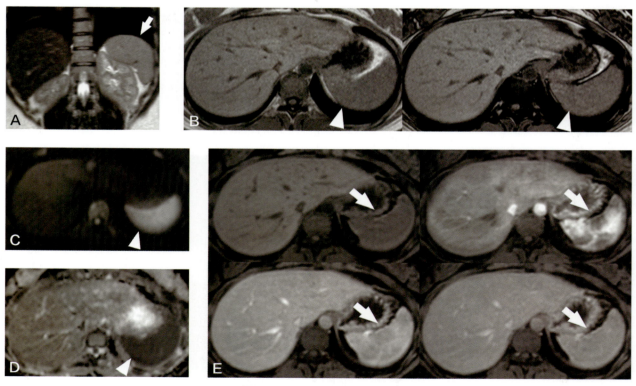

▲ 图 19-2 正常脾脏的 MRI 表现

正常脾脏（箭和箭头）在冠状 T_2 加权图像上呈稍高信号（A）；在轴位同相位 T_1 加权图像上呈低信号，在反相位上没有信号减低（B）；C. 在高 b 值的 DWI 上，脾脏呈高信号；D. 在相应的 ADC 图上呈低信号，表明该器官在正常情况下是生理性扩散受限；E. 在动态增强序列中，脾脏最常见的是在增强早期表现为弓形强化，延迟均匀强化

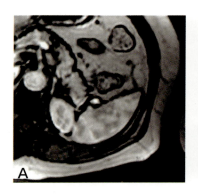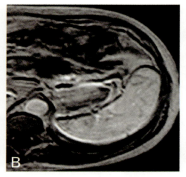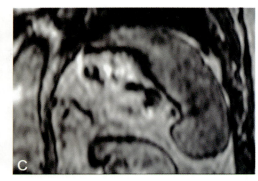

▲ 图 19-3 增强早期脾脏强化的变异

A. 正常脾脏在增强早期通常表现为弓形强化模式；B. 而早期均匀强化更常见于患肝脏疾病的患者中，这个病例则显示为肝脏脂肪变性；C. 增强早期弥漫性的脾脏低信号见于累及脾脏的继发性的输血性铁负荷过载

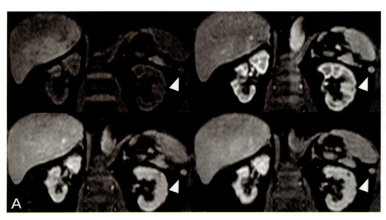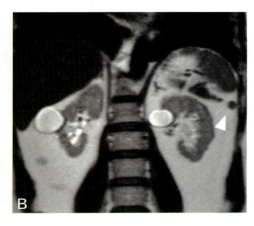

▲ 图 19-4 副脾结节

邻近脾脏下极的一个小的结节状的假病灶（箭头），在所有序列中的信号均与邻近的脾脏信号相同，在轴位 T_2 加权图像（B）上呈高信号，在冠状位 THRIVE 动态增强序列（A）表现为与脾脏相同的强化模式，符合副脾结节的表现

以位于腹部任何地方，但通常位于脾门或胰尾附近[16]。

五、多脾综合征

多脾综合征是一种先天性综合征，伴有完全性内脏转位、多发小脾脏肿块和胸腹部异常（图 19-5）。在该综合征中，脾结节通常沿胃大弯分布[16]。在脾脏切除后和外伤性脾破裂引起的脾组织种植病例中，可能会出现类似的多脾脏表现（图 19-6）。所有这些结节的 MRI 表现与脾脏相似。

六、脾大

脾脏的增大最常见于门静脉高压，尽管也可与多种疾病相关，如恶性肿瘤、感染、血管性和

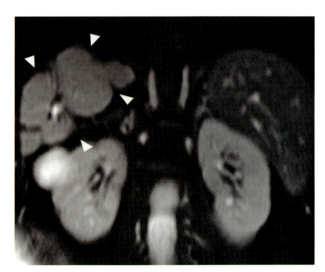

▲ 图 19-5 多脾综合征

冠状位脂肪抑制的 TSE T_2 加权图像显示上腹部内脏和血管的镜像位置表现。右侧季肋部被多个不同大小的脾结节（箭头）占据。该表现是 1 例 3 个月大的女孩的多脾综合征伴内脏转位

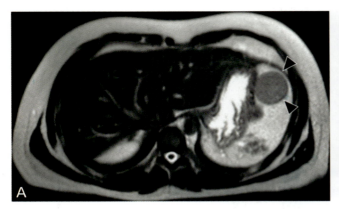
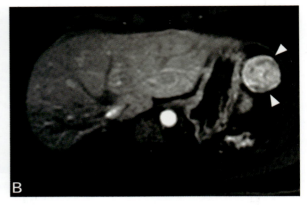

▲ 图 19-6　脾种植

在脾切除术后患者中，靠近脾的前上极可见一个结节状的假性病灶（箭头），在所有序列中的表现均与预期中的脾的表现一致。该结节在轴位 T_2 加权图像（A）上是高信号，并且增强早期图像（B）上显示脾的特征性的匐形强化模式

代谢性疾病。

门静脉高压通常是肝硬化的并发症，进行性肝纤维化导致肝窦水平的血管阻力增加[17]。这种增加的压力梯度导致了侧支循环和脾大的形成。MRI 可以在这种情况下对肝脏和脾脏进行全面评估（图 19-7）。因此，MRI 对于门静脉高压的其他表现也是有用的，例如脾静脉增宽、门体分流以及铁质沉着的脾结节（Gamna-Gandy 体）的形成。虽然对于脾大的诊断，US 是最常见的影像检查手段，MRI 具有可提供精确体积和长度测量的优势，这在需要严格随访的情况下可能是有意义的。

七、血色沉着病（含铁血黄素沉着症和镰状细胞病）

原发性血色沉着病是一种常染色体隐性遗传疾病，导致多器官铁沉积，但脾脏不受累。在继发性血色沉着病（输血相关的含铁血黄素沉着症）中，铁沉积到 RES（脾脏、骨髓和肝脏的 Kupffer 细胞）中，通常是继发于输血或横纹肌溶解[18]。在 MRI 上，由于铁沉积，在 T_1 加权图像和 T_2 加权图像上信号显著下降（图 19-8）。因为原发性和继发性血色沉着病所累及器官的差异[18]，MRI 可以准确区分两者。

镰状细胞病是非洲裔美国人群中常见的疾病，由于输血引起的铁沉积导致所有序列的

脾脏信号强度减低。在纯合子中，可导致脾脏自切除，表现为信号缺失[19]。瘢痕和梗死也是一种常见的表现[6]。

八、外伤

在钝性和穿透性创伤的情况下，脾脏是最常受伤的腹部器官。另一种可能机制是医源性损伤，可在术中发生[20]。脾脏实质可能受到挫伤、裂伤、被膜下或实质内血肿以及血管损伤的影响[6]。在急诊情况下，仍采用 US 和 CT 评估脾脏情况，尽管大多数创伤后脾脏病变可以用 MRI 进行观察。MRI 在检出小的被膜下积液或小灶性亚急性出血方面，甚至在对射线有顾虑的年轻患者或有碘对比剂禁忌证患者的随访中，均可发挥重要的作用。

九、感染性病变（感染）

病毒感染可能导致脾脏增大，但无论是脓肿还是局灶性脾脏受累都并非其他病因感染的常见特征。白色念珠菌、烟曲霉菌和新型隐球菌是大多数免疫低下患者的真菌感染的致病菌[21]。MRI 可以显示肝脾微脓肿，区分急性、亚急性和慢性病变（图 19-9）。急性病变更多见于脾脏，亚急性和慢性病变更多见于肝脏。急性病灶在 T_2 加权图像上表现为非常小的高信号病灶[22]。脂肪抑

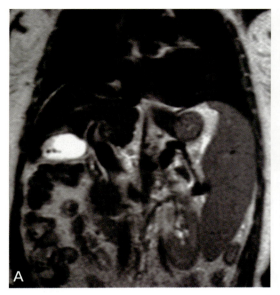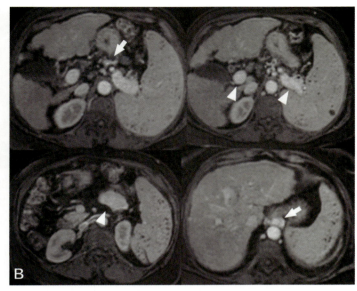

▲ 图 19-7 门静脉高压症

A. 在冠状 T_2 加权图像上可见严重的脾脏增大，继发于肝硬化；B. 注意，肝脏的肝硬化和门静脉及脾静脉（箭头）明显增粗，继发于门静脉高压症，如不同层面的动态增强图像所示。还可见到食管周围和肝胃的侧支循环静脉（白箭），以及散布在脾实质内的多个铁质沉着结节

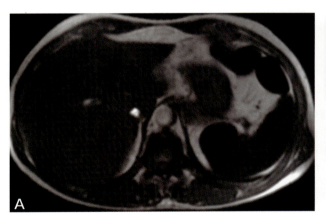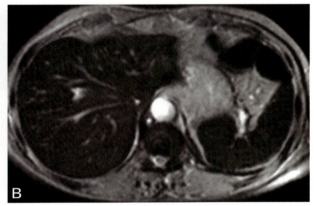

▲ 图 19-8 继发性血色沉着病，累及脾脏

在 GE T_1 加权图像（A）和 TSE T_2 加权图像（B）上，与脊柱旁肌肉相比，脾和肝实质呈现弥漫性低信号，证实为继发性血色沉着病所累及

制的 TSE T_2 加权 TSE 序列可使这些微小病变更易被发现。DWI 也能够检出这些病灶，在高 b 值图像中表现为高信号灶，在 ADC 图上表现为低信号。由于这些患者在急性期免疫功能低下或由于慢性期纤维化改变[23]，微脓肿在所有期相中都通常强化较低。组织胞浆菌病可累及脾脏，最常见于免疫功能低下的患者。在所有序列中，急性和亚急性病变表现为小结节，信号强度低（图 19-10）。与结核一样，在组织胞浆菌病的慢性期，

钙化愈合的肉芽肿也很常见。它们表现为典型的晕状伪影，在 GRE 序列中显示得更明显，反映了这些病灶的钙化性质，这通过 CT 可以很容易地确定[15]。

脾脓肿并不常见，但免疫功能低下患者数量的增加提高了脾脓肿的发病率。由于检出和治疗的延迟，脾脓肿死亡率高[24]。它们反映了全身感染，通常与心内膜炎有关，尽管它也可能是由邻近器官直接感染引起的，或者从菌血症和内源

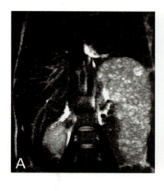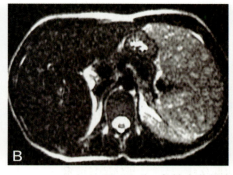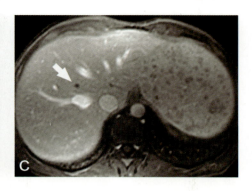

▲ 图 19-9　急性念珠菌病

冠状位和轴位脂肪抑制的 TSE T_2 加权图像上显示脾脏和肝脏上的多个微小高信号病变，代表免疫抑制患者的急性白色念珠菌的微小病变。延迟增强的 GE T_1 加权图像显示肝脏的均匀增强，仅显示了一个病变（C，白箭），以及无强化的脾脏病变。脂肪抑制的 TSE T_2 加权图像使病变显得更加明显

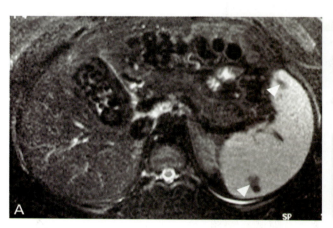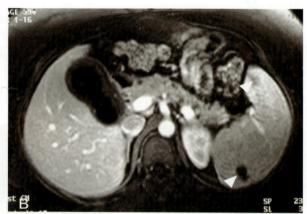

▲ 图 19-10　慢性组织胞浆菌病

1 例曾经感染过组织胞浆菌病的患者的轴位脂肪抑制的 TSE T_2 加权图像（A）和延迟增强 GE T_1 加权图像（B）图像显示 2 个低信号结节（箭头），伴与钙化肉芽肿相关的晕状伪影

性脾脏疾病发展而来[1]。主要病因是需氧菌，其次是真菌（主要是白色念珠菌）和厌氧菌。脓肿可能是单发或多发，相比于脾脏实质，在 T_1 加权图像上表现为稍低或等信号，在 T_2 加权图像上表现为不均匀稍高至中高信号。所有的感染性病灶在增强早期其边缘都表现为轻度强化，反映了包膜的形成，在延迟期也可能表现出周围灌注的变化[2]。在 DWI 上，急性期脓肿与在其他器官中一样表现为扩散受限，高 b 值时为高信号，在 ADC 图上为显著低信号（图 19-11）。如果有气体或囊性成分，信号可能更不均匀[25]。

棘球蚴感染累及脾脏的发生率介于 0.9%～8%[26]。虽然对脾脏包虫病的 MRI 特征认识有限，但它仍被认为是一种合适的评估工具，可监测治疗反应[27]。在 MRI 上，细粒棘球蚴病表现为单发或多发囊肿，伴或不伴囊壁钙化。根据囊性成分的差异，T_1 加权图像的信号可能会有所不同[22]（图 19-12）。

十、囊肿

囊肿是脾脏最常见的良性局灶性病变。它们可分为上皮性囊肿或真性囊肿，25% 的脾脏囊性病变囊壁可见上皮细胞覆盖[28]，以及假性囊肿，无上皮细胞覆盖，通常为创伤所致或为胰腺炎后遗症[21]。囊肿的 MRI 特征包括边界清晰，T_1 加权图像低信号，T_2 加权图像高亮信号（图 19-13）。含蛋白质或出血性成分的复杂性假性囊

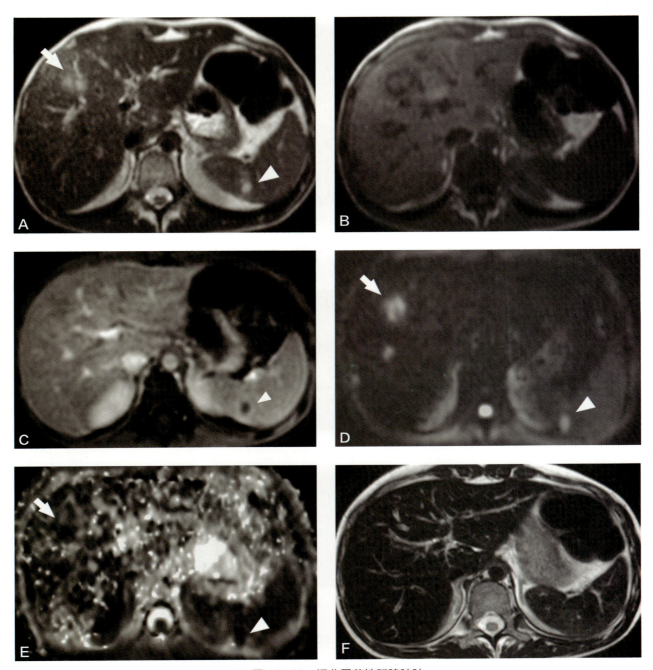

▲ 图 19-11　烟曲霉菌性肝脾脓肿

1 例肱骨骨肉瘤化疗中 14 岁女性患者的烟曲霉菌性肝脾脓肿。A. 在肝脏（白箭）和脾脏（箭头）的轴位 T_2 加权图像上可见多个囊性病变；B. 这些病变在增强前的 GE T_1 加权序列上几乎看不到；C. 在增强后这些脾脏病变表现出外周增强；D、E. 在高 b 值的 DWI 上，肝脏和脾脏病变表现出高信号，代表真正的扩散受限，因为两者在相应的 ADC 图上都是低信号；F. 经过 2 个月的抗真菌治疗后，肝脏和脾脏病变已完全消退，如轴位 TSE T_2 加权图像所示

肿可能表现为 T_1 加权图像高信号、T_2 加权图像混杂信号，或两者皆有（图 19-14）[22,28]。另外，真性囊肿可出现分隔，偶尔会出现囊壁钙化。增强扫描囊肿无强化。这些病变无扩散受限，高 b 值时为低信号，ADC 图为高信号。假性囊肿通常比真性囊肿信号更不均匀[2]。当 US 和 CT 诊断不明确时，或者需要鉴别原发性脾脏囊肿、假性囊肿以及寄生虫感染时，MRI 是一种可见帮助诊断的有效选择[15,29]。

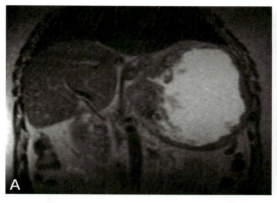
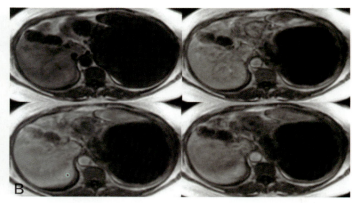

▲ 图 19-12　脾包虫病

大的复杂性囊性肿物占据了大部分脾实质。A. 在冠位 HASTE 上呈高信号，内缘不规则，伴包膜和外周钙化；B. 在动态增强序列中，病变内部未显示任何强化

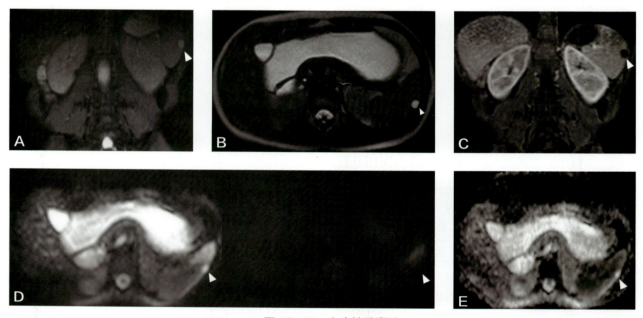

▲ 图 19-13　上皮性脾囊肿

在冠状位脂肪抑制的 SSFP 图像（A）和 HASTE 图像（B）上在脾脏的中部后缘可见一个边界清楚的高信号病灶；C. 增强后该囊肿没有强化；D. 如在囊性病变中所预期的那样，它在 DWI 上没有扩散受限，在 b 值为 0s/mm² （右图）时表现为高信号，在 b 值为 1000s/mm²（左图）时表现为低信号；E. 在 ADC 图上为高信号

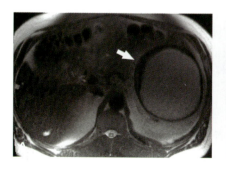
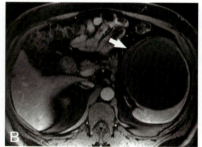
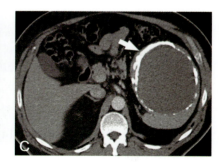

▲ 图 19-14　创伤后假性囊肿

A、B. 轴位 HASTE 和延迟增强的脂肪抑制 GE T₁ 加权图像显示被膜下的一个大的囊性病变。注意在 HASTE 上病灶周围的厚的低信号包膜（白箭），对应于增强 CT（C）所示的外周钙化

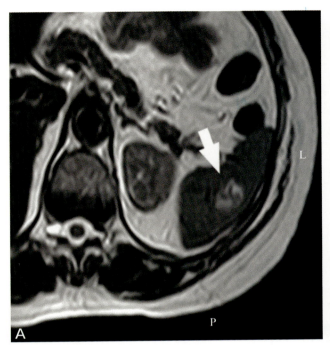 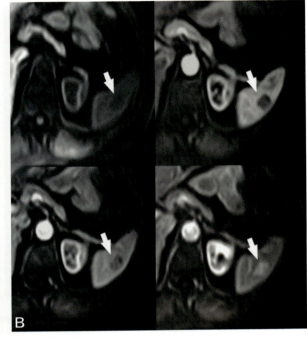

▲ 图 19-15　典型的小血管瘤

A. 在轴位 T_2 加权图像上可见结节状高信号病灶（白箭）；B. 在动态增强序列（白箭）上表现为渐进性向心性强化，在延迟期完全填充，为血管瘤的典型特征

十一、血管源性病变

（一）局灶性血管源性病变

1. 良性肿瘤

（1）血管瘤：血管瘤是脾脏第二常见的局灶性病变和最常见的良性肿瘤[30]。男性略多见，好发于 30—50 岁。它们被认为是先天性的，来自窦状上皮[24]，单发（图 19-15）或多发（图 19-16），可能是广泛性血管瘤病（Klippel-Trenaunay-Weber 和血管瘤综合征）的一部分。根据其血管通道的大小，血管瘤分为海绵状和毛细血管型[31]。

大多数血管瘤小于 2cm，通常无症状。可伴或不伴钙化。大血管瘤可能与贫血、血小板减少和凝血功能障碍（Kasabach-Merritt 综合征）有关。最常见的并发症是肿瘤破裂。其他相关并发症包括梗死、血栓形成、纤维化、脾功能亢进，甚至恶变[32]。它们在 MRI 上的表现因其大小而异。

血管瘤是边界清楚、信号均匀的脾脏病变，在 T_1 加权图像上为低至等信号，在 T_2 加权图像上相对于脾脏背景为稍高信号，其在 T_2 加权图像上也可能为等信号或低信号[30]，其中低信号通常与硬化血管瘤相关（图 19-17）[24]。静脉注射对比剂后，最常见的表现是边缘强化，延迟期对比剂填充至均匀增强，但偶尔会表现为早期均匀强化、延迟期持续强化（图 19-18）。虽然也可以看到典型肝脏血管瘤强化方式，即早期边缘结节状强化、渐进性向心性填充强化，但并不多见[32]。因此，一个小的脾脏病变，在 T_2 加权图像上呈高信号，增强早期均匀强化或边缘强化，高度提示为血管瘤。

较大的血管瘤是异质性更高的病变，部分区域可能存在出血和血栓形成。增强后表现为向心性强化，延迟扫描可有代表中央瘢痕的持续无强化区域或为均匀强化（图 19-19）。较大的血管瘤需要随访或组织学检查以确定其来源，因为血管肉瘤也有类似的表现[33]。

根据经验，脾血管瘤由于为长 T_2 而表现出与肝血管瘤相似的特征。在高 b 值时，它通常是低信号，但由于 T_2 穿透效应偶尔会在高 b 值时表现

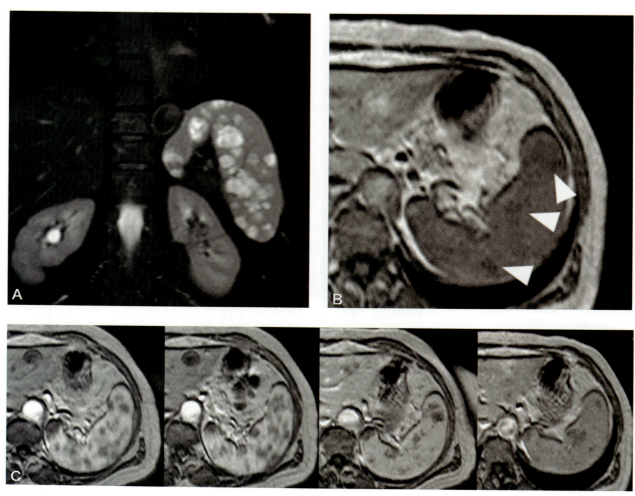

▲ 图 19-16　多发性血管瘤

1例8岁男性患者，常规超声检查发现脾脏增大和多发局灶性脾脏病变。MRI可以更好地显示局灶性脾脏病变：A. 在冠状位脂肪抑制的 T_2 加权图像上可见脾实质中多发散在的高信号结节；B.GE 同相位 T_1 加权图像上显示这些病灶大多数信号与邻近实质相仿，尽管其中一些病灶呈略低信号（箭头）；C. 在增强早期、1min、5min 和 10min 延迟增强图像上，这些病变显示向心性渐进性强化，符合多发血管瘤

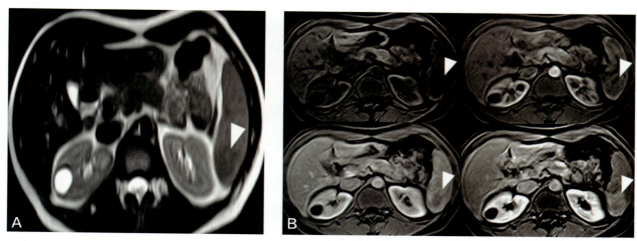

▲ 图 19-17　硬化性血管瘤

A. 轴位 T_2 加权图像（箭头）上可见脾脏后部结节状的低信号；B. 在动态增强序列中，这个病变表现为血管瘤典型的渐进性向心性强化（箭头）

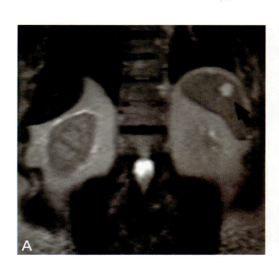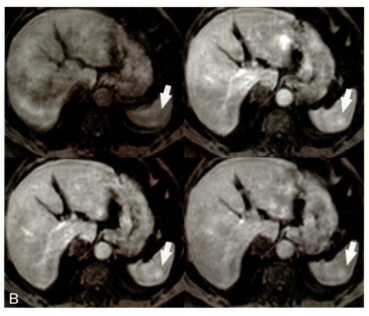

▲ 图 19-18　在增强早期表现为均匀强化的血管瘤

A. 在冠状位 T_2 加权图像（黑箭）上可见一个结节状的高信号病变；B. 其在增强早期、1min 和延迟图像中表现为均匀强化（白箭）

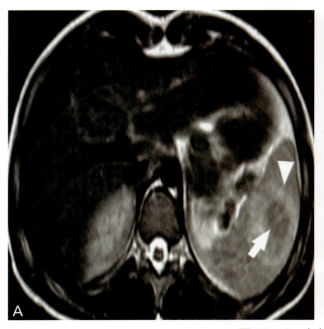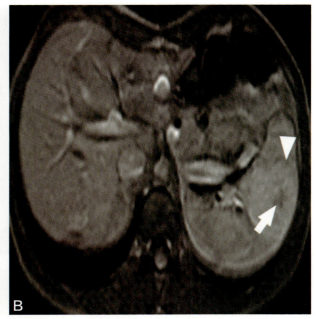

▲ 图 19-19　大血管瘤伴有中央瘢痕

A. 在轴位 TSE T_2 加权图像上可见一个结节状的不均匀高信号病灶（箭头），伴有低信号的中央区域（白箭）；B. 在延迟增强图像上表现为外周均匀强化（箭头），中央瘢痕无强化（白箭）

为高信号，但不变的是，它们在 ADC 图上表现为高信号。因此，脾脏血管瘤并非真正的扩散受限。

（2）窦岸细胞血管瘤：窦岸细胞血管瘤（littoral cell angioma，LCA）是一种罕见的血管源性病变，通常是良性的，能有恶性成分。它起源于沿着红髓的脾窦排列的窦岸细胞，可被认为是一个相对较新的临床病理学类型。该病变还与其他肿瘤相关，包括结直肠癌、肾癌、胰腺癌和脑膜瘤[32]。LCA

患者通常表现出脾功能亢进（贫血和血小板减少）。

LCA 通常表现为多发小结节和脾大。它们的影像表现多样，取决于其组织学特征，解剖上是不规则囊样管腔的血管通道，壁由高的内皮细胞排列覆盖[24]。最常见的是，因肿瘤细胞吞噬血细胞而形成的充满含铁血黄素的融合结节[34]。在 MRI 上，这些结节在 T_1 加权图像为低信号，而在 T_2 加权图像上信号可有差异，由于铁质沉积，它们可表现为低信号（图 19-20）。在动态增强图像上，LCA 在动脉期强化可略不均匀，延迟期均匀强化，代表对比剂池（contrast pooling）[35,36]。脾切除对于明确诊断和治疗通常是必需的。恶性 LCA 在病理上有浸润性或实性生长表现，提示为血管肉瘤。

（3）血管内皮瘤：血管内皮瘤是一种非常罕见的原发性血管源性肿瘤，由内皮细胞覆盖的小血管通道增生形成。它可能是血管瘤和血管肉瘤之间的中间体。脾血管内皮瘤常发生在年轻人，偶尔发生于儿童，表现为可触及疼痛性肿块[32]。

在 MRI 检查中，血管内皮瘤表现为异质性的实性肿块，在 T_1 加权图像和 T_2 加权图像上呈低信号，提示存在含铁血黄素[32]。肝脏血管内皮瘤可常见浸润性改变、坏死或出血，被膜皱缩罕见[37]。

（4）硬化性血管瘤样结节性转化：硬化性血管瘤样结节性转化（sclerosing angiomatoid nodular transformation,SANT）是一种良性血管源性脾脏病变，由多个血管瘤样结节、周围包绕致密的纤维组织形成，纤维组织在中心可能更明显，形成瘢痕。血管瘤样结节可以是通常在红髓中发现的不同类型的血管。它是 2004 年由 Martel 等发现的新病变[38]。其中大多数是影像偶然发现，与

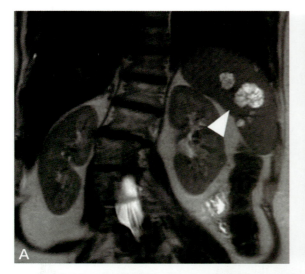
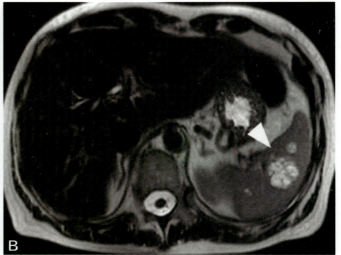
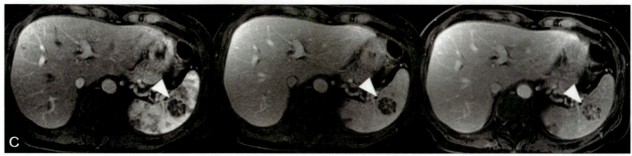

▲ 图 19-20　窦岸细胞血管瘤

A、B. 冠状位和轴位 TSE T_2 加权图像上显示在正常大小的脾脏内可见多个含内部分隔的高信号结节（箭头）；C. 在脂肪抑制的增强早期、1min 和延迟期的 GE T_1 加权图像图像中，这些结节表现出不同程度的内部强化，显示了该肿瘤的血管本质（箭头）

其他部位的恶性肿瘤相关。SANT 发生于中年人，女性略多见[39]。罕见情况下，SANT 会引起诸如腹痛、贫血或脾大等症状。在所有报道的病例中，脾脏切除术都是治愈性的。最近，3 个小型的系列报道在报道有限的病例之前，都更好地描述了 SANT 的影像特征[39-41]。SANT 是单发的结节性病变，无坏死或囊变，伴陈旧性出血灶，陈旧性出血灶在 T_2 加权图像上显示为低信号区域，并可导致化学位移成像中的信号减低[2,5,39,42]。在动态增强序列中最常见的表现是轮辐状改变，即指在动脉期或门静脉期表现为外周强化的放射状线样或边缘强化，在延迟期表现为渐进性或持续强化。强化的辐射线对应于纤维性瘢痕的分支，边缘强化对应于病变边缘的血管瘤样结节，延迟强化则代表了病变内纤维瘢痕和血管瘤样成分。该病变在 T_2 加权图像上主要是低信号，偶尔可出现钙化。因此，SANT 具有特征性的 MRI 表现，有助于与其他良性血管源性脾病变的鉴别。

2. 恶性肿瘤

（1）血管肉瘤：原发性脾脏血管肉瘤是一种非常罕见的血管源性肿瘤，它是最常见的脾脏原发性非淋巴性恶性肿瘤[22]。他们与其他恶性肿瘤的关联并不少见，不像肝脏血管肉瘤那样需要有二氧化钍的暴露史[43]。该病最常发生于老年人，没有性别偏好。血管肉瘤已被报道可见于淋巴瘤化疗患者或乳腺癌放疗患者。脾大几乎总是与脾功能亢进的常见症状相关。该肿瘤在高达 30% 的患者中可增加脾脏自破裂的风险。肝脏、肺、骨、骨髓和淋巴系统转移是常见的转移部位[32]。

在 MRI 上，血管肉瘤通常表现为多发结节或肿物，T_1 加权图像和 T_2 加权图像信号与血液成分和坏死相关（图 19-21）。铁质沉积结节可导致低

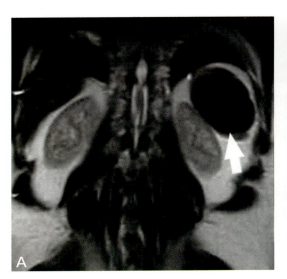
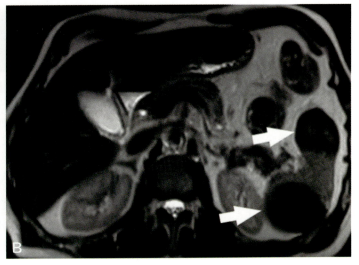
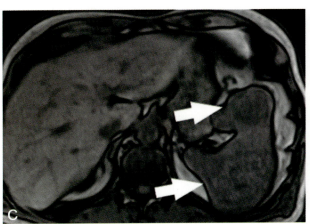
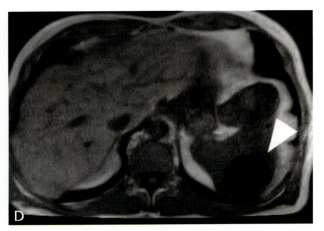

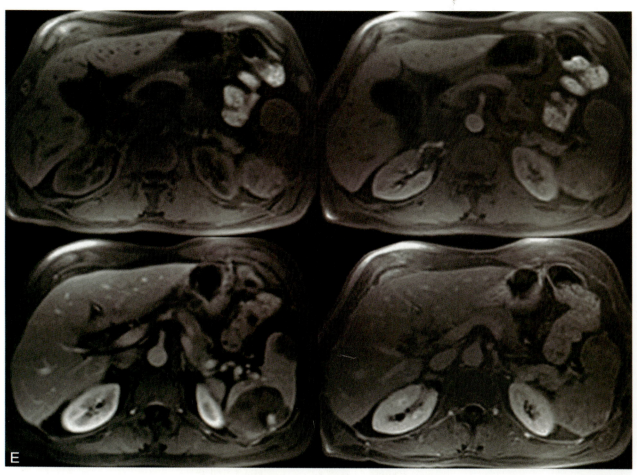

▲ 图 19-21 血管肉瘤

A、B. 在冠状位和轴位 TSE T_2 加权图像图像上可见肿大的脾脏内多发低信号病变（白箭）；C、D. 在轴位的化学位移序列中，这些病变相对于脾脏呈等 - 稍低信号（白箭）。其中一个在同相位序列（箭头）上呈现出重要的信号减低，与含铁血黄素一致；E. 在钆动态增强序列中，这些肿物表现为不均匀的渐进性强化模式

信号[44]。增强后，该病变因其血管本质而表现为明显且不均匀的强化[22]。血管肉瘤由于其内不同阶段的血液成分，因此影像表现存在异质性，这可能与良性病变如血管内皮瘤、血管瘤或窦岸细胞血管瘤难以鉴别。除非血管肉瘤表现出边界不清或脾外受累等侵袭性特征，最终确诊需要依赖脾切除以明确病理诊断。MRI 是评估所有这些病变的最佳影像检查方式，特别是对于血管肉瘤[15]。

（2）血管外皮细胞瘤：血管外皮细胞瘤是一种罕见的血管源性良性肿瘤，具有较高的恶变潜能[45]。此外，在组织学上，很难确定这种肿瘤的生物学侵袭性程度[46]。它很少起源于脾脏，当发生在脾脏时，血管外皮细胞瘤是起源于毛细血管周细胞的富血供肿瘤。它通常无症状，也可能出现与脾大相关的临床症状。文献中仅有少数的脾脏原发性血管外皮细胞瘤的报道[32,45,47-49]。血管外皮细胞瘤表现为脾内多发融合结节，实性成分强化明显，囊性成分无强化。瘤内可见出血。在 MRI 上，血管外皮细胞瘤表现为 T_1 加权图像低信号、T_2 加权图像高信号，实性成分强化明显[32,49]。由于局部复发率高，脾切除术后影像随访是必要的[45]。

3. 非肿瘤性病变

（1）脾梗死：脾梗死常见，最常见原因是心源性的栓子栓塞或者是由脾动脉或其一个分支阻塞引起的。脾梗死也可能由于高凝状态或潜在的血液疾病所致[1]。脾梗死的其他原因是血栓形成、血管炎和脾扭转。脾梗死可伴有急性左上腹痛。

Chapter 19 脾脏磁共振成像新进展
Update in Magnetic Resonance Imaging of the Spleen

急性炎症相关的发热和实验室检查提示为栓子所致。梗死通常为局灶性的，但可以是弥漫性的。

在 MRI 检查中，脾梗死通常表现为外周楔形缺损区，但也可以是圆形或线形。通常，它们在动态增强晚期显示最清楚，表现为无强化的低信号区（图 19-22）。脾被膜表现为边缘线样强化，称为边缘征[50]。脾梗死的信号可以因其成分和时间不同而变化，但通常为 T_1 加权图像低信号，T_2 加权图像不均匀高信号。出血性梗死在 T_1 加权图像和 T_2 加权图像上表现为高信号。在诊断需要十分谨慎，因为 50% 的急性脾梗死无典型影像表现，而是表现为多发结节、边缘不清和信号不均匀[22,51]。在这些情况下，很难与其他病变鉴别，如肿瘤、血肿或脓肿。弥漫性脾梗死可表现为脾脏完全无强化，只有皮质边缘征，表现为一层薄薄的残留被膜强化[52]。慢性脾梗死在所有序列中均为低信号。在这个阶段，梗死可能消失，或者更常见的表现为脾脏边缘无血管区伴被膜皱缩，有时可伴钙化[52]。

（2）血肿：在 MRI 上，由于不同损伤时间的血红蛋白降解产物的顺磁性不同，被膜下或实质内血肿可显示出不同的信号强度。在急性期，血肿 T_1 加权图像呈高信号、T_2 加权图像呈低信号[50]。亚急性出血尤其明显，因为它在 T_1 加权图像和 T_2 加权图像上均呈高信号。慢性期（超过 3 周）通常随着液化而演变为囊性，有时伴有含铁血黄素环（图 19-23）[21]。无血供病灶在增强早期显示最清晰，与正常血供的脾组织的高信号相比，

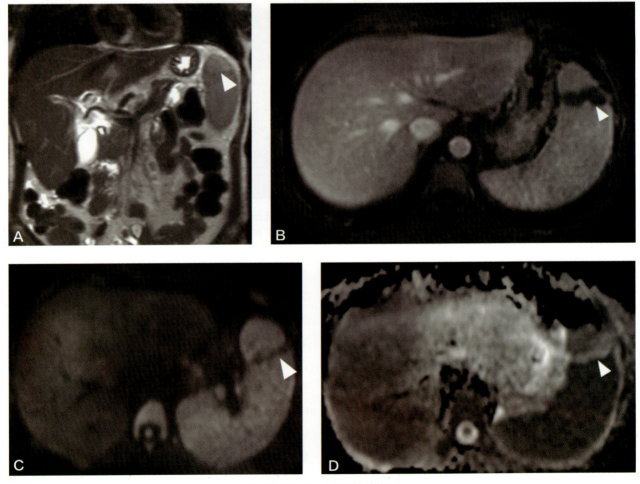

▲ 图 19-22　陈旧性脾梗死

在脾上极可见带状的外周病变（箭头），其在冠状位 HASTE（A）上呈略高信号并且在脂肪抑制的 GE T_1WI 延迟增强图像（B）上没有强化。注意，如高 b 值的 DWI（C）和相应的 ADC 图（D）所示，该病变没有扩散限制

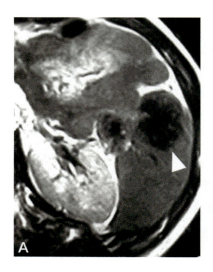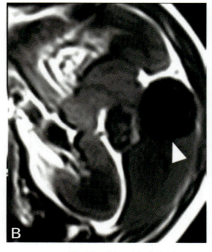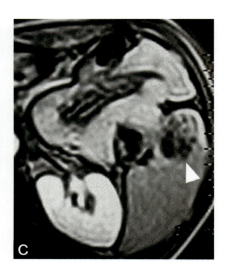

▲ 图 19-23 脾脏血肿

轴位 TSE T_2 加权图像（A）和 GE T_1 加权图像（B）序列显示脾脏前部的一个圆形低信号肿物，代表陈旧性的愈合血肿（箭头）；C. 轴位延迟增强 GE T_1 加权图像图像显示该肿物的边缘和内部不均匀强化（箭头）

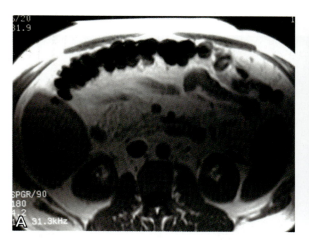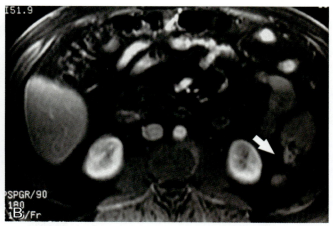

▲ 图 19-24 动静脉畸形

轴位 GE T_1 加权图像（A）和脂肪抑制的增强 VIBE（B）图像上可见脾脏下部的小的信号流空区域，伴迂曲的强化

表现为非常低的信号。在 T_2WI 上，陈旧性血肿通常是低信号。

（二）弥漫性病变

1. 动静脉畸形 脾脏中罕见动静脉畸形和动静脉瘘。动静脉瘘可能是先天性或后天性的，孕妇和多产妇女的风险增加[52]。听诊时通常表现为机械样杂音，主要的临床表现为门静脉高压。MRI 可以提示该诊断，因为所有平扫序列均可见流空效应，在动态增强序列中表现为特征性的早期迂曲样强化（图 19-24）[15]。此外，早期强化的迂曲扩张的脾静脉具有很强的提示性[53]。

2. 血管瘤病 血管瘤病是一种非常罕见的血管肿瘤样病变[54]。在组织病理学上，应将血管瘤病与脾脏的其他表现典型的脾窦内皮特征的肿瘤样血管病变区分开来，如 LCA 或紫癜[55]（图 19-25）。最常见的是，该病变是全身性血管瘤病的一种表现，与 Klippel-Trenaunay-Weber、Turner、Kasabach-Merritt-like、Proteus 和 Beckwith-Wiedemann 综合征相关[15]。其 MRI 表现与血管肉瘤有所重叠[2]。

3. 淋巴管瘤 淋巴管瘤由小的囊性扩张的淋巴管组成。脾淋巴管瘤很少见，是脾脏第三常见的良性肿瘤。淋巴管瘤可以单发，但多发更

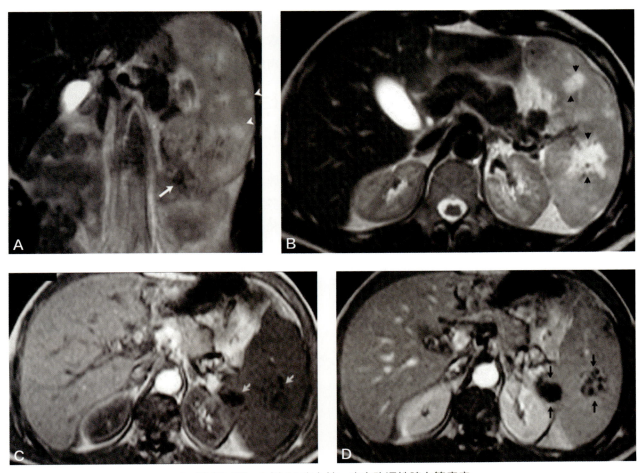

▲ 图 19-25 1 例 41 岁女性，患有弥漫性脾血管瘤病

A、B. 冠状位和轴位 TSE T_2 加权图像图像显示增大的脾脏内可见多发高信号局灶性脾脏病变（箭头）和代表铁质沉积灶的低信号结节（白箭）；C. 轴位平扫的梯度回波 T_1 加权图像图像显示低信号结节，同时存在代表铁质沉积灶的磁敏感伪影（白色箭）；D. 增强后（1min）梯度回波 T_1 加权图像图像显示 2 个结节轻微的边缘强化（黑色箭）。上方的结节表现为内部不均匀强化。在血管肉瘤或窦岸细胞血管瘤的病例中，也可能出现脾脏不均质的表现（经许可引自 Luna, A. 等，AJR Am.J. Roentgenol., 186, 1533, 2006.）

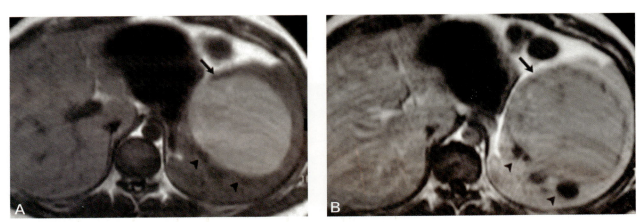

▲ 图 19-26 淋巴管瘤

1 例 27 岁女性，在常规超声检查中检出复杂性囊性肿块，后来在 CT 上确诊。轴位平扫（A）和增强（B）GE T_1 加权图像图像显示可见一多房囊性肿物，伴有低信号（箭头）和高信号（黑色箭）的无强化区域，证实了该病变的囊性特性。高信号区域是由于存在蛋白质成分。脾切除术后确诊（经许可引自 Luna,A. 等，AJR Am.J. Roentgenol., 186,1533,2006.）

常见，可累及多个器官（淋巴管瘤病）。通常无明显临床症状，但目前已有报道部分病例可出现占位效应、出血或脾亢、门静脉高压以及破裂等症状。有症状的肿瘤可能需要部分或完全脾切除。

在 MRI 上，淋巴管瘤表现为多房囊性病变，由纤维分隔隔开，在 T_2 加权图像上为高信号，增强扫描无强化[50]（图 19-26）。囊性部分在 T_1 加权图像上通常为典型的低信号，尽管其中一些可能因为含蛋白质成分，或更少情况下因为出血，表现为 T_1 加权图像高信号[21]。虽然曲线形钙化是淋巴管瘤的一个不常见特征，但它们很难在 MRI 上被观察到[45]。淋巴管瘤的恶变罕见，MRI 能够显示出囊内的实性成分[32]。

4. 紫癜 紫癜是一种罕见疾病，累及脾脏和肝脏的血窦。大多数病例与使用合成类固醇有关，但也可能与再生障碍性贫血、结核、获得性免疫缺陷综合征（acquired immune-deficiency syndrome，AIDS）以及癌症有关。紫癜通常为偶然发现，除非脾脏表面的紫癜破裂导致腹腔内出血。这些病变的破裂可能是自发性的或继发于轻微外伤。其特征性的病理表现为多发椭圆形或圆形明显扩张的囊性病变，内充填血液，主要位于滤泡旁区，需要与充血的脾脏血窦相鉴别[56]。

在 MRI 检查中，可看到多发病灶，T_2 加权图像上为高信号，T_1 加权图像信号多样（图 19-27）。由于存在脱氧血红蛋白和高铁血红蛋白，血栓形成的囊腔表现为 T_2 加权图像混杂信号。液-液平面以及钙化的缺失也常见于该病[32]。最近已有肝脏紫癜在 DWI 上扩散受限的报道[57]。紫癜的影像学鉴别诊断可包括血管瘤病、淋巴管瘤和血管肉瘤。

（三）其他血管源性病变

1. 脾动脉瘤 脾动脉瘤是最常见的内脏动脉瘤。大多数脾动脉瘤较小（小于 2cm），呈囊状，位于脾动脉的中远段。在 20% 的病例中，它们可以是多发的[58]。脾动脉瘤与女性、妊娠（由于雌激素和孕激素对动脉壁的激素作用）和门静脉高压有很强的相关性。其他病因包括动脉粥样硬化、先天性和霉菌性以及肌纤维发育不良。脾动脉假性动脉瘤也是胰腺炎的并发症之一，由于胰酶消化动脉壁，或继发于外伤[15]。最严重的并发症是破裂，死亡率高。

脾动脉瘤通常是偶然的发现。使用增强 3D-GRE 序列或 3D MR 血管成像序列可以有效地诊断和显示脾动脉瘤的特征，后者可以更清晰地显示病变（图 19-28）[59]。上述两个序列均表现为瘤腔的早期强化，该瘤腔在平扫的序列上为低信号。相反，如果存在血凝块，则表现为高信号[52]。

2. 脾静脉血栓形成 脾静脉血栓形成的原因有很多，最常见的是胰腺炎。它可在至少 20% 的慢性胰腺炎患者中出现[15]。在 MRI 检查中，在血管成像序列上表现为脾静脉充盈缺损。急性血栓形成在 T_1 加权图像和 T_2 加权图像上均为高信号，在真稳态进动快速采集图像上表现为低

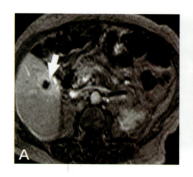
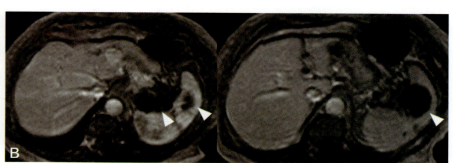

▲ 图 19-27 肝脾紫癜

1 例 72 岁女性，患有播散性结核和肝脾紫癜。A、B. 三个不同层面的动脉期增强 T_1 GE 图像上可见被膜下的多囊性肿块延伸至脾门，伴分隔和边缘强化（箭头），几个肝脏囊性病变也有边缘强化（白箭）

信号[52]。在慢性脾静脉血栓形成的情况下，会形成侧支循环，常见为胃静脉曲张。对比增强和非对比增强的 MR 血管成像技术可以准确地显示这些门体侧支循环的分布情况[60]。

脾静脉血栓形成可以是良性的或恶性的，可以根据其 MRI 特征进行鉴别。良性血栓在 T_2 加权图像上为低信号，且无强化。瘤栓通常见于胰腺癌患者，T_2 加权图像为高信号，增强后可见强化（图19-29）。

十二、非血管源性肿瘤

（一）良性肿瘤

1. 错构瘤 错构瘤是一种罕见的非肿瘤性肿瘤，由不同的脾组织混合组成[30]。它可以发生在任何年龄，发病率无性别差异。该病变通常是偶然发现的，一般表现为边界清楚的、圆形、单发的实性病变[61]。该病变也可以是囊性的，并可伴点状钙化。它们最常发生在脾脏的中部。可分为白髓或红髓型错构瘤，但大多数是这两种细胞类型的混合体。它很少有临床症状，可导致脾大、全血细胞减少、疲劳和厌食。脾脏错构瘤通常与结节性硬化有关，也可能与 Wiskott–Aldrich-like 综合征有关。

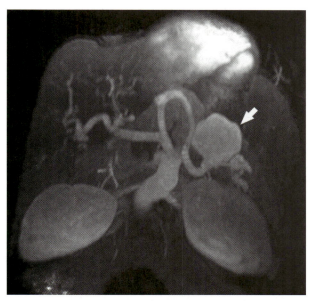

▲ 图 19-28 脾动脉假性动脉瘤
在动脉期的 3D MR 血管成像的斜轴位 MIP 上可以观察到一个大的脾动脉局灶性偏心性扩张（白箭）

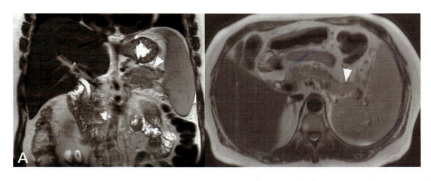

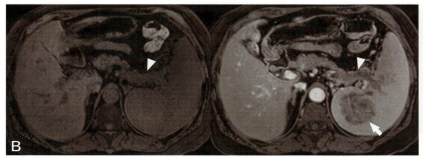 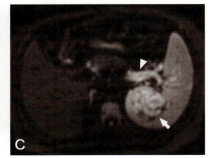

▲ 图 19-29 恶性脾静脉血栓形成
1 例 57 岁女性，有卵巢癌病史；A. 在冠状位和轴位 HASTE 上，脾静脉增厚，伴有高信号的内容物；B. 轴位增强前后脂肪抑制的 GE T_1 加权图像图像显示增强后血栓强化，提示其为瘤栓。此外，还注意到一个脾脏的血行转移瘤（白箭）；C. 在高 b 值的 DWI 上，血栓和转移瘤均显示高信号，即扩散受限，提示其恶性起源

在 MRI 上，典型的脾错构瘤在 T_2 加权图像上表现为混杂高信号，在 T_1 加权图像上为等信号[30]。偶然情况下，错构瘤在 T_2 加权图像上可出现低信号区，代表纤维组织。T_2 加权图像上的这种表现及其典型的增强早期轻度不均匀强化是鉴别错构瘤和血管瘤的关键特征。在增强扫描延迟期，错构瘤表现为相对均匀的明显强化[62]（图 19-30），伴中央低血供的瘢痕或囊性区[30]。尽管错构瘤的影像表现可能与血管瘤和转移有重叠，对放射科医师来说具有挑战，但 MRI 可以更明确地提示错构瘤。

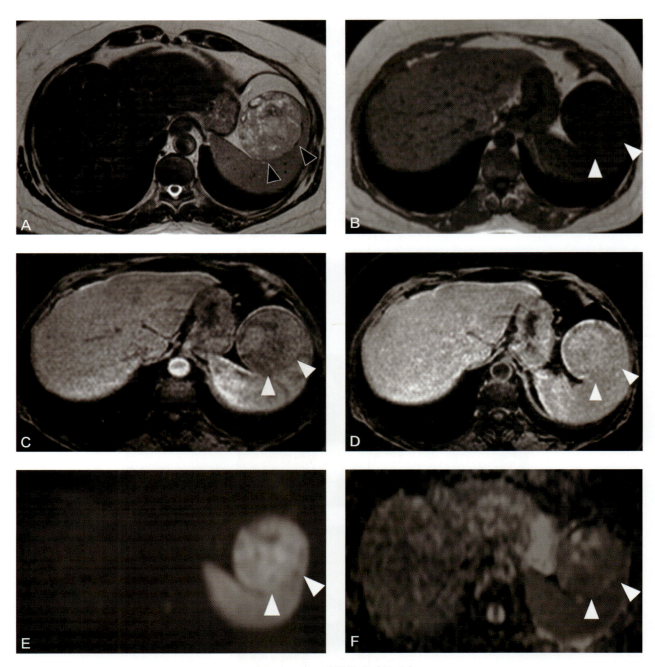

▲ 图 19-30　脾错构瘤（箭头）
A. 轴位 TSE T_2 加权图像显示脾脏前部的不均匀高信号结节样病变；B. 在 GE T_1 加权图像序列上，与脾实质相比，该病变呈略低信号；C. 该肿物在钆增强早期的脂肪抑制 GE T_1 加权图像图像上呈不均匀强化；D. 在延迟增强的脂肪抑制 GE T_1 加权图像图像上表现为相对均匀的明显强化；E. 在高 b 值的 DWI 上，该病变为高信号；F. 在相应的 ADC 图为低信号，提示其细胞密集、扩散受限

2. 脂肪性肿瘤 脂肪瘤和血管平滑肌脂肪瘤、脾脏原发性脂肪性肿瘤非常罕见，尽管已有脂肪瘤[15]和血管平滑肌脂肪瘤[63]的病理学描述，但无相关的影像报道。脂肪瘤是一种罕见的脾脏良性肿瘤，是完全由脂肪组成的软组织肿块[28]。与在身体其他部位的脂肪瘤一样，MRI可以准确地描述其特征。脂肪瘤在所有序列上的信号均与脂肪一样，在 T_1 加权图像和 T_2 加权图像上为高信号，在脂肪抑制序列上信号显著下降。在增强后，典型的单纯性脂肪瘤没有强化[64]。

（二）恶性非血管源性肿瘤

1. 淋巴瘤 脾淋巴瘤是最常见的脾脏恶性肿瘤[1]。霍奇金和非霍奇金淋巴瘤均可发生，可以是原发性的，更常见的是作为全身性（继发性）疾病的一部分[65]。原发性脾淋巴瘤很罕见，在淋巴瘤中比例不足1%[66]；大多数原发性淋巴瘤属于非霍奇金型（图19-31）。高达40%的淋巴瘤患者可出现继发性脾淋巴瘤[22]。这些患者症状无特异性，最常表现为左上腹疼痛或全身症状。常见伴发脾大和腹膜后淋巴结肿大。淋巴瘤可以侵透被膜并侵犯周围器官。

原发性和继发性淋巴瘤累及脾脏有4种表现形式：均匀性脾大，无局灶性病变；弥漫浸润的粟粒性病变，粟粒性病变小于5mm；多发局灶性结节样病变；单发的孤立性大肿物[21,65,67,68]。弥漫性、均匀的浸润性病变是继发性脾淋巴瘤的最常见形式，可表现为正常的脾脏外观或单独的脾大。脾大本身并不具有特异性，因为脾脏在出现肿瘤浸润时大小也可能正常，在没有肿瘤累及时也可能增大。相反，原发性淋巴瘤表现为一个孤立的巨大肿块[22]。脾脏受累的表现形式与细胞类型有关；大的、孤立的肿块通常是大细胞淋巴瘤，多发肿物或粟粒性浸润最常与其他非霍奇金淋巴瘤相关[67,69]。

在MRI上，弥漫性、浸润性脾脏受累难以用平扫图像检出，在增强早期表现为不规则的高低信号混杂区域[22]。局灶性受累也很难被发现，因为大多数结节在 T_1 和 T_2 加权图像上与脾实质信号相仿，部分在 T_2 加权图像上可能表现为低信号，

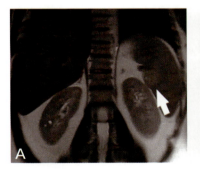
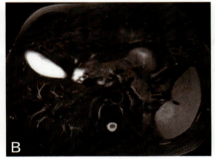
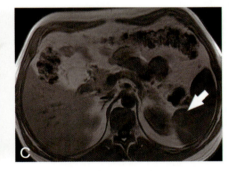
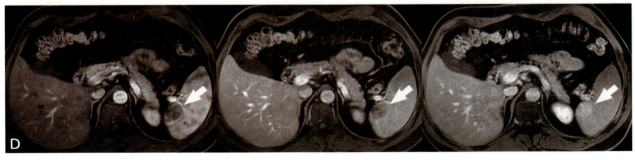

▲ 图 19-31 原发肿块样脾淋巴瘤

1例44岁的患者，进行性脾脏增大和局灶性脾脏病变：A. 在冠状位 TSE T_2 加权图像上，观察到一个略高信号的结节状病变（白箭）；B. 其在轴位脂肪抑制的 FSE T_2 加权图像上更加明显；C. 在 GE T_1 加权图像上，该病变与脾实质信号相仿；D. 在早期、1min 和 5min 延迟增强 THRIVE 图像中，病变表现为渐进性强化，在延迟期为均匀强化。脾切除术证实为原发性脾淋巴瘤

这一点可与转移瘤相鉴别，转移瘤在 T_2 加权图像上罕见低信号[2]。在增强早期，结节表现为低强化，增强后第 1 分钟内强化程度与脾脏实质相仿，延迟期呈渐进性、多样化的强化（图 19-32）[50]。淋巴瘤结节可出现小的不规则异常信号区，提示坏死、纤维化、水肿和出血[67]。在淋巴瘤评估中，早期增强 MRI 扫描优于 CT，然而，MRI 的具体作用还不确定[24]。SPIO 的使用使得脾淋巴瘤更易观察，在 T_2 加权图像上，与低信号的脾实质相比，脾淋巴瘤表现为高信号[7,70]。在 DWI 上，这些病变在高 b 值时为高信号，在相应的 ADC 图上为低信号，如同体内其他部位一样，为明显扩散限制。淋巴瘤在 PET 中表现为重要的 18-氟代脱氧葡萄糖（fluorodeoxyglucose，FDG）摄取，任何脾脏 FDG 浓聚的区域均需怀疑为淋巴瘤[71]。

化疗后，淋巴瘤结节的影像特征可能会改变，在 T_1 和 T_2 加权图像上的信号强度减低，这与化疗诱导的纤维化反应有关，提示治疗有效。

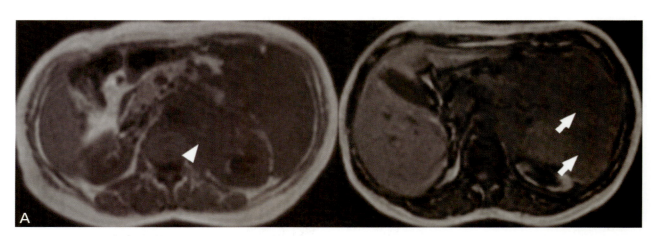

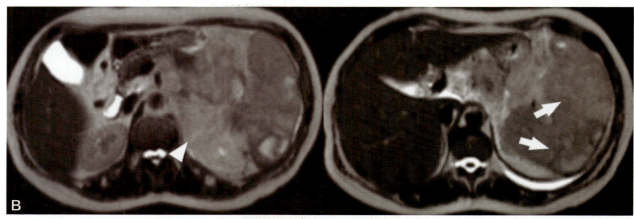

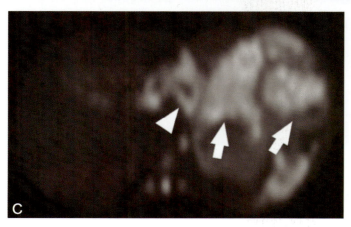

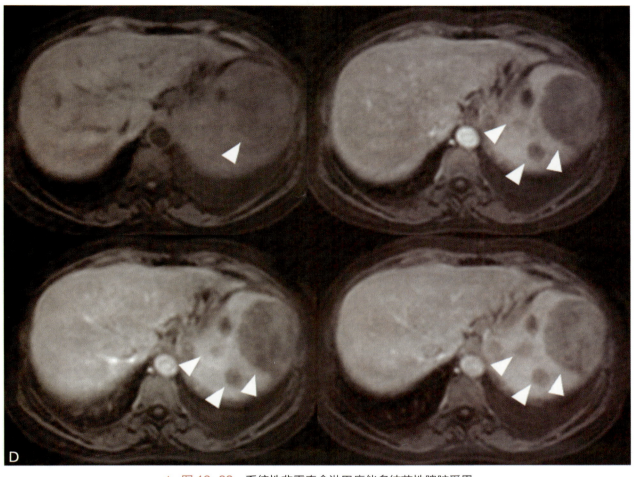

▲ 图 19-32 系统性非霍奇金淋巴瘤伴多结节性脾脏受累

1 例 57 岁女性，有全身症状：两个不同层面的轴位 GE T_1 加权图像（A）和 TSE T_2 加权图像（B）图像显示腹膜后一个大的侵袭性肿块，浸润左肾、胰腺体/尾和胃。此外，可见脾的弥漫性和多结节性受累。脾脏局灶性病变在 T_1 加权图像上为等信号，在 T_2 加权图像上呈高信号；C. 在高 b 值的 DWI 上，腹膜后肿块和脾脏局灶性病变（分别为箭头和白箭）表现出重要的扩散受限；D. 在动态增强序列中，脾脏病变在所有期相均为低血供（箭头），伴有轻度渐进性强化

2. 白血病 急性髓性白血病是最常见的累及脾脏的白血病亚型[64]。白血病的脾脏受累通常无异常的影像表现，或表现为均匀的脾脏增大伴继发于白血病浸润的 T_2 值延长，可伴有腹部淋巴结肿大。在脾脏明显增大的情况下，可能出现自发性脾破裂。在白血病患者中，脾梗死和脾脓肿的发生率增加[22]。

绿色瘤罕见，最常与慢性淋巴细胞性白血病相关，在 MRI 上显示为多发边界不清的肿块，增强早期无强化（图 19-33）[2]。

3. 转移瘤 血源性脾脏转移瘤是罕见的，通常发生在疾病的晚期。最常见的转移到脾脏的原发性肿瘤是乳腺癌、肺癌、卵巢癌、胃癌、黑色素瘤和前列腺癌[21,22]。

在 MRI 上，脾脏转移瘤在 T_1 加权图像上信号与脾实质相仿，在 T_2 加权图像上呈等或高信号[72]。在急性出血或黑色素瘤转移的情况下，在 T_1 加权图像上可能表现为高信号[21]。其他与原发肿瘤相关的特征包括结肠腺癌转移的坏死或囊腺癌转移的钙化[22]。增强扫描的强化程度和特点取决于原发肿瘤的性质。通常情况下，脾脏转移瘤在增强早期为低强化，在延迟期为等强化[10,73]。淋巴瘤在 T_1 加权图像和 T_2 加权图像上无高信号表现，这一点有助于区分淋巴瘤和转移瘤。SPIO 的使用可提高它们的检出率[7]。在 DWI 上，脾转移瘤扩散受限，在高 b 值时为高信号，

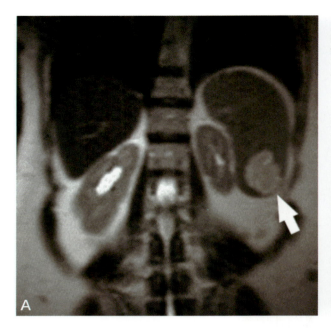
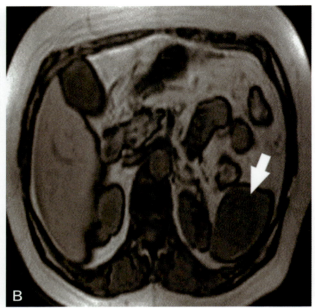
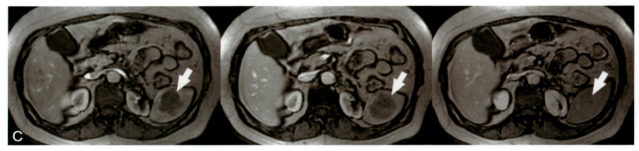

▲ 图 19-33　绿色瘤

1 例患有急性髓性白血病的 5 岁男孩：A. 在冠状位 TSE T_2 加权图像图像上，可见脾脏下极的一个高信号结节（白箭）；B. 在反相位 GE T_1 加权图像上呈略低信号（白箭）；C. 在动态增强图像上（白箭），早期为低强化（左图），在延迟增强信号与脾实质相仿（右图）

在 ADC 图上为低信号（图 19-34）。

在卵巢癌、胃肠道腺癌和胰腺癌的病例中，腹膜种植转移可出现脾脏被膜扇形囊性（腹膜假性黏液瘤）或实性种植转移灶。肿瘤直接侵犯脾脏是罕见的，比起被浸润侵犯，脾脏更容易被邻近恶性肿瘤推挤占位。脾脏的浸润侵犯最常发生在胰腺癌，在恶性间皮瘤、腹膜后肉瘤以及胃、结肠、肾和肾上腺的恶性病变中也可以发生[22]。淋巴瘤也倾向累及脾脏和其他脏器。

4. 脾脏其他原发性肉瘤　脾脏多形性未分化肉瘤，之前称为恶性纤维组织细胞瘤，极为罕见，文献中仅有 15 例报道[74]。这种非常具有侵袭性的肿瘤表现为脾脏增大，无特异性影像学特征（图 19-35）[75]。它可以是囊状、实性或混合性的肿物[76]。

手术切除是确诊及治疗所必需的方法。据报道，更为罕见的原发性纤维肉瘤和脾平滑肌肉瘤的临床和影像特征与多形性未分化肉瘤有重叠[22]。

肝脏卡波西肉瘤与艾滋病有关[77]。这种梭形细胞肿瘤也可能累及脾脏。结节性脾脏增大可见于该肿瘤。在 CT 上，脾结节在延迟期呈等或低密度，与血管瘤相仿[77]。

5. 脾脏囊腺癌　原发性脾脏黏液性囊腺癌是一种极为罕见的肿瘤。患者的主诉通常是上腹部疼痛、左上腹可触及肿物。在轴位图像上，原发性脾囊腺癌表现为大的单房或多房囊性病变，与胰腺的囊腺癌相似[64]。它可能与腹膜假黏液瘤有关，腹腔内可见多发囊性样病灶[78]。只有在手术切除病灶或脾切除术后才能确诊。

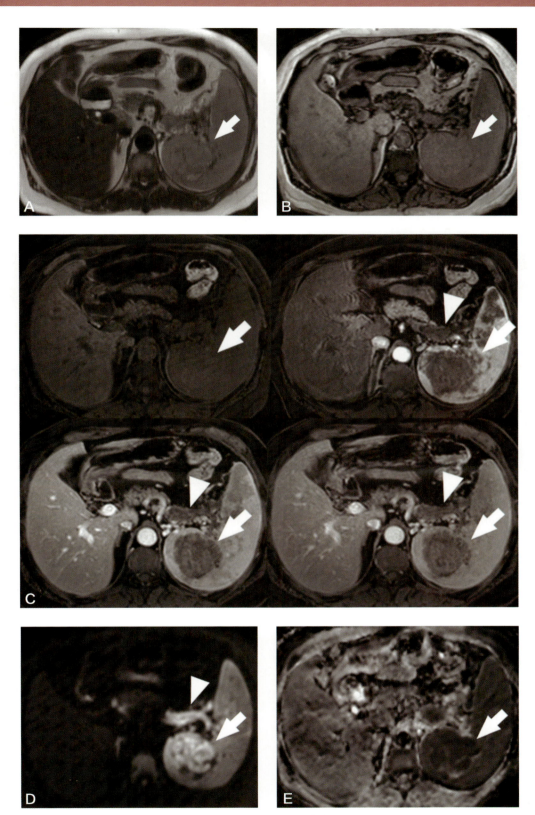

▲ 图 19-34 转移瘤

1 例患有卵巢癌的 57 岁女性：A、B. 在轴位 TSE T_2 加权图像上，脾脏后部可见一个略高信号的肿物（白箭）；B. 其在 GE T_1 加权图像上信号与脾脏相仿；C. 在动态增强序列中，该肿物是低血供的，伴有渐进性不均匀延迟强化；D、E.DWI 和 ADC 图证明其扩散受限，在高 b 值时为高信号，在 ADC 图上为低信号。注意脾静脉恶性血栓形成（箭头），伴有一定程度的强化和扩散受限

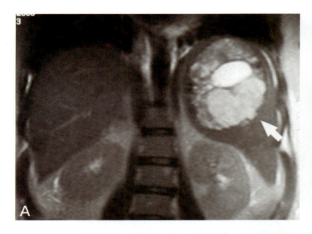
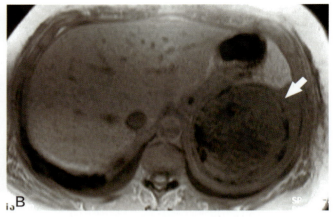
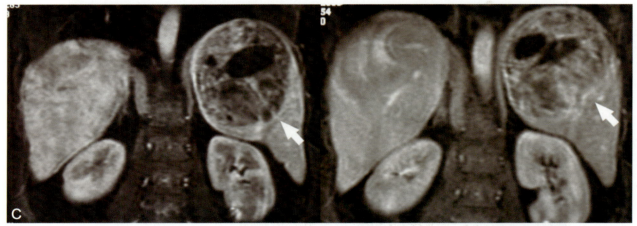

▲ 图 19-35　多形性肉瘤

冠状位 HASTE（A）和轴位 GE T_1 加权图像（B）图像显示位于脾脏上极的一个复杂的不均匀肿物。动脉期和延迟期的冠状位脂肪抑制动态 VIBE 增强图像（C）显示在增强早期不均匀增强，延迟期渐进性强化。持续性无强化区域代表囊变和坏死

十三、其他脾脏病变

（一）贮积性疾病：Gaucher 病和 Niemann-Pick 病

Gaucher 病是一种常染色体隐性溶酶体代谢紊乱疾病，由葡萄糖脑苷脂酶缺乏引起，导致 RES 中糖脂（葡糖脑苷脂）的异常贮积。患者有肝脾大、血小板减少和贫血。在 Hill 等的系列报道中包括 46 名患者，30% 的患者出现脾脏结节[79]。这些结节有红色型和白色型，前者由 Gaucher 细胞和充满血液的扩张血窦形成，后者主要由 Gaucher 细胞形成。在 MRI 上，较常见的白色脾结节在 T_1 加权图像上呈等信号，在 T_2 加权图像上与脾实质相比呈低信号，红色病变在 T_2WI 上呈高信号。这种疾病也可与脾梗死和脾纤维化相关，可能使脾脏形成多灶样的表现[80]。

类似于 Gaucher 病，Niemann-Pick 病导致细胞 RES 中脂质沉积，引起肝脾肿大和脾结节，在 T_2 加权图像上信号多样，增强扫描可见延迟强化[2,81]（图 19-36）。

（二）淀粉样变性

原发性淀粉样变性也可累及脾脏。可表现为弥漫性病变，脾脏 T_2 加权图像信号广泛减低，且为低灌注[82,83]。这些影像特征和多次输血导致 RES 中铁沉积的影像表现相仿[84]。

（三）结节病

结节病是一种全身性的肉芽肿性疾病，可累及许多器官，包括脾脏。24%～59% 的患有这种

全身性疾病的患者在组织学上可见脾结节病，但影像学检查发现的概率要低得多[1]。结节病通常伴发全身症状，如发热、乏力和体重减轻。常常可见到非特异性肝脾肿大和腹部淋巴结肿大[85]。

脾结节病通常表现为弥漫性、可大至3cm的多发小结节，有时可出现点状钙化[86]。在MRI上，这些病变在 T_1 加权图像和 T_2 加权图像上为低信号，增强扫描呈轻度、延迟强化，在延迟期图像中观察不太明显（图19-37）[87]。这些影像特征可与急性脾脏念珠菌病相鉴别。如果存在干酪性肉芽肿，它们在 T_2 加权图像上为高信号病变，伴有外周低信号。

（四）Gamna-Gandy 小体

Gamna-Gandy 小体或铁质沉着结节是由于脾实质中的脾微出血所导致的微小铁沉积灶。这

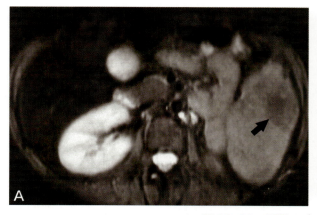
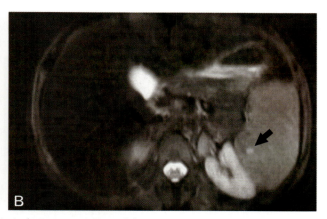

▲ 图 19-36　尼曼－皮克病（Niemann-Pick 病）

1 例患有 Niemann-Pick B 型病的 22 岁女性患者出现脾大：A. 轴位脂肪抑制的 TSE T_2 加权图像显示边界清楚的低信号结节（箭）；B. 另外，还可观察到 T_2WI 图像上的高信号结节（箭）。根据影像学和临床标准，以及肝脏和骨髓活检结果和葡萄糖脑苷脂酶及鞘磷脂酶水平，可确定诊断

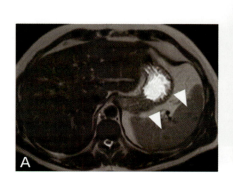
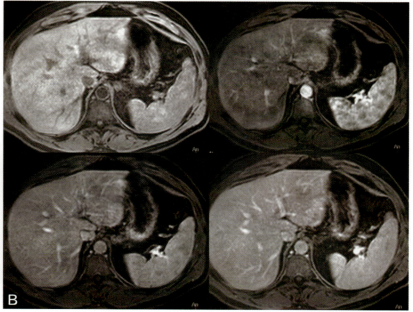

▲ 图 19-37　结节病

1 例患有结节病的 37 岁男性：A. 在 TSE T_2 加权图像上可见多发小的低信号结节（箭头），散布在整个脾实质中；B. 在动态钆增强序列中，这些病变在增强早期为低血供，在延迟期逐渐强化至与脾相等

些病变由纤维组织和含铁血黄素及钙质组成。它们通常发生在肝硬化和门静脉高压症或多次输血的患者中。这些结节小于 1cm，并且在所有 MRI 脉冲序列中表现出特征性的信号缺失[88]（图 19-38）。T_2^* 序列和钆增强扫描无强化是病灶显示更加清晰，因此 MRI 在该病变的检查中优于 US 和 CT[89]。在 GRE 同相位图像中，这些病变可出现磁敏感伪影，称为晕状伪影，对于该病变来说是特征性的。Gamna-Gandy 小体在较短的 TE 序列上看起来更小一些，因为这种磁敏感伪影减少，这一点可与纤维化结节相鉴别，纤维化结节在较短的 TE 序列上大小保持不变。该表现有助于将其与粟粒性结核、组织胞浆菌病和播散性卡氏肺孢子虫感染相关的肉芽肿相鉴别[88]。

（五）炎性假瘤

炎性假瘤是一种极为罕见的脾脏良性病变，男女均可发生，多见于中老年人。它表现为一个边界清楚的孤立性肿块，由局限性的炎症细胞组成。该病变通常是偶然发现的孤立性病变，也

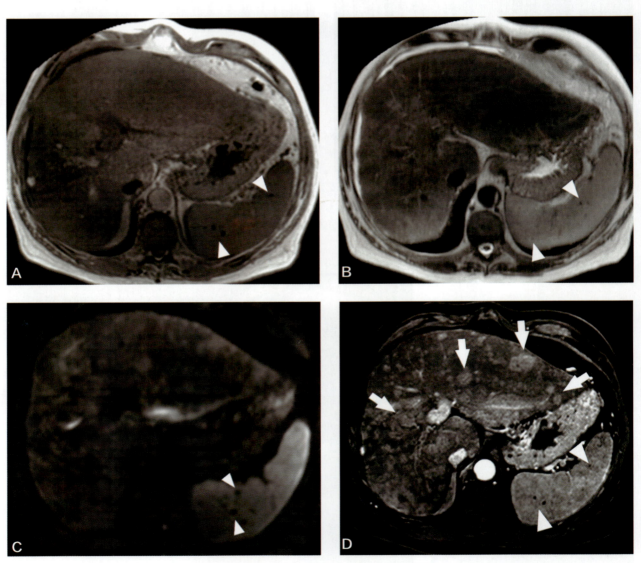

▲ 图 19-38 Gamna-Gandy 小体（箭头）
GE T_1 加权图像（A）和 TSE T_2 加权图像（B）图像上可见脾内多发微小低信号病变。这些病变在钆增强后（D）没有强化并且在高 b 值的 DWI（C）上没有扩散受限，高 b 值时为低信号。在肝实质上可见几个扩散受限的高血供结节（白箭），符合多中心肝细胞肝癌

可能伴有左侧腹痛、发热或脾肿大。在 MRI 上,炎性假瘤在 T_2 加权图像上为低信号,在 T_1 加权图像上为等或低信号,并且在延迟增强图像上表现为不均匀强化,反映了其纤维化的特性[90,91],也有炎性假瘤 T_2 加权图像高信号的报道[92]。MRI 和其他影像检查表现无特异性,因而确诊需要行脾切除。

(六)髓外造血

髓外造血是继发于骨髓造血功能不足的生理代偿现象。髓外造血主要影响脾脏和肝脏,表现为肝脾大,伴有弥漫性的显微镜下可见的微观浸润。罕见情况下可以形成类似于肿块样的造血灶。在 MRI 上,这些肿块的信号强度取决于造血的演变。活动期病变表现为 T_1 加权图像中等信号、T_2 加权图像高信号,在增强后有一定程度的强化。慢性期病变通常在 T_1 和 T_2 加权图像均为低信号,增强扫描无强化[15](图 19-39)。由于存在铁,这些病变在同相位 T_1 加权 GRE 图像中,信号明显低于反相位[93]。因此,在血液病患者中偶然发现脾脏肿块,髓外造血应纳入鉴别诊断[94]。

十四、总结

虽然脾脏局灶性和弥漫性病变并不常见,并且通常为偶然发现,但对于放射科医师来说,研究脾脏病变是具有挑战性的。MRI 是检出局灶性和弥漫性脾脏病变的有用工具,在使用动态增强的情况下,表现优于 CT。在脾大的情况下,MRI 可以全面评估慢性肝病、门静脉高压症及其并发症。最常见的局灶性病变如脾梗死、小血管瘤或囊性病变,可通过 MRI 描述其特性。尽管在许多情况下,MRI 可以区分错构瘤和大血管瘤,但仍需要影像随访或组织学分析。许多不常见的血管源性病变如血管肉瘤、血管瘤病或窦岸细胞血管瘤有相似的 MRI 表现,因此需要活检证实。淋巴瘤和转移瘤在增强早期观察更明显,为低血供结节,但两者 T_2 值和临床病史不同,有助于它们

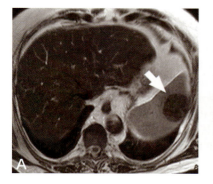
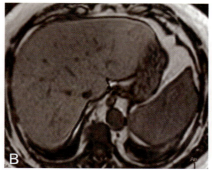
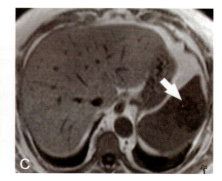
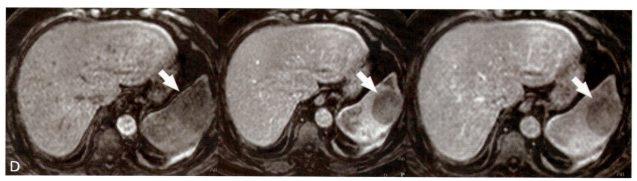

▲ 图 19-39 髓外造血

1 例患有骨髓增生异常综合征的 58 岁男性。轴位 TSE T_2 加权图像(A)上可见一个边界清楚的低信号肿物(白箭),与反相位图像(B)相比,其在同相位图像(C)上的信号减低。在动态增强序列(D)中,这个病变表现出离散的内部强化。手术切除证明是髓外造血

的鉴别诊断。在感染性、炎性和贮积性疾病方面，MRI 也可以改善病变的检出和特征描述。临床情况与病变 MRI 特征的相关性使得绝大多数病例可进行术前诊断，尽管在特征不典型或怀疑恶性肿瘤的情况下，组织学检查仍然是必要的。因此，由于在上腹部评估中 MRI 的使用增加，放射科医师必须了解最常见的脾脏疾病的影像表现。

参考文献

[1] Robertson F, Leander P, Ekberg O. (2001) Radiology of the spleen. *Eur Radiol*; 11:80–95.

[2] Luna A, Ribes R, Caro P et al. (2006) *AJR Am J Roentgenol*; 186:1533–1547.

[3] Benter T, Klühs L, Teichgräber U. (2011) Sonography of the spleen. *JUM*; 30(9):1281–1293.

[4] Gray H. (2000) The spleen. In: Lewis WH (ed.). *Anatomy of the Human Body*. 20th edn. Philadelphia, PA: Bartleby.com: 1282–1286.

[5] Cesta MF (2006) Normal structure, function, and histology of the spleen. *Toxicol Pathol*; 34:455–465.

[6] Altun E, Elias J Jr, Kim YH, Semelka RC. (2010) Spleen. In: Semelka RC (ed.). *Abdominal-Pelvic MRI*. 3rd edn. NJ:Wiley- Blackwell, pp. 677–724.

[7] Weissleder R, Hahn PF, Stark DD et al. (1988) Superparamagnetic iron oxide: Enhanced detection of focal splenic tumors with MR imaging. *Radiology*; 169:399–403.

[8] Harisinghami MG, Saini S, Weissleder R et al. (2001) Splenic imaging with USPIO Ferumoxtran-10 (AMI- 7227): Preliminary observations. *J Comput Assist Tomogr*; 25(5):770–776.

[9] Bremer C, Allkemper T, Baergmig J, Reimer P. (1999) Res-specific imaging of the liver and spleen with iron oxide particles designed for blood pool MR angiography. *J Magn Reson Imaging*; 10(3):461–467.

[10] Semelka RC, Shoenut JP, Lawrence PH. (1992) Spleen: Dynamic enhancement patterns on gradient echo MR imaging enhanced with gadopentetate dimeglumide. *Radiology*; 185:479–482.

[11] Hamed MM, Hamn B, Ibrahim ME, Taupitz M, Mahfouz AE. (1992) Dynamic MR imaging of the abdomen with gadopentate dimeglumide: Normal enhancement patterns of liver, spleen, stomach and pancreas. *AJR Am J Roentgenol*; 158:479–482.

[12] Li G, Xu P, Pan X et al. (2014)The effect of age on apparent diffusion coefficient values in normal spleen: A prelimi nary study. *Clin Radiol*; 69(4):e165–e167.

[13] Klasen J, Lanzman RS, Wittsack HJ et al. (2013) Diffusion-weighted imaging (DWI) of the spleen in patients with liver cirrhosis and portal hypertension. *Magn Reson Imaging*; 31(7):1092–1096.

[14] Storm BL, Abbitt PL, Allen DA, Ros PR. (1992) Splenosis: Superparamagnetic iron oxide enhanced MR imaging. *AJR Am J Roentgenol*; 159:333–335.

[15] Elsayes KM, Narra VR, Mukundan G et al. (2005) MR imaging of the spleen: Spectrum of abnormalities. *RadioGraphics*; 25(4):967–982.

[16] Gayer G, Apter S, Jonas T et al. (1999) Polysplenia syndrome detected in adulthood: Report of eight cases and review of the literature. *Abdom Imaging*; 24(2):178–184.

[17] Brancatelli G, Federle MP, Ambrosini R et al. (2007) Cirrhosis: CT and MR imaging evaluation. *Eur J Radiol*; 61(1):57–69.

[18] Nakamoto DA, Onders RP. (2003) The spleen. In: Haaga JR, Lanzieri CF, Gilkeson RC (eds.). *CT and MRI of the whole body*. Mosby (ed.) *CT and MR Imaging of the Whole Body*, 4th edn. St. Louis, MO: Wiley-Blackwell, pp. 1487–1508.

[19] Adler DD, Glazer GM, Aisen AM. (1986) MRI of the spleen: Normal appearance and findings in sickle cell anemia. *AJR Am J Roentgenol*; 147:843–845.

[20] Taylor FC, Frankl HD, Riemer KD. (1989) Late presentation of splenic trauma after routine colonoscopy. *Am J Gastroenterol*; 84:442–443.

[21] Urrutia M, Mergo PJ, Ros LH, Torres GM, Ros PR. (1996) Cystic masses of the spleen: Radiologic-pathologic correlation. *RadioGraphics*; 16:107–129.

[22] Rabushka LS, Kawashima A, Fishman EK. (1994) Imaging of the spleen: CT with supplemental MR exam ination. *RadioGraphics*; 14(2):307–332.

[23] Semelka RC, Kelekis NL, Sallah S, Worawattanakul S, Ascher SM. (1997) Hepatosplenic fungal disease: Diagnostic accuracy and spectrum of appearances on MR imaging. *AJR Am J Roentgenol*; 169:1311–1316.

[24] Palas J, Matos AP, Ramalho M. (2013) The spleen revisited: An overview on magnetic resonance imaging. *Radiol Res Pract*. doi: 10.1155/2013/219297.

[25] Ng KK, Lee TY, Wan YL et al. (2002) Splenic abscess: Diagnosis and management. *Hepatogastroenterology*; 49: 567–571.

[26] Akhan O, Koroglu M. (2007) Hydatid disease of the spleen. *Semin Ultrasound CT MR*; 28(1):28–34.

[27] von Sinner WN, Stnidbeck H. (1992) Hydatid disease of the spleen: Ultrasonography, CT and MR imaging. *Acta Radiol*; 33:459–446.

[28] Giovagnoni A, Giorgi C, Goteri G. (2005) Tumours of the spleen. *Cancer Imaging*; 5(1):73–77.

[29] Labruzzo C, Haritopoulos KN, El Tayar AR et al. (2002) Posttraumatic cyst of the spleen: A case report and review of the literature. *Int Surg*; 87:152–156.

[30] Ramani M, Reinhold C, Semelka RC. (1997) Splenic hemangiomas and hamartomas: MR imaging characteristics of 28 lesions. *Radiology*; 202:166–172.

[31] Ros PR, Moser RP Jr, Dachman AH, Murari PJ, Olmsted

Chapter 19 脾脏磁共振成像新进展
Update in Magnetic Resonance Imaging of the Spleen

WW. (1987) Hemangioma of the spleen: Radiologic-pathologic correlation in ten cases. *Radiology*; 162:73–77.

[32] Abbott RM, Levy AD, Aguilera NS et al. (2004) From the archives of the AFIP: Primary vascular neoplasms of the spleen: Radiologic–pathologic correlation. *RadioGraphics*; 24:1137–1163.

[33] Ha HK, Kim HH, Kim BK, Han JK, Choi BI. (1994) Primary angiosarcoma of the spleen. CT and MR imaging. *Acta Radiol*; 35(5):455–458.

[34] Levy AD, Abbott RM, Abbondanzo SL. (2004) Littoral cell angioma of the spleen: CT features with clinicopath ologic comparison. *Radiology*; 230:485–490.

[35] Schneider G, Uder M, Altmeyer K, et al. (2000) Littoral cell angioma of the spleen: CT and MR imaging appearance. *Eur Radiol*; 10:1395–1400.

[36] Tatli S, Cizginer S, Wieczorek TJ et al. (2008) Solitary littoral cell angioma of the spleen: Computed tomography and magnetic resonance imaging features. *J Comput Assist Tomogr*; 32:772–775.

[37] Miller WJ, Dodd GD, 3rd, Federle MP, Baron RL. (1992) Epithelioid hemangioendothelioma of the liver: Imaging findings with pathologic correlation. *AJR Am J Roentgenol*; 159:53–57.

[38] Martel M, Cheuk W, Lombardi L, Lifschitz-Mercer B, Chan JK, Rosai J. (2004) Sclerosing angiomatoid nodular transformation (SANT): Report of 25 cases of a distinc- tive benign splenic lesion. *Am J Surg Pathol*; 28:1268–1279.

[39] Lewis RB, Lattin GE Jr, Nandedkar M, Aguilera NS. (2013) Sclerosing angiomatoid nodular transformation of the spleen: CT and MRI features with pathologic correlation. *AJR Am J Roentgenol*; 200(4):353–360.

[40] Raman SP, Singhi A, Horton KM, Hruban RH, Fishman EK. (2013) Sclerosing angiomatoid nodular transformation of the spleen (SANT): Multimodality imaging appearance of five cases with radiology-pathology correlation. *Abdom Imaging*; 38(4):827–834.

[41] Kim HJ, Kim KW, Yu ES et al. (2012) Sclerosing angiomatoid nodular transformation of the spleen: Clinical and radiologic characteristics. *Acta Radiol*; 53(7):701–716.

[42] Thacker C, Korn R, Millstine J, Harvin H, Van Lier Ribbink JA, Gotway MB. (2010) Sclerosing angiomatoid nodular transformation of the spleen: CT, MR, PET, and ^{99m}Tc-sulfur colloid SPECT CT findings with gross and histopathological correlation. *Abdom Imaging*; 35:683–689.

[43] Falk S, Krishnan J, Meis JM. (1993) Primary angiosarcoma of the spleen: A clinic-pathologic study of 40 cases. *Am J Surg Pathol*; 17:959–970.

[44] Vrachliotis TG, Bennett WF, Vaswani KK et al. (2000) Primary angiosarcoma of the spleen—CT, MR and sonographic characteristics: Report of 2 cases. *Abdom Imaging*; 25(3):283–285.

[45] Ferrozzi F, Bova D, Draghi F, Garlaschi G. (1996) CT findings in primary vascular tumors of the spleen. *AJR Am J Roentgenol*; 166(5):1097–1101.

[46] Hatva E, Bohling T, Jaaskelainen J, Persico MG, Haltia M, Alitalo K. (1996) Vascular growth factors and receptors in capillary hemangioblastomas and hemangiopericytomas. *Am J Pathol*; 148:763–775.

[47] Guadalajara Jurado J, Turegano Fuentes F, Garcia Menendez C, Larrad Jimenez A, Lopez de la Riva M. (1989) Hemangiopericytoma of the spleen. *Surgery*; 106(3):575–577.

[48] Hosotani R, Momoi H, Uchida H, et al. (1992) Multiple hemangiopericytomas of the spleen. *Am J Gastroenterol*; 87(12):1863–1865.

[49] Yilmazlar T, Kirdak T, Yerci O et al. (2005) Splenic hemangiopericytoma and serosal cavernous hemangiomatosis of the adjacent colon. *World J Gastroenterol*. 14;11(26):4111–4113.

[50] Ito K, Mitchell DG, Honjo K et al. (1997) MR Imaging of acquired abnormalities of the spleen. *AJR Am J Roentgenol*; 168:697–702.

[51] Goerg C, Schwerk WB. (1990) Splenic infarction: Sonographic patterns, diagnosis, follow-up, and complications. *Radiology*; 174:803.

[52] Vanhoenacker FM, Op de Beeck B, De Schepper AM, Salgado R, Snoeckx A, Parizel PM. (2007) Vascular disease of the spleen. *Semin Ultrasound CT MRI*; 28:35–51.

[53] De Schepper AM, Vanhoenacker F, Op de Beeck B et al. (2005) Vascular pathology of the spleen, part I. *Abdom Imaging*; 30:96–104.

[54] Dufau JP, le Tourneau A, Audouin J, Delmer A, Diebold J. (1999) Isolated diffuse hemangiomatosis of the spleen with Kasabach-Merritt-like syndrome. *Histopathology*; 35(4):337–344.

[55] Ruck P, Horny HP, Xiao JC, Bajinski R, Kaiserling E. (1994) Diffuse sinusoidal hemangiomatosis of the spleen. A case report with enzyme-histochemical, immunohis tochemical, and electron-microscopic findings. *Pathol Res Pract*; 190(7):708–714.

[56] Rege JD, Kavishwar VS, Mopkar PS. (1998) Peliosis of spleen presenting as splenic rupture with haemo- peritoneum—A case report. *Indian J Pathol Microbiol*; 41(4):465–467.

[57] Battal B, Kocaoglu M, Atay AA, Bulakbasi N. (2010) Multifocal peliosis hepatis: MR and diffusion-weighted MR-imaging findings of an atypical case. *Ups J Med Sci*. 115(2):153–156.

[58] Madoff DC, Denys A, Wallace MJ et al. (2005) Splenic arterial interventions: Anatomy, indications, technical considerations and potential complications. *RadioGraphics*; 25:S191–S211.

[59] Kehagias DT, Tzalonikos MT, Moulopoulos LA et al. (1998) MRI of a giant splenic artery aneurysm. *Br J Radiol*; 71:444–446.

[60] Kreft B, Strunk H, Flacke S et al. (2000) Detection of thrombosis in the portal venous system: Comparison of contrast-enhanced MR angiography with intraarterial digital subtraction angiography. *Radiology*; 216:86–92.

[61] Pinto PO, Advigo P, Garcia H et al. (1995) Splenic hamartomas: A case report. *Eur J Radiol*; 5:93–95.

[62] Ohotmo K, Fukoda H, Mori K et al. (1992) CT and MR appearances of splenic hamartoma. *J Comput Assist Tomogr*; 16:425–428.

[63] Tang P, Alhindawi R, Farmer P. (2001) Case report: Primary isolated angiomyolipoma of the spleen. *Ann Clin Lab Sci*; 31(4):405–410. (Abstract).

[64] Gupta S, Deshmukh SP, Ditzler MG, Elsayes KM. (2014) Splenic lesions. In: Luna A et al. (eds.) *Functional Imaging in Oncology*, vol. 2. Berlin, Germany: Springer-Verlag, 2014.

[65] Freeman JL, Jafri SZ, Roberts JL, Mezwa DG, Shirkhoda A. (1993) CT of congenital and acquired abnormalities of the spleen. *RadioGraphics*; 13(3):597–610.

[66] Kamaya A, Weinstein S, Desser TS. (2006) Multiple lesions of the spleen: Differential diagnosis of cystic and solid lesions. *Semin Ultrasound CT MR*; 27:389–403.

[67] Warshauer DM, Hall HL. (2006) Solitary splenic lesions. *Semin Ultrasound CT MR*; 27:370–388.

[68] Peddu P, Shah M, Sidhu PS. (2004) Splenic abnormalities: A comparative review of ultrasound, microbubble-enhanced ultrasound and computed tomography. *Clin Radiol*; 59:777–792.

[69] Lindfors KK, Meyer JE, Palmer EL 3rd, Harris NL. (1984) Scintigraphic findings in large-cell lymphoma of the spleen: Concise communication. *J Nucl Med*; 25:969–971.

[70] Kreft BP, Tanimoto A, Leffler S et al. (1994) Contrast enhanced MR imaging of diffuse and focal splenic disease with use of magnetic starch microspheres. *AJR Am J Roentgenol*; 4:373–379.

[71] Mainenti PP, Iodice D, Cozzolino I et al. (2012) Tomographic imaging of the spleen: The role of morphological and metabolic features in differentiating benign from malignant diseases. *Clin Imaging*; 36:559–567.

[72] Hahn PF, Weissleder R, Stark DD et al. (1988) MR imaging of focal splenic tumors. *AJR Am J Roentgenol*; 150:823–827.

[73] Mirowitz SA, Brown JJ, Lee JKT et al. (1991) Dynamic gadolinium-enhanced MR imaging of the spleen: Normal enhancement patterns and evaluation of splenic lesions. *Radiology*; 179:681–686.

[74] Dawson L, Gupta O, Garg K. (2012) Malignant fibrous histiocytoma of the spleen: An extremely rare entity. *J Cancer Res Ther*. 8:117–119.

[75] Fotiadis C, Georgopoulos I, Stoidis C, Patapis P. (2009) Primary tumors of the spleen. *Int J Biomed Sci*; 5:85–91.

[76] Amatya BM, Sawabe M, Arai T et al. (2011) Splenic undifferentiated high grade pleomorphic sarcoma of a small size with fatal tumor rupture. *J Pathol Nepal*. 1:151–153.

[77] Restrepo CS, Martinez S, Lemos JA et al. (2006) Imaging manifestations of Kaposi sarcoma. *RadioGraphics*; 26:1169–1185.

[78] Ohe C, Sakaida N, Yanagimoto Y et al. (2010) A case of splenic low-grade mucinous cystadenocarcinoma resulting in pseudomyxoma peritonei. *Med Mol Morphol*; 43:235–240.

[79] Hill SC, Damaska BM, Ling A et al. (1992) Gaucher disease: Abdominal MR imaging findings in 46 patients. *Radiology*; 184:561–566.

[80] Poll LW, Koch JA, vom Dahl S et al. (2000) Gaucher disease of the spleen: CT and MR findings. *Abdom Imaging*; 25:286–289.

[81] Omarini LP, Frank-Burkhardt SE, Seemayer TA, Mentha G, Terrier F. (1995) Niemann-Pick disease type C: Nodular splenomegaly. *Abdom Imaging*; 20(2):157–160.

[82] Monzawa S, Tsukamoto T, Omata K, Hosoda K, Araki T, Sugimura K. (2002) A case with primary amyloidosis of the liver and spleen: Radiologic findings. *Eur J Radiol*; 41(3):237–241.

[83] Mainenti PP, Camera L, Nicotra S, et al. (2005) Splenic hypoperfusion as a sign of systemic amyloidosis. *Abdom Imaging*; 30(6):768–772.

[84] Paterson A, Frush DP, Donnelly LF, Foss JN, O'Hara SM, Bisset GS 3rd. (1999) A pattern-oriented approach to splenic imaging in infants and children. *RadioGraphics*; 19(6):1465–1485.

[85] Warshauer DM, Molina PL, Hamman SM et al. (1995) Nodular sarcoidosis of the liver and spleen: Analysis of 32 cases. *Radiology*; 195(3):757–762.

[86] Scott GC, Berman JM, Higgins JL. (1997) CT patterns of nodular hepatic and splenic sarcoidosis: A review of the literature. *J Comput Assist Tomogr*; 21:369–372.

[87] Warshauer DM, Semelka RC, Ascher SM. (1994) Nodular sarcoidosis of the liver and spleen: Appearance on MR images. *J Magn Reson Imaging*; 4(4):553–557.

[88] Sagoh T, Itoh K, Togashi K et al. (1989) Gamna-Gandy bodies of the spleen: Evaluation with MR imaging. *Radiology*; 172:685.

[89] Chan YL, Yang WT, Sung JJ, Lee YT, Chung SS. (2000) Diagnostic accuracy of abdominal ultrasonography compared to magnetic resonance imaging in siderosis of the spleen. *J Ultrasound Med*; 19(8):543–547.

[90] Irie H, Honda H, Kaneko K, et al. (1996) Inflammatory pseudotumors of the spleen: CT and MRI findings. *J Comput Assist Tomogr*; 20(2):244–248.

[91] Ma PC, Hsieh SC, Chien JC, Lao WT, Chan WP. (2007) Inflammatory pseudotumor of the spleen: CT and MRI findings. *Int Surg*; 92(2):119–122.

[92] Noguchi H, Kondo H, Kondo M, Shiraiwa M, Monobe Y. (2000) Inflammatory pseudotumor of the spleen: A case report. *Jpn J Clin Oncol*; 4:196–203.

[93] Granjo E, Bauerle R, Sampaio R et al. (2002) Extramedullary hematopoiesis in hereditary spherocytosis deficient in ankyrin: A case report. *Int J Hematol*; 76:153–156.

[94] Gabata T, Kadoya M, Mori A, Kobayashi S, Sanada J, Matsui O. (2000) MR imaging of focal splenic extramedullary hematopoiesis in polycythemia vera: Case report. *Abdom Imaging*; 25(5):514–516.

Chapter 20
胰腺

Pancrers

Fernanda Garozzo Velloni, Ersan Altun,
Miguel Ramalho, Richard Semelka 著

徐晓娟　马霄虹 译

赵心明　校

目录 CONTENTS

一、正常解剖 / 474

二、MRI 成像技术 / 474

三、发育异常 / 476

四、遗传性疾病 / 476

五、炎症性疾病 / 478

六、胰腺肿瘤 / 485

七、实性肿瘤 / 485

八、囊性肿瘤 / 490

九、外伤 / 492

十、胰腺移植 / 493

十一、总结 / 494

磁共振成像（MRI）是检测和显示胰腺疾病非常有效的一种成像方法。近年来随着其成像技术的不断改进，对于胰腺实质、胰腺导管、胰周软组织、邻近脏器和血管结构的评价能力也进一步提升。

一、正常解剖

胰腺是位于腹膜后区、邻近腹腔主要大血管、同时具有内分泌和外分泌功能的一个具有轻度分叶状外观的脏器。胰腺前方与胃、内侧与十二指肠第二段、后方与腹腔大血管和脊柱毗邻。胰尾部与脾脏毗邻。胰腺后方与双侧肾前筋膜相邻。胰腺前方被覆腹膜。胰腺的解剖结构分为胰头、钩突、颈部、体部和尾部。整个胰头部几乎被十二指肠所形成的 C 形弯曲所包绕。胰腺钩突部是胰头部的延续，形似钩子般位于肠系膜上动脉、静脉之后。胰头和胰体之间是一段轻度狭窄的区域，称为颈部，位于门静脉汇合处水平。

胰腺后方没有腹膜被覆，这是导致胰腺炎时腹水可广泛播散，以及胰腺导管癌早期即可发生腹膜后脂肪侵犯的原因。虽然胰头的大小变异范围较大，但是正常胰头部直径通常在 2～2.5cm，其余部分厚度通常为 1～2cm。

胰腺的主胰管被称作 Wirsung 管，在正常人一般宽度是 1～2mm。它从胰尾部一直延续到胰头，在十二指肠大乳头处开口于十二指肠第二段，周围环绕 Oddi 括约肌。胰腺的另外一根较小的副胰管，被称作 Santorini 管，常常起自胰腺体部，经由颈部单独开口于十二指肠小乳头的近端[1]。

二、MRI 成像技术

新的 MRI 成像技术包括快速采集、不依赖于屏气的序列和并行采集等，降低了腹部扫描的伪影，提高了 MRI 在发现和显示胰腺疾病中的作用。标准的扫描序列包括冠状位和轴位单次激发回波链自旋回波（single-shot echo train spin-echo，SS-ETSE）T_2 加权序列，轴位压脂 SS-ETSE T_2 加权序列，轴位同相位和反相位 2D 或 3D 梯度回波 T_1 加权序列，轴位压脂 3D 梯度回波 T_1 加权序列，以及注射对比剂之后的动态增强压脂 3D 梯度回波序列，包括轴位三个连续期相，以及冠状位和矢状位（最后两个期相，可作为选择性的）。上述序列的联合应用可提高成像质量，有助于观察直径小于 1cm 的胰腺局灶性疾病和弥漫性疾病[2-5]。

使用高空间分辨率的 3.0 T 磁共振扫描仪也可提高对于胰腺局灶小病变的检出能力。磁共振胰胆管成像（MR cholangiopancreatography，MRCP）对于胆管和胰管具有很好的显示能力，可评价胆管梗阻、胆管扩张和胆道异常[6-8]。因此 MRCP 也是胰腺 MR 检查的常规序列之一，对于胰腺疾病可提供全面的评价。MRCP 序列采用重 T_2 加权，采集方式包括 thick-slab 的方式。thick-slab MRCP 是屏气序列，在很短时间（几秒）内采用较厚的层厚（例如 40mm）来采集较大范围包括整个胰腺和胆道系统的图像。该技术获得的图像没有运动伪影，但是空间分辨率较低。thin-slab 技术不依赖屏气，它通过回波门控（更好）或者呼吸触发技术来实现。该序列是 3D 成像，可获得包括胰腺和胆道系统的薄层图像（比如层厚仅为 1mm），并且可进行 3D 最大强度投影（3D maximum intensity projection，3D MIP）重建，有助于临床医师理解胰腺和胆道系统的三维解剖结构。

T_2 加权的 SS-ETSE 序列冠状面显示胆总管（the common bile duct，CBD）和轴位显示胰管结构非常清楚。T_2 加权图像同时能够提供实性病变内部含水量的信息，尤其对于观察伴随出现的慢性胰腺炎，反映囊性病变内部结构诸如分隔和实性成分，以及在感染性疾病出现并发症时能够反映胰腺假囊肿或者胰周积液中的复杂成分[1]。

正常胰腺在 T_1 加权梯度回波序列中显示为高信号，因为胰腺腺泡中富含黏蛋白（aqueous protein），其在 T_1 加权压脂序列图像中尤为显著[2,9,10]（图 20-1）。T_1 加权同相、反相位梯度回波序列对于没有慢性胰腺炎背景的实性病变的

Chapter 20 胰腺
Pancrers

检出以及明确胰腺中的脂肪和铁质成分非常有意义。压脂的 3D 梯度回波序列对于没有慢性胰腺炎背景的胰腺实性肿物的检出尤其重要。对于老年人，胰腺的信号强度会下降，低于肝脏信号[3]。这反映的是继发于老年性改变的胰腺功能的下降，同时伴有或不伴有胰腺纤维化的改变[1]。

胰腺的增强扫描包括 3 个时相：毛细血管期（肝动脉期）、肝静脉期（门静脉期）和间质期，扫描序列采用 3D 梯度回波 T_1 加权压脂序列。肝动脉期表现为对比剂出现在肝动脉和门静脉内，但是尚未进入肝静脉。这一期通常是在注射对比剂之后 35～38s 进行采集。这一期不仅对肝脏富血供病变的评价非常重要，对胰腺实质和胰腺病变的观察也非常重要。正常胰腺在此期表现为显著的增强，与同期肾皮质强化程度相仿，而明显强于同期肝脏实质的强化程度（图 20-1）。另外，胰腺的乏血供病变在此期相非常容易显示，在没有慢性胰腺炎的情况下，表现为明显强化的胰腺实质背景下相对低信号的区域。富血供病变在此期也会得到显著强化。在此期也可进行动脉血管的评价。但是，如果存在慢性胰腺炎，则胰腺实质在此期不会出现显著强化。在肝静脉期，胰腺实质强化程度减低，与同期肝实质强化程度相似（图 20-1）。这一期是注射对比剂之后 60～90s，对于进一步评价病变的强化特点和静脉结构尤其重要。在此期，可评价乏血供病变是否有渐进性的中央强化，富血供病变是否存在对比剂流出，囊性病变中分隔或者实性成分的强化特点，以及含液体病变中壁的是否强化等信息。间质期对于评价病变强化特点也很重要，因为很多病变在间质期具有和肝静脉期相似的强化方式。间质期在注射造影剂后 90～120s 采集。当具有慢性胰腺炎改变时，由于发生纤维化，胰腺会在间质期出现强化。这三个期相都是在轴位采集。接下来可进行冠状面成像。矢状面成像可自由选择，但其对于评价血管侵犯、判断临床手术可切除性和制订手术方案有帮助[5]。

对于不能配合屏气的患者，可选择那些不依赖屏气的序列进行扫描，包括 T_2 加权 SS-ETSE、thick-/thin-slab ERCP、增强前 T_1 加权快速回波序列以及增强前、后采用放射状采集的 T_1 加权压脂 3D 梯度回波序列。

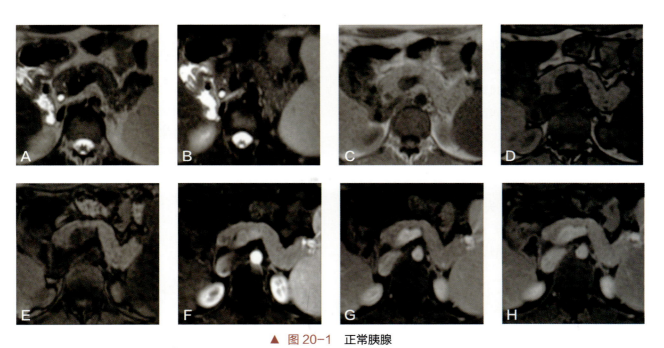

▲ 图 20-1 正常胰腺

T_2 加权 SS-ETSE（A），压脂的 T_2 加权 SS-ETSE（B），T_1 加权同相位（C）和反相位（D）SGE，T_1 加权压脂毁损梯度回波（SGE）（E），T_1 加权增强扫描肝动脉期（F），肝静脉期（G）和间质期（H）。正常胰腺在 T_1 加权 GE 序列上呈高信号，尤其是在 T_1 加权压脂序列图像上，并且在肝动脉期呈明显强化，在肝静脉期和间质期强化程度减退

三、发育异常

（一）胰腺分裂

胰腺分裂是胰腺和胰管系统最常见的解剖变异。传统的胰管结构特点是同时具有主胰管和副胰管。主胰管起自背侧胰腺，在胚胎发育过程中逐渐与腹侧胰管相融合。Wirsung 管是腹侧胰管的一部分，它与背侧胰管在胰头处汇合，并与胆总管共同开口于壶腹部。副胰管（Santorini 管）来源于背侧胰腺，它是背侧胰管的延续，经由十二指肠小乳头引流。这样的解剖结构见于 70% 的病例。有 30% 的病例存在 Santorini 管的退化。

胰腺分裂见于 10% 的正常人群。这是由于胰腺在胚胎发育过程中腹侧和背侧胰管未能融合所致[11]。这种异常会导致腹侧胰芽的胰液经由 Wirsung 管进入十二指肠大乳头，而背侧胰芽（主要的胰腺腺体部分）的胰液通过背侧胰管、经由 Santorini 管进入十二指肠小乳头。形成这种先天畸形的原因，是由于胰腺胚胎发育过程中不同的胰芽有不同的管道系统：一个非常短小的腹侧胰管（Wirsung 管）只引流胰头下方的部分，但是背侧的 Santorini 管引流胰尾、胰体、胰颈和胰头的上部。这种异常是胰腺分裂最常见的类型，据报道会增加胰腺炎的风险。在 MRCP 图像上胰管表现为清晰的高信号管状结构，因此 Wirsung 管和 Santorini 管进入十二指肠不同的开口能够被很好地显示（图 20-2）。

腹侧胰管缺失而 Santorini 管占主导 / 腹侧和背侧胰管功能连接缺失，以及襻样胰管（ansa pancreatica）/ 环状胰管，都是其他比较罕见的胰腺分裂和胰管变异的类型。

（二）环状胰腺

环状胰腺是一种不常见的先天异常，是原始胰芽在旋转过程中提前融合、环绕十二指肠所致。在大部分病例中，环状胰腺包绕十二指肠的第二段。患者会出现十二指肠梗阻 / 狭窄的症状。

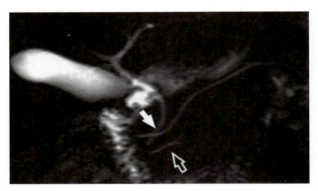

▲ 图 20-2　胰腺分裂

MRCP 图像显示 Santorini 管（白箭）和 Wirsung 管（黑箭）进入十二指肠的不同的开口，两套管道之间没有交通

如果观察到十二指肠被包埋在胰腺实质内，即可明确环状胰腺的诊断，尤其是通过不压脂的 T_2 加权和 T_1 加权增强前、后序列进行观察更为清楚。压脂的 T_1 加权序列也非常有帮助，通过该序列可观察到在相对高信号的胰腺背景实质中被包埋的低信号的十二指肠（图 20-3）[12]。

（三）背侧胰腺先天缺失

背侧胰腺先天缺失是非常罕见的发育异常。在此种情况下，胰头部残端较为圆钝，这与手术切除或者外伤后远端胰腺缺失的不规则、相对锐利的残端有明显不同[1]。

（四）多脾综合征的短胰腺改变

多脾综合征是一种先天异常，表现为多发、出现在异常部位的小的脾脏组织，而没有正常位置的正常脾脏[13]。这种综合征以双侧或左侧多发小的脾脏为特征，并且常常伴发半环状胰腺或者先天性短胰腺改变[1]。

四、遗传性疾病

（一）囊性纤维化

这是一种常染色体隐性多系统疾病，主要表现为所有的外分泌腺的分泌功能障碍和由于黏液纤毛转运功能下降所致的外分泌腺黏液栓形成。

Chapter 20　胰腺
Pancrers

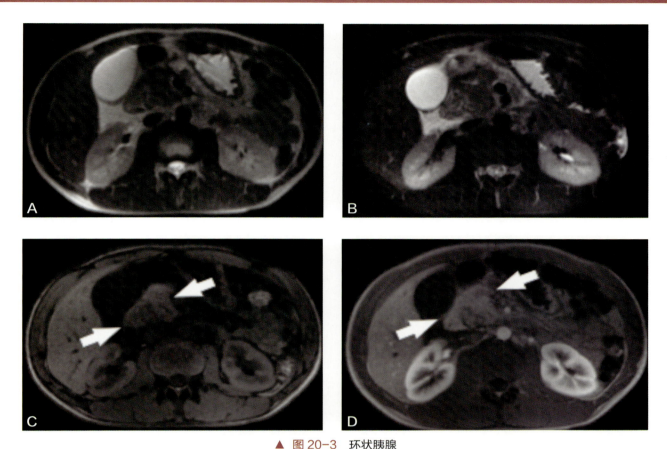

▲ 图 20-3　环状胰腺

T_2 加权 SS-ETSE（A），压脂的 T_2 加权 SS-ETSE（B），T_1 加权压脂 SGE（C），T_1 加权增强的肝动脉期（D）。正常胰腺实质（白箭）包绕十二指肠的第二段，提示环状胰腺的诊断。该疾病在 T_1 加权压脂的平扫序列和增强后即刻扫描观察最为清楚

患者的临床表现常包括：由于反复发生的支气管肺感染导致的慢性肺疾病，胰腺功能不全继发的吸收障碍和汗液中钠含量增高。与之相关的胰腺异常改变的影像学表现分为以下三种类型：胰腺增大完全由脂肪组织来代替（这是最常见的），伴有或者不伴有分叶状外观的缺失（图 20-4）；胰腺萎缩伴有部分脂肪沉积；以及胰腺弥漫性萎缩不伴有脂肪沉积[14-16]。脂肪沉积在 T_1 加权和 T_2 加权图像上表现为高信号，在压脂序列上信号减低。囊性纤维化的另外一个表现是由于胰液分泌梗阻所致的胰腺囊肿。不过该表现非常罕见，并且往往表现为较大的囊肿。

（二）原发血色素沉着病

原发血色素沉着病是一种以铁质过度沉积于不同脏器实质的常染色体隐性遗传疾病。肝脏、胰腺和心脏是主要受累器官。铁质沉积导致 T_2 加权和 T_1 加权同相位梯度回波序列的信号下降。在肝脏、胰腺和心肌中铁质沉积会延长 TE 时间，从而使得 T_1 加权同相位梯度回波序列信号强度比反相位低。与输血之后引起的脾脏铁质沉积不同，原发性血色素沉着病不会导致脾脏的铁质沉积。

（三）von Hippel-Lindau 综合征

von Hippel-Lindau 综合征是一个包含多种不同临床征象的常染色体显性遗传性疾病。它的最主要特点是小脑和视网膜血管网状细胞瘤。患者可出现肝脏和肾脏的囊肿，并具有很强的发展成肾细胞癌的倾向。von Hippel-Lindau 综合征患者还可能出现胰腺囊肿（最常见）、胰岛细胞瘤或者胰腺微囊型囊腺瘤。

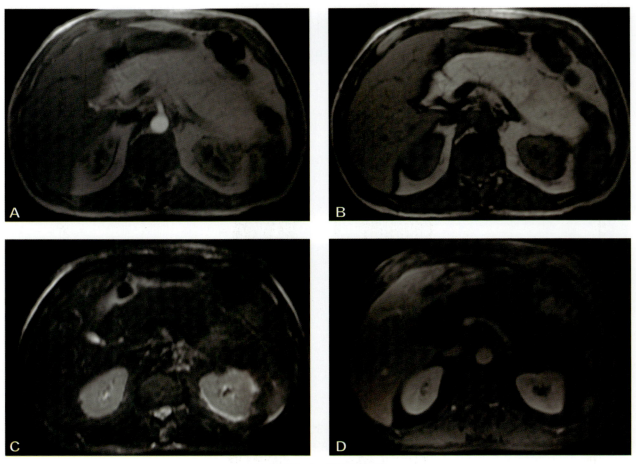

▲ 图 20-4　囊性纤维化

T_1 加权同相位（A）和反相位（B）SGE，压脂的 T_2 加权 SS-ETSE（C）和 T_1 加权增强扫描动脉期（D）。胰腺体积明显增大，在 T_1 加权图像（A、B）上呈高信号，在压脂序列图像（C、D）上呈低信号，反映了胰腺实质被脂肪组织所代替。胰腺完全被脂肪组织所代替是胰腺囊性纤维化最常见的表现

五、炎症性疾病

（一）胰腺炎

胰腺炎是胰腺的炎症性疾病，是成年人和儿童中最常见的胰腺疾病类型。可以是急性，反映胰腺的急性炎症过程，或者是慢性、缓慢进展、持续的炎性损伤[17]。

有超过一半的成年人急性胰腺炎与胆石症或者是过量饮酒有关，而在儿童主要的发病原因是创伤、病毒感染和系统性疾病。在发达国家，过量饮酒是成年人慢性胰腺炎的主要病因（占到 80%），而在全球范围内最主要的原因是营养不良[18]。

1. 急性胰腺炎　急性胰腺炎是由于含有激活的蛋白水解酶的胰液进入了胰腺间质以及渗漏入胰腺周围组织所致。

急性胰腺炎有两个明显的特征性时期：第一期，也就是早期，是疾病发生的第一周内；第二期也就是晚期，发生在发病 1 周之后[19]。

在发病早期或者说第一期（发病 1 周之内），胰腺或者胰周的缺血、水肿可以完全缓解，也可发展成积液或者液体包裹，或是进展成永久的坏死和液化。晚期或者第二期（发病 1 周之后）主要发生在中度或者严重的急性胰腺炎患者，病程可持续数周至数月。它的特点是可出现局部并发症、全身系统性表现（取决于炎症的进展程度）和（或）一过性或持续性脏器功能衰竭[17]。

MRI 在临床怀疑或者鉴别急性胰腺炎时发挥

了很显著的作用。它能够帮助明确胰腺炎的病因：胆囊结石、胆管梗阻或者解剖结构异常。它也能协助对疾病严重程度分级，以及明确胰腺或胰周是否有并发症。

MRI 对于检测急性胰腺炎细微改变尤其是胰腺周围轻度炎症非常敏感，特别是对于 CT 上显示胰腺形态学正常的病例，而这样的病例占到具有急性胰腺炎临床症状病例的 15%～30%[20]。

2. 急性胰腺炎不同的形态学类型

（1）间质水肿型胰腺炎：间质水肿型胰腺炎（interstitial edema pancreatitis,IEP）是胰腺炎较轻的一种类型，通常在发病 1 周之内缓解。IEP 表现为胰腺弥漫性或局部的增大，继发于间质水肿但不伴有坏死。

在 MRI 上，IEP 主要表现为胰腺体积增大，胰腺实质和胰周水肿，以及周围脂肪模糊，这些征象在 T_1 加权和 T_2 加权序列能得到很好地显示。T_2 加权压脂序列对于检测水肿和少量积液非常敏感，因此在观察较轻型的胰腺炎中发挥较大作用[21]（图 20-5）。

（2）坏死性胰腺炎：坏死性胰腺炎是伴有明显的胰腺和胰周组织坏死的胰腺炎症。

在 MRI 上，坏死表现为 T_1 加权图像上低信号区、T_2 加权压脂图像上相应的高信号区，并且在增强扫描后没有见到强化[22-24]。

胰管是否发生破坏是一个重要的预后因素。在坏死性胰腺炎患者中有 30%[25] 的病变累及中央腺体、可发生胰管破坏[26,27]。MRCP 作为一种无创性成像技术，对于检测胰管破坏的准确性较高，因此可帮助患者从早期治疗中获益。

3. 急性胰腺炎的并发症 急性胰腺炎渗出物根据内容分为两大类，一类是单纯液体，另一类是包含坏死物质的复杂液体（表 20-1）。

（1）急性胰周液体积聚：急性胰周液体

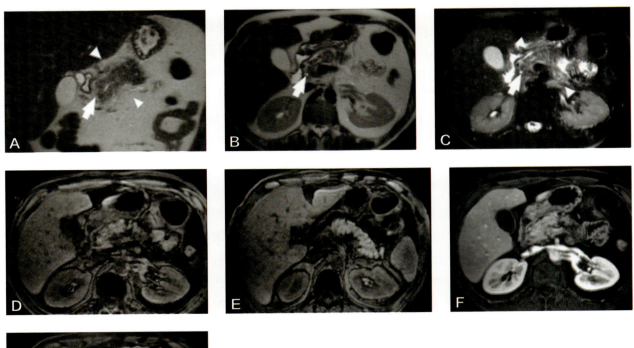

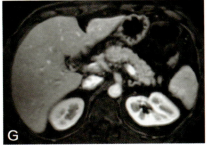

▲ 图 20-5 间质水肿型胰腺炎
冠状位（A）和横轴位（B）T_2 加权 SS-ETSE 图像，压脂的 T_2 加权 SS-ETSE（C），T_1 加权压脂 SGE（D、E），T_1 加权压脂的增强扫描肝动脉期（F、G）。胰腺实质 T_2 信号呈轻度弥漫性降低（白箭），伴有胰周少量积液（箭头），增强扫描胰腺呈正常强化（F、G）

表 20-1 急性胰腺炎之后不同类型渗出物

胰腺炎类型	液体渗出物	影像表现
小于 4 周		
IEP	APFC	均匀，液体密度，没有坏死物碎片，没有包膜
坏死性胰腺炎	ANC	不均匀，有坏死物碎片，分叶，没有包膜
大于 4 周		
IEP	假性囊肿	均匀，液体密度，没有坏死物碎片，有包膜
坏死性胰腺炎	WON	不均匀，有坏死物碎片，分叶，有包膜

积聚（acute peripancreatic fluid collections, APFCs）常常发生在 IEP 后 4 周之内，在胰腺周围区域出现的无壁、均一的含液体的囊性结构，可以单发，也可以多发。

T_2 加权序列对于观察 APFCs 非常敏感，表现为高信号（图 20-5）。在 T_1 加权梯度回波序列图像上，APFCs 表现为在高信号的脂肪背景中低信号改变。在压脂 T_1 加权增强扫描图像上往往看不到强化。

液体聚集的典型部位是小网膜囊和肾前间隙，或者是往下到达盆腔，或者向上到达纵隔[22]。大部分急性液体聚集是无菌性的，通常不经过治疗即可自行吸收缓解[23]。

（2）胰腺假性囊肿：胰腺假性囊肿是指在 IEP 之后发生液体聚集超过 4 周，位于胰腺周围的具有界限清晰的囊壁、不伴有内部实性成分的囊性病变。假性囊肿在 T_1 加权梯度回波图像上表现为低信号，在 T_2 加权图像上表现为相对均匀的高信号。假性囊肿的壁在增强早期无或仅有轻微强化，在间质期由于组织发生纤维化，可表现为渐进性的明显强化（图 20-6）。

假性囊肿有时会与胰管发生沟通，观察到这个征象有助于患者下一步治疗方案的制订。假性囊肿大部分会自愈。发生感染和出血会使单纯的假性囊肿变得复杂。合并有感染的假性囊肿可能会含有气体，从而在 T_1 加权序列图像上出现磁敏感伪影。

（3）急性坏死物积聚：在最初的 4 周，含有液体、坏死物质、出血组织等不同成分的渗出物混合在一起，称作急性坏死物积聚（acute necrotic collection, ANC）。与 APFCs 不同，ANCs 是位于胰腺内部或者胰周的，它常常与主胰管或者其分支胰管相沟通。

在 MRI 上，坏死组织碎片在 T_1 加权和 T_2 加权图像上表现为在坏死物积聚区内不规则的低信号灶。如果发生出血，则可能出现 T_1 和 T_2 信号的增高。这些坏死/出血物质不会发生强化，坏死去积聚区可出现周边强化，但是没有明确的壁（图 20-7）。

（4）无壁坏死：较成熟的 ANC 逐渐形成不含上皮的厚壁，尤其是 4 周之后，称为无壁坏死（walled-off necrosis, WON）。但是，4 周之前的急性坏死渗出液也可以转变成 WON。对于 WON 的处理与假性囊肿不同，因为它含有非液体的坏死物碎片，这需要进行引流或者手术切除。这些液体聚集常常有内部分隔，并且含有坏死/出血物质，因此在 MRI 上根据成分不同，有不同的 T_1 和 T_2 信号表现，增强扫描后可表现为渐进性强化。

（5）胰腺坏死物质合并感染：胰腺和胰周坏死/聚集物质可以保持无菌或者合并感染。胰腺坏死继发感染会增加死亡率[28]。

当出现腔外/壁外气体征象时，应考虑到 ANC 或者 WON 合并感染。这种腔外/壁外气体出现在坏死区，可以合并出现或者不出现气/液平面，这取决于气体与液体量的比例。

4. 瘘管形成 胰管的破坏与液体积聚或者与胃肠道形成的瘘管在 T_2 加权序列、MRCP 和造影增强压脂 3D 梯度回波序列可以得到很好地显示。瘘管在 T_2 加权图像包括 MRCP 上可以很直观显示，也可以通过瘘管边缘的强化来间接观察。

（1）慢性胰腺炎：慢性胰腺炎是病理学上持续的、反复发作的炎症性改变，会导致外分泌腺和内分泌腺不可逆的功能损伤。慢性胰腺炎可以

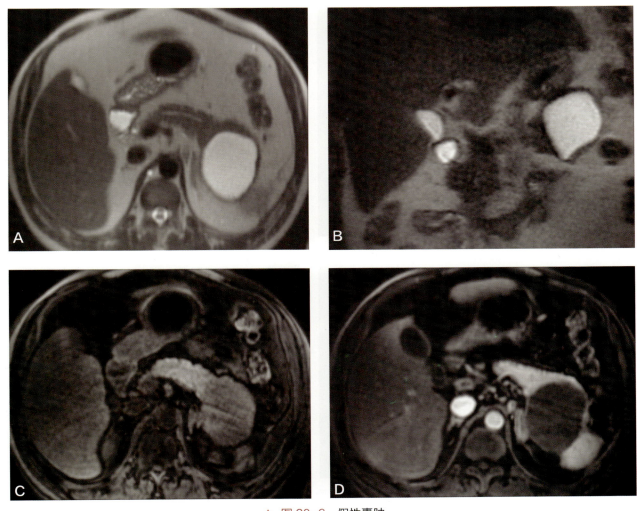

▲ 图 20-6 假性囊肿

横轴位（A）和冠状位（B）T_2 加权 SS-ETSE 图像，T_1 加权压脂 SGE（C），T_1 加权增强扫描肝动脉期（D）。胰腺尾部后方可见一个较大的薄壁囊肿，囊壁有轻度不均匀的强化

由多种因素导致，包括胆石症、过量饮酒、恶性肿瘤、代谢紊乱和各种不同的遗传和环境因素，包括创伤[29]。它可以引起腹痛、体重减轻、脂肪泻和糖尿病。

慢性胰腺炎的组织病理改变，从早期的不均匀分布的纤维化，到病变晚期累及整个胰腺的弥漫纤维化。在进展期，胰腺腺泡实质区大部分被硬化性组织所代替，导致胰腺萎缩改变。胰管异常改变包括狭窄、扩张、分支胰管扩张等都是由于周围组织纤维化所致。其他比较有特征性的慢性胰腺炎改变包括钙化和出现假性囊肿、血管瘤和静脉血栓形成的并发症。

（2）影像学的作用：影像学检查在观察胰腺实质和胰管的异常，帮助鉴别早期和进展期疾病方面发挥重要作用，可以进一步指导临床治疗（表20-2）。

表 20-2 慢性胰腺炎影像表现

早期表现	T_1 压脂序列信号减低
	增强扫描早期强化程度减低
	MRCP 或者动态分泌 MRCP 显示胰管异常
晚期表现	胰腺实质萎缩
	主胰管扩张、呈串珠样改变，分支胰管扩张
	出现并发症：假性囊肿，假性动脉瘤，脾静脉栓塞伴侧支循环形成，胆道梗阻

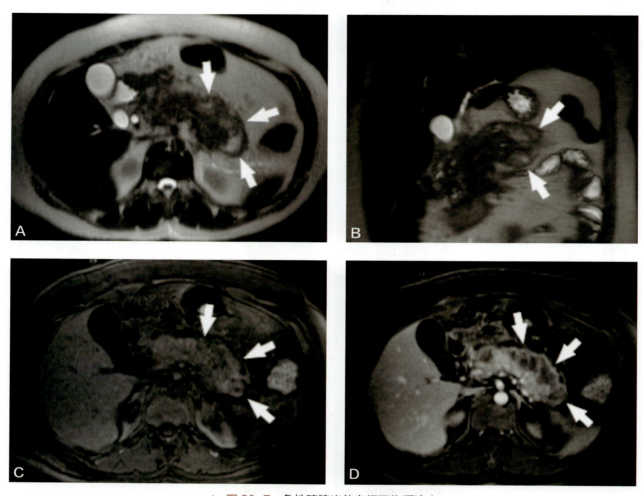

▲ 图 20-7　急性胰腺炎伴有坏死物质渗出

横轴位（A）和冠状位（B）T_2 加权 SS-ETSE 图像，T_1 加权压脂 SGE（C）和 T_1 加权增强扫描肝动脉期（D）。胰腺实质和胰腺周围可见坏死渗出物质（白箭），在 T_1 和 T_2 加权均呈低信号，增强扫描呈周边强化

（3）早期慢性胰腺炎：超声和 CT 对于诊断早期慢性胰腺炎不敏感，往往显示无异常。一项最近研究显示，慢性胰腺炎早期发生实质改变早于胰管改变，因此 MRI 比 MRCP 对于早期慢性胰腺炎的诊断更为重要。

MRI 不仅可以观察胰腺的形态学改变，还可以观察早期纤维化改变。纤维化表现为 T_1 加权压脂序列上的信号减低，以及梯度回波增强扫描早期强化程度的降低[31]（图 20-8）。一些学者研究认为，如果患者 MRI 显示有异常而 MRCP 显示正常，则动态分泌 -MRCP（S-MRCP）对患者有帮助，它可以提高病灶的显示程度，显示出常规 MRCP 不能显示的导管病变[30]。

（4）晚期慢性胰腺炎：晚期或者进展期慢性胰腺炎的表现包括胰腺萎缩，伴有 T_1 加权压脂序列胰腺信号减低，以及增强扫描早期强化程度减低、但间质期出现渐进性实质强化，这与纤维化改变有关。MRCP 可显示主胰管和分支胰管的扩张，并出现胰管狭窄、不规则，以及胰管内低信号充盈缺损的结石（图 20-9）。

早期和晚期慢性胰腺炎的影像学表现总结在表 20-2。

（5）慢性胰腺炎并发症：慢性胰腺炎最常见的非肿瘤性并发症包括假性囊肿、假性动脉瘤（由于动脉壁破坏所致）、脾静脉血栓形成和随之形成的侧支循环、胆系梗阻（由于假性囊肿所致）以及胃肠道并发症，包括胃出口梗阻和小肠缺血[32,33]。慢性胰腺炎比较少见的一种表现是炎性肿块样病变,它可增加胰腺癌的风险。

(二)特殊类型胰腺炎

1. 自身免疫性胰腺炎 自身免疫性胰腺炎(autoimmune pancreatitis,AIP)是一种临床上以梗阻性黄疸(伴或者不伴有胰腺肿物)为特点,组织学上以淋巴浆细胞浸润和纤维化形成为主要表现,对类固醇激素治疗非常敏感的一种特殊类型胰腺炎[34]。它也被认为是IgG4相关疾病谱的一种。IgG4相关疾病是一种以血液中IgG4升高、累及多脏器为特点的系统性疾病,受累脏器包括但并不局限于胰腺、胆管、肾脏、唾液腺和淋巴结。IgG4相关疾病包括但并不局限于AIP、硬化性胆管炎和异常增大的淋巴结。

AIP的MRI表现包括胰腺体积增大,T_1加权信号中等程度减低,T_2加权信号轻度增高,胰

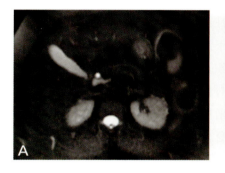
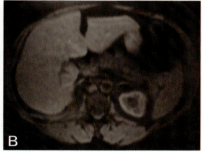
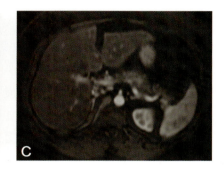

▲ 图 20-8 早期慢性胰腺炎

压脂 T_2 加权 SS-ETSE(A),T_1 加权压脂 SGE(B),T_1 加权增强扫描肝动脉期(C)。纤维化的胰腺实质在 T_1 加权压脂序列上呈信号减低改变(B),在增强扫描肝动脉期强化程度减低(C)。主胰管正常(A)

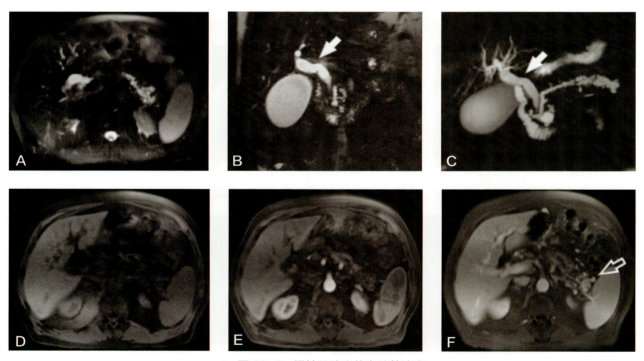

▲ 图 20-9 慢性胰腺炎伴有胰管改变

横轴位(A)和冠状位(B)压脂 T_2 加权 SS-ETSE 序列,MRCP(C),T_1 加权压脂 SGE(D),T_1 加权增强扫描肝动脉期(E)和肝静脉期(F)。胰腺实质萎缩,在 T_1 压脂序列上信号减低(D),并且在增强扫描肝动脉期的强化程度减低(E)。主胰管扩张,伴有副胰管扩张(A、B 和 C)。并发症诸如胆管扩张(白箭),脾静脉栓塞和继发的侧支循环建立(空心箭)也能观察到

腺实质在增强早期强化较弱、但在晚期出现延迟强化。AIP 的其他影像学征象包括：①围绕病变周边的包膜样环状结构，在 T_2 加权序列呈低信号 / 轻度高信号改变，增强扫描呈延迟强化[35]；②没有胰腺实质的萎缩；③在狭窄附近出现胰管串珠状改变和扩张；④胰周无明显积液；⑤病变边界清晰[36]（图 20-10）。

MRCP 上可显示主胰管的弥漫性或者节段性狭窄和不规则改变，是 AIP 的特征性改变。硬化性胆管炎常常与 AIP 合并出现。在这种情况下，肝内外胆管常常呈串珠状狭窄改变，胆管壁增厚伴有异常强化。AIP 根据形态不同分为 3 种类型：弥漫型、局灶型和多灶型。弥漫型是最常见的类型。该型的典型表现是肿胀、如腊肠样的胰腺，边界不清，伴有周边包膜样改变[37]。而弥漫型 AIP 容易误诊为淋巴瘤。

2. 沟槽状 / 十二指肠旁胰腺炎 沟槽状胰腺炎是一种罕见的局灶胰腺炎，它累及位于胰头、十二指肠和胆总管之间的胰腺解剖的沟槽状区域，可以进展为慢性胰腺炎。

该病的病因尚有争议，但有可能是源于副胰管在汇入十二指肠小乳头时发生梗阻所致。它常常常见于有酗酒史的患者[38]。

沟槽状胰腺炎分为两种类型：单纯型，仅仅累及全部沟槽区域；节段型，累及沟槽区域并延伸至胰头[39]。

在副胰管区域出现囊性病灶是该病的一个典型特点，有可能与副胰管梗阻有关[40]。

沟槽状胰腺炎的特点也与炎症反应的时间有关，分为急性或者慢性。单纯型的典型表现包括积液、边界不清的脂肪模糊改变以及胰十二指肠沟内的软组织，伴有因为纤维化改变而出现的延迟强化。有时候能在冠状位图像上观察到内侧十二指肠壁的增厚[39,41]。沟槽状胰腺炎也可以出现类肿物样改变。

3. 遗传性胰腺炎 遗传性胰腺炎是一种常染色体显性遗传疾病，表现为无明显诱因的反复发作胰腺炎。影像学表现包括实质和胰管内的钙化和实质的萎缩。在该类胰腺炎中，影像学可帮助排除那些因为结构异常引起的胰腺炎，以及密

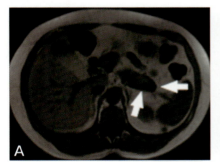
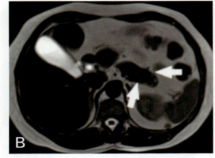
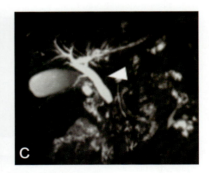
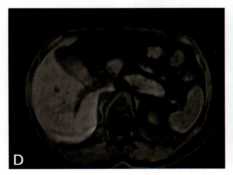
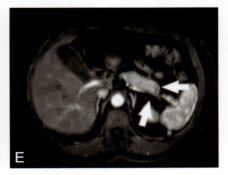

▲ 图 20-10　IgG4 自身免疫性胰腺炎

T_1 加权同相位 SGE（A），T_2 加权 SS-ETSE（B），MRCP（C），T_1 加权压脂 SGE（D）和 T_1 加权增强扫描肝动脉期（E）。胰腺增大，在 T_1 加权序列上信号中等程度降低，在 T_2 加权序列上呈轻度高信号。围绕胰腺实质的低信号包膜样改变（白箭）和胆管扩张（箭头）也可以观察到

切监视是否有向胰腺癌发展的趋势，因为在该类患者当中发生胰腺癌的风险比正常人高很多倍。

六、胰腺肿瘤

根据 WHO 分类，胰腺肿瘤按照细胞来源进行分类，可分为上皮来源或非上皮来源。

胰腺上皮来源肿瘤的来源包括：①外分泌腺导管细胞，包括导管腺癌和黏液性、浆液性囊性肿瘤；②腺泡细胞，包括腺泡细胞癌（ACC）和混合腺泡-内分泌癌；③未知来源，包括实性假乳头状瘤（solid pseudopapillary tumor，SPT）和胰腺母细胞瘤、内分泌肿瘤（功能性和非功能性）。

非上皮来源肿瘤包括原发淋巴瘤，以及来源于间叶细胞的肿瘤（血管瘤、淋巴管瘤、肉瘤、脂肪瘤等）。

也有非胰腺来源的肿瘤累及胰腺，恶性病变包括转移瘤或者继发性淋巴瘤，良性病变包括胰内副脾等。

七、实性肿瘤

（一）胰腺导管腺癌

导管腺癌是最常见的胰腺恶性肿瘤，占到所有胰腺肿瘤的 90%。男性发病率是女性的 2 倍，高峰发病年龄是 70—80 岁[42]。胰腺导管腺癌预后极差，5 年生存率仅有 5%，手术是主要的治疗方法[43]。

典型的导管腺癌表现为不规则、较小的局灶实性肿物（2~3cm），通常不伴有坏死或者出血。肿瘤信号不均，强化较弱，具有明显的局部侵犯、血管包埋侵犯的倾向。

60%～70% 胰腺导管腺癌累及胰头，10%～20% 累及胰体，有 5%～10% 累及胰尾部。全胰腺弥漫受累占到 5%[44]。

在 T_2 加权图像上，肿瘤相对于正常胰腺为稍高信号，观察起来相对困难。在压脂 T_1 加权平扫图像上，肿瘤表现为低信号，与周围正常的高信号胰腺组织分界较清晰（图 20-11 和图 20-12）[5,45-48]。

对胰腺癌的观察在增强扫描早期最有效，此时肿瘤表现为相对于周围正常胰腺组织的低强化（图 20-11 和图 20-12），原因在于肿瘤组织含有丰富的纤维间质，但是肿瘤血管很稀疏。增强扫描间质期（注射造影剂后大于 1min）肿瘤的表现反映了增加的细胞外间隙体积和肿瘤的静脉引流，此期肿瘤与正常胰腺实质的信号差别较小[47]。

由于肿瘤导致的主胰管梗阻会引起肿瘤相关的慢性胰腺炎，尤其是当肿瘤体积较大时。肿瘤病灶远端的胰腺发生萎缩，相比正常胰腺组织信号减低，这是由于进行性的纤维化和胰蛋白分泌减少所致的慢性炎性改变所致（图 20-11）[47]。在这些病例中，T_1 加权压脂平扫序列很难显示病变边界，但是，增强扫描动脉期图像可以很好地显示病变的大小和边界，因为肿瘤病灶强化程度弱于周围的慢性炎性胰腺组织[47,48]。

虽然这是乏血供腺癌最常见的表现，乏血供腺癌也是胰腺癌最常见的类型，但是胰腺癌在极罕见情况下也能表现为与胰腺实质血供相近。这种胰腺癌在增强扫描时很难与正常的胰腺组织区别，尤其是在有慢性胰腺炎、胰腺背景实质强化程度减弱的情况下。在慢性胰腺炎背景下，胰腺实质在 T_1 加权梯度回波序列上信号减低，这使得腺癌小病灶的检出更为困难。这种情况下，联合应用 T_2 加权序列对于明确病灶显得尤为重要。

胰腺癌特征性的影像表现包括胰头增大、胰管和胆总管扩张、胰体和胰尾部萎缩（图 20-11）。但是，胰头的增大伴有胰管和胆总管的扩张，并不是胰腺癌特异性的表现。在少数情况下，局灶性胰腺炎/AIP 也会见到此征象。

放射科医师应该在 MRI 诊断报告中描述如下征象：①远处转移：包括肝脏、腹膜后、肺、主动脉旁淋巴结等；②邻近器官的侵犯：胃、结肠、脾脏等；③胰周动脉的侵犯：包括腹腔干、肝动脉、肠系膜上动脉等；④胰周静脉的侵犯：包

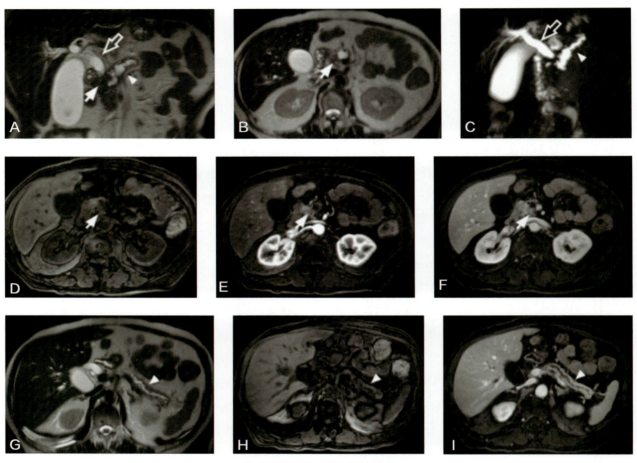

▲ 图 20-11 胰头部胰腺癌

冠状位（A），横轴位（B），T_2 加权 SS-ETSE（G），MRCP（C），T_1 加权压脂 SGE（D、H），T_1 加权增强扫描肝动脉期（E）和肝静脉期（F、I）。胰头部可见一个肿物（白箭），在 T_1 加权（D）和 T_2 加权（A、B）序列上呈低信号。在增强扫描早期（E），肿瘤相对于周围正常胰腺组织是低强化。在压脂的增强扫描肝静脉期（F），因为肿瘤渐进性强化而正常胰腺内对比剂退出，导致肿瘤边界显示欠清晰。MRCP（C）证实胆总管（空心箭）和胰管扩张（箭头），呈现双管征。主胰管梗阻导致远端胰腺组织萎缩，在 T_1 加权压脂序列上呈低信号（H）（肿瘤相关慢性胰腺炎）

括门静脉和肠系膜上静脉[5,46,47]。

目前 MRI 很适合于检出和显示小于 1cm 的局灶性胰腺导管癌[45,46,49]，这种小病灶往往不会导致胰腺轮廓外形的改变。而即使是目前最新的 CT 设备、采用多时相扫描，也很难观察到这样的病变[50,51]。

胰腺癌肝转移的病灶边界不规则，在传统或者压脂 T_1 加权序列上呈现低信号，在 T_2 加权序列上呈现稍高信号，增强扫描早期有明显不均匀环形强化。转移灶本身较低的含水量以及乏血供的特点，使得即使小于 1cm 的病灶也能与囊肿和出血相鉴别。在增强扫描早期可观察到病灶周边一过性边界不清的高强化区[1]（图 20-12）。

淋巴结可以在 T_2 加权压脂序列和增强扫描间质期的 T_1 加权压脂序列上观察。在压脂之后的低信号腹腔背景中，淋巴结显示为轻度高信号。T_2 加权压脂序列对于观察淋巴结和邻近的肝脏组织非常有帮助，因为淋巴结显示为轻度高信号，而肝脏显示为轻度低信号[1]。

肿瘤的血管侵犯和包埋在 3D 薄层梯度回波序列中显示最佳。通过此序列也能获得重建图像。对增强后所有不同平面的图像和增强前图像进行联合评价，对于胰腺癌局部分期非常有帮助。增强扫描动脉期梯度回波序列图像有助于评价动脉是否通畅，动脉期和肝静脉期图像有助于评价静脉是否通畅[1]。胰腺导管腺癌的主要特点列在表 20-3。

Chapter 20 胰腺
Pancrers

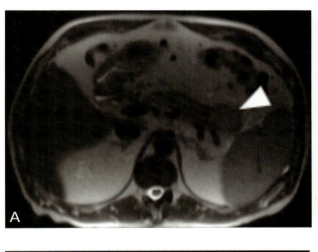
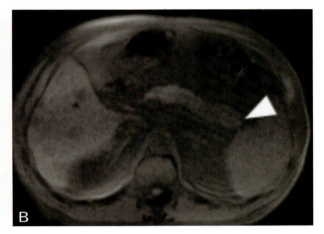
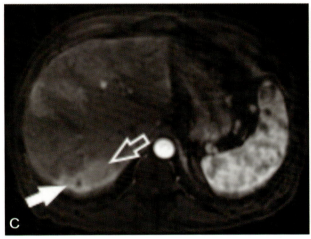
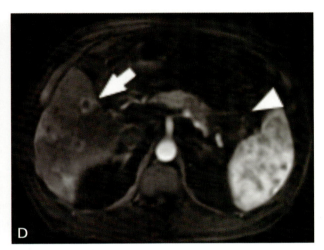

▲ 图 20-12 胰尾部胰腺癌伴有肝脏转移

T_2 加权 SS-ETSE（A），T_1 加权压脂 SGE（B）和 T_1 加权增强扫描肝动脉期（C、D）。胰腺部可见一个肿物（白箭头），在 T_1 加权序列呈低信号（B），在 T_2 加权序列呈轻度高信号（A）。在增强扫描早期（D），与邻近正常强化的胰腺实质相比，肿物呈现低强化。可见到肝脏转移瘤（C、D，白箭），在增强扫描早期显示较明显，为局部低信号肿物伴有环形强化。在增强扫描早期可见到肿物周边一过性、边界不清的强化（C，空心箭）

表 20-3 胰腺导管癌主要特点及影像表现

性别	男性＞女性
高峰发病年龄	70—80 岁
T_2 加权序列	相对于正常胰腺呈轻度高信号
T_1 加权序列	低信号，常常与正常胰腺组织分界清晰
T_1 加权增强序列	相对于正常胰腺呈低强化
其他特点	胰管和胆总管扩张，远端胰腺组织萎缩
转移和播散	远处转移可达肝脏、腹膜、肺和主动脉旁淋巴结；可浸润邻近器官；可侵犯胰周动脉和静脉

（二）胰腺神经内分泌肿瘤

胰腺神经内分泌肿瘤（pancreatic neuroendocrinetumor, pNET）是胰腺第二常见的实性肿瘤，曾被称为胰岛细胞瘤，因为以前认为该类肿瘤起自胰岛细胞。但是最近的证据表明，该类肿瘤起自胰腺导管的多潜能干细胞[52]。大部分病例报道是散发，但是与多种综合征有关系，比如，多发内分泌肿瘤Ⅰ型，von Hippel-Lindau 综合征，神经纤维瘤病Ⅰ型以及结节性硬化。NETs 可分为功能性和无功能性两大类。两者的发病率尚不明确，但是据报道功能性比无功能性更常见。无功能性神经内分泌肿瘤占胰腺内分泌肿瘤的至少 15%～20%，主要临床表现是因为肿瘤较大而引起的压迫症状或者转移。功能性者往往因为激素分泌异常而引起内分泌症状[53]。功能性 NETs 的诊断需要依据生化指标，而影像学的目的主要是精确描述病变的定位。最常见的胰腺功能性神经内分泌肿瘤是胰岛素瘤和胃泌素瘤。前者通常是良性，而后者往往是恶性。总体而言，功能性肿瘤在早期、病灶较小时，即可由于其异常的激素分泌引起临床症状而被发现。肿瘤的形态学特点多种多样。较小的肿瘤往往是实性、密度较均一的，而大的肿瘤通常是不均质同时伴有囊性改变。钙化见于 20% 的病例。

在 MRI 上，神经内分泌肿瘤在 T_1 加权压脂序列上呈现中等程度的低信号，在 T_2 加权图像上呈现中到重度的高信号[54]。胰腺 NET 是典型的富血肿瘤，因此在注射对比剂之后的肝动脉期强化会非常明显（图 20-13）。不过同时也要注意，虽然相对于正常胰腺组织，肿瘤可以较快速、较明显地强化，它们也可以在动脉期表现为与胰腺实质等信号，因为正常胰腺组织也是富血供的。在肝静脉期或者间质期，如果肿瘤小于 2cm，可以表现为对比剂的退出。

胰岛素瘤常常表现为小肿瘤（小于 2cm），伴有快速、明显、均匀强化，而胃泌素瘤常表现为较大病变（3～4cm），常伴有增强后快速的周边环形强化[1,55]。胃泌素瘤常常发生在特定部位，称为胃泌素瘤三角区，即上界位于胆囊与胆总管的汇合处，下界位于十二指肠的第二和第三段，内侧界是胰腺的颈部和体部。

肿瘤的恶性程度大致上与体积相关联，大于 5cm 的病灶往往是恶性的。但即使是恶性，相较于导管腺癌，肿瘤也是缓慢生长、预后较好[42,56]。淋巴结的转移和实质脏器的转移比如肝脏转移瘤，其强化方式与原发肿瘤强化方式相似（图 20-13）。

鉴别 NETs 和胰腺其他肿瘤尤其是导管腺癌非常重要，因为两者的预后和治疗方式非常不同。

鉴别大部分的胰腺内分泌肿瘤和胰腺导管腺癌的主要要点包括 T_2 加权序列上的高信号，注射对比剂之后肝动脉期的明显均匀强化，富血供的肝脏转移瘤，以及不伴有胰管的梗阻和血管的包埋[55]。静脉瘤栓形成、腹膜后和区域淋巴结的增大等胰腺导管腺癌的征象，在内分泌肿瘤当中一般不会出现。

（三）腺泡细胞癌（ACC）

腺泡细胞癌（aciniar cell carcinoma，ACC）是胰腺外分泌腺的极罕见原发肿瘤，虽然腺泡细胞组成了胰腺实质的绝大部分，但是 ACC 仅占胰腺外分泌瘤的 1%。该肿瘤好发于 50—70 岁老年人[1]。

这类肿瘤常常是外生性、卵圆形或者圆形，边界清晰，血供不丰富。较小的肿瘤常常是实性，但是较大肿瘤基本上会不同程度的含有囊变区，代表局部的坏死、出血，偶尔会有无定形的肿瘤内钙化，表现为信号缺失[57,58]。在 MRI 上信号特点主要表现为 T_1 加权图像低信号为主、T_2 加权图像为等到高信号为主。

当看到胰腺较大的乏血供实性肿物伴有内部大小不等的囊变或者是囊性肿物时，需要考虑到 ACC 的诊断[1,57,59]。胰腺的肿瘤标志物 CA19-9 在 ACC 中极少有增高。

（四）实性假乳头状瘤（SPT）

实性假乳头状瘤（solid pseudopapillary tumor of pancreas，SPT）是一种少见、低级别的胰腺外分泌腺上皮恶性肿瘤，好发于青少年和年轻的成年女性[1,44,60]，占所有胰腺肿瘤的 1%～2%[61]。这样的发病年龄在胰腺导管腺癌中非常罕见。该病好发于亚洲和美国黑人妇女，而在儿童和男性中罕见。该肿瘤表现为低度恶性[62,63]，完整的手术切除是首选治疗方案。该肿瘤转移少见，但是局部复发常有报道，在手术切除之后预后较好。

肿瘤好发于胰头或者胰尾。SPT 常常是

偶然发现，表现为较大的边界清晰、有包膜的肿物，周边包膜较厚，内部可见不同比例的实性部分、囊变、出血。在MRI上观察到肿瘤包膜是一个非常普遍的征象，发生率可达到95%～100%[62]。较大肿瘤可以发生血管包埋。

MRI显示病变为边界清晰的不均质信号肿物，反映了肿物内部的成分。T_1加权图像上高信号、T_2加权上低或者不均匀信号代表出血，这一点可以帮助与神经内分泌肿瘤鉴别，后者囊变部分往往不会出血，因此不会在T_1加权图像上出现高信号。

（五）间叶来源肿瘤

胰腺的间叶来源肿瘤非常罕见，仅占所有胰腺肿瘤的1%～2%[64,65]。它们来源于不同的结缔组织，根据组织来源分为不同的类型。

原发胰腺淋巴瘤，虽然很少见，但却是胰腺最常见的恶性间叶肿瘤。良性的间叶来源肿瘤常含有脂肪，比如脂肪瘤或者畸胎瘤，极为罕见，并且在MRI上具有特征性表现，可观察到信号均匀的带有包膜的成熟脂肪组织或者脂-液平面[64,65]。也曾经有过其他的间叶组织肿瘤的报道，比如淋巴管瘤、平滑肌瘤、平滑肌肉瘤、雪旺细胞瘤、血管瘤或者血管内皮瘤，这些更为罕见，仅为散在的个案文献报道。

1. 胰腺淋巴瘤 胰腺淋巴瘤可以是原发性，也可以是继发性。

非霍奇金淋巴瘤可以侵犯胰腺周围淋巴结，或者继发的侵犯胰腺组织。在T_1加权压脂序列上胰腺周围中等信号的淋巴结与高信号的胰腺实质可以区别开来[66]。

需要被的原发胰腺淋巴瘤两种形态学类型认识为局灶型和弥漫型，其中局灶型有80%发生在胰头部，有可能与胰腺癌相混淆。

在MRI上，淋巴瘤在T_1加权图像上表现为低信号，在T_2加权图像表现为中等信号。

胰腺淋巴瘤比导管腺癌的预后要好，因为一线化疗通常有效，使得病灶可以长期处于缓解状态。对于大部分胰腺淋巴瘤患者，不需要进行手术。

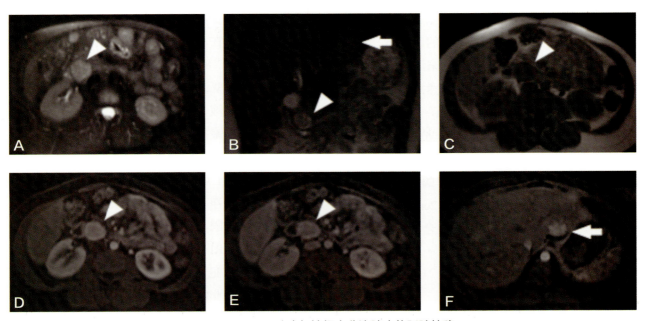

▲ 图20-13 胰头部神经内分泌肿瘤伴肝脏转移

横轴位压脂T_2加权SS-ETSE（A），冠状位T_2加权SS-ETSE（B），T_1加权同相位SGE（C），T_1加权增强扫描肝动脉期（D、F）和肝静脉期（E）。胰头钩突部可见肿物（箭头），在T_1加权序列显示为低信号（C），在T_2加权序列显示为高信号，在肝动脉期呈明显强化（D），并且在肝静脉期持续强化（E）。可见到肝转移瘤（白箭），在T_2加权序列呈轻度高信号（B），增强扫描呈富血供强化模式，与原发肿瘤特点相似（F）

对于鉴别胰腺淋巴瘤和导管腺癌的一些有意义征象包括：胰头部较大的局灶性病变、但是不伴有或仅有非常轻微的主胰管扩张，在肾静脉水平以下的淋巴结肿大，以及腹膜后和上腹部脏器的浸润性改变。血管侵犯在淋巴瘤比腺癌少见[1]。另外，CA19-9升高在原发或者继发胰腺淋巴瘤中均不常见。

2. 非胰腺来源肿瘤

（1）胰腺转移瘤：胰腺转移瘤往往来源于直接侵犯或者血行转移。胃癌、横结肠癌和胃肠道间质瘤（gastrointestinal stromal tumors,GIST）的直接胰腺侵犯虽然罕见，但却是直接侵犯最主要的来源。

血行转移的来源最常见的是肾癌、肺癌，其次是乳腺癌、结肠癌、前列腺癌和恶性黑色素瘤。胰腺转移瘤的3种形态学类型分别是孤立病变（占50%～70%）、多发病灶（5%～10%）和弥漫性病变（15%～44%）[67]。

转移瘤通常在T_1加权图像上表现为低信号，在T_2加权图像上为轻度高信号。强化方式大部分遵循环形强化，强化程度依赖于原发肿瘤的血供特点。即使在肿瘤较大的情况下，导管阻塞也很少见，这是与导管腺癌非常重要的鉴别点[1,67]。

（2）胰腺内副脾：副脾主要来源于实质脏器，尤其要注意胰腺。胰腺是副脾发生的一个相对不常见的部位。病变通常小于2cm，发生在距离胰尾尖端3cm之内[68]。胰尾部末梢发现的圆形、边界清楚、在MRI各个序列上都与脾脏信号相似的实性肿物，提示胰腺内副脾的诊断。一个很重要的鉴别点是，当病变大于2cm时，在增强扫描动脉期病变表现为与脾脏完全一致的花斑样强化[68]。

八、囊性肿瘤

随着近年来断层影像技术应用的不断增多，偶然发现的胰腺囊肿很常见。虽然继发性囊性改变在大部分类型的胰腺肿瘤中都能看到，胰腺囊性病变主要表现为持续不变的囊性外观。

既然囊性病变包括有肿瘤性和非肿瘤性，因此影像学的精确观察有助于鉴别囊性肿瘤和假囊肿。

对胰腺囊性病变的评价包括对于囊肿形态和其内液体成分的具体分析，以及是否与胰管相沟通的详细观察。对于整个胰腺实质的评价可以提供额外的诊断信息[63]。MRI以其在软组织对比方面的优势，是最适合评价上述影像特点的检查方法[69]。

虽然不同组织类型的胰腺囊性肿瘤都在文献中有过报道，但是浆液性囊腺瘤、黏液性囊性肿瘤和胰腺导管内乳头状黏液肿瘤（intraductal papillary mucinous neoplasm，IPMN）占所有胰腺囊性肿瘤的90%[70]。

（一）浆液性囊腺瘤

这类肿瘤更常见于女性（女性比男性为4：1），往往是中老年（60岁之后）。它与von Hippel-Lindau综合征的关系也被发现在逐渐增加[71]。浆液性囊腺瘤最常累及胰头，通常为微囊性、多发改变，表现为直径小于1～2cm的多发微小囊肿。在少见的情况下，浆液性囊腺瘤可以是大囊（2～8cm的囊肿），包括多囊、少囊或者单囊三种亚型。该类病变与胰管不相通。

微囊型浆液性囊腺瘤边界清晰，偶尔内部会含有中央纤维瘢痕。肿瘤大小从1～12cm不等，平均直径约5cm。病变可以表现为光滑或者结节状外观，切面上可见多发小的、紧密排列的囊腔，内部充填了干净、清亮的水（浆液）成分，伴有光整的纤维分隔，形似蜂窝。中央瘢痕有时能看到钙化。在MRI上，肿瘤边界清晰，对脂肪和周围脏器没有侵犯[72]。在T_2加权图像上，小的囊腔和分隔显示非常清晰，形如成簇状的葡萄样高信号。病变内部的分隔在造影增强的早期和晚期可能会出现极轻度的强化，但也有可能出现中等程度强化（图20-14）[1]。中央瘢痕的延迟强化也偶尔会被观察到[2]，这一征象对于较大病变更为典型。上述这些影像学特点足以用来诊断此良性病变。

大囊型浆液性囊腺瘤与微囊型表现截然不同，可能会在影像学上和病理上给诊断带来困难。在 T_2 加权图像上表现为高信号，在 T_1 加权图像上表现为低信号。外观可以表现为多囊、少囊或者单囊。在增强的 T_1 加权图像上，囊壁和分隔可以表现为渐进性轻到中度强化，中央瘢痕不常见[1]。小于 3cm 的病变诊断常常需要依靠随访和（或）囊液抽吸。如果病变大于 3cm，或者出现间断性的增大，则推荐进行手术切除。

胰腺浆液性囊腺瘤的主要特点总结见表 20-4。

表 20-4 胰腺浆液性囊腺瘤主要特点及特征影像

性 别	女性＞男性
高峰发病年龄	60 岁以后
部位	胰头部
影像特征	常常是微囊和多囊 蜂窝状改变 中央瘢痕，伴或不伴有钙化

（二）浆液性囊腺癌

这种恶性肿瘤极为罕见。当出现较厚的分隔和实性成分时，提示有浆液性囊腺癌的可能[1]。它与大囊型浆液性囊腺瘤容易混淆。

1. 黏液性囊腺瘤／囊腺癌 黏液性囊性肿瘤在女性当中更常见（女性比男性为 6 : 1），有 50% 发生在 40—60 岁的人群当中[73]。

这类肿瘤的特点是胰体部和胰尾部较大的单囊或者多囊性肿物，其内充填了丰富的较稠密的凝胶样黏液[1]。它们可以较大（平均直径是 10cm），通常是多囊，并且有包膜[74,75]。在这类肿瘤当中，约有 10% 可以有散在的钙化。这类肿瘤与胰管不相通。

黏液性囊腺瘤具有恶性潜能，在病理检查中需要对囊性病变进行充分的采样，以确定是否伴有局灶异型性或者原位癌[63]。

由于此病变产生黏液，使得原发病灶和肝转移灶可以在 T_1 和 T_2 加权图像上均表现为高信号。病变常常有较厚的壁、分隔和实性成分，在 T_2 加

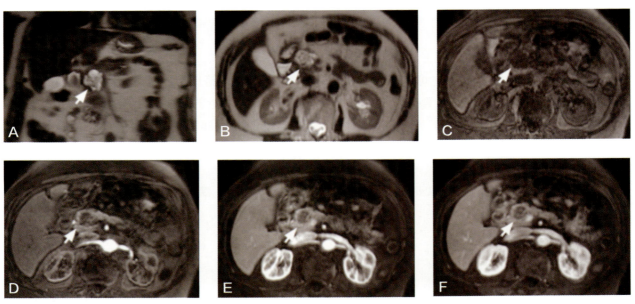

▲ 图 20-14 胰头部浆液性囊腺瘤

冠状位（A）和横轴位（B）T_2 加权 SS-ETSE 序列、T_1 加权压脂 SGE（C）、T_1 加权增强扫描肝动脉期（D）、肝静脉期（E）和间质期（F）。胰头部可见一个囊性肿物（白箭）。病变边界清晰，在 T_1 加权高信号胰腺背景当中显示为低信号病变（C）。T_2 加权序列（A、B）显示高信号形似葡萄的簇状囊腔，囊内分隔较均匀。在增强扫描早期分隔呈轻微强化（D），在延迟期相中呈渐进性强化（E、F）

权图像上显示为低信号，在增强扫描有强化[2]。黏液性囊腺癌的囊壁和分隔通常比黏液性囊腺瘤更厚。黏液性囊腺瘤边界清晰，不会发生周围脏器的侵犯和转移。黏液性囊腺癌可以表现为局部高度侵袭性，并广泛侵犯邻近组织和脏器。但是不伴有周围组织侵犯并不能除外为恶性。

肝脏的转移瘤通常是富血供，表现为较快速、明显的环形强化，并且可以含有黏液，因此在T_1加权和T_2加权图像上表现为混合的低和高信号。

胰腺黏液性囊腺瘤/囊腺癌主要特点总结见表20-5。

2. 导管内乳头状黏液性肿瘤 胰腺的IPMNs是近些年才被发现的，主要发生在男性（平均年龄65岁左右）[63,76]。它是胰腺的一种黏液性囊性肿瘤，但是从临床上和组织病理上都与黏液性囊腺瘤不同。在组织学上，它的特点是胰腺导管上皮发生了黏液转化，并伴有乳头状突起[77,78]。胰管梗阻继发于黏液栓塞、上皮的复杂改变，或者由于囊性肿物压迫所致[79]。

该类疾病包含一系列改变，包括单纯增生、发育不良、乳头状腺瘤以及癌变。这些异常改变可以同时存在，总体来说，增生、发育不良和腺瘤可能会出现恶性转化变成癌[1]。

IPMNs可以根据是否累及主胰管或者孤立的分支胰管来进行分类。它们也可以根据是否导致弥漫性导管扩张或者节段性囊性改变来进行分类[77]。肿瘤的位置是判断预后的重要因素[80]。主胰管IPMNs更容易是恶性，有60%～70%被证实是侵袭性癌[81,82]，而分支胰管IPMNs仅有22%被证实有局灶癌变[83]。IPMNs常常是多发，有5%～10%累及全胰腺[84]。

3. IPMN-主胰管型 主胰管型表现为弥漫性导管扩张，丰富的黏液和形成乳头结节。在MRI上，T_2加权图像或者MRCP可以很好地显示明显扩张的主胰管。在增强图像上可以观察到沿着导管上皮的不规则强化的软组织，证明其是引起导管扩张的原因[1]。

4. IPMN-分支胰管型 累及分支胰管的IPMN表现为主胰管旁卵圆形囊性肿物，最常见于胰头部。常可见内部分隔，表现出簇状葡萄样改变[1]。MRCP在大部分病例中可以显示该囊性病变与主胰管相沟通（图20-15）[85-89]。

结合患者的临床症状（有或无症状）和影像学特点（病变大小，是否有实性成分，主胰管扩张的程度）对于确定是手术切除还是保守治疗非常重要[90]。如果不含有任何实性成分、有较厚的分隔或者是有间断性生长，小于3cm的病变可以随诊观察。导管内乳头状黏液性肿瘤的主要特点总结见表20-6。

九、外伤

胰腺对于挤压伤比较敏感，尤其是在钝性外伤当中，由邻近的脊柱挤压所致。在成年人当中，有超过75%的胰腺钝性挤压伤是由于驾驶摩托车发生车祸所致。在儿童，自行车引起的损伤比较

表20-5 胰腺黏液性囊腺瘤/囊腺癌主要特点及特征影像

性别	女性＞男性
高峰发病年龄	40—50岁
部位	胰腺体部和尾部
影像特征	较大的单囊或多囊 T_1加权图像和T_2加权图像均呈高信号（黏液成分所致） 提示恶性的征象：较厚的壁或者分隔，乳头状实性突起，侵犯周围组织，肝转移

表20-6 胰腺IPMN主要特点及特征影像

性别	男性＞女性
高峰发病年龄	60—70岁
部位	主胰管和（或）分支胰管
影像特征	主胰管：T_2加权序列或者MRCP显示主胰管扩张，乳头状突起，增强扫描可见沿导管上皮呈不规则强化 分支胰管：卵圆形囊性肿物（呈簇状或葡萄状），常位于胰头部，MRCP可显示病变与主胰管相通

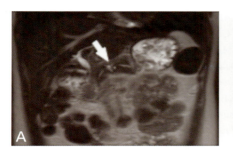
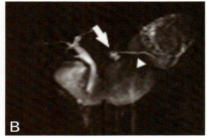
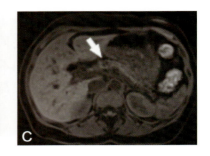
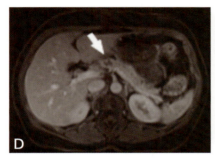
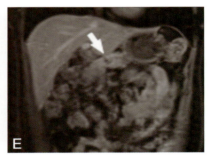

▲ 图 20-15 胰腺颈部分支胰管 IPMN

冠状位 T₂ 加权 SS-ETSE（A）、MRCP（B）、T₁ 加权压脂 SGE（C）、横轴位（D）和冠状位（E）T₁ 加权增强扫描肝静脉期（F）。胰头部表现为呈簇状聚集的小囊（白箭），与主胰管想通，在 MRCP 上显示较为清楚（B，箭头）

常见，在婴幼儿则多见于儿童虐待伤[91]。2/3 的胰腺损伤发生在胰体部，剩余的发生在胰头部、胰颈部和胰尾部的概率相似[92]。孤立的胰腺损伤罕见，在大于 90% 的病例当中往往会合并出现其他脏器损伤，尤其是肝脏、胃、十二指肠和脾脏[92,93]。

由外伤所致的迟发死亡病例主要缘于胰管的破裂，不累及胰管的外伤很少导致死亡[93]。胰管的破裂需要手术治疗或者进行内镜下支架置入术，而不累及胰管的外伤通常采取非手术治疗。正因为如此，利用影像学判断胰管是否有损伤非常重要[94]。

在过去，经内镜逆行性胰胆管造影（endoscopic retrograde cholangiopancreatography, ERCP）是唯一能够评价胰管完整性的方法。MR 胰腺成像现在已经成为取代胰管直接成像的主要技术方法[95]。MR 胰腺成像具有诸多优势，比如非侵袭性、更快速、比 ERCP 更方便应用，并且可以同时评价其他异常改变，比如积液，因此对于评价胰腺实质损伤也很有帮助[96]。

作为损伤的后果，胰管狭窄合并远端胰管的扩张和慢性胰腺炎改变也同时被观察。这种情况并不罕见，尤其是在胰腺中段、脊柱上方发现有较截然的变化，胰头部正常而远端胰腺萎缩和胰管扩张时。诊断时要注意患者的外伤史，尤其是有典型的摩托车车祸，即使在较长时间之前，也需要仔细询问了解[1]。

十、胰腺移植

胰腺移植是对于严重的 I 型糖尿病伴有终末期肾衰竭，或者少见的控制不佳的严重糖尿病患者的明确治疗方案[97]。胰腺移植可以使患者不再使用胰岛素治疗，并且可以降低肾病、视网膜病变和血管病变等并发症的发生率[97]。

移植术后并发症可以分为早期或者晚期，其中早期并发症主要是手术或者技术原因所致。手术相关并发症包括吻合口吻合不良出现的肠内容物渗漏、出血、感染和血管栓塞。非手术性并发症常常是免疫性的，免疫排斥是导致移植失败最主要的原因[97]。

高分辨 3D 造影增强 MR 血管成像是胰腺移植术前精确评价动脉和静脉解剖的技术方法[98-101]。在 T₁ 加权图像上，胰腺实质信号均匀、相对于肝脏是高信号。在 T_2 加权图像上，正常的胰腺移植物显示为介于液体和肌肉之间的信号强度。T_2 加权图像是对于观察胰腺移植术后异常的最敏感序列，因为大部分的病理变化都伴随着含水量的增加[97]。

十一、总结

相比于 CT，结合 MRI 各个可用序列可以实现对各种胰腺病变及其并发症的全面评估。

参考文献

[1] Semelka RC. *Abdominal-Pelvic MRI*, 3rd edn. Hoboken, New Jersey: John Wiley & Sons; 2010.

[2] Semelka RC, Ascher SM. MR imaging of the pancreas. *Radiology*. Sep 1993;188(3):593–602.

[3] Winston CB, Mitchell DG, Outwater EK, Ehrlich SM. Pancreatic signal intensity on T_1-weighted fat satura tion MR images: Clinical correlation. *Journal of Magnetic Resonance Imaging: JMRI*. May–Jun 1995;5(3):267–271.

[4] Mitchell DG, Vinitski S, Saponaro S, Tasciyan T, Burk DL, Jr., Rifkin MD. Liver and pancreas: Improved spin echo T_1 contrast by shorter echo time and fat suppres sion at 1.5 T. *Radiology*. Jan 1991;178(1):67–71.

[5] Semelka RC, Kroeker MA, Shoenut JP, Kroeker R, Yaffe CS, Micflikier AB. Pancreatic disease: Prospective comparison of CT, ERCP, and 1.5-T MR imaging with dynamic gadolinium enhancement and fat suppression. *Radiology*. Dec 1991;181(3):785–791.

[6] Takehara Y, Ichijo K, Tooyama N et al. Breath-hold MR cholangiopancreatography with a long-echo-train fast spin-echo sequence and a surface coil in chronic pancre atitis. *Radiology*. Jul 1994;192(1):73–78.

[7] Bret PM, Reinhold C, Taourel P, Guibaud L, Atri M, Barkun AN. Pancreas divisum: Evaluation with MR cholangiopancreatography. *Radiology*. Apr 1996;199(1):99–103.

[8] Soto JA, Barish MA, Yucel EK et al. Pancreatic duct: MR cholangiopancreatography with a three-dimensional fast spin-echo technique. *Radiology*. Aug 1995;196(2):459–464.

[9] Semelka RC, Simm FC, Recht MP, Deimling M, Lenz G, Laub GA. MR imaging of the pancreas at high field strength: Comparison of six sequences. *Journal of Computer Assisted Tomography*. Nov–Dec 1991;15(6):966–971.

[10] Mitchell DG, Winston CB, Outwater EK, Ehrlich SM. Delineation of pancreas with MR imaging: Multiobserver comparison of five pulse sequences. *Journal of Magnetic Resonance Imaging: JMRI*. Mar–Apr 1995;5(2):193–199.

[11] Cruikshank AH, Benbow EW. *Pathology of the Pancreas*. 2nd edn. Berlin, Germany: Springer; 1995.

[12] Desai MB, Mitchell DG, Munoz SJ. Asymptomatic annular pancreas: Detection by magnetic resonance imaging. *Magnetic Resonance Imaging*. 1994;12(4):683–685.

[13] Applegate KE, Goske MJ, Pierce G, Murphy D. Situs revisited: Imaging of the heterotaxy syndrome. *RadioGraphics: A Review Publication of the Radiological Society of North America, Inc*. Jul–Aug 1999;19(4):837–852; discussion 853–834.

[14] Tham RT, Heyerman HG, Falke TH et al. Cystic fibro sis: MR imaging of the pancreas. *Radiology*. Apr 1991;179(1):183–186.

[15] Ferrozzi F, Bova D, Campodonico F et al. Cystic fibrosis: MR assessment of pancreatic damage. *Radiology*. Mar 1996;198(3):875–879.

[16] King LJ, Scurr ED, Murugan N, Williams SG, Westaby D, Healy JC. Hepatobiliary and pancreatic manifes tations of cystic fibrosis: MR imaging appearances. *RadioGraphics: A Review Publication of the Radiological Society of North America, Inc*. May–Jun 2000;20(3):767–777.

[17] Busireddy KK, AlObaidy M, Ramalho M et al. Pancreatitis-imaging approach. World journal of gastro- intestinal pathophysiology. Aug 15 2014;5(3):252–270.

[18] Shanbhogue AK, Fasih N, Surabhi VR, Doherty GP, Shanbhogue DK, Sethi SK. A clinical and radio logic review of uncommon types and causes of pancreatitis. *Radiographics: A Review Publication of the Radiological Society of North America, Inc*. Jul–Aug 2009;29(4):1003–1026.

[19] Banks PA, Bollen TL, Dervenis C et al. Classification of acute pancreatitis–2012: Revision of the Atlanta classification and definitions by international consensus. *Gut*. Jan 2013;62(1):102–111.

[20] Balthazar EJ. CT diagnosis and staging of acute pancreatitis. *Radiologic Clinics of North America*. Jan 1989;27(1):19–37.

[21] Kim YK, Ko SW, Kim CS, Hwang SB. Effectiveness of MR imaging for diagnosing the mild forms of acute pancreatitis: Comparison with MDCT. *Journal of Magnetic Resonance Imaging: JMRI*. Dec 2006;24(6):1342–1349.

[22] Balthazar EJ, Freeny PC, vanSonnenberg E. Imaging and intervention in acute pancreatitis. *Radiology*. Nov 1994;193(2):297–306.

[23] Lenhart DK, Balthazar EJ. MDCT of acute mild (nonnecrotizing) pancreatitis: Abdominal complications and fate of fluid collections. *AJR American Journal of Roentgenology*. Mar 2008;190(3):643–649.

[24] Matos C, Cappeliez O, Winant C, Coppens E, Deviere J, Metens T. MR imaging of the pancreas: A pictorial tour. *Radiographics: A Review Publication of the Radiological Society of North America, Inc*. Jan–Feb 2002;22(1):e2.

[25] Lau ST, Simchuk EJ, Kozarek RA, Traverso LW. A pancreatic ductal leak should be sought to direct treatment in patients with acute pancreatitis. *American Journal of Surgery*. May 2001;181(5):411–415.

[26] Sandrasegaran K, Tann M, Jennings SG et al. Disconnection of the pancreatic duct: An important but overlooked complication of severe acute pancreatitis. *RadioGraphics: A Review Publication of the Radiological Society of North America, Inc*. Sep–Oct 2007;27(5):1389–1400.

[27] Tann M, Maglinte D, Howard TJ et al. Disconnected pancreatic duct syndrome: Imaging findings and therapeutic implications in 26 surgically corrected patients. *Journal of Computer Assisted Tomography*. Jul–Aug 2003;27(4):577–582.

[28] Petrov MS, Shanbhag S, Chakraborty M, Phillips AR, Windsor JA. Organ failure and infection of pancreatic necrosis as determinants of mortality in patients with acute pancreatitis. *Gastroenterology*. Sep 2010;139(3):813–820.

[29] Peery AF, Dellon ES, Lund J et al. Burden of gastrointestinal disease in the United States: 2012 update. *Gastroenterology*. Nov 2012;143(5):1179–1187 e1171–e1173.

[30] Balci NC, Alkaade S, Magas L, Momtahen AJ, Burton FR. Suspected chronic pancreatitis with normal MRCP: Findings on MRI in correlation with secretin MRCP. *Journal of Magnetic Resonance Imaging: JMRI*. Jan 2008;27(1):125–131.

[31] Semelka RC, Shoenut JP, Kroeker MA, Micflikier AB. Chronic pancreatitis: MR imaging features before and after administration of gadopentetatedimeglumine. *Journal of Magnetic Resonance Imaging: JMRI*. Jan–Feb 1993;3(1):79–82.

[32] Bollen TL. Imaging of acute pancreatitis: Update of the revised Atlanta classification. *Radiologic Clinics of North America*. May 2012;50(3):429–445.

[33] Remer EM, Baker ME. Imaging of chronic pancreatitis. *Radiologic Clinics of North America*. Dec 2002;40(6):1229–1242, v.

[34] Shimosegawa T, Chari ST, Frulloni L et al. International consensus diagnostic criteria for autoimmune pancreatitis: Guidelines of the International Association of Pancreatology. *Pancreas*. Apr 2011;40(3):352–358.

[35] Irie H, Honda H, Baba S et al. Autoimmune pancreatitis: CT and MR characteristics. *AJR American Journal of Roentgenology*. May 1998;170(5):1323–1327.

[36] Van Hoe L, Gryspeerdt S, Ectors N et al. Nonalcoholic duct-destructive chronic pancreatitis: Imaging findings. *AJR American Journal of Roentgenology*. Mar 1998;170(3):643–647.

[37] Takahashi N, Fletcher JG, Fidler JL, Hough DM, Kawashima A, Chari ST. Dual-phase CT of autoimmune pancreatitis: Amultireader study. *AJR American Journal of Roentgenology*. Feb 2008;190(2):280–286.

[38] Chatelain D, Vibert E, Yzet T et al. Groove pancreatitis and pancreatic heterotopia in the minor duodenal papilla. *Pancreas*. May 2005;30(4):e92–e95.

[39] Blasbalg R, Baroni RH, Costa DN, Machado MC. MRI features of groove pancreatitis. *AJR American Journal of Roentgenology*. Jul 2007;189(1):73–80.

[40] Triantopoulou C, Dervenis C, Giannakou N, Papailiou J, Prassopoulos P. Groove pancreatitis: A diagnostic challenge. *European Radiology*. Jul 2009;19(7):1736–1743.

[41] Raman SP, Salaria SN, Hruban RH, Fishman EK. Groove pancreatitis: Spectrum of imaging findings and radiology-pathology correlation. *AJR American Journal of Roentgenology*. Jul 2013;201(1):W29–W39.

[42] Mergo PJ, Helmberger TK, Buetow PC, Helmberger RC, Ros PR. Pancreatic neoplasms: MR imaging and pathologic correlation. *RadioGraphics: A Review Publication of the Radiological Society of North America, Inc*. Mar–Apr 1997;17(2):281–301.

[43] Ros PR, Mortele KJ. Imaging features of pancreatic neoplasms. *JBR-BTR: organe de la Societeroyalebelge de radiologie*. 2001;84(6):239–249.

[44] Low G, Panu A, Millo N, Leen E. Multimodality imaging of neoplastic and nonneoplastic solid lesions of the pancreas. *RadioGraphics: A Review Publication of the Radiological Society of North America, Inc*. Jul–Aug 2011;31(4):993–1015.

[45] Lee ES, Lee JM. Imaging diagnosis of pancreatic cancer: A state-of-the-art review. *World Journal of Gastroenterology: WJG*. Jun 28, 2014;20(24):7864–7877.

[46] Benassai G, Mastrorilli M, Quarto G et al. Factors influencing survival after resection for ductal adenocarcinoma of the head of the pancreas. *Journal of Surgical Oncology*. Apr 2000;73(4):212–218.

[47] Gabata T, Matsui O, Kadoya M et al. Small pancreatic adenocarcinomas: Efficacy of MR imaging with fat suppression and gadolinium enhancement. *Radiology*. Dec 1994;193(3):683–688.

[48] Semelka RC, Kelekis NL, Molina PL, Sharp TJ, Calvo B. Pancreatic masses with inconclusive findings on spiral CT: Is there a role for MRI? *Journal of Magnetic Resonance Imaging: JMRI*. Jul–Aug 1996;6(4):585–588.

[49] Morgan KA, Adams DB. Solid tumors of the body and tail of the pancreas. *The Surgical Clinics of North America*. Apr 2010;90(2):287–307.

[50] Saisho H, Yamaguchi T. Diagnostic imaging for pancreatic cancer: Computed tomography, magnetic resonance imaging, and positron emission tomography. *Pancreas*. Apr 2004;28(3):273–278.

[51] Vellet AD, Romano W, Bach DB, Passi RB, Taves DH, Munk PL. Adenocarcinoma of the pancreatic ducts: Comparative evaluation with CT and MR imaging at 1.5 T. *Radiology*. Apr 1992;183(1):87–95.

[52] Oberg K, Eriksson B. Endocrine tumours of the pancreas. Best practice & research. *Clinical Gastroenterology*. Oct 2005;19(5):753–781.

[53] Mozell E, Stenzel P, Woltering EA, Rosch J, O'Dorisio TM. Functional endocrine tumors of the pancreas: Clinical presentation, diagnosis, and treatment. *Current Problems in Surgery*. Jun 1990;27(6):301–386.

[54] Semelka RC, Custodio CM, CemBalci N, Woosley JT. Neuroendocrine tumors of the pancreas: Spectrum of appearances on MRI. *Journal of Magnetic Resonance Imaging: JMRI*.

Feb 2000;11(2):141–148.

[55] Semelka RC, Cumming MJ, Shoenut JP et al. Islet cell tumors: Comparison of dynamic contrast-enhanced CT and MR imaging with dynamic gadolinium enhancement and fat suppression. *Radiology*. Mar 1993;186(3):799–802.

[56] Sheth S, Hruban RK, Fishman EK. Helical CT of islet cell tumors of the pancreas: Typical and atypical manifestations. *AJR American Journal of Roentgenology*. Sep 2002;179(3):725–730.

[57] Tatli S, Mortele KJ, Levy AD et al. CT and MRI features of pure acinar cell carcinoma of the pancreas in adults. *AJR American Journal of Roentgenology*. Feb 2005;184(2):511–519.

[58] Hsu MY, Pan KT, Chu SY, Hung CF, Wu RC, Tseng JH. CT and MRI features of acinar cell carcinoma of the pancreas with pathological correlations. *Clinical Radiology*. Mar 2010;65(3):223–229.

[59] Hu S, Hu S, Wang M, Wu Z, Miao F. Clinical and CT imaging features of pancreatic acinar cell carcinoma. *La Radiologiamedica*. Aug 2013;118(5):723–731.

[60] Guerrache Y, Soyer P, Dohan A et al. Solid-pseudopapillary tumor of the pancreas: MR imaging findings in 21 patients. *Clinical Imaging*. Jul–Aug 2014;38(4):475–482.

[61] Ng KH, Tan PH, Thng CH, Ooi LL. Solid pseudopapillarytumour of the pancreas. *ANZ Journal of Surgery*. Jun 2003;73(6):410–415.

[62] Cooper JA. Solid pseudopapillary tumor of the pancreas. *RadioGraphics: A Review Publication of the Radiological Society of North America, Inc.* Jul–Aug 2006;26(4):1210.

[63] Kalb B, Sarmiento JM, Kooby DA, Adsay NV, Martin DR. MR imaging of cystic lesions of the pancreas. *RadioGraphics: A Review Publication of the Radiological Society of North America, Inc.* Oct 2009;29(6):1749–1765.

[64] Ferrozzi F, Zuccoli G, Bova D, Calculli L. Mesenchymal tumors of the pancreas: CT findings. *Journal of Computer Assisted Tomography*. Jul–Aug 2000;24(4):622–627.

[65] Carlo Procacci AJM. *Imaging of the Pancreas: Cystic and Rare Tumors*. Berlin, Germany: Springer 2003.

[66] Zeman RK, Schiebler M, Clark LR et al. The clinical and imaging spectrum of pancreaticoduodenal lymph node enlargement. *AJR American Journal of Roentgenology*. Jun 1985;144(6):1223–1227.

[67] Tsitouridis I, Diamantopoulou A, Michaelides M, Arvanity M, Papaioannou S. Pancreatic metastases: CT and MRI findings. *Diagnostic and Interventional Radiology*. Mar 2010;16(1):45–51.

[68] Heredia V, Altun E, Bilaj F, Ramalho M, Hyslop BW, Semelka RC. Gadolinium- and superparamagnetic-iron-oxide-enhanced MR findings of intrapancreatic accessory spleen in five patients. *Magnetic Resonance Imaging*. Nov 2008;26(9):1273–1278.

[69] Martin DR, Semelka RC. MR imaging of pancreatic masses. *Magnetic Resonance Imaging Clinics of North America*. Nov 2000;8(4):787–812.

[70] Fernandez-del Castillo C, Warshaw AL. Cystic tumors of the pancreas. *The Surgical Clinics of North America*. Oct 1995;75(5):1001–1016.

[71] Ros PR, Hamrick-Turner JE, Chiechi MV, Ros LH, Gallego P, Burton SS. Cystic masses of the pancreas. *RadioGraphics: A Review Publication of the Radiological Society of North America, Inc.* Jul 1992;12(4):673–686.

[72] Lewandrowski K, Warshaw A, Compton C. Macrocystic serous cystadenoma of the pancreas: A morphologic variant differing from microcystic adenoma. *Human Pathology*. Aug 1992;23(8):871–875.

[73] Compagno J, Oertel JE. Mucinous cystic neoplasms of the pancreas with overt and latent malignancy (cystadenocarcinoma and cystadenoma). A clinicopathologic study of 41 cases. *American Journal of Clinical Pathology*. Jun 1978;69(6):573–580.

[74] Minami M, Itai Y, Ohtomo K, Yoshida H, Yoshikawa K, Iio M. Cystic neoplasms of the pancreas: Comparison of MR imaging with CT. *Radiology*. Apr 1989;171(1):53–56.

[75] Friedman AC, Lichtenstein JE, Dachman AH. Cystic neoplasms of the pancreas. Radiological-pathological correlation. *Radiology*. Oct 1983;149(1):45–50.

[76] Campbell F, Azadeh B. Cystic neoplasms of the exocrine pancreas. *Histopathology*. Apr 2008;52(5):539–551.

[77] Lack EE. *Pathology of the Pancreas, Gallbladder, Extrahepatic Biliary Tract, and AmpullaryRegion*. New York: Oxford University Press; 2003.

[78] Adsay NV. Cystic neoplasia of the pancreas: Pathology and biology. *Journal of Gastrointestinal Surgery: Official Journal of the Society for Surgery of the Alimentary Tract*. Mar 2008;12(3):401–404.

[79] Silas AM, Morrin MM, Raptopoulos V, Keogan MT. Intraductal papillary mucinous tumors of the pancreas. *AJR American Journal of Roentgenology*. Jan 2001;176(1):179–185.

[80] Terris B, Ponsot P, Paye F et al. Intraductal papillary mucinous tumors of the pancreas confined to secondary ducts show less aggressive pathologic features as compared with those involving the main pancreatic duct. *The American Journal of Surgical Pathology*. Oct 2000;24(10):1372–1377.

[81] Balzano G, Zerbi A, Di Carlo V. Intraductal papillary mucinous tumors of the pancreas: Incidence, clinical findings and natural history. *JOP: Journal of the Pancreas*. Jan 2005;6(1 Suppl.):108–111.

[82] Salvia R, Fernandez-del Castillo C, Bassi C et al. Main-duct intraductal papillary mucinous neoplasms of the pancreas: Clinical predictors of malignancy and long-term survival following resection. *Annals of Surgery*. May 2004;239(5):678–685; discussion 685–687.

[83] Rodriguez JR, Salvia R, Crippa S et al. Branch-duct intraductal papillary mucinous neoplasms: Observations in 145 patients who underwent resection. *Gastroenterology*. Jul 2007;133(1):72–79; quiz 309–310.

[84] Salvia R, Crippa S, Falconi M et al. Branch-duct intraductal

[85] Buetow PC, Rao P, Thompson LD. From the Archives of the AFIP. Mucinous cystic neoplasms of the pancreas: Radiologic-pathologic correlation. *RadioGraphics: A Review Publication of the Radiological Society of North America, Inc*. Mar–Apr 1998;18(2):433–449.

[86] Procacci C, Megibow AJ, Carbognin G et al. Intraductal papillary mucinous tumor of the pancreas: A pictorial essay. *RadioGraphics: A Review Publication of the Radiological Society of North America, Inc*. Nov–Dec 1999;19(6):1447–1463.

[87] Koito K, Namieno T, Ichimura T et al. Mucin-producing pancreatic tumors: Comparison of MR cholangiopancreatography with endoscopic retrograde cholangiopan- creatography. *Radiology*. Jul 1998;208(1):231–237.

[88] Onaya H, Itai Y, Niitsu M, Chiba T, Michishita N, Saida Y. Ductectatic mucinous cystic neoplasms of the pancreas: Evaluation with MR cholangiopancreatography. *AJR American Journal of Roentgenology*. Jul 1998;171(1):171–177.

[89] Irie H, Honda H, Aibe H et al. MR cholangiopancreatographic differentiation of benign and malignant intraductal mucin-producing tumors of the pancreas. *AJR American Journal of Roentgenology*. May 2000;174(5):1403–1408.

[90] Tanaka M, Fernandez-del Castillo C, Adsay V et al. International consensus guidelines 2012 for the management of IPMN and MCN of the pancreas. *Pancreatology: Official Journal of the International Association of Pancreatology*. May–Jun 2012;12(3):183–197.

[91] Ilahi O, Bochicchio GV, Scalea TM. Efficacy of computed tomography in the diagnosis of pancreatic injury in adult blunt trauma patients: A single-institutional study. *The American Surgeon*. Aug 2002;68(8):704–707; discussion 707–708.

[92] Madiba TE, Mokoena TR. Favourable prognosis after surgical drainage of gunshot, stab or blunt trauma of the pancreas. *The British Journal of Surgery*. Sep 1995;82(9):1236–1239.

[93] Bradley EL, 3rd, Young PR, Jr., Chang MC et al. Diagnosis and initial management of blunt pancreatic trauma: Guidelines from a multiinstitutional review. *Annals of Surgery*. Jun 1998;227(6):861–869.

[94] Gupta A, Stuhlfaut JW, Fleming KW, Lucey BC, Soto JA. Blunt trauma of the pancreas and biliary tract: A multimodality imaging approach to diagnosis. *RadioGraphics: A Review Publication of the Radiological Society of North America, Inc*. Sep–Oct 2004;24(5):1381–1395.

[95] Fulcher AS, Turner MA, Yelon JA et al. Magnetic resonance cholangiopancreatography (MRCP) in the assessment of pancreatic duct trauma and its sequelae: Preliminary findings. *The Journal of Trauma*. Jun 2000;48(6):1001–1007.

[96] Soto JA, Alvarez O, Munera F, Yepes NL, Sepulveda ME, Perez JM. Traumatic disruption of the pancreatic duct: Diagnosis with MR pancreatography. *AJR American Journal of Roentgenology*. Jan 2001;176(1):175–178.

[97] Vandermeer FQ, Manning MA, Frazier AA, Wong-You-Cheong JJ. Imaging of whole-organ pancreas transplants. *RadioGraphics: A Review Publication of the Radiological Society of North America, Inc*. Mar–Apr 2012;32(2):411–435.

[98] Dillman JR, Elsayes KM, Bude RO, Platt JF, Francis IR. Imaging of pancreas transplants: Postoperative findings with clinical correlation. *Journal of Computer Assisted Tomography*. Jul–Aug 2009;33(4):609–617.

[99] Hagspiel KD, Nandalur K, Burkholder B et al. Contrast-enhanced MR angiography after pancreas transplantation: Normal appearance and vascular complications. *AJR American Journal of Roentgenology*. Feb 2005;184(2):465–473.

[100] Dobos N, Roberts DA, Insko EK, Siegelman ES, Naji A, Markmann JF. Contrast-enhanced MR angiography for evaluation of vascular complications of the pancreatic transplant. *RadioGraphics: A Review Publication of the Radiological Society of North America, Inc*. May–Jun 2005;25(3):687–695.

[101] Hagspiel KD, Nandalur K, Pruett TL et al. Evaluation of vascular complications of pancreas transplantation with high-spatial-resolution contrast-enhanced MR angiography. *Radiology*. Feb 2007;242(2):590–599.

Chapter 21
肾上腺

The Adrenal Gland

Shaunagh McDermott, Colin J. McCarthy, Michael A. Blake 著

朱永健 译

王 爽 校

目录 CONTENTS

一、MRI 序列 / 500

二、特殊肾上腺病变 / 503

随着医学影像使用的增加，越来越多意外的肿块被发现，肾上腺意外瘤的发现大约占所有腹部 CT 检查的 5%[1,2]。另外，对患有已知的恶性肿瘤的患者进行 CT 检查，9%～13% 会发现肾上腺结节[1]，但是这些病变中转移瘤所占比例不到 36%[3]。放射科医师在基于影像学特征对这些病变进行确定性诊断中起重要作用。本章的目的是回顾目前和新出现的磁共振成像（MRI）技术在肾上腺成像的应用，并阐释常见的肾上腺病变的 MRI 特征。

一、MRI 序列

（一）同相位和反相位化学位移成像

化学位移成像（chemical shift imaging, CSI）利用了脂肪和水不同的共振频率。由于存在较长的化学侧链，脂肪中的氢质子比水中氢质子的进动频率低。对于同相位成像，选择回波时间（echo time, TE），使脂肪和水质子信号是相加的。相反，反相位成像选择的 TE 时间，使得脂肪和水信号呈反相 180°相差，导致信号相消，如果水和脂肪质子存在相同的体素内，会表现为信号下降，这种现象存在于许多腺瘤中。在单个体素中仅含有脂肪或水成分的病变，并不是两者同时存在，不会显示出信号相消。当体素中存在等量的脂肪和水时，在反相位图像上可以看到几乎完全的信号丢失。相反，如果脂质或水质子占主要成分，则反相位图像上的信号强度基本不变，并且病变性质仍不确定。

在 1.5 T，水信号和脂肪信号之间的频移约为 225 Hz，导致在 TE 为 4.4 ms、8.8 ms 和 13.2 ms 时产生同相位信号，在 TE 为 2.2 ms、6.6 ms 和 11.0 ms 时产生反相位信号。在 3T MR 扫描仪上，频率差是标准的 1.5 T 扫描仪的 2 倍，因此 TE 需要调整。在 3T 扫描仪上，脂肪和水同相位分别为 1.1 ms、3.3 ms 和 5.5 ms，反相位分别为 2.2 ms、4.4 ms 和 6.6 ms[4]。

理想情况下，反相位图像应该使用双回波序列的第一回波来获得。在这样做的过程中，同相位图像和反相位图像之间的任何信号丢失都是由于在相同的体素中存在脂质和水的质子造成的。如果使用第二个较长的 TE 获得反相位的图像，信号的丢失可能是由于细胞内脂质的存在或由于 T_2^* 敏感性效应[5,6]或两者的结合而造成的。应该使用同反相位的最小 TE 值，使信噪比最大化，使 T_2^* 敏感性和 T_2 效应最小化。

在肾上腺病变中有不同的方法可以确定脂质存在。我们可以使用相同的窗口设置在工作站上定性地比较同相位和对应的反相位相图像。如果肾上腺病变在反相位图像上显示信号下降，则它包含体素内的脂质和水质子[7]（图 21-1）。另一种方法是从同相位图像中减去反相位图像，从而生成一个减影图像。在减影图像上出现的任何信号都表明在同一体素中存在脂质和水的质子[8]。

也可以对肾上腺病变的脂质进行定量分析，使用多种方法进行内部参考。

肾上腺信号强度（signal intensity, SI）指数计算为

$$\left[\frac{(SI_{同相位} - SI_{反相位})}{SI_{同相位}}\right] \times 100\%$$

肾上腺与脾脏的化学位移比率计算为

$$\left[\frac{(肾上腺 SI_{反相位} / 脾脏 SI_{反相位})}{(肾上腺 SI_{同相位} / 脾脏 SI_{同相位})} - 1\right] \times 100\%$$

由于肝脏经常发生脂肪变性，因此肝脏不能作为内参照，由于胞质内脂肪的存在这也会导致反位相图像的信号丢失。肌肉也可能受到脂肪浸润，因此通常也不用作内参照。

目前尚没有建立最佳的肾上腺 SI 指数，因为对于腺瘤与非腺瘤的鉴别诊断有不同阈值报道，表明肾上腺 SI 指数在 1.5 T 时为 1%～23%[9-13]，在 3.0 T 时为 1.7%～20.2%[6,14,15]。

双回波同反相位成像也可以用来识别宏观脂肪，因为它会在体内脂肪和附近含有水的组织之间产生 *India-ink* 伪影[16]。两点和三点的 Dixon

T_1 脂肪图像可以显示肾上腺病变的体素内脂质质子和宏观脂肪。

(二) 脂肪抑制 T_1 加权成像

通过将同相位 T_1 加权图像与相对应的脂肪抑制 T_1 加权图像进行比较，可以识别病变内的宏观脂肪（图 21-2）。

(三) T_2 加权成像

早期研究发现腺瘤倾向于在 T_2 加权序列上具有与肝脏或肌肉相似的信号强度，而肾上腺转移的 T_2 信号强度更接近于脾脏[17-20]。嗜铬细胞瘤在 T_2 加权序列上具有较高的信号强度（图 21-3）；然而，至少 30% 的患者表现出中等或低 T_2 信号强度，类似于其他肾上腺病变[21]。

(四) 动态对比增强成像

动态增强研究中肿瘤的强化模式取决于其血管系统、血管通透性和细胞外间隙的大小。肾上腺皮质的正常血供具有丰富的网状毛细血管窦。与腺瘤和正常肾上腺皮质相比，肾上腺癌血管化程度减低，且正常动脉系统受到恶性肿瘤细胞侵犯，因

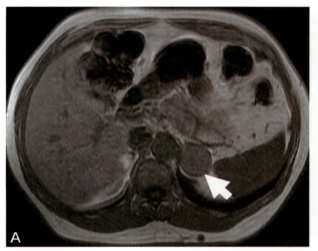

▲ 图 21-1 肾上腺病变
57 岁男性，左肾上腺结节（箭），富含脂肪的腺瘤，同相位（A）和反相位（B）之间的信号明显下降

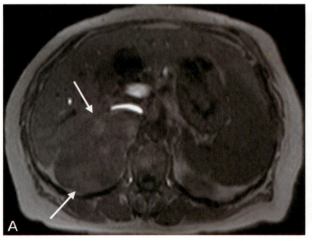 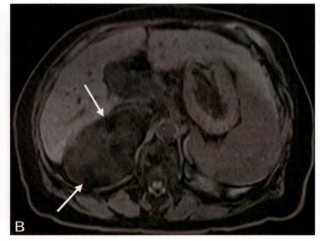

▲ 图 21-2 肾上腺肿块
80 岁男性，右侧肾上腺巨大肿块，T_1 加权序列（A）信号强度高的区域在脂肪抑制序列（B，箭）显示出信号下降，符合含脂肪成分的髓样脂肪瘤

此肾上腺癌的强化程度较低且强化速度较慢。

较早的研究表明，延迟对比增强 MRI 可能有助于区分腺瘤和非腺瘤，大多数腺瘤显示出比转移更快的对比剂廓清[19,20,22]。然而，通常不会延迟对比增强的 MR 图像上对病变的对比剂廓清模式进行评估，因为特定的延迟扫描通常不包括在肾上腺 MR 扫描方案中。

最近，有研究着眼于肾上腺病变的早期强化模式来解决这个问题。一项研究发现，大多数腺瘤在增强后即刻（第 18s）会出现毛细血管显影，在第 45s 出现消退。相比之下，恶性病变在第 18s 表现为可忽略的或微弱强化，在第 45s 时仍表现为不规则或边缘强化[23]。另一项研究发现，与恶性病变的斑片状或边缘强化相比，腺瘤在增强早期通常是均匀的或点状的强化。增强晚期图像上，所有恶性病变表现为不均匀强化，而超过半数的腺瘤表现为边缘强化。腺瘤的对比剂流入率明显高于恶性肿物，因此，恶性病变的强化达峰时间明显长于腺瘤[24]。

（五）扩散加权成像

扩散加权成像（diffusion-weighted imaging，DWI）基于水分子在微观层面的运动生成图像对比。最常用的序列是基于两个大小相同的梯度

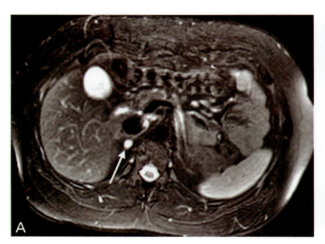
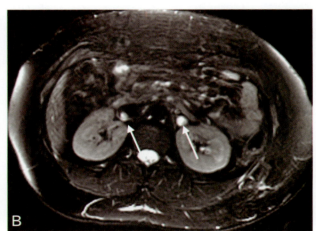

▲ 图 21-3　嗜铬细胞瘤

24 岁男性 VHL（von Hippel-Lindau）患者，右侧（A）和左侧（B）肾上腺可见 T_2 明显高信号的肾上腺结节（箭），符合嗜铬细胞瘤

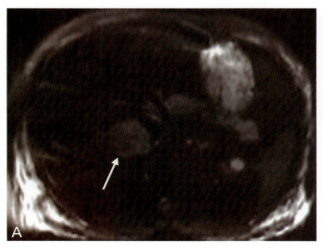
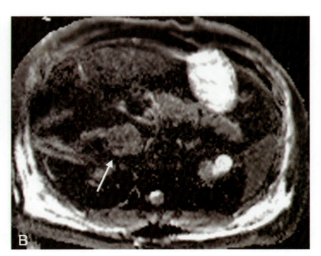

▲ 图 21-4　肾上腺肿块

53 岁男性，右侧肾上腺肿块（箭），DWI 高信号（A），ADC 低信号（B）。活检证实为肾上腺皮质癌

在 180°的自旋回波序列的重新聚焦脉冲。这两个梯度对水分子的影响取决于它们的运动。在两个梯度之间没有明显移动的固定水分子中，这些梯度脉冲的作用是完全的复相位，同时保留信号。相反，在非静止的水分子中，在第一个和第二个梯度之间移动的分子会导致信号的失相位和信号丢失。信号损失的程度与水分子运动的程度成正比。

通过使用至少两个不同的 b 值进行 DWI 成像，可以通过计算表观扩散系数（apparent diffusion coefficient，ADC）进行定量分析。ADC 是独立于磁场的，可以克服 T_2 穿透效应的影响。扩散受限的区域在 DWI 上表现为亮的，而 ADC 图上表现为暗的（图 21-4）；这与简单的 T_2 延长（T_2 穿透）相反，在 DWI 和 ADC 图上均显示高信号强度。

虽然 DWI 已被证明对身体其他体部肿瘤的定性诊断有帮助，但现有文献表明，DWI 及评估肾上腺病变的 ADC 对区分良性和恶性肾上腺病变都没有帮助[13,25-28]。

（六）磁共振波谱

在磁共振波谱（MR spectroscopy, MRS）中，应用射频脉冲后组织的信号频率被用来分离和表征一个体素内的实际代谢产物或化学物质。信号强度和线宽可以用来确定化学物的相对数量。迄今为止，在肾上腺病变的定性诊断中使用 MRS 的经验很有限。一个 MRS 可能的作用是将腺瘤与非腺瘤区分，因为研究发现腺瘤与非腺瘤相比，脂质峰更高[29]，其脂质/肌酐峰更高[30]。MRS 的另一种可能的应用是鉴别嗜铬细胞瘤。一项关于病理证实的嗜铬细胞瘤的小样本研究发现，嗜铬细胞瘤在 6.8 ppm 处具有特征性的波谱峰，与病变内部儿茶酚胺的存在一致[31]。

然而，肾上腺的 MRS 是具有挑战性的，因为病灶较小且存在由于膈肌运动引起呼吸伪影。

（七）PET/MR

随着越来越多的 PET/MR 系统进入日常临床实践，它的作用或比目前常规影像检查手段相比的额外益处目前还尚不明确。

二、特殊肾上腺病变

（一）含脂肪的病变

1. 肾上腺腺瘤 肾上腺腺瘤的患病率与年龄有关，一项研究表明 20—29 岁的患者患病率为 0.14%，70 岁以上的患者患病率为 7%[32]。大约 70% 的肾上腺腺瘤富含脂质，并含有足够数量的细胞胞质内脂肪，导致 CSI 上的信号丢失（图 21-1 和图 21-5）。一项研究表明，在平扫 CT 上不确定的肾上腺病变（例如 HU 值 10～30）的患者中，化学移位 MRI 对腺瘤的诊断有 89% 的敏感性和 100% 的特异性[33]。因为多达 30% 的

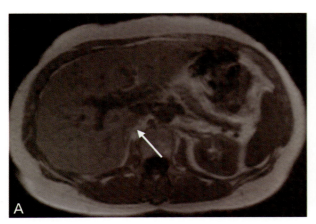 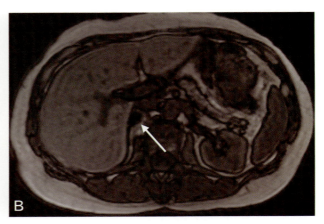

▲ 图 21-5 肾上腺腺瘤

63 岁女性，右侧肾上腺小结节（箭），显示在同相位（A）和反相位（B）图像之间的信号明显下降，与富含脂肪的腺瘤相符

肾上腺腺瘤是缺乏脂质的，化学移位 MRI 对这些病变的评估的作用有限。然而，需要注意的是，除了腺瘤以外的病变，如肾上腺皮质癌、嗜铬细胞瘤、透明细胞肾细胞癌和肝细胞癌转移，有时也可以在反位相图像上显示信号丢失。

2. 髓脂肪瘤 髓脂肪瘤是一种良性肿瘤，由成熟的脂肪组织和散在的造血成分组成。髓脂肪瘤占偶然发现的肾上腺病变的 6%[2]。髓脂肪瘤的影像学诊断基于宏观脂肪的检出。脂肪成分在非脂肪抑制 T_1 加权图像上表现为高信号，在脂肪抑制图像上表现为信号强度的下降（图 21-2）。在反相位图像上病变 - 肾上腺交界面或肾上腺病变中出现 India ink 伪影，则提示为髓脂肪瘤。

MRI 的表现是基于病变内的脂肪含量。如果主要是由脂肪组成，病变在 T_1 加权像上是均匀的高信号，在 T_2 加权像上有中等信号强度。如果是由脂肪和髓质成分混合组成的，病变是不均匀的，包含局灶的脂肪信号强度，并且在 T_2 加权和对比增强 T_1 加权图像上呈高信号。然而，如果病变主要由髓样细胞构成，那么在 T_1 加权像上病变会相对于肝脏呈低信号，T_2 加权序列上病变相对于肝脏呈高信号，增强扫描后有强化（图 21-6）。

尽管宏观脂肪的存在是髓脂肪瘤的特征，但它不是诊断性的，因为病例报告已经描述了其他肿瘤的宏观脂肪。其他影像学特征，如边缘、异质性和侵犯，都应被考虑以排除少脂肪的恶性肿瘤。

（二）囊性肿块

1. 单纯囊肿 单纯性囊肿在 T_2 加权像上表现为高信号，T_1 加权像上表现为低信号，没有软组织成分或内部增强（图 21-7）。

2. 假性囊肿 假性囊肿通常是出血或梗死的后遗症。肾上腺假性囊肿的外观更复杂，包括有膈膜、血液成分，甚至是出血或透明血栓形成的软组织成分（图 21-8）。

3. 淋巴管瘤 肾上腺的囊性淋巴管瘤很少见。在 MRI 上，这些病变是薄壁囊性结构，在 T_1 加权序列上呈低信号强度，在 T_2 加权序列上呈高信号强度，并没有明显的内部强化。

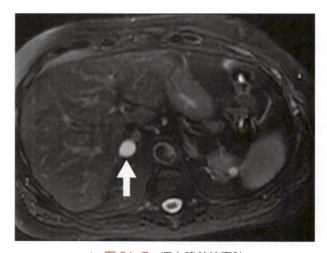

▲ 图 21-7 肾上腺单纯囊肿
61 岁男性，右侧肾上腺结节（箭），T_2 呈高信号。T_1 呈低信号，增强扫描未见强化（未显示）。符合肾上腺囊肿

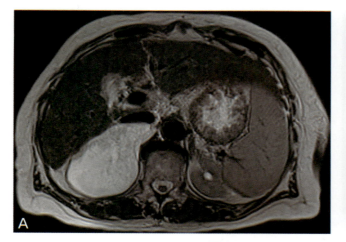
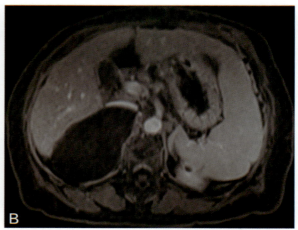

▲ 图 21-6 肾上腺脂肪瘤（同图 21-2 患者）
80 岁男性，右侧肾上腺髓脂肪瘤，在 T_2 加权序列上（A）呈高信号，增强扫描呈不均匀强化（B）

（三）富血供病变

嗜铬细胞瘤

嗜铬细胞瘤是由嗜铬细胞组成的肿瘤，分泌儿茶酚胺。在 MRI 上，嗜铬细胞瘤在 T_1 加权序列上呈低信号；但是，如果病变内存在脂肪或出血，则表现为高信号强度。典型的嗜铬细胞瘤表现为在 T_2 加权序列上明显的高信号强度（灯泡征），与其他病变形成对比（图 21-3 和图 21-9）。然而，最近发现高达 30% 的嗜铬细胞瘤可以在 T_2 加权序列上显示低信号强度。不典型的影像学特征在遗传相关的嗜铬细胞瘤中尤其普遍。但是，在没有局部侵袭或转移的情况下，没有特定的特征来预测肿瘤的恶性程度（图 21-9 和图 21-10）。

直到最近，只有 10% 的嗜铬细胞瘤被认为与遗传相关；然而，分子遗传学的最新进展表明，至少有 1/3 的嗜铬细胞瘤患者存在基因突变[34,35]。

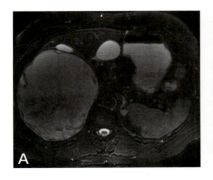 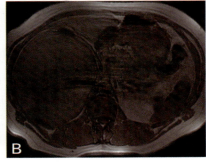 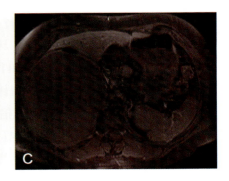

▲ 图 21-8 肾上腺假性囊肿

46 岁男性，右侧肾上腺巨大肿物，在 T_2 加权序列信号不均匀（A），且在增强扫描前（B）和后（C）未显示强化。切除后证实为假性囊肿

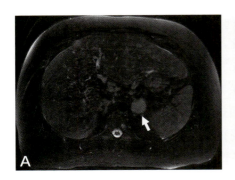 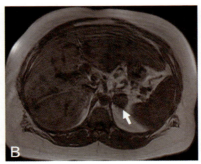 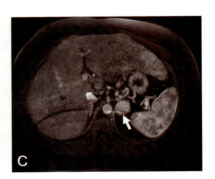

▲ 图 21-9 嗜铬细胞瘤伴肝转移

61 岁女性，左侧肾上腺肿物（箭），T_2 呈轻度高信号（A），T_1 低信号（B），并有明显的强化（C）。本例被证实为嗜铬细胞瘤，伴有多发肝转移

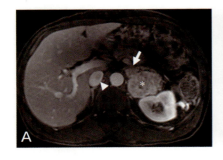 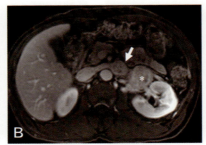 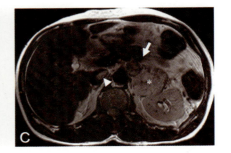

▲ 图 21-10 嗜铬细胞瘤

52 岁男性，左侧肾上腺巨大肿物（星号），增强后呈不均匀强化，延伸至左肾静脉（箭）及下腔静脉（箭头，A 和 B）。在 T_2 加权序列（C）上也有类似的发现。本例被证实为嗜铬细胞瘤

嗜铬细胞瘤可在多种的综合征中发现，包括多发内分泌肿瘤（MEN）综合征Ⅱa型和Ⅱb型、神经纤维瘤型 1 型、von Hippel–Lindau 综合征、结节性硬化、Sturge-Weber 综合征、琥珀酸脱氢酶（succinate dehydrogenase, SDH）突变 B、C、D 和 Carney 三联征（图 21-3）。

（四）恶性病变

1. 肾上腺皮质癌 肾上腺皮质癌（adrenocortical carcinoma, ACC）是一种起源于肾上腺皮质的恶性肿瘤。由于存在脂肪和（或）坏死，ACCs 在 MRI 上通常是异质性的（图 21-11）。在 T_1 加权序列上，这些肿瘤通常与肝脏相比呈等低信号，在某些区域或出血中表现为 T_1 高信号。这些肿瘤也可能含有胞质内脂肪，这可能导致反位相序列的信号下降。ACCs 有侵犯静脉的倾向。

2. 淋巴瘤 淋巴瘤偶尔也会原发或继发性地侵犯肾上腺。原发性肾上腺淋巴瘤极为罕见。原发性肾上腺淋巴瘤通常保持肾上腺的形态；然而，坏死或囊性成分的存在不均匀的强化使它们很难与其他肿瘤如 ACC、嗜铬细胞瘤或转移性区分开来[36]。继发性肾上腺受侵典型出现在非霍奇金淋巴瘤中。早期的继发性累及可能只导致弥漫性肾上腺增大，而腺体结构没有改变。进展期疾病中可见更多的结节性肿大，MR 表现是非特异性的，类似于转移。通常情况下，病变是在 T_1 加权序列上相对于肝脏是低信号的，并在 T_2 加权序列上相对于肝脏呈不均匀的高信号。

3. 转移 肾上腺是仅次于肺、肝和骨的第四大转移部位。肺癌、乳腺癌、结肠癌、黑色素瘤和甲状腺癌通常与肾上腺转移有关[37]。肾上腺转移可以表现为软组织肿物，也可以表现为腺体的弥漫性肿大。转移灶往往表现为巨大、不均匀性和边界不清（图 21-12 和图 21-13）。少数情况下，原发恶性肿瘤的转移瘤含有胞质内脂肪，如透明细胞肾细胞癌或肝细胞癌，会导致反相位图像上的信号丢失，因此可能误诊为腺瘤（图 21-14）。

4. 碰撞瘤 碰撞瘤定义为并存的两个相邻但组织学上不同的肿瘤，两者都可以是良性的，也可以是恶性的[38]。

（五）儿童肿瘤

1. 神经母细胞瘤 神经母细胞瘤是儿童第三常见的恶性肿瘤；然而在成年人中却很罕见。肾上腺受累表现为软组织肿物，通常伴有钙化。在 MRI 上，神经母细胞瘤通常是异质性的，增强呈不均匀强化，T_1 加权图像呈低信号，T_2 加权图像呈高信号[39,40]（图 21-15）。神经母细胞瘤可以包绕和（或）压缩邻近血管，很少有血管侵犯。与其他横断面技术相比，MRI 的一个优点是能够检测椎管内侵犯和（或）骨髓受累。

2. 神经节细胞瘤 神经节细胞瘤是一种罕见的良性神经源性肿瘤，由 Schwann 细胞和交感

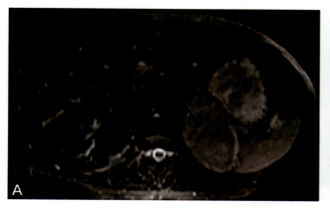
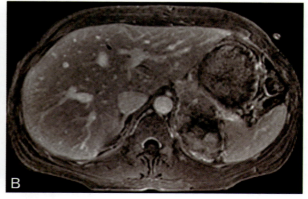

▲ 图 21-11　肾上腺皮质癌

42 岁女性，左侧肾上腺肿物，在 T_2 加权上呈不均匀信号（A），增强后表现为不均匀强化（B）。该肿物被证实为 ACC

神经节来源的神经节细胞组成。神经节细胞瘤在 T_1 加权序列上是均有低信号，在 T_2 加权序列上呈不同的信号强度，这取决于黏液、细胞和胶原成分的比例（图 21-16）。MRI 的特征之一是 T_2 加权序列上的低信号强度曲线带，使肿瘤呈现扭曲的表现[41]。在动态对比增强 MRI 上，神经节细胞瘤通常表现为渐进性强化而不是早期强化[42]。

3. 神经节母细胞瘤 神经节母细胞瘤是一种中等级别的肿瘤，具有良性神经节神经瘤和恶性的神经母细胞瘤的特征。影像学的表现各不相同，从实性肿物为主，到囊性肿物为主，伴少许条带状实性组织成分。

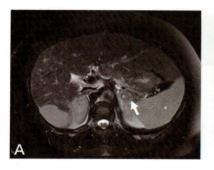 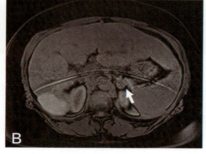 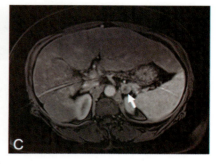

▲ 图 21-12 肝细胞癌的肾上腺转移灶

63 岁女性，患有肝细胞癌（hepatocellular carcinoma, HCC），左侧肾上腺结节（箭）。表现为 T_2 高信号（A），（B）和（C）显示增强前后的强化程度。本例经活检证实为肝癌转移

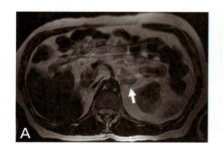 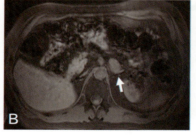 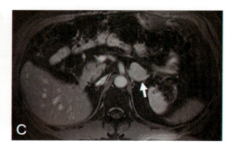

▲ 图 21-13 肾细胞癌的肾上腺转移灶

74 岁男性，既往有肾细胞癌（renal cell carcinoma, RCC）病史，左侧肾上腺结节状增大（箭）。表现为 T_2 高信号（A），并显示增强扫描前（B）和后（C）的序列。本例经活检证实 RCC 转移

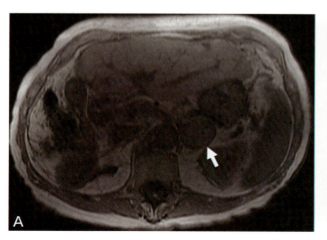 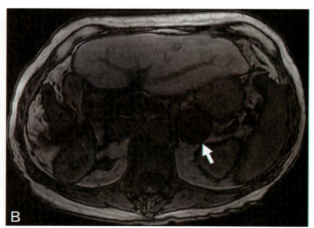

▲ 图 21-14 肾上腺结节

78 岁 HCC 患者，左肾上腺结节（箭）迅速增大，显示同相位（A）和反相位（B）有信号降低。然而，由于它的生长迅速，被认为是转移

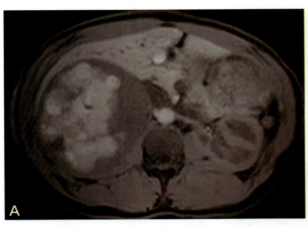 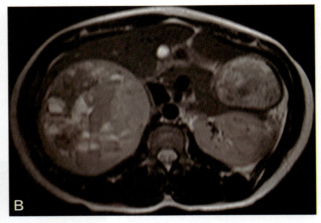

▲ 图 21-15 神经母细胞瘤

24 岁女性，右肾上腺大肿物，在 T_1（A）和 T_2 加权序列（B）上均为异质性。该肿物在切除后证实为神经母细胞瘤

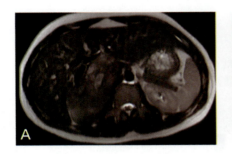 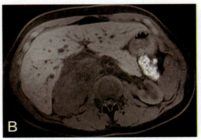 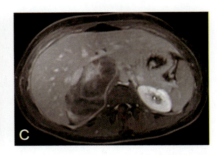

▲ 图 21-16 神经节细胞瘤

20 岁女性，右侧肾上腺巨大肿物，在 T_2 加权序列（A）上呈异质性，T_1 加权序列上呈高信号（B），钆增强后序列上呈不均匀强化（C）。该肿物在切除后被证实为神经节细胞瘤

（六）其他

1. 肾上腺出血 肾上腺出血可继发于外伤性和非外伤性病因。在右侧肾上腺更常见，有 20% 的病例发生于双侧。非创伤性病因包括凝血病、压力、静脉高压和出血性肿瘤。

MRI 表现取决于出血的阶段。在急性期，小于 7d，血肿在 T_1 加权序列上表现为等或稍低信号，在 T_2 加权序列上表现为显著低信号。在亚急性期，1~7 周，血肿在 T_1 和 T_2 加权序列上均表现为高信号（图 21-17）。T_1 高信号出现在血肿周围，并在数周内向中央填充。在慢性阶段，7 周后，T_1 和 T_2 加权序列上都出现了一个低信号环，它是由血铁血黄素沉积引起的，显示在梯度回波序列上。

对于没有外伤性或非外伤性出血危险因素的患者，需要进行对比增强，并可能需要的影像学随诊，以排除潜在的肿物。

2. 感染 结核、组织胞质菌病和其他肉芽肿病可以累及肾上腺，通常累及双侧。影像学特征是非特异性的，可能包括软组织肿物、囊性改变和钙化[43]。

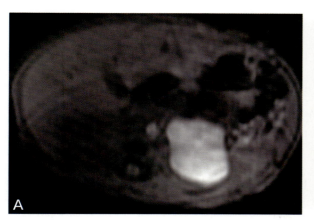
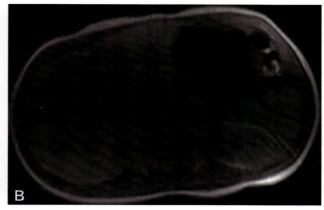

▲ 图 21-17　1 例 10d 大的脓毒症女性患儿
左侧肾上腺巨大 T_1 高病变（A）。5 个月后随访 MRI 显示出血完全吸收（B）

参考文献

[1] Bovio S, Cataldi A, Reimondo G et al. (2006) Prevalence of adrenal incidentaloma in a contempo rary computerized tomography series. *J Endocrinol Invest* 29:298–302.

[2] Song JH, Chaudhry FS, Mayo-Smith WW (2008) The incidental adrenal mass on CT: Prevalence of adrenal disease in 1,049 consecutive adrenal masses in patients with no known malignancy. *AJR Am J Roentgenol* 190:1163–1168.

[3] Oliver TW, Jr., Bernardino ME, Miller JI et al. (1984) Isolated adrenal masses in nonsmall-cell bronchogenic carcinoma. *Radiology* 153:217–218.

[4] Chang KJ, Kamel IR, Macura KJ et al. (2008) 3.0-T MR imaging of the abdomen: Comparison with 1.5 T. *Radio-Graphics* 28:1983–1998.

[5] Tsushima Y, Dean PB (1995) Characterization of adrenal masses with chemical shift MR imaging: How to select echo times. *Radiology* 195:285–286.

[6] Schindera ST, Soher BJ, Delong DM et al. (2008) Effect of echo time pair selection on quantitative analy sis for adrenal tumor characterization with in-phase and opposed-phase MR imaging: Initial experience. *Radiology* 248:140–147.

[7] Mayo-Smith WW, Lee MJ, McNicholas MM et al. (1995) Characterization of adrenal masses (< 5 cm) by use of chemical shift MR imaging: Observer performance versus quantitative measures. *AJR Am J Roentgenol* 165:91–95.

[8] Savci G, Yazici Z, Sahin N et al. (2006) Value of chemi cal shift subtraction MRI in characterization of adrenal masses. *AJR Am J Roentgenol* 186:130–135.

[9] Tsushima Y, Ishizaka H, Kato T et al. (1992) Differential diagnosis of adrenal masses using out-of-phase FLASH imaging. A preliminary report. *Acta Radiol* 33:262–265.

[10] Namimoto T, Yamashita Y, Mitsuzaki K et al. (2001) Adrenal masses: Quantification of fat content with dou ble-echo chemical shift in-phase and opposed-phase FLASH MR images for differentiation of adrenal adeno mas. *Radiology* 218:642–646.

[11] Fujiyoshi F, Nakajo M, Fukukura Y et al. (2003) Characterization of adrenal tumors by chemical shift fast low-angle shot MR imaging: Comparison of four methods of quantitative evaluation. *AJR Am J Roentgenol* 180:1649–1657.

[12] Israel GM, Korobkin M, Wang C et al. (2004) Comparison of unenhanced CT and chemical shift MRI in evaluat ing lipid-rich adrenal adenomas. *AJR Am J Roentgenol* 183:215–219.

[13] Sandrasegaran K, Patel AA, Ramaswamy R et al. (2011) Characterization of adrenal masses with diffusion- weighted imaging. *AJR Am J Roentgenol* 197:132–138.

[14] Marin D, Soher BJ, Dale BM et al. (2010) Characterization of adrenal lesions: Comparison of 2D and 3D dual gradi-ent-echo MR imaging at 3 T—Preliminary results. *Radiology* 254:179–187.

[15] Nakamura S, Namimoto T, Morita K et al. (2012) Characterization of adrenal lesions using chemical shift MRI: Comparison between 1.5 Tesla and two echo time pair selection at 3.0 Tesla MRI. *J Magn Reson Imaging* 35:95–102.

[16] Hood MN, Ho VB, Smirniotopoulos JG et al. (1999) Chemical shift: The artifact and clinical tool revisited. *Radio-Graphics* 19:357–371.

[17] Baker ME, Blinder R, Spritzer C et al. (1989) MR evaluation of adrenal masses at 1.5 T. *AJR Am J Roentgenol* 153:307–312.

[18] Kier R, McCarthy S (1989) MR characterization of adrenal masses: Field strength and pulse sequence considerations. *Radiology* 171:671–674.

[19] Krestin GP, Freidmann G, Fishbach R et al. (1991) Evaluation of adrenal masses in oncologic patients: Dynamic contrast-enhanced MR vs CT. *J Comput Assist Tomogr* 15:104–110.

[20] Slapa RZ, Jakubowski W, Januszewicz A et al. (2000) Discriminatory power of MRI for differentiation of adrenal non-adenomas vs adenomas evaluated by means of ROC analysis: Can biopsy be obviated? *Eur Radiol* 10:95–104.

[21] Blake MA, Kalra MK, Maher MM et al. (2004) Pheochro-

mocytoma: An imaging chameleon. *RadioGraphics* 24(Suppl. 1):S87–S99.

[22] Krestin GP, Steinbrich W, Friedmann G (1989) Adrenal masses: Evaluation with fast gradient-echo MR imaging and Gd-DTPA-enhanced dynamic studies. *Radiology* 171:675–680.

[23] Chung JJ, Semelka RC, Martin DR (2001) Adrenal adenomas: Characteristic postgadolinium capillary blush on dynamic MR imaging. *J Magn Reson Imaging* 13:242–248.

[24] Inan N, Arslan A, Akansel G et al. (2008) Dynamic contrast enhanced MRI in the differential diagnosis of adrenal adenomas and malignant adrenal masses. *Eur J Radiol* 65:154–162.

[25] Tsushima Y, Takahashi-Taketomi A, Endo K. (2009) Diagnostic utility of diffusion-weighted MR imaging and apparent diffusion coefficient value for the diagnosis of adrenal tumors. *J Magn Reson Imaging* 29:112–117.

[26] Miller FH, Wang Y, McCarthy RJ et al. (2010) Utility of diffusion-weighted MRI in characterization of adrenal lesions. *AJR Am J Roentgenol* 194:W179–W185.

[27] Cicekci M, Onur MR, Aydin AM et al. (2013) The role of apparent diffusion coefficient values in differentiation between adrenal masses. *Clin Imaging* 38:148–153.

[28] Halefoglu AM, Altun I, Disli C et al. (2012) A prospective study on the utility of diffusion-weighted and quantitative chemical-shift magnetic resonance imaging in the distinction of adrenal adenomas and metastases. *J Comput Assist Tomogr* 36:367–374.

[29] Leroy-Willig A, Roucayrol JC, Luton JP et al. (1987) In vitro adrenal cortex lesions characterization by NMR spectroscopy. *Magn Reson Imaging* 5:339–344.

[30] Faria JF, Goldman SM, Szejnfeld J et al. (2007) Adrenal masses: Characterization with in vivo proton MR spectroscopy—Initial experience. *Radiology* 245:788–797.

[31] Kim S, Salibi N, Hardie AD et al. (2009) Characterization of adrenal pheochromocytoma using respiratory triggered proton MR spectroscopy: Initial experience. *AJR Am J Roentgenol* 192:450–454.

[32] Kloos RT, Gross MD, Francis IR et al. (1995) Incidentally discovered adrenal masses. *Endocr Rev* 16:460–484.

[33] Haider MA, Ghai S, Jhaveri K et al. (2004) Chemical shift MR imaging of hyperattenuating (>10 HU) adrenal masses: Does it still have a role? *Radiology* 231:711–716.

[34] Neumann HP, Bausch B, McWhinney SR et al. (2002) Germ-line mutations in nonsyndromic pheochromocytoma. *N Engl J Med* 346:1459–1466.

[35] Benn DE, Gimenez-Roqueplo AP, Reilly JR et al. (2006) Clinical presentation and penetrance of pheochromocytoma/paraganglioma syndromes. *J Clin Endocrinol Metab* 91:827–836.

[36] Kato H, Itami J, Shiina T et al. (1996) MR imaging of primary adrenal lymphoma. *Clin Imaging* 20:126–128.

[37] Taffel M, Haji-Momenian S, Nikolaidis P et al. (2012) Adrenal imaging: A comprehensive review. *Radiol Clin North Am* 50:219–243, v.

[38] Schwartz LH, Macari M, Huvos AG et al. (1996) Collision tumors of the adrenal gland: Demonstration and characterization at MR imaging. *Radiology* 201:757–760.

[39] Lonergan GJ, Schwab CM, Suarez ES et al. (2002) Neuroblastoma, ganglioneuroblastoma, andgan glioneuroma: Radiologic-pathologic correlation. *RadioGraphics* 22:911–934.

[40] Hiorns MP, Owens CM. (2001) Radiology of neuroblastoma in children. *Eur Radiol* 11:2071–2081.

[41] Rha SE, Byun JY, Jung SE et al. (2003) Neurogenic tumors in the abdomen: Tumor types and imaging characteristics. *RadioGraphics* 23:29–43.

[42] Zhang Y, Nishimura H, Kato S et al. (2001) MRI of ganglioneuroma: Histologic correlation study. *J Comput Assist Tomogr* 25:617–623.

[43] Wilson DA, Muchmore HG, Tisdal RG et al. (1984) Histoplasmosis of the adrenal glands studied by CT. *Radiology* 150:779–783.

Chapter 22
上消化道和小肠疾病

Diseases of the Upper Gastrointestinal Tract and Small Bowel

Davide Bellini, Carlo Nicola De Cecco, Domenico De Santis, Marco Rengo, Justin Morris, Andrea Laghi 著

朱永健 译

冯 冰 校

目录 CONTENTS

一、解剖 / 512
二、MRI 技术 / 513
三、上消化道病理学 / 515
四、小肠病理学 / 519
五、总结 / 526

横断面成像技术越来越多地应用于上消化道和小肠疾病的无创性评估中。计算机断层扫描（computed tomography, CT）仍是食管恶性肿瘤和胃恶性肿瘤研究的首选研究方法，而钡餐检查是评价食管运动功能障碍的首选方法。无论如何，磁共振成像（magnetic resonance imaging, MRI）的应用正在向通过单一的成像技术同时获取解剖学和功能学的信息方面扩展。此外，磁共振小肠造影检查不仅在克罗恩病（Crohn's disease, CD）中起着重要作用，而且在各种良性及恶性肿瘤、乳糜泻、感染性疾病和小肠梗阻的评估中也起着重要作用。与 CT 相比，MRI 的优点包括对比度高、无辐射暴露以及应用的静脉对比剂更加安全。磁共振小肠造影检查还可以提供功能学方面的信息，包括动态评估小肠蠕动情况和管腔狭窄处的可扩张性情况。另一方面，MRI 也有一些局限性，包括费用较高，以及检查的质量依赖于患者的配合程度和屏住呼吸的能力。

本章的目的是概述 MRI 在上消化道和小肠疾病中的实际作用，并阐述说明临床指征、采集方案及最常见疾病的经典影像学表现。

一、解剖

（一）食管

食管是消化道的一部分，上接咽部，向下与胃部相连。

食管上段位于颈部，约第 6 颈椎水平。然后向下进入胸腔，穿过膈肌进入腹部，总长度为 25～26cm。

在食管颈段，食管与气管、甲状腺及左右喉返神经相邻。

再往下，食管位于后纵隔，并与左主支气管相交叉。

在纵隔内，食管位于气管和纵隔淋巴结的后方。食管后壁与胸椎及 C_4 以下颈椎紧密贴邻，然后缓慢向前弯曲，与奇静脉、半奇静脉、胸导管和降主动脉相邻。食管侧面与纵隔胸膜和迷走神经纤维相邻。

再向下，食管通过膈肌的食管裂孔进入腹腔并与胃连接。食管的腹腔部分的前壁被腹膜所覆盖。

（二）胃

胃是消化道的囊状扩张部分，位于横膈下的腹腔内，与食管及十二指肠相连。它在成人体内的平均容量约为 1200 ml，胃的位置随姿势、胃内容物的多少和小肠的状况而变化。

胃由下列结构组成。

（1）两壁：前下壁和后上壁。

（2）两弯：胃小弯形成胃部的右或后缘，胃大弯向后、向上及向左形成弓形结构。在胃小弯的幽门侧有一个明显的切迹，为胃角切迹。

（3）两口：上面的贲门和下面的幽门。

通过胃小弯的胃角切迹及胃大弯相对扩张的左侧缘平面，将胃部分成上部或体部，以及下部或幽门部。胃体的上部被称为胃底，经贲门口的水平面将胃底与剩余的胃体区分开来。幽门部由幽门窦和幽门管依次组成。

（三）小肠

小肠位于胃和大肠之间，包括十二指肠、空肠（近端）和回肠（远端）。它的长度为 3～10 m 不等，平均长度为 6 m。十二指肠通过 Treitz 韧带固定到腹膜后，在十二指肠空肠曲延续为空肠。空肠和回肠的界限不是很清楚。空肠约占小肠的 1/3，壁较厚，腔较回肠宽，主要位于左上腹部。空肠的典型形态特征是环状黏膜皱襞。相对于回肠，环状黏膜皱襞在空肠更明显，在 MR 小肠造影检查中很容易辨认。回肠约占小肠的 2/3，位于中腹部、右下腹部和盆腔。

在 MR 小肠造影检查中，在未使用解痉药的情况下，空肠和回肠肠腔的正常直径必须小于 25 mm，且两者壁厚通常均小于 2 mm。

回肠在回结肠交界处延续为大肠。

小肠和大肠之间的主要区别之一是肠系膜的存在。它的根部从左侧 L_2 延伸到右骶髂关节，长

Chapter 22 上消化道和小肠疾病
Diseases of the Upper Gastrointestinal Tract and Small Bowel

度只有 15 cm。

消化道解剖如图 22-1 所示。

二、MRI 技术

（一）食管

食管是一个受图像伪影影响的器官，这些伪影由呼吸心脏搏动而产生，导致在扰相梯度（spoiled gradient-echo，SGE）回波序列上图像质量差且有运动伪影。

目前，纵隔和食管的 MRI 已经通过钆增强的 3D 梯度回波（Gd-enhanced 3D gradient-echo，GRE）序列得到改善，该序列在非常短的屏气时间内获得，可以使运动伪影最小化，并获得纵隔和食管壁的优质图像[1]。

与传统的快速自旋回波序列相比，3D GRE T_1 的特点是具有较短的回波时间（echo time, TE）和重复时间（repetition time, TR），可以减少典型的气体与组织界面的顺磁性伪影。除了 T_1 加权成像外，T_2 加权单次激发快速自旋回波序列在检测游离液体或囊性病变方面也很有帮助。

还可以使用平衡梯度回波序列；利用这些同时具有 T_1 和 T_2 加权特性的序列，可以获得超快（大约每层 1s）和具有良好的液体/组织对比度和信噪比的优质图像。采用稳态自由进动序列的磁共振电影成像技术可以通过计算收缩幅度和频率来评估运动功能。

然而，这些序列对食管常规评估的作用仍未确定。

（二）胃

胃壁扩张和低张可以使胃部 MRI 获得更好的结果。通过口服对比剂，可以使胃壁扩张。它们可以分为阳性（在 T_1 和 T_2 加权图像上产生高信号）、阴性（在 T_1 和 T_2 加权图像上产生低信号）和双相对比剂（在 T_1 和 T_2 加权图像上产生相反的信号强度）[2]。水是双相对比剂，也是最简单的对比剂。必须在 MRI 检查前 5 min 内口服对比剂（800～1000 ml）。水在避免磁敏感伪影方面优于空气或其他阴性对比剂，特别是在扩散加权成像（diffusion-weighted imaging，DWI）中。

胃部低张是通过注射解痉药获得的，通常在进行这项检查之前不久进行静脉注射；临床常规应用的两个主要的解痉药为丁基东莨菪碱（Buscopan®）和胰高糖素（GlucaGen®）。

患者在接受 MR 检查前必须进行正常呼吸和屏气的训练。

MRI 扫描方案应包括屏气 T_1 加权 2D、T_2 加权快速自旋回波（TSE）（脂肪抑制和非脂肪抑制）、DWI 序列和脂肪抑制对比增强 T_1 加权序列。

（三）小肠

良好的小肠评价需要结合两个重要的条件：快

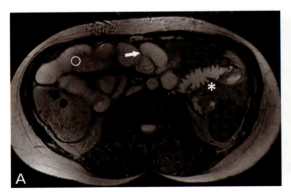
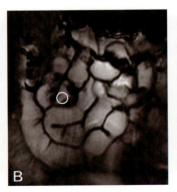
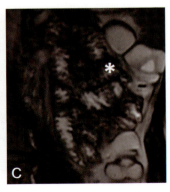

▲ 图 22-1 1 例 27 岁男性，正常的 MRI 小肠造影表现

T_2 加权轴位（A）和冠状位（B、C）口服双相对比剂的正常小肠扩张的图像。注意小肠壁很薄，仅有 1～2 mm（箭）。空肠的正常皱襞（星号）与回肠的正常皱襞不同，回肠的皱襞（圆）较少

速成像技术和应用对比剂使肠腔充分扩张。此外，静脉注射对比剂对于评估肠壁、病变强化和肠系膜血管情况是必需的[4]。

1. 对比剂　介绍几种肠内对比剂，包括普通水、甲基纤维素以及含有刺槐豆胶、甘露醇、硫酸钡和聚乙二醇的溶液[5]。这些药物的作用是抑制肠道内水分的吸收，并可导致轻度腹泻。

肠对比剂可根据其对于肠腔信号强度的作用分为阳性（肠腔呈高亮信号）、阴性（肠腔呈低信号）或双相（肠腔在 T_2 上呈高亮信号，T_1 上呈低信号）。单一对比剂的选择有优点也有缺点。放射科医师应根据临床需求、MRI 经验、药物的可用性和患者的耐受性选择适当的对比剂。

阳性对比剂可导致 T_1 弛豫时间的缩短；因此，这些药物可以增加肠腔 T_1 加权图像的信号强度。这类对比剂在很大程度上已被弃用。

阴性对比剂以超顺磁粒子为基础，通过诱导局部磁场的不均匀性而发挥作用，从而缩短 T_1 和 T_2 弛豫时间。T_2 加权效应占主导地位，对评估肠壁水肿有所帮助。

双相对比剂是在不同序列上具有不同信号强度的物质，这取决于给药的浓度。这些对比剂包括一些产生水样效应的不可吸收的溶液；它们在 T_2 加权图像上是高信号的，在 T_1 加权的图像上是低信号的。在静脉注射对比剂后，肠腔与壁之间的差异得到提高，这是评估不同强化模式的理想条件。

在 MR 小肠造影检查前小肠充盈的理想方案仍存在争议；肠对比剂可以口服（口服法 MR 小肠造影检查）或通过鼻空肠管注入（插管法 MR 小肠造影检查）。一般情况下，插管法 MR 小肠造影检查仅用于轻度小肠梗阻的评估和无法通过口服对比剂行 MR 小肠造影检查的患者。一些研究表明，插管法 MR 小肠造影检查中肠道扩张得更好，因此插管法比口服法 MR 小肠造影检查能更好地显示肠黏膜异常[6]。但是，对于充分地评估小肠的其他疾病，并不需要这种程度的扩张。事实上，其他研究已经表明，口服法 MR 小肠造影检查在检测 CD 患者活性炎症方面的敏感性与插管法 MR 小肠造影检查相似[7,8]。

2. 口服法 MR 小肠造影检查　目前，已有几种不同的剂量计算方法被推荐，并由所使用的药物种类和用量决定[7,9]。最普遍接受的充盈肠腔的方法是在检查前禁食 6h，检查前 40min 内给予大量对比剂（1500～2000 ml）。解痉药对减少肠蠕动和运动伪影很有帮助。

3. 插管法 MR 小肠造影检查　在透视下将鼻胃管插入至十二指肠空肠结合处远端。基线图像 [真实稳态进动快速成像（true fast imaging with steady state precession, TrueFISP）] 用来评估肠道充盈程度。以 80 ml/min 的速度手动注入约 1500 ml 肠对比剂，每 2 分钟监测一次小肠的充盈情况。整个过程必须由放射科医师监控，并相应地调整流量。当对比剂到达结肠时，可静脉注射解痉药（20 mg Buscopan® 或 0.3 mg GlucaGon®）[5]。

4. MRI 扫描方案　患者可在采用仰卧位或俯卧位扫描。

通常，使用双相肠对比剂时，T_2 加权序列和对比增强梯度回波 T_1 序列最有帮助。

首先，我们获得基于稳态进动（TrueFISP）的冠状位和轴位 T_2 加权序列图像，以便对整个腹部的肠管充盈情况进行评估。如果充盈足够，则在冠状位和轴位上获得基于单次激发技术（半傅里叶采集单次激发快速自旋回波序列，half-Fourier acquisition single-shot turbo spin echo, HASTE）的 T_2 加权序列[5]。

稳态进动序列图像上可能出现化学移位和磁敏感伪影，可能使得肠壁厚度评估的复杂化；然而，它们对运动伪影相对不敏感，可以更好地显示肠系膜血管和淋巴结。另一方面，HASTE 序列上肠腔和肠壁之间对比度高，可以良好地显示肠壁厚度和黏膜皱襞形态变化情况。脂肪抑制 T_2 加权图像对于改善炎症时高信号的肠壁和肠周脂肪的显示情况很重要。

采用稳态自由进动序列的电影 MR 成像可以

用来对小肠运动功能进行监测和评估,计算小肠的收缩幅度和频率。电影 MR 成像可以提供额外的信息,特别是对于不明确的肠段,也可以帮助确认真正的狭窄。

为了减少小肠蠕动,静脉注射 0.5mg 胰高血糖素。1min 后,应用钆双胺(Dotarem;Guerbet,Roissy,France;注射速率为 2 ml/s,0.2 mg/kg)前和 70 s 后分别采集冠状位和轴位二维或三维 T_1 加权 SGE 序列。

可以应用 DWI 序列。但是,在临床应用中,目前尚没有达成共识的理想 b 值。活动性疾病或肿瘤都可表现为扩散受限,DWI 序列可帮助识别病变肠段。

显然,在对 1.5 T 的脉冲序列进行足够的修改后,也可以用更高的场强(3T 系统)对小肠进行 MRI 检查。

三、上消化道病理学

(一)失弛缓症

1. 临床表现 失弛缓症是一种以食管下端括约肌(lower esophageal sphincter, LES)功能丧失为特征的慢性食管运动障碍。其结果是摄入食物在胃食管交界处下行进入胃腔困难、食物停滞,以及由此引起的食管扩张。主要症状为吞咽困难[10]。

2. 病理生理学 该疾病的发病机制与食管下 1/3 的肠肌间(Auerbach)神经丛的神经元死亡有关,这将导致 LES 的张力减退和缺乏运动协调,原发性(吞咽诱导)和继发性(扩张诱导)蠕动消失,出现不协调、无推动力的节段性收缩(第三蠕动)。原发性失弛缓症可能由感染等原因引起,如 Chagas 病,但也可能继发于肿瘤。

3. MRI 表现 MRI 可显示食管远端和贲门壁的软组织情况。

主要表现是远端食管狭窄,伴和(或)不伴壁增厚,进展期会出现狭窄上方食管的节段扩张。典型的表现呈鸟嘴样外观。电影 MRI 序列可以显示扩张的食管和无功能的 LES。通常伴随食团通过时间的延长(> 20s)[11]。

4. 鉴别诊断 恶性肿瘤,正常蠕动,不对称狭窄,胃食管反流疾病所致的狭窄。

(二)弥漫性食管痉挛

1. 临床表现 弥漫性食管痉挛(diffuse esophageal spasm, DES)的患者在吞咽食团时可能会出现吞咽困难、胸痛、反胃和胃灼热,尤其是吞咽那些富含胶原纤维(如肉类)的食物、冷饮或碳酸饮料时。痉挛通常独立于吞咽发生,引起一种收缩感,有时剧烈,或胸骨后不适。

2. 病理生理学 主要的病因是由于抑制性神经的损伤,导致远端食管出现过早及迅速的推进性收缩。

在远端食管,收缩是由胆碱能(兴奋性)和一氧化氮(抑制性)神经节细胞介导的。此外,神经梯度的存在使得远端的抑制性神经节神经元的比例越来越大。因此,吞咽反应引起远端食管出现一段时间的静止(吞咽抑制),并逐渐延伸至 LES[12]。远端收缩的潜伏期,即测量从咽部吞咽开始到食管远端出现收缩的时间。同时收缩的患者的远端收缩潜伏期比正常蠕动向远端推进的患者的短。在 DES 患者中,食管平滑肌厚度也有所增加[13]。最后,还有一些 DES 患者(如失弛缓症)的特点是 LES 松弛功能的受损。

3. MRI 表现 在 DES 中,功能性改变影响食管的下 1/3 段。食团的通过引起食管肌肉的痉挛和不协调收缩,从而改变了食管腔的形态,使其类似于螺旋状或串珠状。由于下段食管过早地收缩,导致食团移动时间不够,因此阻塞在痉挛节段的食管中。

显然,并不是每次进食时都会出现痉挛,因此需要患者重复数次这个过程。

(三)胃食管反流病

1. 临床表现 胃食管反流病(gastroesophageal reflux disease, GERD)是西方国家最常见的胃肠

疾病之一[14]，定义为胃部，有时也包括十二指肠的内容物反流进入食管。

胃灼热和胃酸反流是主要症状，被认为是诊断 GERD 相当特异的症状。

GERD 也可与哮喘、肺炎病史、非典型性胸痛、慢性咳嗽、声音嘶哑、咽部异物感、消化不良和吞咽困难（非典型症状）有关。

胃灼热是由反流物质与敏感或溃疡的食管黏膜接触而产生的。持续的吞咽困难提示发生了消化道的狭窄。许多消化性狭窄的患者都有数年胃灼热的临床病史。

GERD 可能与出血、狭窄、Barrett 食管及食管腺癌等并发症有关。

2. 病理生理学 正常的抗反流机制包括 LES 和食管胃交界处的解剖位置；当 LES 和胃之间的压力梯度消失时就会发生反流（由于硬皮病样疾病、其他肌病、食管裂孔疝、肥胖、药物、手术损伤及胃潴留等引起的 LES 减弱）。

胃内容物的反流导致食管损伤和食管炎症。

症状是由黏膜内化学敏感的痛觉感受器激活而引起的，与此同时，腔内胃酸扩散到组织中产生炎症级联反应[15]。最近有人提出胃液反流并不直接损伤食管黏膜，而是刺激食管上皮细胞分泌趋化因子，吸引并激活免疫细胞，对食管鳞状上皮细胞造成损伤[16]。

随着幽门螺杆菌感染率的降低，消化性溃疡的患病率也随之降低，这与 GERD 患病率的增加有关。有迹象表明，幽门螺杆菌感染可能保护食管免受反流性食管炎的侵害，这可能是因为感染会引起慢性胃炎，从而降低胃酸分泌[17]。

然而，幽门螺杆菌的根除与 GERD 的发展之间的联系仍然存在疑问[18]。

3. MRI 表现 常见的 MRI 表现为食管壁增厚。静脉注射钆对比剂后，炎症和纤维化的管壁在延迟期图像上可见强化。

（四）食管裂孔疝

1. 临床表现 食管裂孔疝是指部分胃通过横膈的食管裂孔向上脱位进入胸腔。根据贲门、横膈和疝入的部分胃之间的关系，食管裂孔疝可分为四类[19]。

Ⅰ型——滑动型裂孔疝，是目前最常见的类型。它的特征是胃-食管交界处和部分胃底滑动到纵隔。

Ⅱ型、Ⅲ型和Ⅳ型——均为食管旁型裂孔疝。Ⅱ型发生于食管胃交界仍处于正常位置，而胃底通过裂孔疝出；Ⅲ型是Ⅰ型和Ⅱ型的混合疝，包括胃底/胃体疝出；Ⅳ型的特征是胃与其他器官一起疝入胸腔。

2. 病理生理学 滑动疝可能是由于胃-食管交界处固定于横膈作用的减弱、食管的纵向收缩或腹内压力的增加而引起的。

3. MRI 表现 食管裂孔的扩大及胃-食管交界部向横膈上方脱位。

（五）憩室

憩室是食管壁的囊袋状结构。相对于消化道的其他部位，憩室在食管中并不常见。

根据定位憩室可分为三组：食管上段出现的憩室，典型的 Zenker 憩室；发生在食管中段的憩室；膈上憩室，发生于 LES 上面。

Zenker 憩室位于下咽后壁（Killian 裂）的自然薄弱区，位于食管上括约肌的近端，会导致口臭、唾液和几天前摄入食物颗粒的反流。当它变大并充满食物时，会压迫食管，导致吞咽困难或完全梗阻。

食管中段憩室和膈上憩室可能是由陈旧性粘连或与食管运动异常相关的推进性蠕动引起的牵拉所导致。中小型憩室通常无症状。

MRI 显示了食管壁的囊袋状突起的轮廓，也可以测量大小、定位及显示与其他纵隔结构的关系。

（六）肿瘤

1. 食管癌

（1）病理生理学：食管癌是一种严重的恶性

肿瘤，死亡率高、预后差。这是全球第八常见的恶性肿瘤，其发病率正迅速增加[20]。尽管在诊断和治疗方面取得了许多进展，但所有被诊断为食管癌的患者5年生存率仅有15%～20%[21]。

食管癌最常见的两种组织学类型包括鳞状细胞癌（squamous cell carcinoma，SCC）和腺癌。

SCC是世界上最常见的食管癌类型，在食管中下段的发生概率相同。烟草和乙醇的使用是SCC的主要危险因素，并且两者在同一患者身上具有复合效应。

在大多数国家，腺癌是第二大食管恶性肿瘤。然而，在过去的几十年里，一些西方国家食管腺癌的发病率急剧上升。大约3/4的食管腺癌发生在远端食管，与Barrett食管有关。Barrett食管被定义为食管上皮的胃黏膜化生，继发于慢性胃反流[22]。食管腺癌有明显经胃食管连接部直接侵犯胃贲门和胃底的趋势[23]。

（2）临床表现：SCC最常见的症状是进行性吞咽困难、吞咽疼痛和体重减轻。吞咽困难最初发生于固体食物，逐渐发展为包括半固体和液体食物。肿瘤侵犯纵隔的患者可能伴有胸痛。不幸的是，有症状的患者在诊断时通常已为进展期疾病[24]。

大多数食管腺癌的患者在出现症状时已为进展期，其症状与SCC患者相似。无论分期如何，食管腺癌预后均优于SCC[25]。

（3）MRI表现：诊断性检查通常包括超声内镜（endoscopic ultrasonography，EUS）和CT。EUS可以有效地区分T_1、T_2期及T_3、T_4期病变。CT在评估周围组织浸润程度和检测远处转移中起着重要作用[26]。腔内MRI是正在被开发用于局部分期的一种潜在方法[27]，尽管这种技术在评估狭窄性肿瘤中仍存在困难。

高分辨MRI可以显示食管壁的三层结构：黏膜层呈中等信号强度，被高信号强度的黏膜下层及中低信号强度的黏膜肌层所包围[28]。

T_1期肿瘤难以与周围正常管壁区分。

T_2期肿瘤表现为包括黏膜下层的中等信号强度，向固有肌层延伸，但不超过固有肌层。

固有肌层外缘不光滑或中等信号强度的结节延伸至其内，表明肿瘤已扩展到外膜（T_3）。结节状的中等信号强度向食管周围组织侵犯也提示T_3。肿瘤扩散到不同的器官表明病变为T_4期[29]。

MRI在确定肿瘤的可切除性方面比CT（软组织对比有限）更准确。MRI确定可切除性的标准为在手术时不切除的组织边缘距离肿瘤必须≥1mm[30]。

术前准确地评估淋巴结转移情况至关重要。无淋巴结转移的患者在手术切除后的整体5年生存率为70%～92%，而有淋巴结转移的患者为18%～47%[31]。

食管癌的淋巴转移发生率高于其他任何胃肠道肿瘤。这些转移的淋巴结分布非常广泛，从颈部延伸到腹部，淋巴结转移的大小通常都很小[32]。基于T_1或T_2弛豫时间的淋巴结特征的价值有限；淋巴结大小通常并不是可信赖的预测因素，因为大的淋巴结可以是良性的，而小的淋巴结可以是恶性的[33]。食管癌分期系统见表22-1[34]。

2. 胃腺癌

（1）病理生理学：胃癌是世界上第四常见的恶性肿瘤，仅次于肺癌、乳腺癌和直肠癌。超过70%的胃癌病例发生在发展中国家，全世界一半的病例发生在东亚。总体来说，胃癌的发病率和死亡率在过去几十年里急剧下降。尽管最近有所下降，但它仍是全球癌症致死的第二大原因[35]。

幽门螺杆菌感染是胃癌的一个危险因素。这种细菌引起慢性胃炎和萎缩性胃炎，其特点是胃黏膜慢性炎症，导致胃黏膜肠上皮化生和不典型增生[36]。

胃癌通过胃壁向胃周组织直接扩散，有时与相邻器官粘连，如胰腺、结肠或肝脏。该疾病也通过淋巴管扩散或腹膜表面种植转移。肝脏是肿瘤血源性扩散最常见的部位。

（2）临床表现：胃癌早期通常无症状。随着肿瘤的进展，患者可能会出现上腹部不适，从隐约餐后的饱胀到严重的持续疼痛。厌食和恶心很

表 22-1 《AJCC 癌症分期手册》（第 7 版）的食管癌分期系统

原发肿瘤（T）	
T_X	原发肿瘤无法评估
T_0	无原发肿瘤证据
Tis	高度不典型增生
T_1	肿瘤侵及黏膜固有层、黏膜肌层或黏膜下层
T_{1a}	肿瘤侵及黏膜固有层或黏膜肌层
T_{1b}	肿瘤侵及黏膜下层
T_2	肿瘤侵及固有肌层
T_3	肿瘤侵及纤维膜
T_4	肿瘤侵及邻近器官
T_{4a}	可切除肿瘤侵及胸膜、心包或膈肌
T_{4b}	不可切除肿瘤侵及其他邻近结构，如主动脉、椎体、气管等
区域淋巴结（N）	
N_X	区域淋巴结无法评估
N_0	无区域淋巴结转移
N_1	1～2 个区域淋巴结转移
N_2	3～6 个区域淋巴结转移
N_3	≥7 个区域淋巴结转移
远处转移	
M_0	无远处转移
M_1	有远处转移

常见。最终会出现体重下降。恶心和呕吐在幽门肿瘤的患者中很常见。如果病变侵犯贲门，吞咽困难可能是主要症状。

Borrmann 分型基于形状和浸润边缘，将进展期胃癌分为四类：1 型，息肉型；2 型，局限溃疡型；3 型，浸润溃疡型；4 型，弥漫浸润型。

人们普遍认为 Borrmann 4 型胃癌的预后比其他三种类型差[37]。

（3）MRI 表现：MRI 可以显示胃壁内层的局限性增厚和强化，或不规则肿物伴不均匀强化。

病变组织在 T_1 加权像上主要表现为等信号，T_2 加权像表现为高信号，但并非所有病例都存在这些特征，因此导致信号的一致性较差。然而，在 DWI 上肿瘤表现为高信号，因此在 T_2 加权和动态增强 MRI 的基础上增加弥散加权 MRI，可以显著提高胃癌 T 分期的整体准确性。与 T_2 加权和 CE MRI 相比，DWI 更容易识别淋巴结转移。

进展期胃癌的分期有两个困难。首先，由于肿瘤边界模糊，pT_2 期病变可能被高估。第二，在靠近肝脏、胰腺和横膈处胃部的 pT_3 期病变容易被高估为 T_4 期，这是由于这些结构被一层薄薄的内脏周围脂肪所包绕[3]。

在 DW 图像上可以广泛和肯定地观察到三明治征的特征性表现，提示分期 $\geq pT_3$。这个影像特征是指黏膜/黏膜下层呈高信号，固有肌层呈中低信号和浆膜下层/浆膜层呈高信号[38]。

与 MDCT 相比，胃癌患者的 MRI 研究较少。尽管 MRI 的软组织对比良好，但是目前研究提示 MDCT 和 MRI 在 T 分期和 N 分期的诊断准确率方面价值相近[39]。胃癌分期系统见表 22-2[34]。

3. 胃间质瘤

（1）病理生理学：胃肠道间质瘤（gastrointestinal stromal tumors, GISTs）是最常见的胃肠道间叶源性肿瘤，其特点是表达一种特定的免疫组化标记物：c-kit[40]。GISTs 可以发生在胃肠道的任何部位，但最常见的发生部位是胃部（60%～70%）[41]。大约 20% 的 GISTs 是恶性的，最常见的转移部位是肝脏和腹膜；淋巴结转移罕见[42]。治疗首选是手术切除。对于出现转移的患者应保留联合化疗的方法。

（2）临床表现：GISTs 在临床上通常是无症状的。如果有症状，胃 GISTs 最常见的症状是出血、消化不良、厌食和腹痛。

（3）MRI 表现：GISTs 的影像学特征因肿瘤大小而异。它们通常表现为外生性的生长方式，表现为明显突出胃轮廓的肿物。壁内和腔内肿物并不常见。

小肿瘤往往边界清楚，信号均匀，而大肿瘤

往往边缘呈分叶状、有黏膜溃疡、中央坏死、出血、空洞和不均匀的强化[43]；尽管肿瘤很大，但很少出现梗阻[44]。生长方式的特点是邻近器官和血管的移位，直接侵犯邻近结构较为少见，有时可以出现在进展期肿瘤中。

在 MRI 上，肿瘤通常在 T_1 加权像上表现为低信号，T_2 加权像上表现为中高信号，注射钆对比剂后可见强化。在《AJCC 癌症分期手册》（第 7 版）（表 22-3）中首次出现了针对 GISTs 的正式分期系统[34]。

四、小肠病理学

（一）先天畸形

胚胎学上，小肠和近端大肠由中肠发育而来。中肠由肠系膜动脉供血，从十二指肠襻的起始部延伸至横结肠的后 1/3。

在发育的早期阶段，中肠通过卵黄肠（脐肠）管与卵黄囊相通，后者随后消失。分化在 1 个月内按照从头到尾的顺序发生（31～59d）。

在 MRI 检查中可以发现的两种常见先天畸形是肠旋转不良和 Meckel 憩室。

1. 小肠旋转不良 小肠旋转不良是一种先天性异常，导致小肠和（或）大肠的位置异常。它的发生是由于中肠在发育过程中未能完成所需的 270° 逆时针旋转。

表 22-2 《AJCC 癌症分期手册》（第 7 版）的胃腺癌分期系统

原发肿瘤（T）	
T_X	原发肿瘤无法评估
T_0	无原发肿瘤证据
Tis	原位癌：上皮内肿瘤，未侵及固有层
T_1	肿瘤侵及黏膜固有层、黏膜肌层或黏膜下层
T_{1a}	肿瘤侵及黏膜固有层或黏膜肌层
T_{1b}	肿瘤侵及黏膜下层
T_2	肿瘤侵及固有肌层
T_3	肿瘤穿透浆膜下结缔组织，而尚未侵犯脏腹膜或邻近结构。T_3 期肿瘤也包括那些侵犯胃结肠或胃肝韧带，或进入大或小网膜的肿瘤，没有穿透覆盖这些结构的脏腹膜
T_4	肿瘤侵犯浆膜（脏腹膜）或邻近结构
T_{4a}	肿瘤侵犯浆膜（脏腹膜）
T_{4b}	肿瘤侵犯邻近结构，如脾脏、横结肠、肝脏、膈肌、胰腺、腹壁、肾上腺、肾脏、小肠或腹膜后
区域淋巴结（N）	
N_X	区域淋巴结无法评估
N_0	无区域淋巴结转移
N_1	1～2 个区域淋巴结转移
N_2	3～6 个区域淋巴结转移
N_3	≥7 个区域淋巴结转移
远处转移	
M_0	无远处转移
M_1	有远处转移

表 22-3 《AJCC 癌症分期手册》（第 7 版）胃肠道间质的分期系统

原发肿瘤（T）	
T_X	原发肿瘤无法评价
T_0	无原发肿瘤的证据
T_1	肿瘤 ≤ 2 cm
T_2	肿瘤 > 2 cm 但 ≤ 5 cm
T_3	肿瘤 > 5 cm 但 ≤ 10 cm
T_4	肿瘤最大径 > 10 cm
区域淋巴结	
N_X	区域淋巴结无法评价
N_0	无区域淋巴结转移
N_1	有区域淋巴结转移
远处转移	
M_0	无远处转移
M_1	有远处转移

通常，小肠旋转不良是孤立的，但也可能与先天性心脏病或内脏转位有关。

在成年人中，这通常是无症状的和偶然发现的；极少数情况下，会因为肠扭转而导致急性结肠梗阻。

这种情况的诊断相对简单。典型表现为空肠位于右下腹部、左侧位盲肠、胰腺钩突部发育不全、肠系膜上动脉与静脉关系异常。

2. Meckel 憩室 Meckel 憩室是胃肠道最常见的先天性异常，发生在 2%～3% 的人群中，占所有卵黄管畸形的 90%[45,46]。它是一个真正的憩室，由肠壁的全层组成，是由卵黄管不完全退化造成的[47-49]。

Meckel 憩室起始处通常位于距回盲瓣 100cm 以内的末端回肠的系膜对侧缘。发病率无性别差异，一般是无临床症状，通常在影像检查或外科手术过程中偶然发现。大约 25% 的 Meckel 憩室病例会出现临床症状。临床症状继发于并发症，最常见并发症的是出血、憩室炎以及肠套叠、肠扭转引起的肠梗阻。

（二）肿瘤

小肠肿瘤相对少见。MRI 对小肠病变的良恶性鉴别可能有困难，特别是当病变较小的时候[50,51]。

1. 良性肿瘤 GIST 是最常见的小肠良性肿瘤。它现在被认为起源于 Cajal 间质细胞的前体，通常存在于肠壁肌间神经丛。GIST 可发生在胃肠道的任何部位，33% 的病例累及小肠。

典型的原发性 GIST 是大的类圆形肿物，在注射对比剂后呈明显强化。由于坏死、出血或囊性变，信号往往是不均质的。

较小的肿瘤（＜2cm）通常被认为是良性的，复发风险非常低，并且可能具有更均匀的信号。它们可以是外生性、肌壁间或向腔内生长。

脂肪瘤通常是 MRI 检查中偶然发现的。在大多数情况下无临床症状，但有时可能导致肠套叠。最常累及的是回肠和空肠，由于含有脂肪成分，MRI 可以很容易识别。

其他良性的小肠肿瘤包括腺瘤、错构瘤、增生性息肉和神经纤维瘤。所有这些类型的肿瘤都没有典型的 MRI 特征。家族性腺瘤性息肉病综合征（familial adenomatous polyposis syndrome, FAP）和多发性错构瘤（Peutz-Jeghers 综合征患者）中可见多发腺瘤（图 22-2）。

2. 恶性肿瘤 小肠恶性肿瘤占所有胃肠道肿瘤的 1%～2%，经常会被误诊[52]。腺癌是小肠最常见的原发性肿瘤。70% 的小肠腺癌发生在十二指肠和空肠。通常是在肿瘤处于晚期时，患者才会出现症状。常表现为息肉样肿物或壁环周

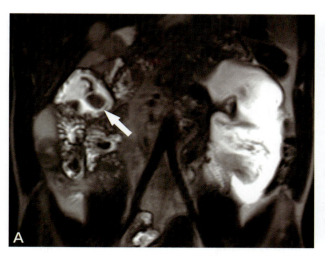
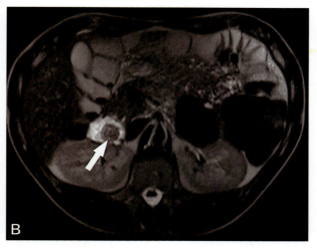

▲ 图 22-2 1 例 35 岁的 Peutz-Jeghers 综合征患者
MR 小肠造影检查的冠状位 HASTE（A）和轴位 HASTE（B）图像显示小肠内有一个大的低信号息肉（箭）

增厚伴肠腔狭窄，从而导致肠梗阻。

类癌通常是恶性的，是小肠最常见的原发肿瘤。它们起源于黏膜下层的神经内分泌细胞，通常很小。当肠系膜根部出现典型的转移淋巴结时应考虑类癌的诊断，类癌典型转移淋巴结的表现为毛刺状肿块，中心通常有钙化。肿瘤可以产生血管活性胺、5-羟色胺和色氨酸，从而引起局部肠系膜收缩、小肠襻的弯曲和邻近壁增厚的一系列促结缔组织增生性反应。这些肿瘤可局部直接侵犯或通过淋巴系统转移。患者可能出现面色潮红、头痛、腹泻、恶心和呕吐的类癌综合征表现[53]。

小肠的淋巴瘤中约2/3的病例是B细胞淋巴瘤，通常发生在远端回肠，1/3的病例为T细胞淋巴瘤，通常发生在十二指肠和空肠。淋巴瘤可表现为圆形、空洞样或息肉样肿物[54]。通常伴随肠系膜及腹膜后的淋巴结肿大。血管通常不受累。

小肠的浆膜和肠系膜是腹膜转移的常见部位，最常见的是卵巢癌、结肠腺癌和胃腺癌的转移。MRI对诊断腹膜小结节具有良好的敏感性。

（三）炎性疾病

1. 克罗恩病

（1）临床表现：CD是炎症性肠病的一种，可影响从口腔到肛门的胃肠道任何部分。它主要发生在发达国家。

通常发病年龄在15—30岁，但可以在任何年龄发病。

这种疾病的病程特点是缓解和反复发作。症状因病变部位、严重程度和疾病行为而异。最常见的临床症状是慢性腹泻（粪便浓度下降超过6周）。其他症状包括腹痛、体重减轻、不适、厌食或发热。多达40%～50%的克罗恩肠炎患者中会出现粪便中带血和（或）黏液。

当病变累及末端回肠时，可能会发生急性症状，并可能被误诊为阑尾炎。患者还可能出现肠外表现，包括肌肉骨骼系统、眼、胆囊、皮肤和内分泌系统。

CD诊断没有单一的金标准；临床评估、内镜检查、组织学检查、生化检查和影像检查的联合，是对于明确诊断是非常重要的。

（2）病理生理学：CD的确切病因尚不清楚。越来越多的证据表明，炎症性肠病（inflammatory bowel diseases, IBD）是由遗传易感宿主对肠道微生物的不恰当炎症性反应引起的。肠道黏膜免疫的改变导致细胞因子分泌过多，肠道壁白细胞浸润增多。嗜中性粒细胞和单核细胞浸润隐窝，导致炎症（隐窝炎）或脓肿（隐窝脓肿）。

病理和组织学标本显示透壁性炎症（炎症累及肠壁全层），未受累组织和受累组织之间不连续（跳跃式的病变）；溃疡和肉芽肿是CD常见的表现。

疾病晚期病理表现为慢性黏膜损伤，以化生和纤维化为特征。

（3）MRI表现：MR小肠造影检查可以用来评价CD的表现[4]。它可以全面地观察腔内、外的病变情况，能够评估疾病的活动性和并发症，为临床决策提供有效的帮助。这种疾病通常从黏膜内壁开始，再扩展到肠壁，包括肠周结构。最常用的影像学分类系统将CD分为三种亚型：活动性炎症型、纤维狭窄型和瘘管/穿孔型。每一种情况都包括典型的影像学表现。

①活动性炎症型

- 肠壁增厚：肠壁增厚3mm或以上，与疾病活动程度相关。肠壁增厚是由于水肿和炎性细胞浸润所致。
- 增强扫描后肠壁明显强化：活动性炎症是透壁性或分层样强化。这种分层样强化的表现是指内层为强化的黏膜，中间层代表黏膜下水肿，外层是强化的浆膜和肠壁肌层结构。
- T_2加权信号增高：这是由于肠壁水肿的存在。
- 肠系膜血供增加：被称为梳状征，与炎症的活动程度密切相关。在炎症和纤维脂肪增生的背景下，由于血流增加而使血管弓十分明显。
- 淋巴结肿大：位于活动性炎症肠段附近；轴位直径为 5mm 或以上。
- 黏膜溃疡。

这些典型的表现如图 22-3 所示。

②纤维狭窄型。纤维狭窄型的影像表现更多地依赖于缺乏与活动性炎症相关的影像表现，而不是直接显示纤维组织。影像学很难区分炎症和纤维化。然而，有以下表现时需要考虑纤维狭窄型（图 22-4）。
- 肠壁增厚（由于胶原沉积）：>3mm。
- 均匀的肠壁强化。
- 肠腔狭窄伴上方肠管扩张：即狭窄可能继发于炎症、纤维化或两者兼而有之。

③瘘管 / 穿孔型。在穿孔型中，透壁性炎症延伸到肠壁之外，包括邻近的肠系膜、器官或肠襻。典型的表现（图 22-5）如下。
- 瘘管：炎症侵蚀进入邻近的肠襻。给予对比剂后可显示强化。
- 窦道：连接肠管与肌肉或肠系膜之间的盲端。
- 相邻肠襻的异常弯曲：高度指示瘘管。

通常，患有长期 CD 的患者可能有混合型表现，即在纤维狭窄型的基础上叠加活性炎症表现（图 22-6）。然而，准确评估组织纤维化是困难的；在这种情况下，描述影像表现时最好采用以下两种报告方法：肠管狭窄时伴有炎症相关的影像学征象，或肠管狭窄时无炎症相关的影像学征象。

2. 乳糜泻

（1）临床表现：乳糜泻是一种麦胶敏感性肠病，它影响基因易感个体的小肠。通常被认为是儿科疾病，在 40 岁和 60 岁也有两个发病高峰。

乳糜泻现在被认为是一种常见疾病，大约每 200 个人中就有 1 人患有乳糜泻。常见的症状包括腹痛、缺铁性贫血和便潜血阳性。然而，乳糜泻的症状是非特异性的，包括腹泻（20%）、便秘（15%）、脂肪泻、腹痛、腹胀和呕吐。体重下降较为少见，只有 5% 的患者会出现[55,56]。

长期并发症包括营养不良，这可能导致贫血、骨质疏松和流产，以及其他问题，如肝脏疾病、小肠淋巴瘤和小肠癌。当以前无症状的乳糜泻患者出现肠道习惯的快速改变时，应该怀疑小肠癌可能。

乳糜泻可通过小肠活检确诊。MR 小肠造影的应用对于非特异性肠道疾病的评估和肠套叠等并发症的检测具有重要意义。

（2）病理生理学：乳糜泻主要累及十二指肠和近端空肠。

组织学的表现主要是 Marsh 分级系统，涉及自身免疫性炎症浸润和绒毛萎缩。在 0 期（静止期），无明显变化，活检结果正常。1 期和 2 期（活动期）的特点是淋巴细胞浸润增多伴十二指肠和空肠皱襞增厚。

3 期（破坏期）具有典型表现：出现表面上皮内淋巴细胞浸润，部分绒毛萎缩和隐窝增生。4 期（萎缩期）是非常少见的，经常发生在非常严重的乳糜泻中。有完全绒毛萎缩和肠壁变薄。

随着疾病的进展，回肠皱襞变得红肿增厚，产生空回肠皱襞逆转（回肠皱襞增加，空肠皱襞减少）。

淋巴结逐渐增大，表现为大的、低信号、甚至空洞样、含有脂肪的淋巴结。

（3）MRI 表现：在 75% 的患者中，可以通过 MRI 检查发现乳糜泻相关表现。典型表现（图 22-7）包括以下各项。
- 小肠襻扩张（>3cm）
- 空回肠皱襞逆转：正常空回肠皱襞模式逆转，空肠皱襞数量减少（$n < 3$ 个皱襞，2.5 cm），回肠皱襞数量增加（$n > 4$ 个皱襞，2.5cm）。
- 肠壁的炎性增厚：淋巴细胞浸润使空肠皱襞和肠壁增厚。随着炎症过程的进展（3 期和 4 期），肠壁和皱襞的增厚发展至回肠。

Chapter 22 上消化道和小肠疾病
Diseases of the Upper Gastrointestinal Tract and Small Bowel

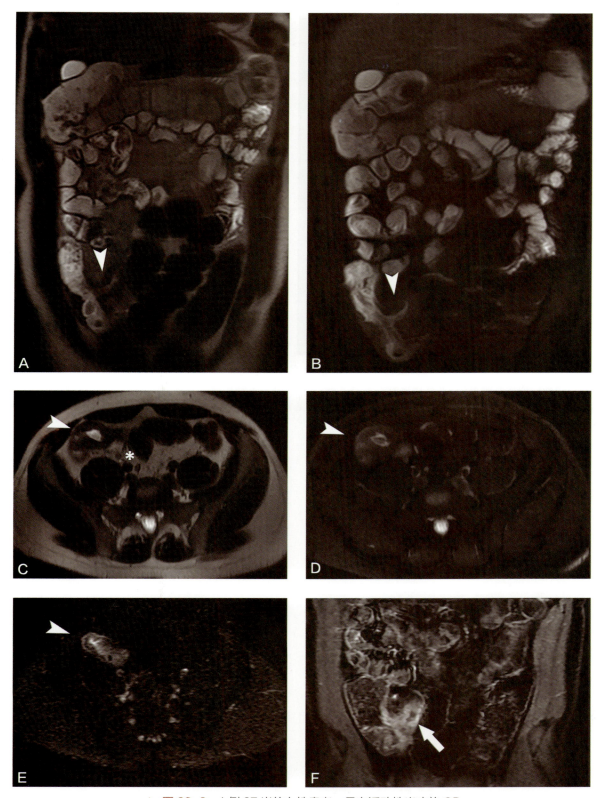

▲ 图 22-3 1 例 27 岁的女性患者，具有活动性炎症的 CD

冠状位（A）和轴位（C）T_2 加权单次激发快速自旋回波成像，显示了受累的末端回肠壁环状增厚。冠状位（B）和轴位（D）T_2 加权脂肪抑制成像，显示肠壁信号强度增加，提示肠壁水肿（箭头）；E. 轴位 DWI 图像显示因扩散受限而使信号强度增加（箭头）；F. 冠状位 T_1 加权对比增强 GRE 图像显示肠壁分层样强化（箭），肠系膜血管扩张，与炎性疾病的活动程度相符

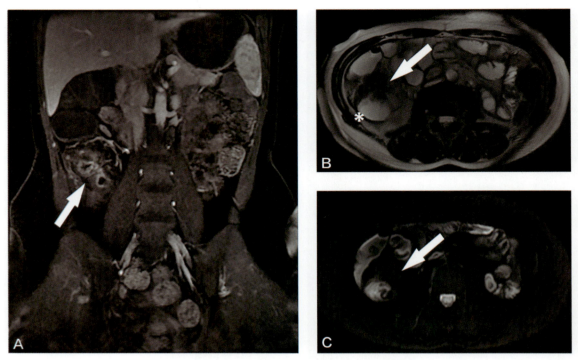

▲ 图 22-4　1 例 20 岁的 CD 患者，慢性炎症

A. 冠状位增强扫描延迟期 3D T_1 加权图像显示末端回肠壁增厚，其异常强化局限于黏膜层（箭），提示出现了肠壁纤维化；B. 相应节段的轴位 T_2 加权图像，可以清楚地看到狭窄近端肠管扩张（星号）；C. 脂肪抑制轴位 T_2 加权图像显示肠壁信号强度低，说明肠壁无水肿

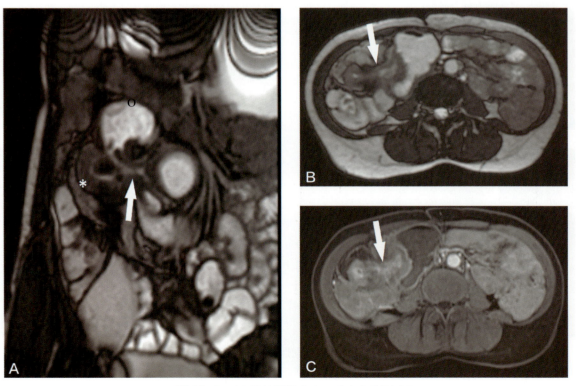

▲ 图 22-5　30 岁的男性患者，患有穿孔型 CD

A. 冠状位 T_2 加权 SSFSE 成像显示环形肠壁增厚（星号），累及回肠末端，伴有肠腔狭窄及狭窄近端水平出现瘘道（A、B，箭）。可清楚地看到狭窄近端肠管扩张（A，圆）；C. 轴位增强 T_1 GRE 图像显示强化的瘘管（箭）

Chapter 22 上消化道和小肠疾病
Diseases of the Upper Gastrointestinal Tract and Small Bowel

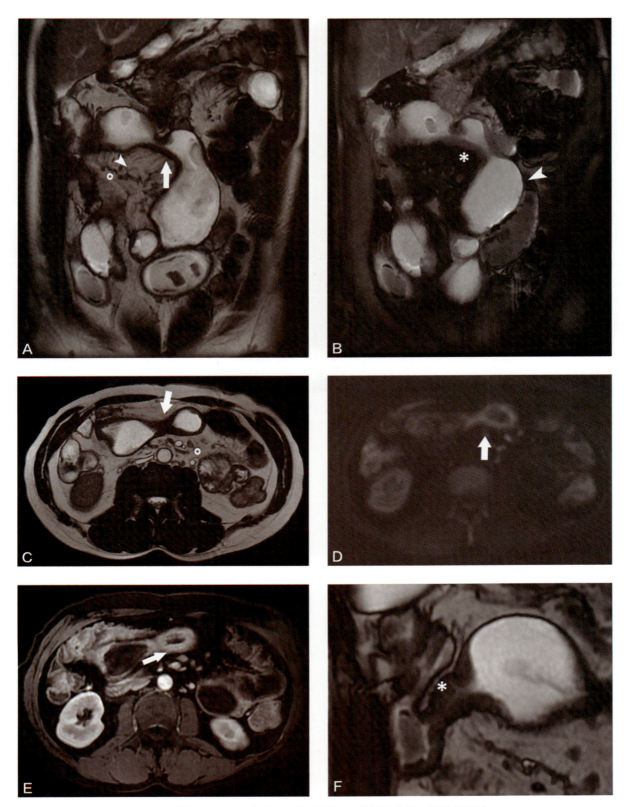

▲ 图 22-6 26 岁男性，狭窄型 CD 的基础上伴有活动性炎症

冠状位（A）和轴位（C）T_2 加权（FIESTA）图像显示环形肠壁增厚，累及末端回肠（箭）、病变肠段有明显的肠系膜血管供血（箭头）和肿大的淋巴结（圆）；B. 脂肪抑制冠状位 T_2 加权图像显示肠壁信号强度增加，提示肠壁水肿（星号）伴狭窄近段肠管扩张（箭头）；D.DW 图像显示肠壁扩散受限（箭）；E. 轴位 T_1 加权对比增强（GRE）图像显示肠壁分层强化（箭），肠系膜血管充血，与活动性炎症病变相符；F. 黏膜溃疡在邻近肠段清晰可见（星号）

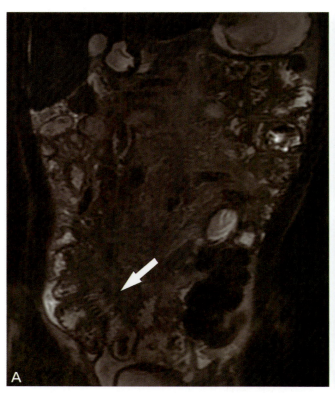
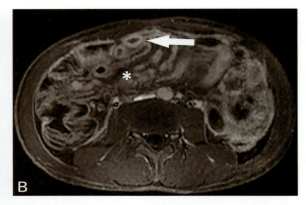
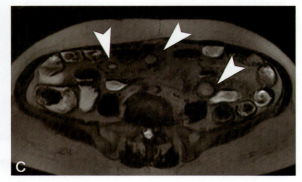

▲ 图 22-7 1 例 23 岁男性乳糜泻患者

A.MR 小肠造影冠状位 T_2 图像显示回肠襻的皱襞数量增加（箭）；B. 经静脉注射对比剂后的轴位 GRE T_1 图像显示肠壁增厚及强化（箭）。肿大的淋巴结也清晰可见（星号）；C.36 岁女性患者，空洞性肠系膜淋巴结综合征，伴有肿大坏死性淋巴结（箭头）

- 壁内脂肪：可在十二指肠壁或空肠壁中发现；这被认为是慢性炎症刺激脂肪沉积的结果。
- 淋巴结肿大：由于反应性 B 淋巴细胞和 T 淋巴细胞增殖引起的滤泡增生，导致上部肠系膜淋巴结肿大。当淋巴结的累积轴位面积大于相邻血管的轴位面积时，可认为淋巴结明显肿大。
- 肠系膜血管充血：小肠系膜可能出现血管充血、肿大；肠系膜脂肪可能出现水肿，信号增高（模糊肠系膜）。
- 非梗阻性肠套叠：在相邻肠襻的管腔内可见肠系膜脂肪和肠襻的血管。
- 脾脏萎缩。
- 空洞性肠系膜淋巴结综合征：以淋巴结内出现脂肪 - 液平面为特征，较为少见，可以在晚期症状性疾病的患者中出现。

五、总结

MRI 是临床上用于小肠研究的一种技术。特别是，它提供了一个全面的评估腔内和腔外病变的方法。因此，它被认为是评价 CD 的可选择的成像技术，能够评价疾病活动度和相关并发症。MRI 对上消化道疾病的评价有重要作用，尤其是对食管运动的动态评价。

参考文献

[1] Kulinna-Cosentini C, Schima W, Lenglinger J et al. Is there a role for dynamic swallowing MRI in the assessment of gastroesophageal reflux disease and oesophageal motility disorders? *EurRadiol*.2011;22(2):364–370.

[2] Yang DM, Kim HC, Jin W et al. 64 multidetector-row computed tomography for preoperative evaluation of gastric cancer: Histological correlation. *J Comput Assist Tomogr*. 2007;31(1):98–103.

[3] Liu S, He J, Guan W et al. Added value of diffusion weighted MR imaging to T2-weighted and dynamic contrast-enhanced MR imaging in T staging of gastric cancer. *JClin Imaging*: Elsevier Inc., 2014;38(2):122–128.

[4] Anupindi SA, Terreblanche O, Courtier J. Magnetic resonance enterography: Inflammatory bowel disease and beyond. *MagnReson Imaging Clin N Am*. 2013;21(4):731–750.

[5] Fidler JL, Guimaraes L, Einstein DM. MR imaging of the small bowel. *RadioGraphics*. 2009;29(6):1811–1825.

[6] Masselli G, Casciani E, Polettini E, Gualdi G. Comparison of MR enteroclysis with MR enterography and conventional enteroclysis in patients with Crohn's disease. *EurRadiol*. 2008;18(3):438–447.

[7] Negaard A, Paulsen V, Sandvik L et al. A prospective randomized comparison between two MRI studies of the small bowel in Crohn's disease, the oral contrast method and MR enteroclysis. *EurRadiol*. 2007;17(9):2294–2301.

[8] Schreyer AG, Geissler A, Albrich H et al. Abdominal MRI after enteroclysis or with oral contrast in patients with suspected or proven Crohn's disease. *ClinGastroenterolHepatol*. 2004;2(6):491–497.

[9] Frokjaer JB, Larsen E, Steffensen E, Nielsen AH, Drewes AM. Magnetic resonance imaging of the small bowel in Crohn's disease. *Scand J Gastroenterol*. 2005;40(7):832–842.

[10] O'Neill OM, Johnston BT, Coleman HG. Achalasia: A review of clinical diagnosis, epidemiology, treatment and outcomes. *World J Gastroenterol*. 2013;19(35):5806–5812.

[11] Richter JE. Oesophageal motility disorders. *Lancet*. 2001;358(9284):823–828.

[12] Roman S, Kahrilas PJ. Management of spastic disorders of the esophagus. *GastroenterolClin North Am*. 2013;42(1):27–43.

[13] Pehlivanov N, Liu J, Kassab GS et al. Relationship between esophageal muscle thickness and intraluminal pressure in patients with esophageal spasm. *Am J PhysiolGastrointest Liver Physiol*. 2002;282:1016.

[14] Dent J, El-Serag HB, Wallander MA, Johansson S. Epidemiology of gastro-oesophageal reflux disease: A systematic review. *Gut*. 2005;54(5):710–717.

[15] Altomare A. Gastroesophageal reflux disease: Update on inflammation and symptom perception. *WJG*. 2013;19(39):6523.

[16] Tutuian R, Castell DO. Review article: Complete gastro-oesophageal reflux monitoring—Combined pH and impedance. *Aliment PharmacolTher*. 2006;24(Suppl. 2):27–37.

[17] Koike T, Ohara S, Sekine H et al. Helicobacter pylori infection prevents erosive refluxoesophagitis by decreasing gastric acid secretion. *Gut*. 2001;49(3):330–334.

[18] Malfertheiner P, Sipponen P, Naumann M et al. Helicobacter pylori eradication has the potential to prevent gastric cancer: A state-of-the-art critique. *Am J Gastroenterol*. 2005;100(9):2100–2115.

[19] Kahrilas PJ, Kim HC, Pandolfino JE. Approaches to the diagnosis and grading of hiatal hernia. *Best Pract Res Clin Gastroenterol*. 2008;22(4):601–616.

[20] van Hagen P, Hulshof MC, van Lanschot JJ et al. Preoperative chemoradiotherapy for esophageal or junctional cancer. *N Engl J Med*. 2012;366(22):2074–2084.

[21] Pennathur A, Gibson MK, Jobe BA, Luketich JD. Oesophageal carcinoma. *Lancet*. 2013;381(9864):400–412.

[22] Zhang Y. Epidemiology of esophageal cancer. *World J Gastroenterol*. 2013;19(34):5598–5606.

[23] Levine MS, Caroline D, Thompson JJ, Kressel HY, Laufer I, Herlinger H. Adenocarcinoma of the esophagus: Relationship to Barrett mucosa. *Radiology*. 1984;150(2):305–309.

[24] Lewis RB, Mehrotra AK, Rodriguez P, Levine MS. From the radiologic pathology archives: Esophageal neoplasms: Radiologic-pathologic correlation. *RadioGraphics*. 2013;33(4):1083–1108.

[25] Siewert JR, Stein HJ, Feith M, Bruecher BL, Bartels H, Fink U. Histologic tumor type is an independent prognostic parameter in esophageal cancer: Lessons from more than 1,000 consecutive resections at a single center in the Western world. *Ann Surg*. 2001;234(3):360–367; discussion 368–369.

[26] Sakurada A, Takahara T, Kwee TC et al. Diagnostic performance of diffusion-weighted magnetic resonance imaging in esophageal cancer. *EurRadiol*. 2009;19(6):1461–1469.

[27] Dave UR, Williams AD, Wilson JA et al. Esophageal cancer staging with endoscopic MR imaging: Pilot study. *Radiology*. 2004;230(1):281–286.

[28] Riddell AM, Hillier J, Brown G et al. Potential of surface-coil MRI for staging of esophageal cancer. *AJR Am J Roentgenol*. 2006;187(5):1280–1287.

[29] Riddell AM, Allum WH, Thompson JN, Wotherspoon AC, Richardson C, Brown G. The appearances of oesophageal carcinoma demonstrated on high-resolution, T2-weighted MRI, with histopathological correlation. *EurRadiol*. 2007;17(2):391–399.

[30] Lehr L, Rupp N, Siewert JR. Assessment of resectability of esophageal cancer by computed tomography and magnetic resonance imaging. *Surgery*. 1988;103(3):344–350.

[31] Kayani B, Zacharakis E, Ahmed K, Hanna GB. Lymph node metastases and prognosis in oesophageal carcinoma—A systematic review. *Eur J SurgOncol*. 2011;37(9):747–753.

[32] Nishimura H, Tanigawa N, Hiramatsu M, Tatsumi Y, Matsuki M, Narabayashi I. Preoperative esophageal cancer staging: Magnetic resonance imaging of lymph node with ferumoxtran-10, an ultrasmall superparamagnetic iron oxide. *J Am Coll Surg*. 2006;202(4):604–611.

[33] Lahaye MJ, Engelen SME, Kessels AGH et al. USPIO-enhanced MR imaging for nodal staging in patients with primary rectal cancer: Predictive criteria 1. *Radiology*. 2008;246(3):804–811.

[34] Washington K. 7th edition of the AJCC cancer staging manual: Stomach. *Ann SurgOncol*. 2010;17(12):3077–3079.

[35] Rahman R, Asombang AW, Ibdah JA. Characteristics of gastric cancer in Asia. *World J Gastroenterol*.

2014;20(16):4483–4490.

[36] Lechago J, Correa P. Prolonged achlorhydria and gastric neoplasia: Is there a causal relationship? *Gastroenterology*. 1993;104(5):1554–1557.

[37] An JY, Kang TH, Choi MG, Noh JH, Sohn TS, Kim S. Borrmann type IV: An independent prognostic factor for survival in gastric cancer. *J Gastrointest Surg*. 2008;12(8):1364–1369.

[38] Zhang XP, Tang L, Sun YS et al. Sandwich sign of Borrmann type 4 gastric cancer on diffusion-weighted magnetic resonance imaging. *Eur J Radiol*. 2012;81(10):2481–2486.

[39] Tokuhara T, Tanigawa N, Matsuki M et al. Evaluation of lymph node metastases in gastric cancer using magnetic resonance imaging with ultrasmallsuperparamagnetic iron oxide (USPIO): Diagnostic performance in postcontrast images using new diagnostic criteria. *Gastric Cancer*. 2008;11(4):194–200.

[40] Chourmouzi D, Sinakos E, Papalavrentios L, Akriviadis E, Drevelegas A. Gastrointestinal stromal tumors: A pictorial review. *J Gastrointestin Liver Dis*. 2009;18(3):379–383.

[41] De Vogelaere K, Aerts M, Haentjens P, De Grève J, Delvaux G. Gastrointestinal stromal tumor of the stomach: Progresses in diagnosis and treatment. *ActaGastroenterol Belg*. 2013;76(4):403–406.

[42] Gong J, Kang W, Zhu J, Xu J. CT and MR imaging of gastrointestinal stromal tumor of stomach: A pictorial review. *Quant Imaging Med Surg*. 2012;2(4):274–279.

[43] Lee NK, Kim S, Kim GH et al. Hypervascularsubepithelial gastrointestinal masses: CT-pathologic correlation. *RadioGraphics*. 2010;30(7):1915–1934.

[44] Sandrasegaran K, Rajesh A, Rushing DA, Rydberg J, Akisik FM, Henley JD. Gastrointestinal stromal tumors: CT and MRI findings. *EurRadiol*. 2005;15(7):1407–1414.

[45] Moore TC. Omphalomesenteric duct malformations. *SeminPediatr Surg*. 1996;5(2):116–123.

[46] Bauer SB, Retik AB. Urachal anomalies and related umbilical disorders. *UrolClin North Am*. 1978;5(1):195–211.

[47] Yahchouchy EK, Marano AF, Etienne JC, Fingerhut AL. Meckel's diverticulum. *J Am Coll Surg*. 2001;192(5):658–662.

[48] Mackey WC, Dineen P. A fifty year experience with Meckel's diverticulum. *SurgGynecol Obstet*. 1983;156(1):56–64.

[49] Ymaguchi M, Takeuchi S, Awazu S. Meckel's diverticulum. Investigation of 600 patients in Japanese literature. *Am J Surg*. 1978;136(2):247–249.

[50] Kamaoui I, De-Luca V, Ficarelli S, Mennesson N, Lombard-Bohas C, Pilleul F. Value of CT enteroclysis in suspected small-bowel carcinoid tumors. *AJR Am J Roentgenol*. 2010;194(3):629–633.

[51] Van Weyenberg SJ, Meijerink MR, Jacobs MA et al. MR enteroclysis in the diagnosis of small-bowel neoplasms. *Radiology*. 2010;254(3):765–773.

[52] Masselli G, Polettini E, Casciani E, Bertini L, Vecchioli A, Gualdi G. Small-bowel neoplasms: Prospective evaluation of MR enteroclysis. *Radiology*. 2009;251(3):743–750.

[53] Horton KM, Kamel I, Hofmann L, Fishman EK. Carcinoid tumors of the small bowel: Amultitechnique imaging approach. *AJR Am J Roentgenol*. 2004;182(3):559–567.

[54] Lohan DG, Alhajeri AN, Cronin CG, Roche CJ, Murphy JM. MR enterography of small-bowel lymphoma: Potential for suggestion of histologic subtype and the presence of underlying celiac disease. *AJR Am J Roentgenol*. 2008;190(2):287–293.

[55] Schuppan D, Dennis MD, Kelly CP. Celiac disease: Epidemiology, pathogenesis, diagnosis, and nutritional management. *NutrClin Care*. 2005;8(2):54–69.

[56] Dickey W, Kearney N. Overweight in celiac disease: Prevalence, clinical characteristics, and effect of a gluten-free diet. *Am J Gastroenterol*. 2006;101(10):2356–2359.

Chapter 23
腹膜后磁共振成像

MRI of the Retroperitoneum

Abed Ghandour, Verghese George, Rakesh Sinha, Prabhakar Rajiah 著

朱　正 译

冯　冰 校

目录　CONTENTS

一、腹膜后磁共振成像的检查序列 / 530

二、病理情况 / 530

三、腹部大血管 / 543

四、总结 / 553

磁共振成像（MRI）已成为腹部疾病的一种重要成像方式。腹膜后病变少见，其诊断和特征具有一定挑战性。磁共振成像在这些疾病的评估中具有如下优点，包括固有的高对比分辨率有助于组织定性、良好的空间分辨率、宽视野和多平面成像能力。然而，该检查费用较高，尚未广泛应用，并有一些禁忌证和局限性，后者包括患者幽闭恐惧症。此外，应谨慎对待钆对比剂可能对严重肾功能不全患者带来的潜在肾源性系统性纤维化（nephrogenic systemic fibrosis, NSF）的风险。

在本章中，我们将讨论评估腹膜后疾病的不同磁共振成像序列，以及腹膜后病变的磁共振成像特征。

一、腹膜后磁共振成像的检查序列

一些磁共振成像序列可用于评估腹膜后间隙。T_1加权成像用于判断有无脂肪或出血（高信号强度），评估淋巴结肿大和血管侵犯。双回波T_1加权成像的同、反相位可检测微观脂肪及交界面处脂肪，在反相位图像中表现为信号下降。有无脂肪抑制的T_2加权成像在评估淋巴结肿大、疾病进展中向邻近侵犯、囊性变或坏死、积液和骨髓水肿时有很大帮助。单次激发涡流（half-Fourier acquisition single-shot turbo spin-echo, HASTE）/快速自旋回波（single-shot turbo spin echo, SSTSE）和稳态自由旋进（steady-state free precession, SSFP）是快速序列，液体表现为高亮信号。扩散加权成像与表观扩散系数图有助于评估由腹膜后疾病引起的扩散受限；扩散受限提示细胞结构，常见于肿瘤和炎症过程中。T_1和T_2加权的三点dixon序列能够一次采集即可获得四组相位，即同相位、反相位、水相和脂相，因此可快速定性病变。腹膜后病变的对比增强使用体积、脂肪饱和的T_1加权梯度回波序列（volume interpolated body examination, VIBE；THRIVE或LAVA）。对比增强有助于区分实性与非增强的囊性或坏死病变，评估病变范围，以及有无血栓或血管侵犯并明确其性质。如果需要血管成像（例如，制订外科手术计划时），磁共振血管成像（MR angiography, MRA）常应用T_1加权三维扰相梯度回波序列。对于严重肾功能不全的有NSF风险的患者，可应用非增强磁共振血管成像技术，包括SSFP、VIPR和NATIVE SPACE。最近腹膜后有潜在应用前景的技术是PET/MRI，它能同时采集两种模式。这种融合成像技术结合了由磁共振成像提供的良好的形态学和组织特征信息以及正电子发射断层扫描（positron emission computed tomography, PET）所提供的代谢信息。FDG（18-氟-脱氧葡萄糖）是最常用的PET放射性药物，是葡萄糖的一种类似物，在炎性细胞和肿瘤细胞中积聚，从而过度表达葡萄糖转运蛋白的细胞受体。

二、病理情况

表23-1列出了腹膜后肿瘤和非肿瘤病变的总结，表23-2总结了常见磁共振成像表现和相关的鉴别诊断。

（一）肿瘤性病变

腹膜后肿瘤的四大类是：中胚层肿瘤、生殖细胞和性索间质肿瘤、神经源肿瘤和淋巴组织肿瘤。原发腹膜后肿瘤起源于腹膜后间隙，但非腹膜后器官。提示原发腹膜后起源的特征是：腹膜后器官的向前移位；鸟嘴征阴性（毗邻腹膜后器官的圆形边缘）；器官包埋征阴性（肿瘤造成的新月形改变）；以及缺乏明确器官起源（器官隐匿征）[1,2]。根据影像学特征和人口统计资料，一些原发腹膜后肿物可进一步定性，但通常需要组织学明确。

1. 中胚层肿瘤 肉瘤占恶性腹膜后病变的1/3，常见于60—70岁，常因症状出现晚而肿瘤体积较大[3,4]。肿瘤依细胞起源不同而种类繁多。常通过手术切除治疗[5]。

（1）脂肪肉瘤：脂肪肉瘤是起源于原始间叶

表 23-1　常见腹膜后肿瘤的起源和非肿瘤病变

病　变	肿瘤类型
	肿瘤类病变
中胚层起源	
脂肪组织	脂肪瘤，脂肪肉瘤
平滑肌	平滑肌瘤，平滑肌肉瘤
结缔组织	纤维瘤，恶性纤维组织细胞瘤，软骨肉瘤，滑膜细胞肉瘤
横纹肌	横纹肌肉瘤，横纹肌肉瘤
血管	血管瘤，血管肉瘤
血管周上皮样细胞	血管周上皮样细胞瘤（perivascular epithelioid cell tumor，PEComa）组（如血管平滑肌脂肪瘤、淋巴管平滑肌瘤病），血管周细胞肉瘤
其他	纤维瘤病
不确定	黄色肉芽肿
神经源性	
神经鞘	神经鞘瘤，神经纤维瘤，恶性神经鞘瘤，神经源性肉瘤，神经纤维肉瘤
交感神经	节细胞神经瘤，神经节细胞母细胞瘤，神经母细胞瘤
嗜铬组织	副神经节瘤，嗜铬细胞瘤，恶性副神经节瘤，嗜铬细胞瘤
生殖细胞、性索间质和间质细胞来源肿瘤	成熟畸胎瘤，未成熟畸胎瘤，恶性畸胎瘤，混合生殖细胞肿瘤
淋巴组织或造血系统肿瘤	淋巴瘤，髓外浆细胞瘤
	非肿瘤性病变
	假瘤性脂肪瘤病，腹膜后纤维化，Erdheim–Chester 病和髓外造血

表 23-2　常见磁共振成像表现及其相关的鉴别诊断

纯脂肪肿物	脂肪瘤，高分化脂肪肉瘤
不均质肿物伴脂肪成分	去分化脂肪肉瘤，血管平滑肌脂肪瘤
脂 - 液平面	畸胎瘤，高分化脂肪肉瘤
黏液基质	黏液样脂肪肉瘤，神经源性肿瘤，黏液样恶性纤维组织细胞瘤
大肿物、广泛坏死、侵犯下腔静脉	平滑肌肉瘤
出血引起的液 - 液平面	副神经节瘤
低血供	淋巴瘤，低级别脂肪肉瘤，良性肿瘤
T_2 低信号	淋巴瘤，硬纤维瘤，腹膜后纤维化，Erdheim- Chester 病
主动脉或下腔静脉旁肿物	淋巴瘤，腹膜后纤维化，Erdheim- Chester 病
主动脉漂浮征或 CT 血管造影征象	淋巴瘤

细胞的恶性肿瘤[6]，占腹膜后肉瘤的 40%[4,5,7,8]。35% 的肿瘤起源于肾周脂肪[8,9]。有 5 种亚型：高分化型、黏液型、去分化型、圆形细胞型和多形性型[10]。常表现为巨大肿物。转移率低于 10%，局部复发是最常见的发病率和死亡率原因[4,5,8,11,12]。

高分化脂肪肉瘤是最常见的脂肪肉瘤（图 23-1），其信号强度与大体脂肪相似，即 T_1 加权图像上高信号，T_2 上等高信号和脂肪抑制图像上的信号缺失。它通常边界光滑清晰、分叶状，脂肪成分轻度或无强化。鉴别诊断包括脂肪瘤或血管平滑肌脂肪瘤。高分化脂肪肉瘤与脂肪瘤的影像学鉴别具有挑战性。体积大（> 10cm）、结节状或球状成分、厚分隔（> 2mm）、软组织成分和较少的脂肪部分（< 75%）倾向脂肪肉瘤而非脂肪瘤的诊断。此瘤生长缓慢，局部复发和转移少见。25% 的肿瘤可以发生去分化为级别更高的肿瘤[14]。

黏液型脂肪肉瘤由于黏液样基质中黏多糖成分而呈假囊肿样表现，T_1 加权成像为低信号，T_2 加权成像为高信号。可见到 T_1 加权图像上高信号和 T_2 加权图像上等信号的花边状、线性或不规则的瘤内脂肪成分[1,15]。由于细胞外间隙中对比剂的缓慢逐渐积累，肿瘤具有渐进性、不均匀、不完全强化[13]。它具有侵袭性的临床进程和明显的转移倾向，常转移至罕见部位如骨和皮肤[8]。

去分化脂肪肉瘤（图 23-2）可以原发，或由先前存在的高分化脂肪肉瘤进展而来，因此含有高分化的脂质成分和去分化的非脂质成分。在磁共振成像上常表现为一种等信号的非脂肪性软组织肿物，以及肿块内、邻近或包含脂肪肿物的强化[16,17]。它生长迅速且易转移[8]。

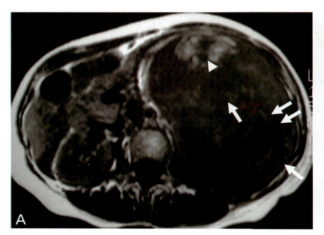
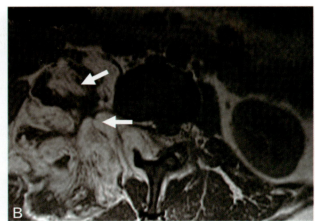

▲ 图 23-1 高分化脂肪肉瘤
A.T_1 加权的横轴位磁共振成像示左侧腹部等信号大肿物（箭），其内前部高信号区域（箭头）提示脂肪。肿块推压肾脏使之向前移位；B. 另一位患者的横轴位 T_1 加权磁共振成像示含大面积脂肪（箭）的高分化脂肪肉瘤，使右肾向前移位。可见肿物通过右侧神经孔进入椎管

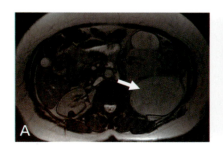
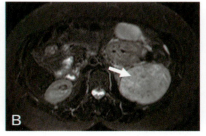
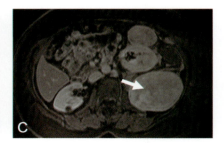

▲ 图 23-2 去分化脂肪肉瘤
横轴位 T_2（A）、STIR（B）和 VIBE 增强序列（C）图像示 T_2 和 STIR 高信号的边界清晰的软组织肿块，增强后明显强化（箭）。肿物是含有大量实性成分的去分化脂肪肉瘤

多形性型脂肪肉瘤常发生在老年人中，具有高度转移潜力[8]。常表现为不均质肿瘤，少量或无可检测到的脂肪，常无法与其他恶性软组织肿块鉴别[13]。

圆细胞型脂肪肉瘤表现为不均质软组织肿块伴坏死。

（2）平滑肌肉瘤：平滑肌肉瘤是腹膜后第二常见的肉瘤（30%），2/3 发生于女性[5,11]，常见于 60 岁[18]（图 23-3 和图 23-4）。临床表现取决于位置和下腔静脉的受侵情况，肿瘤可以完全位于下腔静脉腔外，即有腔内和腔外成分，或纯腔内。肿瘤通常界限清楚，并且可有广泛的坏死区域（T_1 加权图像上为等低信号，T_2 加权图像上为不均质等高信号），以及依肌肉和纤维成分多少表现为不同程度的强化[17,19-21]。当发生在下腔静脉内时，鉴别诊断包括血栓、肾细胞癌、淋巴瘤、脂肪肉瘤和平滑肌瘤病的延伸[22]。

（3）恶性纤维组织细胞瘤：恶性纤维组织细胞瘤（malignant fibrous histiocytoma，MFH）是第三常见的腹膜后肉瘤（15%）[11]，男性多见[23]。病理类型为多形性（最常见）、黏液样、巨细胞及炎症性[10,24]。在磁共振成像上，MFH 在 T_1 上呈低至中等信号，相对于肌肉而言，T_2 信号呈不同程度的增加（图 23-5）[11,17]。T_2 上混合低、

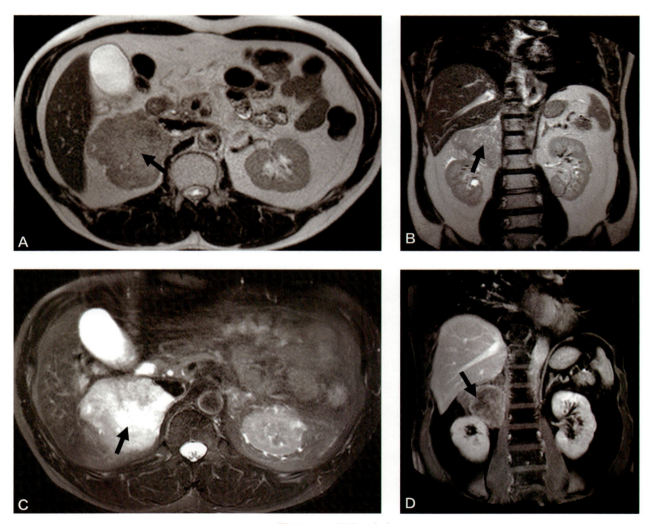

▲ 图 23-3 平滑肌肉瘤

A. 横轴位 T_1 加权磁共振成像示腹膜后等信号大肿物侵犯右肾（箭）；B. 冠状位 T_2 单次激发（HASTE）图像示不均匀等高信号肿物（箭）；C. 横轴位 T_2 脂肪饱和加权图像示高信号肿物，下腔静脉凹陷但未受侵（箭）；D. 冠状位三维 T_1 加权磁共振成像示不均匀强化肿物，活检证实为平滑肌肉瘤（箭）

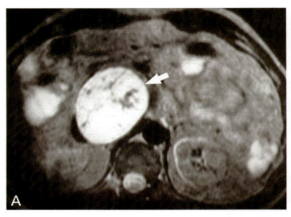
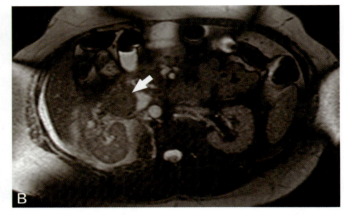

▲ 图 23-4　腔内平滑肌肉瘤

A. 一位患者的 T_2 加权 STIR 图像示平滑肌肉瘤部分延伸到下腔静脉（箭）；B. 另一位患者的 T_2 加权图像示平滑肌肉瘤延伸到下腔静脉（箭）

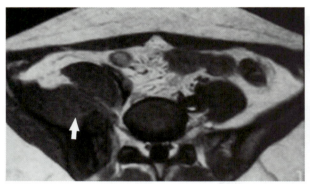

▲ 图 23-5　恶性纤维组织细胞瘤

横轴位 T_1 加权磁共振成像示右侧髂窝等信号肿物（箭），为恶性纤维组织细胞瘤

中、高信号马赛克样分布的表现，与瘤内实性成分、囊性变、出血、黏液样基质和纤维组织成分有关，形成"果盘征"[25]。增强扫描为不均匀强化。

（4）少见的肉瘤：有几种其他类型的肉瘤，其中大部分没有明确的磁共振成像特征表现。横纹肌肉瘤常见于儿童，7% 的病例累及腹膜后[26]。有多种组织学类型，通常为等信号的磁共振成像且具有不同的强化[27]。血管肉瘤是一种侵袭性肿瘤，表现为肿物累及血管（图 23-6），并由于坏死而不均匀强化[28]。软骨肉瘤 2% 见于骨外，平均年龄 50 岁[29]。典型软骨瘤的磁共振成像特征，T_2 加权像上为高亮信号，对比增强后仅轻度外周或间隔强化。间质软骨肉瘤具有较低的水含量，

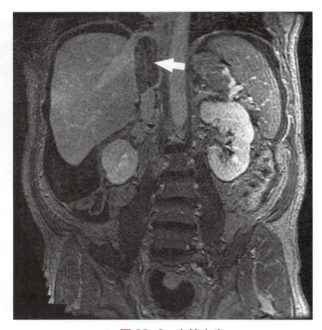

▲ 图 23-6　血管肉瘤

增强后冠状位 T_1 加权磁共振成像示延伸和扩张下腔静脉的低信号肿物（箭）

因此 T_2 加权上为等信号，增强后表现为弥漫性不均匀强化[30]。滑膜细胞肉瘤无特异性磁共振成像表现，但在 T_2 加权成像上可表现为具有特征性三重信号强度（散在高、等、低信号区）的多囊性肿物[31]。此外，MRI 表现为边界清晰的不均质的出血性病变，也应考虑滑膜肉瘤的诊断。T_2 加权序列上的液-液平面也支持诊断[32]。

（5）血管周上皮细胞瘤：血管周上皮细胞瘤

（PEComas）是表达黑色素细胞（HMB 45，黑色素-A）和肌源性标记物（SM-actin，SMA；肌间线蛋白）的血管周围间叶肿瘤[33]；包括血管平滑肌脂肪瘤、肺透明细胞糖瘤、淋巴管平滑肌瘤病和跖/镰状韧带的透明细胞肌黑色素瘤。通常，肿瘤体积大，侵袭性强，可复发转移[33]。磁共振成像上，在T_1加权像上呈等低信号，T_2加权图像上呈不均质高信号，呈不均匀强化（图23-7）。出血在体积大的肿瘤中更常见[34]。扩张的血管穿行于病变、动脉瘤和出血等是与脂肪肉瘤的鉴别点[35]。

（6）硬纤维瘤：硬纤维瘤（深部纤维瘤病，侵袭性纤维瘤病）由梭形细胞组成，由肌肉结缔组织、筋膜和腱膜组成。硬纤维瘤是雌激素依赖性，因此在年轻女性中更常见，30岁为发病高峰[36,37]。它们与家族性息肉病和Gardner综合征相关，可单发或多发。在MRI上边界清晰，但偶尔浸润性生长。信号特征取决于组织成分（梭形细胞、胶原和黏液样基质）和血管，并可随时间而改变。病变早期为细胞，呈T_2高信号，病变晚期细胞减少而胶原沉积导致T_2低信号（图23-8）[38]。由于致密的胶原带的存在也可呈低信号轨道样改变[39]。增强为中度至明显强化[40]。即使广泛切除仍具有较高的局部复发率（50%）[41]。

（7）脂肪瘤：脂肪瘤是由边界清晰的脂肪细胞组成的良性肿瘤。脂肪瘤在腹膜后罕见，应谨慎得出此诊断，因为大多数腹膜后含脂肪的病变不是脂肪瘤，而是脂肪瘤样的分化良好的脂肪肉瘤。然而，如果被证明是脂肪瘤，是否值得再次确定患者脂肪瘤可能恶性变为脂肪肉瘤尚无统一定论[35]。症状通常是由于肿物占位效应和压迫邻近组织器官产生。在磁共振成像上，脂肪瘤具有脂肪信号强度，并且很少有任何分隔。脂肪瘤不强化，也没有软组织成分[35]。

2. 生殖细胞与性索间质肿瘤 生殖细胞和性索间质肿瘤在腹膜后少见。

（1）原发性腹膜后外生殖细胞瘤：原发性腹膜后外生殖细胞肿瘤（extragonadal germ cell tumors,EGCTs）起源于在胚胎发育中未能迁移的生殖嵴的原始中线生殖细胞，没有明显的性腺原发病变[11,42,43]。由于转移性生殖细胞肿瘤较常见，因此应慎重诊断。腹膜后是仅次于纵隔的性腺外生殖细胞瘤的第二常见部位。男性患病率较高[42]。腹膜后EGCTs可以是精原细胞瘤或非精原细胞瘤（如胚胎癌、卵黄囊瘤、绒毛膜癌、畸胎瘤和混合生殖细胞瘤）。在磁共振成像上，原发EGCTs体积大、位于中线、可见强化，相对于骨骼肌而言在T_1上呈等低信号，在T_2上为等高信号。精原细胞瘤表现为均匀的实性分叶状肿物伴纤维血管间隔，增强后明显强化。非精原性GCTs表现为不均质肿物，伴坏死、出血或囊性变的区域[43]。

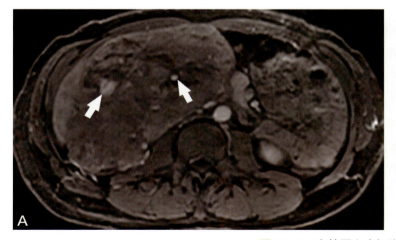 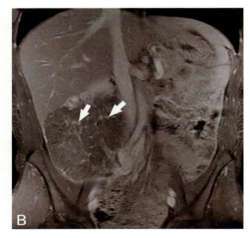

▲ 图23-7 血管周上皮细胞瘤

横轴位（A）和冠状位（B）增强磁共振成像示含强化血管的腹膜后大肿物，活检证实为PEComa（箭）

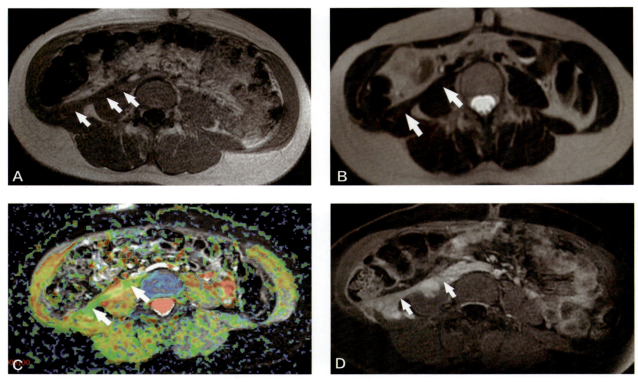

▲ 图 23-8　硬纤维瘤

A. 横轴位 T_1 加权图像示右侧腹膜后区域右侧腰大肌前缘边界不清的等信号软组织肿物（箭）；B. 同一层面横轴位 T_2 加权磁共振成像示病变等低信号（箭）；C. 横轴位 T_2 加权图像上叠加的 ADC 伪彩图显示病变轻中度扩散受限（箭）；D. 对比剂注射 5min 后增强 T_1 图像示明显延迟强化（箭），与腹膜后硬纤维瘤（纤维瘤病）相符

（2）原发性腹膜后畸胎瘤：畸胎瘤是由源自三个生殖细胞层混合而成[44]。原发性腹膜后畸胎瘤占腹膜后肿瘤的 1%～11%[45]。畸胎瘤可按组织学分类为成熟（分化良好）、未成熟（分化不良）和恶性（非生殖细胞恶性肿瘤，起源于三种胚胎学成分中的一种）。宏观上，有两种变型：囊状畸胎瘤由完全成熟的成分组成；它们含有皮脂腺物质和毛发，通常是良性的；实性畸胎瘤更可能是恶性的，由未成熟的成分组成[46]。在磁共振成像上，肿瘤内脂肪或液平面高度提示畸胎瘤的诊断。钙化在磁共振成像上为低信号。对比增强是强化方式多种多样且不均质的（图 23-9）。

（3）原发性索间质肿瘤：原发性索间质肿瘤在腹膜后少见，女性常见。颗粒细胞瘤是最常见的，而 Sertoli–Leydig 细胞瘤、卵泡膜细胞瘤和其他类型的肿瘤较少。在颗粒细胞瘤和卵泡膜细胞瘤中可见雌激素升高。磁共振成像表现非特异性，为不均质的实性肿瘤，增强后不均匀强化[34]。

3. 神经源性肿瘤

（1）神经鞘瘤：神经鞘瘤是起源于周围神经雪旺细胞，有报道在腹膜后间隙肿瘤中，0.7% 为良性神经鞘瘤，1.7% 为恶性神经鞘瘤[47,48]。靶征——中央等低 T_2 信号的纤维组织被外周高信号黏液组织包绕[49]，束状征提示存在纤维束[50]，是神经鞘瘤的特征性影像表现，但在腹膜后神经鞘瘤中少见。磁共振成像上另一个重要的特征是邻近骨结构的破坏[51]。增强扫描强化不均匀，伴有不强化的囊性成分和强化的实性成分。

（2）神经纤维瘤：神经纤维瘤是良性神经鞘肿瘤，男性常见，尤其是 20—40 岁[49]，并与神经纤维瘤病 -1（neurofibromatosis type1, NF-1）有很强的相关性。神经纤维瘤伴有 NF-1 表现为年龄小，通常多灶、体积大（> 5cm），更易出现症状。常恶性变，特别是神经纤维瘤病的患者[49]。腹膜后神经纤维瘤常位于腰大肌旁或骶前区，双侧对称并沿腰骶神经丛分布[52]。在 T_1 加权磁共振成像中，中央部分具有比周边更高的信号强度，而在 T_2 加权图像上，由于中央神经组织和外周黏液样变性，外周信号强度较高[53]。增强后强化方式多样。脊神经根出神经纤维瘤穿过神经孔并使神经孔扩大，呈哑铃形[17,25,54]。丛状神经纤维瘤外观看起来犹如一袋蠕虫，为大量的浸润性肿物伴神经弥漫性增厚[10]。

（3）恶性外周神经鞘肿瘤：恶性外周神经鞘肿瘤（malignant peripheral nerve sheath tumors，MPNST）是指恶性神经鞘瘤、神经源性肉瘤和神经纤维肉瘤[55]。MPNST 可见于伴有或不伴有神经纤维瘤病的患者[49]。男女性均常见，仅见于成人[49]。磁共振成像表现非特异性，但不规则的肿瘤边缘和内部不均质提示其诊断[49]（图 23-10）。肿瘤快速增大和疼痛是可疑的临床体征[49,56,57]。

（4）神经节细胞瘤：神经节细胞瘤是由神经纤维和成熟神经节细胞组成的良性肿瘤。通常在 20 岁以前，男性更常见，32%～52% 发生在腹膜后间隙[58]。一些神经节细胞瘤功能活跃并且分泌儿茶酚胺、血管活性肠肽或雄激素，可以解释如高血压、腹泻和男性化的症状[49]。在磁共振成像上，它们表现为主要血管周围的比较清晰

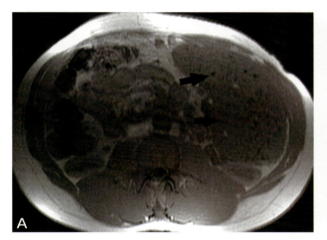
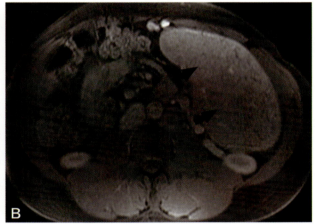

▲ 图 23-9 畸胎瘤
A. 横轴位 T_1 加权图像示 T_1 等信号（箭）的腹膜后大肿物；B. 对比增强图像示肿物不均匀强化（箭）

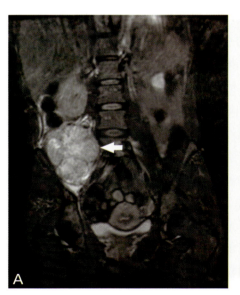
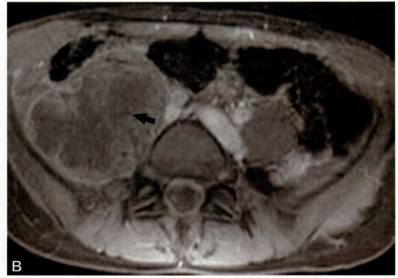

▲ 图 23-10 MPNST
A. 冠状位 STIR 图像示腹膜后邻近椎体的不均匀高信号肿物（箭）；B. 横轴位增强 T_1 加权图像示肿物不均匀强化（箭）

的椭圆形、新月形或分叶状的肿块，但对管腔轻微或没有压迫[49]。神经节细胞瘤具有均质 T_1 低信号和不同强度的 T_2 信号。在 T_2 加权磁共振图像上具有等高信号的肿瘤含有丰富的细胞和纤维成分以及少量黏液基质。具有明显 T_2 加权高信号的肿瘤含有明显的黏液样基质以及少量的细胞和纤维成分[49]。与 MPNST 一样，T_2 加权像上的曲线样条带状低信号使该肿瘤呈螺旋状表现，并与 MPNST 鉴别困难[49]。

神经母细胞瘤是一种中间级别肿瘤，有良性神经细胞瘤和恶性神经母细胞瘤的成分。发生于 2—4 岁，男女孩之间无差异。其预后和对治疗的反应比神经母细胞瘤更好[59]。在磁共振成像上，它可以是实性的或囊性伴实性成分[34,49]。

（5）神经母细胞瘤：神经母细胞瘤是一种由原始神经母细胞组成的恶性肿瘤，常见于 10 岁左右，女孩多见[60]，并位于交感神经丛的任何部位或肾上腺髓质。在磁共振成像上，神经母细胞瘤是不规则的、分叶状、不均匀的，并可能显示邻近器官的侵犯和对血管造成管腔压迫[34,49]。

（6）副神经节瘤：副神经节瘤是起源于副交感神经节的嗜铬细胞瘤，通常比起源于肾上腺髓质的嗜铬细胞瘤更有侵袭性。大多数副神经节瘤活跃（高达 60%）并分泌肾上腺素或去甲肾上腺素，激素活性与恶性的相关性较低。在磁共振成像上，它们表现出 T_1 低等信号强度和中等程度高 T_2 信号强度。它们是高血供且明显强化[2]（图 23-11 到图 23-13）。在 T_2 上呈高亮信号，称为灯泡征，见于 80% 的患者[61]。

4. 淋巴组织肿瘤

（1）淋巴瘤：淋巴瘤是最常见的恶性腹膜后肿瘤，约占 1/3。腹部霍奇金淋巴瘤倾向于局限在脾脏和腹膜后间隙，可依次侵及邻近淋巴结；而非霍奇金淋巴瘤可累及不连续的淋巴结群和结外部位[62,63]。在磁共振成像上，淋巴瘤在 T_1 加权图像上信号相对均质，低于脂肪信号并轻度高于肌肉信号强度。但在 T_2 加权图像上却是与脂肪呈等信号、高于肌肉信号强度（图 23-14）。

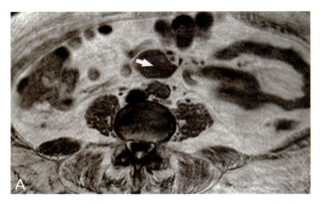
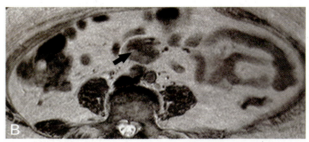

▲ 图 23-11 副神经节瘤

横轴位 T_1（A）和 T_2（B）磁共振成像示腹膜后主动脉旁体附近的不均质肿物（箭），证实为副神经节瘤

（2）转移性淋巴结肿大：淋巴结转移常见于腹膜后。通常使用大小进行诊断，使用 1cm 作为界值。然而依据大小诊断并不具有非特异性，有时在非肿大的淋巴结中可发现肿瘤成分。转移性淋巴结肿大典型表现为球形结节，伴有分叶状，由于坏死而出现不均匀强化和 T_2 信号不均。另一方面，良性结节呈椭圆形，轮廓光滑，T_2 信号均匀，增强后均匀强化。应用超小的超铁磁性氧化铁颗粒，恶性淋巴结信号比良性结节低[64]。腹膜后转移可由其他原因引起，包括其他器官的原发实体瘤。在肌肉组织中可见转移瘤（图 23-15）。

（3）髓外浆细胞瘤：髓外浆细胞瘤的特征是在髓外部位浆细胞的单克隆增殖，可以是原发性或继发性的多发性骨髓瘤[65]。常见于 60—70 岁男性[66]。原发性浆细胞瘤仅可在排除了骨髓多发性骨髓瘤而无骨髓浆细胞增多症，并且血清或尿副蛋白水平低于 2g/dl[67]。磁共振成像表现为实体瘤，T_1 加权像上表现为等信号，T_2 加权像表现为等高信号，增强后轻至中度强化。较大的肿瘤可显示坏死区域[68]。

Chapter 23　腹膜后磁共振成像
MRI of the Retroperitoneum

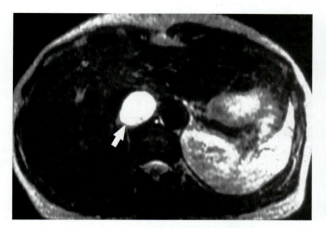

▲ 图 23-12　肾上腺外嗜铬细胞瘤

横轴位 T_2 加权 STIR 图像示下腔静脉后明显高信号肿物（箭）并使之向前移位

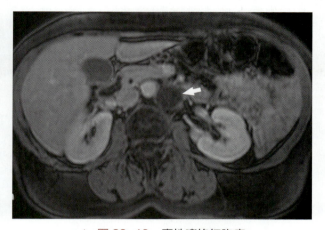

▲ 图 23-13　囊性嗜铬细胞瘤

囊性嗜铬细胞瘤的横轴位 T_1 加权像示腹膜后低信号肿物（箭）

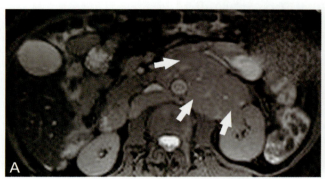

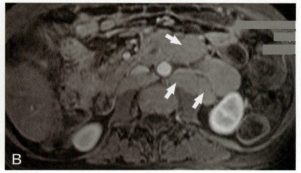

▲ 图 23-14　淋巴瘤

横轴位 T_2 加权像（A、B）示一个包绕腹主动脉并使之向前移位的融合成团的不均质的大肿物，与淋巴瘤（箭）相符

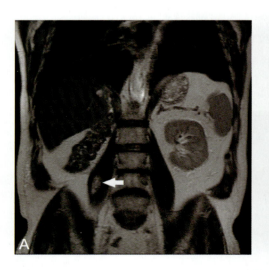

▲ 图 23-15　转移

A. 肾癌患者的冠状位单次快速自旋回波图像示右侧腰大肌高信号肿物（箭）；B. 同一患者的横轴位 STIR 图像示腰大肌中病变为高信号（箭）。这与肾细胞癌腰大肌转移相符

539

（二）非肿瘤性疾病

1. 腹膜后纤维化 特发性腹膜后纤维化（retroperitoneal fibrosis, RPF）是指腹膜后以慢性炎症组织伴纤维化为特征，并可以扩展到腹腔内各种器官，最常见的是输尿管。RPF 现在被认为是 IgG4 相关硬化性疾病的重要腹部组成成分[69]。其他原因包括动脉瘤、药物（甲硫氨酸、LSD、溴隐亭、β受体阻断药、甲基多巴和肼屈嗪）、感染和炎症过程、腹膜后出血[70]、吸烟和石棉暴露[71]。恶性肿瘤表现为腹膜后促纤维增生性反应，可与高达 8% 的病例有关；原发性肿瘤包括乳腺癌、肺癌、甲状腺癌、胃肠道癌和泌尿生殖系统癌，以及淋巴瘤和一些肉瘤[70,72]。大多数患者 50—70 岁，男性是女性的 2～3 倍[72,73]。

在磁共振成像上，RPF 在 T_1 加权图像上表现为低信号。然而，T_2 信号随着疾病活动程度的不同而变化，受炎症和水肿的影响。慢性、非活动期纤维化含少量水肿因此在 T_1 和 T_2 上均为低信号，而活动期在 T_2 上为高信号，并显示与疾病活动相关的明显强化[69,74]（图 23-16 至图 23-19）。RPF 通常是以一个融合的纤维斑块开始，常位于主动脉分叉低于 $L_{4\sim5}$ 水平。然后沿中线连续性延伸，通常是向上，包裹主动脉、下腔静脉和输尿管。通常，不超过腰大肌外侧缘向外侧延伸[70]。

2. 腹膜后积液

（1）出血/血肿：虽然外伤是最常见的原因，但腹膜后出血可能与出血倾向、抗凝治疗、动脉瘤漏、肾上腺和肾脏疾病（尤其是肿瘤性）以及创伤相关[75]。血肿可能发生在任何腹膜后间隙，并且部位可能提示其病因。自发性出血通常始于肾旁后间隙，并延伸至腹膜外脂肪、骨盆、腰大肌或腹壁肌肉[76]。主动脉瘤或移植物漏出的血首先围绕主动脉，然后延伸到肾旁前间隙并经常进入腰大肌[75]。肾上腺和肾脏出血通常局限在肾周间隙[77]。磁共振成像信号随时间而变化。T_1 加权像上的高信号归因于血肿内高铁血红蛋白的存在[78]。对比剂的主动外渗提示动脉持续出血，需要立即支持治疗、血管造影介入或外科手术干预[79]（图 23-20）。

（2）淋巴囊肿：淋巴囊肿是指充满液体的而无上皮内衬的囊肿，通常发生在骨盆或腹膜后淋巴结清扫术或肾移植手术后。腹膜后淋巴囊肿可引起静脉阻塞，并伴有相应的水肿和血栓栓塞并发症[55]。它们也可能导致周围结构如膀胱和输尿管的压迫，并可能导致进一步的并发症，如肾功能不全或输尿管积水[80]。通常它们是与手术夹相邻的边界清晰的水样信号强度结节。

（3）尿性囊肿：尿性囊肿是在肾脏集合系统之外的尿液包裹性积聚，最常见的是阻塞性尿路疾病导致集合系统破裂。其他原因是腹部创伤、手术或诊断性操作[81]。大多数尿性囊肿位于肾周间隙[82]。在磁共振成像上，尿性囊肿是一种水样

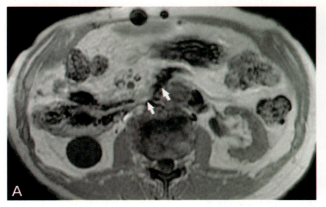 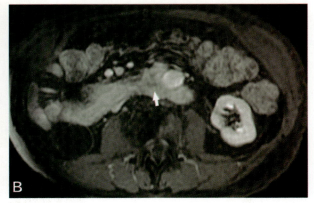

▲ 图 23-16 腹膜后纤维化

A. 横轴位 T_1 磁共振图像示腹膜后等信号软组织肿物（箭）；B. 延迟期图像示腹膜后肿物明显强化，提示该病处于活动期（箭）

信号强度的集合，增强扫描延迟期可见明显的对比剂渗漏其内。经皮抽吸引流术可明确诊断并进行治疗[55]。

（4）炎性液体积聚：大多数炎性液体积聚始于肾旁前间隙，由消化道腹膜外部分（胰腺、升降结肠、十二指肠和腹膜后阑尾）引起[76,83]，其中胰腺是最常见原因。肾周炎性液体积聚比肾旁前间隙少见。它们多继发于肾脏的直接蔓延。易感因素比较常见的有糖尿病、肾创伤、尿路梗阻或肾结石，尽管有时并无明确原因[77]。炎性渗出液在肾旁后间隙罕见，因为这个间隙没有器官，因此大多数的渗出液继发于其他间隙的严重感染。腹膜前脂肪和腰大肌可继发受侵[77]。液体积聚可以是边界清晰，也可以不规则的，取决于腹膜后间隔的不同形态。邻近的结构可因炎性液体积聚而显示不清或移位，并且周围软组织有明显增厚。暴发性感染可通过横筋膜播散[77]。在磁共振成像上，炎性液体聚积可呈不同程度的 T_1 信号强度，中高的 T_2 信号强度，以及厚的边缘强化方式[84]。

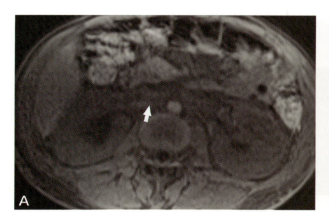
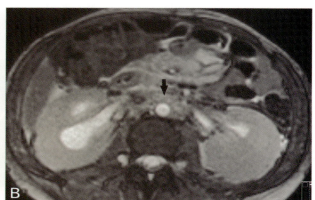
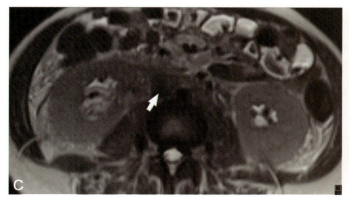
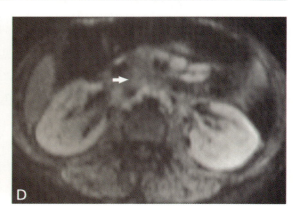
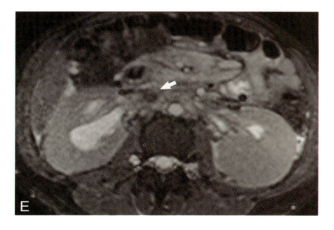

▲ 图 23-17　IgG4 相关的纤维化疾病和小血管白细胞碎裂性血管炎
A. T_1 加权图像示包裹主动脉和下腔静脉的低信号软组织肿物（箭）；B. SSFP 图像示肿物高信号（箭）；C. T_2 加权图像（T_2 FSE）示肿物等信号（箭）；D. 扩散加权图像示轻度受限扩散（箭）；E. 可见不均匀强化（箭）

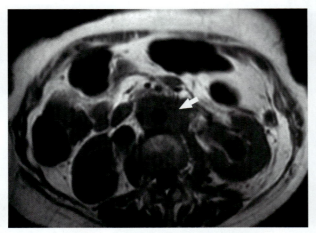

▲ 图 23-18　腹膜后纤维化非活动期

横轴位 T_1 加权图像示包绕腹主动脉的低信号肿物（箭）。STIR（此处无）示低信号且无强化

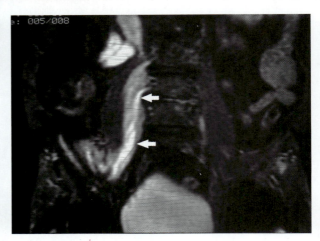

▲ 图 23-20　腰大肌血肿

脂肪抑制 T_1 加权图像示右侧腰大肌高信号区域（箭），与血肿相符

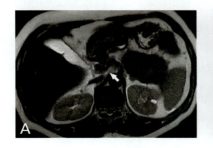
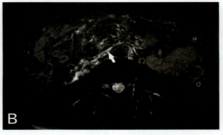
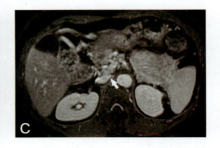

▲ 图 23-19　变异性腹膜后纤维化

A.HASTE 图像示腹膜后软组织肿物（箭）；B.STIR 图像示等高信号肿物（箭）；C.可见不均匀明显强化（箭）

（5）腰大肌脓肿：腰大肌脓肿是一种罕见的疾病，在发展中国家其病因通常是结核性的，而在发达国家是非结核性的，最常见的是金黄色葡萄球菌[85]。它可与多种感染相关，如胃肠道（最常见）、肾脏或腰椎骨髓炎蔓延[10]。腰大肌脓肿的临床诊断可能非常困难，而典型症状如侧腹疼痛、发热和跛行可能并不总是出现[86]。在图像中，它表现与其他的炎性液体积聚相似。治疗采用导管引流，而外科手术仅为经皮穿刺失败后进行[86]。

（三）其他腹膜后疾病

1. 黄色肉芽肿 /Erdheim-Chester 病

黄色肉芽肿是非朗格汉斯载脂组织细胞聚集形成的类肿瘤性病变；Erdheim-Chester 病是指多系统黄色肉芽肿。该病与骨硬化、骨膜炎、部分骨骺受累、长骨骨髓梗死相关[87]。组织学上，黄色肉芽肿伴泡沫状组织细胞被纤维化组织包绕，无 Birbeck 颗粒或 S-100 免疫染色。在磁共振成像上（图 23-21），黄色肉芽肿病表现为浸润性的强化软组织肿物，伴相对于骨骼肌的 T_1 和 T_2 信号中度增强[88,89]。腹膜后受累的特点是产生包绕肾脏及输尿管的软组织周围的肾周炎，可导致肾衰竭[90]。主动脉周围受累伴双侧对称性肾周间隙受累，但未侵犯下腔静脉和盆腔输尿管有助于鉴别 Erdheim-Chester 病与特发性腹膜后纤维化[88]。

2. 髓外造血

髓外造血（extramedullary hematopoiesis，EMH）是机体对骨髓造血功能缺乏的反应，它指的是红细胞前体在骨髓外的部位沉积。EMH 在腹膜后间隙少见[91]。在磁共振成像上，T_2 加权像上低信号和轻度强化以及血液学情况提示该病[91]（图 23-22）。输血治疗后，病变趋于消退最终导致强化消失[92]。图像中可显示由于慢性疾病导致的肝脏和脾脏肿块以及骨骼的变化，导致骨髓衰竭[91]。

3. 脂肪过多症 脂肪过多症是成熟脂肪的良性过度生长，常见于黑人男性。患者表现为尿路和胃肠道症状，腰背痛和胁痛[35]。在磁共振成像上，骨盆因为过于丰富的对称性分布的脂肪及偶尔可见的带状纤维组织而显得拥挤[35]。脂肪不强化且骨盆的软组织平面可被显示[93]。

4. 脂肪坏死 腹膜后脂肪坏死最常见的原因是急性胰腺炎[94-97]。磁共振成像上表现为脂肪信号强度病变，伴有周围软组织。由于与胰腺炎相关，其分布主要在胰周，但也可延伸至其他地方[98]。脂肪坏死在时间上体积大小趋于稳定或者缩小。

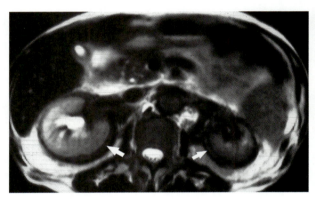

▲ 图 23-21 Erdheim-Chester 病
横轴位 T_2 加权图像示双侧包绕肾脏的低信号软组织肿物（箭）

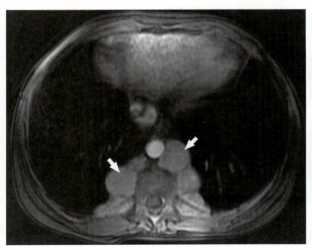

▲ 图 23-22 髓外造血
横轴位增强后图像示分叶状明显强化肿物（箭），邻近肋骨膨隆，符合髓外造血

（四）腹膜后非实质性囊肿和囊性病变

1. 淋巴管瘤 淋巴管瘤是一种由腹膜后淋巴组织与主要淋巴管血管和淋巴系统的其余部分所引起的发育畸形[99]。是一种单房或多房囊肿含透明或乳白色液体，内衬单层或扁平内皮细胞[99]。男性常见[99,100]。淋巴管瘤在 T_1 上信号不定（与蛋白含量相关的），在 T_2 上等高信号。

2. 淋巴管瘤病 弥漫性淋巴管瘤病的特点是不规则的淋巴管增生，包括软组织、内脏、腹膜后、眼和骨骼系统[101]，最常见于儿童和青少年。磁共振成像上，T_1 加权序列呈低信号，T_2 加权像上呈高信号或等信号（图 23-23）。一些淋巴管瘤在 T_1 加权图像上也显示高信号，可能是因为蛋白、脂肪或血液成分。磁共振扩散加权成像有助于诊断非典型腹部淋巴管瘤病[102]；磁共振淋巴管造影也可在应用对比剂后用重 T_2 加权 3D-TSE 序列和 T_1 加权 3D-VIBE 序列获得。该病的并发症可能包括乳糜胸、乳糜性心包积液、肝脾大、乳糜性腹水、蛋白质缺失性肠病以及淋巴水肿、淋巴漏和感染的发展[101,103]。

3. 非胰源性假性囊肿 非胰源性假性囊肿起源于肠系膜和网膜[104]，有一个厚的纤维壁并且通常含出血、脓或浆液。它们与囊液中淀粉酶或脂肪酶的高水平无关，这使得它们与胰腺假性囊肿不同。磁共振成像表现为单房或多房厚壁伴液体肿物[55]。

三、腹部大血管

（一）主动脉

1. 动脉粥样硬化 动脉粥样硬化是一种广泛的炎症过程，以脂质和纤维产物在动脉壁上的沉积为特点。动脉粥样硬化斑块的主要成分包括了部分：①结缔组织细胞外基质，包括胶原、蛋白多糖和纤维粘连弹性纤维；②胆固醇结晶、胆固醇酯和磷脂；③细胞如单核细胞来源的巨噬细胞、T 淋巴细胞和平滑肌细胞[105]。不稳定斑块具有薄纤维帽、大的脂质核心和显著的炎性细胞浸润[106]。腹主动脉斑块与年龄增长和血压相关,并且在冠状动脉和心脏疾病的患者中更严重[107]。在常规磁共振成像上,斑块表现为沿主动脉壁的不规则病变。脂质成分表现为 T_1 加权高信号和 T_2 加权低信号。纤维细胞成分在 T_1 和 T_2 上为高信号。钙沉积为 T_1 和 T_2 低信号区域[107]。靶向磁共振对比剂(超顺磁性铁氧铁)在动脉粥样硬化斑块中被巨噬细胞吞噬,是对不稳定斑块成像的有效方法[106](图 23-24 和图 23-25)。

2. **主髂动脉闭塞病** 主髂动脉闭塞病见于慢性动脉粥样硬化性疾病,发生在动脉分叉。症状取决于侧支循环血流的情况,包括间歇性大腿、髋部或臀部跛行和阳痿(30%～50%)[108,109]。磁共振血管成像有助于评估受累区域的长度和多样性、狭窄程度、侧支程度以及合并的股骨头疾病(图 23-26 和图 23-27)。有多种治疗方式包括血管内介入治疗如球囊血管成形术和支架置入术,或外科手术如主动脉双股动脉旁路术或腋动脉股动脉伴股股旁路术[108]。

3. **动脉瘤** 动脉瘤是腹主动脉节段的局部扩张大于其正常直径的 50%(或 > 3cm)。患病率男性 4%～8%,女性 1%[108]。危险因素包括年龄增长、吸烟、男性和家族史[110]。动脉瘤形成的理论包括促炎症介质触发酶消化细胞外基质并损害其随后的修复或湍流产生剪切力,导致动脉瘤扩张甚至破裂[108,111]。大多数动脉瘤是无症状的直到破裂,但有些也可出现背痛、腹痛或可触及的腹部肿物。在磁共振成像上,动脉瘤表现为腹主动脉的囊状或梭形扩张。当动脉瘤 > 5.5cm 时建议手术。术前评估的特征包括动脉瘤囊的最大前后径;动脉瘤颈的横轴长度(肾最下动脉与动脉瘤开始之间的距离);颈部的形状和角度;髂动脉直径(进入腹股沟处)和远端髂动脉的潜在长度和状态(图 23-28)。动脉瘤可以通过手术或血管内修复治疗(表 23-3)。

假性动脉瘤没有动脉壁完整的三层结构,通常与内膜和中膜破裂相关,通过外膜或周围组织贮存血液。它们是由创伤、感染(图 23-29)、外科手术或穿透性动脉粥样硬化溃疡引起。它们在腹主动脉肾上段更常见的原因是主动脉在这个位置与周围组织固定紧密,因而有更大的填塞可能性[112]。假性动脉瘤因其有破裂的风险和高死亡率而推荐外科手术治疗[113]。

4. **动脉瘤破裂** 破裂是腹主动脉瘤的并发症之一,可以是包含的或游离的,急性或慢性。破裂见于动脉瘤 > 5.5cm 或随访 6 个月扩张 > 0.5cm[114]。大于 5cm 的动脉瘤 5 年累积

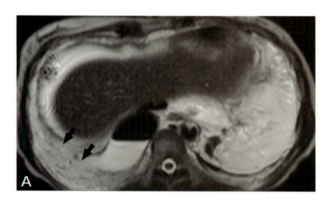
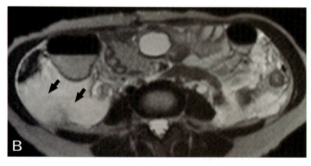
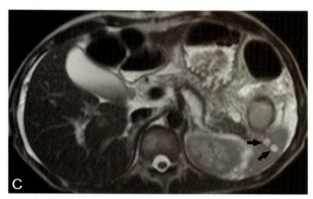

▲ 图 23-23 淋巴管瘤病
A. 横轴位 T_2 加权像示腹膜后弥漫浸润生长不均匀高信号病变(箭);B. 低层面图像证实诊断(箭);C. 在高层面图像示脾淋巴管瘤(箭)

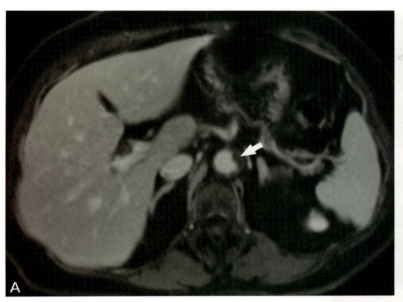 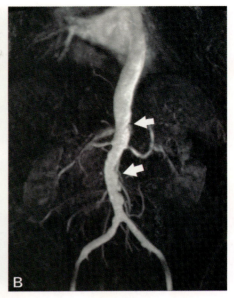

▲ 图 23-24 严重主动脉粥样硬化斑块

A. 横轴位增强 VIBE 图像示腹主动脉外周一个大的不规则低信号斑块（箭）；B. 磁共振血管成像示腹主动脉轮廓不规则，与严重动脉粥样硬化性疾病相符（箭）

破裂率为 25%～40%，而直径 4～5cm 动脉瘤为 1%～7%[115,116]。破裂表现为腹部搏动性肿物的患者突发腹部或背部疼痛伴低血压。其他表现有晕厥、便秘、尿潴留和排便。只有约 50% 腹主动脉瘤（abdominal aortic aneurysms，AAA）破裂患者到医院后仍活着；其中 50% 没有机会通过修复而幸存[117]。AAA 破裂预后不良，社区死亡率约 79%，围术期死亡率约 40%[118]。

AAA 破裂最常见的是通过后外侧壁进入腹膜后间隙[119]，血液延伸到肾周间隙、肾旁间隙或腰大肌。腹腔破裂较少见[108]。磁共振成像不是 AAA 破裂的常规检查，但可以显示出血从破裂部位延伸到腹膜后间隙。轻微的破裂表现为环周钙化的不连续[120]。即将破裂的征象包括新月征，即附壁血栓出血区域[120]和披挂征即主动脉后壁是不规则的，并且向后贴临椎体而无明显的脂肪间隙[121]。具有腹主动脉瘤病史、疼痛缓解、血流动力学稳定、血细胞比容正常、腹膜后出血的患者，诊断为慢性破裂[122]。

5. 主动脉肠瘘 主动脉肠瘘是一个腹主动脉和肠管之间的连接，这可以是由于一个穿透性溃疡、憩室、异物、主动脉炎、阑尾炎和胃肠道恶性肿瘤所造成的原发性[123-126]，或更多常见于继发于外科手术或介入。移植物周围慢性感染或移植物对肠管的持续压迫是继发性瘘常见的发病原因[127]。瘘的经典位置（60%）是十二指肠水平段。不常见位置包括余段十二指肠，空肠和回肠、胃、乙状结肠和升/降结肠[123]。症状包括胃肠道出血的预示，随后伴随大量出血。其他症状可包括疼痛、搏动性肿物和腹股沟肿物。主动脉肠瘘的磁共振成像结果包括主动脉旁周围脂肪间隙的

表 23-3 内漏类型

类型	描述
I	支架移植物在主动脉壁附着处的渗漏 IA——近端附着处 IB——远端附着处
II	由于相连的分支血管中的反向血流渗漏至动脉瘤囊内
III	由于移植物机械性故障而泄漏（连接处泄漏、中间移植孔、连接断开及分裂）
IV	移植物多孔渗漏
V	内张力（动脉瘤扩张而无明显可见的渗漏→排除诊断）

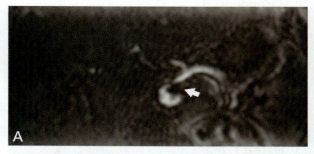
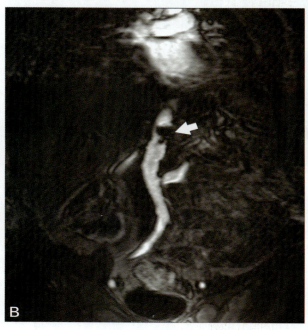

▲ 图 23-25　钙化斑块

A. 横轴位磁共振血管成像示接近腹腔干起源的主动脉壁的低信号无强化病变，与致密钙化斑块相符（箭）；B. 冠状位磁共振血管成像示胸主动脉广泛的粥样硬化改变，伴低信号大斑块，可能有钙化（箭）

消失，局部增厚，主动脉紧密相邻的肠襻拴系，主动脉旁游离液体和软组织增厚，移植物的断裂或明显的移植物移位。少见表现包括异常气体和对比剂从主动脉外渗至肠腔内[128]。鉴别诊断包括移植物感染、主动脉炎、真菌性动脉瘤和动脉瘤旁纤维化[129]。主动脉肠瘘的治疗方法是去除感染的移植物、肠切除术和建立额外的解剖旁路移植[124]。近来的趋势是使用血管内技术[128]。

6. 主动脉 - 腔静脉瘘　原发性主动脉 - 腔静脉瘘是腹主动脉瘤的一种罕见并发症，累及不到 1% 的所有 AAAs，但累及 2%～6.7% 的破裂动脉瘤[130]。这些瘘中 80% 是动脉粥样硬化动脉瘤的自发破裂直接进入邻近的腔静脉；余者为创伤（15%）或医源性（5%）[131]。男性更常见，平均年龄为 64 岁[132]。急性瘘可表现为搏动性腹部肿块、持续性腹部杂音或震颤和高输出充血性心力衰竭。主动脉腔静脉瘘的慢性表现为高输出性心力衰竭、腹部杂音和颤动、可触及的腹部动脉瘤、少尿和相应的区域性静脉高血压[133]。在磁共振血管成像上，下腔静脉和髂总静脉出现早期和明显的强化并且与腹主动脉强化相同[134]。可以证明瘘管的交通。不同于主动脉破裂，下腔静脉是膨胀的。无阻塞性病变可区别瘘与其他原因的下腔静脉扩张。治疗是通过外科修复或血管内排除腹主动脉瘤[133]。

7. 主动脉夹层　夹层是主动脉壁的破裂，导致内膜和内层基质与外层基质和外膜的分离，导致形成内膜片围成的真腔，以及具有血流或栓子的假腔[135]。腹主动脉夹层通常是胸主动脉夹层的延伸，但是局部腹主动脉夹层亦可见，在肾动脉和肠系膜下动脉（inferior mesenteric artery, IMA）（33%）的近端或腹腔干和肾动脉（23%）的远端至髂总动脉终止。它通常是由高血压引起的，但其他原因包括结缔组织疾病如 Marfan 综合征和 Ehler-Danlos 综合征、纤维发育不良、吸烟、糖尿病、高胆固醇血症和之前的动脉瘤手术[136]。在局部的夹层病变中，近端范围在肾动脉和肠系膜下动脉（IMA）之间（33%），或腹腔干和肾动脉之间（23%），远端范围位于髂总动脉的近端[136]。临床特征是急性发作的腹部、胸部或背部疼痛。其他表现包括肠系膜缺血、肾血管性高血压或肢体缺血[108,136]。

在磁共振成像上，在主动脉腔内可见一个可延伸到分支血管的皮瓣（图 23-30）。假腔往往较大，有一个鸟嘴征，因为在假腔蔓延的前缘有楔形血肿；蜘蛛网征代表了由不完全剪切的基质形成的低信号线性区域。分支血管的闭塞可能是由于内膜片撕脱延伸至分支血管或内膜片动态脱垂覆盖分支血管起始处[137]。夹层的鉴别诊断包括动脉瘤内的血栓：血栓有不规则的边界，与主

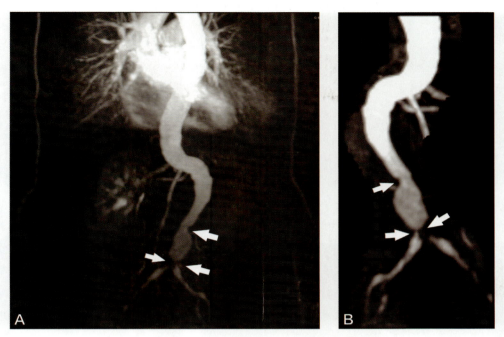

▲ 图 23-26 严重的主髂动脉狭窄疾病

A. 冠状位磁共振血管成像示腹主动脉肾下部分的严重狭窄（箭）和双侧髂总动脉起源处严重狭窄（箭）；B. 同一患者的矢状斜位磁共振血管成像示腹主动脉远端和双侧髂总动脉近端狭窄（箭）

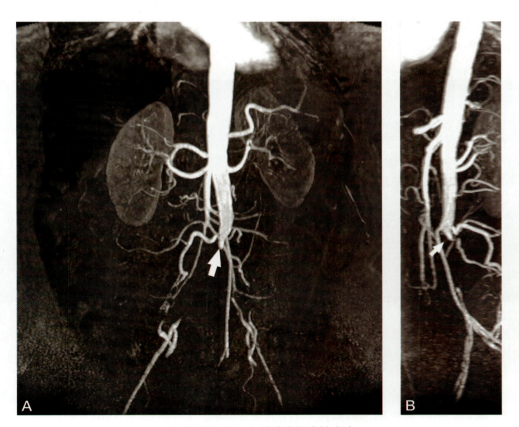

▲ 图 23-27 主髂动脉闭塞性疾病

冠状面（A）和矢状面（B）MIP 图像显示腹主动脉远端（箭）和髂总动脉全长广泛的动脉粥样硬化性改变，导致动脉完全闭塞。重建图像显示髂外动脉及近端髂内动脉通过侧支循环供血

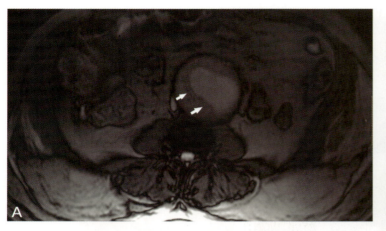
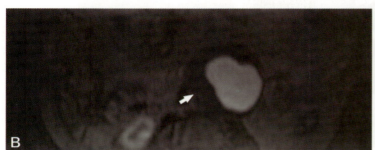
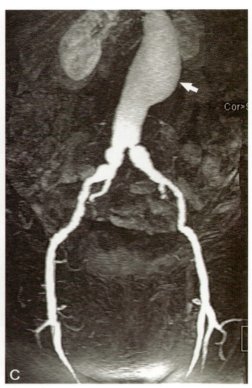

▲ 图 23-28 动脉瘤

横轴位 SSFP（A）、横轴位增强 MRA（B）和冠状位增强 MRA（C）图像示腹主动脉肾下部分的大动脉瘤，最大截面约 7.2cm×4.6cm（箭）

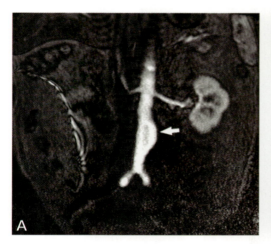
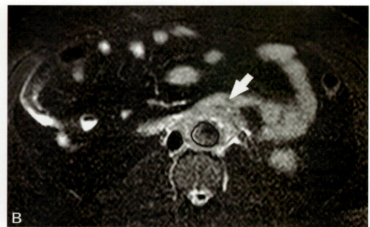

▲ 图 23-29 炎性动脉瘤

A. 磁共振血管成像的冠状位 MIP 图像示腹主动脉肾下区域局灶性动脉瘤（箭）；B. 同一患者的横轴位 T_2 加权 STIR 图像示高信号的主动脉壁增厚（箭）与炎性主动脉瘤相符

动脉和血栓深部的钙化形成固定的圆周关系，而夹层具有螺旋结构、平滑的内部边界和假腔表面的钙化[138,139]。虽然开放修复用于主动脉夹层和创伤的治疗，但是血管内技术越来越受欢迎，包括主动脉开窗术或支架移植物修复[140]。

8. 主动脉壁内血肿 壁内血肿（aortic intramural hematoma, IMH）的形成是由于主动脉壁内的出血，导致壁薄弱，没有内膜破裂或主动脉夹层内膜片的形成。高血压和动脉粥样硬化在主动脉 IMH 形成中起重要作用[141]。形成的理论

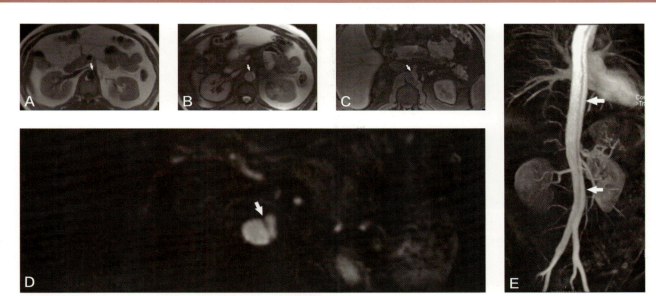

▲ 图 23-30 夹层

横轴位 HASTE（A），SSFP（B），增强 VIBE（C），横轴位磁共振血管成像（D）和冠状位磁共振血管成像（E）图像示急性胸痛患者贯穿腹主动脉的内膜片

包括主动脉血管瘤自发破裂，病理性新生血管，内膜微撕裂或穿透性主动脉溃疡的延伸[142,143]。IMH 常见于 70 — 90 岁，表现为急性胸/腹痛。在磁共振成像上，可以用黑血显像和 T_1、T_2 加权序列检测主动脉壁中的血肿。在 T_1 加权成像中，由于高铁血红蛋白而出现高信号[144]并且无强化或内膜片（图 23-31）。内膜的存在和连续性以及内膜片的出现有助于鉴别急性主动脉夹层与 IMH 和穿透性动脉粥样硬化性溃疡。然而，急性主动脉夹层的血栓性假腔、内膜钙化或主动脉壁动脉粥样硬化斑块，很难与 IMH 区分[143]。

9. 穿透性动脉粥样硬化性溃疡 穿透性主动脉溃疡是穿透内弹力膜和血管中层的动脉粥样硬化性溃疡[145]。它通常与主动脉壁的中层血肿形成相关[146]。这种溃疡可能发展成囊状动脉瘤、主动脉夹层或主动脉破裂[147]。它经常呈现伴有急性腹痛，类似于主动脉夹层的表现。磁共振成像有助于诊断，因为在 T_1 和 T_2 加权图像上主动脉壁的信号强度增加了溃疡的显示[148]。增强后，可见到一个通过内膜延伸到主动脉壁的局部溃疡病灶，由于 IMH，也可观察到一个厚的强化的主动脉壁（图 23-32）。穿透性溃疡应与内膜粥样硬化性溃疡鉴别，它局限于内膜，无症状，并且无

IMH[138]。需要外科手术治疗[147]。

10. 外伤性主动脉损伤 钝性腹主动脉损伤罕见，约占钝性腹部创伤的 0.05%[149]。腹主动脉损伤需要很大的力量，常见于机动车事故[150]。多数损伤（33%）发生在肠系膜下动脉水平，24% 接近肾动脉，19% 在肠系膜下动脉和主动脉分叉之间，其余位于其他位置[151]。虽然多数患者无症状，但有症状的患者可有急腹症、神经功能缺损、终末期器官和肢体缺血[152]。在磁共振成像上，内膜片、血栓或假性神经瘤的出现提示此诊断[151]。治疗包括外科手术或血管内修复[153]。

11. 主动脉炎 主动脉炎是主动脉壁的炎症，可以是感染性的或非感染性的。感染的原因包括细菌或病毒。非感染性原因包括大、中、小血管血管炎、特发性炎性动脉瘤或 RPF。

（1）非感染性主动脉炎：Takayasu 动脉炎（也称为无脉病和主动脉弓综合征）是最常见的胸腹主动脉血管炎，是一种常见于年轻亚洲女性的大血管血管炎。1 型疾病局限于主动脉弓及分支；2 型累及胸腹区域的降主动脉和腹主动脉内脏分支；3 型包括 1、2 型；4 型包括 1、2 或 3 合并相关肺动脉血管炎。Takayasu 动脉炎中主动脉中层、

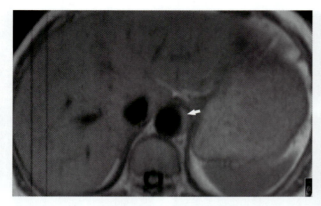

▲ 图 23-31 主动脉壁内血肿
（译者注：原著有误，已修改）

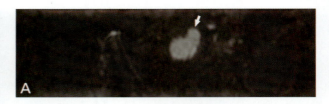

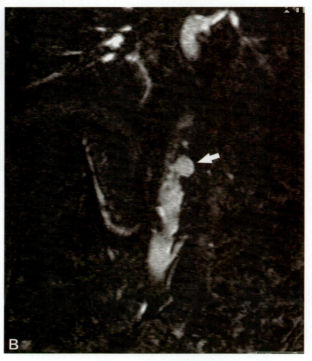

▲ 图 23-32 穿透性溃疡
A. 横轴位磁共振血管成像示腹主动脉上部的前部的局灶性穿透性溃疡（箭）；B. 冠状位磁共振血管成像示腹主动脉上部的穿透性溃疡（箭）

外膜和滋养血管又都会有炎性细胞浸润，主要为淋巴细胞、巨噬细胞和多核巨细胞。随着时间的推移，主动脉中层瘢痕形成和弹性层破坏[154,155]。发病机制不明，但有可能是一种抗原驱动的细胞介导的自体免疫过程[156]。平均诊断年龄25—30岁，75%～97%为女性。常见症状是由主动脉、主动脉弓和大血管的动脉闭塞性疾病［主动脉或肾动脉闭塞性疾病造成的高血压,脉搏障碍和（或）血管杂音，以及上肢和/或下肢跛行］[157,158]。腹主动脉是最常见的受累部位，主动脉上的狭窄病变常被检测到，尽管主动脉瘤也常见[157-160]。磁共振成像显示主动脉壁增厚。活动性动脉炎表现为STIR高信号（图23-33）和增强后强化[161]。慢性动脉炎表现为壁增厚、无水肿或对比增强、动脉狭窄、闭塞或动脉瘤形成[108]。

巨细胞动脉炎是一种大中型血管系统性肉芽肿性动脉炎，其特征是与Takayasu动脉炎相似的病理组织学和类似的自身免疫病因学[156]，但与高龄和高加索妇女相关[162]。通常表现为头痛、体格检查时颞动脉异常、炎症标志物升高、风湿性多肌痛、头皮压痛、嚼暂停、视野改变[163]。磁共振成像表现与Takayasu动脉炎相似。一些研究表明巨细胞动脉炎与腹主动脉瘤风险增加相关[164]。

特发性炎性动脉炎的特点是壁增厚和与周围结构粘连的纤维化。炎症局限于主动脉和主动脉周围组织，而不是广泛性血管炎的表现[156]。斑块状坏死的主动脉中层是主要的组织学发现，并伴有炎性细胞浸润，可包括多核巨细胞[165]。通常为亚临床表现，在回顾主动脉瘤手术后的组织病理学时偶然诊断[166]。磁共振成像显示动脉瘤伴主动脉旁炎性壁增厚、外膜纤维化和湍流。

（2）感染性主动脉炎：感染性主动脉炎常由沙门菌、葡萄球菌或肺炎链球菌肺炎造成，通常是从已感染的主动脉壁的细菌播散而来[154,167]。可见中层和外膜血管的慢性炎性浸润，最终导致中层坏死[154]。磁共振成像表现与非感染性主动脉炎相似，影像学表现为菌血症和软组织扩张的临床征象。通常推荐强化抗生素治疗和手术清创术，如果需要行动脉瘤修复[167,168]。

（3）真菌性（感染性）动脉瘤：真菌性动脉瘤是一种感染性动脉瘤，可能是感染性主动脉炎

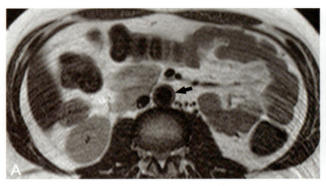
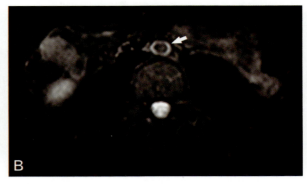

▲ 图 23-33　主动脉炎

A. 横轴位 T₂ 加权图像示主动脉壁的环周增厚（箭）；B. 同一患者同一层面的 STIR 图像示增厚壁中的高信号（箭），表明活动性动脉炎出现水肿

的后遗症，动脉粥样硬化表面的重复感染，或是邻近神经血管结构的蔓延。葡萄球菌和沙门菌是最常见的致病源[165]。真菌性动脉瘤的磁共振成像表现为囊状动脉瘤、动脉瘤周围软组织肿块、对比剂渗漏或进展明显[165]。并发症包括椎体破坏、腰大肌脓肿、肾脓肿、破裂、出血、脓毒症和死亡。治疗包括延长全身抗生素或手术切除，疾病严重时可行清创术和脓肿引流[169]。

12. 主动脉肿瘤　主动脉的原发性肿瘤罕见且多数为恶性[170]。它们分为内膜的原发肿瘤表现为血栓栓塞，和起源于中层和外膜的肿瘤表现为肿物占位效应[171]。在磁共振成像上，血流的移动在血管腔内和血管壁或周围软组织之间提供了天然的对比，从而能够更好地诊断。治疗方式不明确但常涉及手术[170]。

13. 腹主动脉发育不良　腹主动脉发育不良是腹主动脉的一种弥漫狭窄，通常是由于原始背侧主动脉的过度融合，包括主动脉后支起源引起的一种发育性缺陷[172]。其他病因包括病毒感染或炎性改变如动脉炎[173]。辐射或创伤也能产生相似的表现。女性常见，常见于 20—30 岁[174]。症状包括高血压、下肢跛行和主动脉髂动脉分布的动脉粥样硬化的早期进展[173]。当所有症状出现时，诊断为中段主动脉综合征。磁共振血管成像上有一段很长的环周形狭窄。磁共振成像也可评估血管炎症的存在。治疗是外科血管重建术，切除受累节段和端端吻合或放置替代移植物[173]。

（二）下腔静脉

1. 先天性异常　下腔静脉由后主静脉、下主静脉、上主静脉按顺序汇合形成，这些静脉的异常存在或退化导致多种先天性异常。这些异常大多是无症状的，在影像学检查中偶然发现。

左侧下腔静脉由于右侧上主静脉的退化和左侧上主静脉的持续存在。发病率为 0.2%～0.5%[175]。这种畸形的主要临床意义是可能被误诊为左侧主动脉旁淋巴结肿大[176]。当放置 IVC 过滤器时，这种畸形也很重要，尤其是通过颈静脉途径[177]（图 23-34）。

双下腔静脉是由于右侧和左侧上主静脉的同时持续存在。发病率为 1%～3%[175]。这种畸形最常见的类型是两个不同的下腔静脉从各自的髂静脉起源而无正常汇合[178]。放置下腔静脉过滤器后反复肺栓塞应怀疑此诊断。IVC 过滤器应放置在两个 IVC 或汇合处。

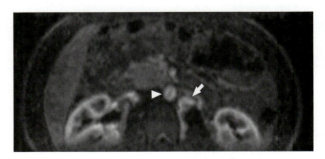

▲ 图 23-34　左侧下腔静脉

横轴位增强磁共振图像示位于腹主动脉（箭头）左侧的左下腔静脉（箭）

IVC 的离断是由于右下主静脉-肝静脉吻合失败和右下主静脉萎缩所致。因此，血液从下腔静脉上方吻合通过奇静脉分流，其部分来源于右侧上主静脉的胸段。发病率为 0.6%[179]。IVC 的肝段中断，但下腔静脉以奇静脉扩张连接到胸廓右侧的上腔静脉。其本身无病理后果，但这种异常与心脏畸形有关，如内脏异位综合征、多脾、房室隔缺损、部分肺静脉异位连接和肺动脉闭锁。另外，手术中奇静脉的意外结扎可能致命[180]（图 23-35）。

主动脉后左肾静脉是由于环主动脉环的背侧持续存在和腹侧退化所致[181]。其患病率为 0.8%～3.7%[182]。主动脉后左肾静脉有时可引起临床症状，如血尿和腹/胁痛[183]。当考虑左肾移植和（或）脾肾分流术时，有必要认识这种异常。未能识别这种异常可能导致严重出血[184]（图 23-36）。

环主动脉左肾静脉，是由于环主动脉环的背侧和腹侧持续存在。主要临床意义是在肾切除术前的术前计划和经肾静脉插管取血时要注意识别。应注意避免误诊为腹膜后淋巴结肿大[177]。

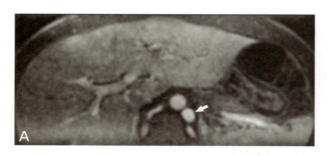

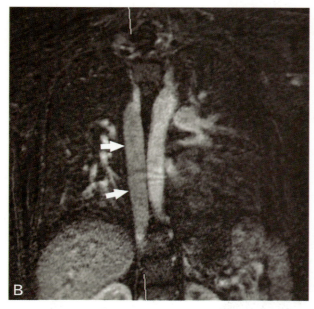

▲ 图 23-35 下腔静脉的中断
A. 横轴位增强磁共振图像示左下腔静脉（箭）。此外，下腔静脉的肝内段缺如，与下腔静脉离断相符；B. 胸部冠状位磁共振血管成像示大的扩张的奇静脉（箭）汇入上腔静脉

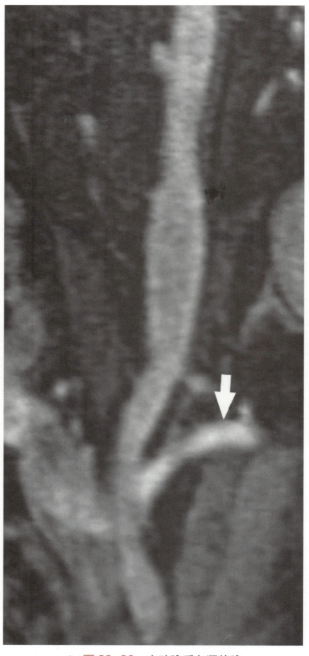

▲ 图 23-36 主动脉后左肾静脉
冠状位磁共振血管成像示主动脉后左肾静脉（箭），延伸到腹主动脉（abdominal aorta，AA）后方

类似于主动脉后左肾静脉，主动脉压迫肾静脉引起临床症状，如血尿和腹/胁痛[183]。

腔静脉后输尿管是由于 IVC 由后主静脉形成而非正常的上主静脉。这使得右输尿管位于 IVC 后内侧，导致输尿管受压伴并发症如肾积水或复发性尿路感染[177]。据报道尸检中 0.06%~0.17% 可见[185]。在图像上，其表现为腰椎椎弓根水平的近端输尿管的鱼钩或倒 J 形外观[186]。

2. 下腔静脉血栓与肿瘤 Bland 血栓常见于下肢或盆腔静脉血栓的延续。急性血栓使下腔静脉扩张，而慢性血栓不扩张下腔静脉。Bland 血栓具有不均质的 T_1 和 T_2 等低信号，且增强后无强化，而肿瘤血栓强化，并且常与原发肿瘤相邻。

下腔静脉的肿瘤是继发性肿瘤，较原发多见。平滑肌肉瘤是最常见的下腔静脉原发恶性肿瘤。常见于 50—60 岁女性[187]。肿瘤可以完全为腔内，也可兼有腔外、腔内成分，预后较差[187]。从邻近结构延伸到下腔静脉的继发恶性肿瘤包括肾细胞癌、肝细胞癌和肾上腺皮质癌[188]。延伸到下腔静脉的良性肿瘤包括嗜铬细胞瘤、血管平滑肌脂肪瘤和血管内平滑肌瘤病[189]。影像学检查决定手术方法：血栓延伸到膈上段下腔静脉需要体外循环手术，伴发病率和死亡率增加[188]（图 23-37）。

四、总结

磁共振成像是一种有价值的成像工具，用于评估腹膜后病变，包括主动脉和下腔静脉的血管异常。磁共振成像的优点包括其对组织的定性能力和无电离辐射对病变范围的评估。磁共振成像序列应优化，用以评估和定性腹膜后病变。

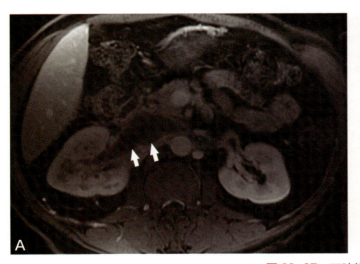 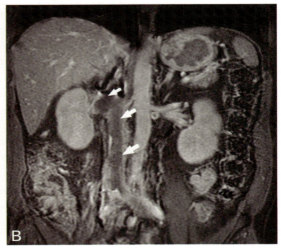

▲ 图 23-37 下腔静脉血栓
横轴位（A）和冠状位（B）增强 T_1 加权成像示从右肾癌延伸到下腔静脉和髂静脉的大血栓（箭）

参考文献

[1] Nishino M, Hayakawa K, Minami M et al. Primary retroperitoneal neoplasms: CT and MR imaging findings with anatomic and pathologic diagnostic clues. *RadioGraphics* 2003;23(1):45–57.

[2] Sanyal R, Remer EM. Radiology of the retroperitoneum: Case-based review. *AJR Am J Roentgenol* 2009;192(6Suppl.):S112–S127; (Quiz S118–S121).

[3] Jemal A, Siegel R, Ward E et al. Cancer statistics, 2006. *CA Cancer J Clin* 2006;56(2):106–130.

[4] Shibata D, Lewis JJ, Leung DH et al. Is there a role for incomplete resection in the management of retroperitoneal liposarcomas? *J Am Coll Surg* 2001;193(4):373–379.

[5] Lewis JJ, Leung D, Woodruff JM et al. Retroperitoneal soft-tissue sarcoma: Analysis of 500 patients treated and followed at a single institution. *Ann Surg* 1998;228(3):355–365.

[6] Sung MS, Kang HS, Suh JS et al. Myxoid liposarcoma: Appearance at MR imaging with histologic correlation. *RadioGraphics* 2000;20(4):1007–1019.

[7] Cormier JN, Pollock RE. Soft tissue sarcomas. *CA Cancer J*

[8] Vijay A, Ram L. Retroperitoneal liposarcoma: A comprehensive review. *Am J Clin Oncol* 2015;38(2):213–219.

[9] DasGupta TK. Tumors and tumor-like conditions of adipose tissue. *Curr Probl Surg* 1970;7:1–60.

[10] Torigian DA, Ramchandani P. The retroperitoneum. In: Haaga JR, Dogra VS, Forsting M et al. (eds.), 5th edn., *CT and MRI of the whole body*. Philadelphia, PA: Mosby Elsevier, 2009: 1953–2040.

[11] Engelken JD, Ros PR. Retroperitoneal MR imaging. *Magn Reson Imaging Clin N Am* 1997;5(1):165–178.

[12] Lane RH, Stephens DH, Reiman HM. Primary retroperitoneal neoplasms: CT findings in 90 cases with clinical and pathologic correlation. *AJR Am J Roentgenol* 1989;152(1):83–89.

[13] Kim T, Murakami T, Oi H et al. CT and MR imaging of abdominal liposarcoma. *AJR Am J Roentgenol* 1996;166:829–833.

[14] Henricks WH, Chu YC, Goldblum JR et al. Dedifferentiated liposarcoma: A clinicopathological analysis of 155 cases with a proposal for an expanded definition of dedifferentiation. *Am J Surg Pathol* 1997;21:271–281.

[15] Jelinek JS, Kransdorf MJ, Shmookler BM et al. Liposarcoma of the extremities: MR and CT findings in the histologic subtypes. *Radiology* 1993;186(2):455–459.

[16] Tateishi U, Hasegawa T, Beppu Y et al. Primary dedifferentiated liposarcoma of the retroperitoneum. Prognostic significance of computed tomography and magnetic resonance imaging features. *J Comput Assist Tomogr* 2003;27:799–804.

[17] Neville A, Herts BR. CT characteristics of primary retroperitoneal neoplasms. *Crit Rev Comput Tomogr* 2004;45(4):247–270.

[18] Kieffer E, Alaoui M, Piette JC et al. Leiomyosarcoma of the inferior vena cava: Experience in 22 cases. *Ann Surg* 2006;244(2):289–295.

[19] McLeod AJ, Zornoza J, Shirkhoda A. Leiomyosarcoma: Computed tomographic findings. *Radiology* 1984;152(1):133–136.

[20] Hartman DS, Hayes WS, Choyke PL et al. From the archives of the AFIP. Leiomyosarcoma of the retroperitoneum and inferior vena cava: Radiologic-pathologic correlation. *RadioGraphics* 1992;12(6):1203–1220.

[21] La Fianza A, Alberici E, Meloni G et al. Extraperitoneal pelvic leiomyosarcoma. MR findings in a case. *Clin Imaging* 2000;24(4):224–226.

[22] Ganeshalingam S, Rajeswaran G, Jones RL, Thway K, Moskovic E. Leiomyosarcomas of the inferior vena cava: Diagnostic features on cross-sectional imaging. *Clin Radiol* Jan 2011;66(1):50–56.

[23] Kransdorf MJ. Malignant soft-tissue tumors in a large referral population: Distribution of diagnoses by age, sex, and location. *AJR Am J Roentgenol* 1995;164(1):129–134.

[24] Ko SF, Wan YL, Lee TY et al. CT features of calcifications in abdominal malignant fibrous histiocytoma. *Clin Imaging* 1998;22(6):408–413.

[25] Nishimura H, Zhang Y, Ohkuma K et al. MR imaging of soft-tissue masses of the extraperitoneal spaces. *RadioGraphics* 2001;21(5):1141–1154.

[26] Maurer HM, Beltangady M, Gehan EA et al. The Intergroup Rhabdomyosarcoma Study-I. A final report. *Cancer* Jan 15, 1988;61(2):209–220.

[27] Kransdorf MJ, Murphey MD. Muscle tumors. In: Kransdorf M, Murphey M (eds.), *Imaging of Soft Tissue Tumors*. Philadelphia, PA: WB Saunders, 1997, pp. 3–36 and 57–102.

[28] Best AK, Dobson RL, Ahmad AR. Cardiac angiosarcoma. *RadioGraphics* 2003;23(Spec Issue): S141–S145.

[29] Enzinger FM, Shiraki M. Extraskeletal myxoid chondrosarcoma: An analysis of 34 cases. *Hum Pathol* 1972;3:421–435.

[30] Murphey MD, Walker EA, Wilson AJ, Kransdorf MJ, Temple HT, Gannon FH. From the archives of the AFIP: Imaging of primary chondrosarcoma: Radiologic-pathologic correlation. *RadioGraphics* Sep–Oct 2003;23(5):1245–1278.

[31] Nakanishi H, Araki N, Sawai Y, Kudawara I, Mano M, Ishiguro S, Ueda T, Yoshikawa H. Cystic synovial sarcomas: Imaging features with clinical and histopathologic correlation. *Skeletal Radiol* Dec 2003;32(12):701–707.

[32] Jones BC, Sundaram M, Kransdorf MJ. Synovial sarcoma: MR imaging findings in 34 patients. *AJR Am J Roentgenol* Oct 1993;161(4):827–830.

[33] Wu JH, Zhou JL, Cui Y, Jing QP, Shang L, Zhang JZ. Malignant perivascular epithelioid cell tumor of the ret roperitoneum. *Int J Clin Exp Pathol* Sep 15, 2013;6(10):2251–2256. eCollection 2013.

[34] Rajiah P, Sinha R, Cuevas C et al. Imaging of uncommon retroperitoneal masses. *RadioGraphics* 2011;31(4):949–976.

[35] Craig WD, Fanburg-Smith JC, Henry LR, Guerrero R, Barton JH. Fat-containing lesions of the retroperitoneum: Radiologic-pathologic correlation. *RadioGraphics* 2009;29(1):261–290.

[36] Castellazzi G, Vanel D, Le Cesne A et al. Can the MRI signal of aggressive fibromatosis be used to predictits behavior? *Eur J Radiol* 2009;69(2):222–229.

[37] Kreuzberg B, Koudelova J, Ferda J et al. Diagnostic problems of abdominal desmoid tumors in various locations. *Eur J Radiol* 2007;62(2):180–185.

[38] Vandevenne JE, De Schepper AM, De Beuckeleer L et al. New concepts in understanding evolution of desmoid tumors: MR imaging of 30 lesions. *Eur Radiol* 1997;7:1013–1019.

[39] Kransdorf MJ, Jelinek JS, Moser Jr RP et al. Magnetic resonance appearance of fibromatosis: A report of 14 cases and review of the literature. *Skeletal Radiol* 1990;19:495–499.

[40] Lee JC, Thomas JM, Phillips S, Fisher C, Moskovic E. Aggressive fibromatosis: MRI features with pathologic correlation. *AJR Am J Roentgenol* 2006;186:247–254.

[41] Dinauer PA, Brixey CJ, Moncur JT et al. Pathologic and MR imaging features of benign fibrous soft-tissue tumors in adults. *RadioGraphics* 2007;27(1):173–187.

[42] Choyke PL, Hayes WS, Sesterhenn IA. Primary extragonadal germ cell tumors of the retroperitoneum: Differentiation of primary and secondary tumors. *RadioGraphics* 1993;13(6):1365–1375; quiz 1377–1378.

[43] Ueno T, Tanaka YO, Nagata M et al. Spectrum of germ cell tumors: From head to toe. *RadioGraphics* 2004;24(2):387–404.

[44] Gatcombe HG, Assikis V, Kooby D et al. Primary retroperitoneal teratomas: A review of the literature. *J Surg Oncol* 2004;86(2):107–113.

[45] Wang RM, Chen CA. Primary retroperitoneal teratoma. *Acta Obstet Gynecol Scand* 2000;79(8):707–708.

[46] Bruneton JN, Diard F, Drouillard JP et al. Primary retroperitoneal teratoma in adults: Presentation of two cases and review of the literature. *Radiology* 1980;134:613–616.

[47] Hayasaka K, Tanaka Y, Soeda S et al. MR findings in primary retroperitoneal schwannoma. *Acta Radiol* 1999;40(1):78–82.

[48] Li Q, Gao C, Juzi JT et al. Analysis of 82 cases of retroperitoneal schwannoma. *ANZ J Surg* 2007;77(4): 237–240.

[49] Rha SE, Byun JY, Jung SE et al. Neurogenic tumors in the abdomen: Tumor types and imaging characteristics. *RadioGraphics* 2003;23(1):29–43.

[50] Kinoshita T, Naganuma H, Ishii K, Itoh H. CT features of retroperitoneal neurilemmmoma. *Eur J Radiol* 1998;27:67–71.

[51] Wong CS, Chu TY, Tam KF.Retroperitoneal Schwannoma: A common tumor in an uncommon site. *Hong Kong Med J* 2010;16:66–68.

[52] Bass JC, Korobkin M, Francis IR et al. Retroperitoneal plexiform neurofibromas: CT findings. *AJR Am J Roentgenol* 1994;163(3):617–620.

[53] Sakai F, Sone S, Kiyono K et al. Intrathoracic neurogenic tumors: MR-pathologic correlation. *AJR Am J Roentgenol* 1992;159:279–283.

[54] Hughes MJ, Thomas JM, Fisher C et al. Imaging features of retroperitoneal and pelvic schwannomas. *Clin Radiol* 2005;60(8):886–893.

[55] Yang DM, Jung DH, Kim H et al. Retroperitoneal cystic masses: CT, clinical, and pathologic findings and literature review. *RadioGraphics* 2004;24(5):1353–1365.

[56] Hrehorovich PA, Franke HR, Maximin S et al. Malignant peripheral nerve sheath tumor. *RadioGraphics* 2003;23(3):790–794.

[57] Korf BR. Malignancy in neurofibromatosis type 1. *Oncologist* 2000;5(6):477–485.

[58] Felix EL, Wood DK, Das Gupta TK. Tumors of the retroperitoneum. *Curr Probl Cancer* Jul 1981;6(1):1–47.

[59] Kilton LJ, Aschenbrener C, Burns CP. Ganglioneuroblastoma in adults. *Cancer* 1976;37:974–983.

[60] Bousvaros A, Kirks DR, Grossman H. Imaging of neuroblastoma: An overview. *Pediatr Radiol* 1986;16:89–106.

[61] Francis IR, Korobkin M. Pheochromocytoma. *Radiol Clin North Am* 1996;34:1101–1112.

[62] Blackledge G, Best JJ, Crowther D et al. Computed tomography (CT) in the staging of patients with Hodgkin's Disease: A report on 136 patients. *Clin Radiol* 1980; 31(2):143–147.

[63] Neumann CH, Robert NJ, Canellos G et al. Computed tomography of the abdomen and pelvis in non-Hodgkin lymphoma. *J Comput Assist Tomogr* 1983;7(5):846–850.

[64] Froehlich JM, Triantafyllou M, Fleischmann A, Vermathen P, Thalmann GN, Thoeny HC. Does quantification of USPIO uptake-related signal loss allow differentiation of benign and malignant normal-sized pelvic lymph nodes? *Contrast Media Mol Imaging* May–Jun 2012;7(3):346–355.

[65] Alexiou C, Kau RJ, Dietzfelbinger H et al. Extramedullary plasmacytoma: Tumor occurrence and therapeutic concepts. *Cancer* 1999;85:2305–2314.

[66] Monill J, Pernas J, Montserrat E et al. CT features of abdominal plasma cell neoplasms. *Eur Radiol* 2005;15:1705–1712.

[67] Galieni P, Cavo M, Avvisati G et al. Solitary plasmacytoma of bone and extramedullary plasmacytoma: Two different entities? *Ann Oncol* 1995;6:687–691.

[68] Oh D, Kim CK, Park BK, Ha H. Primary extramedullary plasmacytoma in retroperitoneum: CT and integrated PET/CT findings. *Eur J Radiol Extra* 2007;62:57–61.

[69] George V, Tammisetti VS, Surabhi VR, Shanbhogue AK. Chronic fibrosing conditions in abdominal imaging. *RadioGraphics* Jul–Aug 2013;33(4):1053–1080.

[70] Amis ES Jr. Retroperitoneal fibrosis. *AJR Am J Roentgenol* 1991;157(2):321–329.

[71] Uibu T, Oksa P, Auvinen A et al. Asbestos exposure as a risk factor for retroperitoneal fibrosis. *Lancet* 2004;363(9419):1422–1426.

[72] Lepor H, Walsh PC. Idiopathic retroperitoneal fibrosis. *J Urol* 1979;122(1):1–6.

[73] Cronin CG, Lohan DG, Blake MA, Roche C, Mc-Carthy P, Murphy JM. Retroperitoneal fibrosis: A review of clinical features and imaging findings. *AJR Am J Roentgenol* 2008;191(2):423–431.

[74] Mehta A1, Blodgett TM. Retroperitoneal fibrosis as a cause of positive FDG PET/CT. *J Radiol Case Rep* 2011;5(7):35–41.

[75] Sagel SS, Siegel MJ, Stanley RJ, Jost RG. Detection of retroperitoneal hemorrhage by computed tomography. *AJR Am J Roentgenol* Sep 1977;129(3):403–407.

[76] Meyers MA. *Dynamic Radiology of the Abdomen*. New York: Springer-Verlag, 1976, pp.I 13–95.

[77] Alexander ES, Colley DP, Clark RA. Computed tomography of retroperitoneal fluid collections. *Semin Roentgenol* Oct 1981;16(4):268–276.

[78] Syuto T, Hatori M, Masashi N, Sekine Y, Suzuki K. Chronic expanding hematoma in the retroperitoneal space: A case report. *BMC Urol* Nov 18, 2013;13:60.

[79] Shanmuganathan K, Mirvis SE, Sover ER. Value of contrast-enhanced CT in detecting active hemorrhage in patients with blunt abdominal or pelvic trauma. *AJR Am J Roentge-

nol 1993;161(1):65–69.

[80] Thaler M, Achatz W, Liebensteiner M, Nehoda H, Bach CM. Retroperitoneal lymphatic cyst formation after anterior lumbar interbody fusion: A report of 3 cases. *J Spinal Disord Tech* Apr 2010;23(2):146–150.

[81] Kawashima A, Sandler CM, Corriere JN Jr, Rodgers BM, Goldman SM. Ureteropelvic junction injuries secondary to blunt abdominal trauma. *Radiology* 1997;205:487–492.

[82] Gore RM, Balfe DM, Aizenstein RI, Silverman PM. The great escape: Interfascial decompression planes of the retroperitoneum. *AJR Am J Roentgenol* Aug 2000; 175(2):363–370.

[83] Altemeier WA, Alexander JW. Retroperitoneal abscess. *Arch Surg* 1961;83:512–524.

[84] Callen PW. Computed tomographic evaluation of abdominal and pelvic abscesses. *Radiology* 1979; 131(1):171–175.

[85] Wells RD, Bebarta VS. Primary iliopsoas abscess caused by community-acquired methicillin-resistant *Staphylococcus aureus*. *Am J Emerg Med* 2006;24: 897–898.

[86] Charalampoulos A, Macheras A, Charalabopoulos A, Fotiadis C, Charalabopoulos K. Iliopsoas abscesses: Diagnostic, aetiologic and therapeutic approach in five patients with a literature review. *Scand J Gastroenterol* 2009;44(5):594–599.

[87] Dion E, Graef C, Miquel A et al. Bone involvement in Erdheim-Chester disease: Imaging findings including periostitis and partial epiphyseal involvement. *Radiology* 2006;238(2):632–639.

[88] Dion E, Graef C, Haroche J et al. Imaging of thoracoabdominal involvement in Erdheim-Chester disease. *AJR Am J Roentgenol* 2004;183(5):1253–1260.

[89] Fortman BJ, Beall DP. Erdheim-Chester disease of the retroperitoneum: A rare cause of ureteral obstruction. *AJR Am J Roentgenol* 2001;176(5):1330–1331.

[90] Gottlieb R, Chen A. MR findings of Erdheim-Chester disease. *J Comput Assist Tomogr* 2002;26(2): 257–261.

[91] Mesurolle B, Sayag E, Meingan P, Lasser P, Duvillard P, Vanel D. Retroperitoneal extramedullary hematopoiesis: Sonographic, CT, and MR imaging appearance. *AJR Am J Roentgenol* Nov 1996;167(5):1139–1140.

[92] Tsitouridis J, Stamos S, Hassapopoulou E et al. Extramedullary paraspinal hematopoiesis in thalassemia: CT and MRI evaluation. *Eur J Radiol* 1999;30(1):33–38.

[93] Waligore MP, Stephens DH, Soule EH, McLeod RA. Lipomatous tumors of the abdominal cavity: CT appearance and pathologic correlation. *AJR Am J Roentgenol* 1981;137:539–545.

[94] Andac N, Baltacioglu F, Cimsit NC et al. Fat necrosis mimicking liposarcoma in a patient with pelvic lipomatosis. CT findings. *Clin Imaging* 2003;27(2):109–111.

[95] Haynes JW, Brewer WH, Walsh JW. Focal fat necrosis presenting as a palpable abdominal mass: CT evaluation. *J Comput Assist Tomogr* 1985;9(3):568–569.

[96] Ross JS, Prout GR, Jr. Retroperitoneal fat necrosis pro ducing ureteral obstruction. *J Urol* 1976;115(5):524–529.

[97] Takao H, Yamahira K, Watanabe T. Encapsulated fat necrosis mimicking abdominal liposarcoma: Computed tomography findings. *J Comput Assist Tomogr* 2004;28(2):193–194.

[98] Jeffery GM, Theaker JM, Lee AH et al. The growing teratoma syndrome. *Br J Urol* 1991;67(2):195–202.

[99] Davidson AJ, Hartman DS. Lymphangioma of the retroperitoneum: CT and sonographic characteristic. *Radiology* 1990;175(2):507–510.

[100] Konen O, Rathaus V, Dlugy E et al. Childhood abdominal cystic lymphangioma. *Pediatr Radiol* 2002;32(2):88–94.

[101] Foeldi M, Foeldi E, Kubik S. *Textbook of Lymphology*. 2nd edn. Munich, Germany: Elsevier, 2007.

[102] Humphries PD, Wynne CS, Sebire NJ, Olsen ØE. Atypical abdominal paediatric lymphangiomatosis: Diagnosis aided by diffusion-weighted MRI. *Pediatr Radiol* 2006;36:857–859.

[103] Lohrmann C, Foeldi E, Langer M. Assessment of the lymphatic system in patients with diffuse lymphangiomatosis by magnetic resonance imaging. *Eur J Radiol* Nov 2011;80(2):576–581.

[104] Ros PR, Olmsted WW, Moser RP, Dachman AH, Hjermstad BH. Mesenteric and omental cysts: Histologic classification with imaging correlation. *Radiology* 1987;164:327–332.

[105] Fayad ZA, Fuster V. Clinical imaging of the high-risk or vulnerable atherosclerotic plaque. *Circ Res* Aug 17, 2001;89(4):305–316.

[106] Kramer CM. Magnetic resonance imaging to identify the high-risk plaque. *Am J Cardiol* Nov 21, 2002;90(10C):15L–17L.

[107] Momiyama Y, Fayad ZA. Plaque imaging and monitoring atherosclerotic plaque interventions. *Top Magn Reson Imaging* 2007;18:349–355.

[108] Budovec JJ, Pollema M, Grogan M. Update on multidetector computed tomography angiography of the abdominal aorta. *Radiol Clin N Am* 2010;48:283–309.

[109] Brewster DC. Clinical and anatomical considerations for surgery in aortoiliac disease and results of surgical treatment. *Circulation* 1991;83(2 Suppl.):I42–I52.

[110] Pande RL, Beckman JA. Abdominal aortic aneurysm: Populations at risk and how to screen. *J Vasc Interv Radiol* 2008;19(Suppl. 6):S2–S8.

[111] Khanafer KM, Bull JL, Upchurch GR Jr et al. Turbulence significantly increases pressure and fluid shear stress in an aortic aneurysm model under resting and exercise flow conditions. *Ann Vasc Surg* 2007;21(1):67–74.

[112] Veith FJ, Gupta S, Daly V. Technique for occluding the supraceliac aorta through the abdomen. *Surg Gynecol Obstet* 1980;151:426–428.

[113] Chase CW, Layman TS, Barker DE et al. Traumatic abdominal aortic pseudoaneurysm causing biliary obstruction: A case report and review of the literature. *J Vasc Surg* 1997;25(5):936–940.

[114] Hirsch AT, Haskal ZJ, Hertzer NR et al. ACC/AHA 2005 Practice Guidelines for the management of patients with peripheral arterial disease (lower extremity, renal, mesenteric, and abdominal aortic): AU. *Circulation* 2006;113(11):e463.

[115] Nevitt MP, Ballard DJ, Hallett JW, Jr. Prognosis of abdominal aortic aneurysms. A population-based study. *N Engl J Med* 1989;321:1009–1014.

[116] Lederle FA, Johnson GR, Wilson SE et al. Rupture rate of large abdominal aortic aneurysms in patients refusing or unfit for elective repair. *JAMA* 2002;287:2968–2972.

[117] Harris LM, Faggioli GL, Fiedler R, Curl GR, Ricotta JJ. Ruptured abdominal aortic aneurysms: Factors affecting mortality rates. *J Vasc Surg* 1991;14:812–818.

[118] Yankelevitz DF, Gamsu G, Shah A et al. (2000) Optimization of combined CT pulmonary angiography with lower extremity CT venography. *AJR Am J Roentgenol* 174(1):67–69.

[119] Schwartz SA, Taljanovic MS, Smyth S et al. CT findings of rupture, impending rupture, and contained rupture of abdominal aortic aneurysm. *AJR Am J Roentgenol* 2007;188:W57–W62.

[120] Siegel CL, Cohan RH, Korobkin M et al. Abdominal aortic aneurysm morphology; CT features in patients with ruptured and non-ruptured aneurysms. *AJR Am J Roentgenol* 1994;163:1123–1129.

[121] Rakita D, Newatia A, Hines JJ et al. Spectrum of CT findings in rupture and impending rupture of abdominal aortic aneurysms. *RadioGraphics* 2007;27:497–507.

[122] Jones CS, Reilly MK, Dalsing MC et al. Chronic contained rupture of abdominal aortic aneurysms. *Arch Surg* 1986;121:542–546.

[123] Sevastos N, Rafailidis P, Kolokotronis K et al. Primary aortojejunal fistula due to foreign body: A rare cause of gastrointestinal bleeding. *Gastroenterol Hepatol* 2002;14:797–800.

[124] Tse DML, Thompson ARA, Perkins J et al. Endovascular repair of a secondary aorto-appendiceal fistula. *Cardiovasc Interv Radiol* 2011;34(5):1090–1093.

[125] Kappadath SK, Clarke MJ, Stormer E, Steven L, Jaffray B Primary aortoenteric fistula due to a swallowed twig in a threeyear-old child. *Eur J Vasc Endovasc Surg* 2010;39:217–219.

[126] Skourtis G, Papacharalambous G, Makris S et al. Primary aortoenteric fistula due to septic aortitis. *Ann Vasc Surg* 2010;24(6):825.e7–825.e11.

[127] Hagspiel KD, Turba UC, Bozlar U et al. Diagnosis of aortoenteric fistulas with CT angiography. *J Vasc Interv Radiol* 2007;19:497–504.

[128] Raman SP, Kamaya A, Federle M, Fishman EK. Aortoenteric fistulas: Spectrum of CT findings. *Abdom Imaging* Apr 2013;38(2):367–375.

[129] Vu QDM, Menias CO, Bhalla S, Peterson C, Wang LL, Balfe DM. Aortoenteric fistulas: CT features and potential mimics. *RadioGraphics* 2009;20:197–209.

[130] Schmidt R, Bruns C, Walter M, Erasmi H. Aorto-caval fistula—An uncommon complication of infrarenal aortic aneurysms. *Thorac Cardiovasc Surg* 1994;42:208–211.

[131] Abbadi AC, Deldime P, Van Espen D, Simon M, Rosoux P. The spontaneous aortocaval fistula: A complication of the abdominal aortic aneurysm. Case report and review of the literature. *J Cardiovasc Surg (Torino)* 1998;39:433–436.

[132] Miani S, Giorgetti PL, Arpesani A, Giuffrida GF, Biasi GM, Ruberti U. Spontaneous aorto-caval fistulas from ruptured abdominal aortic aneurysms. *Eur J Vasc Surg* 1994;8:36–40.

[133] Brightwell RE, Pegna V, Boyne N. Aortocaval fistula: Current management strategies. *ANZ J Surg* Jan 2013;83(1–2):31–35.

[134] Alexander JJ, Imbembo AL. Aorta-vena cava fistula. *Surgery* 1989;105:1–12.

[135] Liu PS, Platt JF. CT angiography in the abdomen: A pictorial review and update. *Abdom Imaging* Feb 2014;39(1):196–214.

[136] Jonker FH, Schlosser FJ, Moll FL et al. Dissection of the abdominal aorta. Current evidence and implications for treatment strategies; a review and meta analysis of 92 patients (comment). *J Endovasc Ther* 2009;16(1):71–80.

[137] Sebastia C, Pallisa E, Quiroga S et al. Aortic dissection:Diagnosis and follow-up with helical CT. *RadioGraphics* 1999;19:45–60.

[138] Cataner D, Andreu M, Gallardo X et al. CT in nontraumatic acute thoracic aortic disease: Typical and atypical features and complications. *RadioGraphics* 2003;23:S93–S110.

[139] Cambria RP, Brewster DC, Gertler J et al. Vascular complications associated with spontaneous aortic dissection. *J Vasc Surg* 1988;7:199–209.

[140] Barnes DM, Williams DM, Dasika NL et al. A single-center experience treating renal malperfusion after aortic dissection with central aortic fenestration and renal artery stenting. *J Vasc Surg* 2008;47(5):903–910.

[141] Ganaha F, Miller DC, Sugimoto K, Do YS, Minamiguchi H, Saito H, Mitchell RS, Dake MD. Prognosis of aortic intramural hematoma with and without penetrating atherosclerotic ulcer: A clinical and radiological analysis. *Circulation* 2002;106:342–348.

[142] Coady MA, Rizzo JA, Elefteriade JA. Pathologic variants of thoracic aortic dissections:Penetrating atherosclerotic ulcer and intramural hematoma. *Cardiol Clinic* 1999;17:637–657.

[143] Alomari IB, Hamirani YS, Madera G, Tabe C, Akhtar N, Raizada V. Aortic intramural hematoma and its complications. *Circulation* Feb 11, 2014;129(6):711–716.

[144] Chao CP, Walker TG, Kalva SP. Natural history and CT appearances of aortic intramural hematoma. *RadioGraphics* 2009;29:791–804.

[145] Stanson AW, Kazmier FJ, Hollier LH. Ulceres atheroma-

teux penetrants de l'aorte thoracique: Histoire naturelle et correlations anatomo-cliniques. *Ann Chir Vasc* 1986;1:15–23.

[146] Georgiadis GS, Trellopoulos G, Antoniou GA, Georgakarakos EI, Nikolopoulos ES, Pelekas D, Pitta X, Lazarides MK. Endovascular therapy for penetrating ulcers of the infrarenal aorta. *ANZ J Surg* Oct 2013;83(10):758–763.

[147] Sato M, Imai A, Sakamoto H, Sasaki A, Watanabe Y, Jikuya T. Abdominal aortic disease caused by penetrating atherosclerotic ulcers. *Ann Vasc Dis* 2012;5(1):8–14.

[148] Tsuji Y, Tanaka Y, Kitagawa A. Endovascular stent-graft repair for penetrating atherosclerotic ulcer in the infrarenal abdominal aorta. *J Vasc Surg* 2003;38:383–388.

[149] Teruya TH, Bianchi C, Abou-Zamzam AM, Ballard JL. Endovascular treatment of a blunt traumatic abdominal aortic injury with a commercially available stent graft. *Ann Vasc Surg* 2005;19(4):474–478.

[150] Rosengart MR, Zierler RE. Fractured aorta—A case report. *Vasc Endovascular Surg* 2002;36(6):465–467.

[151] Nucifora G, Hysko F, Vasciaveo A. Blunt traumatic abdominal aortic rupture: CT imaging. *Emerg Radiol* 2008;15(3):211–213.

[152] Gunn M, Campbell M, Hoffer EK. Traumatic abdominal aortic injury treated by endovascular stent placement. *Emerg Radiol* 2007;13(6):329–331.

[153] Lock JS, Huffman AD, Johnson RC. Blunt trauma to the abdominal aorta. *J Trauma* 1987;27(6):674–677.

[154] Virmani R, Burke A. Nonatherosclerotic diseases of the aorta and miscellaneous disease of the main pulmonary arteries and large veins. In: Silver M, Gotlieb A, Schoen F (eds.), *Cardiovascular Pathology*, 3rd edn. Philadelphia, PA: Churchill Livingstone, 2001, pp. 107–137.

[155] Gravanis MB. Giant cell arteritis and Takayasu aortitis: Morphologic, pathogenetic and etiologic factors. *Int J Cardiol* 2000;75(Suppl. 1):S21–33. discussion S35–S36.

[156] Gornik HL, Creager MA. Aortitis. *Circulation* 2008;117(23):3039–3051.

[157] Kerr GS, Hallahan CW, Giordano J, Leavitt RY, Fauci AS, Rottem M, Hoffman GS. Takayasu arteritis. *Ann Intern Med* 1994;120:919–929.

[158] Mwipatayi BP, Jeffery PC, Beningfield SJ, Matley PJ, Naidoo NG, Kalla AA, Kahn D. Takayasu arteritis: Clinical features and management: Report of 272 cases. *ANZ J Surg* 2005;75:110–117.

[159] Sueyoshi E, Sakamoto I, Hayashi K. Aortic aneurysms in patients with Takayasu's arteritis: CT evaluation. *AJR Am J Roentgenol* 2000;175:1727–1733.

[160] Matsumura K, Hirano T, Takeda K, Matsuda A, Nakagawa T, Yamaguchi N, Yuasa H, Kusakawa M, Nakano T. Incidence of aneurysms in Takayasu's arteritis. *Angiology* 1991;42:308–315.

[161] Flamm SD, White RD, Hoffman GS. The clinical application of 'edema-weighted' magnetic resonance imaging in the assessment of Takayasu's arteritis. *Int J Cardiol* 1998;66(Suppl. 1):S151–S159.

[162] Salvarani C, Crowson CS, O'Fallon WM, Hunder GG, Gabriel SE. Reappraisal of the epidemiology of giant cell arteritis in Olmsted County, Minnesota, over a fifty-year period. *Arthritis Rheum* 2004;51:264–268.

[163] Salvarani C, Cantini F, Boiardi L, Hunder GG. Polymyalgia rheumatica and giant-cell arteritis. *N Engl J Med* 2002;347:261–271.

[164] Evans JM, O'Fallon WM, Hunder GG. Increased incidence of aortic aneurysm and dissection in giant cell (temporal) arteritis. A population-based study. *Ann Intern Med* 1995;122:502–507.

[165] Miller DV, Isotalo PA, Weyand CM, Edwards WD, Aubry MC, Tazelaar HD. Surgical pathology of noninfectious ascending aortitis: A study of 45 cases with emphasis on an isolated variant. *Am J Surg Pathol* 2006;30:1150–1158.

[166] Rojo-Leyva F, Ratliff NB, Cosgrove DM, 3rd, Hoffman GS. Study of 52 patients with idiopathic aortitis from a cohort of 1,204 surgical cases. *Arthritis Rheum* 2000;43:901–907.

[167] Foote EA, Postier RG, Greenfield RA, Bronze MS. Infectious aortitis. *Curr Treat Options Cardiovasc Med* 2005;7:89–97.

[168] Reddy DJ, Ernst CB. Infected aneurysms. In: Rutherford RB (ed.), *Vascular Surgery*, 4th edn. Philadelphia, PA: WB Saunders, 1995, pp. 1139–1153.

[169] Restrepo CS, Ocazionez D, Suri R, Vargas D. Aortitis: Imaging spectrum of the infectious and inflammatory conditions of the aorta. *RadioGraphics* 2011;31:435–451.

[170] Daas AK, Reddy KS, Suwanjindar P, Fulmer A, Siquiera A, Floten S, Starr A. Primary tumors of the aorta. *Ann Thorac Surg* 1996;62:1526–1528.

[171] Mason MD, Wheeler JR, Gregory RT et al. Primary tumors of the aorta: Report of a case and review of the literature. *Oncology* 1982;39:167–172.

[172] Graham LM, Zelenock GB, Erlandson EE, Coran AG, Lindenauer SM, Stanley JC. Abdominal aortic coarctation and segmental hypoplasia. *Surgery* 1979;86:519–529.

[173] Terramani TT, Salim A, Hood DB, Rowe VL, Weaver FA. Hypoplasia of the descending thoracic and abdominal aorta: A report of two cases and review of the literature. *J Vasc Surg* Oct 2002;36(4):844–848.

[174] Bashour T, Jokhadar M, Cheng TO, Nasri M, Kabbani S. Hypoplasia of descending aorta as a rare cause of hypertension. A report of 5 cases. *Angiology* 1982;33:790–799.

[175] Phillips E. Embryology, normal anatomy, and anomalies. In: Ferris EJ, Hipona FA, Kahn PC, Phillips E, Shapiro JH (eds.), *Venography of the Inferior Vena Cava and Its Branches*. Baltimore, MD: Williams & Wilkins, 1969, pp. 1–32.

[176] Siegfried MS, Rochester D, Bernstein JR, Milner JW. Diagnosis of inferior vena cava anomalies by computerized tomography. *Comput Radiol* 1983;7:119–123.

[177] Bass JE, Redwine MD, Kramer LA, Huynh PT, Harris JH

Jr. Spectrum of congenital anomalies of the inferior vena cava: Cross-sectional imaging findings. *RadioGraphics* May–Jun 2000;20(3):639–652.

[178] Pineda D, Moudgill N, Eisenberg J, DiMuzio P, Rao A. An interesting anatomic variant of inferior vena cava duplication: Case report and review of the literature. *Vascular* Jun 2013;21(3):163–167.

[179] Ginaldi S, Chuang VP, Wallace S. Absence of hepatic segment of the inferior vena cava with azygous continuation. *J Comput Assist Tomogr* 1980;4:112–114.

[180] Mazzucco A, Bortolotti U, Stellin G, Gallucci V. Anomalies of the systemic venous return: A review. *J Card Surg* 1990;5(2):122–133.

[181] Karaman B, Koplay M, Ozturk E, Basekim CC, Ogul H, Mutlu H, Kizilkaya E, Kantarci M. Retroaortic left renal vein: Multidetector computed tomography angiography findings and its clinical importance. *Acta Radiol* Apr 2007;48(3):355–360.

[182] Karkos CD, Bruce IA, Thomson GJ, Lambert ME. Retroaortic left renal vein and its implications in abdominal aortic surgery. *Ann Vasc Surg* 2001;15:703–708.

[183] Cuellar i Calabria H, Quiroga Gomez S, Sebastia Cerqueda C, Boye de la Presa R, Miranda A, Alvarez- Castells A. Nutcracker or left renal vein compression phenomenon: Multidetector computed tomography findings and clinical significance. *Eur Radiol* 2005;15:1745–1751.

[184] Brancatelli G, Galia M, Finazzo M, Sparacia G, Pardo S, Lagalla R. Retroaortic left renal vein joining the left common iliac vein. *Eur Radiol* 2000;11:1724–1725.

[185] Uthappa MC, Anthony D, Allen C. Retrocaval ureter: MR appearances. *Br J Radiol* 2002;75:177–179.

[186] Talner LB, Reilly PHO, Wasserman NF. Specific causes of obstruction. In: Pollack HM, McClennan BL (eds.), *Clinical Urography*, 2nd edn. Philadelphia, PA: WB Saunders, 2000,pp. 1967–2136.

[187] Jenkins S, Marshall GB, Gray R. Leiomyosarcoma of the inferior vena cava. *Can J Surg* 2005;48(3):252–253.

[188] Kaufman LB, Yeh BM, Joe BN, Qayyum A, Coakley F. Inferior vena cava filling defects on CT and MRI. *AJR Am J Roentgenol* 2005;185:717–726.

[189] Kutcher R, Rosenblass R, Mitsudo S, Goldman M, Kogan S. Renal angiomyolipoma with sonographic demonstration of extension into the inferior vena cava. *Radiology* 1982;143:755–756.

Chapter 24
腹壁和疝

Abdominal Wall and Hernias

Sonja M.Kirchhoff 著

朱 正 译

张红梅 校

目录 CONTENTS

一、磁共振成像序列 / 562

二、腹壁 / 562

三、疝 / 567

四、总结 / 568

腹内粘连常见，主要累及腹壁，可以是一种不可预防的术后改变。约93%的腹部或盆腔大手术后的患者发生粘连[1]。这些粘连主要由纤维带连接腹壁和腹膜内器官[2,3]。尽管出现粘连的患者中多数无症状；然而，仍有相当一部分患者存在与粘连相关的症状。粘连性小肠梗阻的发生率为65%～75%[4]。一般来说，下腹部和盆腔的手术或介入治疗或这些治疗导致腹膜表面大面积损伤往往会使患者发生粘连的风险更高[5]。再次手术的预期粘连程度最高。

因此，在手术或再手术治疗前必须要对粘连情况做出正确诊断。在这种情况下，可用的成像方式应准确确定粘连部位和程度。

通常情况下，计算机断层扫描（CT）和（或）超声（US）是在急诊情况下进行的，但磁共振成像（MRI）包括功能性电影成像提供了一种更有价值的选择方式。

一、磁共振成像序列

磁共振成像序列一般应适应患者的临床条件且采集时间应尽量缩短。

在目前的文献中，并无标准的腹部磁共振成像序列，尤其是用于诊断粘连和（或）疝。然而，除了妊娠和已知的肾损伤患者外，通常使用钆对比剂。可以从自由呼吸或屏气序列中选择。总之，一个典型的评估腹部的磁共振成像方案可包括如下各项。

1. 使用所谓的半傅里叶单脉冲自旋回波（HASTE）技术的轴位和冠状位 T_2 加权图像。

2. T_1 加权屏气梯度回波序列，包括同、反相位。

3. 屏气非增强或增强的轴位和冠状三维 T_1 加权脂肪压脂图像。

4. 冠状位上结合平衡稳态自由进动序列。

功能性电影磁共振成像

功能性电影磁共振成像不应被误认为是使用静脉或动脉对比剂进行动态磁共振成像，而是被解释为呼吸冻结运动时采集连续磁共振图像。为了克服其他技术甚至3D磁共振成像技术对内脏层面可视化的影响，Lienemann等研发了一种特殊的磁共振成像序列[6]。

功能磁共振成像检查需在高于1.5 T的高场强上进行。患者仰卧用体部表面线圈覆盖腹部。无需对比剂或任何检查前用药。首先，用一个叠加的网格获取冠状定位相，用于参考定位矢状和轴位相上整个腹部，覆盖从膈肌到盆腔的区域。紧接着，在网格的每个点上完成一个由10个连续测量组成的周期（图24-1）。在每一个检查位置，患者被要求通过紧张增加腹内压力，随后在每个周期中放松，以诱导内脏滑动能够诊断或排除粘连（图24-2）。网格中两个连续位置之间的平均距离是3cm，从而获得300～400个图像，检查时间约30min。

为了方便不同机构中粘连的定位，腹部采用九分格图进行定位，即腹直肌两侧外缘的两条线、一条横跨下肋缘的横线和另一条横跨髂嵴线将腹部划分为9格（图24-3）。

二、腹壁

（一）粘连

一般来说，粘连可能是先天性或获得性的，尽管大多数粘连是在腹膜损伤、感染或腹盆腔手术后获得的。幸运的是，大多数粘连患者没有表现任何严重的临床症状，而对于某些人，粘连可能会导致显著增高的发病率和死亡率[7]。

粘连是使用腹腔镜套管针（trocar）再次手术时腹腔内脏器损伤的易感因素。因此，在曾手术的患者中计划腹部手术入路的外科医师必须考虑粘连的可能性，因此准确诊断腹腔粘连是非常有必要的[8]。关于成像方式，文献已提出实时超声评估粘连，也观察腹腔镜下针或套管针（trocar）放置的位置以避免内脏损伤[9]。然而，超声也存在一些严重的缺点，如检查者相关结果、因患者体型造成的检查条件困难、肠气遮挡。

Chapter 24 腹壁和疝
Abdominal Wall and Hernias

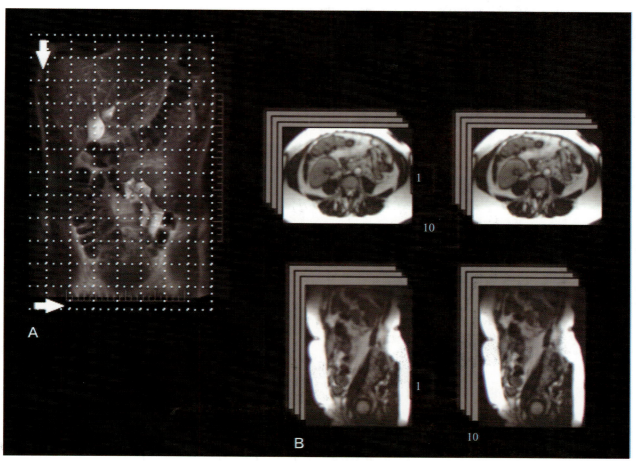

▲ 图 24-1 冠状位 MRI

定位相（A）叠加的网格显示精确的定位。在检查期间，患者的整个腹部是从右向左、从颅骨到尾部扫描（箭），每层之间约 3cm 的层间隔。在每个检查序列，横轴位和矢状位（B）由 10 幅连续的图像组成

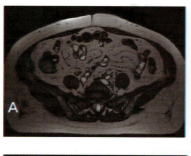
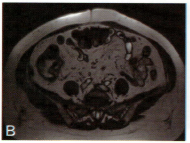
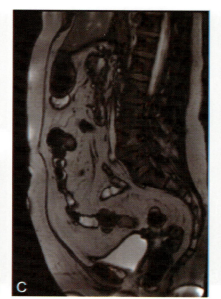
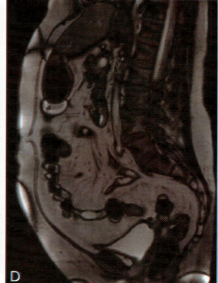

▲ 图 24-2 内脏 MRI

这些图像显示了在休息期（A）和用力期间（B）轴位正常内脏滑动的情况。图（C）和（D）也显示了矢状位正常内脏滑动的方向，以及在休息（C）和（D）用力期间肠管在头尾方向的来回移动

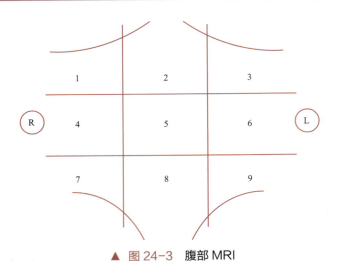

▲ 图 24-3 腹部 MRI

该图显示了腹部的九分格图，以充分准确地定位腹部的粘连

除了超声，其他成像方法如小肠灌肠对表现为管腔狭窄或未能通过手动施加腹部压力分离相邻肠襻的纤维束带的检测相当不敏感[9]。2000 年 Leulnman 等[6]介绍功能性电影磁共振成像显示内脏滑动，以可靠、准确、无创的方法检测粘连。我们的结果[10]表明，功能性电影磁共振成像是检测腹腔粘连最佳的成像方式。在这项最近的研究中，89 例术后粘连相关患者的功能性电影磁共振成像结果与手术结果进行了比较，敏感性 93%，准确性 90%，磁共振成像阳性预测值 96%。另一项腹腔粘连和手术结果的相关性研究[11]显示，71 个粘连中小肠肠襻和腹壁之间粘连是最常见的类型（图 24-4 至图 24-6），其次是小肠肠襻和盆腔器官之间的粘连（图 24-7）。

包括 Valsalva 动作中肠襻在内的相邻器官移位变形的征象被认为是粘连的另一直接征象。

（二）肿瘤

硬纤维瘤也称为侵袭型纤维瘤病，是良性伴局部侵袭性的软组织肿瘤，可发生在各种解剖部位，依据位置分为腹内、腹壁或腹外肿瘤[12]。这些肿瘤起源于筋膜、腱膜和肌肉的结缔组织，并且在初次切除后呈现高复发趋势，但通常不转移。腹壁硬纤维瘤通常发生在妊娠期或妊娠后的第一年。硬纤维瘤的磁共振成像表现依其组成成分不同而不同。随着演变，硬纤维瘤倾向于少量细胞成分和多量纤维成分，因此在早期为 T_2 高亮信号，随着演变发展 T_2 加权像上随着胶原蛋白程度的增加信号强度逐渐变低。通常，硬纤维瘤在钆对比剂增强后表现为中度至明显强化（图 24-8）。

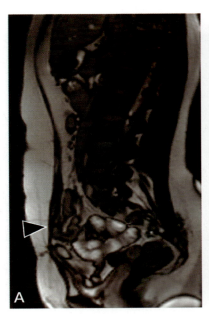
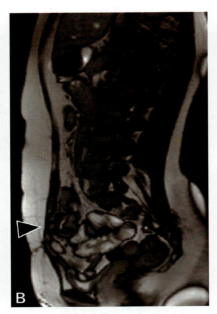
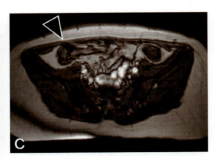
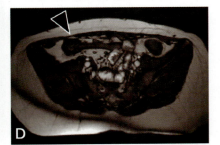

▲ 图 24-4 手术后患有非特异性腹部疼痛的 34 岁女性

分别在矢状位和横轴位的休息（A、C）和 Valsalva 动作（B、D）的功能性电影磁共振（TrueFISP）。几个小肠襻在用力时似乎附着腹侧腹壁（黑箭头），肠襻的分离和偏移显示不清

Chapter 24　腹壁和疝
Abdominal Wall and Hernias

育龄妇女的一个比较常见的妇产科问题是子宫内膜异位症。腹壁是子宫内膜异位症最常见的盆腔外位置，尽管它可能发生在几乎所有的体部腔隙和器官[13]。通常腹壁子宫内膜异位症与先前手术切开子宫和相应细胞的散布相关[14]。大多数患者在最大的压痛部通常是手术瘢痕的区域出现可触及

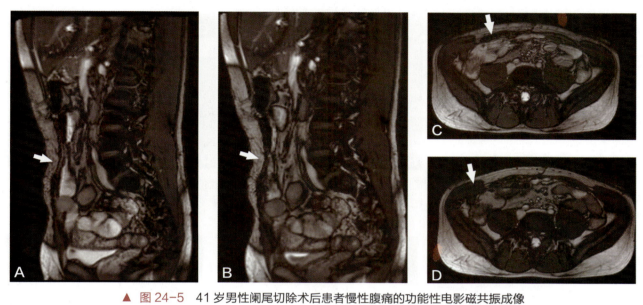

▲ 图 24-5　41 岁男性阑尾切除术后患者慢性腹痛的功能性电影磁共振成像
矢状位（A、B）及横轴位（C、D）的休息（A、C）及 Valsalva 动作（B、D）（箭）显示几个小肠襻黏附在腹壁上。同时亦可见盆腔区域的小肠襻间的粘连

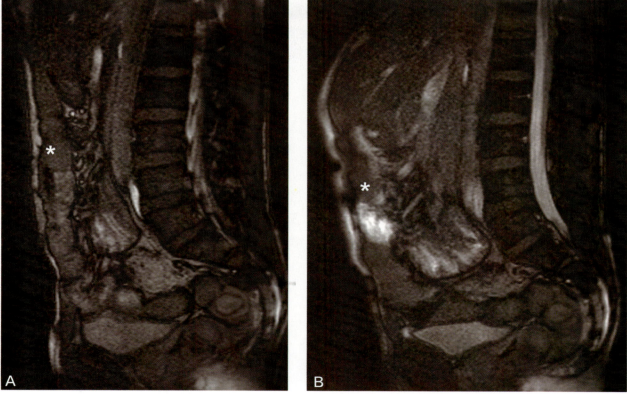

▲ 图 24-6　矢状位休息（A）和用力（B）的功能电影磁共振成像
图像显示用力时术后瘢痕旁几个小肠襻（星号）没有发生任何移位

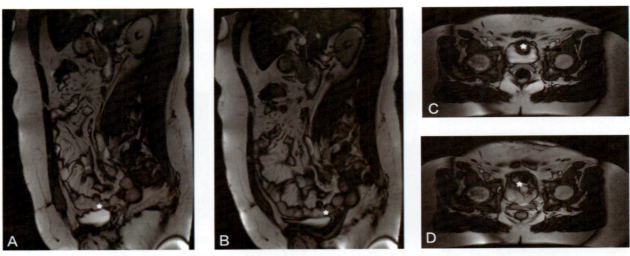

▲ 图 24-7　46 岁女性子宫切除术后急性下腹疼痛的在横轴位和矢状位的功能性电影磁共振成像

休息（A、C）及 Valsalva 动作（B、D）的图像示小肠襻与骨盆器官如膀胱和子宫之间无偏移或分离（星号）

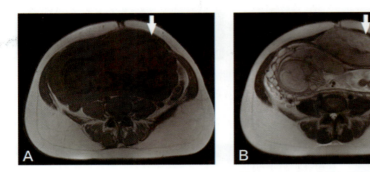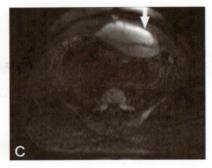

▲ 图 24-8　36 岁孕妇腹部的磁共振成像

左侧腹壁 T_1 加权序列（A）较肌肉低信号和 T_2 加权 HASTE 序列（B）以及正扩散（C）高信号肿物。这些影像表现与腹壁硬纤维瘤的诊断相符

肿块。腹壁子宫内膜异位症具有广泛的形态改变，从单纯巧克力囊肿到实性肿物或纤维化[15]。腹壁子宫内膜异位症的磁共振成像表现无特异性，因此磁共振成像通常不是为诊断而进行的，而是在术前评估疾病的程度。然而，腹壁子宫内膜异位症的磁共振成像表现，与卵巢子宫内膜异位不同，可为 T_1 和 T_2 加权像上的等或轻度高于肌肉的信号。静脉注射钆对比剂后，它们通常均匀强化。

出现腹壁肿块时，转移灶也应被考虑为鉴别诊断，因为许多恶性肿瘤可能会播散到浅表软组织。乳腺癌是女性腹壁最常见的原发恶性肿瘤。对于男性，恶性黑色素瘤是最常见的转移到此的原发肿瘤，表现为皮下结节。转移病灶通常是 T_1 加权像低信号，T_2 加权像等低信号，钆对比剂增强后表现为边缘强化（图 24-9）。

当腹侧腹壁发生皮下软组织病变时，尤其是在以前的切口处，鉴别诊断应包括血肿，尤其是有典型的外伤史、凝血疾病或剧烈运动。血肿的磁共振成像表现随红细胞降解产物的不同而不同。在 T_1 加权图像上，急性血肿倾向于比肌肉更高的信号且 T_2 加权序列上低信号。在血肿的演变过程中，T_2 加权像上的信号可能根据细胞内脱氧血红蛋白和含铁血黄素的浓度而变化，导致低信号（图 24-10）。血肿增强后强化不明显。

臀部外上象限皮下脂肪在频繁注射后可出现肉芽肿，但注射后出现的肉芽肿也可出现在腹壁的任何注射部位，而是偶然发现。典型表现为 T_1 加权低信号，而 T_2 加权图像上信号强度取决于肉芽肿的演变，所以信号有炎症反应时为高信号，或纤维特征反应时低信号[16]。

Chapter 24 腹壁和疝
Abdominal Wall and Hernias

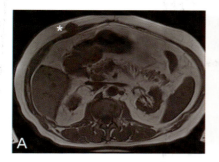 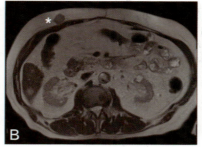 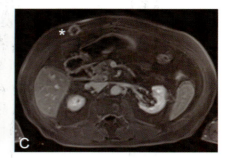

▲ 图 24-9　85 岁男性原发恶性黑色素瘤患者的腹部磁共振图像

横轴位 T_1 加权图像（A）显示位于皮下脂肪的右侧腹壁的周围组织低信号肿物（星号）；相应的 T_2 加权成像 HASTE 序列图像（B）显示在静脉注射钆对比剂后的等高信号肿物；T_1 加权图像（C）上显示环形强化肿物。根据原发肿瘤病史，诊断为腹壁转移

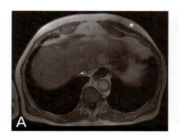 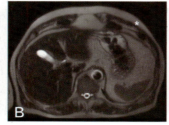 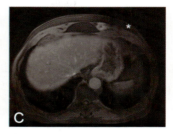 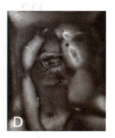

▲ 图 24-10　65 岁腹部外伤患者

横轴位 T_1 加权图像（A）示左侧腹壁（星号）等高信号，横轴位 T_2 加权图像（B）低信号，横轴位（C）和冠状位（D）的 T_1 加权脂肪饱和序列表现出弥漫的对比强化的病变。综上所述，这些影像表现与腹壁血肿相符

三、疝

腹壁疝的诊断通常是在体检期间进行的，然而，诊断可能是困难的，尤其是在肥胖、疼痛或腹壁瘢痕的患者中。在这些情况下，腹部影像学检查可为正确诊断提供第一线索。在过去的疝诊断中，主要应用传统的 X 线片或钡餐的检查。目前，CT 在大多数急诊救治中应用广泛，但磁共振成像是一种有价值的选择方案。

尤其功能性电影磁共振成像也有助于检测肥胖患者或手术后患者，以及不典型部位或非可疑部位疝的情况。在 2009 年，我们的研究[17] 能可靠地检测和评估 43 例疝修补术后植入的网状物和典型的并发症如网状物脱位。

根据解剖起源及其孔道，疝通常可分为外部（例如腹股沟的和股骨的）和内部（例如十二指肠旁）。

（一）外疝

对于外疝，疝孔主要位于先天性薄弱或先前手术的特殊部位。因此，腹壁缺损是最常见的外疝类型[18]。

腹股沟疝：腹股沟疝可分为直疝和斜疝；斜疝是目前美国最常见的腹壁疝[19]，是疝囊穿过腹壁下血管外侧潜在的鞘状突而形成。斜疝通常是获得性的，且由腹股沟环扩张引起的[20]。相反，直疝是由腹横筋膜薄弱引起的，因此位于腹壁下血管内侧。

然而，股疝较腹股沟疝明显少见。这种类型的疝是由于附着于耻骨的腹横筋膜缺陷，因此发生在股静脉内侧和腹股沟韧带后方。股疝具有较高的嵌顿倾向，往往难以与腹股沟疝鉴别。

腹部疝（包括所有的通过前腹壁 / 腹侧壁的疝）：脐、上腹、下腹部疝被认为是中线缺损。

在儿童中，这种疝通常是先天性的，而成人中，这种疝通常是获得性的，多次妊娠、腹水和肥胖是危险因素[20]。嵌顿和绞窄的高发病率与脐疝有关，并且它们通常不会自发减少。

侧腹壁缺损：侧腹壁最常见的缺损，即半月线缺损发生的疝——Spigelian 疝。这些疝多继发于腱膜或手术切口的后天性薄弱，通常部分网膜和短肠部分突入此处，因而具有较高的嵌顿倾向[18]。

切口疝：一般情况下，腹盆腔手术的延迟并发症包括切口疝，多在手术后的第 1 个月发生。这些疝多沿垂直切口而不是横向切口发生；然而，它们也可发生在小的腹腔镜切口[20]。年龄、肥胖、术后切口感染、腹水被认为是切口疝发生的典型危险因素（图 24-11）。

如果疝发生在造口附近，就会出现所谓的造口旁疝，被认为是切口疝的一种形式。肥胖和慢性咳嗽等因素加速了这种疝的发展[20]。

（二）内疝

一般来说，肠襻疝通过腹膜的发育或手术造成的腹膜、网膜或肠系膜的缺损被认为是内疝。这些类型的疝比外疝少见。诊断通常以影像学检查为基础，因内疝常常出现急诊情况，所以主要基于 CT 图像诊断。

四、总结

腹腔粘连的检测常基于临床检查，主要表现为急性或更多见的慢性腹痛。然而，为了能够精确地计划和调整治疗，必须考虑成像方法。当然，在急诊情况下，超声或 CT 是最合适的成像方式，但对于亚急性情况，磁共振成像包括功能性电影磁共振成像提出了一种无创的选择方案，目前部分文献已证明可用于检测和评估粘连和疝。相较实时超声，功能性电影磁共振成像提供了几个显著的优点，例如评估整个腹部及盆腔的可行性。不依赖于检查者经验，以及检查肥胖患者或气体严重影响的可行性。

一般来说，放射科医师还应通过功能性电影磁共振检查评估临床是否有隐匿性疝。如果发现疝，重要的是描绘它的大小、内容、形状、位置和相关的并发症。功能电影磁共振为腹部解剖提供了一个广阔的视角，显示腹壁缺损，并为尤其是手术的相关治疗提供了有关计划的重要信息。

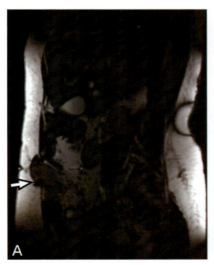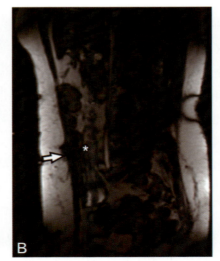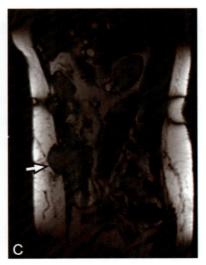

▲ 图 24-11　45 岁男性疑似偶发疝的功能电影磁共振成像

Valsalva 动作的矢状位（A、C）示肠管进入疝囊的腹壁疝（箭），而在放松时（B）可见裂孔，腹壁和肠襻无偏移 / 分离（星号）

参考文献

[1] Menzies D, Ellis H (1990) Intestinal obstruction from adhesions: How big is the problem? *Ann R Coll Surg Engl* 72:60–63.

[2] Levrant SG, Bieber EJ, Barnes RB (1997) Anterior abdominal wall adhesions after laparotomy or laparoscopy. *J Am Assoc Gynecol Laparosc* 4:353–356.

[3] Cox MR, Gunn IF, Eastman MC, Hunt RF, Heinz AW (1993) The operative aetiology and types of adhesions causing small bowel obstruction. *Aust N Z J Surg* 63:848–852.

[4] Ellis H (1998) The magnitude of adhesion-related problems. *Ann Chir Gynaecol* 87:9–11.

[5] Dijkstra FR, Nieuwenhuijzen M, Reijnen MM et al. (2000) Recent clinical developments in pathophysiology, epidemiology, diagnosis, and treatment of intraabdominal adhesions. *Scand J Gastroenterol Suppl* 232:52–59.

[6] Lienemann A, Sprenger D, Steitz HO et al. (2000) Detection and mapping of intraabdominal adhesions by using functional cine MR imaging: Preliminary results. *Radiology* 217:421–425.

[7] Ellis H, Moran BJ, Thompson JN et al. (1999) Adhesion-related hospital readmission after abdominal and pelvic surgery: A retrospective cohort study. *Lancet* 353:1476–1480.

[8] Freys SM, Fuchs KH, Heimbucher J, Thiede A (1994) Laparoscopic adhesiolysis. *Surg Endosc* 8:1202–1207.

[9] Bartram CI (1980) Radiologic demonstration of adhesions following surgery for inflammatory bowel disease. *Br J Radiol* 53:650–665.

[10] Lang RA, Buhmann S, Hopman A et al. (2008) Cine-MRI detection of intraabdominal adhesions: Correlation with intraoperative findings in 89 consecutive cases. *Surg Endosc* 22:2455–2461.

[11] Buhmann S, Lang RA, Kirchhoff C et al. (2008) Functional cine MR imaging for the detection and mapping of intraabdominal adhesions: Methods and surgical correlation. *Eur Radiol* 18:1215–1223.

[12] Goldblum J, Fletcher JA (2002) Desmoid-type fibromatoses. In: Fletcher CD, Unni KK, Mertens F (eds) *World Health Organization Classification of Tumours: Pathology and Genetics of Tumours of Soft Tissue and Bone*. Lyon, France: IARC Press.

[13] Ideyi SC, Schein M, Niazi M et al. (2003) Spontaneous endometriosis of the abdominal wall. *Dig Sur* 20:246–248.

[14] Blanco RG, Parithivel VS, Shah AK et al. (2003) Abdominal wall endometriosis. *Am J Surg* 185:596–598.

[15] Woodward PJ, Sohaey R, Mezzetti TP (2001) Endometriosis: Radiologicpathologic correlation. *RadioGraphics* 21:193–216.

[16] Salgado R, Alexiou J, Engelhorn JL (2006) Pseudotumoral lesions. In: De Schepper AM, Vanhoenacker F, Gielen J, Parizel PM (eds) *Imaging of Soft Tissue Tumors*. Berlin, Germany: Springer Verlag.

[17] Kirchhoff S, Ladurner R, Kirchhoff C et al. (2010) Detection of recurrent hernia and intraabdominal adhesions following incisional hernia repair: A functional cine MRI study. *Abdom Imaging* 35:224–231.

[18] Miller PA, Mezwa DG, Feczko PJ et al. (1995) Imaging of abdominal hernias. *RadioGraphics* 15:333–347.

[19] Rutkow IM (2003) Demographic and socioeconomic aspects of hernia repair in the United States in 2003. *Surg Clin North Am* 83:1045–1051.

[20] Harrison LA, Keesling CA, Martin NL et al. (1995) Abdominal wall hernias: Review of herniography and correlation with cross sectional imaging. *RadioGraphics* 15:315–322.

Chapter 25
结肠和直肠疾病

Diseases of the Colon and Rectum

Maria Ciolina, Carlo Nicola De Cecco, Marco Rengo, Justin Morris, Franco Iafrate, Andrea Laghi 著

杨 阳 译

张红梅 校

目录 CONTENTS

一、结肠疾病 / 572
二、直肠疾病 / 576

在过去的几十年中，随着诊断技术的提高与计算机断层扫描（CT）和磁共振（MR）仪器的广泛使用，横断面成像模式越来越多地应用于下消化道的无创评估。CT 仍然是评估急性结肠炎、结直肠恶性肿瘤转移性疾病和结直肠癌筛查的首选检查；在上述情况下，CT 结肠镜（CT colonography，CTC）可对结肠的内表面提供良好的评价。由于优越的采集速度，更高的空间分辨率和卓越的图像质量稳健性，多层螺旋 CT 似乎比 MR 更适合用于结直肠癌筛查。然而，由于没有电离辐射，MR 结肠成像（MR colonography，MRC）可以成为结肠无创性检查的一种很好的替代方法，特别是在年轻患者中。

尽管 CT 在结肠评估中优先于 MR 成像（MRI），但 MRI 无疑是评估直肠和会阴疾病的金标准。MRI 能够提供盆腔高空间分辨率和高对比分辨率的图像，是直肠癌初次分期、放化疗后再分期（chemoradiotherapy，CRT）以及肿瘤随访的金标准，特别是还在标准流程中加入其他 MR 生物标记物 [如扩散加权成像（diffusion weighted imaging，DWI）和灌注 MRI]。MRI 在瘘道研究的评估中也起着关键作用，为不同治疗方案的选择提供详细的放射学信息。

本章概述了 MRI 在下消化道研究中的实际应用，特别阐明了 MRI 在常见疾病中的实际临床适用范围，图像采集的方案和经典影像学表现。

一、结肠疾病

（一）结肠解剖

大肠从回盲瓣延伸到肛门。在成年人中长约 1.5m，但存在相当大的变异[1]。

结肠的外部结构包括三种，结肠带（teniae）、结肠袋（haustra）和肠脂垂（appendices epiploicae）。

结肠带是纵行的带状结构，宽约 8mm，沿结肠全长延伸，代表外层纵行肌层。我们可以根据不同位置区分三种结肠带：结肠系膜带（tenia mesocolica）位于横结肠壁的后缘，为横结肠系膜的附着处，在升结肠和降结肠肠壁的后内侧缘，位于肠管和腹后壁相连接处；网膜带（tenia omentalis 或 epiploic tenia）位于横结肠壁的前上缘，对应于大网膜附着处，在升结肠和降结肠，位于肠壁的后侧外缘；独立带（tenia libera），位于横结肠壁的下缘，升结肠和降结肠的前缘。

在阑尾与盲肠连接处和直肠乙状结肠交界处，三条结肠带汇合形成一层均匀的纵行肌层。

结肠袋是在结肠带之间的空间形成的袋状结构，它们之间由深浅不同的圆形凹槽相互分开。它们的凸出程度取决于结肠带的收缩。

肠脂垂是由浆膜下脂肪组织构成的小突起。它们具有类似葡萄的外观，大小根据个体的营养状况不同而存在差异。在升结肠和降结肠中，它们通常分布成两排。在横结肠上，它们沿着独立结肠带形成一排。在肠腔内观察，凹槽对应的皱襞称为半月襞（plicae semilunaris）。这些皱襞的长度对应于两个结肠带之间的距离。

在回盲部交界处，回肠末端凹入大肠，形成括约肌，即回盲瓣（valvula Bauhini）[2]（图 25-1D）。

回盲瓣可呈现为具有上、下唇的唇形瓣膜结构。在瓣膜的末端，两个黏膜襞在大肠腔内水平延伸，类似于结肠的半月形皱襞。这些黏膜襞即为瓣膜瓣，形成盲肠和升结肠之间的分界面。回盲瓣还可以表现为大乳头状并突入结肠中，瓣口呈星状。

阑尾的位置（图 25-1D）在体表投影在髂前上棘至脐连线的外、中 1/3 交界处（McBurney 点）。

在胎儿发育早期，盲肠尾部延伸形成一个锥形突起，其尖端形成蚓状阑尾。之后随着盲肠壁的不对称发育，阑尾出现的位置转移到盲肠内后侧壁，即三条结肠带汇合形成一层均匀的纵行肌层的地方[2]。

升结肠长约 15cm（图 25-1A），起于盲肠，上行至肝右叶下方转向左前方形成结肠肝曲。升结肠位于腹膜后，三面被腹膜覆盖。升结肠管腔较盲肠管腔窄，在 1/3 的病例中可由有狭长的结

Chapter 25 结肠和直肠疾病
Diseases of the Colon and Rectum

肠系膜形成。

结肠肝曲连接升结肠和横结肠（图25-1C），它的位置可变。在解剖关系上右肾位于其后方，肝右叶在其外上方，十二指肠降段在其内侧，胆囊在其内上方，其后方没有被腹膜覆盖，而是直接贴邻肾周筋膜。

横结肠连接结肠肝曲和脾曲（图25-1B），它的长度和位置是可变的，长约50cm。它通常形态类似于向后、向上凹陷的倒拱形。横结肠几乎完全被腹膜覆盖。

横结肠由横结肠系膜悬吊在腹腔内。胃结肠韧带连接横结肠及胃大弯，并延续为大网膜[1,2]。

脾曲（图25-1E）连接横结肠和降结肠，位于左季肋部，解剖关系上左肾和胰尾位于其后方，脾脏在其后上方外侧。与肝曲相比，脾曲更靠上、靠后，通过膈结肠韧带附着于左侧膈肌。

降结肠（图25-1E、F）从左季肋部向下延伸约25cm，通过腰部至髂嵴水平。在此处向内下移行为乙状结肠。

乙状结肠（图25-1F）是起自左髂嵴下方（真骨盆入口）水平，下端接直肠，活动度大，成人展开长40～50cm，儿童长约18cm。

乙状结肠的位置和形状因其长度和结肠系膜的长度及活动性不同而存在差异。它的位置和形状还取决于肠腔处于空虚还是充盈状态，以及邻近器官如膀胱（充盈或空虚）和子宫的状态。乙状结肠系膜通常由腹膜覆盖。它呈现倒置的V形附着于后腹壁。

乙状结肠系膜根部的左侧份起自左侧腰大肌内缘，绕过左侧髂外血管和左侧输尿管。乙状结肠系膜附着处的右侧份穿过左侧髂总血管，位于动脉分叉处上方。在直肠乙状结肠交界处，环形

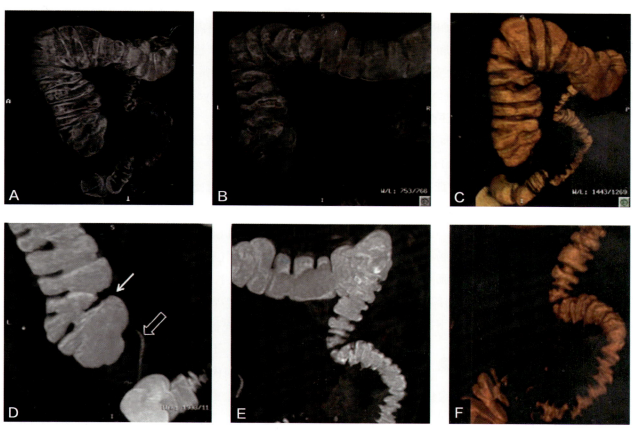

▲ 图25-1 结肠解剖图

冠状位单次激发MR结肠成像图像（A～C）、MR虚拟结肠镜图像（C）显示正常盲肠、升结肠、结肠肝曲（A～C）和横结肠（B），冠状位单次激发MR结肠成像（D）显示回盲瓣（箭）和阑尾（空心箭）。冠状位单次激发MR结肠成像（E）显示结肠脾曲和降结肠。MR虚拟结肠镜（F）显示降结肠和乙状结肠

肌层形成一个突出部位，称为 O'Beirne 第三括约肌，它位于直肠上瓣上方 2～3cm 处；在这个水平，直肠肠腔缩小至匹配乙状结肠的口径（直肠乙状结肠交界处）。它不是一个真正的括约肌，但在作用上类似[1,2]。

结肠血供

大肠的动脉起自肠系膜上动脉和肠系膜下动脉。盲肠、升结肠和 2/3 的横结肠（起源于中肠的部分）由回结肠动脉、右结肠动脉和中结肠动脉供血，上述动脉亦是肠系膜上动脉的所有分支。横结肠左侧部分、降结肠和乙状结肠以及上段直肠（起源于后肠的部分）由左结肠动脉和乙状结肠动脉及直肠上动脉供血，即肠系膜下动脉的所有分支。

边缘动脉（marginal artery 或 Drummond）是最靠近并与结肠壁平行的血管，由回结肠、右结肠、中结肠和左结肠动脉的动脉弓形成。

Riolan 动脉弓（The arc of Riolan）是存在于横结肠右侧和降结肠上部之间肠系膜的吻合弓[1]。它由中结肠动脉的一个大的分支形成，该分支在横结肠系膜中平行且向后延伸至中结肠动脉，并与左结肠动脉的一个上行分支吻合。它提供了肠系膜上动脉和肠系膜下动脉之间的直接连接。

终末动脉（terminal arterial）分为长支（vasa longa）和短支（vasa revia），直接进入结肠壁或走形于浆膜下。这些血管穿过环形平滑肌层，形成网膜动脉。

静脉引流如下：起源于中肠者（盲肠、阑尾、升结肠和右 2/3 的横结肠）引流入肠系膜上静脉。起源于后肠者（横结肠的左侧部分、降结肠、直肠和上段肛管）引流入肠系膜下静脉[1]。

（二）磁共振结肠成像

MRC 是一种无创诊断成像模式，于 20 世纪 90 年代后期首次引入，它可以评估结肠和结肠疾病，类似 CTC。

该采集不受电离辐射的影响，为研究结肠壁提供了极好的对比度分辨率，与其他腹部 MR 检查相比，完成时间（20～23min）是可接受的[3]。与常规结肠镜检查（conventional colonoscopy, CC）相比，MRC 报道的穿孔率（约 0.0009%）较低，而 CC 约为 0.3%[4,5]，这是由于较低的液体充盈所产生的压力以及与 CC 和 CTC 相比，MRC 所需检查次数较少。

MRC 的主要缺点包括此技术尚未普及，仅限于少数专科医疗中心，与 CT 相比成本更高，与 CC 相比没有治疗功能。

MRC 常见的禁忌证与普通 MRI 相同（幽闭恐惧症、心脏起搏器或其他植入金属器械、肾衰竭和造影剂过敏）。

实际上，关于检查前所需最佳的肠道准备、腔内对比剂、双重或单一定位以及是否应使用粪便标记目前还没有达成共识。

1. 肠道准备、钡灌肠分类及粪便标记 肠道清洁是必需的，用以消除残留的粪便，否则可能会被误解为腔内的充盈缺损，如息肉或癌。

接受 MRC 检查的患者需要进行正确的肠道清洁，通常在检查前一天口服聚乙二醇（polyethylene glyco, PEG）和磷酸钠液体，分别为 1L 和 4L。

清洁肠管后，可以使用以下 3 种方法之一进行结肠扩张。

（1）阳性对比剂（亮腔 MRC）是指将钆标记灌肠剂（1.5～2L），通过混合钆和水得到浓度为 5～10 mmol/L 的制剂灌入结肠。通常需要双重定位来置换空气和粪便，粪便会根据重力移动。结肠腔在 T_2 和 T_1 加权序列上都呈现高信号。在充满对比剂的亮腔背景下，息肉和肿块表现为 T_1 加权图像低信号充盈缺损。有时，充盈缺损，如空气或压紧的粪便，不会随着定位的改变而移位，可能被误诊为腔内息肉，导致检查结果出现假阳性。这项技术的另一个重要缺点是难以区分强化的息肉和亮的内腔[6]。对于应用亮腔 MRC 进行结肠癌筛查的患者，敏感性仅为 75%，特异性较好为 95%[7]。

（2）阴性造影剂（黑腔 MRC）是指阴性的腔内对比剂如室内空气、二氧化碳或水。空气比水灌肠能更好地扩张结肠，这通常不会增加磁敏感伪影[8]。然而，磁敏感伪影可能发生在空气/组织交界面处，降低了图像质量和检查的灵敏度，但短回波时间可能限制这种伪影。黑腔 MRC 不会有直肠对比剂溢出的风险。关于黑腔 MRC 对结肠癌筛查结果的准确性存在争议，对于测量小于 5mm 的病变，单个息肉/病变检出的敏感性为 10.5%，对于 5mm 和 10mm 之间的息肉，息肉/病变的检出的敏感性为 57.6%，对于大于 10mm 的病变，检出敏感性为 73.9%。而且，很多漏诊的息肉是增生性息肉，这些并不是大肠癌筛查的对象。

（3）双相腔内对比剂指在水溶液中加入 PEG 的灌肠剂。使用这种方法，结肠腔在 T_2 加权图像上呈高信号，在 T_1 加权图像上呈低信号。在检查过程中使用水的缺点是直肠对比剂溢出（或需要排便）[9]，以及在 T_2WI 上难以鉴别结肠腔内出现液体是否为腹腔内脓肿（特别是克罗恩病或憩室炎）。

可以添加粪便标记来减少甚至取代导泄性肠道清洁[10]。粪便标记可改变粪便残留物的信号强度，使其不可见并且具有与使用的灌肠剂相同的信号强度（亮的粪便用于亮腔 MRC，黑色粪便用于黑腔 MRC）。对于亮腔 MRC，通常使用的标记物是钆，但这意味着成本的增加并可能导致便秘[11]。对于黑腔 MRC，通常使用含有小颗粒铁的口服造影剂，名为 ferumoxsil（Lumirem, Guerbet Group, Paris, France）[12]。

另一种用于改变黑腔 MRC 残留粪便信号强度的方法是使粪便碎裂。应用乳果糖和多库酯钠直肠灌肠剂（0.5%）的组合可使粪便的含水量增加，从而使得其在黑腔 MRC 中信号强度下降[13]。

2. MRC 技术　一个或两个表面线圈可与内置相控阵线圈一起用于信号接收。一旦完成肠道的充盈并使整个结肠充分扩张，就可以在俯卧位和仰卧位获得三维（3D）扰相梯度回波（GRE）序列。每个成像序列在冠状位扫描，单次屏气时间小于 30s。成像方法还包括 2D 单次激发快速自旋回波（SS-FSE 或 HASTE）脉冲序列和对比增强的 2D 扰相梯度回波序列以评估结肠外情况（即肝转移和淋巴结病变）。

这些序列优先选择冠状位成像。特定的软件可以进行多平面重建和使用腔内顺行及逆行飞越程序。然而，腔内飞越程序（fly-through）对于检出息肉比评估炎性肠病更有帮助。对于可疑的息肉样病变，推荐直接比较平扫 T_1 加权图像和增强后 SE T_1 加权序列，以区别粪便。T_2 加权图像可以更好地评估 IBD、憩室炎和结肠炎中的黏膜下水肿和结肠周围的炎性改变。

3. MRC：临床应用

（1）结肠癌筛查：MRC 在能够准确地检出结肠癌（100% 敏感）和大于 10 mm 的息肉（癌前病变）（每名患者敏感性为 88%）（图 25-2 和图 25-3）。检测 6～9mm 的息肉目前报道有多种敏感性和特异性的结果[14]。由于 MRC 提供包含整个腹部和盆腔的数据，因此可以在早期检测到偶发的结肠外异常和潜在的严重病变。应根据发现的严重程度，以标准方式报道这些偶然发现的结果，类似于 CTC 中使用的 CTC 报告和数据系统（C-RADS）[15]。

（2）不能完成全程结肠镜检查：由于狭窄段（进行 CC 检查的患者中发生率高达 13%[16]）结肠镜无法通过，而导致不能完成全程结肠镜检查时，只有空气或液体可以通过狭窄段使近端结肠充盈扩张。因此，MRC 能够评估是否存在双原发灶或是结肠外疾病所引起的外源性压迫，从而通过形态学评估、增强扫描序列和 DWI，区分良性狭窄和恶性狭窄[17]。

（3）结肠吻合术的评估：MRC 用于评估结肠吻合口的敏感性为 84%，特异性为 100%[18]，并且可用于吻合口处炎症、炎症性肠病（inflammatory bowel disease，IBD）复发或肿瘤复发的鉴别诊断。

（4）炎症性肠病

① MRC 在评估慢性疾病方面尤其具有吸引力，因为其可以在没有电离辐射的情况下对病情进行更为密切的评估，特别是年轻患者。MRC 可用于评估肠壁增厚、透壁性和腔外疾病、肠管

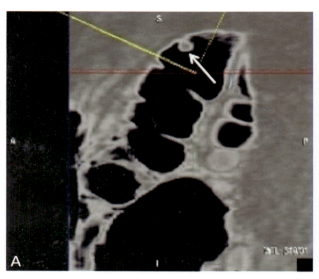

▲ 图 25-2　结肠息肉

冠状位 T_1 加权 MR 结肠成像图像（A）显示结肠脾区一枚 8mm 无蒂息肉样病变（箭），通过 MR 仿真图像（B）亦可显示

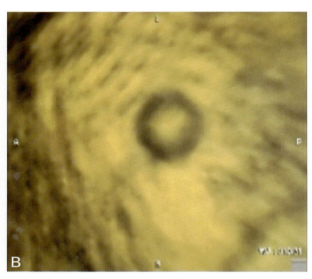

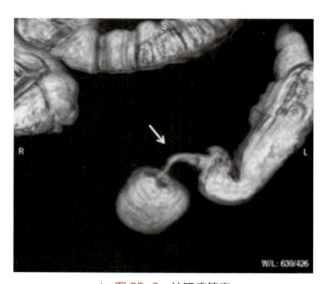

▲ 图 25-3　结肠癌筛查

MR 虚拟结肠镜显示由环周性癌变引起的严重肠腔狭窄进而导致的近端乙状结肠苹果核样改变（箭）

强化情况（全壁强化或靶征）（图 25-4）、黏膜下水肿、狭窄、肠系膜血管充血增粗（木梳征）、肠系膜淋巴结强化、纤维脂肪增生性瘘和脓肿，或用于评估药物治疗反应，尤其是在急性炎症性肠病中[19]。

② MRC 还可以鉴别炎症活动性 CD 和纤维狭窄性 CD，因为这两种疾病需要不同手术和内科治疗方法的疾病，所以鉴别两者具有重要的临床意义。

③ Ajaj 等报道了 MRC 用于检出炎症具有 87% 的敏感性和 100% 的特异性[20]。尽管如此，在 CD 和 UC 中，MRC 对检出轻度炎症的敏感性似乎不如重度炎症，在 CD 中仅为 31.6%，在 UC 中为 58.8%[21]。

（5）憩室炎：虽然怀疑憩室炎腹部 CT（非 CTC）仍然是最常用的检查技术，但研究发现 MRC 能准确检出憩室病（图 25-5）和急性憩室炎[22]，黑腔 MRC 中总体敏感性为 86%，特异性为 92%，有 3 例能够更准确地区分急性憩室炎和结肠癌[23]。

（6）子宫内膜异位症：高分辨率盆腔 MRI 相比时，对于有经验的 MR 阅片者，MRC 发现直肠子宫内膜异位症的敏感性和特异性分别从 76% 和 96% 增加到 95% 和 97%[24]。

二、直肠疾病

（一）直肠肛管解剖

1. 直肠解剖　直肠从第 3 骶椎椎体（S_3）水平延伸到肛直肠线，肛直肠线位于尾骨尖稍下方和男性前列腺尖的连线处[1]（图 25-6）。

直肠通常是自肛缘向上延伸 15～20cm，可分为三部分：下段（肛缘上方 0～6cm）、中段（肛缘上方 7～11cm）和上段（肛缘上方 12～15cm）[1,25]。

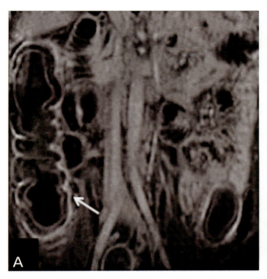
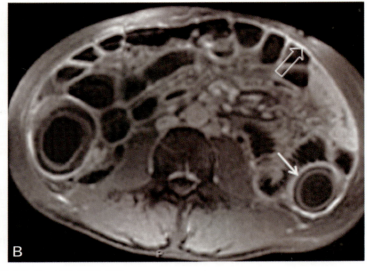

▲ 图 25-4　MR 结肠成像

T_1 加权序列使用钆对比剂后冠状位（A）和轴位（B）图像，显示结肠壁弥漫增厚（箭）伴分层强化形成的靶征，可见因充血水肿而呈低信号的黏膜下层和由于炎症而明显强化的浆膜（空心箭）

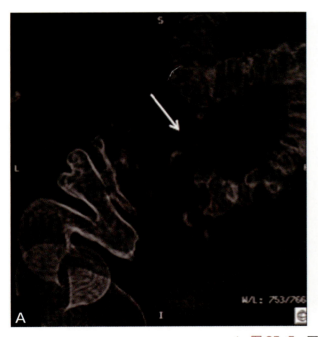
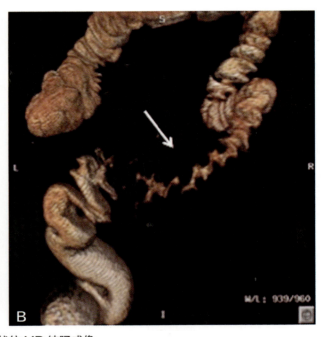

▲ 图 25-5　冠状位 MR 结肠成像

A、B. 示结肠憩室病导致的乙状结肠肠腔狭窄伴其壁上多发囊袋状突起（箭）

内径可从直肠乙状结肠交界处的 1.5cm 变化大到其壶腹部最宽处的 3.5cm 或更大[1,2]。

直肠外缘有 3 个侧曲，上：向右凸出；中（最突出）：向左凸出；下：向右凸出。直肠的两端位于正中矢状面[2]（图 25-7）。

直肠没有袋状结构，但通常有 3 个半月形横襞，又叫 Houston 瓣（Houston valves）：上、中、下瓣（图 25-8）。上直肠横襞位于直肠腔一侧或环周，在腔内标志着直肠和乙状结肠的转折点。在直肠乙状结肠交界处，约 S_3 水平，直肠的管腔内径减小，与乙状结肠（直肠乙状结肠交界）相匹配[1,2]。除了内径之外，乙状结肠与直肠的区别还在于乙状结肠纵行肌层形成的结肠带。中直肠横襞最厚，位于直肠壶腹部的正上方，起源于

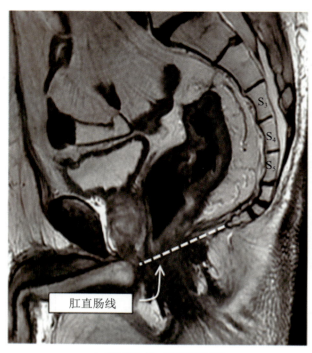

▲ 图 25-6　直肠解剖图

矢状位 T₂ 加权图像示直肠通常从第 3 骶椎椎体（S₃）水平延伸到肛直肠线，肛直肠线位于尾骨尖稍下方与男性前列腺尖的连线处。同时显示了该患者直肠中段和上 1/3 段肿瘤性肠壁环周性增厚（星号）和直肠系膜淋巴结（箭）

前壁和右壁，也被称为 Kohlraush 瓣。下直肠横襞通常在左侧，中直肠横襞下方约 2.5cm 处[2,25]。

直肠大部分属于腹膜外位器官，除了直肠上段在前面和侧面覆盖着一层薄薄的脏腹膜。腹膜反折通常位于距肛缘 7～9cm 处，但在女性中可能较低，为 5～7.5cm[26]（图 25-9）。

2. 肛管解剖　成人肛管从肛门直肠连接处（在耻骨直肠肌悬吊的水平）至肛缘，平均长度为 4.2cm。上面是外科学肛管的定义，而解剖学肛管是指从齿状线到肛缘，平均长度约为 2.1cm[25]（图 25-10）。肛管与直肠呈现出一定的角度，由于耻骨直肠肌的悬吊而形成肛管直肠角。在后方，肛管通过肛尾韧带连接到尾骨，该韧带为肛门外括约肌浅部向后延伸与尾骨相连形成[1,3]（图 25-11）。肛尾韧带与肛提肌中缝汇合。

在前方，肛管的中间 1/3 通过致密的结缔组织连接到会阴中心腱（perineal body），它将肛管与尿道膜部及男性的阴茎球或女性的阴道下段分隔开（图 25-12）。

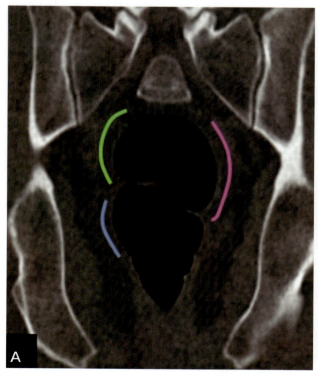 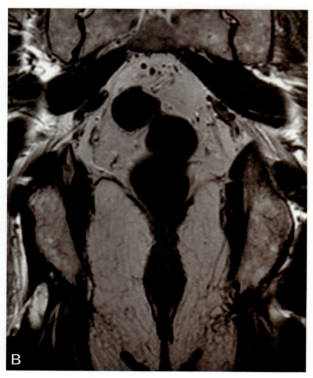

▲ 图 25-7　冠状位 CT 结肠成像

A. 非常好地显示了直肠三个侧曲：上，向右凸出（绿线）；中（最突出，粉线），向左凸出；下，向右凸出（蓝线）；B. 冠状位 MR 示直肠的两端均位于正中矢状面

Chapter 25 结肠和直肠疾病
Diseases of the Colon and Rectum

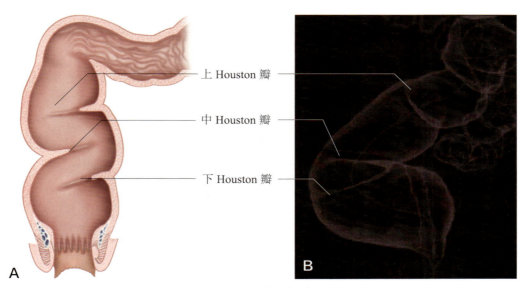

▲ 图 25-8 直肠与结肠结构

绘制的呈现出"类似钡灌肠"的 3D 立体视图（A）和 CT 结肠成像图像（B）示直肠通常有 3 个半月形横襞，又叫 Houston 瓣：上、中、下瓣。上直肠横襞在腔内标志着直肠和乙状结肠的转折点。中直肠横襞位于直肠壶腹部的正上方，起源于前壁和右壁，也被称为 Kohlraush 瓣。下直肠横襞通常在左侧，中直肠横襞下方约 2.5cm 处

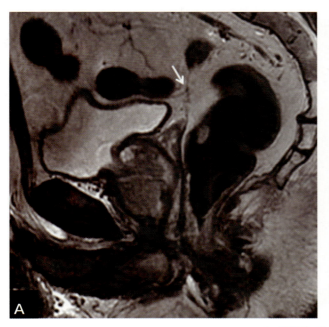 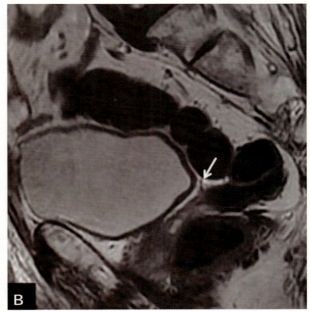

▲ 图 25-9 腹膜反折

矢状位 T_2 加权图像（A）示膀胱直肠窝的腹膜反折表现为距肛缘 7～9cm 处直肠前方等信号的细线。矢状位 MR 图像（B）示腹膜反折的位置可以更低，位于距肛缘 5cm 处

在外后方，肛管被坐骨肛门窝内的疏松脂肪组织包绕[1]（图 25-12）。

肛门括约肌是由平滑肌组成的肛门内括约肌和由骨骼肌组成的肛门外括约肌复合体共同构成（图 25-12）。肛门内括约肌即固有肌层，是直肠环形肌层的延续。而直肠纵行肌层与肛提肌远端的横纹肌纤维在耻骨直肠肌悬带水平汇合，然后形成肛门外括约肌（图 25-13）。肛门外括约肌复合体（external sphincter complex）是指肛提肌的最下部、耻骨直肠肌悬带和肛门外括约肌[26]。

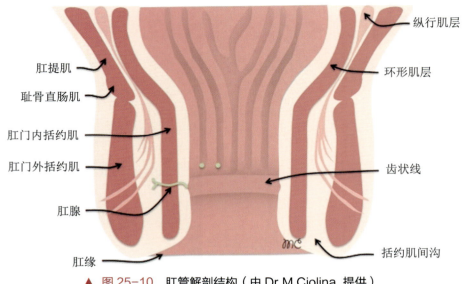

▲ 图 25-10　肛管解剖结构（由 Dr.M Ciolina. 提供）

在耻骨直肠肌悬带水平，直肠外膜与肛门内外括约肌之间的薄层结缔组织即括约肌间隙融合[27]（图 25-12）。

肛管黏膜近端由约 10mm 的柱状上皮样直肠黏膜组成，其下 15mm 是柱状上皮和复层扁平上皮之间的过渡区，包括肛门瓣和齿状线。肛管最远端的 5～10mm 是有毛的皮肤复层扁平上皮[26]。

3. 直肠血供　直肠的上 2/3 是由胚胎期后肠的远端部分发育而来，由直肠上动脉供血，直肠上动脉是由肠系膜下动脉的分支。在 S_3 水平，直肠上动脉分成两支，即右支和左支。右支是较粗大的一支，供应直肠的后部和侧面。左支提供直肠前壁的血供。直肠中动脉可能缺如，通常起源于双髂内动脉前支或下部内脏血管，与直肠上、下动脉吻合[26]。

直肠下动脉起自阴部内动脉，供应肛门内、外括约肌并最终到达肛管黏膜层和黏膜下层[4]。

直肠上 2/3（后肠）由直肠上静脉引流，通过肠系膜下静脉汇入门静脉系统。

直肠下 1/3 的静脉通过直肠中、下静脉引流入髂内静脉。这种静脉引流解释了直肠下段和肛管的肿瘤会在没有肝转移的情况下直接导致肺转移的原因[28,29]。

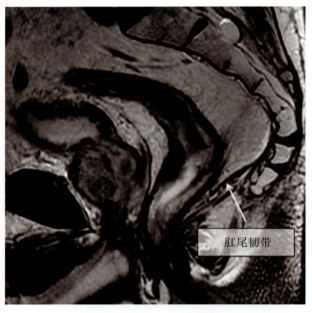

▲ 图 25-11　肛尾韧带

矢状位 T_2 加权图像示肛管在后方通过肛尾韧带连接到尾骨，该韧带为肛门外括约肌浅部向后延伸与尾骨相连形成。肛尾韧带沿中线与肛提肌中缝汇合

4. 直肠系膜　直肠系膜位于腹膜下间隙，从腹膜反折延伸至耻骨直肠肌。直肠系膜包含直肠上动脉及其分支、直肠上静脉及其属支、淋巴管、淋巴结、肠系膜下静脉丛的分支以及松散的脂肪结缔组织和分隔[1,2]。结缔组织在靠近耻骨直肠肌侧变得越来越薄至消失。在耻骨直肠肌处实际上已经没有淋巴管或淋巴结组织[27]。

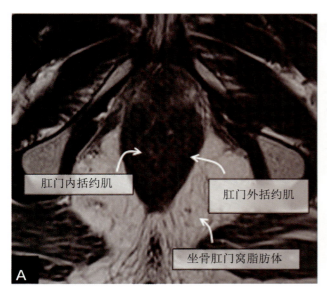
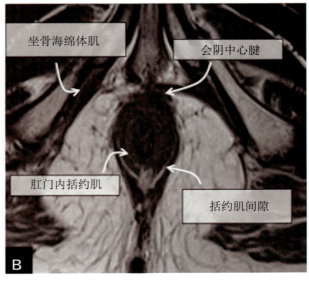

▲ 图 25-12　肛门括约肌

A、B. 横轴位 T_2 加权图像示固有肌层的内环形肌层构成了肛门内括约肌和外层横纹肌纤维形成肛门外括约肌。肛门内括约肌与肛门外括约肌之间的薄层结缔组织为括约肌间隙

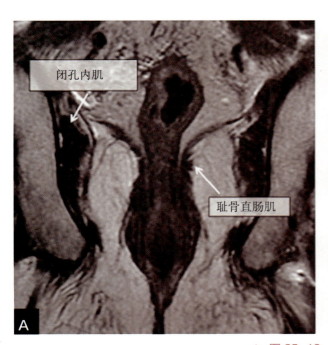
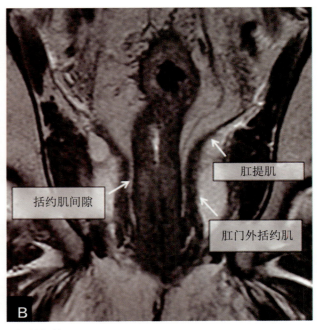

▲ 图 25-13　肛门外括约肌

A、B. 冠状位 T_2 加权图像示肛门外括约肌复合体指肛提肌的最下部、耻骨直肠肌悬带和肛门外括约肌。直肠纵行肌层与肛提肌远端的横纹肌纤维在耻骨直肠肌悬带水平汇合，然后形成肛门外括约肌

　　来源于脏腹膜的直肠系膜筋膜覆盖直肠系膜。直肠系膜筋膜是盆内筋膜的脏层。直肠系膜筋膜向后连接直肠系膜与骶前筋膜，骶前筋膜是盆内筋膜的壁层，覆盖骶骨、尾骨、骶正中动脉和骶前静脉。直肠系膜筋膜向上与乙状结肠系膜的结缔组织融合；向两侧包绕直肠和直肠系膜并延伸向前方形成更致密的筋膜组织。在男性中，前筋膜又叫 Denonvillier 直肠膀胱筋膜，分隔精囊腺与直肠系膜；在女性中，形成直肠阴道隔筋膜（图 25-14）。在第 4 骶椎（S_4）以下，

直肠系膜筋膜与直肠骶骨筋膜紧密融合，称为 Waldeyer 筋膜，这是骶前筋膜向前下方形成的筋膜反折[1,26]。

（二）直肠癌 MR 检查

1. 临床方面和适应证 在工业化国家中，直肠腺癌是最常见的肿瘤之一，患病率约 40 人 /10 万人，男性稍多，且在 20 世纪 50 年代后患病率稳定增长[30]。其他直肠肿瘤相对罕见，包括类癌（0.1%）、淋巴瘤（1.3%）和胃肠道间质瘤（<1%）[31]。在直肠肿瘤的术前评估中，MRI 起着至关重要的作用，主要是因为内镜和超声检查（US）不能全面评估肿瘤侵犯范围和淋巴结受累情况，而这些都是直肠癌术前治疗的重要预后因素[32-36]。

直肠全系膜切除术（total mesorectal excision，TME）结合 / 不结合新辅助 CRT 治疗是直肠癌的主要治疗方法。在过去的几十年中，TME 的普及使局部复发率从 38% 快速下降至不到 10%[37]。手术沿直肠系膜筋膜平面整体切除原发肿瘤和直肠系膜，直肠系膜筋膜平面则代表环周切缘（circumferential resection margin, CRM）[37]。

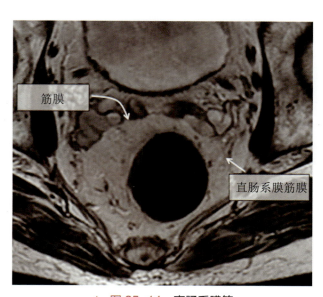

▲ 图 25-14 直肠系膜筋
轴位 T_2WI 示覆盖直肠系膜的系膜筋膜。在男性中，前筋膜又叫 Denonvillier 直肠膀胱筋膜；在女性中，形成直肠阴道隔筋膜

在距离 CRM 1mm 内存在肿瘤或恶性淋巴结仍然是局部复发的重要预后因素[38]。

MRI 在直肠癌术前分期中的主要作用如下。

（1）对可能从新辅助 CRT（进展期 T_3 和 T_4 肿瘤）中获益的患者进行分层[39,40]。

（2）确定可以从局部治疗中获益的患者（例如，经肛门切除术和经肛门内镜显微外科手术），从而避免由于延长 CRT 疗程导致的过度治疗和毒性。这些患者通常是 T_1 期患者[41-43]和符合 TME 适应证的患者（主要是 T_2 期和 T_3 早期）[44]。

（3）通过结构化报告制订具体的手术计划[38]。

（4）评估 CRT 治疗期间及治疗后的肿瘤再分期[39,40]。

需要短程或长程新辅助 CRT 患者的分层主要基于肿瘤分期（T）、淋巴结（N）分期、固有肌层外肿瘤浸润深度（早期与晚期 T_3 期肿瘤）以及肿瘤与潜在 CRM 的关系。最近有研究表明，高分辨率 MRI 可以获得关于肿瘤与 CRM 关系以及固有肌层外肿瘤浸润的深度，其结果具有可重复性及较高的特异性（92%），可用于预测 CRM 阴性病例[45-47]。

2. 技术方面 MR 检查通常需要使用高场强（使用至少 1.5T 扫描仪进行）和相控阵表面线圈，患者仰卧位扫描[31]。建议进行直肠清洁以减少图像误判，因为残留的粪便可能改变肿瘤与直肠系膜筋膜之间的距离并可能留下残留物，在某些情况下使用少量直肠内注射的超声凝胶（60～120ml，用量取决于肿瘤位置）可以更好地显示息肉样病变、小的直肠病变（>2～3cm），或新辅助 CRT 后的残存肿瘤[38,48]。然而，不建议使用大于上述量的直肠内凝胶以及直肠内阵列（特别是在评估低位直肠肿瘤时），因为直肠的扩张会改变肿瘤与 CRM 之间真实距离的测量。此外，它会过度压缩直肠周围脂肪，使淋巴结和血管浸润显示模糊[31,38]。患者仰卧位，盆腔扫描范围建议从 L_3 椎体水平的肠系膜下动脉的起始处到会阴皮肤水平[31,38,48]。

扫描方案包括矢状位、与肿瘤主轴平行和垂

直的斜冠状位及斜轴位的高分辨率 T_2 加权快速自旋回波序列（图 25-15）。这种多平面成像方法提高了评估肿瘤分期的准确性，因为可以在 3 个平面中确认肿瘤与 CRM 及其他结构的关系。这对于评价扭曲的直肠肿瘤非常有帮助[31]。

与肿瘤主轴垂直的高空间分辨率轴位图像可以对直肠系膜筋膜和 CRM 进行更好的评估。需特别注意的是，不正确的斜轴位平面会导致前方固有肌层模糊或直肠壁的假性毛刺状外观，这可能导致肿瘤的过度分期[48,49]（图 25-16）。

高分辨率矢状图像提供了关于 CRM 的额外信息，并能更好地评估肿瘤与腹膜反折的位置，这是一个重要的预后因素，因为侵及腹膜反折的肿瘤分期会升级到 T_4 期[38]（图 25-17）。

与肿瘤主轴平行的方向可获得高分辨率斜冠状位图像（如之前的几篇文章所述），但正冠状位似乎可更好地确定肛门括约肌解剖结构以及括约肌与肿瘤关系。还有助于评估肿瘤与盆腔侧壁和腹膜反折的关系及盆腔侧壁淋巴结形态[49]。

高分辨率多平面成像还可对所有直肠系膜结

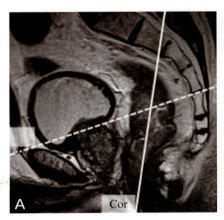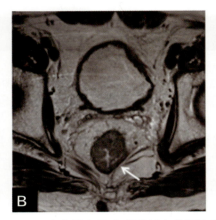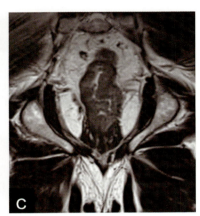

▲ 图 25-15 高分辨率 T_2 加权快速自旋回波序列

先获得矢状位图像（A），在矢状位 T_2 加权图像基础上可获得与肿瘤主轴垂直的斜轴位（B）及与肿瘤主轴平行的斜冠状位（C）图像，可清晰地显示固有肌层的外侧轮廓（箭）

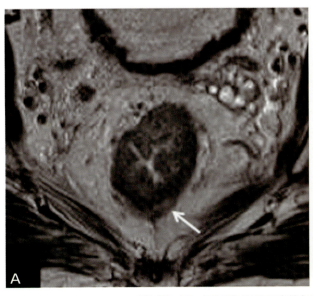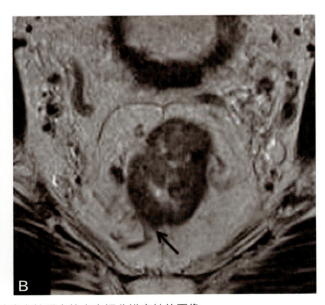

▲ 图 25-16 不正确的和正确的与肿瘤主轴垂直的高空间分辨率轴位图像

A. 在不正确的平面获得的轴位 T_2 加权图像示模糊的固有肌层可能导致肿瘤的过度分期；B. 正确的与肿瘤主轴垂直的斜轴位 T_2 加权 MR 图像可更好地显示固有肌层的外侧轮廓（黑色箭），没有模糊伪影

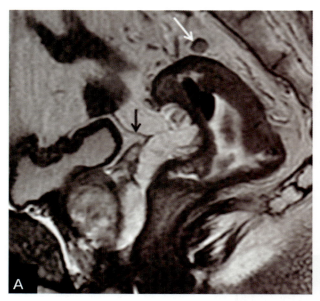 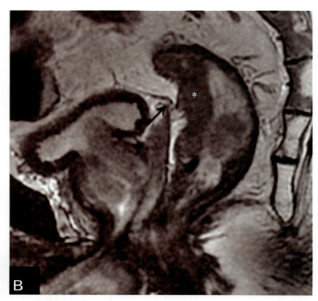

▲ 图 25-17 高分辨率矢状图像

A. 矢状位 T_2 加权 MR 图像示直肠上 1/3 段 T_{3b} 期直肠癌伴肠系膜淋巴结转移，图像可清晰地显示腹膜反折（黑色箭）；B. 如图所示，在直肠上 1/3 段肿瘤（星号）病例中，矢状位 T_2 加权 MR 扫描是更好地显示腹膜受累（黑色箭）的基础

节和盆腔结节进行形态和大小的评价，并可通过它们来评价 N 分期[50]。

DWI 通过增加肿瘤及淋巴结与周围正常组织之间的对比度，有助于肿瘤和淋巴结的定位。然而，由于表面扩散系数（ADC）值在恶性与良性增生性淋巴结之间存在重叠，因此对于这些结节的定性价值有限[51]。在最近的一项研究中，低 ADC 值与肿瘤侵袭性的生物学行为相关，ADC 值在局限于肠壁的肿瘤较高，而在伴有直肠系膜筋膜受累和中或低分化的 T_3N_2 期肿瘤中较低[52]。此外，DWI 可能在用 ADC 值预测化疗反应方面有所应用。一些研究结果显示，低 ADC 值肿瘤对 CRT 的反应良好，因为高度富含细胞的肿瘤似乎比坏死和血管化的病变对 CRT 反应更好[53-56]。因此，ADC 值似乎是肿瘤对放化疗反应的早期 MR 生物标志物：由于细胞的死亡，ADC 值的增高先于肿瘤体积的缩小[53-56]。注射钆对比剂后的 GRE T_1 压脂序列在直肠癌的术前 MR 分期中不是强制要求的，但是最近的研究已经证明了这些序列在化疗或肿瘤复发后检测残存肿瘤中的作用。另外动态对比增强 MR 灌注成像中的 K_{trans} 值与 CT 灌注成像中的 K_{trans} 值具有可比性[57]，并且将作为一种生物成像标记物，在开始治疗之前预测肿瘤对化疗的反应[58]（表 25-1 和表 25-2）。

3. 疗前计划 用 MRI 评估原发肿瘤包括以下几方面[59-61]：形态和肿瘤下缘至肛缘皮肤的距离；T 分期；肛门括约肌复合体、耻骨直肠肌和肛提肌；淋巴结分期；壁外血管侵犯；CRM：手术层面的安全性（TME 平面或更广泛的切除）。

（1）直肠癌形态学特征和位置：直肠癌在形态上可描述为（图 25-18）以下内容。

① 环状或半环状病变，伴广泛和较大的边缘浸润。

② 息肉样病变通过蒂突入腔内，并侵犯直肠周围脂肪，通常比环状或半环状病变短[61]。

③ 溃疡性病变，典型表现为深溃疡，恶性肿瘤细胞可浸润直肠系膜[61]。

直肠癌的定位是通过从肛缘到肿瘤隆起边缘的最尾端的距离来表示（图 25-19）。传统上直肠划分为三部分，这对确定肿瘤位置进而影响手术方式是有帮助的[59,61]（图 25-20）。

高位：肿瘤的下缘距肛缘大于 10cm。在这个水平上，直肠的前壁被腹膜反折覆盖，要对腹

Chapter 25 结肠和直肠疾病
Diseases of the Colon and Rectum

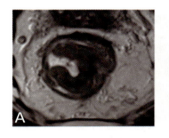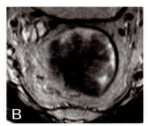
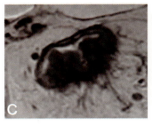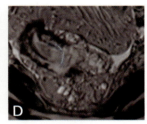

▲ 图 25-18 直肠癌的形态学特征

A. 环状或半环状病变：特征为广泛的浸润；B. 息肉样病变：特征为息肉蒂处有小范围浸润；C. 溃疡性病变：深溃疡处出现肿瘤浸润；D. 黏液性病变：示含有黏蛋白的黏液湖在 T_2 加权图像上为高信号，是具有高侵袭性生物学行为和不良预后的组织类型

膜侵袭或穿孔进行仔细评估，并提示外科医师肿瘤外侵的风险。然而，腹膜反折附着处的位置存在多发变异，特别是在女性中。

中位：肿瘤下缘位于距肛缘 5～10 cm。这段直肠位于腹膜反折的下方，完全被直肠系膜和直肠系膜筋膜覆盖，这是 TME 手术中的解剖平面。

低位：肿瘤下缘距肛缘小于 5cm。在这一水平上，直肠系膜变薄，在肛提肌平面下方，耻骨直肠肌标志着肛门直肠连接处，对应外科学肛管。直肠低位肿瘤发生于耻骨直肠肌悬带下方，可侵犯肛门固有肌层，对应的是肛门内括约肌和肛门外括约肌复合体，肛门外括约肌包括肛提肌的最下部、耻骨直肠肌和肛门外括约肌，它与肛门内括约肌之间由薄层脂肪组织隔开，形成括约肌间隙平面。

表 25-1 基于 3.0T 系统的初始直肠癌分期的 MRI 标准化扫描方案

	序列	加权（W）	平面（Plane）	TE（ms）	TR（ms）	FA	矩阵（Matrix）	激励次数（NEX）	层厚（mm）
必选	2D FRFSE	T_2	矢状面	119.5	4172	—	512×512	2	4
	2D FRFSE	T_2	横断面	122.3	3056		512×512	2～4	3
	2D FRFSE	T_2	冠状面	111.4	2086		512×512	2～4	4
可选	3D GRE	T_1	横断面	3.3	13.6	15	512×512	2	2
可选	SSEPI	DW	横断面	81.4	4400	—	256×256	2	2
可选	Dyn3D FSPGR	T_1	横断面	3.3	13.6	15	512×512	2	2

表 25-2 基于 1.5T 和 3.0T 系统的直肠癌再分期的 MRI 扫描方案

	序列	加权（W）	平面（Plane）	TE（ms）	TR（ms）	FA	矩阵（Matrix）	激励次数（NEX）	层厚（mm）
必选	2DFRFSE	T_2	矢状面	119.5	4172	—	512×512	2	4
	2D FRFSE	T_2	横断面	122.3	3056		512×512	2～4	3
	2D FRFSE	T_2	冠状面	111.4	2086		512×512	2～4	4
可选	3D GRE	T_1	横断面	3.3	13.6	15	512×512	2	2
可选	SSEPI	DW	横断面	81.4	4400	—	256×256	2	2
必选	Dyn3D FSPGR	T_1	横断面	3.3	13.6	15	512×512	2	2

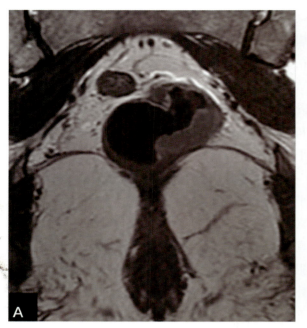
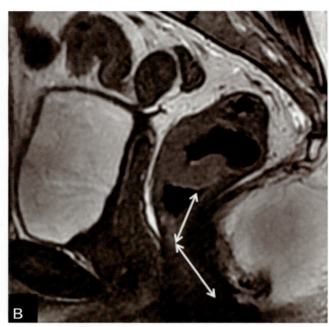

▲ 图 25-19 直肠癌定位

肿瘤距肛缘的距离是测量肛缘至肿瘤隆起边缘的最尾端的距离

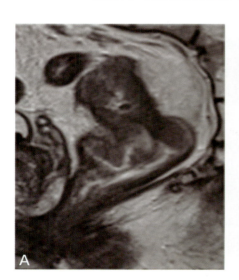
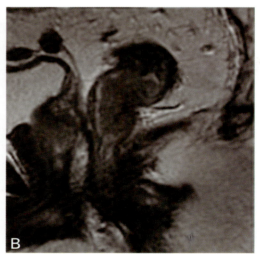
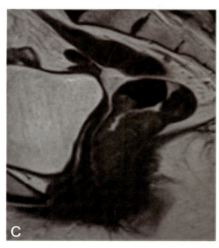

▲ 图 25-20 直肠肿瘤的定位

也可以根据传统直肠分段方法分为三段：A. 上 1/3，肿瘤下缘距肛缘距离大于 10cm，腹膜浸润的风险更高；B. 中 1/3，肿瘤下缘距肛缘 5～10cm，完全被直肠系膜包绕；C. 下 1/3，肿瘤下缘距肛缘的距离小于 5cm，括约肌浸润的风险更高

（2）T 分期：MERCURY 临床试验证明，众多机构提供的可重复结果显示 MRI 似乎是一种可以准确进行直肠癌分期的影像检查方式[45]。依据美国癌症联合委员会[肿瘤-淋巴结-转移（TNM）]的指南，发布了原发性直肠肿瘤分期的 MRI 标准（表 25-3）。这些 MRI 标准在 T 分期评估中的真正目标不是区分 T_2 期肿瘤与早期 T_3 期肿瘤（具有与 T_2 期相同的良好预后），而是对 T_3 期肿瘤进行分层，其肿瘤外侵犯范围以毫米计（图 25-21），并因此对三个风险类别的人群进行了细分：低风险、中等风险及疾病复发和预后不良的高风险（表 25-4）。

5 年生存率很大程度上取决于固有肌层外肿瘤浸润的深度。根据生存率，早期 T_3 期肿瘤（<5 mm 浸润）和 T_2 期肿瘤可归为低风险类别，5 年生存率约为 85%，局部复发率为 3%，可能仅能从手术治疗中获益。然而，固有肌层外浸润深度超过 5 mm 的肿瘤，不管是否有淋巴结受累，5 年生存率降至 54%。这些患者应分为中度和高度风险类别，并且是术前新辅助 CRT 的受益群体。

评估 T 分期方面，放射科医师需记住以下建议。

①采集平面必须严格垂直于肿瘤，以避免固有肌层产生模糊伪影，导致过度分期。

②壁外侵犯深度是一个独立的预后因素，固有肌层以外必须以毫米为单位进行测量，以区分局部复发风险低（<5 mm）的患者与复发风险较高的患者（>5 mm）（图 25-22）。

③肿瘤浸润到直肠系膜表现为组织增厚、为中等信号，呈宽基底凸起或结节状外观（图 25-23）。

④肿瘤性促结缔组织增生反应是直肠周围脂肪的典型炎症反应，与真正的肿瘤浸润有时难以

表 25-3 直肠癌 TNM 分期指南

Tis	原位癌
T_1	肿瘤侵犯黏膜下层
T_2	肿瘤侵犯固有肌层
T_3	肿瘤穿透固有肌层到达浆膜下层，或侵犯无腹膜覆盖的直肠旁组织
T_{3a}	肿瘤侵出固有肌层 < 5mm*
T_{3b}	肿瘤侵出固有肌层 5～10mm*
T_{3c}	肿瘤侵出固有肌层 > 10mm*
T_{3d}	肿瘤侵出固有肌层 > 15mm*
T_{4a}	肿瘤穿透脏层腹膜
T_{4b}	肿瘤直接侵犯或粘连于其他器官或结构

分级改编自 American Joint Committee on Cancer（AJCC）Cancer Staging Manual 7th edition. New York, Springer, 2010.

*. 临床分期基于 Smith and Brown（*Acta. Oncol.*, 2008），与 AJCC 分期略有不同。T_{3a} < 1 mm; T_{3b} ≥ 1～5 mm; T_{3c} > 5～15 mm, T_{3d} > 15 mm

表 25-4 考虑复发风险及不良预后的直肠癌三种风险分层[62,63]

风险因子	低	中	高
壁外侵犯	≤ 5mm	> 5mm	> 5mm
淋巴结情况	N_0	N_1～N_2	N_2
CRM	无风险	无风险	有风险
肿瘤位置	高	高或低	低
EMVI	无	有	有

CRM. 环周切缘；EMVI. 壁外血管受累

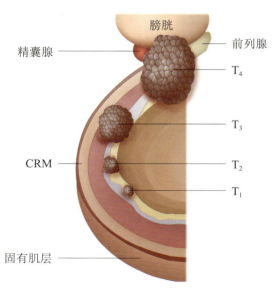

▲ 图 25-21 新 MRI 的 T 分期标准

根据测量壁外浸润深度（精确到 mm）对 T_3 期肿瘤进行分层（由 Dr. M Ciolina 提供）

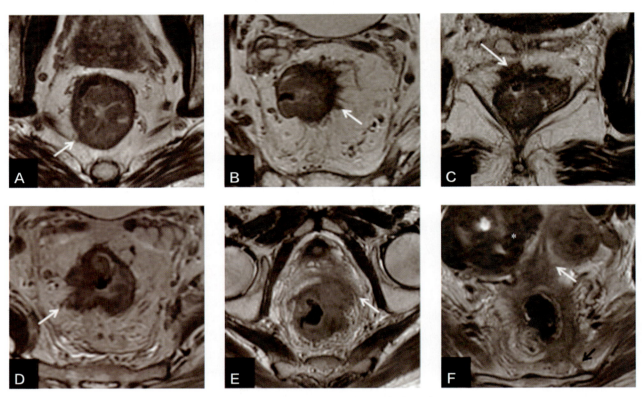

▲ 图 25-22 壁外侵犯深度区别复发风险

A. 横轴位 T_2 加权图像示直肠壁环周弥漫性增厚，直肠周围脂肪右后方可见微小浸润（箭）（<5 mm, T_{3a}）；B. 示环周性直肠癌左侧壁浸润深度 5～10mm（T_{3b}）；C. 横轴位 T_2WI 示低位直肠癌向前浸润直肠系膜（箭）> 10mm（T_{3c}）；D. 横轴位 T_2WI 示直肠癌假结节样浸润（箭）突入直肠系膜脂肪 > 15mm（T_{3d}）；E. 横轴位 T_2WI 示巨大直肠癌浸润直肠系膜筋膜（箭）因此累及环周切缘（CRM）（T_{4a}）；F. 横轴位 T_2WI 示直肠癌侵犯腹膜及子宫后壁（T_{4b}），同时可见子宫后壁较大平滑肌瘤（星号）

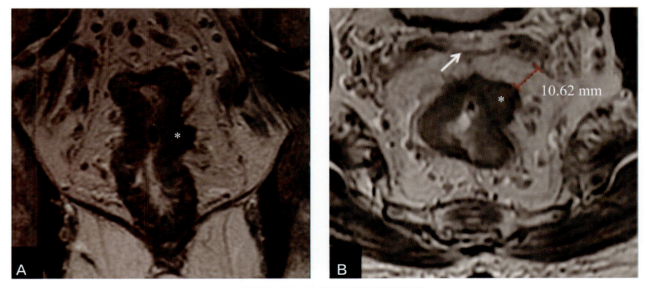

▲ 图 25-23 肿瘤浸润直肠系膜表现

A. 冠状位 T_2 加权图像示肿瘤浸润直肠系膜，表现为宽基底的隆起组织（星号）或中等信号的结节状组织。肿瘤与 CRM 之间 > 1 mm 与局部复发率下降相关；B. 轴位 T_2 加权图像图像显示肿瘤与直肠系膜筋膜之间的距离（箭）

区分，在 T_2 加权图像上表现为沿肿瘤边界的低信号细针样结构。

⑤在高位直肠肿瘤中，腹膜反折必须使用矢状位 T_2 加权图像进行评估，表现为从膀胱穹窿后部到直肠腹侧的线样低信号结构（图 25-17）。

⑥腹膜受累必须分为 T_{4a} 期，但并不一定累及 CRM。

（3）与肛门括约肌的关系：由于更复杂的解剖关系，低位直肠肿瘤的阳性切缘率和局部复发率通常较高，因此预后较差[66]。MR 在低位直肠癌中起着至关重要的作用，决定病变是否局限于肛门括约肌复合体，仅需部分肛门括约肌切除并进行结肠肛管重建，或者累及范围更广，需要 CRT 治疗或括约肌切除[67-69]。

对于低位直肠癌 T 分期的评估，放射科医师需记住以下几点建议：①使用高空间分辨率 T_2 加权快速自旋回波冠状和轴位图像，以更好地显示肿瘤与肛提肌、耻骨直肠肌、肛门括约肌复合体和括约肌间隙平面的关系。②耻骨直肠肌悬带对应于肛管的上缘；如果在矢状位和冠状位图像上，肿瘤的下缘位于耻骨直肠肌悬带上方，则可以容易地排除肛门括约肌受累。③如果在矢状位和冠状位图像上，肿瘤的下缘位于耻骨直肠肌悬带上方，那么根据 Shihab 等的低位直肠癌 T 分期[70,71]可分为：部分浸润固有肌层，局限在距肛门内括约肌外缘 1 mm 以内区域（1 期）；累及肛门内括约肌的全层（2 期）；累及肛门括约肌间隙平面（3 期）；侵犯肛门外括约肌复合体（肛门外括约、肛提肌和耻骨直肠肌，4 期）（图 25-24）。

这种 MRI 分期由 Shihab 等提出。对于低位直肠癌，可以确定所需切除的平面对肿瘤来说是否是足够的，阳性和阴性预测值分别为 57% 和 96%[70]。Zhang 等使用 3T MRI 图像预测是否可行保留括约肌的手术，准确率可达到 96.9%[72]。

1 期，肿瘤局限于肠壁，肌层外缘完整

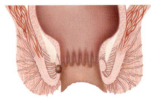

2 期，肿瘤侵透全肌层但未侵及括约肌间隙

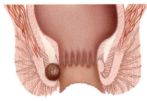 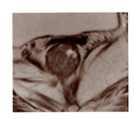

3 期，肿瘤侵犯括约肌间隙并距肛提肌 1 mm 以内

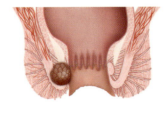 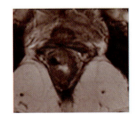

4 期，肿瘤侵犯肛门外括约肌并超过肛提肌伴或不伴有周围器官的受累

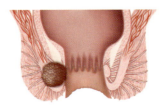 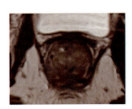

▲ 图 25-24　低位直肠癌分期方法（由 Dr.M Ciolina 提供）

然而，分期的准确性严格来说取决于放射科医师的专业知识，具有一定的过高或过低分期的可能性[70]。通过这种分期方式提供的信息，外科医师可以选择以下 3 种低位直肠癌手术方式之一（图 25-25）：①适用于没有括约肌浸润的低位直肠肿瘤的低位前切除术（AR）。完整切除直肠和直肠系膜至盆底水平（即 TME）。②经括约肌间隙平面的低位前切除术。适用于累及括约肌间隙平面的低位直肠肿瘤，为了保证切缘阴性，应选择肿瘤局限于固有肌层，与肛门内括约肌的外缘相距 1 mm 以内（1 期）的病例。③肛提肌外腹会阴直肠癌联合切除术（abdominoperineal excision, APER）。它与传统的 APER 不同，此术式将肛提肌与直肠下段和肛管整体切除。与常规 APER 相比，这种外科手术保证了低阳性切缘率和患者更好的预后[73]。此术式适用于肿瘤侵犯固有肌层全层、括约肌间隙、侵犯肛提肌或超过肛提肌的情况（2、3 或 4 期）。

（4）N 分期：术前评估直肠癌患者的淋巴结情况很重要，因为它会影响患者的预后。特别是，尽管手术切缘干净，但直肠系膜筋膜（传统手术 CRM）附近的转移性淋巴结和直肠系膜筋膜外的恶性淋巴结可能仍未切除，使得复发风险增加[50]。

①必须评估以下各组淋巴结：直肠系膜、直肠上、肠系膜下；髂内、髂外、髂总；腹膜后；腹股沟浅表淋巴结（图 25-26）。

②根据淋巴结的位置和大小，放疗科医师可选用适当的放疗野，外科医师可对直肠系膜外淋巴结进行扩大切除。特别是盆壁转移淋巴结可显著减低无病生存率，可以通过术前辅助治疗来改善预后。MERCURY 研究小组发现，与没有可疑盆壁淋巴结转移的患者（70%）相比，MRI 上存在可疑盆壁淋巴结转移患者的 5 年无病生存率仅为 42%[74]。

③淋巴结大小标准（即淋巴结 > 5 mm）在鉴别恶性和非恶性淋巴结方面的作用有限；直肠癌 30%～50% 转移性淋巴结大小在 2～5 mm[75,76]。

④提示恶性的征象包括淋巴结边缘不规则或呈毛刺状和淋巴结信号不均（斑驳的信号强度）（图 25-27）。Brown 等的研究得出了一个有趣的结果：MR 图像上评估直肠周围淋巴结时，淋巴结边缘特征和混杂的信号强度具有高特异性（97%）和中等程度的敏感性（85%）[77]。目前没有已知的强化特征能可靠地鉴别转移淋巴结和反应性淋巴结[60,78]。

⑤ DWI 有利于淋巴结的检出，比 T_2WI 检出

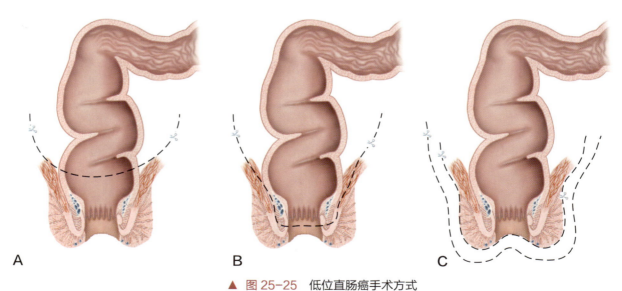

▲ 图 25-25　低位直肠癌手术方式
低位前切除术（A），经括约肌间隙平面的低位前切除术（B），腹会阴联合切除术（APER）（C，蓝线）肛提肌外 APER（C，红线）（由 Dr. M Ciolina 提供）

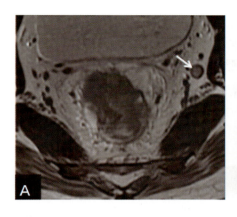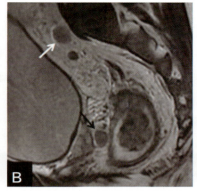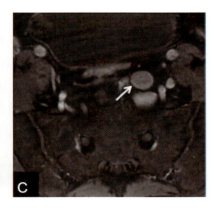

▲ 图 25-26　淋巴结转移

轴位 T_2 加权图像（A）和矢状位 T_2 加权图像显示直肠癌伴周围脂肪间隙浸润及左髂内血管（A，箭）、直肠上动脉（B，箭）和直肠系膜（B，黑色箭）转移淋巴结。轴位钆对比剂 T_1 加权压脂图像（C）也显示沿左髂总动脉存在转移淋巴结（箭）

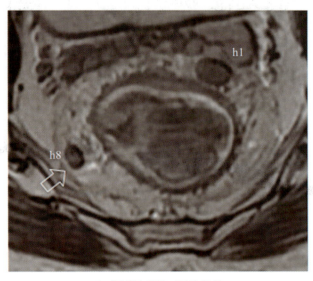

▲ 图 25-27　恶性征象

横轴位 T_2 加权图像（A）示 2 个淋巴结（8 点和 1 点方向）表现为恶性征象包括淋巴结边缘不规则或呈毛刺状，信号不均，呈斑点状高、低混杂信号；当转移淋巴结距离系膜筋膜（空心箭）≤ 1mm 时，需要考虑 CRM 受累

率高 6%，但单独应用 DWI 区分良性和恶性淋巴结并不可靠[79]（图 25-28）。单独使用 ADC 无法识别转移淋巴结，甚至比 MRI 更差[80]。

⑥如果恶性淋巴结距离 CRM 不到 1 mm，则需要怀疑累及 CRM（图 25-28）[81]。

（5）壁外血管侵犯：血管侵犯不影响临床治疗，但它是局部和远处复发的独立危险因素，具有不良预后。在 10%～ 54% 直肠癌患者中在病理上会出现血管侵犯[82]。MR 评估外壁血管侵犯（extramural vascular invasion, EMVI）的敏感性和特异性分别为 62% 和 88%[60]。

对于 T_3 期肿瘤应进行 EMVI 评估，在血管与肿瘤非常靠近的情况下均应怀疑 EMVI。一般来说，小血管受累很难评估，而较大血管的受累则表现为血管的迂曲和扩张，可能的影像表现包括[38]：在扩张和迂曲的血管内存在稍高信号的实性组织成分；在大小正常的血管腔内存在异常信号；血管扩张，管壁破坏呈假结节样形态（图 25-29）。

（6）何时需要考虑 CRM 侵犯：肿瘤与直肠系膜筋膜之间的关系对手术计划至关重要，也是一个重要的预后因素[83]。Taylor 等报道，MRI 显示未累及 CRM 的患者 5 年总生存率和 5 年无病生存率分别为 62.2% 和 67.2%，而 MRI 显示 CRM 受累的患者分别为 42.2% 和 47.3%[81]。肿瘤与 CRM 之间距离 > 1mm 与局部复发率降低相关。当肿瘤距直肠系膜筋膜 ≤ 1mm 时，必须考虑累及 CRM。

直肠系膜筋膜与以下所有结构的距离均需测量：肿瘤边缘、直肠系膜中的肿瘤种植结节、血管内的瘤栓或恶性淋巴结。与病理结果相比，MR 用于预测 CRM 的准确度在 92% 和 100% 之间[47,84]，具有较高的观察者间一致性[47]。直肠前方的直肠系膜脂肪可以很薄，因而直肠可能与 CRM 距离非常近，在这种情况下，对放射科医师而言，评估 CRM 具有一定的挑战性。

（7）与腹膜反折及盆腔器官的关系：腹膜反折最好在矢状或冠状高分辨率 T_2 加权图像上观察。如果肿瘤侵犯腹膜反折，则必须将其视为 T_{4a} 期病变。原发性直肠癌向前最易侵犯的盆腔结构是子宫、阴道、前列腺和精囊（图 25-22F）。

在侧后方，邻近直肠的其他盆壁结构包括髂内外血管及髂总血管、输尿管、梨状肌、闭孔内肌以及有骶神经根穿出的坐骨大孔区域。这些结构被盆内筋膜的壁层覆盖，并在直肠上段水平与盆内筋膜的脏层（直肠系膜筋膜）融合。在后部，盆腔筋膜壁层与骶前筋膜融合，通过潜在的直肠后

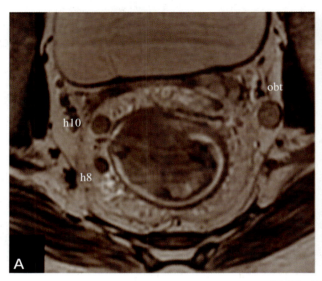 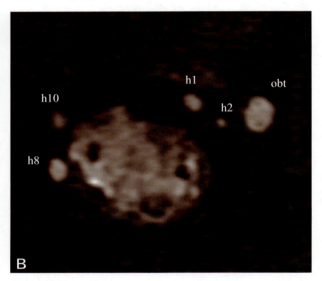

▲ 图 25-28 CRM 受累

DWI 因其高对比度分辨率有利于淋巴结的检出，横轴位 T_2 加权图像（A）可见一闭孔区淋巴结（obt）和 2 个主要的直肠系膜淋巴结（一个在 10 点方向，一个在 8 点方向）。DWI 图像（B）可显示更多淋巴结，另可见一个淋巴结位于 1 点方向，一个淋巴结位于 2 点方向

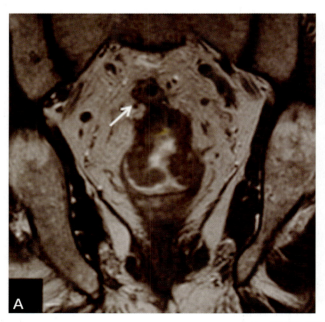 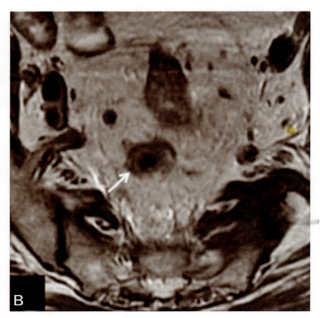

▲ 图 25-29 环状直肠癌

冠状位（A）和横轴位（B）T_2 加权图像显示一例环状直肠癌，可见结节样中等信号强度软组织（箭）包绕壁外直肠系膜血管，血管由于流空现象呈管状低信号

间隙与直肠系膜筋膜分开，也就是 TME 的解剖平面。在直肠中间 1/3 的水平，盆内筋膜的脏层和壁层通常为线样低信号结构；在 MR 图像上是独立分开、显示清晰。然而，相同的结构在直肠下段和直肠上段的水平上可能是难以区分的，并且直肠系膜筋膜在这些区域受累可能对应于盆壁受累。

评估肿瘤与盆壁之间关系最好在冠状或矢状位高分辨率图像上进行。如果肿瘤侵犯到骶骨近端或累及 S_2 椎体水平以上的神经根可能导致其无法切除[38]。

4. CRT 治疗后评估 CRT 可使直肠肿瘤降期、提高可切除性并保留括约肌以及使局部和远处复发低风险的患者数量增加，从而改善预后。在一些研究中，CRT 治疗后的肿瘤完全缓解率为 10%~20%[39,85]。CRT 的主要适应证：局部进展 T_3 期直肠肿瘤，超过固有肌层外浸润 > 5 mm；与 CRM 距离 ≤ 1mm 的肿瘤；存在肛门括约肌受累风险；淋巴结受累；EMVI。

（1）MR 表现

①纤维化区域的信号强度非常低，与固有肌层的信号强度相似，而残存肿瘤呈中等信号与基线肿瘤信号相似[86]（图 25-30）。

②促纤维增生反应是一种反应性纤维化，通常表现为直肠周围脂肪间隙中背离肿瘤方向的放射状毛刺或索条样低信号。将这种毛刺状纤维增生误认为是残存肿瘤会导致分期过高[86]（图 25-31）。

③在某些情况下，肿瘤坏死可导致黏液变性，在残存肿瘤内出现 T_2WI 高信号黏液湖[86]。

④对于原发性黏液性肿瘤，T_2 加权图像上高信号黏液湖的存在可能对 CRT 无反应的表现，预后较差，局部复发风险增加[87]。

⑤在 CRT 之前，肿瘤附近的非肿瘤性黏膜由于反应性炎症而肿胀凸出到腔内，呈假瘤样外观。在 CRT 后，由于黏膜下水肿，肿瘤附近的正常黏膜假瘤样反应更加明显，呈中等信号（图 25-32）。这些陷阱可能导致误诊，可以通过比较治疗前和治疗后的 MR 图像，注意基线肿瘤的定位并确定呈假瘤样表现的直肠壁是否位于 CRT 前肿瘤所在的肠壁区域[86]。

（2）CRT 治疗后评估肿瘤大小：肿瘤长度常常是定量评估肿瘤治疗反应的手段，但缺乏观察者间的可重复性。然而，就肿瘤降期和肿瘤退缩分级（tumor regression grade，TRG）而言，肿瘤体积与 MR 上肿瘤形态变化相结合似乎与病理上肿瘤治疗反应密切相关[88-90]。然而，体积测量需要在横轴位高空间分辨率 T_2 加权 MR 图像上用特定的软件手动勾画并计算每一层肿瘤体积再求和。许多作者认为 CRT 后肿瘤体积减小 70% 或更多，与病理中肿瘤消退具有良好相关性，并且无病生存率更高[91,92]。然而，CRT 后在 MR 的形态学图像上，癌症体积的测量并不简单。特别是，很难确定哪些纤维化区域仍然有可疑的残存肿瘤，有可以肿瘤残存的纤维化区域应包含在测量范围内，而无残存肿瘤纤维化区域则不应包括在测量范围内。最近，Curvo-Semedo 等研究发现，应用 DWI 结合 MR 形态学图像（T_2WI）进行肿瘤体积的评估，可提高 MRI 评估治疗反应的效果，总体准确率达到 88%[93]。

必须评估的还包括肛缘与治疗后肿瘤的距离，并与基线扫描的高度进行比较。

（3）T 分期：据报道应用 MRI 评估直肠癌（未放疗）T 分期的整体准确率为 71%~91%（平均值 =85%）。CRT 后，由于放疗后组织出现治疗后改变，T 分期评估通常很困难；治疗后应用 MRI 进行 T 分期的总体准确度降低至 50%[94]。

对于基线扫描，必须记录 CRT 后壁外侵犯的最大深度，据此对肿瘤超过固有肌层小于 1mm（预后与 T_2 期相同）和广泛浸润生长的肿瘤进行分层。在 CRT 后，低信号区域通常代表纤维化瘢痕，但仍难以与残存肿瘤区分。

增加应用 DWI 在区分残存肿瘤和纤维化方面具有进一步的作用[95,96]。纤维化通常具有低细胞密度，因此在高 b 值 DWI 上显示低信号，而残留肿瘤具有相对高的细胞密度，因而在高 b 值 DWI

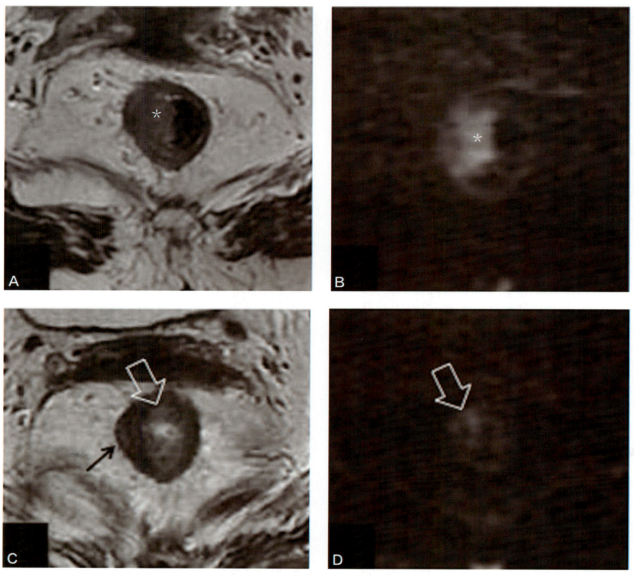

▲ 图 25-30 纤维化

A. 横轴位 T_2 加权图像示直肠癌壁偏心性增厚（白色星号）；B.DWI 上可见水分子明显扩散受限（白色星号）；C.CRT 后，横轴位 T_2 加权图像示直肠右侧壁由于纤维化改变而呈弥漫低信号（黑色箭）；D.CRT 后 DWI 可检测小肿瘤残存灶（空心箭），由于扩散受限呈稍高信号，在 T_2 加权图像上呈等信号

上呈高信号[97,98]（图 25-31 和图 25-33）。与单独应用 T_2 加权图像相比（敏感性，82%～84%；特异性，85%～90%），T_2 加权图像联合 DWI 评估 CRT 后直肠癌的敏感性为 93%～95%，特异性为 95%～100%[99]。

此外，考虑到对 CRT 反应的具有显著的个体差异（9%～25% 的患者表现出完全的病理缓解，54%～75% 的患者表现为肿瘤降期，而其他患者则没有反应）[100,101]，DWI 似乎是一种有前景的无创性技术，可作为影像生物标志物用于预测和监测直肠癌患者的早期治疗反应[102]。早期的检出和评估可能有助于在治疗前或 CRT 的第一周内识别出对治疗无反应者，从而可以强化或调整治疗方案[102]。最近的研究表明，直肠癌 CRT 疗前低 ADC 平均值和治疗中 ADC 平均值早期升高与最终良好的治疗反应相关。对 CRT 最终治疗反应良好和最终肿瘤降期的患者，其基线 ADC 值低于无反应患者组[96]。在 CRT 期间肿瘤

Chapter 25 结肠和直肠疾病
Diseases of the Colon and Rectum

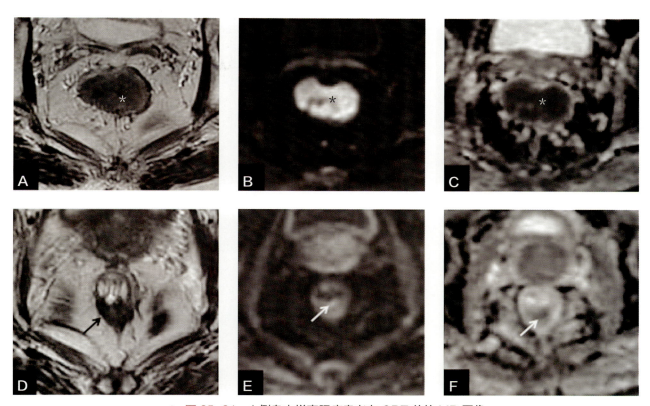

▲ 图 25-31 1 例息肉样直肠癌患者在 CRT 前的 MR 图像

横轴位 T₂ 加权图像（A，星号）呈中等信号，在 DWI 和 ADC（B、C，星号）上可见扩散受限。同一个病变 CRT 后 MR 图像示由于反应性纤维化直肠周围脂肪内可见背离肿瘤方向低信号放射状毛刺（D，黑色箭）。DWI（E）和 ADC（F）示只有局部肿瘤残存区域（白色箭）扩散受限，在 DWI 上呈高信号，ADC 图上呈低信号

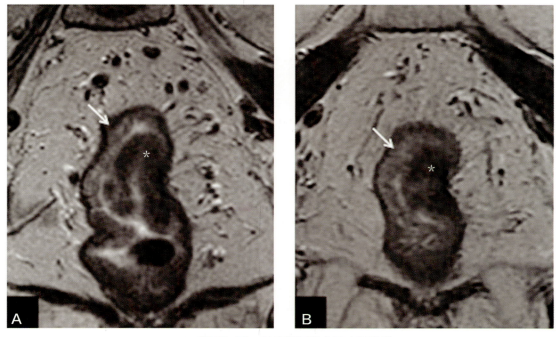

▲ 图 25-32 肿瘤附近的非肿瘤性黏膜

在 CRT 前（冠状位 T₂ 加权图像，A），肿瘤（星号）附近的非肿瘤性黏膜（箭）似乎是由于反应性炎症而呈假瘤样外观凸入腔内。在 CRT 之后（冠状位 T₂ 加权图像，B），由于黏膜下水肿肿瘤（星号）附近正常黏膜（箭）的假瘤样反应更加明显而在 T₂ 加权图像上呈中等信号

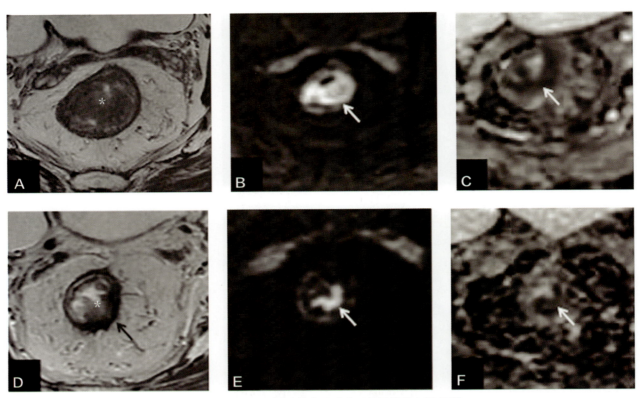

▲ 图 25-33　1 例环状直肠癌在 CRT 前的 MR 图像

A. 横轴位 T_2 加权图像（星号）上呈中等信号；B.DWI 上由于水分子扩散受限呈高信号（箭）；C. 相应 ADC 呈低信号（箭）；D.CRT 后相同病变的 MR 图像（横轴位 T_2 加权图像）示由于反应性纤维化在治疗后肿瘤周围脂肪间隙可见背离肿瘤方向的低信号放射毛刺状（黑色箭），其内组织呈中等信号（星号），可能是残存肿瘤或水肿的黏膜；E.DWI 可解决关于残存肿瘤的疑问，它可以很好地显示直肠壁残存肿瘤呈半月形高信号（箭）；F. 相应 ADC 上呈半月形低信号（箭）

降期组及未降期组均可观察到 ADC 值升高，但这一结果似乎更适用于肿瘤降期组。所有患者在 CRT 结束时均观察到肿瘤 ADC 平均值减低，主要是因为 CRT 导致间质纤维化和放射性炎症逐渐消退[96]。

Kim 等报道，CRT 后区分完全反应者与非完全反应者的 ADC 临界值（cut-off 值）为 1.20×10^{-3}，阴性预测值为 100%。然而在 CRT 前预测患者治疗反应的 ADC 值的 cut-off 值尚未确定，需要更大规模的人群中研究[103]。

此外，对于黏液性肿瘤的患者，ADC 的测量结果在确定肿瘤是否完全缓解方面仍是一个挑战，因为难以区分残存肿瘤与无肿瘤活性的高信号黏液湖[95]。

（4）肿瘤退缩分级：CRT 后，应用 MR 评估肿瘤退缩分级（TRG）和 T 分期有助于将可行局部切除的有小残存肿瘤灶（$ypT_{1-2}N_0$）的患者与可暂时等待观察的完全缓解（ypT_0N_0）的患者进行分层[104,105]。

MERCURY 研究表明，依据病理上 Dworak 肿瘤退缩分级系统[106]，即基于肿瘤组织与纤维化组织的定量病理学分析，应用斜位高空间分辨率图像可以得到基于 MRI 的肿瘤退缩分级系统。在影像上，需要对比 CRT 前及 CRT 后的高空间分辨率斜位 MR 图像，旨在评估低信号纤维化组织和中等信号的残存肿瘤组织的比例[86]（图 25-34）。在 T_2 加权图像上评估的肿瘤退缩分级的量表如下。

1 级：病理学完全缓解，100% 低信号纤维组织，没有肿瘤残存。

2 级：病理学良好反应，> 75% 的低信号纤维化组织和 < 25% 的中等信号肿瘤组织。

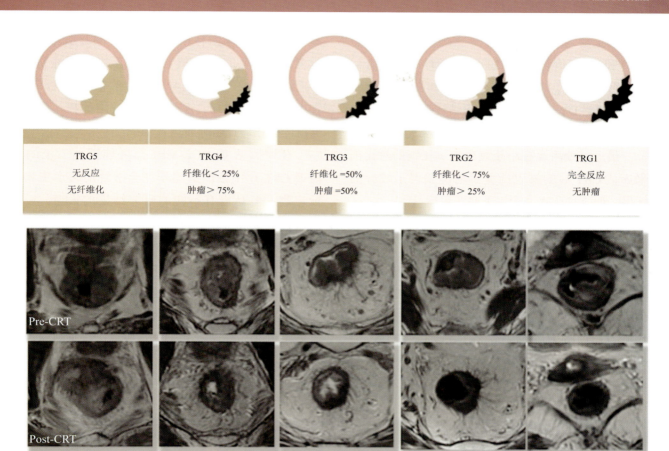

▲ 图 25-34 肿瘤退缩分级图示
Pre-CRT. CRT 前；Post-CRT. CRT 后

3 级：病理学中度反应，50% 低信号纤维组织和 50% 中等信号肿瘤组织。

4 级：病理学轻度反应，< 75% 的低信号纤维组织和 > 25% 的中等信号肿瘤组织。

5 级：病理学无反应，无纤维化组织，100% 中等信号肿瘤组织。

在 MERCURY 研究中，TRG 的 MRI 评估被证明是一个重要的独立预后预测因子。CRT 后，良好的 TRG（1～3 级）患者的平均总生存率为 72%，平均 5 年无病生存率为 64%，平均局部复发率为 14%。另一方面，最终差的 TRG（4 级和 5 级）患者的平均总生存率为 27%，平均 5 年无病生存率为 31%，平均局部复发率为 29%[86]。

(5) N 分期：放化疗后准确的淋巴结再分期可能对治疗决策产生重大影响。当患者在 MR 图像上显示淋巴结阴性和原发肿瘤的良好反应或完全缓解时，可以考虑微创手术治疗（局部切除）或等待观察。CRT 后 MR 评估淋巴结的准确度在 64%～68%[94]。仅凭淋巴结大小不可能准确地区分恶性淋巴结和反应性淋巴结。10 mm 的 cut-off 值具有高特异度和低灵敏度，而 3 mm 的 cut-off 值则相反[50]。使用形态学标准而不是大小，可以更好地区分 CRT 后 MR 图像上的转移性淋巴结与正常淋巴结。这些形态学标准是淋巴结边缘轮廓（边界清楚或边缘不规则）和信号不均匀（图 25-35）。

Koh 等[107] 报道，新辅助治疗后，使用以上标准检出恶性淋巴结，MRI 的阴性预测值 90%，准确率为 88%。

在 MERCURY 研究[108] 中，治疗后 MRI 检出淋巴结转移患者的 5 年无病生存率为 46%，而无恶性淋巴结的患者为 63%。诊断中有两大陷阱，其一是纤维化可能在 T_2 加权图像上表现为低信号的毛刺状的边缘，其二是淋巴结呈稍高信号可能是由 CRT 诱导的黏液性变性引起的。如一些研究所示（主要为头颈部和子宫/宫颈癌[109,110]），将 DWI 和 ADC 值与影像上的形态学标准相结合似乎可用于区分小的（1cm 以下）恶性和良性淋巴结。

最近，DWI 检出区域淋巴结转移的灵敏度为 80%，特异性为 76.9%，准确度为 78.3%[102]。

最近，使用含超小超顺磁性氧化铁的对比剂来评估 CRT 后的淋巴结受累情况获得了较好的结果，但这种药物尚未用于商业用途[111]。

（6）CRT 治疗后评价 CRM：由于难以区分肿瘤浸润与附着于直肠系膜筋膜的纤维化瘢痕，因此 MR 预测放疗后直肠癌 CRM 受累的准确度为 66%[112]。然而，MERCURY 研究组使用 MRI 预测 CRT 后 CRM 阴性的特异度可达 92%[86]。

（7）动态增强 MRI 的作用：动态增强 MRI（DCE-MRI）最近被用来评估肿瘤组织的灌注特征，灌注特征反映了肿瘤微血管状态，其主要参数是跨内皮细胞转移常数 K_{trans}，动态增强 MR 与灌注 CT 中的 K_{trans} 值具有显著的可比性[57]。肿瘤组织微循环增加与异常血管的存在有关，血管内皮通透性增加、血管生成活性增加和动静脉分流的存在，提示肿瘤更具侵袭性。

有研究表明 DCE-MRI 有可能成为在 CRT 前或 CRT 疗中预测病理学完全缓解的影像生物标志物，但是也有不同的研究结果的报道。一些研究人员发现反应良好者的初始流量/通透性较高[113]（图 25-36），而另一些研究者则发现初始流量/通透性较低[114,115]。

DCE-MRI 也可以作为 CRT 后有用的评估手段，有助于评估患者是否需要传统外科手术或微创手术（局部切除）干预，或者可以采取避免手术的等待观察的策略。在这方面，Gollub 等报道，治疗前和治疗后 DCE-MRI 的流量/通透性的显著

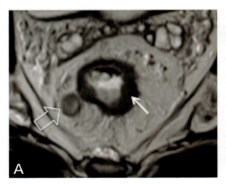
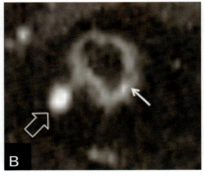
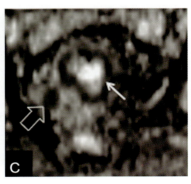

▲ 图 25-35 CRT 后环周性直肠癌的 MR 图像

A. 横轴位 T_2 加权图像示直肠壁外层弥漫性低信号，内层由于残存肿瘤呈中等信号（箭），相应在 DWI（B）和 ADC（C）上可见扩散受限。治疗后的直肠系膜区恶性淋巴结（空心箭）在 T_2 加权图像上边缘不规则，信号不均匀；在 DWI（B）和 ADC（C）上（空心箭）由于细胞密集可见扩散受限，但这个特征不能区分转移性淋巴结和反应性淋巴结

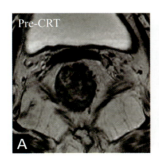
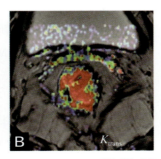
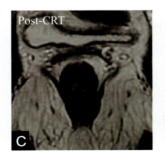
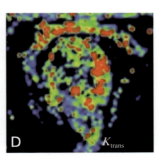

▲ 图 25-36 1 例直肠癌病例

A.（横轴位 T_2 加权图像）CRT 后完全缓解，术后分期 pTx；B. 在 CRT 之前，这种肿瘤呈现出较高的初始流量/通透性，如灌注 MR 图像中几个红色斑点所示；C. CRT 后，在横轴位 T_2 加权图像上没有肿瘤的证据；D. 并且发现低灌注 K_{trans} 值，可见红色斑点减少

下降与对 CRT 的良好反应或完全缓解相关[58]。

5. 疗效评价和随访

（1）直肠癌手术方式的分类：AR（直肠前切除术）：距离齿状线上方超过 8 cm 的直肠癌需行这种类型的外科手术[116]，包括以下三种术式：高位 AR：切除远端降结肠、乙状结肠和腹膜内的上段直肠（图 25-37A）；标准低位 AR：切除直肠乙状结肠交界处、上段直肠和腹膜反折以下的中段直肠，包括直肠系膜，即 TME（图 25-37C）；扩大低位 AR：还包括切除远端乙状结肠和远端直肠（图 25-37B）。

部分直肠系膜切除术可用于高位直肠癌，而 TME 是中低位直肠癌所必需的[117,118]。这种手术与局部复发率相关[119]。吻合术可以是结肠 - 直肠或结肠 - 肛管吻合，同时行临时近端结肠造口术或回肠造口术。吻合术式包括：端端吻合；端侧吻合；结肠"J"形储袋：降低吻合口并发症的发生率，增加新建直肠的容积，但解剖结构复杂，进行 CT 评估更为困难。它是通过直线切割闭合器将结肠缝合成两个平行的环，这个双环形结肠就构成 J 形的储袋结构[120]（图 25-38）。

在 pT_4 肿瘤（直接侵犯其他器官或结构和 / 或穿透脏腹膜的肿瘤）中，必要时需进行扩大切除邻近器官。

外科手术后的正常 MRI 表现[121]（图 25-39）：术后水肿导致吻合部位肠壁增厚；骶前间隙正中积液或少量纤维组织，通常比正常情况厚约 2cm；髂血管周围有少量腹膜外气体或液体。

当软组织厚度＞ 5 cm 时应怀疑吻合口漏或肿瘤复发[122]。

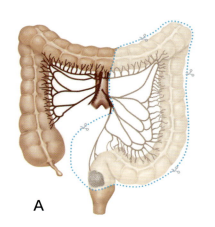
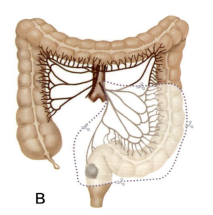
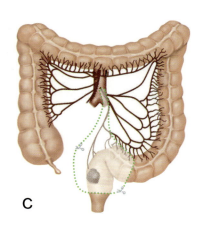

▲ 图 25-37　直肠癌外科手术方式类型
A. 高位前切除；B.TME 扩大低位前切除；C.TME 标准低位前切除（由 Dr. M Ciolina 提供）

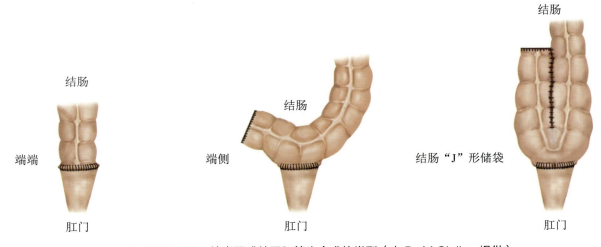

▲ 图 25-38　结直肠或结肠肛管吻合术的类型（由 Dr.M Ciolina 提供）

APER（经腹会阴联合直肠癌根治术）：此类手术的适应证为：直肠肿瘤距离齿状线上方不到8cm，侵犯括约肌或肛提肌，在狭窄的骨盆内有体积大的肿瘤；肛门恶性肿瘤。

这种类型的外科手术干预包括经腹部会阴入路，切除一部分乙状结肠，整个直肠和肛门，不保留括约肌，并进行永久性结肠造口术[117,120]。通过臀肌[123]和腹直肌皮瓣（泰勒皮瓣）或使用网膜[124]来对会阴切口进行简单的闭合。

MRI可以显示以下解剖学变化[125]（图25-40）：括约肌缺如，结肠造口术通常位于左髂窝；膀胱、精囊腺、子宫和小肠向后移位填充骶前或尾骨前的位置；骶前软组织通常代表术后纤维化或肉芽组织，初始评估时最大直径为3～5cm，随着时间的推移变得边界不清呈浸润状。另外，1～2年无生长、临床稳定和正常的癌胚抗原水平可帮助确认肿块为正常的术后变化[126]。如果怀疑复发，正电子发射断层扫描（PET）/CT可区分良性和癌性病变，灵敏度为100%，特异性为96%[127]。

①术后早期并发症——漏、瘘管和脓肿

吻合口漏（anastomotic leak）：吻合口漏通常在术后前2周出现，是最常见的术后并发症，发生率为5%～10%，如果没有进行诊断和治疗，死亡率约为50%[128]。吻合口漏可能导致的并发症包括腹膜炎和败血症。与手术有关的危险因素

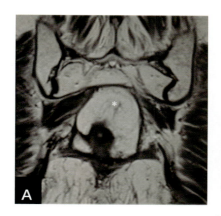 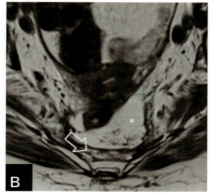 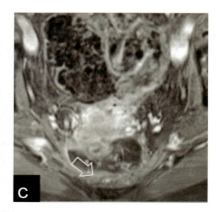

▲ 图25-39 外科手术后的正常MRI表现

前切除术的MR表现是骶前间隙增宽（星号），可见少量软组织影（空心箭），通常比正常情况厚约2cm，如冠状位（A）和横轴位（B）T_2加权图像所示。钆对比剂增强后横轴位T_1加权图像（C）示骶前组织没有明显强化（空心箭）

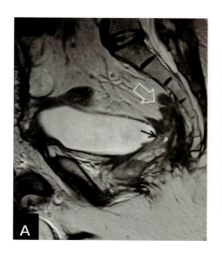 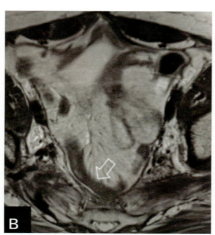 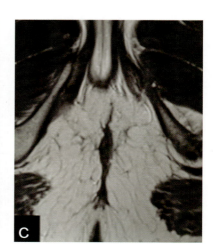

▲ 图25-40 术后解剖学变化

APER术后矢状位（A）和横轴位（B）T_2加权图像示膀胱向后移位（黑色箭）和向后移位到骶骨的小肠（空心箭）以及骶前低信号的纤维性组织（星号）。横轴位T_2加权图像（C）示会阴部括约肌缺如

包括手术：败血症、围术期活动性出血和吻合张力过大。低位前直肠切除术后吻合口漏的风险最高。据报道 CT 可确诊 48%～100% 的吻合口漏，而术后早期通常不行 MR 检查[129,130]。吻合口漏可在临床上分为症状性和无症状[121]：临床吻合口漏：术后 4d 内出现发热、白细胞增多、剧烈腹痛、反跳痛、里急后重和便秘等症状；亚临床吻合口漏：此类包括在术后常规影像检查中发现的隐匿性漏，占 5.7%～10.7%，可手术后 6 个月或更长时间持续存在。

吻合口漏的影像学表现[121]：吻合钉线不连续；肠壁内或肠壁附近出现气体；通常位于吻合口后方的腹腔积气或游离液体。

在直肠吻合口漏中，通常可以看到双直肠征，因为前方直肠与后方积液在 T_2 加权序列上呈不均匀高信号，或者为后方含气腔，可能伴有或不伴有边缘强化[122,130]（图 25-41）。

放射科医师应该描述是吻合口漏是局限性的还是游离的。

对比剂灌肠检查和使用直肠内对比剂的 CT 是评估术后积液的一线检查。MRI 不是术后常规进行的，但它可作为其他成像技术的替代方法，尤其是在怀疑瘘管形成需要显示感染并发症和炎症时应用[128]。低位吻合口漏通常局限在盆腔内，而高位 AR 或更近端结肠吻合口的漏通常会游离进入腹腔，因而具有更高的发病率[121]。

吻合口漏的处理包括手术引流或影像引导下引流，用于低位和近端局限性吻合口漏，最后采用全肠外营养。然而，如果没有出现脓毒症及随后瘘管形成，则没有紧急再次手术的指征。

肠内容物严重漏入腹腔内需要立即手术和腹腔冲洗。手术修复吻合口并通过临时造口来保护吻合口[121]。疑似吻合口漏的主要鉴别诊断是正常的端侧吻合的 MR 表现。多平面图像对帮助避免误诊吻合口漏至关重要，而没有症状、手术干预的细节以及积液没有明显强化可排除吻合口

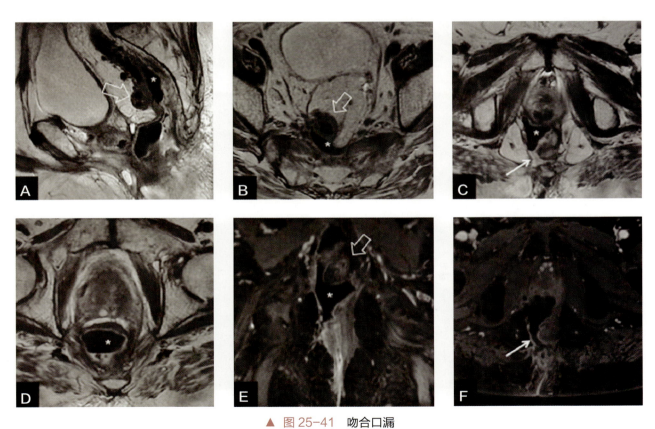

▲ 图 25-41　吻合口漏

A～D. 矢状位和横轴位 T_2 加权图像示吻合口漏，可见积气（星号）和积液（箭），结肠腔后方（空心箭）可见双直肠征；E、F. 使用对比剂后获得的冠状位和横轴 T_1 加权图像示由于炎症和瘘道（箭）的存在可导致含气腔边缘强化

开裂（图 25-42）。

瘘管（fistulae）：瘘管由吻合口漏引起，可与皮肤或泌尿生殖道连通，特别是阴道，或可与骶前间隙连通形成慢性积液。一个活动性的瘘道在 T_2WI 上表现为高信号线样结构，在钆对比剂增强的 T_1 加权压脂图像中，可与脓肿或积液相通（图 25-43）[131]。此外，脓肿在 STIR 和 T_2 加权图像上呈现高信号，在对比剂增强的 T_1 加权图像上呈现环形强化[131]。瘘管的治疗包括脓肿引流、改道术和抗生素治疗，处理方式包括肠道休息和肠外营养[121]。

②术后晚期并发症：会阴疝、腹腔包裹性囊肿、吻合口狭窄和局部复发

会阴疝（perineal hernia）：由于盆腔器官（小

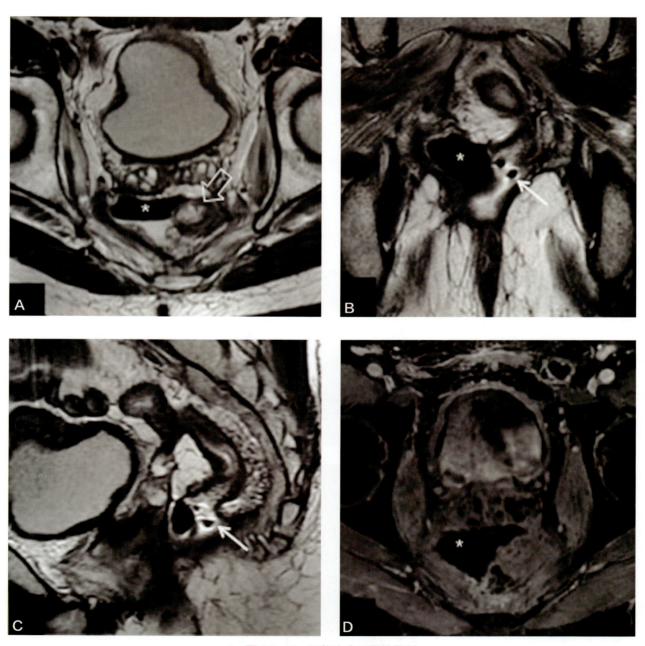

▲ 图 25-42　疑似吻合口漏的鉴别

A~C. 横轴位、冠状位和矢状位 T_2 加权图像示结肠（空心箭）和直肠（星号）之间的正常的端侧吻合（箭指示缝线铁磁性伪影）。多平面图像是避免误诊吻合口漏的基础，患者没有临床症状，钆对比剂后轴位 T_1 加权图像（D）中未见可疑漏（星号）的明确强化，可认为是正常的术后表现

肠和网膜）脱垂而造成的会阴疝是一种罕见的并发症，通常 APER 术后晚期出现[132]。症状包括会阴压迫感、胀、疼痛或像坐在肿块上的感觉。

腹腔包裹性囊肿（peritoneal inclusion cyst）：腹腔内包裹性囊肿通常见于经过结直肠切除贮袋成形术治疗溃疡性结肠炎的绝经后妇女，但其他盆腔手术干预或炎症并发症可能会出现腹膜粘连并形成包裹性积液。MRI 是诊断腹腔包裹性囊肿的首选方法，表现为局限性积液，在腹腔内并环绕卵巢[133]。

吻合口狭窄（anastomotic stricture）：定义为患者存在无法通过 12mm 直径的乙状结肠镜的狭窄区域[118]，这是一种罕见的并发症，在手术后 2～12 个月内由于吻合口漏或局部缺血引起的纤维化改变而导致吻合口狭窄[121]。患者可能出现便秘、里急后重、污粪、尿急、腹泻以及大肠梗阻的体征和症状，但也可能无症状，特别是在行近端造口旷置吻合口的情况下。除非怀疑肿瘤复发是导致狭窄的原因，否则应用 MRI 评估吻合口狭窄的价值不大。狭窄上方的结肠会扩张。吻合口狭窄的治疗包括连续球囊扩张、经直肠内修复或侵入性外科修复。

肿瘤局部复发：直肠癌根治性手术后的局部复发率差异很大（3%～30%）。约 80% 的病例，术后 2 年内出现复发，影响因素包括 T 分期和肿瘤分化程度、淋巴血管侵犯 CRM 受累肿瘤位于直肠下 1/3 段、肿瘤导致穿孔或梗阻、术前新辅助治疗和手术情况[121]。

直肠癌复发的影像学：由于盆腔解剖结构的术后改变，以及残留纤维化组织与肿瘤复发鉴别困难，使得直肠癌盆腔复发的放射学评估变得复杂。

大多数吻合口复发通常起源于肠腔外，不能通过内镜检查到，需要 CT 引导下的活检。

MRI 对于复发性直肠癌的评估至关重要，因为 T_2 加权的轴位梯度回波序列提供了盆腔的解剖细节信息，并且通常可区分呈低信号的纤维组织和稍高信号的病理组织。在所有三个平面中动态采集增强前后 DWI 和 T_1 加权压脂序列是评估肿瘤与盆壁关系的基础（图 25-44）。强化的方式有助于区分肿瘤组织与纤维化，因为肿瘤强化通常是不均匀的或边缘强化。而纤维化通常具有均匀的延迟强化。使用动态采集的原理是基于复发的肿瘤中血供增多而使得强化的峰值出现得更早。

肿瘤复发的报告中应描述以下内容[134]：
前部：与膀胱及女性的阴道、子宫颈、子宫以

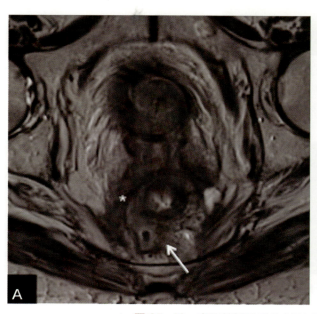
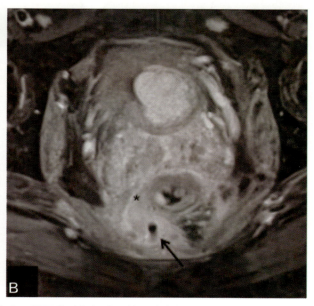

▲ 图 25-43 直肠前切除后的 MRI 示吻合口周围脂肪组织弥漫性不均匀增厚
A. 横轴位 T_2 加权图像（星号）；B. 对比增强的 T_1 加权图像上（星号），并可见由于吻合口裂开形成的瘘管（箭）

及男性的前列腺和精囊腺的关系；侧面：与盆腔侧壁、坐骨大孔的关系，评估输尿管受累情况；后部：与盆底肌肉、髂窝、骶前筋膜和骶骨的关系。

在临床实践中，应使用对检出局部复发非常敏感的 PET/CT 来补充 MRI 对肿瘤复发的评估。然而，PET/CT 中的假阴性结果可发生于黏液性肿瘤、小的腹膜转移灶或小的肝转移灶，由于 FDG 摄取水平低以及 PET 扫描仪探测器的特殊分辨率有限[127]。

（2）局部切除：经肛门内镜下显微外科手术。

越来越多的科学证据表明对于局部切除可以适用于那些病灶位于直肠中下段、具有良好的组织学特征且术前 MR 未显示淋巴结受累的早期直肠癌患者[135]。经肛内镜显微手术于 20 世纪 80 年代由德国图宾根的 Gehard Buess 教授引入。操作设备包括手术直肠镜（12～20cm 长）和用于解剖、切除和缝合的长柄器械。内镜装置提供二氧化碳（CO_2）注入、抽吸、冲洗和直肠内压的连续监测[136]。

① TEM 的适应证：TEM 适用于切除良性病变，如腺瘤、GIST 或高位肛门直肠瘘，TEM 的其他现有适应证包括治疗以下几种恶性病变[136]：治疗早期直肠癌（CRT 后 T_1N_0 和 T_1/T_2N_0）；拒绝根治性切除的患者进展期直肠癌的姑息治疗或不适合手术的患者；息肉切除术后意外发现癌灶的患者，担心切缘阳性时。

对于恶性病变的根治性切除术，直肠腔内超声和 MRI 均可用于确定病变侵犯的深度，而淋巴结的评估只适用于 MRI。TEM 后，MRI 示 T_2 加权图像上术区可见背离直肠壁方向的多发纤维性低信号毛刺（图 25-45）。

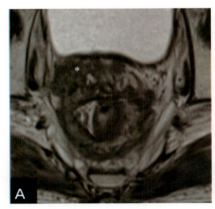 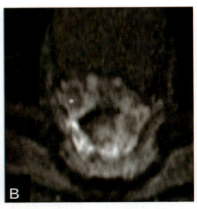 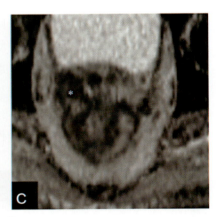

▲ 图 25-44　MRI 对于复发性直肠癌的评估

A. 轴位 T_2 加权图像，2 年后行直肠前切除，可见吻合口周围中等信号强度（星号）的弥漫性软组织影；B、C. 在 DWI 和 ADC 图上由于细胞密集而表现为扩散受限（星号）。这些表现提示肿瘤复发

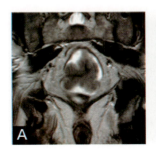 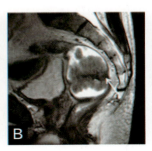 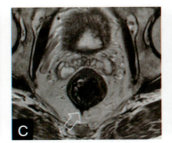 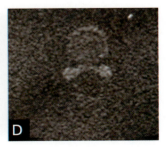

▲ 图 25-45　MRI 术后应用

A、B. 冠状位和矢状位 T_2 加权图像示 1 例息肉型直肠癌，可见血管蒂（箭）附着于直肠后壁；C. TEM 术后，在轴位 T_2 加权图像上，在直肠周围后方术区可见一些低信号纤维性毛刺（空心箭）；D. 在 DWI 上没有出现可疑肿瘤残存的高信号区

② TEM 的并发症：据报道 TEM 后总体并发症的发生率为 6%～31%[137-147]。围术期并发症包括出血和肠穿孔，其发生率为 0%～9%[137,141,144]。据报道，术后出血发生率为 1%～13%[137,140,145,148-152]，TEM 后大多数出血可自发缓解或需要输血保守治疗[152-154]。在几项随机试验中，TEM 术后的其他早期和晚期并发症的发生率与接受开放性切除的患者相似或更低（图 25-46）。特别是，Lezoche 及其同事发现新辅助治疗后随机接受 TEM（$n=35$）或腹腔镜 TME（$n=35$）治疗的 T_2N_0 直肠癌患者并发症的发生率无显著性差异[104]。

Wind 及其同事发现，TEM 组早期并发症发生率为 21%，而 AR 组早期并发症发生率为 35%。并且 TEM 手术平均手术时间更短（103min 对 149min，$P<0.05$），出血量更少（$P<0.001$），住院时间更短 [5.7d 标准差（SD），1.8d 相比于 15.4d[（SD 1.5d），$P<0.0001$] 且具有较低的术后镇痛要求[152]。

③ 复发：使用 TEM 作为确定性的根治性治疗方式应仅限于早期 T_1N_0 期病变。T_1 期病变 TEM 术后的复发率为 0%～11%[139,144-146,152]，TEM 与根治性手术相比，复发率或生存率无统计学差异[151,152]。如果在 TEM 切除后发现不利的组织学特征（pT_2，淋巴血管侵犯或累及切缘），应立即进行根治性手术（图 25-47）。

然而，已经证明使用新辅助疗法或辅助疗法可显著降低局部复发率，因此，对于接受新辅助治疗的 T_2 期病变患者，可考虑 TEM 局部切除。Duek 及其同事发现 TEM 后接受放疗的患者局部复发率为 0%，而 TEM 后拒绝辅助放疗的患者复发率为 50%[154]。Lezoche 等发现，在接受 CRT 治疗的人群中，TEM 和腹腔镜 TME 的最少 5 年随访期间局部复发或无病生存率无显著差异[104]。

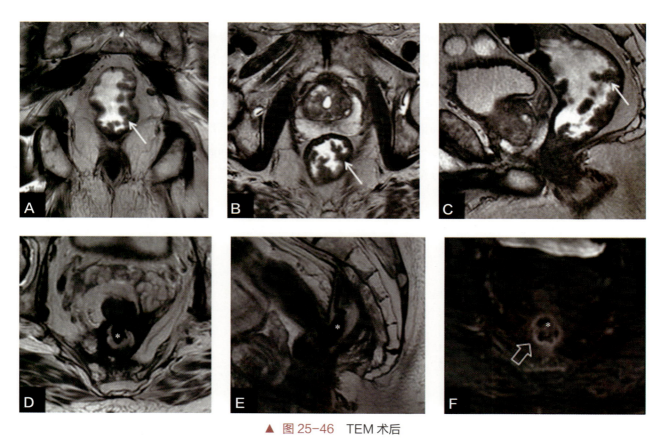

▲ 图 25-46　TEM 术后

A～C. 冠状位、轴位和矢状位 T_2 加权图像示直肠黏膜的多发结节样增厚（箭），肿瘤发生壁内扩散（pT_2）；D、E. 在 TEM 后，轴位和矢状位 MR 图像示直肠腔后方包裹性积液、积气，提示漏；F. 横轴位 T_1 加权 MR 图像示包裹积液壁呈中等强化（空心箭）

T_3 期病变患者不能进行 TEM，因为局部复发及淋巴结转移风险高，并且在肿瘤预后方面没有足够的证据。

（3）等待观察策略：在 CRT 后肿瘤降期的患者中，有 10%～30% 的患者[155-160]在可获得病理学上的完全缓解（定义为切除标本进行全面的病理检查后无存活的肿瘤细胞 $pT_0N_0M_0$）。在这种情况下，称为 0 期疾病，患者可以进行临床、内镜和放射学的密切随诊，无须立即手术，避免不必要的手术并发症。在 Habr-Gama 等进行的一项研究中，71 名患者（26%）在 CRT 后获得临床完全缓解，仅进行随访观察。在这些人群中，只有 2 名患者出现了晚期直肠内复发并通过经肛门全层切除术（pT_1）或近距离放射治疗获得了成功的治疗，而 3 名患者发生了全身转移接受了全身化疗[161]。选择等待观察策略患者需要在 CRT 后和随访期间评估原发肿瘤治疗反应和淋巴结情况。应始终使用 T_2 加权序列联合 DWI 评估原发肿瘤的治疗反应。有报道显示，应用 T_2 加权序列评估 CRT 后肿瘤残留或局部复发情况的阳性预测值（positive predictive value, PPV）为 50%～56%[95,97,162]，而 DWI 似乎将 MRI 预测 CRT 后的肿瘤残留或随访期间的局部复发敏感性提高了 17%～46%，PPV 为 66%～92%[95,97]。然而，MRI 结合内镜检查仍然十分重要，可将检出残存肿瘤或局部复发的概率增加 36%，并有助于 DWI 图像的解释。CRT 后或随访期间需应用 MRI 高空间分辨率 T_2 加权像对单个淋巴结的信号强度和形态进行评估［见二、（二）4.（5）］。如前所述，根据淋巴结大小判断仅有 64%～68% 的准确度[94]，因为转移也可发生在 2～3mm 淋巴结中。由于高对比度分辨率，DWI 更易检出淋巴结，但不能区分 N^+ 与 N_0。然而，在 DWI 上对应区域没有高信号的淋巴结可认为是 N_0（图 25-48）。

（三）直肠瘘的 MR 检查

1. 临床方面和 MR 适应证 瘘管的定义为连接两个上皮覆盖的器官或是连接有上皮覆盖的器官与体表间的异常管道；肛周瘘管指肛管与肛周区域的皮肤相通，累及括约肌复合体。肛瘘的患病率为 0.01%，主要发生在年轻男性中，男女比例为 2:1。症状包括流脓（65%）和炎症导致的肛周疼痛[163]。肛瘘可能会导致肛周脓毒症，需要手术治疗。术前需要详细的 MR 评估瘘管与肛门括约肌复合体的解剖关系，以帮助外科医师选择最佳的手术方式[164]。肛周瘘管手术治疗的成功与复发的概率密切相关[165]。

肛管的上半部分被纵行黏膜褶皱中的柱状上皮覆盖，即 Morgagni 肛柱。每个 Morgagni 肛柱的远端通过肛瓣上端的半月襞相连。肛瓣形成波

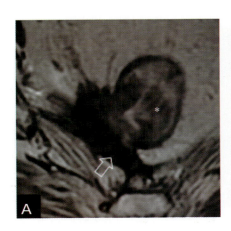 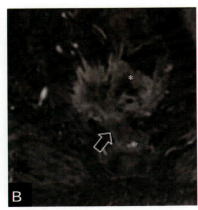 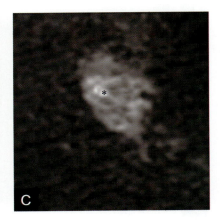

▲ 图 25-47　TEM 术后 1 年

A. 横轴位 T_2 加权图像示局部切除后形成的低信号纤维组织（空心箭）上方可见中等信号的结节状软组织影（星号）；B. 这种结节状软组织影为肿瘤复发，表现为强化不均匀（星号）；C. 在 DWI 上由于细胞密集而扩散受限（星号）；术后纤维化改变通常不会明显强化（B，空心箭）

浪形的黏膜隆起，构成齿状线（dentate /pectinate line）即移行区的远端（距肛缘 2cm），柱状上皮移行为鳞状上皮[164]。

肛瓣的上缘反折过来形成一些袋状结构，称为 Morgagni 隐窝。在 Morgagni 隐窝底部，有肛腺的开口，沿齿状线分布在肛管周围被覆柱状上皮。这些肛腺是由 6～10 个分支的腺体结构组成，面积约 1cm^2。大多数肛腺位于上皮下，另外一些肛腺的分支位置更深，穿过肛门内括约肌并最终进入括约肌间隙。感染可以沿位置较深的腺体分支形成的管道从肛门腔向深部扩散至括约肌平面，并由此到达皮肤或盆腔。如果脓肿累及上皮下腺体，则感染自发地排入肛管。同样，如果脓肿累及深部腺体，腺体分支穿过内括约肌，内括约肌可以充当屏障，感染则沿着阻力最小的路径播散，沿着括约肌的平面或穿过外括约肌并进入坐骨肛门窝[166]。

2. 直肠瘘的 MR：技术方面 MRI 扫描方案包括用相位阵列线圈覆盖盆腔行高空间分辨率多平面成像。在定位之后，第一次扫描必须是矢状位快速自旋回波（urbo spin echo，TSE）T$_2$ 加权图像，这有助于了解盆腔的概况并显示肛管的延伸和走向[164]。

从肛管的延伸方向，可以得到其他序列的正确位置。在垂直于肛管长轴平面的采集可获得斜轴位 T$_2$ TSE 序列，在平行于肛管的长轴方向采集可获得斜冠状位 T$_2$ TSE 序列。其他序列也应采集这些平面：脂肪抑制的斜轴位 T$_2$ TSE 加权图像和斜冠状 T$_2$ TSE 加权图像、无脂肪抑制的斜轴位 T$_1$ TSE 加权图像、钆对比剂增强前后的斜轴位和斜冠状位 T$_1$ GRE 脂肪抑制序列[167,168]。脂肪抑制的 T$_2$ 加权序列可使得由于水肿和肉芽组织存在而呈高信号的瘘管与周围脂肪形成明显对比[169,170]。T$_2$ 加权序列中的脂肪抑制通常通过频率选择性脂肪饱和（Fat Saturation，FAT SAT）技术以获得具有高空间分辨率的图像[171]。然而这种脂肪抑制方法更容易受到铁磁性伪影的影响，并且在这些情况下不能保证脂肪抑制的均匀性。为了解决这个问题，在瘘管中存在缝线伪影或挂线时，STIR 序列可作为有效的替代方案，其可以提供良好且均匀的脂肪抑制并且在存在磁敏感性伪影时更稳定[172-174]。

新 3D T$_2$ 加权序列可仅需在单次采集 3D T$_2$ 序列后将获得数据进行处理重建得到矢状位、斜轴位和斜冠状位的高分辨率图像，可以明显缩短采集时间，从而可获得更薄扫描层面并减少技术操作人员所产生的误差[175-177]。

肛周瘘使用 MRI 的其他优点包括：T$_1$ 加权增强后图像的数字减影技术，可获得活动性瘘管

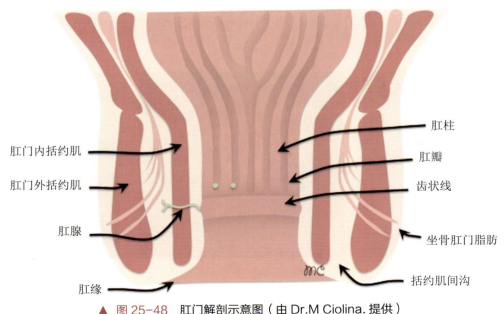

▲ 图 25-48 肛门解剖示意图（由 Dr.M Ciolina. 提供）

或脓肿的 MR 瘘管造影图像；使用 DWI 获得化脓瘘道的扩散受限的信号并更好地显示脓肿，尤其是在先前有对造影剂的过敏反应或其他禁忌证的情况下[178]。

3. 直肠瘘的 MR：术前影像学表现　活动性肛瘘在 T_2 加权图像上表现为高信号的瘘管，瘘管周围水肿在脂肪抑制的 T_2 加权图像上更易观察，可与周围信号被抑制的脂肪组织和低信号括约肌形成更好的对比。在钆对比剂增强的 T_1 加权脂肪抑制序列，瘘管和脓肿由于活动性炎症及肉芽组织表现出明显的边缘强化，而瘘管或脓肿中心仍然是低信号[164]。

肛瘘影像报告中应重点描述肛瘘内口的准确位置、径向方向和瘘管路径[165]。

根据肛门钟点位置来描述内口位置和径向方向，其中前会阴位于 12 点位置，臀沟位于 6 点位置，左侧壁位于 3 点位置，右侧壁位于 9 点位置[179]。

肛瘘的路径根据 Park 分类（1976）[180]可描述为 4 种类型：①括约肌间型，经过肛门内括约肌到括约肌间隙并与会阴沟通，占肛瘘的 70%（图 25-49 和图 25-50）；②经括约肌型，通过肛门内、外括约肌到达坐骨肛门窝并与会阴沟通，占肛瘘的 25%（图 25-51）；③括约肌上型，通过括约肌间隙，在耻骨直肠肌上方向上延伸到坐骨直肠窝，再到会阴部，约占肛瘘的 5%；④括约肌外型，从直肠腔到肛周皮肤，穿过肛提肌，完全在肛门外括约肌以外，占肛瘘的 1%（图 25-52）。

放射科医师提出的另一种分类方法是圣詹姆斯大学医院（St James's University Hospital）分类（表 25-5），其中包括一些重要的 MR 表现，以区分单纯瘘管和具有脓肿或继发性瘘道的复杂瘘管[179]。

这种分类主要是将 Park 分型中每类肛瘘划分为无并发症的单纯型瘘和伴有脓肿或次级瘘道的

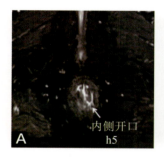
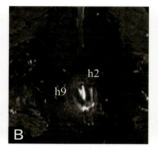
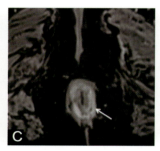
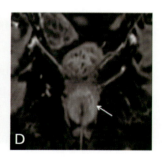

▲ 图 25-49　括约肌间型
横轴位压脂肪抑制 T_2 加权 MR 图像（A、B）可见括约肌间线样高信号结构，即瘘管，从 2 点延伸到 9 点方向，呈马蹄形态，并在 5 点处见内口。使用对比剂后获得的轴位（C）和冠状位（D）T_1 加权图像示瘘管壁由于活动性炎症可见强化（箭）

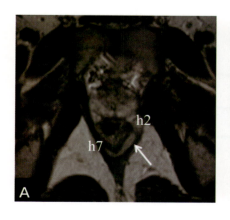
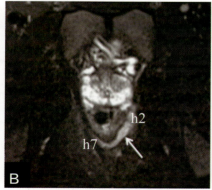
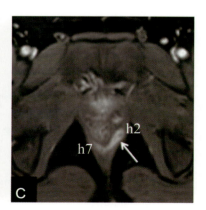

▲ 图 25-50　括约肌间型
横轴位 T_2 加权图像和脂肪抑制的 T_2 加权 MR 图像（A、B）可见高信号管状结构，代表括约肌间瘘，瘘管从 2 点延伸到 7 点方向。使用对比剂后获得的轴位（C）T_1 加权图像示瘘管壁由于活动性炎症可见强化（箭）

Chapter 25 结肠和直肠疾病
Diseases of the Colon and Rectum

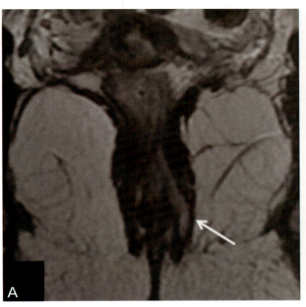 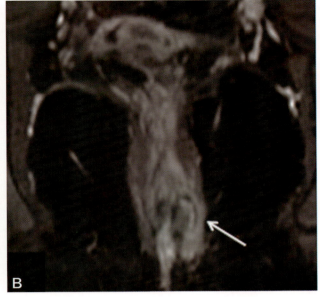

▲ 图 25-51 经括约肌型

冠状位 T_2 加权 MR 图像（A）可见高信号管状结构，代表括约肌间瘘，瘘管在肛管下段水平穿过左侧肛门外括约肌。使用对比剂后获得的冠状位（B）T_1 加权图像示瘘管壁由于活动性炎症可见强化（箭）

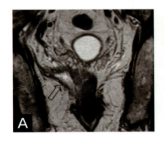 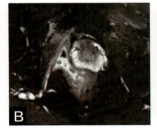 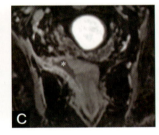 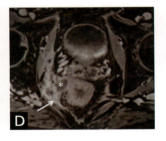

▲ 图 25-52 括约肌外型

冠状位 T_2 加权图像（A）和横轴位 T_2 加权脂肪抑制 MR 图像（B）示右侧肛提肌上方（空心箭）的包裹性积气积液（星号）形成的气-液平面，为肛提肌上瘘形成的脓肿。使用对比剂后获得的冠状位（C）和轴位（D）T_1 加权图像示脓肿、瘘管壁和轴位脂肪组织（箭）由于活动性炎症可见强化（箭）

表 25-5 圣詹姆斯大学医院提出的肛瘘分类

分级	类型	描述
1	单纯线形括约肌间瘘	局限在括约肌间的 Parks A 型，不伴有脓肿或次级瘘道
2	括约肌间瘘伴脓肿或次级瘘道	局限在括约肌间的 Parks A 型，伴有脓肿、同侧括约肌间隙的次级分支或延伸至对侧括约肌间隙呈马蹄状
3	经括约肌瘘	经过括约肌间隙穿过肛门外括约肌的 Parks B 型，不伴有脓肿或坐骨直肠窝/坐骨肛门窝的次级瘘道
4	经括约肌瘘伴脓肿或坐骨直肠窝/坐骨肛门窝的次级瘘道	经过括约肌间隙穿过肛门外括约肌的 Parks B 型，但为伴有脓肿或坐骨直肠窝/坐骨肛门窝次级瘘道的复杂型
5	肛提肌上瘘或经肛提肌瘘	经括约肌间平面上方，越过肛提肌和耻骨直肠肌交点的顶部，在坐骨直肠窝和坐骨肛门窝向下达肛周皮肤

复杂型瘘[179]。

4. 治疗和术后MRI表现 肛瘘患者的处理需要通过MRI进行准确的术前评估，以描述瘘道与肛门括约肌的关系，从而保持括约肌复合体和肛门控制排便功能。

根据不同类型的瘘道，治疗方法不同。肛瘘的术式如下。

（1）瘘管切开术（fistulotomy）：切开整个瘘道，将其开放，以便进行后续治疗。应用探针穿过内口及外口，可应用于大多数肛瘘（括约肌间和低位经括约肌肛瘘），特别是在低位肛管水平，其中肛门内外括约肌纤维可以在不影响排便功能的情况下以直角分开。这些在女性患者的前位肛瘘中不适用。

（2）瘘管切除术（core fistulectomy）：不分离肌肉直接切除瘘管。通过穿过内口和外口的探针切除瘘管，然后可以封闭内口（可结合直肠推移皮瓣）。

（3）挂线手术：在瘘管中放置异物（通常是不可吸收的缝合线或橡皮筋）以引流脓性液体或缓慢地切开括约肌，缓慢刺激肌肉纤维化，同时保持括约肌功能的完整性。它适用于高位、复杂、复发性或多发性瘘管，以及括约肌压力较差的患者或患有前位肛瘘的女性患者。如果瘘管具有更复杂的向上的分支，它也可以与瘘管切开术联合进行。

（4）黏膜推移皮瓣：瘘管切除术切除或刮除瘘管并通过黏膜皮瓣封闭内口。它适用于由于复杂疾病导致的传统的瘘管切开术及挂线失败或不当的情况。

（5）纤维蛋白胶或胶原蛋白填塞：瘘管经挂线引流并为后续治疗准备好。然后用纤维蛋白胶或胶原蛋白塞填充以形成瘢痕。

在克罗恩病相关瘘管患者中，抗生素是一线治疗，而嘌呤类似物（硫唑嘌呤、6-巯基嘌呤）用于维持缓解[181]。

最近引入了抗坏死因子（tumor necrosis factor，TNF）抗体（英夫利昔单抗），具有良好的临床效果可诱导瘘管孔的快速闭合。然而，尽管开口闭合，但瘘道持续存在可导致慢性炎症、瘘管反复发作和脓肿[182]。

MRI在确认和评估术后复发性疾病以及评估对药物治疗反应方面也发挥着重要作用[183]。在手术治疗后，MRI仍然是最好的诊断工具，优于直肠腔内超声，因为其对肛周区域的评估范围更广，并且能够区分活动性瘘管和愈合的瘘管。基于这些原因，对于肛瘘疾病患者的随访，超声检查的作用非常有限，仅在MRI禁忌的情况下适用。

成功治疗的瘘管在T_2和T_1加权图像上显示为低信号的线性结构，即瘢痕组织，在使用对比剂增强后没有强化。在挂线治疗后，重点在于识别挂线穿过高信号瘘管的中心低信号灶[169]。

肛瘘手术治疗后的早期并发症包括尿潴留和出血。在未增强的T_1加权图像上手术部位的出血可以表现为高信号。在晚期并发症中，低位和单纯性瘘管复发率为20%，高位复杂瘘管复发率为40%。由于既往手术或药物治疗的纤维化改变，复发性瘘管在T_2加权图像中表现为高信号管道边缘包绕低信号毛刺。活动性复发性瘘管或脓肿在增强后脂肪抑制的T_1加权图像上表现为瘘管壁强化，脓液和炎性液体是瘘管中心呈低信号[121]。

失禁通常只需要临床诊断，肛门括约肌的损伤可能有轻微症状（高达50%），主要表现为不自主的排气，或是有更严重的实质性损伤（3%～5%的病例），表现为大便失禁。另一种不常见的晚期并发症是继发于愈合过程中纤维化改变导致的肛门狭窄[121]。

参考文献

[1] Standring S (2008) *Gray's Anatomy: The Anatomical Basis of Clinical Practice*, 40th edn. Churchill, Livingston, Scotland.

[2] Netter F (1973) In: Oppenheimer E, ed. *The CIBA Collection of Medical Illustrations*, volume 3: Digestive system.

[3] Achiam MP, Chabanova E, Løgager V et al. (2007) Implementation of MR colonography. *Abdom Imaging* 32(4):457–462.

[4] Korman LY, Overholt BF, Box T et al. (2003) Perforation during colonoscopy in endoscopic ambulatory surgical centers. *Gastrointest Endosc* 58(4):554–557.

[5] Pickhardt PJ (2006) Incidence of colonic perforation at CT colonography: Review of existing data and implications for screening of asymptomatic adults. *Radiology* 239(2):313–316.

[6] Debatin JF, Lauenstein TC (2003) Virtual magnetic resonance colonography. *Gut* 52(Suppl 4):iv17–22.

[7] Florie J, Jensch S, Nievelstein RA et al. (2007b) MR colonography with limited bowel preparation compared with optical colonoscopy in patients at increased risk for colorectal cancer. *Radiology* 243(1):122–131.

[8] Ajaj W, Lauenstein TC, Pelster G et al. (2004) MR colonography: How does air compare to water for colonic distention? *J Magn Reson Imaging* 19(2):216–221.

[9] Bakir B, Acunas B, Bugra D et al. (2009) MR colonography after oral administration of polyethylene glycolelectrolyte solution. *Radiology* 251(3):901–909.

[10] Rodriguez-Gomez S, Pages Llinas M, Castells Garangou A et al. (2008) Dark-lumen MR colonography with fecal tagging: A comparison of water enema and air methods of colonic distension for detecting colonic neoplasms. *Eur Radiol* 18(7):1396–1405.

[11] Lauenstein T, Holtmann G, Schoenfelder D et al. (2001) MR colonography without colonic cleansing: A new strategy to improve patient acceptance. *AJR Am J Roentgenol* 177(4):823–827.

[12] Achiam MP, Chabanova E, Løgager VB et al. (2008) MR colonography with fecal tagging: Barium vs. barium ferumoxsil. *Acad Radiol* 15(5):576–583.

[13] Ajaj W, Lauenstein TC, Schneemann H et al. (2005a) Magnetic resonance colonography without bowel cleansing using oral and rectal stool softeners (fecal cracking)—A feasibility study. *Eur Radiol* 15(10):2079–2087.

[14] Zalis ME, Barish MA, Choi JR et al. (2005) CT colonography reporting and data system: A consensus proposal. *Radiology* 236(1):3–9.

[15] Zijta FM, Bipat S, Stoker J et al. (2010) Magnetic resonance (MR) colonography in the detection of colorectal lesions: A systematic review of prospective studies. *Eur Radiol* 20(5):1031–1046.

[16] Shah HA, Paszat LF, Saskin R et al. (2007) Factors associated with incomplete colonoscopy: A population-based study. *Gastroenterology* 132(7):2297–2303.

[17] Achiam MP, Holst Andersen LP, Klein M et al. (2009a) Preoperative evaluation of synchronous colorectal cancer using MR colonography. *Acad Radiol* 16(7):790–797.

[18] Ajaj W, Goyen M, Langhorst J et al. (2006) MR colonography for the assessment of colonic anastomoses. *J Magn Reson Imaging* 24(1):101–107.

[19] Rottgen R, Herzog H, Lopez-Häninnen E et al. (2006) Bowel wall enhancement in magnetic resonance colonography for assessing activity in Crohn's disease. *Clin Imaging* 30(1):27–31.

[20] Ajaj WM, Lauenstein TC, Pelster G et al. (2005c) Magnetic resonance colonography for the detection of inflammatory diseases of the large bowel: Quantifying the inflammatory activity. *Gut* 54(2):257–263.

[21] Schreyer AG, Rath HC, Kikinis R et al. (2005) Comparison of magnetic resonance imaging colonography with conventional colonoscopy for the assessment of intestinal inflammation in patients with inflammatory bowel disease: A feasibility study. *Gut* 54(2):250–256.

[22] Schreyer AG, Furst A, Agha A et al. (2004) Magnetic resonance imaging based colonography for diagnosis and assessment of diverticulosis and diverticulitis. *Int J Colorectal Dis* 19(5):474–480.

[23] Ajaj W, Ruehm SG, Lauenstein T et al. (2005b) Darklumen magnetic resonance colonography in patients with suspected sigmoid diverticulitis: A feasibility study. *Eur Radiol* 15(11):2316–2322.

[24] Scardapane A, Bettocchi S, Lorusso F et al. (2011) Diagnosis of colorectal endo-metriosis: Contribution of contrast enhanced MR-colonography. *Eur Radiol* 21:1553–1563.

[25] Salerno G, Sinnatambi C, Branagan G et al. (2006) Defining the rectum: Surgically, radiologically and anatomically. *Colorectal Dis* 8:5–9.

[26] Jorge JM, Wexner SD (1997) Anatomy and physiology of the rectum and anus. *Eur J Surg* 163:723–731.

[27] Schäfer A-O, Langer M (2010) *MRI of Rectal Cancer Clinical Atlas*. Springer, New York.

[28] Aigner F, Trieb T, Öfner D et al. (2007) Anatomical considerations in TNM staging and therapeutical procedures for low rectal cancer. *Int J Colorectal Dis* 22:1339–1342.

[29] Sakorafas GH, Zouros E, Peros G (2006) Applied vascular anatomy of the colon and rectum: Clinical implications for the surgical oncologist. *Surg Oncol* 15:243–255.

[30] Maier A, Fuchsjager M (2003) Preoperative staging of rectal cancer. *Eur J Radiol* 47:89–97.

[31] Iafrate F, Laghi A, Paolantonio P et al. (2006) Preoperative staging of rectal cancer with MR Imaging: Correlation with surgical and histopathologic findings. *RadioGraphics* 26(3):701–714.

[32] Harrison JC, Dean PJ, el Zeky F et al. (1994). From Dukes through Jass: Pathological prognostic indicators in rectal cancer. *Hum Pathol* 25: 498–505.

[33] Jass JR, Love SB (1989) Prognostic value of direct spread in Dukes' C cases of rectal cancer. *Dis Colon Rectum* 32:477–480.

[34] Tang R, Wang JY, Chen JS et al. (1995) Survival impact of lymph node metastasis in TNM stage III carcinoma of the colon and rectum. *J Am Coll Surg* 180:705–712.

[35] Willett CG, Badizadegan K, Ancukiewicz M et al. (1999) Prognostic factors in stage T3N0 rectal cancer: Do all patients require postoperative pelvic irradiation and chemotherapy? *Dis Colon Rectum* 42:167–173.

[36] Wolmark N, Fisher B, Wieand HS (1986) The prognostic

value of the modifications of the Dukes' C class of colorectal cancer. *Ann Surg* 203:115–122.

［37］Heald RJ, Moran BJ, Ryall RD et al. (1998) Rectal cancer: The Basingstoke experience of total mesorectal excision, 1978–1997. *Arch Surg* 133(8):894–899.

［38］Kaur H, Choi H, You YN et al. (2012) MR imaging for preoperative evaluation of primary rectal cancer: Practical considerations. *RadioGraphics* 32(2):389–409.

［39］Sauer R, Becker H, Hohenberger W et al. (2004) Preoperative versus postoperative chemoradiotherapy for rectal cancer. *N Engl J Med* 351(17):1731–1740.

［40］Kapiteijn E, Marijnen CA, Nagtegaal ID et al. (2001) Preoperative radiotherapy combined with total mesorectal excision for resectable rectal cancer. *N Engl J Med* 345(9):638–646.

［41］Akasu T, Kondo H, Moriya Y et al. (2000) Endorectal ultrasonography and treatment of early stage rectal cancer. *World J Surg* 24:1061–1068.

［42］Blair S, Ellenhorn JD (2000) Transanal excision for low rectal cancers is curative in early-stage disease with favorable histology. *Am Surg* 66:817–820.

［43］Gao JD, Shao YF, Bi JJ et al. (2003) Local excision carcinoma in early stage. *World J Gastroenterol* 9:871–873.

［44］Langer C, Liersch T, Markus P et al. (2002) Transanal endoscopic microsurgery (TEM) for minimally invasive resection of rectal adenomas and *low-risk* carcinomas (uT1, G1–2). *Z Gastroenterol* 40:67–72.

［45］MERCURY Study Group (2007) Extramural depth of tumor invasion at thin-section MR in patients with rectal cancer: Results of the MERCURY study. *Radiology* 243(1):132–139.

［46］MERCURY Study Group (2006) Diagnostic accuracy of preoperative magnetic resonance imaging in predicting curative resection of rectal cancer: Prospective observational study. *BMJ* 333(7572):779.

［47］Beets-Tan RG, Beets GL, Vliegen RF et al. (2001) Accuracy of magnetic resonance imaging in prediction of tumourfree resection margin in rectal cancer surgery. *Lancet* 357(9255):497–504.

［48］Ho M-L, Liu J, Narra V (2008) Magnetic resonance imaging of rectal cancer. *Clin Colon Rectal Surg* 21:178–187.

［49］Brown G, Daniels IR, Richardson C et al. (2005) Techniques and trouble-shooting in high spatial resolution thin slice MRI for rectal cancer. *Br J Radiol* 78(927):245–251.

［50］Brown G, Richards CJ, Bourne MW et al. (2003) Morphologic predictors of lymph node status in rectal cancer with use of high-spatial-resolution MR imaging with histopathologic comparison. *Radiology* 227(2):371–377.

［51］Figueiras RG, Goh V, Padhani AR et al. (2010) The role of functional imaging in colorectal cancer. *AJR Am J Roentgenol* 195(1):54–66.

［52］Curvo-Semedo L, Lambregts DM, Maas M et al. (2012) Diffusion-weighted MRI in rectal cancer: Apparent diffusion coefficient as a potential noninvasive marker of tumor aggressiveness. *J Magn Reson Imaging* 35(6): 1365–1371.

［53］Dzik-Jurasz A, Domenig C, George M et al. (2002) Diffusion MRI for prediction of response of rectal cancer to chemoradiation. *Lancet* 360(9329): 307–308.

［54］Hein PA, Kremser C, Judmaier W et al. (2003) Diffusion-weighted magnetic resonance imaging for monitoring diffusion changes in rectal carcinoma during combined, preoperative chemoradiation: Preliminary results of a prospective study. *Eur J Radiol* 45(3):214–222.

［55］Jung SH, Heo SH, Kim JW et al. (2012) Predicting response to neoadjuvant chemoradiation therapy in locally advanced rectal cancer: Diffusion-weighted 3 Tesla MR imaging. *J Magn Reson Imaging* 35(1):110–116.

［56］Gu J, Khong PL, Wang S et al. (2011) Quantitative assessment of diffusion-weighted MR imaging in patients with primary rectal cancer: Correlation with FDG-PET/CT. *Mol Imaging Biol* 13(5):1020–1028.

［57］Kierkels RG, Backes WH, Janssen MH et al. (2010) Comparison between perfusion computed tomography and dynamic contrast-enhanced magnetic resonance imaging in rectal cancer. *Int J Radiat Oncol Biol Phys* 77(2):400–408.

［58］Gollub MJ, Gultekin DH, Akin O et al. (2012) Dynamic contrast enhanced-MRI for the detection of pathological complete response to neoadjuvant chemotherapy for locally advanced rectal cancer. *Eur Radiol* 22(4):821–831.

［59］Nougaret S, Reinhold C, Mikhael HW et al. (2013) The use of MR imaging in treatment planning for patients with rectal carcinoma: Have you checked the "DISTANCE"? *Radiology* 268(2):330–344.

［60］Tudyka V, Blomqvist L, Beets-Tan RG et al. (2014 Apr) EURECCA consensus conference highlights about colon & rectal cancer multidisciplinary management: The radiology experts review. *Eur J Surg Oncol* 40(4):469–475.

［61］Taylor F, Mangat N, Brown G et al. (2010) Proformabased reporting in rectal cancer. *Cancer Imaging* 10 Spec no A:S142–S150.

［62］Moon SH1, Kim DY, Park JW et al. (2012) Can the new American Joint Committee on Cancer staging system predict survival in rectal cancer patients treated with curative surgery following preoperative chemoradiotherapy? *Cancer* 118(20):4961–4968.

［63］Taylor FG, Quirke P, Heald RJ et al. (2011) Preoperative high-resolution magnetic resonance imaging can identify good prognosis stage I, II, and III rectal cancer best managed by surgery alone: A prospective, multicenter, European study. *Ann Surg* 253(4):711–719.

［64］Merkel S, Mansmann U, Siassi M et al. (2001) The prognostic inhomogeneity in pT3 rectal carcinomas. *Int J Colorectal Dis* 16(5):298–304.

［65］Shirouzu K, Akagi Y, Fujita S et al. (2011) Clinical significance of the mesorectal extension of rectal cancer: A Japanese multi-institutional study. *Ann Surg* 253(4):704–710.

［66］Nagtegaal ID, van de Velde CJ, Marijnen CA et al. Low rectal cancer: A call for a change of approach in abdominoperineal resection. *J Clin Oncol* 2005;23(36):9257–9264.

［67］Kao PS, Chang SC, Wang LW et al. (2010) The impact of

preoperative chemoradiotherapy on advanced low rectal cancer. *J Surg Oncol* 102(7):771–777.

[68] Weiser MR, Quah HM, Shia J et al. (2009) Sphincter preservation in low rectal cancer is facilitated by preoperative chemoradiation and intersphincteric dissection. *Ann Surg* 249(2):236–242.

[69] Rouanet P, Saint-Aubert B, Lemanski C et al. (2002) Restorative and nonrestorative surgery for low rectal cancer after high-dose radiation: Long-term oncologic and functional results. *Dis Colon Rectum* 45(3):305–313.

[70] Shihab OC, How P, West N et al. (2011) MRI staging system for low rectal cancer aid surgical planning? *Dis Colon Rectum* 54(10):1260–1264.

[71] Shihab OC, Moran BJ, Heald RJ et al. (2009) MRI staging of low rectal cancer. *Eur Radiol* 19(3):643–650.

[72] Zhang XM, Zhang HL, Yu D et al. (2008) 3-T MRI of rectal carcinoma: Preoperative diagnosis, staging, and planning of sphincter-sparing surgery. *AJR Am J Roentgenol* 190(5):1271–1278.

[73] West NP, Anderin C, Smith KJ et al. (2010) European extralevator abdomino-perineal excision study group. Multicentre experience with extralevator abdominoperineal excision for low rectal cancer. *Br J Surg* 97(4):588–599.

[74] MERCURY Study Group, Shihab OC, Taylor F et al. (2011) Relevance of magnetic resonance imaging-detected pelvic sidewall lymph node involvement in rectal cancer. *Br J Surg* 98(12):1798–1804.

[75] Kim JH, Beets GL, Kim MJ et al. (2004) High-resolution MR imaging for nodal staging in rectal cancer: Are there any criteria in addition to the size? *Eur J Radiol* 52(1):78–83.

[76] Koh DM, George C, Temple L et al. (2010) Diagnostic accuracy of nodal enhancement pattern of rectal cancer at MRI enhanced with ultra-small superparamagnetic iron oxide: Findings in pathologically matched mesorectal lymph nodes. *AJR Am J Roentgenol* 194(6): W505–W513.

[77] Brown G, Richards CJ, Bourne MW et al. (2003) Morphologic predictors of lymph node status in rectal cancer with use of high-spatial-resolution MR imaging with histopathologic comparison. *Radiology* 227(2):371–377.

[78] Moran B, Brown G, Cunningham D et al. (2008) Clarifying the TNM staging of rectal cancer in the con text of modern imaging and neo-adjuvant treatment: 'y' 'u' and 'p' need 'mr' and 'ct'. *Colorectal Dis* 10(3):242–243.

[79] Heijnen LA, Lambregts DM, Mondal D et al. (2013) Diffusion-weighted MR imaging in primary rectal cancer staging demonstrates but does not characterise lymph nodes. *Eur Radiol* 23(12):3354–3360.

[80] Lambregts DM, Maas M, Riedl RG et al. (2011) Value of ADC measurements for nodal staging after chemoradiation in locally advanced rectal cancer-a per lesion validation study. *Eur Radiol* 21(2):265–273.

[81] Taylor FG, Quirke P, Heald RJ et al. (2014) Preoperative magnetic resonance imaging assessment of circumferential resection margin predicts disease-free survival and local recurrence: 5-year follow-up results of the MERCURY study. *J Clin Oncol* 32(1):34–43.

[82] Smith NJ, Barbachano Y, Norman AR et al. (2008) Prognostic significance of magnetic resonance imagingdetected extramural vascular invasion in rectal cancer. *Br J Surg* 95(2):229–236.

[83] Lahaye MJ, Engelen SM, Beets-Tan RG et al. (2005) Imaging for predicting the risk factors—The circumferential resection margin and nodal disease—of local recurrence in rectal cancer: A meta-analysis. *Semin Ultrasound CT MR* 26(4):259–268.

[84] Brown G, Radcliffe AG, Newcombe RG et al. (2003) Preoperative assessment of prognostic factors in rectal cancer using high-resolution magnetic resonance imaging. *Br J Surg* 90:355–364.

[85] Madoff RD (2004) Chemoradiotherapy for rectal cancer—When, why, and how? *N Engl J Med* 351(17):1790–1792.

[86] Patel UB, Blomqvist LK, Taylor F et al. (2012) MRI after treatment of locally advanced rectal cancer: How to report tumor response-the MERCURY experience. *AJR Am J Roentgenol* 199(4):W486–W495.

[87] Nagtegaal I, Gaspar C, Marijnen C et al. (2004) Morphological changes in tumour type after radiotherapy are accompanied by changes in gene expression profile but not in clinical behaviour. *J Pathol* 204:183–192.

[88] Yeo SG, Kim DY, Kim TH et al. (2010) Tumor volume reduction rate measured by magnetic resonance volumetry correlated with pathologic tumor response of preoperative chemo-radiotherapy for rectal cancer. *Int J Radiat Oncol Biol Phys* 78(1):164–171.

[89] Kim YC, Lim JS, Keum KC et al. (2011) Comparison of diffusion-weighted MRI and MR volumetry in the evaluation of early treatment outcomes after preoperative chemoradiotherapy for locally advanced rectal cancer. *J Magn Reson Imaging* 34(3):570–576.

[90] Kang JH, Kim YC, Kim H et al. (2010) Tumor volume changes assessed by three-dimensional magnetic reso- nance volumetry in rectal cancer patients after preoperative chemoradiation: The impact of the volume reduction ratio on the prediction of pathologic complete response. *Int J Radiat Oncol Biol Phys* 76(4):1018–1025.

[91] Barbaro B, Fiorucci C, Tebala C et al. (2009) Locally advanced rectal cancer: MR imaging in prediction of response after preoperative chemotherapy and radiation therapy. *Radiology* 250(3):730–739.

[92] Torkzad MR, Lindholm J, Martling A et al. (2007) MRI after preoperative radiotherapy for rectal cancer; correlation with histopathology and the role of volumetry. *Eur Radiol* 17(6):1566–1573.

[93] Curvo-Semedo L, Lambregts DM, Maas M et al. (2011) Rectal cancer: Assessment of complete response to preoperative combined radiation therapy with chemotherapy—Conventional MR volumetry versus diffusion-weighted MR imaging. *Radiology* 260(3):734–743.

[94] Kim DJ, Kim JH, Lim JS et al. (2010) Restaging of rectal cancer with MR imaging after concurrent chemotherapy and radiation therapy. *RadioGraphics* 30(2):503–516.

[95] Kim SH, Lee JM, Hong SH et al. (2009) Locally advanced rectal cancer: Added value of diffusion-weighted MR imaging in the evaluation of tumor response to neoadjuvant chemo- and radiation therapy. *Radiology* 253(1):116–125.

[96] Sun YS, Zhang XP, Tang L et al. (2010) Locally advanced rectal carcinoma treated with preoperative chemotherapy and radiation therapy: Preliminary analysis of diffusion-weighted MR imaging for early detection of tumor histopathologic downstaging. *Radiology* 254(1):170–178.

[97] Lambregts DM, Vandecaveye V, Barbaro B et al. (2011) Diffusion-weighted MRI for selection of complete responders after chemoradiation for locally advanced rectal cancer: A multicenter study. *Ann Surg Oncol* 18(8): 2224–2231.

[98] Kim SH, Lee JY, Lee JM et al. (2011) Apparent diffusion coefficient for evaluating tumour response to neoadjuvant chemoradiation therapy for locally advanced rectal cancer. *Eur Radiol* 21(5):987–995.

[99] Rao SX, Zeng MS, Chen CZ et al. (2008) The value of diffusion-weighted imaging in combination with T2-weighted imaging for rectal cancer detection. *Eur J Radiol* 65(2):299–303.

[100] Feliu J, Calvilio J, Escribano A et al. (2002) Neo-adjuvant therapy of rectal carcinoma with UFT-leucovorin plus radiotherapy. *Ann Oncol* 13(5):730–736.

[101] Fernandez-Martos C, Aparicio J, Bosch C et al. (2004) Preoperative uracil, tegafur, and con-comitant radiotherapy in operable rectal cancer: A phase II multicenter study with 3 years' follow-up. *J Clin Oncol* 22(15):3016–3022.

[102] Barbaro B, Vitale R, Leccisotti L et al. (2010) Restaging locally advanced rectal cancer with MR imaging after chemoradiation therapy. *RadioGraphics* 30(3):699–716.

[103] Prasad DS, Scott N, Hyland R et al. (2010) Diffusion-weighted MR imaging for early detection of tumor histopathologic downstaging in rectal carcinoma after chemotherapy and radiation therapy. *Radiology* 256(2):671–672; author reply 672.

[104] Lezoche G, Baldarelli M, Guerrieri M et al. (2008) A prospective randomized study with a 5-year minimum follow-up evaluation of transanal endoscopic microsurgery versus laparoscopic total mesorectal excision after neoadjuvant therapy. *Surg Endosc* 22:352–358.

[105] Habr-Gama A, Perez RO, Proscurshim I et al. (2006) Patterns of failure and survival for nonoperative treatment of stage c0 distal rectal cancer following neoadjuvant chemoradiation therapy. *J Gastrointest Surg* 10:1319–1328.

[106] Dworak O, Keilholz L, Hoffmann A et al. (1997) Pathological features of rectal cancer after preoperative radiochemotherapy. *Int J Colorectal Dis* 12(1):19–23.

[107] Koh DM, Chau I, Tait D et al. (2008) Evaluating mesorectal lymph nodes in rectal cancer before and after neo-adjuvant chemoradiation using thin-section T2-weighted magnetic resonance imaging. *Int J Radiat Oncol Biol Phys* 71:456–461.

[108] Patel UB, Taylor F, Blomqvist L et al. (2011) Magnetic resonance imaging-detected tumor response for locally advanced rectal cancer predicts survival outcomes: MERCURY experience. *J Clin Oncol* 29:3753–3760.

[109] King AD, Ahuja AT, Yeung DK et al. (2007) Malignant cervical lymphadenopathy: Diagnostic accuracy of diffusion-weighted MR imaging. *Radiology* 245:806–813.

[110] Nakai G, Matsuki M, Inada Y et al. (2008) Detection and evaluation of pelvic lymph nodes in patients with gynecologic malignancies using body diffusion-weighted magnetic resonance imaging. *J Comput Assist Tomogr* 32:764–768.

[111] Lahaye MJ, Beets GL, Engelen SM et al. (2009) Locally advanced rectal cancer: MR imaging for restaging after neoadjuvant radiation therapy with concomitant chemotherapy. Part II. What are the criteria to predict involved lymph nodes? *Radiology* 252(1):81–91.

[112] Vliegen RF, Beets GL, Lammering G et al. (2008) Mesorectal fascia invasion after neoadjuvant chemotherapy and radiation therapy for locally advanced rectal cancer: Accuracy of MR imaging for prediction. *Radiology* 246(2): 454–462.

[113] George ML, Dzik-Jurasz ASK, Padhani AR et al. (2001) Non-invasive methods of assessing angiogenesis and their value in predicting response to treatment in colorectal cancer. *Br J Surg* 88:1628–1636.

[114] Kremser C, Trieb T, Rudisch A et al. (2007) Dynamic T1 mapping predicts outcome of chemoradiation therapy in primary rectal carcinoma: Sequence implementation and data analysis. *J Magn Reson Imaging* 26:662–671.

[115] Sahani DV, Kalva SP, Hamberg LM et al. (2005) Assessing tumor perfusion and treatment response in rectal cancer with multi-section CT: Initial observations. *Radiology* 234:785.

[116] Zissin R, Gayer G (2004) Postoperative anatomic and pathologic findings at CT following colonic resection. *Semin Ultrasound CT MR* 25(3): 222–238.

[117] Tytherleigh MG, McC Mortensen NJ (2003) Options for sphincter preservation in surgery for low rectal cancer. *Br J Surg* 90:922–933.

[118] Corman M (2005) Carcinoma of the rectum. In: Corman M, ed. *Colon and Rectal Surgery*, 5th ed. Lippincott Williams & Wilkins, Philadelphia, PA, pp. 905–1061.

[119] Goldberg S, Klas JV (1998) Total mesorectal excision in the treatment of rectal cancer: A view from the USA. *Semin Surg Oncol* 15(2):87–90.

[120] Dehni N, Tiret E, Singland JD et al. (1998) Long-term functional outcome after low anterior resection: Comparison of low colorectal anastomosis and colonic J-pouch-anal anastomosis. *Dis Colon Rectum* 41:817–822.

[121] Brittenden J, Tolan DJM (2012) *Radiology of the Post Surgical Abdomen*. Springer, London.

[122] Weinstein S, Osei-Bonsu S, Aslam R et al. (2013) Multidetector CT of the postoperative colon: Review of normal appearances and common complications. *RadioGraphics* 33(2):515–532.

[123] Bell SW, Dehni N, Chaouat M et al. (2005) Primary rectus abdominis myocutaneous flap for repair of perineal and vaginal defects after extensive abdominoperineal resection. *Br J Surg* 92:482–486.

[124] Taylor GI, Corlett R, Boyd JB (1983) The extended deep inferior epigastric flap: A clinical technique. *Plast Reconstr Surg* 72:751–765.

[125] Lee JK, Stanley RJ, Sagel SS et al. (1981) CT appearance of the pelvis after abdomino-perineal resection for rectal carcinoma. *Radiology* 141:737–741.

[126] Kelvin FM, Korobkin M, Heaston DK et al. (1983) The pelvis after surgery for rectal carcinoma: Serial CT observations with emphasis on nonneoplastic features. *AJR Am J Roentgenol* 141(5):959–964.

[127] Even-Sapir E, Parag Y, Lerman H et al. (2004) Detection of recurrence in patients with rectal cancer: PET/CT after abdomino-perineal or anterior resection. *Radiology* 232(3):815–822.

[128] Scardapane A, Brindicini D, Fracella MR et al. (2005) Post colon surgery complications: Imaging findings. *Eur J Radiol* 53(3):397–409.

[129] DuBrow RA, David CL, Curley SA (1995) Anastomotic leaks after low anterior resection for rectal carcinoma: Evaluation with CT and barium enema. *AJR Am J Roentgenol* 165:567–571.

[130] Nicksa GA, Dring RV, Johnson KH et al. (2007) Anastomotic leaks: What is the best diagnostic imaging study? *Dis Colon Rectum* 50(2):197–203.

[131] Hoeffel C, Arrivé L, Mourra N (2006) Anatomic and pathologic findings at external phased-array pelvic MR imaging after surgery for anorectal disease. *RadioGraphics* 26(5):1391–1407.

[132] So JB, Palmer MT, Shellito PC (1997) Postoperative perineal hernia. *Dis Colon Rectum* 40:954–957.

[133] Jain KA (2000) Imaging of peritoneal inclusion cysts. *AJR Am J Roentgenol* 174:1559–1563.

[134] Messiou C, Chalmers AG, Boyle K (2006) Surgery for recurrent rectal carcinoma. The role of magnetic resonant imaging. *Clin Rad* 61:250–258.

[135] Heidary B, Phang TP, Raval MJ, Brown CJ (2014) Transanal endoscopic microsurgery: A review. *Can J Surg* 57(2):127–138.

[136] Kunitake H, Abbas MA (2012) Transanal endoscopic microsurgery for rectal tumors: A review. *Perm J* 16(2):45–50.

[137] Guerrieri M, Baldarelli M, Morino M et al. (2006) Transanal endoscopic microsurgery in rectal adenomas: Experience of six Italian centres. *Dig Liver Dis* 38(3):202–207.

[138] Guerrieri M, Baldarelli M, Organetti L et al. (2008) Transanal endoscopic microsurgery for the treatment of selected patients with distal rectal cancer: 15 years experience. *Surg Endosc* 22(9):2030–2035.

[139] Floyd ND, Saclarides TJ (2006 Feb) Transanal endoscopic microsurgical resection of pT1 rectal tumors. *Dis Colon Rectum* 49(2):164–168.

[140] Bach SP, Hill J, Monson JR et al. (2009) Association of coloproctology of Great Britain and Ireland Transanal Endoscopic Microsurgery (TEM) Collaboration. A predictive model for local recurrence after transanal endoscopic microsurgery for rectal cancer. *Br J Surg* 96(3):280–290.

[141] Endreseth BH, Wibe A, Svinsås M et al. (2005) Postoperative morbidity and recurrence after local excision of rectal adenomas and rectal cancer by transanal endoscopic microsurgery. *Colorectal Dis* 7(2):133–137.

[142] Baatrup G, Elbrønd H, Hesselfeldt P et al. (2007) Rectal adenocarcinoma and transanal endoscopic microsurgery. Diagnostic challenges, indications and short term results in 142 consecutive patients. *Int J Colorectal Dis* 22(11):1347–1352.

[143] Kreissler-Haag D, Schuld J, Lindemann W et al. (2008) Complications after transanal endoscopic microsurgical resection correlate with location of rectal neoplasms. *Surg Endosc* 22(3):612–616.

[144] Stipa F, Burza A, Lucandri G et al. (2006) Outcomes for early rectal cancer managed with transanal endoscopic microsurgery: A 5-year follow-up study. *Surg Endosc* 20(4):541–545.

[145] Maslekar S, Pillinger SH, Monson JR (2007) Transanal endoscopic microsurgery for carcinoma of the rectum. *Surg Encosc* 21(1):97–102.

[146] Lezoche E, Guerrrieri M, Paganini AM et al. (1998) Transanal endoscopic microsurgical excision of irradiated and non-irradiated rectal cancer. *Surg Laparosc Endocsc* 8(4):249–256.

[147] Serra-Aracil X, Vallverdù H, Bombardó-Junca J et al. (2008) Long-term follow-up of local rectal cancer surgery by transanal endoscopic microsurgery. *World J Surg* 32(6):1162–1167.

[148] Lezoche E, Guerrrieri M, Paganini AM et al. (2005) Long-term results in patient with T2 - 3 N0 distal rectal cancer undergoing radiotherapy before transanal endoscopic microsurgery. *Br J Surg* 92(12):1546–1552.

[149] Gavagan JA, Whiteford MH, Swanstrom LL (2004) Full-thickness intraperitoneal excision by transanal endoscopic microsurgery does not increase short-term complications. *Am J Surg* 187(5):630–634.

[150] Said S, Stippel D (1995) Transanal endoscopic microsurgery in large, sessile adenomas of the rectum. A 10-year experience. *Surg Endosc* 9(10):1106–1112.

[151] Lee W, Lee D, Choi S et al. (2003) Transanal endoscopic microsurgery and radical surgery for T1 and T2 rectal cancer. *Surg End* 17(8):1283–1287.

[152] Winde G, Nottberg H, Keller R et al. (1996) Surgical cure for early rectal carcinomas (T1). Transanal endoscopic microsurgery vs anterior resection. *Dis Colon Rectum* 39(9):969–976.

[153] Lezoche E, Guerrieri M, Paganini AM et al. (2005) Transanal endoscopic versus total mesorectal laparoscopic resections of T2-N0 low rectal cancers after neoadjuvant treatment: A prospective randomized trial with 3-years 40.

[154] Duek SD, Issa N, Hershko DD et al. (2008) Outcome of transanal endo-scopic microsurgery and adjuvant radiotherapy in patients with T2 rectal cancer. *Dis Colon Rectum* 51(4):379–384.

[155] Habr-Gama A, de Souza PM, Ribeiro U Jr et al. (1998) Low rectal cancer: Impact of radiation and chemotherapy on surgical treatment. *Dis Colon Rectum* 41:1087–1096.

[156] Luna-Perez P, Rodriguez-Ramirez S, Rodriguez-Coria DF et al. (2001) Preoperative chemo-radiation therapy and anal sphincter preservation with locally advanced rectal adenocarcinoma. *World J Surg* 25:1006–1011.

[157] Medich D, McGinty J, Parda D et al. (2001) Preoperative chemoradiotherapy and radical surgery for locally advanced distal rectal adenocarcinoma: Pathologic findings and clinical implications. *Dis Colon Rectum* 44:1123–1128.

[158] Grann A, Minsky BD, Cohen AM et al. (1997) Preliminary results of preoperative 5-fluorouracil, low-dose leucovorin, and concurrent radiation therapy for clinically resectable T3 rectal cancer. *Dis Colon Rectum* 40:515–522.

[159] Janjan NA, Khoo VS, Abbruzzese J et al. (1999) Tumor downstaging and sphincter preservation with preoperative chemoradiation in locally advanced rectal cancer: The M. D. Anderson Cancer Center experience. *Int J Radiat Oncol Biol Phys* 44:1027–1038.

[160] Hiotis SP, Weber SM, Cohen AM et al. (2002) Assessing the predictive value of clinical complete response to neoadjuvant therapy for rectal cancer: An analysis of 488 patients. *J Am Coll Surg* 194:131–135.

[161] Habr-Gama A, Perez RO, Nadalin W et al. (2004) Operative versus nonoperative treatment for stage 0 distal rectal cancer following chemoradiation therapy: Long-term results. *Ann Surg* 240(4):711–717.

[162] Suppiah A, Hartley JE, Monson JR (2009) Advances in radiotherapy in operable rectal cancer. *Dig Surg* 26(3):187–199.

[163] Sainio P (1984) Fistula-in-ano in a defined population: Incidence and epidemiological aspects. *Ann Chir Gynaecol* 73(4):219–224.

[164] de Miguel Criado J, del Salto LG, Rivas PF et al. (2012) MR imaging evaluation of perianal fistulas: Spectrum of imaging features. *RadioGraphics* 32(1):175–194.

[165] Lilius HG (1968) Fistula-in-ano, an investigation of human foetal anal ducts and intramuscular glands and a clinical study of 150 patients. *Acta Chir Scand Suppl* 383:7–88.

[166] Parks AG (1961) Pathogenesis and treatment of fistula-in-ano. *BMJ* 1(5224):463–469.

[167] Halligan S, Buchanan G (2003) MR imaging of fistula-in-ano. *Eur J Radiol* 47(2):98–107.

[168] Ziech M, Felt-Bersma R, Stoker J (2009) Imaging of perianal fistulas. *Clin Gastroenterol Hepatol* 7(10):1037–1045.

[169] Halligan S, Stoker J (2006) State of the art: Imaging of fistula in ano. *Radiology* 239(1):18–33.

[170] Bartram C, Buchanan G (2003) Imaging anal fistula. *Radiol Clin North Am* 41(2):443–457.

[171] Delfaut EM, Beltran J, Johnson G et al. (1999) Fat suppression in MR imaging: Techniques and pitfalls. *RadioGraphics* 19(2):373–382.

[172] Haggett PJ, Moore NR, Shearman JD et al. (1995) Pelvic and perineal complications of Crohn's disease: Assessment using magnetic resonance imaging. *Gut* 36(3): 407–410.

[173] Haramati N, Penrod B, Staron RB et al. (1994) Surgical sutures: MR artifacts and sequence dependence. *J Magn Reson Imaging* 4(2):209–211.

[174] Yang RK, Roth CG, Ward RJ et al. (2010) Optimizing abdominal MR imaging: Approaches to common problems. *RadioGraphics* 30(1):185–199.

[175] Kim H, Lim JS, Choi JY et al. (2010) Rectal cancer: Comparison of accuracy of local-regional staging with two- and three-dimensional preoperative 3-T MR imaging. *Radiology* 254(2):485–492.

[176] Lichy MP, Wietek BM, Mugler JP et al. (2005) Magnetic resonance imaging of the body trunk using a single-slab, 3-dimensional, T2-weighted turbo-spin-echo sequence with high sampling efficiency (SPACE) for high spatial resolution imaging: Initial clinical experiences. *Invest Radiol* 40(12): 754–760.

[177] Proscia N, Jaffe TA, Neville AM et al. (2010) MRI of the pelvis in women: 3D versus 2D T2-weighted technique. *AJR Am J Roentgenol* 195(1):254–259.

[178] Schaefer O, Lohrmann C, Langer M et al. (2004) Assessment of anal fistulas with high-resolution subtraction MR-fistulography: Comparison with surgical findings. *J Magn Reson Imaging* 19(1):91–98.

[179] Morris J, Spencer JA, Ambrose NS (2000) MR imaging classification of perianal fistulas and its implications for patient management. *RadioGraphics* 20(3):623–635; discussion 635–637.

[180] Parks AG, Gordon PH, Hardcastle JD (1976) A classification of fistula-in-ano. *Br J Surg* 63(1):1–12.

[181] Bell SJ, Halligan S, Windsor AC et al. (2003) Response of fistulating Crohn's disease to infliximab treatment assessed by magnetic resonance imaging. *Aliment Pharmacol Ther* 17(3):387–393.

[182] Karmiris K, Bielen D, Vanbeckevoort D et al. (2011) Long-term monitoring of infliximab therapy for perianal fistulizing Crohn's disease by using magnetic resonance imaging. *Clin Gastroenterol Hepatol* 9(2):130–136.

[183] Keighley M, Williams N (2007) *Surgery of the Colon, Rectum and Anus*, 1st ed. Elsevier, London.

Chapter 26 创伤后及术后的腹部影像

Posttraumatic and Postsurgical Abdomen

Jose Luis Moyano-Cuevas, Juan Maestre-Antequera, Diego Masjoan, José Blas Pagador, Francisco Miguel Sánchez-Margallo 著

朱 正 译

冯 冰 校

目录 CONTENTS

一、术后 MRI 应用 / 618

二、创伤后 MRI 的应用 / 635

多个系统（肌肉骨骼、脑和髓质等）已普遍证明了MRI作为外科手术干预的非侵入性诊断和引导工具的有用性。主要来说，MRI的这些重大成果归因于其高对比分辨率，以及可使用多个序列以获得优异的组织特征的潜能。然而，在MRI序列已经不断优化、改善了性能、减少了其暴露时间，并增加了空间分辨率的情况下，其技术在腹部的应用直到最近几年才发展起来。如今，MRI的这些改进已经可以检测和分析大部分腹部器官和结构，这些器官和结构是高度可变形的，并且通常在腹腔内经历了复杂的形态变化和运动。出于这个原因，MRI技术在手术后的应用，随着对腹部干预的兴趣日益增加，在一些手术方案中得到了充分实施，在其他手术方案中的应用也越来越多。在这个意义上，根据外科专业，一些特定的MRI技术已被开发使用，例如MR尿路成像术、MR胰胆管成像术和MR血管成像术。

本章分为两个主题。首先，分析了术后MRI的应用，分为肝脏和肾脏术后两部分。此外，在每个部分中首先描述了MRI技术的术中辅助作用。其后，描述了对可能的并发症的术后监测。最后，目前创伤后MRI的应用非常有限，主要是因为严重创伤患者就医检查时间紧迫，本章末尾将简要介绍该主题。

传统上，MRI被用于肝脏局灶性病变和弥漫性疾病的诊断和特征描绘。其中，肝硬化可能是最常见的可使用MRI检测和诊断的肝脏弥漫性疾病之一。然而，由于MRI对肝细胞癌（hepatocellular carcinoma，HCC）和转移瘤的重要指导作用，本章的肝脏部分将主要集中在这两种疾病。此外，还分析了一些关于胆石症的问题，比较了内镜逆行胰胆管造影术（endoscopic retrograde cholangiopancreatography，ERCP）和MR胰胆管成像术（MR cholangiopancreatography，MRCP）。

在临床实践中，肾脏中最常见的影像技术是超声（ultrasound，US）和计算机断层扫描（computed tomography，CT），因为它容易获得、诊断结果良好和可承受的低成本。然而，当传统技术（US和CT）获得非结论性诊断时，MRI会被用来鉴别肿瘤。此外，在不能使用碘对比剂的情况下，MRI可作为替代的检查方法，并且是完美的术后监测技术。因此，在一（二）章节中将重点关注肾脏肿瘤和肾衰竭。

根据微创手术对不同腹部器官的影响，每个部分都会介绍一些关于手术期间气腹所引起的变化的最新发现。因此，在这些内容分析了肝脏和肾脏微创手术的几种形态学、血流动力学和功能变化。

最后，提高治疗质量和安全性的其他重要进展是影像引导治疗（image-guided therapy，IGT）。这种治疗方法促进了提高患者手术效果的所有进展。因此，MRI是目前应用于不同IGT的主要医学影像技术之一。尽管一些术中问题（包括图像配准和软组织变形等）在技术上很难解决且仍未解决，但IGT在几个特定领域的应用正在不断增加。本章不涉及这些技术方面，但本章将展示不同IGT中的MRI应用。

一、术后MRI应用

与开放手术相比，微创手术——更具体地说是腹腔镜手术——减小了手术切口，从而缩短了患者住院时间并优化了医疗费用[1-4]。尽管这些手术技术提高了患者的安全性，但术后可能出现多种并发症，这些并发症很大程度上取决于手术过程[5,6]。因此早期发现这些并发症对于确保患者安全至关重要，因为这些患者经常需要再次手术。从这个意义上讲，MRI在软组织分析中起着关键的作用（由于它的高对比度和更好的清晰度），可用于不同病变的早期诊断和特征描绘，以及手术结果和术后并发症的分析。因此，由于其在检测病变的高灵敏度和高特异性，MRI的作用已超过CT或US等其他诊断技术。在其他应用中，还可用于评估腹部一些脏器的肿瘤手术切缘、术后内出血的检测或胆道梗阻的识别。

本节描述MRI在腹部术后随访监测中的一些

最重要的功能和优点，主要聚焦于肝脏和肾脏。

（一）肝脏

肝脏是人体第二大器官，只有皮肤比肝脏更大更重。肝脏具有许多与消化、代谢、免疫和体内营养物质储存相关的基本功能。这些功能使它成为一个重要的器官，没有它，身体组织很快就会因缺乏能量和营养而死亡。

由于肝脏的这些特征，MRI被认为是诊断其病变的关键技术。虽然刚开始MRI并未完全被接受，但最近的研究已经证明了它的实用性和有效性[7]。与其他医学影像诊断技术（如CT）相比，MRI在检测和表征肝脏病变时更敏感。此外，MRI可对胆道系统进行无创观察，具有和其他诊断技术如内镜ERCP相似的灵敏度[8,9]。

屏气的T_1和T_2加权序列被用于肝脏的观察（图26-1）。屏气扫描是为了减少呼吸运动导致的图像伪影。需根据检查目的使用不同的扫描序列。

1. MRI在手术中的应用 介入和影像技术及其相关技术的快速发展带动了可改善手术结果的新治疗方法的出现。介入MRI就是其中的一个例子。介入MRI指代的是所有MRI引导的操作[10]。这些手术可以是微创的或是开放手术。由于传统磁共振空间有限，这些影像引导技术通常在开放式的磁共振中进行。在开放式磁共振中，由于它们的特性，很难获得高场强，这对图像质量有直接影响。由于这些局限性和手术室所需的特殊条件（非铁磁仪器和设备），这些影像引导的技术尚未被标准化。

在肝脏手术中，介入性MRI可应用于不同肿瘤（例如HCC）的热消融，因为它们是具有安全性高和恢复快的微创技术。这些技术通过经皮穿刺到达肿瘤位置并给予适当的治疗，例如射频（radio frequency，RF）、低温或微波，进而导致组织坏死。通过使用热能或低温来凝固或使肿瘤组织失活但不将其从患者体内移除，所产生的效果与手术切除的效果相当[11]。在该手术中，介入MRI为外科医师提供了肿瘤定位的信息，以及其他一些优势，例如治疗效果监测、高对比度软组织观察、成像平面自由选择、不需要碘对比剂、无电离辐射等。此外，MRI引导的HCC消融的有效性已在科学研究中得到证实[7,13]，在某些情况下，其性能优于其他引导技术，如US或CT。Clasen等[12]分析了56例HCC中RF治疗的有效性。他们比较了使用MRI和CT作为引导的消融技术的有效性，MRI引导的消融技术的结果更好。在冷冻消融治疗时，CT不能提供覆盖肿瘤的冰球的清晰图像，这限制了它的安全性和有效性。US引导被广泛用于消融治疗，但它有一些缺点，例如因为蒸发产生的气泡可能影响肿瘤组织的观察和热效应的监测[13]。这些缺点导致了肝脏肿瘤需重复进行RF治疗，因为在一次

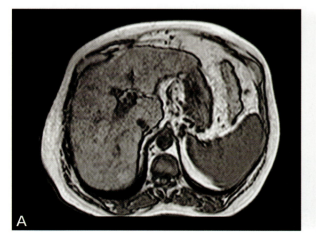
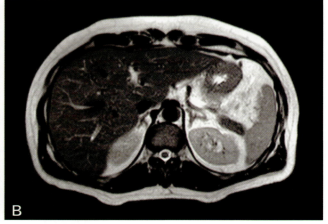

▲ 图26-1 腹部MRI的示例
A.45岁女性，肝脏屏气T_1加权图像；B.63岁男性，肝脏屏气T_2加权图像

消融过程中无法精确地了解治疗的程度[14]。

（1）气腹的作用：MRI 在微创手术中作为影像引导技术是有用的，同时它还增加了对腹腔镜手术期间腹部器官的了解。尽管腹腔镜手术具有优势[15]，但由于这种手术技术的性质，它也存在一定的困难和并发症。手术所需的气腹的负面影响就是其中一种并发症。

在腹腔镜手术中，增加腹内压以获得足够的腹部空间是必要的[15]。对于肝脏来说，气腹可引起肝脏的正常功能的改变，在腹腔镜手术后不同肝酶如丙氨酸氨基转移酶或天冬氨酸氨基转移酶的产生发生改变[16,17]。由于气腹的产生，也可导致肝动脉和门静脉的血流动力学变化。然而，关于这些变化仍有一些争论，因为一些作者显示在气腹期间门静脉的流量减少[18,19]，而其他人则描述了门静脉流量的增加[20]。因此，科学家们仍然在继续研究这些变化以及其导致的变化和事件链。

有一些技术可用于分析这些形态和功能变化，如食管探针和 US 探针以分析动脉血流，或基于患者通路的监测设备。它们都是侵入性技术。另一方面，MRI 可以非侵入性地分析腹部结构的形态学和血流动力学变化。

屏气 T_2 加权序列可用于分析肝脏的形态变化，T_1 加权序列同样可用于此目的。合适的层厚为 1～4mm，层之间没有间距，以便提取观察形态的变化。在气腹吹入前后分别进行 MRI 扫描，可分析肝脏的形态变化[21]。图 26-2 为 MRI 扫描的几个断层，显示了肝脏和腹部解剖结构在用气腹增加腹内压力后的变化。这些选定的层面显示了肝脏和其他腹部结构的压缩以及腹壁的扩张，以产生进行腹腔镜手术所需的空间。

在使用猪模型的实验条件下，当腹腔内压力增加至 14 mmHg，腹腔镜手术期间肝脏的平均体积显著增加了 57.67 cm^3 [21]。这种体积增加的原因尚不清楚，因为本研究没有分析门静脉血流。其他研究分析了猪模型在 15 mmHg 压力下的血流动力学变化，显示全身血管阻力增加，这可能使得静脉回流情况复杂化[22]。此外，一些作者显示当压力增加时，猪门静脉血流减少[18,19]。因此，静脉淤滞可能导致肝脏体积增加。

几个 DICOM 文件的图像处理软件可用于检索与 MRI 相关的信息并分析特定器官的参数，例如计算所选结构的体积。为此，需要预先在该序列的每个层面中用感兴趣区域（rigion of interest，ROI）勾画肝脏结构（图 26-3）。

当腹内压增加时也观察到肝脏的变形[21]。在这种情况下，猪肝的内外径增加、在腹内的基底

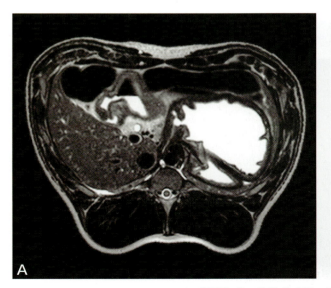
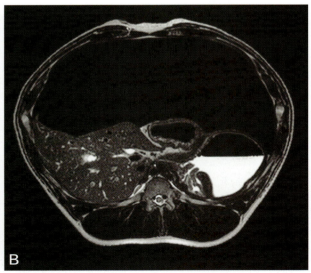

▲ 图 26-2　仰卧位 35kg 猪模型的 T_2 加权 MRI 图像
在气腹产生之前（A）和以 14mmHg 的压力产生气腹后（B）获得的图像。观察到腹部结构的变形

位置发生变化。图 26-4 显示了在气腹吹气之前和之后相同受试者（猪模型）的冠状位，其中可以观察到肝脏的内外侧径向左侧延伸。这种反应是由于压力的增加。因此，通过计算矢状位图像上肝脏出现的层数、相应厚度、层间距，可以获得这些参数。

腹腔镜手术所需的腹内压增加引起血流动力学变化，这已在科学文献中被广泛描述。MRI 序列期相对比可以用非侵入性方式分析血流量和其他血流动力学参数，这一点已经使用其他金标准技术进行过验证[23]。虽然尚无在腹腔镜肝脏手术期间腹部血流情况的分析，但 MRI 可分析肝脏的大血管（例如门静脉）的形态学变化。为此目的，可以使用高分辨率 T_2 加权序列来获得门静脉管腔的图像，以此观察其在手术期间的形态变化。图 26-5 为猪模型在压力增加前后的图像。这些图像显示背侧 - 腹侧轴上的门静脉管腔变窄。在这项研究中，沿着血管测量了 3 次，从腹腔干（第一次测量）到腹腔干上方 4cm 的位置（第三次测量）。

2. 术后表现 术后与患者安全相关的主要有两个方面：监测手术的疗效和早期识别手术导致的并发症。从这个意义上讲，MRI 在手术治疗后的肿块监测或肝移植术后的术后问题的鉴定中起着至关重要的作用。随后的部分将描述 MRI 观察到的情况和并发症，并根据肝脏的病变进行分类。

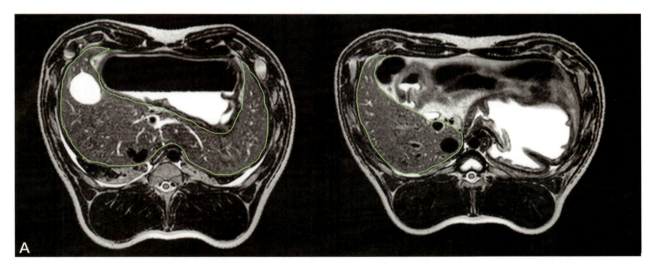

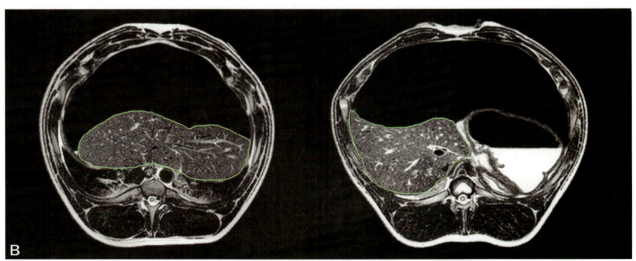

▲ 图 26-3　仰卧位 35kg 猪模型的 T_2 加权 MRI 图像
在气腹产生前（A）后（B）用 OXiris 可视化 DICOM 软件进行肝脏手动分割，以评估肝脏体积的变化

（1）肝脏肿瘤

① HCC：根据美国的数据，近年来原发性肝癌的发病率有所增加：从 1999 年的 2.3 人/100 000 人增加到 2008 年的 4.2 人/100 000 人[24]。HCC 是最常见的原发性肝癌，占 80%。HCC 分别是成年男性和女性中排名第五和第七的最常见癌症，也是全球癌症死亡的第二大原因[25]。

可以使用 T_2 加权序列确定 HCC 的初始诊断（图 26-6）。顺磁性钆对比剂增强的动态 T_1 加权序列可排除一些良性病变（如血管瘤），了解病变的血供，以及是否存在无强化区域，无强化区域可能意味着瘤内坏死。这些动态增强序列的每个层面均由四个不同图像组成：增强前以及动脉期、门静脉期和静脉期的图像（图 26-7）。血管瘤表现为向心性渐进性强化，强化持续存在，是血管瘤的特征性增强模式，因为这些病变是由

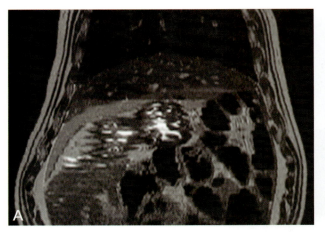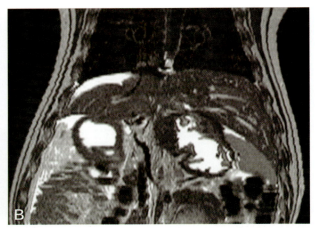

▲ 图 26-4　仰卧位 35kg 猪模型的冠状位 T_2 加权图像

通过将压力增加至 14 mmHg 来分析肝脏所经历的内 - 外侧扩张

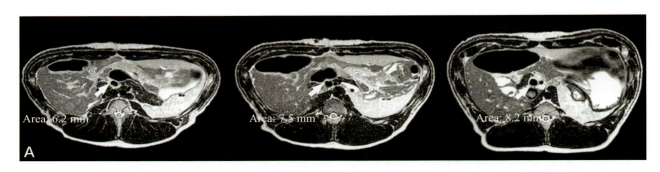
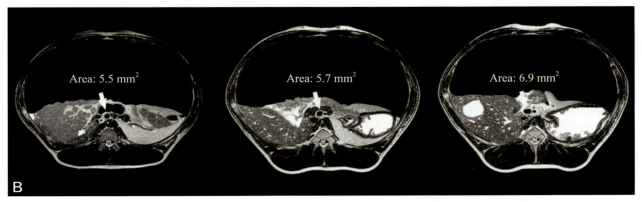

▲ 图 26-5　仰卧位 33kg 猪模型的 T_2 加权图像

分析气腹创建前（A）和后（B）不同位置的门静脉管腔的情况。将压力增加至 14mmHg，观察到静脉管腔的缩小

Chapter 26 创伤后及术后的腹部影像
Posttraumatic and Postsurgical Abdomen

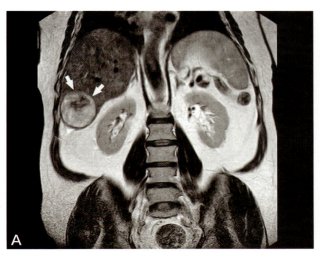 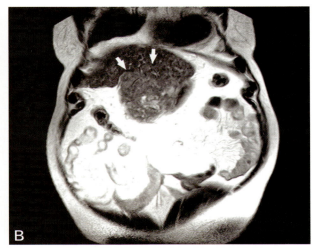

▲ 图 26-6　1 例 70 岁男性患者，有 2 个肝细胞肝癌的病灶，肿瘤病灶的冠状位 T$_2$ 加权图像

A. 最大病灶位于肝Ⅲ和Ⅳ段的交界处，直径为 8.9 cm；B. 最小病变的直径为 5.9 cm，位于肝Ⅴ和Ⅵ段。两者都是实性病变

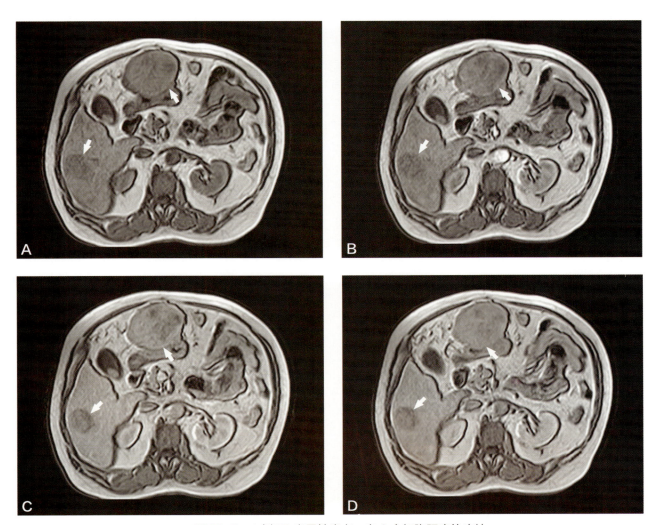

▲ 图 26-7　1 例 70 岁男性患者，有 2 个细胞肝癌的病灶

2 个病灶在增强前（A）、动脉期（B）、门静脉期（C）和静脉期（D）的 T$_1$ 加权图像。2 个病灶在 4 个时相，相对于肝实质均为低信号，在动脉期可见小区域的强化

血管的细胞组成，肿瘤内部流动缓慢[26]。另一方面，HCC 病变与肝实质相比，各期均为低信号，在动脉期有小的高信号灶，而在其后期的各期中信号减低。此外，肿瘤的中心区域在各期强化均减低。不典型增生结节（HCC 的前驱病变）在癌变过程中，随着新生的动脉血管（窦壁毛细血管化现象），动脉血供逐渐取代静脉血供[27]。如前所述，所研究的两个期相中的那些无强化区可能与肿瘤坏死区域相关。

此外，建议使用具有脂肪抑制的 T_2 加权序列来完成诊断，排除脂肪性病变，并确认初始假设（图 26-8）。

根据肿瘤的特征和位置不同，HCC 有不同类型的手术治疗方法。尽管肝切除术是首选的治疗方法，但由于以下几个原因，它在很大一部分的病例中并不适用：肿瘤的位置、切除后残余肝脏体积不足，或可能导致肿瘤扩散。另一方面，肝移植治疗效果好，但临床应用受限，主要是由于受体选择的标准非常苛刻，成本高，并且供体有限[28]。其他技术，例如微创消融治疗，为患者提供了许多获益，但对技术需求和临床医师的手术技巧要求高。这些微创疗法基于不同的物理原理来实现肿瘤坏死。其中一些使用高温（射频和微波消融），而另一些使用低温（冷冻消融）或高强度聚焦超声（high intensity focused ultrasound, HIFU）或聚焦超声（focused ultrasound surgery, FUS）。尽管所有这些疗法都相应的优点和缺点，但 RF 和微波消融对于小于 5cm 的 HCC 非常有效，术后并发症发生率低。另一方面，冷冻消融和 HIFU 分别具有并发症发生率高和暴露时间长的缺点，这限制了它们目前的可应用性[29]。冷冻消融治疗最常见的并发症为出血、邻近器官的

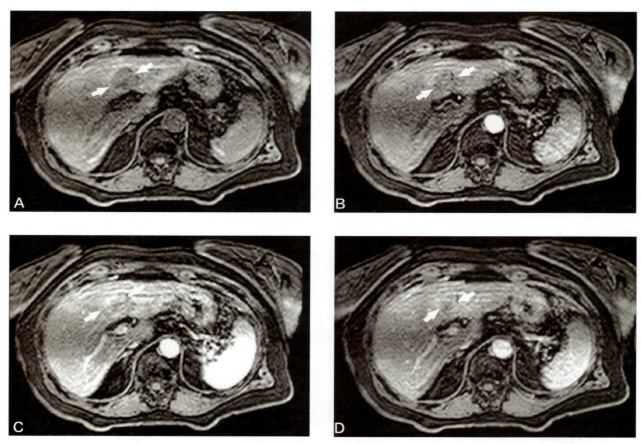

▲ 图 26-8　1 例 70 岁女性患者，患有肝血管瘤
血管瘤在钆增强前（A）和钆增强动脉期（B）、门静脉期（C）和静脉期（D）的屏气动态 T_1 加权图像。病变位于肝Ⅳ段，直径为 20～25mm

冷伤、肝破裂。然而，最近的研究表明，冷冻消融和 RF 治疗两者并发症的数量没有显著的统计学差异（图 26-9）[30]。

在治疗之后肝脏肿瘤的监测对于评估肿瘤体积（肿瘤缩小）、是否需要额外的疗程（重复治疗）或者定位相同或相邻器官中的新的肿瘤区域至关重要。因此，需经常进行多期增强 CT 或 MRI 以确定肿瘤消融成功。

MRI 用于评估的另一个重要用途是用于肿瘤栓塞的动脉内治疗。这些疗法包括用不同的方法，如经动脉栓塞、药物洗脱微球或放射性栓塞，阻断或减少供给病变的血管[31]。当由于肿瘤的位置或大小而不能进行受损区段的切除和其他消融技术时，肝肿瘤栓塞是常见的治疗方法。术后影像学检查，核实血管是否栓塞成功是明确治疗后肿瘤反应的基本措施。

栓塞后监测以评估治疗效果是至关重要的。MRI 可确定病变的营养血管的阻塞程度并分析肿瘤的大小变化。在这些情况下，扩散加权（diffusion-weighted，DW）序列是最佳选择。具体而言，DWI 测量游离水分子的微观迁移情况，可以通过表观扩散系数来量化[32]。因此，该医学影像技术可无创测量肿瘤营养血管的动脉阻塞情况以及病变的大小（血管阻塞和肿瘤缩小是所期望的），因为注射对比剂后不同时期的病变摄取的减少和病变表现的变化均可通过 DWI 序列轻易地被检测出来。因此，使用和不使用对比剂所获得的图像之间没有差异，意味着准确的动脉栓塞。在这种情况下，通过血管系统的对比剂不能到达肿瘤，从而导致了肿瘤组织的坏死（图 26-10 和图 26-11）。尽管肿瘤本身表现为低强化，存在与不存在对比剂时，其信号没有差异，并不能证明肿瘤成分的减少（图 26-12B）。

除 DWI 外，另一个常见的用于评估栓塞治疗结果的序列，是脂肪抑制的 T_2 序列（图 26-12）。该 T_2 序列同样可以观察肿瘤大小的变化并评估治疗后肿瘤的变化。

②转移瘤：肝脏是胃肠原发性肿瘤的常见转移部位[33]。大多数来源于结直肠癌，高达 55% 的结直肠癌患者最终会出现肝转移。其他原发癌症由于位置邻近或其他转移途径（如血行转移）也可能引起肝转移。其中最常见的是乳腺癌、胰腺癌、胃癌或神经内分泌癌。Weinrich 等展示了一个例子，他们回顾性地分析了乳腺癌与肝转移的相关性，相关率为 2%～12%[34]。

肝转移瘤切除术可提高不同原发癌患者的生存率。根据文献，乳腺癌转移瘤切除的第一年存活率为 77%～100%；第二年为 50%～86%；第

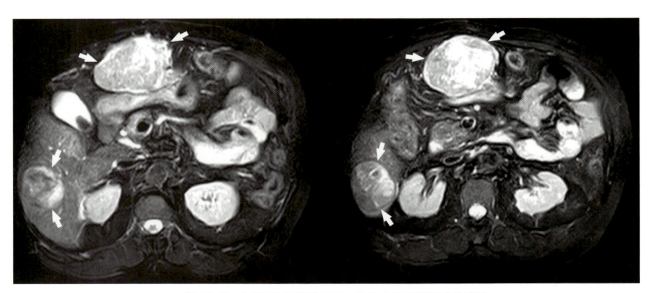

▲ 图 26-9 1 例 70 岁男性患者，有 2 个肝细胞肝癌的病灶
脂肪抑制的 T_2 加权图像可确认肿瘤的诊断。在图像中可以看到病变的非脂质性质

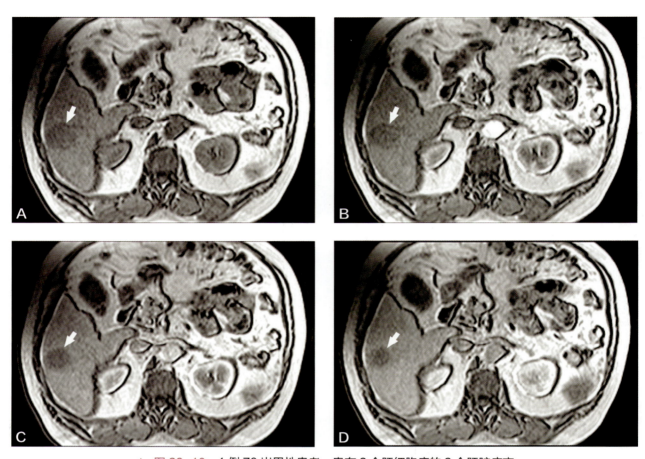

▲ 图 26-10 1 例 70 岁男性患者，患有 2 个肝细胞癌的 2 个肝脏病变

这名男性接受了动脉内栓塞治疗。在栓塞治疗 2 个月后获得位于 Ⅴ 和 Ⅵ 段病变的图像。增强前（A）、钆增强动脉期、门静脉和静脉期（B～D）的病变图像没有区别。表明动脉阻塞是足够的，因为使用钆不会使肿瘤强化

五年为 9%～61%[34]。另一方面，结直肠癌的肝转移切除术使患者的生存率从 0%～1% 提高到 31%～58%[35]。

影像学检查对于肝转移切除术的计划和监测来说是必需的。出于这个原因，一些作者评估了这些检查技术的有效性。Floriani 等[34] 对 6030 例临床病例进行了大量回顾，分析了不同成像方式识别和表征肝脏肿瘤的能力，结果为 US（63%～97%）、CT（74.8%～95.6%）和 MRI（80.1%～97.2%）。根据这些结果，MRI 的有效性似乎是最高的，仅次于研究中 FDG-PET（fluorodeoxyglucose-positron emission tomography）的 93.8%～98.7% 的灵敏度。然而，术前化疗所引起的肝实质改变可导致肿瘤轮廓的变化，在这些病例中，MRI 的敏感性高于 FDG-PET[36]。由于这些原因以及 Legou 等的观点[37]，MRI 是鉴别和表征肝转移的最佳影像学技术。

至于其他干预措施，肝转移切除术需要进行随访监测，以确定切缘是否合适、肿瘤组织是否被完全切除（图 26-13）。为了安全、非侵入性地实现这一目的，MRI 序列可用于区分健康和恶性组织以及术后的积液。手术后，T_2 序列可用于识别原转移瘤所在区域的术后积液，以评估手术治疗的有效性（图 26-14）。因此，这些序列可用于区分肝脏术区积液与囊肿。囊肿信号均匀，但是术后积液信号不均匀，由信号有差异的不同的液体成分组成。

③ 胆石症：很大比例的人群都有胆囊结石[38]，其中一些患者也患有胆总管结石[39,40]。其病理是指胆总管中出现结石，可引起其他更危险的问题如胆管炎或急性胰腺炎，严重影响患者健康。传统上，内镜下 ERCP 被认为是诊断和治

Chapter 26 创伤后及术后的腹部影像
Posttraumatic and Postsurgical Abdomen

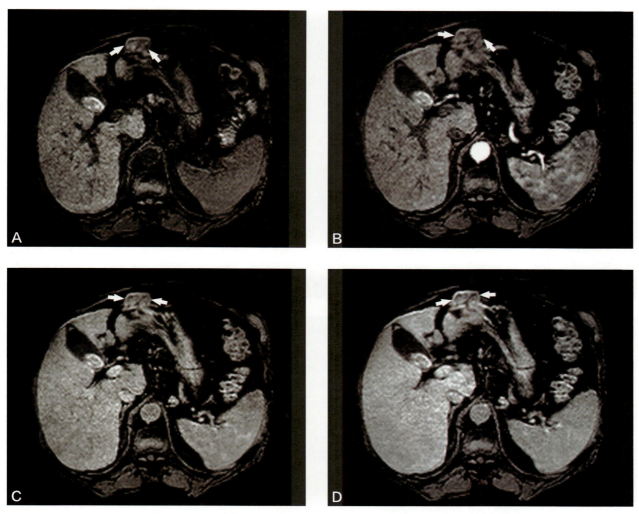

▲ 图 26-11　1 例 70 岁男性患者，患有 2 个肝细胞癌的 2 个肝脏病变

这名 70 岁男性接受了动脉内栓塞治疗。在栓塞治疗 2 个月后获得位于肝Ⅲ和Ⅳ段的病灶的图像。增强前（A）、钆增强动脉期、门静脉和静脉期（B～D）的病变图像没有区别。然而，肿瘤的大小并没有缩小

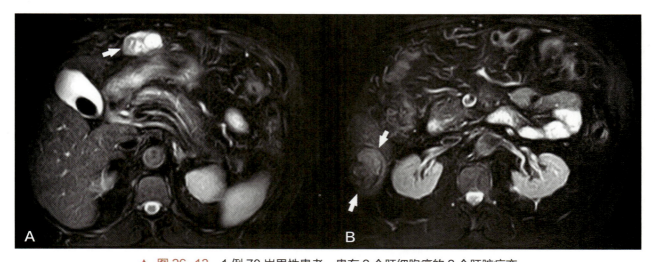

▲ 图 26-12　1 例 70 岁男性患者，患有 2 个肝细胞癌的 2 个肝脏病变

这名 70 岁男性接受了动脉内栓塞治疗。栓塞后的 T_2 加权脂肪抑制图像。相对于图 3-10B 的大小，我们观察到位于Ⅲ段和Ⅳ段的 4cm 病灶的缩小。与诊断时的图像相比，位于Ⅵ段的病变没有明显的缩小（图 3-10A）

627

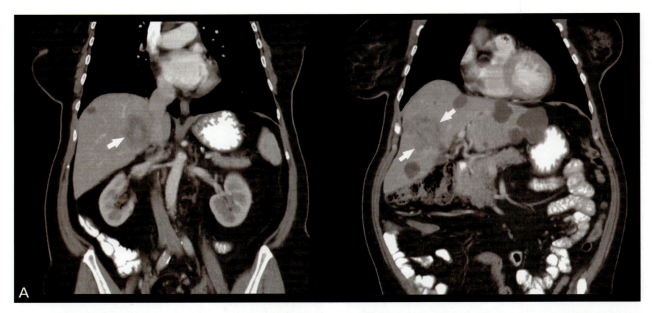

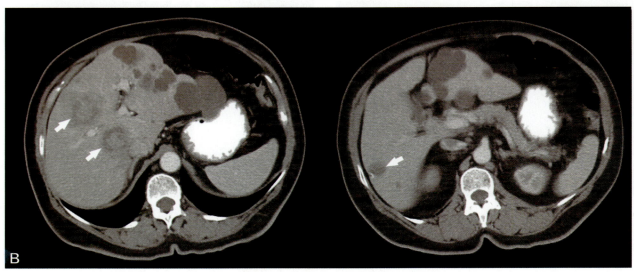

▲ 图 26-13　1 例 69 岁女性患者，伴有单纯囊肿和肝转移瘤

肝冠状位（A）和轴位（B）的 CT 证实了肝左、右叶囊肿的诊断，最大的囊肿位于肝Ⅱ段，直径为 5.3 cm。此外，在这些图像中，我们可以看见位于肝Ⅷ段的 5cm 的转移瘤和其后的 4cm 的转移瘤，伴有边缘强化。这些是来源于结直肠癌的转移瘤

疗胆总管结石的金标准。它们的应用范围很广，一些作者计划将 MRCP 纳入胆总管结石诊断规范中[41-43,44]。尽管其具有最高的灵敏度和诊断效能，均为 95% 左右[39,44,45]，但它可能会导致严重的并发症。此外，另外一些作者认为其应用受限，主要是由于其成本和可获得性[46]。

MRCP 在将背景和其他液体如血液饱和后，可获得静态液体信号，不需要使用对比剂。该技术的敏感性和特异性分别为 85%～92% 和 93%～97%[47,48]。然而，CT 胆管成像与 MRCP 具有相似的敏感性和特异性，但 CT 需要使用对比剂，并且患者暴露于电离辐射下，从而阻碍了 CT 胆管成像成为胆总管结石的最终诊断方法。

MRCP 的其他常见非术前应用是评估胆囊切除术后的并发症。其中，该手术最常见的并发症是由胆石症引起的胆漏或胆管阻塞。这些问题通常在手术后几天出现。具体来说，胆石症可以来自胆囊切除术，在术前检查中观察到结石或者

Chapter 26 创伤后及术后的腹部影像
Posttraumatic and Postsurgical Abdomen

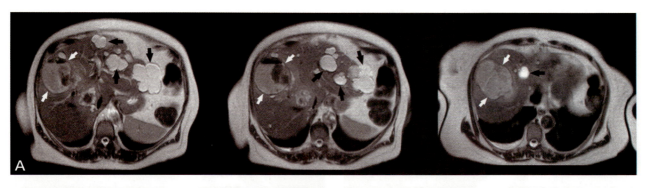

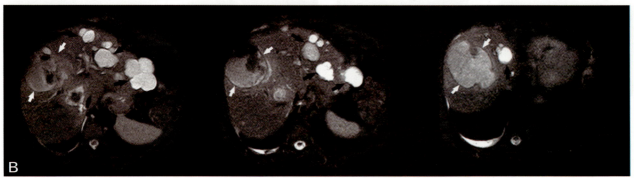

▲ 图 26-14 1 例 69 岁女性患者，肝 VIII 段转移瘤切除术后

术后获得 T₂ 加权（A）和 T₂ 加权脂肪抑制（B）图像。图像中未见残留病变，术后仅可见 8cm 的积液（白色箭）。相比于诊断时的图像（图 3-14），囊肿（黑色箭）没有变化

在外科手术之后在胆总管内形成胆结石。在这些情况下，建议使用 MRCP 代替 ERCP 作为进行胆囊切除术后的首选监测方法，主要是基于它的高精确度[49]。胆总管扩张是 MRCP 常观察到的并发症（图 26-15），是胆囊切除术后常见的并发症。此外，当和轴位 T₂ 加权序列联合使用时，MRCP 可以评估胰管的轻度扩张（图 26-16）、分析胰腺炎的性质[50]。这项工作描述了几项研究中胆总管的不同扩张程度。Pavone 等[51]证实了这项技术的准确性，也显示了所有研究的慢性胰腺炎病例的胰管扩张和管腔狭窄。其他可以用 MRCP 分析的并发症是腹水（腹部液体积聚）。T₂ 加权图像和压脂的 T₂ 加权图像可以鉴别腹水和其他物质如脂肪（图 26-17）。

（二）肾脏

肾脏是一个豆状的腹膜后器官，位于第 12 胸椎和第 4 腰椎之间的脊柱两侧。该器官的主要功能是血液过滤和清除废物及过量的成分。

肾脏 MRI 的研究增加了其诊断用途，可以用来评估不同的疾病。它们相对于其他影像技术的主要优点是可用于评估肿瘤分期和病变特征，可用于鉴别囊实性病变，甚至可用于术后病变监测。此外，它可以进行尿路成像检查以了解肾功能。

下面将讲述一些 MRI 的术中辅助应用，以及肾脏切除术后并发症的评估和监测作用。

1. MRI 的术中应用 MRI 可引导不同的肾脏手术操作，可提供具有高对比度和清晰软组织的图像。介入性 MRI 的研究更侧重在其他手术领域，如肝脏或前列腺肿瘤消融。

（1）引导工具：虽然 MRI 在肾脏手术中的应用并没有扩展，但有一些肾脏介入的病例使用 MRI 作为引导工具。影像引导的经皮肾造瘘术是一种成熟的微创手术，该手术是将导管放入尿路梗阻患者的肾集合系统中以引流尿液。该外科手术通常在 US 和透视的联合双成像技术的引导下进行。然而，这两种技术都存在一些局限性，例

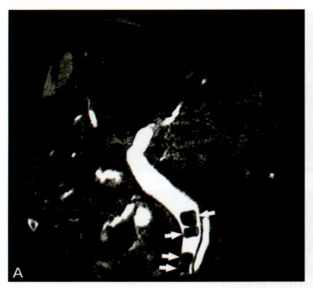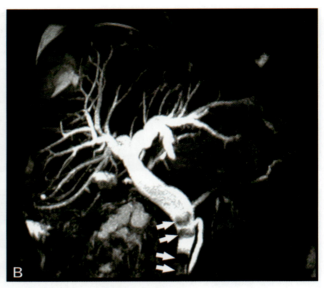

▲ 图 26-15　1 例 60 岁男性患者在胆囊切除术后出现胆总管结石

术后获得 MRCP（A）和 MRCP 的 MIP 重建（B）图像。可以观察到由于 4 块直径在 6～10mm 的结石所导致的 17mm 的胆总管扩张

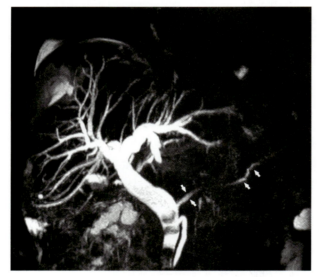

▲ 图 26-16　1 例 60 岁男性患者在胆囊切除术后出现胆总管结石

术后获得 MRCP 的 MIP 重建图像。可以观察到由于四块直径在 6～10mm 的结石所导致的 17mm 的胆总管扩张

如肠内气体可降低 US 的图像质量、透视检查需使用静脉内对比剂及电离辐射。另一方面，MRI 引导下的肾造瘘术是一种可行且安全的手术，在肾盂扩张[52] 和无肾盂扩张时均可进行[53]。从这个意义上说，Fischbach 等[53] 的研究表明这项技术的实用性超过了 US，本研究的所有患者由于以下几个原因不适合用 US 进行引导：一般状况非常差，只可以在 US 引导不常使用的仰卧或半侧卧位下进行操作，无肾盂扩张或肥胖；在这些情况下可用 MRI 进行引导。此外，MRI 引导还具有其他优点，例如图像不受肠气的干扰或不需要对比剂。

肾肿瘤的消融治疗也可以在 MRI 引导下进行。与肝脏肿瘤一样，MRI 引导的肾肿瘤消融治疗优于其他引导技术，例如 US 或 CT。这些优点包括高对比度的图像、多平面成像能力以及对温度和血流的敏感性。此外，对于 RF、微波或冷冻消融等基于热能的技术，MRI 可以在治疗期间监测热组织破坏的区域，并有助于根据术中的情况进行调整[54]。在冷冻消融治疗时，MRI 可以识别产生的冰球，从而可以更准确地评估肿瘤切除边缘，以确保所有切缘都在治疗的工作区域内。一些作者已经对这些 MRI 引导的操作进行了分析，结果表明这些技术的效率很高（手术干预成功率为 91%～100%）[55,56]。通常，用于规划或辅助外科手术的 MRI 序列因消融技术和肿瘤的性质不同而有所差异。手术规划通常使用 T_2 加权、T_1 加权或快速回波序列进行。另一方面，术中 MRI 引导需用短回波时间的梯度回波序列（西门子的 FSIP 序列或飞利浦的 FFE 序列）[55]。

Chapter 26　创伤后及术后的腹部影像
Posttraumatic and Postsurgical Abdomen

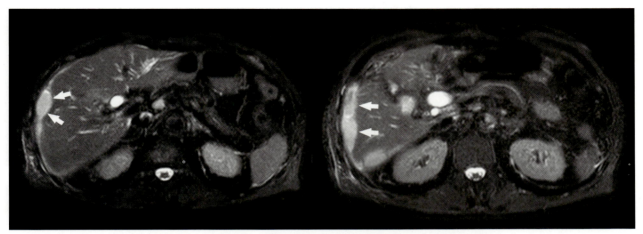

▲ 图 26-17　1 例 60 岁男性患者在胆囊切除术后出现胆总管结石
术后的 T_2 加权脂肪抑制图像，可以观察到腹水的存在

（2）气腹的作用：肾脏是腹膜后器官，因此腹腔镜手术期间所需的腹内压力的变化对它的影响是间接的。尽管如此，压力的增加引起肾功能的不同改变，其中肾血流量的显著减少和产生尿量的改变是最重要的[57]。

这些变化的分析是通过不同的技术完成的，例如静脉导管和尿量监测或活检[57]。所有这些技术都是在外科手术过程中进行的，因此外科手术本身的操作也会对观察到的效果产生影响。虽然这些变化已被广泛分析，但研究并未集中于评估可能的形态变化。与肝脏一样，MRI 是一种非侵入性的、无害的工具，可用于分析腹腔镜手术过程中肾脏的形态和功能变化，这要归功于其高对比度和对软组织的敏感性。这种方法已被用于分析动物实验中的变化[58]，但尚未应用于人类试验。

建议使用 T_2 加权序列来分析这些形态变化，因为它能够清晰观察双肾。层厚越小越好，但是由于需要考虑到成像时间，并且由于肾脏表面信号是均匀的，层厚可以达到 4～5mm。评估变化的方法需要采集 2 个 T_2 序列。第一个应该在患者静息状态下采集，第二个应该在气腹期间，在稳定 20min 后进行采集。

在腹腔镜检查腹腔压力增高达 12 mmHg 后，腹部结构的位置会发生重大变化（图 26-18）。由于肾脏比肝脏结构更紧密，因此图像中不会感觉到变形。但在对图像进行详细分析后，可观察到肾脏体积显著缩小。首先，在可观察到肾脏的每个层面手动完成肾脏的轮廓分割勾画。然后，使用 DICOM 可视化软件如 Osirix，获得分割区域的体积（图 26-19）。在气腹形成后，5 只实验动物肾脏体积的平均值从（75.71±11.73）cm^3 降至（73.14±12.39）cm^3 [58]。这种体积的缩小可能是由内脏承受的挤压造成的，也可能是由其他作者所描述的血管阻力引起的静脉怒张导致的[22]。关于肾脏的位置，因为它们是腹膜后器官，并没有可观察到的变化。最大面积也受到了压力增加的影响。

此外，除了对腹部器官的形态变化的分析，MRI 还可以无创性地分析动脉和静脉（例如肾动脉）中的血流。在气腹期间，使用 MRI 进行血流分析，有可能将气腹本身的影响与手术过程所造成的变化相区分开来。相位对比序列可用于此目的。该序列不需要使用对比剂，并且在处理之后，它可以分析血流量、血流速度或每搏输出量以及其他血流动力学参数。该序列的有效性已经在不同的血管血流中进行了科学的分析验证[59]。例如，该序列的作用已经在参数预知如人体模型的门静脉血流的分析中得到了验证。使用 MRI 获得的数值与流量的实际值之间显示出高度相关性[60]。通过将获得的结果与其他已验证的方法进行比较，相位对比序列的血流分析在肾动脉中应用也得到了验证[61-63]。尽管 MRI 的效用

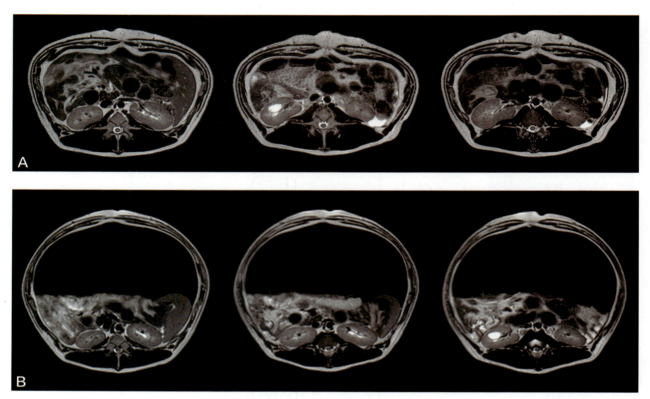

▲ 图 26-18　对体重 30kg 的猪模型进行 MRI 检查
T_2 加权图像显示了肾脏在气腹前和气腹后的变化

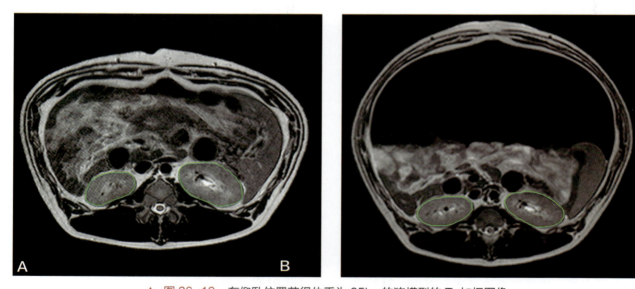

▲ 图 26-19　在仰卧位置获得体重为 35kg 的猪模型的 T_2 加权图像
用 Oxiris 可视化 DICOM 软件对肾脏进行人工分割，以评价在气腹生成前（A）和后（B）肾脏体积的变化

已经在正常结构的血管中得到了证实，但是当存在解剖变异或当动脉高度弯曲或扭曲时，结果会产生变化。因此，由于肾动脉尺寸缩小，进行血管造影以准确地设置该序列是很重要的（图 26-20）。

图 26-21 是在气腹产生前后所采集的动物模型的相位对比序列图像。腹内压的增加导致肾血流量的减少和肾动脉腔的缩小（图 26-22）。这些变化与文献中的其他发现一致，文献中，使用侵入性的方法，如在动脉周围放置超声探头或放置静脉导管，测量得到肾血流量的减少[57,64]。此外，

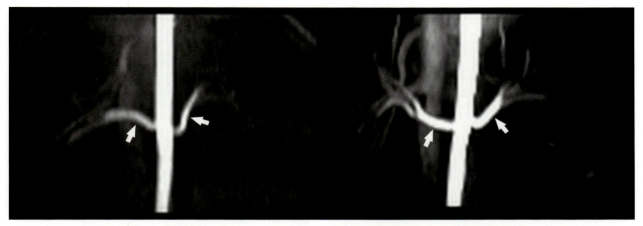

▲ 图 26-20　在体重为 33kg 和 32kg 的猪模型中获得的无对比剂主动脉和肾动脉血管成像
这些图像可以用于充分规划肾动脉的相位对比序列

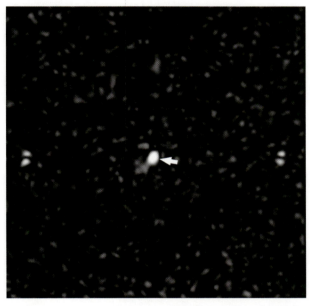

▲ 图 26-21　在体重为 31kg 的猪模型中获得的肾动脉的相位对比图

如文献中所述，肾动脉血流的减少可能导致腹腔镜期间肾功能的改变，例如尿液产生减少[57]。观察到的肾脏体积的增加也可能是肾动脉流量减少的一种结果。

(3) 手术后 MRI 的应用：肾脏手术的术后监测对于诊断和评估不同的并发症（例如出血的鉴定）至关重要，作为一项无创且无害的技术，MRI 是一种有用的诊断和监测方法，适用于多种外科手术如肿瘤切除术和术后并发症，例如肾移植术后。下一部分描述了几种肾脏疾病，MRI 作为诊断工具的优势以及外科手术可能引起的并发症。

① 肾脏肿瘤：肾细胞癌（renal cellcar cinoma，RCC）是成人中第八位最常见的恶性肿瘤[65]，也是肾脏中最常见的恶性肿瘤[66]。由于 US、CT 和 MRI 等医学影像技术的改进，近年检测到的 RCC 总数有所增加。

肾癌治疗的金标准是全肾切除术。然而，根据患者的肿瘤大小和肾脏状况，也可以进行肾部分切除术。肾部分切除术需要进行定期随访监测，以评估和控制病变的复发。由于这些原因，MRI 的监测应用正在增加，这得益于其图像的高对比度和可以区分肿瘤和囊性组织的特征。T_2 和 T_1 加权序列可以显示手术后肿瘤组织的缺失并区分单纯囊肿（图 26-23）。此外，尽管肾脏是腹膜后器官，但在切除肾脏后可引起腹部的一些解剖学变化，肾区可被腹部器官占据，例如胰尾或小肠襻（图 26-23）。

② 肾衰竭：肾衰竭指的是肾脏滤过功能及水电解质平衡的能力降低。当肾功能达到严重功能障碍且患者需要接受血液透析时，唯一的治疗方法就是肾移植。肾移植是目前最常用的方法之一，但也会出现并发症。具体而言，术后并发症非常危险，并且可能需要在术后早期再次介入以解决问题。不幸的是，很大一部分的再干预会导致移植肾功能的丧失[67]。根据文献，血管和泌尿系统

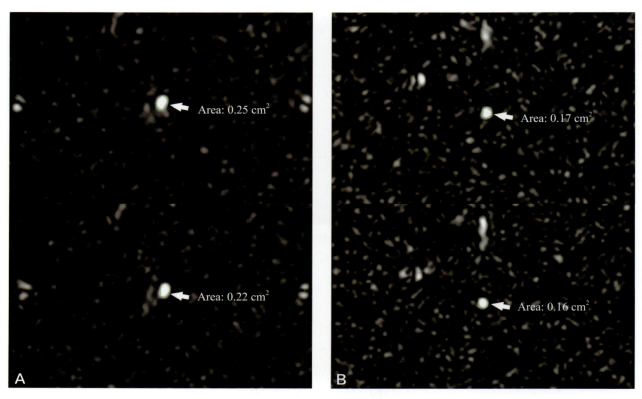

▲ 图 26-22　在仰卧位获得 30kg 的猪模型的相位对比图像
在气腹形成前（A）和后（B）人工分割肾动脉管腔。腹腔内压力增加到 14mmHg 后，肾动脉管腔缩小

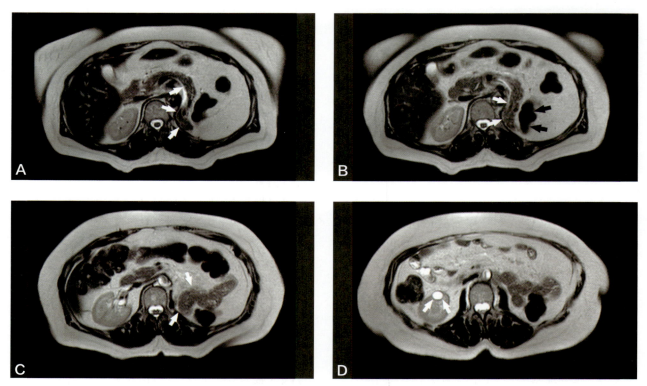

▲ 图 26-23　1 例 55 岁的女性肾细胞癌患者
这名患者接受了左肾的全肾切除。采用 T_2 加权图像评估手术结果。在图像中未见病变复发征象。此外，在肾切除术后，肾区被胰腺尾部（A、B）和小肠（B，黑箭和 C）占据。右肾可见大小为 16mm 的单纯囊肿（D）

问题是最常见的并发症[68,69]。由于这些原因，在术后早期阶段需要对患者进行详尽的监测诊断，以避免可能的并发症并提高移植肾的存活率。

肾动脉狭窄、肾静脉血栓形成、肾动脉血栓形成和术后出血是肾移植术后最常见的并发症。其中，肾动脉狭窄是最常见的[70]。评估这些血管并发症的金标准是数字减影血管造影（digital subtraction angiography, DSA），尽管其他成像技术如MR血管成像正在逐渐取代DSA；由于在MR血管成像中不需要使用碘对比剂，因此肾毒性降低。对于肾功能不全的患者来说，这是一个很大的优势，因为使用碘对比剂对他们损害过大。另一方面，MRI是一种非侵入性检查方法，可以避免使用导管，减少了术后早期再干预的需要。增强MR血管成像是一项基于MRI的技术，可获得与DSA相仿的效率，并且通过在若干研究中有效地分析血管解剖结构的状态已经证实了其有用性[71,72]。特别是，Huber等[73]设计了一项对比研究，比较MR血管成像和DSA的作用，以确定MR血管成像作为血管术后并发症监测工具的有用性和有效性。发现动脉血管上的显著狭窄的敏感性和特异性分别为100%和95%。最近的其他研究显示了在肾移植术后早期使用MR血管成像的一些发现[74]。通过这种方法，MR血管成像可以识别非常常见的术后并发症——肾血管吻合的轻度狭窄。

MR血管成像可观察肾移植相关的血管并发症。同样，MRI可观察到肾静脉压迫、肾同种异体移植和髂外静脉吻合术中的狭窄[73]或肾静脉血栓形成[75]。

尽管由于钆对比剂的损害小于离子对比剂，MRI在监测血管并发症和减少辐射剂量上具有优势，但最近也出现了一些肾源性系统性纤维化（nephrogenic systemic fibrosis, NSF）病例[76,77]。这些情况提示，在使用这些技术之前需要评估其使用的风险和益处。

尽管泌尿系统并发症的发生频率低于血管并发症，但它们对肾移植患者的存活率的影响也很大（图26-24）。根据文献报道，并发症发生率在2.5%~27%[67,78-80]。最常见的泌尿系统并发症是膀胱输尿管连接部狭窄、尿瘘、肾积水或结石等。早期发现这些并发症对于确保患者安全至关重要。从这个意义上讲，不同的医学影像检查在提高患者安全性方面发挥着重要作用。静脉US被认为是监测泌尿道并发症的金标准。然而，该技术需要离子型对比剂，并且这些对比剂对某些患者可能是有毒性的。因此，MRI检查是另一个可以在肾移植术后早期分析泌尿系统并发症的技术。增强MR尿路成像已被证明可在标准条件下观察尿路并识别肾移植后可能的并发症。其中一些并发症是由于输尿管压迫引起的输尿管狭窄或肾积水（图26-24）。此外，增强MR尿路成像通过对肾移植物和移植物区域进行最大密度投影重建，提供了比其他成像技术更高的图像质量。因此，MR尿路造影的灵敏度和特异性分别达到95.8%和93.3%[81]，其中尿路囊肿是比较难以检出的并发症之一。尽管其肾毒性低于碘化对比剂，但钆对比剂的使用可能会引起其他问题，例如NSF。由于这些原因，另一种可用于观察肾并发症的序列是重T_2加权MR尿路成像。该序列是非侵入性的，不需要造影剂并且可以在无肾毒性风险的情况下观察移植输尿管的解剖结构。然而，由于该序列是基于检测静态液体，因此只可以监测伴有肾积水的并发症。在这种情况下，重T_2加权序列和增强MR尿路成像在识别狭窄和输尿管梗阻的敏感性和特异性之间没有显著差异[81]。

二、创伤后MRI的应用

高性能MR梯度系统与快速梯度回波序列相结合，主要为屏气序列，缩短了图像采集时间。尽管如此，MRI在腹部创伤患者诊断中的应用是有限的。这是由于急救中心的MRI检查不易获得，图像采集时间较长，诊断检查成本较高[82]。

然而，在对碘对比剂过敏的情况下或在对肝、

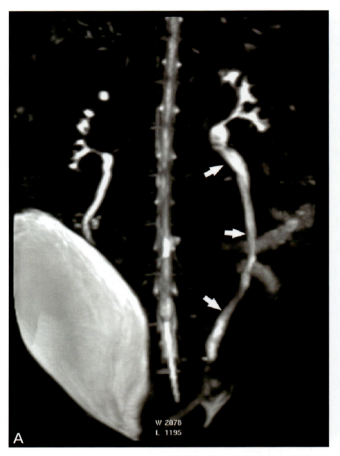 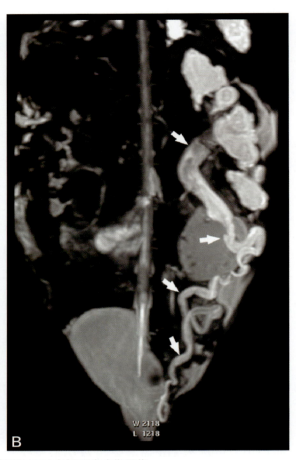

▲ 图 26-24　体重 33kg 猪模型中获得的无对比剂尿路成像图像
A、B. 由于膀胱输尿管梗阻，在两幅图像中均可观察到肾盂积水

脾、胰、肾损伤保守治疗的情况下，可用钆增强的 MRI 进行检查监测。此外，没有电离辐射是 MRI 的一个优点，特别适合儿科患者出现腹内实质性脏器损伤在保守治疗中需要反复检查的情况[83]。

在肝外伤中，MRI 在检测创伤后血管分流中的应用已被证实。使用静脉对比剂，在动脉和静脉期应用、屏气 3D 序列采集，提示创伤后血管分流的 3 个标志是分流的流入和流出血管的扩张、肝实质的短暂强化以及同侧流出血管的早期增强[84]。

对于脾脏中的创伤后囊肿，通过 T_1 序列中的高信号，MRI 能够比 CT 和超声更好地鉴别囊肿内的新鲜出血，并且与继发性囊肿（例如寄生虫囊肿）区分开[85]。

在胰腺损伤中，CT 是常用的诊断方法。MRI 已被证明优于其他诊断方法，因为它能够显示实质病变和主胰管的病变（Wirsung 管）[86]。为实现此目的，使用特定的 3D-MIP 重建的 MRCP 序列。使用这些序列，可以看到 Wirsung 管的破坏。此外，脂肪抑制的 T_1 和 T_2 序列，可以观察实质的损伤和相关的积液。

MRI 应用于产科病变的评估已有 20 余年，在高达 1.5T 的磁场中没有热损伤证据。关于高场强设备（超过 3T 的场）的文献非常有限[87]。腹部创伤妊娠患者建议不要使用电离辐射进行诊断，因此建议使用 US 或 MRI。US 通常是首选的影像方法，CT 是次选的，对于电离辐射，需谨记 ALARA（As Low As Razonable Achievable）标准。关于在急诊病例中使用腹腔盆 MRI 检查，虽然理论上可行，但并没有足够的研究支持该应用[87]。

参考文献

[1] Wang MY, Cummock MD, Yu Y, Trivedi RA (2010) An analysis of the differences in the acute hospitalization charges following minimally invasive versus open posterior lumbar interbody fusion. *J Neurosurg Spine* 12(6):694–699.

[2] Da Luz Moreira A, Kiran RP, Kirat HT et al. (2010) Laparoscopic versus open colectomy for patients with American Society of Anesthesiology (ASA) classifications 3 and 4: The minimally invasive approach is associated with significantly quicker recovery and reduced costs. *Surg Endosc* 24(6):1280–1286.

[3] Lazzarino AI, Nagpal K, Bottle A et al. (2010) Open versus minimally invasive esophagectomy: Trends of utilization and associated outcomes in England. *Ann Surg* 252(2):292–298.

[4] Wei B, Qi CL, Chen TF et al. (2011) Laparoscopic versus open appendectomy for acute appendicitis: A metaanalysis. *Surg Endosc* 25(4):1199–1208.

[5] Yin J, Hou X (2014) Complications of laparoscopic versus open bariatric surgical interventions in obesity management. *Cell Biochem Biophys* 70(2):721–728. doi:10.1007/ s12013-014-0041–2.

[6] Sajid MS, Ahamd A, Miles WF et al. (2014) Systematic review of oncological outcomes following laparoscopic vs open total mesorectal excision. *World J Gastrointest Endosc* 166(5):209–219.

[7] Wu B, Xiao YY, Zhang X et al. (2010) Magnetic resonance imaging-guided percutaneous cryoablation of hepatocellular carcinoma in special regions. *Hepatobiliary Pancreat Dis Int* 9(4):384–392.

[8] Jendresen MB, Thorbøll JE, Adamsen S et al. (2002) Preoperative routine magnetic resonance cholangiopancreatography before laparoscopic cholecystectomy: A prospective study. *Eur J Surg* 168:690–694.

[9] Nebiker CA, Baierlein SA, Beck S et al. (2009) Is routine MR cholangiopancreatography (MRCP) justified prior to cholecystectomy. *Langenbecks Arch Surg* 394:1005–1010.

[10] Blanco RT, Ojala R, Kariniemi J et al. (2005) Interventional and intraoperative MRI at low field scanner—A review. *Eur J Radiol* 56(2):130–142.

[11] Ni Y, Chen F, Mulier S et al. (2006) Magnetic resonance imaging after radiofrequency ablation in a rodent model of liver tumor: Tissue characterization using a novel necrosis-avid contrast agent. *Eur Radiol* 16(5):1031–1040.

[12] Clasen S, Rempp H, Boss A et al. (2011) MR-guided radiofrequency ablation of hepatocellular carcinoma: Long-term effectiveness. *J Vasc Interv Radiol* 22(6):762–770.

[13] Kim JE, Kim YS, Rhim H et al. (2011) Outcomes of patients with hepatocellular carcinoma referred for percutaneous radiofrequency ablation at a tertiary center: Analysis focused on the feasibility with use of ultrasonography guidance. *Eur J Radiol* 79(2):e80–84.

[14] Tateishi R1, Shiina S, Teratani T (2005) Percutaneous radiofrequency ablation for hepatocellular carcinoma. An analysis of 1000 cases. *Cancer* 103(6):1201–1209.

[15] Usón J, Sánchez FM, Sánchez MA, Pérez FJ, Hashizume M (2007) Principios básicos. In: Usón J, Sanchez FM, Pascual S, Climent S, (eds) *Formación en Cirugía Laparoscópica Paso a Paso*, 3rd edn. Centro de Cirugía de Mínima Invasión, Cáceres, Spain.

[16] Guven HE, Oral S (2007) Liver enzyme alterations after laparoscopic cholecystectomy. *J Gastrointestin Liver Dis* 16(4):391–394.

[17] Atila K, Terzi C, Ozkardesler S et al. (2009) What is the role of the abdominal perfusion pressure for subclinical hepatic dysfunction in laparoscopic cholecystectomy? *J Laparoendosc Adv Surg Tech A* 19(1):39–44.

[18] Sáenz Medina J, Asuero de Lis MS, Galindo Alvarez J et al. (2007) Modification of the hemodynamic parameters and peripheral vascular flow in a porcine experimental of model of laparoscopic nephrectomy. *Arch Esp Urol* 60(5):501–518.

[19] Smith MK, Mutter D, Forbes LE et al. (2004) The physiologic effect of the pneumoperitoneum on radiofrequency ablation. *Surg Endosc* 18(1):35–38.

[20] Alexakis N, Gakiopoulou H, Dimitriou C et al. (2008) Liver histology alterations during carbon dioxide pneumoperitoneum in a porcine model. *Surg Endosc* 22(2):415–420.

[21] Sánchez-Margallo FM, Moyano-Cuevas JL, Latorre R et al. (2011) Anatomical changes due to pneumoperitoneum analyzed by MRI: An experimental study in pigs. *Surg Radiol Anat* 33(5):389–396.

[22] Bickel A, Loberant N, Bersudsky M, Goldfeld M, Ivry S, Herskovits M, Eitan A (2007) Overcoming reduced hepatic and renal perfusion caused by positive-pressure pneumoperitoneum. *Arch Surg* 142(2):119–124.

[23] Gouya H, Vignaux O, Sogni P et al. (2011) Chronic liver disease: Systemic and splanchnic venous flow mapping with optimized cine phase-contrast MR imaging validated in a phantom model and prospectively evaluated in patients. *Radiology* 261(1):144–155.

[24] Simard EP, Ward EM, Siegel R, Jemal A (2012) Cancers with increasing incidence trends in the United States: 1999 through 2008. *CA Cancer J Clin* 62(2):118–128. doi:10.3322/caac.20141.

[25] Jemal A, Bray F, Center MM (2011) Global cancer statistics. *CA Cancer J Clin* 61(2):69–90.

[26] SERAM (2009) *Actualizaciones Seram. Imagen en Oncología*. Médica Panamericana, Buenos Aires, Argentina.

[27] Siegelman ES (2008) *Resonancia Magnetica Tórax Abdomen y Pelvis. Aplicaciones clínicas*. Médica Panamericana, Buenos Aires, Argentina.

[28] Figueras J, Jaurrieta E, Valls C et al. (2000) Resection or transplantation for hepatocellular carcinoma in cirrhotic patients: Outcomes base on indicated treatment strategy. *J Am Coll Surg* 190:580–587.

[29] McWilliams JP, Yamamoto S, Raman SS et al. (2010) Percutaneous ablation of hepatocellular carcinoma: Current status.

J Vasc Interv Radiol 21(8 Suppl):204–213.
[30] Dunne RM, Shyn PB, Sung JC et al. (2014) Percutaneous treatment of hepatocellular carcinoma in patients with cirrhosis: A comparison of the safety of cryoablation and radiofrequency ablation. Eur J Radiol 83(4):632–638.
[31] Guo Y1, Yaghmai V, Salem R (2013) Imaging tumor response following liver-directed intra-arterial therapy. Abdom Imaging 38(6):1286–1299.
[32] Malayeri AA, El Khouli RH, Zaheer A et al. (2011) Principles and applications of diffusion-weighed imaging in cancer detection, staging, and treatment followup. RadioGraphics 31(9):1773–1791.
[33] Chatzifotiadis D, Buchanan JW, Wahl RL (2006) Positron emission tomography and cancer. In: Chang A, Ganz PA, Hayes DF et al. (eds) Oncology: Ab Evidenced-Based Approach, 1st edn. Springer, New York.
[34] Weinrich M, Weiß C, Schuld J et al. (2014) Liver resections of isolated liver metastasis in breast cancer: Results and possible prognostic factors. HPB Surg 2014(4):1–6. doi:10.1155/2014/893829.
[35] Floriani I, Torri V, Rulli E et al. (2010) A performance of imaging modalities in diagnosis of liver metastases from colorectal cancer: A systematic review and meta- analysis. J Magn Reson Imaging 31(1):19–31.
[36] Van Kessel CS, Buckens CF, Van den Bosch MA et al. (2012) Preoperative imaging of colorectal liver metastases after neoadjuvant chemotherapy: A meta-analysis. Ann Surg Oncol 19(9):2805–2813.
[37] Legou F, Chiaradia M, Baranes L et al. (2014) Imaging strategies before beginning treatment of colorectal liver metastases. Diagn Interv Imaging 95:505–512.
[38] Shaffer EA (2006) Gallstone disease: Epidemiology of gallbladder stone disease. Best Pract Res Clin Gastroenterol 20(6):981–996.
[39] Oneill CJ, Gillies DM Gani JS (2008) Choledocholithiasis: Overdiagnosed endoscopically and undertreated laparoscopically. ANZ J Surg 78:487–491.
[40] Petelin JB (2003) Laparoscopic common bile duct exploration. Surg Endosc 17:1705–1715.
[41] Jendresen MB, Thorbøll JE, Adamsen S et al. (2002) Preoperative routine magnetic resonance cholangiopancreatography before laparoscopic cholecystectomy: A prospective study. Eur J Surg 168:690–694.
[42] Nebiker CA, Baierlein SA, Beck S et al. (2009) Is routine MR cholangiopancreatography (MRCP) justified prior to cholecystectomy. Langenbecks Arch Surg. 394:1005–1010.
[43] Dalton SJ, Balupuri S, Guest J (2005) Routine magnetic resonance cholangiopancreatography and intra-operative cholangiogram in the evaluation of common bile duct stones. Ann R Coll Surg Engl 87:469–470.
[44] Dumot JA (2006) ERCP: Current uses and less-invasive options. Cleve Clin J Med 73:418–425.
[45] Mori T, Sugiyama M, Atomi Y (2006) Gallstone disease: Management of intrahepatic stones. Best Pract Res Clin Gastroenterol 20:1117–1137.
[46] Al-Jiffry BO, Elfateh A, Chundrigar T et al. (2013) Non-invasive assessment of choledocholithiasis in patients with gallstones and abnormal liver function. World J Gastroenterol 19(35):5877–5882.
[47] Romagnuolo J, Bardou M, Rahme E et al. (2003) Magnetic resonance cholangiopancreatography: A meta-analysis of test performance in suspected biliary disease. Ann Intern Med. 139(7):547–557.
[48] Verma D, Kapadia A, Eisen GM et al. (2006) EUS vs MRCP for detection of choledocholithiasis. Gastrointest Endosc. 64(2):248–254.
[49] ASGE Standards of Practice Committee, Maple JT, Ben-Menachem T et al. (2010) The role of endoscopy in the evaluation of suspected choledocholithiasis. Gastrointest Endosc 71(1):1–9.
[50] Wang DB, Yu J, Fulcher AS et al. (2013) Pancreatitis in patients with pancreas divisum: Imaging features at MRI and MRCP. World J Gastroenterol 19(30):4907–4916.
[51] Pavone P, Laghi A, Catalano C et al. (1996) Non-invasive evaluation of the biliary tree with magnetic resonance cholangiopancreatography: Initial clinical experience. Ital J Gastroenterol. 28(2):63–69.
[52] Kariniemi J, Sequeiros RB, Ojala R, Tervonen O (2009) MRI-guided percutaneous nephrostomy: A feasibility study. Eur Radiol 19(5):1296–1301.
[53] Fischbach F1, Porsch M, Krenzien F, Pech M, Dudeck O, Bunke J, Liehr UB, Ricke J (2011) MR imaging guided percutaneous nephrostomy using a 1.0 Tesla open MR scanner. Cardiovasc Intervent Radiol. 34(4):857–863.
[54] Nour SG, Lewin JS (2012) MRI-guided RF ablation in the kidney. In: Kahn T, Busse H (eds), Interventional Magnetic Resonance Imaging, 1st edn. Springer, Berlin, Germany.
[55] Boss A, Clasen S, Kuczyk M et al. (2005) Magnetic resonance-guided percutaneous radiofrequency ablation of renal cell carcinomas: A pilot clinical study. Invest Radiol 40(9):583–590.
[56] Grasso RF, Luppi G, Faiella E (2012) Radiofrequency ablation of renal cell carcinoma in patients with a solitary kidney: A retrospective analysis of our experience. Radiol Med. 117(4):606–615.
[57] Demyttenaere S, Feldman LS, Fried GM (2007) Effect of pneumoperitoneum on renal perfusion and function: A systematic review. Surg Endosc. 21(2):152–160.
[58] Sánchez Margallo FM, Moyano Cuevas JL, Maestre Antequera J et al. (2013) Efectos del neumoperitoneo en la morfología y hemodinámica renal analizado mediante resonancia magnética. In: Proceeding Congreso Nacional de Urología, Mexico.
[59] Pelc LR, Pelc NJ, Rayhill SC et al. (1992) Arterial and venous blood flow: Noninvasive quantitation with MR imaging. Radiology 185(3):809–812.
[60] Gouya H, Vignaux O, Sogni P et al. (2011) Chronic liver disease: Systemic and splanchnic venous flow mapping with

optimized cine phase-contrast MR imaging validated in a phantom model and prospectively evaluated in patients. *Radiology* 261(1):144–155.

[61] De Haan MW, van Engelshoven JM, Houben AJ et al. (2003) Phase-contrast magnetic resonance flow quantification in renal arteries: Comparison with 133Xenon washout measurements. *Hypertension* 41:114–118.

[62] Park JB, Santos JM, Hargreaves BA et al. (2005) Rapid measurement of renal artery blood flow with ungated spiral phase-contrast MRI. *J Magn Reson Imaging* 21:590–595.

[63] Bax L, Bakker CJ, Klein WM (2005) Renal blood flow measurements with use of phase-contrast magnetic resonance imaging: Normal values and reproducibility. *J Vasc Interv Radiol* 16:807–814.

[64] Wiesenthal JD, Fazio LM, Perks AE et al. (2011) Effect of pneumoperitoneum on renal tissue oxygenation and blood flow in a rat model. *Urology* 77(6):1508. e9–1508.e15.

[65] Jemal A, Siegel R, Ward E et al. (2007) Cancer statistics, 2007. *CA Cancer J Clin* 57:43–66.

[66] Ng CS, Wood CG, Silverman PM (2008) Renal cell carcinoma: Diagnosis, staging, and surveillance. *AJR Am J Roentgenol* 191:1220–1232.

[67] Barba Abad J, Rincón Mayans A, Tolosa Eizaguirre E et al. (2010) Surgical complications in kidney transplantation and their influence on graft survival. *Actas Urol Esp* 34(3):266–273.

[68] Greco F, Fornara P, Mirone V (2014) Renal transplantation: Technical aspects, diagnosis and management of early and late urological complications. *Panminerva Med* 56(1):17–29.

[69] Karam G, Maillet F, Braud G, Battis S (2007) Surgical complications of renal transplantation. *Annales d'urologie* 41:261–275.

[70] Bruno S, Remuzzi G, Ruggenenti P (2004) Transplant renal artery stenosis. *J Am Soc Nephrol* 15:134–141.

[71] Von Knobelsdorff-Brenkenhoff F, Gruettner H, Trauzeddel RF et al. (2014) Comparison of native high-resolution 3D and contrast-enhanced MR angiography for assessing the thoracic aorta. *Eur Heart J Cardiovasc Imaging* 15(6):651–658.

[72] Makowski MR, Botnar RM (2013) MR imaging of the arterial vessel wall: Molecular imaging from bench to bedside. *Radiology* 269(1):34–51.

[73] Huber A, Heuck A, Scheidler J, Holzknecht N, Baur A, Stangl M, Theodorakis J, Illner WD, Land W, Reiser M (2001) Contrast-enhanced MR angiography in patients after kidney transplantation. *Eur Radiol* 11(12):2488–2495.

[74] Gufler H, Weimer W, Neu K et al. (2009) Contrast enhanced MR angiography with parallel imaging in the early period after renal transplantation. *J Magn Reson Imaging*. 29(4):909–916.

[75] Di Felice A, Inguaggiato P, Rubbiani E (2002) Magnetic resonance in renal transplantation: Evaluation of postsurgery complications. *Transplant Proc* 34(8):3193–3195.

[76] Cohan RH, Ellis JH, Hussain HK et al. (2008) Nephrogenic systemic fibrosis: Report of 29 patients. *AJR Am J Roentgenol* 190:736–741.

[77] Marckmann P, Skov L, Rossen K et al. (2006) Nephrogenic systemic fibrosis: Suspected etiological role of gadodiamide used for contrast-enhanced magnetic resonance imaging. *J Am Soc Nephrol* 17:2359–2362.

[78] Behzadi AH, Kamali K, Zargar M (2014) Obesity and urologic complications after renal transplantation. *Saudi J Kidney Dis Transpl* 25:303–308.

[79] Kamali K, Zargar MA, Zargar H (2003) Early common surgical complications in 1500 kidney transplantations. *Transplant Proc* 35(7):2655–2656.

[80] Koçak T, Nane I, Ander H (2004) Urological and surgical complications in 362 consecutive living related donor kidney transplantations. *Urol Int* 72(3):252–256.

[81] Blondin D, Koester A, Andersen K et al. (2009) Renal transplant failure due to urologic complications: Comparison of static fluid with contrast-enhanced magnetic resonance urography. *Eur J Radiol* 69(2):324–330.

[82] Weishaupt D, Grozaj AM, Willmann JK et al. (2002) Traumatic injuries: Imaging of abdominal and pelvic injuries. *Eur Radiol* 12(6):1295–1311.

[83] Sivit CJ (2008) Contemporary imaging in abdominal emergencies. *Pediatr Radiol* 38(Suppl 4):S675–S678.

[84] Semelka RC, Lessa T, Shaikh F et al. (2009) MRI findings of posttraumatic intrahepatic vascular shunts. *J Magn Reson Imaging* 29(3):617–620.

[85] Acar M, Dilek ON, Ilgaz K, Çalışkan G, Kirpiko O, Tokyol C (2008) Posttraumatic splenic cyst Diagnostic value of MRI. *Eur J Gen Med* 5(4):242–244.

[86] Yang L, Zhang XM, Xu XX (2010) MR imaging for blunt pancreatic injury. *Eur J Radiol* 75(2):97–101.

[87] Katz DS, Klein MA, Ganson G et al. (2012) Imaging of abdominal pain in pregnancy. *Radiol Clin North Am* 50(1):149–171.

中国科学技术出版社
影像学经典译著推荐

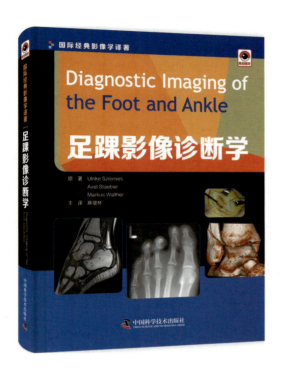

足踝影像诊断学

引进地：德国 Thieme 出版社
定价：178.00 元（大 16 开精装）
原著：Ulrike Szeimies 等
主译：麻增林

全书共 11 章，对踝关节及前、中、后足的损伤，以及慢性、损伤后、退行性改变的疾病进行详细介绍，同时还对足底软组织疾病、足踝部代谢性疾病、神经性疾病、系统性疾病、肿瘤样病变、解剖变异等进行了阐述，其最主要的精华部分就是影像诊断，由于 MRI 在显示足踝部软组织及骨组织方面有非常大的优势，因此介绍尤为详细，同时配有大量 MRI 图像，图文并茂，有助于读者深刻理解。

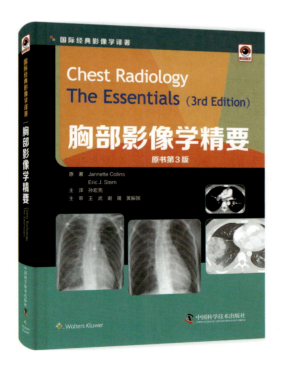

胸部影像学精要：原书第 3 版

引进地：荷兰 Wolters Kluwer 出版社
定价：248.00 元（大 16 开 精装）
原著：Jannette Collins 等
主译：孙宏亮

本书是引进自 Wolters Kluwer 出版社的一部高质量医学影像学著作。全书共分 19 章，全面讲解了胸部常见与罕见疾病的影像学诊断与鉴别诊断，包括间质性肺疾病、肺泡性肺疾病、纵隔肿块、肺结节、肺不张、胸部创伤、上肺疾病、感染和免疫性疾病、外周性肺病等。采用大量临床典型病例图片，辅以文字说明，易学易懂。每章末尾还附有该章节重要知识点的自测题，利于读者巩固记忆本章知识点。本书实为胸部疾病影像诊断的精华，但内容又足够详细，既可以用于住院医师或影像执业医师的快速学习，也可以用来指导胸部影像教学，适用于实习医师、呼吸科医师、胸外科医师、重症监护医师、家庭医生等阅读参考。

中国科学技术出版社
影像学经典译著推荐

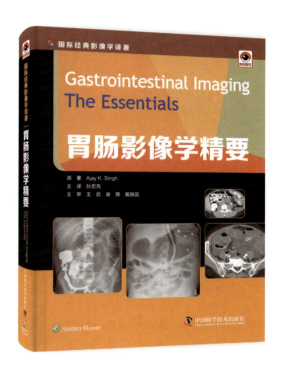

胃肠影像学精要

引进地：荷兰 Wolters Kluwer 出版社
定　价：178.00 元（大 16 开精装）
原　著：Ajay K. Singh
主　译：孙宏亮

　　本书是引进自 Wolters Kluwer 出版社的一部高质量医学影像学著作。由于影像技术的快速发展，影像医师不但要熟悉传统的荧光影像技术，还要熟悉断层影像技术。影像学在胃肠道疾病的早期诊断和治疗中扮演着重要角色，影像领域的快速发展使医生诊断胃肠道疾病的水平显著提高。原著者汇集了一批胃肠道影像领域的知名专家，共同编写了本书，对胃肠常规影像和影像学进展进行了详细说明，对钡餐、MR 成像等内容也做了介绍，还对胃肠道不同器官的常见疾病影像学表现及鉴别诊断进行了具体阐述。书中每章章首均列有学习目标，章末均附有自测题，书末还附有自我测评，帮助读者检验整体学习情况。本书内容紧凑实用，讲解系统详细，可作为放射科医师或临床医师的参考书，也可作为高年资医生指导住院医师和实习医师的教学用书。

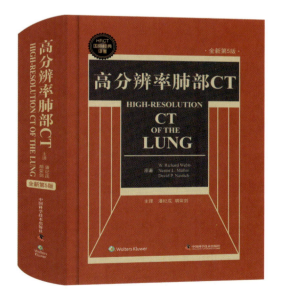

高分辨率肺部 CT：全新第 5 版

引进地：荷兰 Wolters Kluwer 出版社
定　价：295.00 元（大 16 开精装）
原　著：W. Richard Webb 等
主　译：潘纪戍　胡荣剑

　　本书是由三位美国著名胸部影像学家联合编著的国际权威名著，自 1991 年初版以来，已多次再版。
　　本书是最新的第 5 版，内容更加丰富、完善。全书共三部分，从正常解剖、病理生理到常见病、罕见病，对每一种肺部疾病都系统地从术语、影像表现、鉴别诊断、病理、临床、鉴别要点等方面做了详尽描述。对常见 HRCT 征象也分类做了详细阐述，罗列了每一征象的常见疾病，对鉴别诊断非常有帮助。书末还附有 HRCT 回顾的相关介绍。原著思路清晰、重点突出，译文准确流畅，易于通读。本书权威、前沿、实用，具有很强的临床和研究参考价值，可供广大影像科、呼吸科、胸外科医师及医学院校师生学习参考。

中国科学技术出版社

影像学经典译著推荐

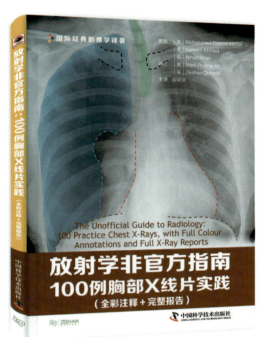

放射学非官方指南：100 例胸部 X 线片实践（全彩注释 + 完整报告）

引进地： 英国 Zeshan Qureshi 出版社
定　价： 98.00 元（大 16 开 平装）
原　著： Mohammed Rashid Akhtar 等
主　译： 胡荣剑

　　本书引进自英国 Zeshan Qureshi 出版社，由 3 位英国放射学家联合编写，并得到英国放射学会、英国皇家放射医师学会等权威机构的认可，是一部新颖、独特的胸部 X 线诊断参考书。

　　为了便于读者学习，著者选择病例从易至难，每个病例都从临床病史、常规检查介绍开始，并配以大幅高质量胸部 X 线片图像，然后在次页展示该图像的全彩注释，帮助读者快速、清晰地了解各种胸部 X 线片影像表现、诊断及临床处理意见，让读者轻松融入真实临床情境，提高 X 线片解读技能，摆脱以往其他放射诊断教科书的局限性。

　　本书编写特点鲜明，图像质量优良，全彩注释清晰，译文准确流畅，非常适合广大影像科临床医师阅读参考。

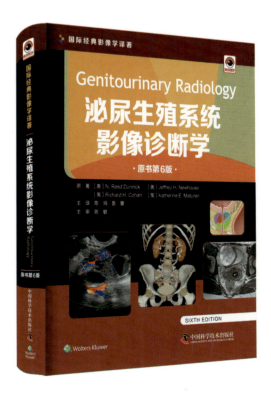

泌尿生殖系统影像诊断学：原书第 6 版

引进地： 荷兰 Wolters Kluwer 出版社
定　价： 248.00 元（大 16 开 精装）
原　著： N. Reed Dunnick 等
主　译： 陈　涓　姜　蕾

　　本书是引进自 Wolters Kluwer 出版社的一部高质量医学影像学著作，综合介绍了超声、放射、核医学等各种影像学检查方法在泌尿生殖系统的应用。开篇先阐述了泌尿道及男性和女性生殖系统的先天发育异常及影像表现；阐释了肾脏的功能解剖、生理及对比剂的不良反应，这是后续阐释肾脏疾病影像表现的基础。接下来，阐述了肾上腺的功能亢进疾病和非功能亢进疾病的影像表现，腹膜后疾病的影像诊断及鉴别诊断，肾脏囊性疾病、肾脏肿瘤、肾脏炎性疾病、肾脏血管性疾病、尿石症及肾钙盐沉积症、肾盂肾盏输尿管疾病、膀胱疾病的影像诊断及肾衰竭和肾移植相关问题的影像表现。在生殖系统方面，详细阐述了前列腺与精囊、尿道与阴茎、阴囊与内容物及卵巢与附件、子宫（包括宫颈）、女性会阴与阴道的正常和异常影像表现。本书内容系统、翔实，可供泌尿生殖亚专业影像科医师和临床医师参考阅读。